VETERINARY

PATHOLOGY

HILTON ATMORE SMITH, D.V.M., M.S., Ph.D.

Late Research Associate, Baylor University College of Medicine; Consultant to the Armed Forces Institute of Pathology; Lecturer (Pathology) University of Texas Medical Branch, Formerly Professor of Veterinary Pathology at (successively) Washington State University, Colorado State University, Iowa State University, Texas A & M University; Consultant to Stanford Research Institute

THOMAS CARLYLE JONES, B.S., D.V.M., D.Sc. (Hon).

Professor of Comparative Pathology and Associate Director, New England Regional Primate Research Center, Harvard Medical School; Formerly: Director of Pathology, Angell Memorial Animal Hospital; Lt. Col. U.S. Army Veterinary Corps; Chief, Veterinary Pathology Section, Armed Forces Institute of Pathology.

RONALD DUNCAN HUNT, B.S., D.V.M.

Associate Professor of Comparative Pathology and Chairman, Division of Comparative Pathology, New England Regional Primate Research Center, Harvard Medical School; Associate Director, Animal Research Center, Harvard Medical School; Lecturer, Department of Nutrition and Food Science, Massachusetts Institute of Technology; Affiliate Pathologist, Angell Memorial Animal Hospital.

FOURTH EDITION

510 Figures and 2 Color Plates

Lea & Febiger
Philadelphia

ISBN 0-8121-0364-5

Library of Congress Catalog Card Number. 73-157473

Printed in the United States of America

Print number: 5   4

Preface to Fourth Edition

Following the death of Hilton Atmore Smith, this edition of *Veterinary Pathology* was prepared with the welcome addition of Ronald Duncan Hunt as an author. As in previous editions, each author assumed responsibility for revising individual chapters and also read and criticized the entire text. Our aims were to encompass as much new information as possible, correct or modernize concepts whenever necessary and still keep the book manageable as a single volume.

A large amount of new information on specific aspects of veterinary pathology has been produced since the third edition was completed and knowledge related to general pathology has expanded greatly. Concepts of general pathology, particularly at the molecular and cellular levels, have been revolutionized over the past decade, making it exceedingly difficult to condense even the most firmly established principles in part of one volume. We have attempted to include many new ideas, particularly when they apply generally or specifically to animal disease problems. We may have succeeded in some aspects and failed in others. We ask our colleagues to communicate with us in reference to those areas which are incomplete, in error, or poorly supported by evidence.

The recent growth of knowledge in veterinary pathology is due to the research productivity of many contemporary persons whose work we have acknowledged in the text or in the list of references. We would also like to acknowledge the contributions of certain veterinary pathologists, now deceased or retired, whose life work has contributed to the soundly based position of this speciality and whose ideas have been used frequently in this book. We acknowledge especially: Hilton Atmore Smith, whose skill as a teacher and writer gives him special prominence; William H. Feldman, pioneer in the study of animal neoplasms and chemotherapy of tuberculosis; Frank A. Schofield, original discoverer of the toxic principle in sweet clover which eventually proved to be dicoumarin; Charles L. Davis, whose enthusiasm inspired many young pathologists and who described for the first time so many pathologic entities in food-producing animals; Evan L. Stubbs, contributor of many fundamental concepts of disease of poultry; Erwin Jungherr, expert in diseases of poultry and many other species, first to recognize leptospira in swine; Peter Olafson, whose incisive mind penetrated many problems, one of which was bovine hyperkeratosis; Hadleigh Marsh, innovative investigator of diseases of sheep; Hans Schlumberger, a medical pathologist with unbounded enthusiasm which he applied to the elucidation of many problems in fish, birds, invertebrates and mammals; Albert Hjarre, the brilliant Swedish veterinary pathologist whose initial descriptions of disease problems in many species have stood the test of time; Paul Cohrs, a stalwart of veterinary pathology in Germany for many years; E. A. Benbrook, early worker on the effects of helminth and arthropod parasites on domesticated animals; Raymond A. Kelser, discoverer of the arthropod-transmission of the virus of equine encephalomyelitis; Russell A. Runnells, dedicated teacher; and James Robert Maitland Innes, pioneer contributor to neuropathology.

These are some of the men who have influenced the writing of this book and were or are personal friends of one or both of the authors.

As a textbook, this volume is not intended to replace the instructor, who should exercise his role in shifting emphasis, reorganizing the order of presentation, correcting errors and clarifying obscure or poorly explained points. We hope that those who use this book in instruction will point out deficiencies to us.

Electron micrographs have been added in those situations in which they help to make a point or to present new data. Although we have tried to be accurate and reasonably current, details are sometimes omitted in order to keep the book within one volume. Additional references have been added throughout the book and some have been deleted. In most cases, the references lead to more detail than could be included in the text.

We are indebted to many for help but are especially grateful for the support and understanding of Dr. Bernard F. Trum, Harvard Medical School, Director of the New England Regional Primate Research Center. We are also grateful for the help in typing the manuscript and assembling references, ably given by Mrs. Anne Marie Bloch and Mrs. Mary Dorman. We also acknowledge the assistance of Mrs. Patricia Lavin, Mrs. Lorraine Schrader, Miss Laura Chalifoux and Miss Beverly Blake. Dr. Leonard C. Marcus helped us particularly by his critical and detailed study of the manuscript. The efficient work of the staff of Lea & Febiger is particularly acknowledged. The intelligent and supporting role of Mr. Christian C. F. Spahr, Jr., was unusually helpful to the authors.

Boston and   THOMAS CARLYLE JONES
Southborough, Massachusetts   RONALD DUNCAN HUNT

Preface to First Edition

In offering this book to our colleagues in the various medical sciences we venture to hope that it may be useful not only as a textbook for the student in veterinary medicine, but also as a source of reference for the veterinary practitioner who may wish to renew his familiarity with the fundamental features of a disease confronting him. We should like to think that those in the fields of human and comparative pathology would find in it the answers to some of their questions about diseases in domestic and other animals. Conversely, we hope that the student in veterinary pathology may gain an acquaintance with the fundamentals of many human diseases, which is appropriate as a part of his general educational background.

While the scope of the text itself has necessarily been limited, we have endeavored to include reference lists sufficient to provide a starting point for more exhaustive study of the various diseases known to current literature. As far as possible, references have been selected from standard periodicals commonly available in veterinary medical libraries, bulletins and similar restricted publications being used only when there was no substitute. In the case of a few periodicals more or less inaccessible to the English-speaking investigator, reference has been made to published abstracts.

In an effort to conserve space and economize on the expense which falls heavily upon the student, we have kept repetition to a minimum, relying upon numerous cross-references to lead the reader to all the different approaches to a particular subject. Since current information is already available in other textbooks, comprehensive coverage of avian diseases was not undertaken.

For the omissions of subjects or significant references, of which there must be some, we hasten to apologize. For the statements which time proves to be fallacious we offer deep regret. We certainly have not espoused a new concept merely because it was new, but have endeavored to support ideas which seemed well founded in relation to available evidence and the general principles of pathology. Important controversial views have received only momentary consideration lest the student be confused rather than enlightened. Adherence to the most recently proposed nomenclatures of bacteria and parasites has not been attempted because many names have changed so rapidly that there is no assurance of a given term continuing in favor. We have tried, therefore, to use the names that have been well established and are generally understood, giving synonyms as needed.

It is a pleasure to acknowledge the assistance of several persons who have helped with the book in many ways. We are deeply indebted to Mrs. Helen K. Steward and her assistants, Miss Flora Treut and Mrs. Charlotte Flom, for editing those chapters emanating directly from the Armed Forces Institute of Pathology, to Mr. Herman Van Cott, Chief of the Medical Illustration Service, A.F.I.P., whose staff prepared many of the illustrations, to Lieutenant Colonel Daniel P. Sasmore, Majors C. N. Barron and J. A. Rehkemper, and Captains

Donald H. Yost and James E. Cook, all of the A.F.I P., for help in preparation of photomicrographs, and to Dr. P. W. Burns of the Texas School of Veterinary Medicine for providing data used in the preparation of the chapter on Poisons. Mrs. Mary Anderson, Mrs. Leatrice Smith, Mrs. Carole Speck, Mrs. Nancy Osborne and Mrs. Lynda Bankard were faithful and effective assistants in the preparation of the manuscript. Don C. Jones and Dorotha A. Jones assisted by gathering and verifying references. Chapter 9 was reviewed by Lieutenant Colonel Fred D. Maurer of the A.F.I.P. staff, and Chapter 13 by Dr. R. D. Turk of the Texas School of Veterinary Medicine. In those instances in which illustrations were prepared from cases in the Registry of Veterinary Pathology, the contributors are named in the captions. Illustrations supplied by others are acknowledged individually. The tireless efforts of the Publishers to provide a book of high quality at a reasonable cost are deeply appreciated by the authors.

College Station, Texas   HILTON ATMORE SMITH
Washington, D.C.   THOMAS CARLYLE JONES

Contents

Chapter

1

Introduction, the Cell, Death of Cells and Tissues

Pathology is the study of the molecular, cellular, tissue or organismal response of the living body (animal or plant) when exposed to injurious agents or deprivations. Many of these injurious agents are chemical compounds, either inorganic or, more frequently, the product of living organisms, the most conspicuous of which are the disease-producing bacteria and viruses. Others consist of energy in such forms as heat and mechanical trauma applied to a harmful degree. While most pathological conditions arise as a result of the exposure of body tissues to injurious substances, failure of access to various necessary materials such as proteins, minerals, vitamins, water and oxygen can have equally deleterious effects. Inherited factors also play an important role in pathology.

To the extent that our limited knowledge permits any biological science to be precise, pathology is that branch of medical studies which attempts to relate specific effects to definite causes. When, if ever, our understanding of the laws of pathology becomes perfect, then it will be possible to predict the effect of a disease-producing agent with just as much certainty as it is now possible to measure the force of gravity and predict the course of a falling body. Under what appear to be entirely comparable conditions one animal survives an infection and one succumbs, one person develops a malignant neoplasm and another escapes. We pass these things off as biological variations or differences in resistance and tell ourselves that such irregularities must be expected even in carefully conducted biological experiments. But let no one suppose that each unexplained event is in reality without adequate and finite cause; it is only because of our incomplete information and knowledge of pertinent facts that we try to group such variable outcomes according to the laws of chance. Too much time has been wasted in considering pathology as a long list of separate observations upon diseased animals and tissues. The things that occur in health and disease are fully related to each other and are founded upon chemical and physical laws as constant as any in science.

The pathologist may approach the study of pathologic processes at any of several different levels. At the **population** level, the interaction of organisms to each other and to the environment under various adverse conditions may contribute to pathologic states. At the level of the **organism,** or individual, pathologic states are manifest by overt clinical signs (observable objectively) or by symptoms subjectively recognized by the human patient and are the result of interaction of changes in one or more organ systems. Specific pathologic changes in **organs** or **tissues** may be recognized by inspection of the gross specimen or by study of preparations under the light microscope. At the **cellular** level, some pathologic features may be recognized with the light microscope; others, involving intracellular organelles, may be visualized only with the electron microscope. At the **molecular** level, the chemical reactions which underlie all pathologic processes may be studied, using the techniques of chemistry and to some extent electron microscopy. Study of pathologic changes at the molecular level is the latest approach to emerge and offers the most promise toward understanding the fundamental processes of pathology.

The careful anatomic study of gross and microscopic preparations (pathologic anatomy) has yielded a great deal of useful information about disease processes and still is valuable as a method of recognizing disease states. It is expected that the techniques and approaches of pathologic anatomy will continue to be useful in arriving at a diagnosis or for limiting the possible diagnoses and therefore are emphasized in this book. Skill and judgment in the use of these tools are not easily acquired but are currently necessary to the specialist in pathology. Deeper elucidation of pathologic problems, old and new, increasingly depend upon use of modern techniques, including those of electron microscopy and biochemistry.

We like to think of each injurious agent as causing a specific sort of injury and provoking a specific reaction on the part of the tissues and, in general, this is the case. The products of the tubercle bacillus (p. 625), for instance, evoke a tissue response which is readily distinguishable from that resulting from the canine hepatitis virus (p. 447). It is by virtue of these differences that it is possible to diagnose the type of disease to which the body is being subjected. On the other hand, if the young child falls and hurts his knee, or if he receives a spanking from his parent, the loud reaction is likely to be identical in both cases for the reason that a child of early age has only one way of expressing dissatisfaction, whatever its cause. Likewise, body cells and tissues have only a limited number of ways of reacting to a considerable variety of injurious agents. This is especially true in the central nervous system, where it is particularly difficult to decide from the type of reaction what the injurious agent may have been.

Death of Cells.—Cellular death has been defined by Majno (1960) as a process during which the cell loses its integrity as a functional unit. A "point of no return" is visualized as a singular point beyond which damage to the cell is no longer reversible and which leads inevitably to necrosis, a state which is recognizable by light (optical) microscopy. Necrosis will be discussed more fully later because it still has pragmatic application to the recognition of disease.

Since a fixative, such as a 10 per cent solution of formalin, promptly puts a stop to lytic or other changes in body cells, it is customary in microscopic pathology to speak of a cell or tissue as living if its characteristics are those of cells which were living when placed in the fixative, and as dead if it shows any of the series of changes about to be discussed as occurring after death. These, if present, must have developed between the time of actual death of the cells and their fixation. As will be shown, it becomes a matter of prime importance for the pathologist to know whether he is dealing with "living" or "dead" cells and tissues.

The fact is that there is no way of saying exactly when the death of a cell occurred but about six to twelve hours lapse between the onset of cell death and incontroversial recognition that the cell is dead by light microscopy. As soon as life has in reality departed, a series of chemical decompositions begins which, in the case of all but very dry tissues, will end only when the complicated organic structures are reduced to simple inorganic compounds including water, carbon dioxide, nitrates, hydrogen disulfide and other substances. Details of the process are readily available in books on chemistry and will not be elaborated here, but before long, with the gas formation, swelling of the cadaver, the foul odors and numerous other changes, it becomes only too clear that the creature is dead. Microscopic changes accompany those noticed grossly and will shortly be described. It remains to point out that while the decomposition of dead bodies is largely due, under ordinary circumstances, to the action of putrefactive bacteria, the same end will be achieved although the tissues are kept sterile. This is because of enzymatic substances within the cells themselves, called autolytic enzymes, and the process is called **post-mortem autolysis.**

The changes in the dead cells and tissues are essentially the same whether they have died with the animal as a whole, which constitutes post-mortem autolysis, or whether this particular group of cells died within the living animal, which, by definition, is necrosis. But, while the gross and microscopic appearances of dead cells remain the same regardless of which way they died, the significance to the pathologist is quite another matter. If it can be established that the observed changes occurred after the death of the patient, they have no connection with disease and are of no concern to the physician, pathologist or biologist. But if the cells underwent necrosis, a process occurring within the living body, obviously abnormal and unhealthy, this becomes something of great interest and concern in the study of disease and to anyone undertaking to combat it. We propose first to describe the observable changes incident to death of cells and then to see how necrosis can be distinguished from post-mortem autolysis.

THE CELL

Within the past decade, concepts concerning the structural and functional aspects of the cell have been drastically changed. This has been due to the use of new techniques and instruments, particularly the electron microscope. This instrument makes it possible to clearly visualize many organelles whose existence within the cell heretofore were only speculative. It is now possible to demonstrate the structural basis for functions which biochemical techniques reveal at the molecular level. Many of these events underlie the processes which can be recognized as disease in the cell, tissue or organism. Many structures which are recognized as components of normal cells and whose function is at least partially understood, are most certainly involved in disease processes. However, relatively few of the morphologic changes at the ultrastructural level have been clearly established in relation to disease in the organism, although the list of ultra-microscopic lesions is growing rapidly. It is now important to understand the structural and functional components of the cell at the magnifications of the electron microscope in order to appreciate current research in pathology. In some particular disease problems this understanding is also necessary to arrive at a definitive diagnosis. A brief review of the current status of knowledge of the ultrastructure of cells is therefore considered pertinent in an introduction to pathology.

The **cell membrane** is not visible by the light microscope but has been presumed

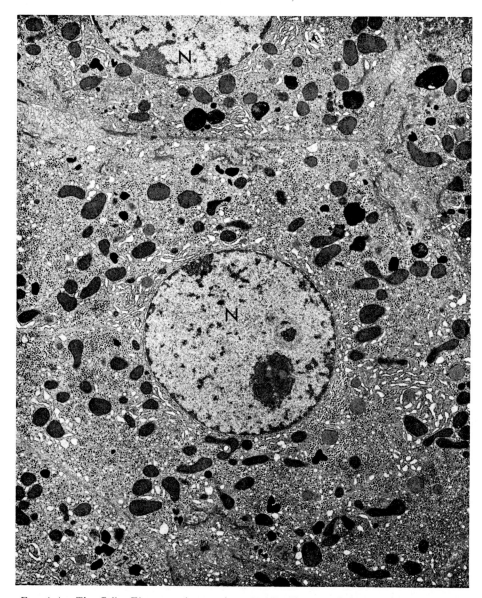

FIG. 1–1.—The Cell. Electron micrograph × 10,350, of parts of three liver cells of an owl monkey (*Aotus trivirgatus*). Note: nucleus (N), mitochondria—(membrane bound irregularly ovoid structures), lysosomes—(electron dense bodies), glycogen—(smallest dense granules) cell membranes—(separating adjacent cells). (Courtesy of Dr. Norval W. King.)

to surround the cytoplasm because of indirect indications: cytoplasm would flow from the cell after it was pricked by a micro-dissection needle; cells would shrink in hypertonic solution and swell in hypotonic solution; the cell is highly permeable to lipid-soluble substances and less permeable to ions—suggesting that the cell membrane consists of lipid or lipoprotein. Ultra thin sections of cells disclosed that the limiting membrane has a remarkably constant structure, consisting of two electron-dense lines, each about 30 Å thick separated by a light line of about the same thickness. (Å or Au is the Ångström unit, equivalent to

0.0001 micron, and is named after the Swedish physicist, Anders J. Ångström [1814–1874].)

This trilaminar arrangement is remarkably similar in most animal cells and has been referred to by some as the "unit membrane." The two outer layers are currently believed to consist of protein, the intermediate layer of lipid. The membrane is not always smooth but may be evaginated to produce specialized structures such as **microvilli** which increase absorptive surfaces on such cells as the epithelial cells lining intestinal villi. The brush border of some cells of the renal tubules is made up of similar microvilli. The cell membrane may also be invaginated into the cytoplasm probably as a part of the process known as **pinocytosis.** This process results in the engulfing of a minute droplet of fluid from the interstitium. This fluid contains inorganic ions such as sodium which in part are eliminated by a process which requires energy (the "sodium pump"). The cell membrane also acts as a semipermeable membrane permitting the passive transfer of substances, varying in molecular size, chemical composition and electrical charge. Active transport also occurs across the cell membrane, requiring energy and probably enzyme systems-processes which are as yet incompletely understood.

Many modifications of the cell membrane structure occur in different situations such as between adjoining cells, or over free surfaces, which are interesting but will not be considered further here.

The **cytoplasm** of the normal cell, seen with the light microscope to consist of eosinophilic, homogeneous to granular ground substance containing various inclusions and vesicles, is seen in electron micrographs to contain an amazing array of organelles. The number of each organelle varies with the type of cell and with its functional state. Among the most conspicuous are the **mitochondria,** which are discrete structures, visible with the light microscope, usually measuring 2 to 3 microns in length but often much longer. They vary in number, size and shape but usually appear as slender tubules with blind ends and are occasionally bent or folded. Often they are found in close proximity to structures which require energy such as cardiac or skeletal muscle fibers, or lipid globules. They were recognized in cells as early as 1850 but Benda, in 1898, was the first to use the term "mitochondrion." Each mitochondrion is outlined by an outer membrane, about 70 A thick, separated by a clear space about 80 Å wide from a similar inner membrane. This inner membrane extends into the mitochondrion as lamellae, or tubular arrays called **cristae.** These cristae may be few in number, extending only a short distance into the matrix of the mitochondrion or may be numerous, closely packed and bridge the width of the mitochondrion.

The more complex arrays of cristae appear to be associated with increased oxidative capacity. Differential centrifugation has been used to isolate mitochondria in quantities suitable for chemical analysis and to demonstrate that they are the principal sites of the oxidative reactions which make the energy in foodstuff available for cell metabolism. The necessary enzymes are situated for the most part in the membranes, presumably with spatial arrangements which permit the sequential events in the cytochrome chains linked to the Krebs cycle. Oxidative phosphorylation leads to the transfer of the energy released by oxidation to adenosine diphosphate and its eventual storage in the form of adenosine triphosphate.

A complex system of membranes which traverse the cytoplasm to form canaliculi, cisternae, vesicles or parallel arrays is known as the **endoplasmic**

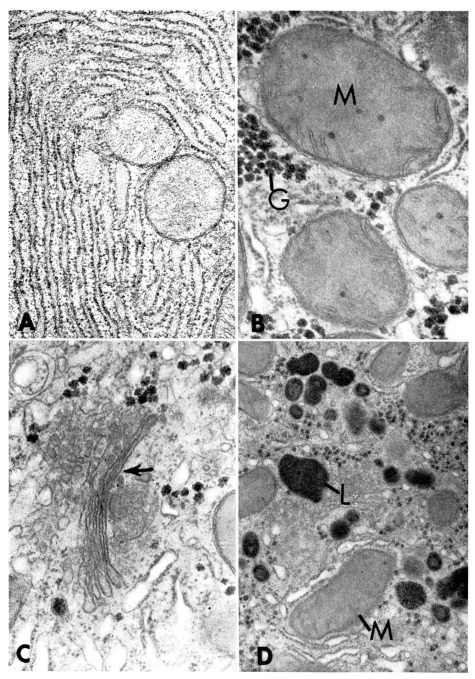

Fig. 1–2.—Intracellular organelles in electron micrographs. *A*, Rough endoplasmic reticulum in a plasma cell (× 36,000). *B*, Mitochondria (M) and glycogen (G) (× 44,500). *C*, Golgi apparatus. Each preparation from owl monkeys (*Aotus trivirgatus*). *D*, Lysosomes (largest at L) and mitochondria (M) (× 22,900). (Courtesy of Dr. Norval W. King.)

reticulum or ergastoplasm. Some of the membranes are smooth and are usually referred to as the **smooth surfaced,** or **agranular endoplasmic reticulum.** Others are studded with distinct granular bodies, **ribosomes,** and are therefore referred to as rough-surfaced or **granular endoplasmic reticulum.** This type has its greatest development in glandular cells which produce a secretion containing protein. However, synthesis of protein is known to be associated with ribosomes which may function adequately in the absence of endoplasmic reticulum. The endoplasmic reticulum appears to be necessary as a system of pathways which segregate the cell product, transport it to the Golgi region, store it temporarily and later move it to the exterior of the cell.

The granular reticulum usually appears in electron micrographs as thin profiles of membranes which form flat sacular expanses called **cisternae,** from a pair of membranes 300 to 600 Å apart. These membranes are continuous with one another at the end of their profile. These may be single or more often aggregated together and form intercommunicating tubules as well as cisternae. Vesicles may also be formed in isolated portions of the endoplasmic reticulum.

Smooth surfaced (agranular) endoplasmic reticulum often appears to be continuous with the rough variety—differing only in the absence of ribosomes. This type of membrane is richest in cells of the endocrine glands but may be caused to increase in liver cells by administration of certain drugs such as barbiturates. Thus, agranular reticulum is believed to be involved in the production of hormones and possibly have a role in detoxification.

The endoplasmic reticulum cannot be clearly visualized with the light microscope but it was probably demonstrated many years ago in preparations of muscle cells impregnated with metal. Basic dyes stain structures in the cytoplasm which probably are cisternae, and have been called basophilic bodies, Nissl substance, chromophilic substance or ergastoplasm. The electron microscope was required to demonstrate the canalicular nature, reticular formation and widespread occurrence of the endoplasmic reticulum.

The **Golgi complex,** or Golgi apparatus, was discovered by Golgi in 1898 in nerve cells which had been treated for a prolonged period in a solution of osmium tetroxide. Golgi called this structure the "internal reticular apparatus." Prolonged immersion in osmium tetroxide ("postomication") is necessary to stain this structure although it may be demonstrated by light microscopy following negative staining with toluidine blue. A long controversy over the actual existence of this structure, in part due to the failure to demonstrate it in living cells, was resolved by the use of the electron microscope. The complex is usually located near the nucleus and, in glandular cells, at the apical pole of the nucleus. Secreting granules are usually in close proximity.

In ultra thin sections, the Golgi complex is made up of aggregations of closely packed membrane-bound elements, arranged parallel to one another and joined at their ends. These packets vary in length, are usually about 150 Å wide and may be flat or curved. Clustered around the ends of these packets are many small vesicles 400 to 800 Å in diameter. On the inner, or concave, surface of the complex the cisternae are often distended and contain secretory products. Secretory granules are usually adjacent and surrounded by a membrane apparently arising from the Golgi complex.

The functions of the Golgi complex are not entirely known but it is believed that it functions to assemble secretory products brought to it through the endoplasmic reticulum after synthesis by the ribosomes. Polysaccharides may be added by the Golgi complex to the protein brought to it. Lipid absorbed by cells of the small intestine may accumulate in the Golgi complex of intestinal epithelial cells but the exact nature of the chemical events at this site is not known. It is possible that other functions may be found for this structure.

Lysosomes were originally found by differential centrifugation of tissue suspensions and defined as membrane-bound particles containing one or more hydrolytic enzymes. Structures meeting this chemical definition are found with difficulty in electron micrographs by demonstrating, with cytochemical staining, the presence of acid phosphatase. Bodies containing this enzyme are found to have diverse morphologic features in different tissues. The specific granules of neutrophils and eosinophils contain acid hydrolases and are therefore clearly lysosomes. Certain membrane limited dense bodies which are found in relation to the Golgi complex and in bile canaliculi in the liver also meet the criteria for lysosomes. Morphologic criteria alone are not sufficient to identify lysosomes, hence much confusion will probably continue in connection with these structures within the cytoplasm of cells except in cases in which electron microscopic and biochemical methods are used in concert.

The **centrioles** may be resolved with the light microscope as a pair of deeply stained short rods (sometimes called the diplosome). They are often adjacent to the nucleus in a zone known as the centrosome or cell center. Cytologists often refer to a line projected through the nucleus and the centrosome as the "cell axis." In some cells, the centrioles are surrounded by the Golgi complex, in others are located immediately beneath the cell membrane. One to forty pairs may occupy a single cell. The functions of the centrioles are not clear but apparently include the organization of the cell, particularly during cell division. Their position, after they have replicated, at opposite poles of the nucleus during mitosis is significant in the movement of the chromosomes to opposite poles of the cytoplasm. The chromosomes are connected to dense bodies (satellites) adjacent to the centriole by means of the spindle fibers which in electron micrographs are seen to be **microtubules.** In ciliated cells, reduplicated centrioles form the "basal bodies" which give rise to the cilia and serve as their kinetic centers.

Structurally, the electron microscope reveals each centriole to consist of a hollow cylinder, 0.15 micron in diameter and up to 0.5 micron long. One end of this cylinder is open, the other closed. The pair are often arranged with each long axis perpendicular to the other. The wall of the cylinder is made up of nine evenly spaced, hollow fibrils or tubules, each in triplicate. In some cells, ill defined, often spherical bodies up to 700 Å in diameter are seen adjacent to the centriole. These pericentriolar structures are the satellites to which the "spindle fibers" are attached.

Electron micrographs of the **nucleus** confirm the presence of structures seen by light microscopy and resolve many details, but discloses few new organelles, in contrast to the rich lode found in the cytoplasm. The **nuclear envelope** consists of two membranes, each about 75 A thick, separated by a space about 400 to 700 Å wide, the **perinuclear cisterna.** The outer membrane of the envelope is studded with ribosomes and often is continuous with endoplasmic reticulum of the cytoplasm. The nuclear envelope has its origin from these membranes. The inner and outer membranes of the nuclear envelope are diverted at intervals around circular structures called **nuclear pores.** These are not freely communicating fenestrations but under high resolution appear to be closed by a characteristic membrane. These so called pores may be the means of transfer of materials to and from the cytoplasm under enzymatic control. The perinuclear cisterna appears to be the means of exchange of most materials with the cytoplasm. Some cells have a third membrane on the inner surface of the nuclear envelope. This is a filamentous structure, moderately dense, about 300 Å thick and is called the **fibrous lamina.** It appears to function as a supportive skeleton for the cell.

Most of the content of the nucleus is made up of basophilic material called **chromatin.** Its distribution and structure depends upon the type of cell, its functional state and the fixation and staining procedures used. The most dense granular component forms masses of various sizes, is called **heterochromatin** and is considered to be relatively inactive metabolically. One specific mass of chromatin located adjacent to the nuclear envelope in cells of females is the **sex chromatin,** representing the inactive X chromosome (page 327). The more loosely arranged chromatin granules make up the **euchromatin** and are considered to be in the metabolically active state. Both stain characteristically with Feulgen reagent, demonstrating the principal component to be deoxyribonucleic acid, DNA (see Chapter 9).

The **nucleolus,** readily recognized with the light microscope, also has characteristic ultrastructure. This organelle appears to have a key role in synthesis of protein and in metabolism of nucleic acids. It consists of a rounded mass of chromatin, usually eccentrically placed, basophilic and stains specifically for ribonucleic acid, RNA. It disappears during mitosis but in the interphase nucleus has two ultrastructural components. The **nucleolonema** appears as branching coarse strands that form a network. Under higher magnification these strands are seen to consist of a matrix in which are embedded dense granules resembling ribosomes. These granules are judged to be made up of ribonucleoprotein. The nucleolonema usually surrounds a spherical, apparently structureless, component of the nucleolus, the **pars amorpha.**

The nucleus is not essential for the life of some cells, such as the mature erythrocyte and the epithelial cells in the interior of the lens, but is necessary for the cell to divide or carry out complex metabolic activities. Present concepts have the DNA of the nucleus responsible for the character of the enzymes which control all functions of the cell and, by exact replication of the DNA and its distribution to daughter cells in the chromosomes, determine the characteristics of each cell generation. This is discussed further in Chapter 9.

Many **cell inclusions** are resolved in the cytoplasm in more detail with the electron microscope although most have been recognized with the light microscope. These include secretory products such as are found in anterior pituitary cells, pancreatic islets and other endocrine cells. Similar inclusions are found in exocrine gland cells, such as in salivary, goblet, mucous, chief, pancreatic acinar and Brunner's gland cells. Neurosecretory granules are another important cell inclusion. Pigments, such as melanin and lipofuscin are included in this category as are glycogen, lipid and crystalline inclusions. These will be described in detail in the appropriate chapters.

DEATH OF CELLS AND TISSUES

Microscopic Appearance of Dead Tissue. — (Note to the Student: We frequently give the microscopic description before giving the gross characteristics.

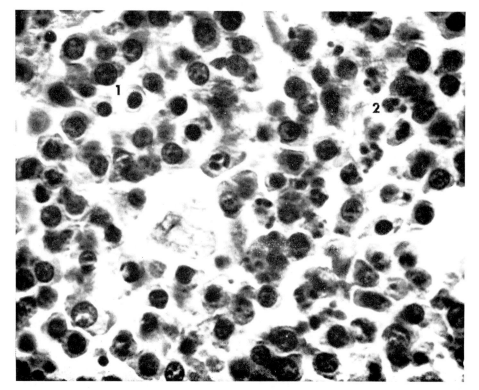

Fig. 1–3.—Necrosis, evidenced by pyknosis and karyorrhexis of nuclei in neoplastic cells of a canine malignant lymphoma after treatment with nitrogen mustard. Pyknotic nuclei (1) are round, decreased in size and homogeneous; nuclei undergoing karyorrhexis (2) are fragmented into several pieces. H & E, × 600.

One reason for doing this is to impress upon him the fact that if the microscopic appearances are known, the gross picture can usually be deduced with considerable accuracy; the converse is not necessarily true. A part of the student's training should involve practice in these deductions.)

1. Changes in the Nucleus:

a. **Pyknosis.**—This is one of the common manifestations of death of the cells, although it must not be supposed that pyknosis will be seen in every dead cell. The pyknotic nucleus is **decreased in size** but **round**, more perfectly so than it was during life. The nucleus is **black** or nearly so when stained by ordinary stains such as hematoxylin and eosin. This is because it is more acid in its reaction and attracts the basic hematoxylin; its nucleic acid is being set free. The pyknotic nucleus is **homogeneous**; it lacks the nucleolus, chromatin granules and internal structure characteristic of most kinds of nuclei during life. Pyknosis is best seen in epithelial cells, leukocytes and nerve cells. The elongated nuclei of connective tissue and muscle, of course, do not become round, but the loss of internal structure and the shrinking are conspicuous features of the dead smooth-muscle nucleus. Pyknosis is one of the earlier changes in point of time; ultimately the dead nucleus disappears altogether.

b. **Karyorrhexis.**—Literally a flowing of the nucleus, this term is used to designate the dead nucleus which is reduced to many tiny fragments, barely

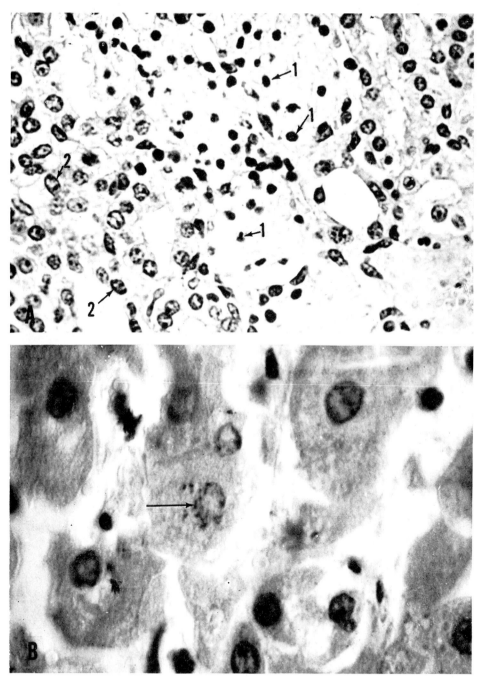

FIG. 1–4.—A, Pyknosis. Small, round, densely staining nuclei (1) at the margin of an infarct in the kidney of a pig. Compare with the nuclei (2) of unaffected renal tubules. (Courtesy of Armed Forces Institute of Pathology.) × 490. Contributor: Lt. Col. F. D. Maurer.

B, Karyorrhexis. Fragmentation of nuclear chromatin (arrow) in a liver cell of a dog. × 800. (Courtesy of Armed Forces Institute of Pathology.)

visible, and these may remain to mark the original position of the nucleus or they may be scattered over a considerable space. It is seen occasionally and is a step in the development of caseous necrosis to be described later.

c. **Karyolysis.**—This is a dissolution of the nuclear material. When complete the nucleus naturally is not seen, but the term is used to refer to the incomplete stages, when the nucleus appears as a hollow sphere, a ghost with only the nuclear membrane remaining.

A corollary process to karyolysis is **chromatolysis.** The stainable material of the nucleus including the nucleolus, the chromosomes, and other visible structures, is known as **chromatin** because it gives the nucleus its color (blue by ordinary stains). In karyolysis it is the chromatin which is dissolved. The dissolved chromatin does not necessarily vanish but is in solution in the intercellular fluids of the vicinity, carrying its blue color with it. This accounts for a diffuse bluish discoloration in some unusual locations, for instance if there is fibrin in the neighborhood it will absorb the chromatin and become blue instead of its usual magenta.

d. **Absence of the Nucleus.**—All of the preceding nuclear changes terminate in complete destruction of the nucleus. If the nucleus is absent, the cell is dead. The erythrocyte may be considered an exception but it has lost, with its nucleus, its reproductive power and other characteristics of life.

2. **Changes in the Cytoplasm :**

In some cases the cytoplasm may reveal relatively little change, but if changes in the nucleus indicate death the cell should be considered dead. The following abnormalities of cytoplasm may be present.

a. **Unusually Acidophilic Cytoplasm.**—The cytoplasm is acidophilic because its reaction is more basic than during life, hence it takes the acid stain, which is usually red (eosin). The cytoplasm is, then, a deeper red than usual. Cytoplasmic structure is obscured. This sign of death is prominent when the more delicate epithelial cells such as those of renal tubules and liver undergo the condition called coagulation necrosis, the nuclei being concomitantly pyknotic. The cytoplasm of dead polymorphonuclear neutrophils is also often conspicuously red-staining, as seen in pus. This acidophilia is believed to be largely the result of loss of nucleoproteins (ribonucleoprotein and deoxyribonucleoprotein) from the cytoplasm and nucleus.

b. **Cytoplasmolysis.**—As the changes of death progress, the cytoplasm tends to become less and less dense and ultimately disappears completely. It is possible for much of the cytoplasm to disappear while the cell remains alive, however, and therefore the decision whether the cell is living or dead under circumstances of partial lysis of cytoplasm should depend on the condition of the nucleus.

3. **More advanced changes—the cell as a whole :**

a. **Loss of Cell Outline.**—When the changes of death are well advanced, it may be impossible to see the form and outline of the cells although the material of which they are made is obviously still present. In applying this criterion, one must not be misled by failure to identify cell outlines which are often indistinct in normal histology, such as those in stratified squamous epithelium and smooth muscle. The condition under consideration may be illustrated by the cells of an inflammatory exudate in which the nucleus, or remains of it, may still be visible but the shape and nature of the cell quite undeterminable. Complete loss of cell outline will be seen when the student studies the caseous necrosis of a tubercle.

b. **Loss of Differential Staining.**—There are situations when tissue can still be

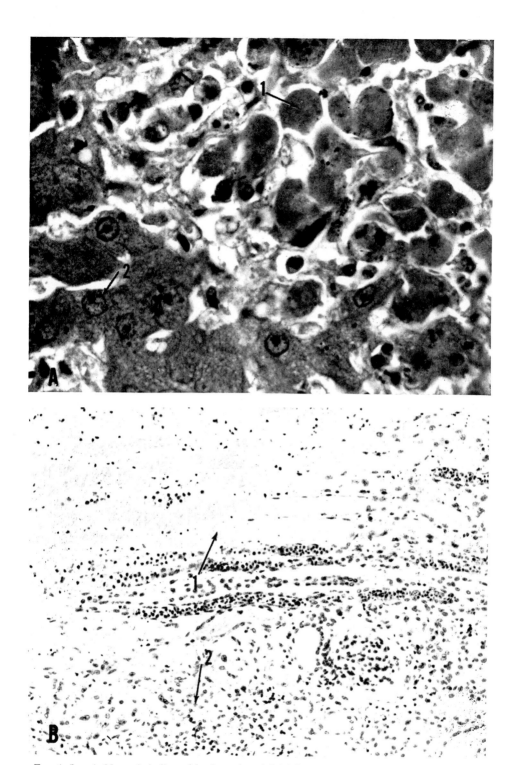

FIG. 1–5.—A, Necrosis indicated by loss of nuclei (1) from liver cells of a dog. Compare with vesicular nuclei (2) containing nucleoli, in unaffected liver cells. × 600. Contributor: Dr. D. J. Carren.

B, Necrosis, indicated by loss of differential staining in renal tubules (1) at the margin of an anemic infarct in the kidney of a pig. Normal renal tubules at (2). (Courtesy of Armed Forces Institute of Pathology.) × 125. Contributor: Lt. Col. F. D. Maurer.

seen but the colors of nuclei and cytoplasm, as well as the colors characteristic of the different histological tissues, cannot be distinguished. Chromatolysis will be found to have had an important part in producing this condition. As an example one may look at the mucosa of an intestine involved either in necrosis or post-mortem autolysis. There is a stage in which the villi and glands are fairly well outlined, but not a single individual cell or structure can be identified. This represents both loss of differential staining and loss of cell outline.

c. **Absence of Cell.**—If the cell cannot be found, it must be assumed to have died. Absence of cells that should be present has practical importance both within organs and tissues and on their surfaces. If the number of hepatic cells in a liver lobule, for instance, is less than we know to be normal, it can be concluded that the missing ones have died, no doubt through necrosis, and have undergone **autolysis** and disappeared, one by one. On a surface, such as the intestinal mucosa and the skin, when a cell dies there is commonly nothing to hold it in its place and it disappears through the process of **desquamation,** or sloughing. If one sees a body surface without its normal epithelial covering, that epithelium has died, either through necrosis or post-mortem autolysis. In the intestine such desquamated cells may often be seen mixed with fecal material and still showing rather satisfactory staining qualities. Those cells are dead by virtue of being desquamated if there is nothing else to show it. If one sees the lining epithelium of a gland or duct, or the endothelium of a blood vessel free in the lumen, those cells must be considered dead even though they may stain rather well. Usually if they still stain well, the desquamation and death is a matter of post-mortem autolysis and therefore of no significance, but if they come off during life they will never be reunited to their base and the process is one of necrosis. This is not an infrequent occurrence; the sloughing of the bronchial epithelium in bronchitis is an example, as well as the loss of alveolar epithelium in mastitis.

Gross Characteristics of Dead Tissue.—This subject will be discussed further under Differentiation between Necrosis and Post-mortem Autolysis, but the following general characteristics may be pointed out:

1. **Loss of Color.**—Dead tissue is regularly paler than living, except when it is well filled with blood, which makes it black. Hemolyzed blood is blackish-red and if large amounts are present in the tissue, this will be the dominant color. Spotting with black and white usually has no other significance than this. Areas of necrosis are often quite conspicuous by their change in color.

2. **Loss of Strength.**—Dead tissue has little strength, especially tensile strength. In lifting the intestine out of the cadaver at autopsy, a length of intestine, necrotic because of obstruction, or infarction, or the whole intestine in case of advanced post-mortem autolysis, may be too weak to support its own weight and it pulls apart as it is raised. The finger may be thrust with little resistance into a liver or lung which has undergone these changes.

3. Odors of putrefaction appear if the dead tissue was exposed to air-borne bacteria in gangrene (p. 26) or post-mortem autolysis.

4. Such changes as caseation, liquefaction and coagulation will be discussed under Necrosis, although most of them develop also during the process of post-mortem autolysis. As an example, one sees brains which have been sent without preservative arrangements to the laboratory for examination for Negri bodies. In warm weather they sometimes arrive in a state of complete liquefaction.

DIFFERENTIATION BETWEEN NECROSIS AND
POST-MORTEM AUTOLYSIS

Microscopically the following considerations assist in deciding whether tissue died ante mortem or post mortem, that is, in distinguishing between necrosis and post-mortem autolysis:

1. If one finds both living and dead tissue within the same microscopic section, it seems obvious that the dead part represents necrosis and not post-mortem autolysis but unfortunately things are not always so simple. Post-mortem autolysis sometimes shows a decidedly patchy distribution which is deceptive and justifies reliance on other criteria to decide between ante-mortem and post-mortem death of tissue.

2. The erythrocytes *within the blood vessels* should be examined for sharpness of outline and for the degree to which they take the stain. Hemolysis of the blood cells in the blood stream, if present, took place after death, thus indicating a certain degree of post-mortem autolysis of the whole specimen. Formalin-fixed erythrocytes stained with hematoxylin and eosin should stain a bright copper-red; with mercuric chloride fixation they are a rose-red. Alcohol fixation hemolyzes erythrocytes to empty circles, whatever stain is used. Erythrocytes separated by hemorrhage from the circulation and their source of oxygen undergo hemolysis within the living body. Hence they are not of value in determining the presence or absence of post-mortem autolysis.

3. Necrotic tissue left in the body usually acts as an irritant, hence there should be at least a slight inflammatory zone of leukocytes and hyperemia in the living tissue which immediately surrounds the dead tissue, if the process was one of necrosis.

4. A knowledge of the relative rate at which different tissues of the body tend to show the effects of post-mortem autolysis may be of material assistance. The mucosa of the digestive tract shows these changes early because the usual autolysis is abetted by the action of the no longer inhibited digestive juices. Even earlier the lining of the gallbladder succumbs to autolysis intensified by the destructive action of bile. The medulla of the adrenal undergoes early post-mortem liquefaction so that it is not unusual to examine an otherwise rather well-preserved adrenal and find only a collapsed space where the medulla should be. The neurons are probably next to show the changes of post-mortem autolysis; connective tissue is among the last to do so.

Grossly the problem is usually to decide at the start of an autopsy how long the animal has been dead. Both autolysis and putrefaction are greatly slowed by refrigerator temperature. At summer temperatures the post-mortem deterioration which occurs in hours may almost equal the effect of as many days in the refrigerator. Sheep show serious post-mortem changes very early because the insulating effect of the fleece prevents dissipation of the body heat, and the same is true of larger swine because of the insulating layer of fat. Post-mortem changes proceed with unusual rapidity when the body temperature is very high at the time of death, as in heat stroke, and when it continues to rise even after death, as in tetanus, and when potentially putrefactive organisms are disseminated through the blood at the time of, or possibly before death (*Clostridium septicum*). An example of the latter phenomenon has at times resulted in a post-mortem picture so startling as to have been called "black disease" (p. 573), a name attrib-

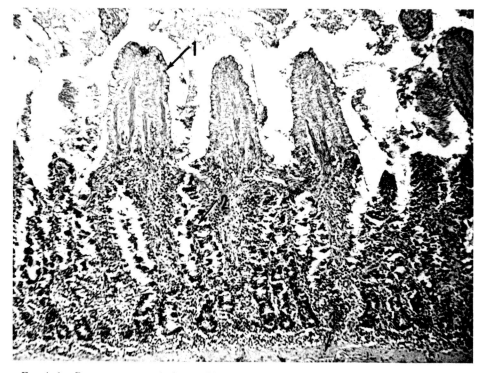

FIG. 1–6.—Post-mortem autolysis, small intestine of a dog. The villi (*1*) are denuded of epithelium which, however, is still present in the crypts (*2*). Muscularis mucosae at (*3*). (Courtesy of Armed Forces Institute of Pathology.) × 90. Contributor: Dr. R. O. Delano.

uted to the almost universal blackish discoloration of congested, autolyzed tissues seen upon removal of the animal's skin. "Pulpy-kidney disease" (p. 1211) has been described in sheep when autolytic and putrefactive softening have involved the kidneys especially. With or without more specific changes, such kidneys are severely congested and contain large numbers of clostridial organisms.

If the digestive tract of herbivorous animals is well filled with ingesta, fermentation and gas formation may within a very few hours cause great distention of the digestive tract and consequently of the torso, and also press bloody foam out the nostrils and cause the rectal lining to protrude in a pseudo-prolapse. The distention due to post-mortem fermentation has to be distinguished from ante-mortem bloating (tympanites), a frequent cause of death in ruminants. Signs of anoxia (p. 121) usually accompany the bloating which occurred during life.

When post-mortem changes are far advanced, the muscles are softened, pale red, watery, and resemble meat that has been cooked slightly. When post-mortem autolysis is only moderately advanced, an important indication is **post-mortem imbibition**. This is the result of the previously mentioned hemolysis of erythrocytes in the blood vessels. Their hemoglobin is released to go into solution in the blood plasma, and at the same time the walls of the blood vessels become more permeable to fluids as the result of post-mortem autolysis and weakening. Consequently the red-tinged plasma leaks out into the surrounding tissues, or, as it is customarily expressed, is "imbibed" by them. The result is a distinct dark red fringe along the course of each vessel which is easily seen on white tissues such as the mesentery or omentum. "Imbibition of bile" is a similar leaking of bile through the autolyzed wall of the gallbladder to stain adjacent liver tissue a greenish hue to a varying depth, which is sharply delimited.

Further information is gained upon opening the heart. Ordinarily rigor mortis contracts the left ventricle strongly and empties it of blood. The right ventricle remains more or less filled with blood and when this blood is hemolyzed a few hours post mortem, the lining of the ventricle assumes a lusterless but strong red color which does not wash off. If the left ventricle does contain blood, and this is unclotted, it indicates that rigor mortis has not yet taken place, death being quite recent. However, after a lapse of some twenty-four to seventy-two hours post mortem, depending upon temperature, the rigor has come and gone, allowing dark, hemolyzed blood from the disintegrating clot to run back into the ventricle. This latter indicates prolonged post-mortem autolysis. If the left ventricle contains clotted blood, the body forces were too low at the time of death for rigor mortis to develop, as is often the case with lingering illness.

In the rumen, reticulum and omasum of ruminants an impressive sign of post-mortem autolysis is desquamation of the epithelium. Within a surprisingly short time after death this comparatively thick surface layer is completely displaced by the slightest touch.

The **cause of post-mortem autolysis** is obvious and its importance to the pathologist is only that it be avoided if possible and that it be distinguished accurately from necrosis.

NECROSIS

Necrosis has already been defined as death of cells or tissues while the body as a whole still lives. The term *necrobiosis* is used as a synonym by some although to others it signifies merely the death of cells at the end of their life-span as is natural in most healthy tissues.

The **gross** and **microscopic appearances** are, in general, those stated for dead tissue.

The **causes of necrosis** can be summarized under the following headings:

1. **Poisons.**—It is difficult to state exactly what is meant by the term, poison. Included is the idea of a definite chemical structure, simple or complex, known or unknown, and that it is a substance which produces injury when taken into, or applied to the animal body. The injury may result through a number of mechanisms varying with the kind of poison, but many act to produce necrosis either locally by direct contact or remotely when distributed in the blood. It is convenient to divide poisons into four classes according to their origin.

a. **"Chemical poisons"** are chemical preparations, usually articles of commerce such as drugs, insecticides and a great variety of substances used in the industries. The insecticide, lead arsenate, is a good example; when ingested in large amount and in somewhat concentrated form, it kills many of the cells with which it comes in contact, producing intestinal ulceration; taken in small amount and suitably diluted over a period of time, it slowly destroys the delicate parenchymal cells of the liver, which it reaches via the blood stream. Strong acids and strong alkalies also belong in this group.

b. The toxins, or **poisons of pathogenic micro-organisms** are the principal means by which such organisms produce disease, necrosis of delicate parenchymatous cells often being a prominent feature. The necrophorus bacillus is outstanding for its ability to kill the tissues around it wherever it may localize. The blackleg organism kills the muscle tissue where it localizes.

c. Poisons produced by certain plants and animals cause necrosis, either locally or in the cells of parenchymatous organs such as the liver and kidney. Even the common "chigger" (*Trombicula sp.*) causes necrosis of a zone around its tiny bite in susceptible humans. Hypersensitization may be a factor in this case. Slow death of hepatic or renal epithelium is a feature of many plant poisonings.

d. Toxins or **poisons produced by decomposition** processes in the body are well illustrated in the necrosis of liver cells which follows severe burns in any part of the body. Absorbed toxic products from decomposing tissue at the site of the burn are considered responsible.

2. **Lack of Proper Blood Supply.**—Not all tissues require the same amount of blood, but the minimum must be met or the tissue will die. The immediately critical requirement is that of oxygen. The arterial flow to a part can be partially or completely obstructed by lodged emboli and thrombosis (p. 113) within the artery, by compression of the artery by ligatures, tourniquets (which should be temporarily released at intervals of twenty minutes) or the pressure of nearby tumors or abscesses. The blood vessels of the bowel are obstructed by twisting or compression of the mesentery in which they run, such as occurs in intestinal volvulus or intussusception (p. 1215). Ergotism (poisoning by ergot, the "smut" of grains and grasses) causes death of the extremities because its contractile effect on smooth muscle constricts the arteries until the more distal ones are obliterated. Poisoning by tall fescue grass (*Festuca arundinacea*) has a similar effect (p. 928). Stagnation of the flow of blood in venous congestion (p. 131) is a factor in the necrosis of the central cells of the hepatic lobules whenever there is prolonged impairment of cardiac function (see Toxic Hepatitis, p. 1223).

3. **Lack of Nerve Supply.**—It is still unsettled to what extent "trophic" nerve fibers are essential for proper nutrition of the tissues, but it is known that limbs and other parts suffer atrophy and necrosis of many cells when deprived of normal innervation. The best example is seen in "sweeney" of the horse. The animal, when put to heavy work without gradual conditioning, is prone to develop a sudden shoulder lameness and in a very few days the supraspinatus or the infraspinatus muscle, or both, waste away until the skin lies almost in direct contact with the scapula. It is found that the collar has put undue pressure on the suprascapular nerve where it passes over the anterior edge of the scapula, impairing the continuity of many of its fibers. In the resultant paralyzed state of these muscles, many or most of their fibers disappear. In the case of some, the necrosis becomes complete, in others the sarcoplasm is destroyed but the sarcolemma persists. These latter muscle fibers are capable of regeneration concurrently with the nerve fibers.

4. **Pressure.**—Severe pressure suddenly applied would be classed as trauma, to be treated below. Pressure necrosis is that which occurs as the result of long-continued pressure, often relatively mild. Spectacular examples are seen in bedsores (decubitus) and at the site of casts or bandages. An animal, recumbent for some days, even though carefully bedded, will often suffer slow death of the skin and all soft tissues over the bony prominences of the body, such as the tuber

coxae and the zygomatic arch. In spite of the best of nursing, the same unfortunate complications arise with even greater frequency in humans for the reason that life commonly continues longer for the bed-fast human patient. Casts and bandages applied too tightly may be removed only to reveal an ulcerated and necrotic skin beneath. This is not to be confused with death of a whole limb which sometimes results from shutting off its circulation (lack of blood supply) by a tight cast or bandage. Slower in development but no less sure is the necrosis of the parenchymal cells of soft organs as they yield to the continuous pressure of encroaching tumors or chronic abscesses. In these cases, the necrosis proceeds so insidiously that few dead cells may be seen at any given moment, an example of necrosis detected by "absence of cell" as mentioned earlier.

5. **Mechanical and Thermal Injuries.**—Any number of forms of physical trauma can be severe enough to kill body cells in the area involved. This is readily believed by almost anyone whose thumb has accidentally borne the brunt of a hammer-blow intended for a nail. In addition to such purely mechanical injuries, heat and the various related forms of energy can have a similar effect. The latter include light rays, ultraviolet rays, roentgen rays, radiations from radium and other radioactive substances, and electric currents. All tend to coagulate protoplasm, thus killing the cells, and, if sufficiently severe, to carbonize it.

The milder **burns** may not immediately kill even the epidermis but cause only erythema. They are known as burns of the **first degree,** however the epidermis usually desquamates a week later, as in the case of sunburns and mild burns by ultraviolet light. Burns of the **second degree** also produce a serous inflammatory exudate in the form of vesicles (blisters) between the epidermis and the dermis. **Third degree** burns kill the tissue outright to an appreciable depth.

Freezing kills cells directly by bursting their walls as well as by disarranging the colloidal suspensions of the protoplasm. However, extremities can suffer necrosis and gangrene without actually being frozen, for at near-freezing temperature the blood becomes a sludge and stops flowing, and the tissues die from lack of blood supply.

We now wish to discuss briefly certain special manifestations of necrosis to which custom and tradition have given special names.

COAGULATIVE (OR "COAGULATION") NECROSIS

Occurrence.—Coagulative necrosis occurs in a variety of situations especially the following:

1. In connection with diphtheritic (fibrinous, p. 156) inflammations of mucous membranes. The epithelium and, to some extent, the deeper layers under such circumstances undergo necrosis of this type. If the layer of fibrin is removed, the underlying necrotic cells are detached with it. The necrophorus organism is responsible for this lesion in many instances, especially the "necrotic" enteritis of swine (p. 1206). The same type of change occurs in the throat in human diphtheria

2. In infarcts (p. 28), which are circumscribed areas of necrosis caused by stoppage of the blood supply.

3. In "Zenker's necrosis" of muscle (p. 22).

Microscopically such tissue structures and cellular outlines as existed previously are still discernible. The nuclei are generally pyknotic but still readily visible. The cytoplasm is often strongly acidophilic.

Grossly the necrotic tissue is gray or white (unless filled with blood), firm, dense and often depressed as compared with surrounding living tissue.

Causes especially tending to produce this variety of necrosis include (1) local ischemia (p. 28) as in infarcts, (2) the toxic products of certain bacteria, as in calf diphtheria, necrophorus enteritis and other forms of necrobacillosis, (3) certain locally acting poisons, such as mercuric chloride, and (4) the milder burns, whether produced by heat, electricity or roentgen rays.

Significance.—Tissue undergoing this type of necrosis ultimately passes on to loss of nuclei, loss of differential staining and complete absence of the tissue due to slow and imperceptible liquefaction. In these later stages, it is not different from simple necrosis. However, in its typical form, its recognition as a separate type affords useful diagnostic indications as is evident from the causes.

CASEOUS NECROSIS

Occurrence.—Caseous necrosis occurs as part of the typical lesions of tuberculosis, syphilis (humans), ovine caseous lymphadenitis and other granulomas (p. 615).

Microscopically there is loss of cell outline and loss of differential staining. Cell walls and other histological structures disappear, the tissue disintegrating to form a finely granular mass which has a purplish color (hematoxylin and eosin stain) resulting from the mixture of blue chromatin granules with red ones derived from the cytoplasm. Any pre-existing fibrillar structure will have disappeared.

The gross appearance is suggestive of "milk curds," or "cottage" cheese, hence the name, caseous. The necrotic tissue is dry but slightly greasy, firm but without

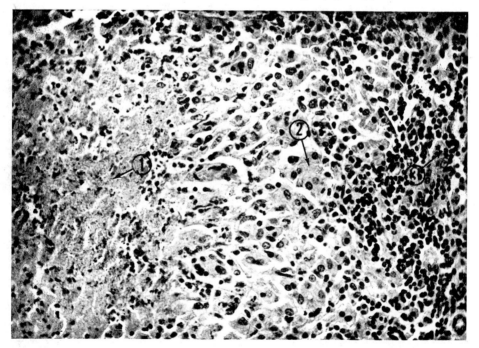

FIG. 1–7.—Caseous necrosis (1) in the center of a tubercle in the lung of a monkey (*Macacus rhesus*). Epithelioid granulation tissue (2), and lymphocytes (3) surround the caseous center. (Courtesy of Armed Forces Institute of Pathology.)   × 260.   Contributor: Army Veterinary School.

any cohesive strength, so that it can be easily separated into granular fragments by a blunt instrument. The color is white, grayish or yellowish.

Causes of caseous necrosis are the locally acting toxins of the specific microorganisms of the diseases already mentioned.

Significance.—The caseous material often remains in position for a long time, especially when encapsulated by fibrous tissue as is commonly the case. It is prone to undergo calcification, as in tubercles. However, liquefaction and disappearance is not impossible.

LIQUEFACTIVE (OR "LIQUEFACTION") NECROSIS

While most necrotic tissue slowly disappears by a process of insidious and imperceptible liquefaction, there are situations in which this change proceeds rapidly with accumulation of measurable amounts of fluid and without any noticeable precursor change in the dying cells. This process is known as liquefaction necrosis.

Occurrence.—There are two principal situations in which noticeable liquefaction of dying tissue is encountered. The first is in the central nervous system; the second, in abscesses. Areas of liquefactive necrosis sometimes occur in tuberculous lungs, producing cavities of considerable size.

Microscopically the necrotic area, be it large or small, appears as an empty space. The space not only is without any definitive lining, but its edges are frayed and irregular and usually the cells on the edge show some of the evidences of necrosis. A pink-staining proteinaceous precipitate may or may not remain from the liquid. The actual water was removed in the process of dehydration of the tissue preparatory to sectioning. In the case of an abscess the liquid is represented by pus, which leaves a dehydrated residue of polymorphonuclear neutrophils, fragments of destroyed tissue cells, fibrin and nondescript débris.

Grossly this lesion is represented by a cavity, small or large, containing a fluid which is usually clear. Assuming that the process is still in progress, the walls of the cavity are frayed and irregular and more or less softened. Such a fluid-filled space is not generally considered a cyst since a true cyst involves the accumulation of fluid, usually a secretion, in a cavity which has a natural and permanent type of lining, usually epithelial. In liquefaction necrosis, the liquid usually is drained away by the lymphatics and the wall is merely the pre-existing tissue in the process of disintegration. In an abscess, the liquefaction is a minor aspect, the accumulation of inflammatory exudate being of transcendent importance.

The **causes** of liquefactive necrosis are included in those already given for necrosis in general. The reason that the tissue liquefies in the brain and spinal cord almost as soon as it dies is considered to be the high content of lipoids and the small amount of coagulable albumin present in these tissues. It has also been shown that an acid reaction of the tissue is essential. In the case of abscesses, the liquefaction of tissue is attributable to liquefying toxins (lysins) which have been demonstrated for most of the bacteria responsible. The leukocytes which comprise most of the inflammatory exudate also produce liquefying enzymes. The liquefaction of old pulmonary tubercles may be regarded as an end stage of the caseous necrosis which is typically encountered, since all necrotic tissue tends ultimately to disappear by a slow process of liquefaction. However, it is probable that secondary pyogenic infection and lytic substances produced by the bacteria play an important part in these tubercles.

NECROSIS OF FAT

When adipose tissue undergoes necrosis, the fat is not infrequently decomposed, perhaps slowly, into its two constituent radicals, fatty acid and glycerin. The fatty acid then combines in various proportions with the metallic ions present, chiefly sodium, potassium and calcium. The result is the formation of a soap within what was a fat cell, and the soap is not dissolved out, as fat is, by the fat solvents (xylene, etc.) used in the sectioning technique.

Microscopically one sees the same adipose-connective-tissue cells as in the normal tissue, but the fat is replaced by a solid, opaque material, nearly homogeneous but sometimes pervaded by minute clear slits marking the site of dissolved fatty-acid crystals. It takes a bluish or a pinkish tinge depending on the presence of sodium or potassium respectively, or a purple if calcium has been deposited. The nuclei tend to be pyknotic but are histologically not of a type to show this change clearly.

Grossly adipose tissue that has undergone this change loses its shiny and semi-translucent character to become opaque, whitish and solid or slightly granular. It retains its previous position and extent indefinitely.

Causes.—Two types of causative mechanism are recognized. The traditional **pancreatic necrosis of fat** occurs only in the abdominal cavity and is the result of the fat-splitting action of pancreatic juice which has escaped from its proper ducts and channels because of some other lesion in the ductal system of the pancreas, such as invasion by a neoplasm. But the same type of change occurs outside the abdominal cavity due to pressure and mechanical trauma. It is known as **traumatic necrosis of fat** and is well exemplified in the subcutaneous and intermuscular fat in the sternal region of a cow which has been for some time in a position of sternal recumbency.

Significance.—In the abdominal cavity one searches for a pancreatic lesion, although the non-pancreatic type can be found here. While the condition is known as necrosis, it appears that at times the condition is reversible, the cells still retaining life.

ZENKER'S NECROSIS

This condition, which is also known as **Zenker's degeneration,** occurs only in striated muscle. It is essentially a coagulation of proteins of the sarcoplasm.

Microscopically the individual fibers are swollen, often markedly, and are homogeneous and hyaline in texture. The sarcoplasm is unusually acidophilic (red by ordinary stains), the myofibrils cannot be seen and the nuclei are small and dark (see Fig. 20–1, p. 1047).

Grossly, if the involved area is large enough to be seen, the muscle is white or pale, rather shiny and somewhat swollen. The term **hyaline degeneration** has been used by some for this change in muscle but will be reserved in this work for certain more specific lesions to be described later.

The **causes** are considered usually to be toxins of pathogenic micro-organisms

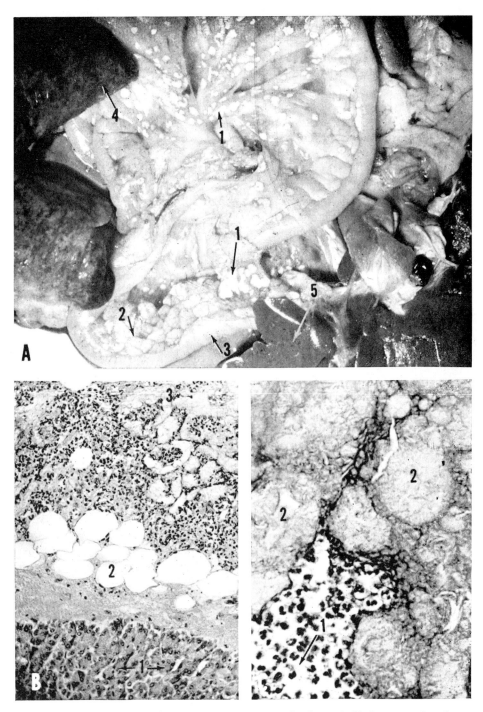

FIG. 1–8.—Pancreatic necrosis of fat in the mesentery of a dog. *A*, Chalky appearing plaques (*1*), pancreas (*2*), duodenum (*3*), lung (*4*), and liver (*5*). *B*, Pancreas (*1*), normal fat cells (*2*) and necrotic fat (*3*) surrounded by leukocytes. × 165. *C*, Higher magnification of polymorphonuclear leukocytes (*1*) and necrotic (saponified) fat (*2*). (*B* and *C*, Courtesy of Armed Forces Institute of Pathology.) × 440. Contributor: Dr. Samuel Pollock.

2

since it occurs in connection with various systemic or local infections but white-muscle diseases (p. 1049) present a similar change.

Significance.—The affected fibers are dead. Regeneration of other fibers may possibly be seen in the vicinity, although this is not usual.

THE OUTCOME OF NECROSIS

Under exceptional circumstances, necrotic tissue may remain in the body for quite some time but ultimately its disposal is accomplished along one of the following routes.

1. Liquefaction and removal of the fluid via the blood and lymph streams. This is the usual termination when the number of dead cells in a given area at a given time is small, and larger masses may gradually follow the same course. As already stated it is the rule in the central nervous system.

2. Liquefaction and formation of a cyst-like accumulation of fluid is an occasional occurrence, the fluid accumulating faster than it is drained away.

3. Liquefaction with abscess formation occurs when necrosis is part of the damage inflicted by pyogenic bacteria. It is accompanied by formation of a purulent exudate. The tendency is for abscesses to rupture, the pus making its way to the nearest free surface along a path of subsequently developing necrosis in the overlying tissue. (p. 21).

4. Encapsulation Without Liquefaction.—When there is little moisture in the part, dead tissue may remain with little change, usually in the form of caseous or coagulative necrosis. It then acts as an irritant to surrounding living tissue and incites a cellular (leukocytic) inflammatory reaction around it. Before many days have passed, the reaction involves fibrosis and the formation of a fibrous capsule. Enclosed in this fibrous capsule it may persist for a long time, doing the patient little or no harm. In addition to tubercles (p. 629), dead parasites within the tissues are commonly encapsulated in this manner.

5. Desquamation or Sloughing.—If on an external or internal body surface, dead cells regularly lose their attachment to the underlying living tissue. Thin layers, such as an epithelial covering, are said to desquamate, that is, to come off in flat, scale-like fragments. Larger and deeper masses of tissue are said to "slough off." The desquamated epithelial cells are often seen clumped together in the lumen of glands, ducts, bronchi, or renal tubules or in the lumen of an intestine. The endothelial cells lining blood vessels behave similarly. Post-mortem sloughing (p. 17) must be excluded.

6. Replacement by scar tissue ultimately follows as the terminal stage of abscesses, encapsulated areas, cyst-like cavities, infarcts or diffuse loss of tissue such as occurs in the kidney and liver.

7. Calcification (p. 54) converts the dead tissue into a sandy mass. It is thus rendered inert and harmless, unless in such a location that the hard and irregular material interferes mechanically with movement or other function of the nearby structures.

8. Gangrene supervenes when parts exposed directly or indirectly to the external air and its saprophytic bacteria have become necrotic. This will presently be treated in detail.

9. Atrophy (p. 90) of the organ, tissue or part is naturally an accompaniment of the necrosis and loss of any considerable number of cells.

10. Regeneration, the formation of new cells like those which were lost, is a fortunate termination in some cases. The regenerated cells are produced by subdivision and multiplication of remaining cells which escaped or withstood the original necrotizing agent. This is seen commonly on epithelial surfaces, in the lining cells of pulmonary alveoli and bronchi, and in the parenchymatous cells of the liver and kidneys.

Cytochemical Alterations.—During the process of degeneration leading to necrosis, several biochemical alterations occur. The capacity of oxidative-phosphorylation is one of the earliest manifestations, and can be measured by a drop in ATP level. This results in a decrease in intracellular pH to about 6.0 (presumably due to the accumulation of lactate derived from glycolysis) and lack of available energy for the energy-dependent cation pump working against normal electro-chemical gradients. Failure of the latter and loss of integrity of the cell membrane results in an influx of sodium, chloride, calcium and water leading to acute cellular swelling, to be discussed in the next chapter (p. 42). The damaged cell membranes also allow the leaking of intracellular ions (such as potassium) proteins and soluble enzymes. The leaking of soluble enzymes provides an important diagnostic aid for the recognition of dead or dying tissues in the living patient. The measurement of serum levels of such enzymes as glutamic oxalo-acetic acid transaminase, glutamic pyruvic transaminase, lactic dehydrogenase and creatine phosphokinase only allows recognition of necrosis, but by character-

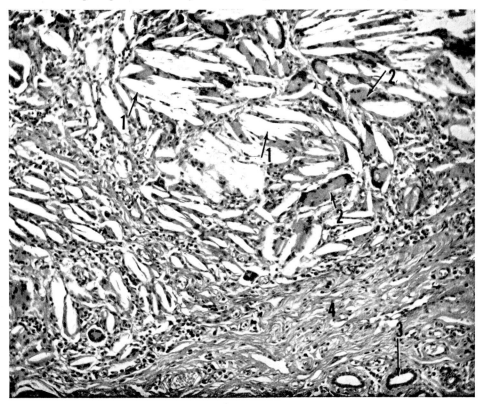

FIG. 1–9.—Cholesterol clefts (*1*) at the site of old hemorrhage and necrosis in the mammary gland of a dog. Giant cells of foreign body type (*2*), mammary acini (*3*), connective tissue (*4*). (Courtesy of Armed Forces Institute of Pathology.) × 115. Contributor: Dr. W. H. Riser.

ization of these enzymes by electrophoretic separation, exacting localization of the necrosis to a specific tissue is possible.

Cholesterol clefts are encountered not infrequently as by-products of necrosis. They are the empty spaces left by crystals of cholesterol dissolved out by the solvents used in preparation of the tissue. The crystals are readily recognized by their special shape which is that of a flat, thin rhomboid plate with one corner cut out along lines parallel to the outer edges of the crystal. The dimensions of length and breadth commonly fall between 50 and 100 microns, with a thickness of 5 to 10 microns. Since the crystal is dissolved in preparation of the tissue, what one sees in a microscopic section is the cleft-like empty space of approximately the same size and shape. Since the probability of this narrow slit being cut transversely is much greater than of its happening to lie in the plane of the section, one usually sees a narrow cleft perhaps 50 microns in length and bulging slightly at the middle. The crystals are anisotropic (birefringent) when seen in frozen sections.

The cholesterol is not usually seen grossly, but when in large amount it is visible as shiny, yellowish, granular or flaky material.

Since the cholesterol which crystallizes in the tissues comes from the decomposed protoplasm of cells that have died, it is obvious that these clefts are found in regions where there has been considerable necrosis of cells relatively rich in that substance. Such situations include the sites of old hemorrhages, old abscesses, atheromas and sometimes dermoid and sebaceous cysts. Cholesterol also appears in the tissue of the liver and gallbladder when, for any reason, bile is entrapped there.

GANGRENE

Gangrene is a condition in which necrotic tissue is invaded by saprophytic, and usually putrefactive, bacteria. Necrotic tissue accessible to air-borne bacteria regularly suffers such invasion; hence, we seldom speak of necrosis of limbs, ears, tails, lungs, intestines or udder, but rather of gangrene of those organs.

Microscopically the condition is recognized as a necrotic part or area in which large **bacilli** (rod-shaped bacteria) are demonstrated. They need not be numerous. By the ordinary hematoxylin-eosin stain, bacteria are bluish, but much less so than nuclei, and hazy in outline as compared with results achieved by the bacterial stains. Since many species of saprophytic bacteria are gas-formers, the gangrenous tissue may contain gas-bubbles, recognizable as empty spaces of various sizes, having no wall of their own and tending to be spherical but subject to distortion by the pressure of adjoining histological structures.

From the standpoint of **gross appearance,** two kinds of gangrene exist. In **moist gangrene** the affected part, be it a limb or an area of lung or intestine, is swollen, soft, pulpy and usually dark or black in color. Depending on the kinds of bacteria present, it is likely to have a foul, putrefactive odor. During life, it is without body heat and insensible to touch or pain. This, the more frequent type, occurs in those tissues which are well filled with blood at the time the necrosis begins.

Dry gangrene occurs in tissues which have a more limited content of blood and fluid or in which the necrosis has developed slowly with retardation of the natural circulation. Since dry tissue is not a favorable culture medium, the multiplication and spread of the bacteria is slow.   In appearance the part is shrivelled and leather-like, usually light in color.

All areas of gangrene are separated from the adjoining living tissue by **a line of demarcation** which is readily seen in the gross, either during life or after death, as a swollen, reddish or bluish zone of hyperemia and inflammation.

The **causes** of gangrene are the causes of necrosis plus the exposure to air-borne bacteria.   In the extremities, interference with the blood supply is the outstanding cause, as it is also in the intestine.   In the lungs and udder, the toxic products of highly lethal bacteria are the usual causes.   In the lungs, irritant medicines intended to be swallowed, but unskillfully allowed to pass down the trachea, set the stage for the growth of airborne micro-organisms, both pathogens and saprophytes.

Significance and Effect.—The principal therapeutic efforts are usually directed toward stopping the spread of the gangrenous process and this involves stopping the spread of necrosis, whatever its cause.   Highly toxic substances are produced as steps in the decomposition of proteins, in gangrenous tissue and elsewhere. These tend to be absorbed into the circulating blood of the adjacent living areas with disastrous consequences to the patient.   Indeed, in a weakened and moribund patient we sometimes see **sapremia**, a condition in which the saprophytic bacteria, ordinarily growing only in dead organic matter, are able to survive in the blood-stream and be disseminated by it through the living body.   For all of these

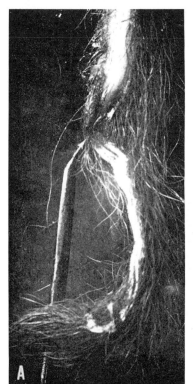
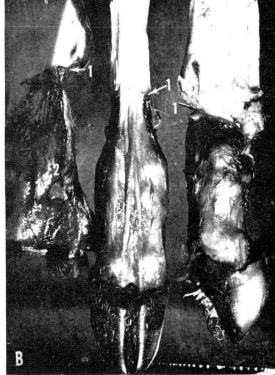

FIG. 1–10.—*A*, Dry gangrene, ear (longitudinal section) of a calf (arrow) following ergot poisoning. *B*, Moist gangrene involving feet of same calf. Note sharp line of demarcation between black gangrenous and white living tissue (*1*), the skin, inside out, after removal (*2*).

considerations, amputation of an extremity, even of the udder, is often necessary. In the case of the intestine, early surgical removal of the gangrenous portion with anastomosis of the healthy segments is the only hope.

But with good resistance nature does have her own remedy for gangrene. The line of demarcation is an inflammatory zone of combat in which all of the body's protective devices, humoral and cellular, are drawn up in battle array to resist the entrance of harmful substances, living or otherwise, into the healthy tissues. Often these are successful, in which case separation of the dead tissue, even of bone, eventually causes the gangrenous extremity to drop off, and the stump slowly heals. In dry gangrene, this is the usual outcome and the process may involve no startling changes in the general bodily health.

Gangrene of the uterus is possible on the basis of the definitions above set forth, and is occasionally seen. This is principally because a gangrenous uterus from its size and location, leads to a quickly fatal peritonitis by spread of the toxic products and pathogenic organisms. Superficial necrosis of the uterine lining, most often from too irritant medicine, is quite possible, as it is on other mucous surfaces.

Gas Gangrene.—Several species of anaerobic spore-forming bacteria, classified by Bergey (at this writing) in the genus Clostridium, have the faculty of growing both in dead organic matter and in living tissues. Hence they are both saprophytes and pathogens. They are able to kill animal tissue and then continue to multiply in it as saprophytes. They produce gas from constituents of the dead tissue, which appears as bubbles in the affected tissue. The group of diseases so produced are known as the gas gangrenes, including specifically malignant edema and blackleg in animals and nonspecific wound infections in the human (p. 575). They constitute examples of gangrene and necrosis occurring without the previous action of some other necrotizing agent.

INFARCTION, INFARCTS

Infarcts are localized areas of necrotic tissue resulting from sudden deprivation of their blood supply. The necrosis is coagulative in type, but the affected tissue eventually passes through the whole series of changes described for dead tissue with ultimate complete disappearance. The area involved is ordinarily that supplied by a single "end-artery," whose flow has been arrested, and the boundaries are, therefore, sharply delimited.

As the tissue dies, its capillary network obviously dies with it and there must be a line somewhere with dead capillaries on one side and living on the other. A certain amount of blood diffuses back from the living into the dead capillaries and these latter, being dead and without normal strength and resistance, permit escape of the blood into the surrounding necrotic tissue. Blood in the efferent veins doubtless flows back into the necrotic area in a similar way. Consequently a recent infarct tends to fill with blood. Indeed it is this feature that gives the lesion its name, which is derived from the Latin *infarcire*, meaning to fill fully or to stuff.

Some infarcts, then, if seen before the stranded erythrocytes have undergone hemolysis (see Post-Mortem Autolysis, p. 15), are filled with blood. These are called **hemorrhagic,** or **red infarcts.** In other cases, the escaped blood never gets beyond a thin peripheral zone, leaving the bulk of the lesion with the pale color which is characteristic of necrosis (p. 17). These are called **anemic** or **pale infarcts.** The existence of the two types has been explained by some as dependent on the length of time which elapsed between formation of the infarct and examination of the tissue, it having been theorized that all infarcts are hemorrhagic before disappearance of the blood cells by autolytic processes, usually a matter of two to three days. Others believe that the amount of blood which escapes into the necrotic area is determined by the denseness or perviousness of the tissue in question. Certain it is that infarcts seen in the kidney, a dense and solid organ, are almost always anemic, those in the pervious and lace-like tissue of the lung are invariably hemorrhagic.

Microscopic Appearance.—The picture is that of coagulative necrosis (p. 19) with or without the filling of the tissue spaces with blood as above described. The shape of the necrotic area is that of the part supplied by the obstructed vessel below the point of obstruction. In sections of most organs this is a triangular or wedge-shaped area with its apex near the place of obstruction and its base at or just inside the organ's wall or capsule, which may have a sufficient blood supply of its own. Since necrotic tissue regularly constitutes an irritant to adjacent living tissues (p. 15), an infarct has more or less of an inflammatory zone (hyperemia and leukocytes) surrounding it. Unfortunately for the diagnos-

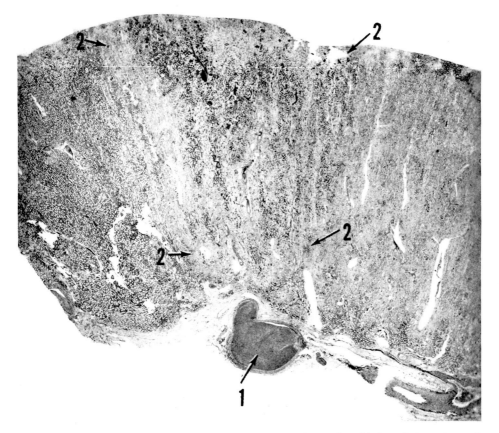

FIG. 1–11.—Infarct in the kidney of a pig infected experimentally with hog cholera virus. A thrombus is seen in an arciform artery (*1*), the margins of the infarct are indicated by arrows (*2*). (Courtesy of Armed Forces Institute of Pathology.) × 6. Contributor: Lt. Col. F. D. Maurer.

tician, this is sometimes slight. The smaller leukocytes must be carefully distinguished from the dark, angular fragments of nuclei of pre-existing parenchymatous cells, which, in the peripheral zone of an infarct, may remain for some time in a state of karyorrhexis (p. 10) rather than disappearing promptly by karyolysis. Old infarcts are chiefly fibrous as will be seen shortly. In case a trifling amount of blood continues to flow, any structure having prior access to it may survive as living oases in the necrotic desert. Renal glomeruli, for instance, may persist indefinitely, although other microscopic components of the kidney have long since disappeared.

Gross Appearance.—The red or white color has already been described. Hemorrhagic infarcts may protrude slightly above the surrounding tissues; the pale ones tend to be slightly depressed. Old infarcts are decidedly sunken on the surface. In all cases they are sharply demarcated. In the three-dimensional view the triangular shape seen microscopically becomes pyramidal or conical; the affected area, as seen on the surface of the organ, is likely to be very irregular. The pale infarct is a little denser and tougher than the surrounding tissue; the hemorrhagic one may be softer.

Cause.—By definition (on which there is practically universal agreement) an infarct is an area of necrosis and the cause of the necrosis is lack of proper blood supply. The cause of the lack of blood is ordinarily an obstruction in an artery or vein as a result of a lodged embolus.

Possibly there is some lack of precision in applying the name of infarct to areas which become filled with blood because of external pressure sufficient to prevent the venous outflow, but not sufficient to obstruct completely the stiffer-walled arteries. However, if the exit of blood is impossible that which accumulates in a part soon becomes stagnant, no more oxygen or other nutrients can be brought in and necrosis ensues. In this way venous obstruction can be admitted as a cause, chiefly in the case of a strangulated intestine and possibly in rare cases of occluding venous thrombi in other organs. It would seem proper, nevertheless, to insist on the demonstration of necrosis in any true infarct, since it is the death of the tissue, rather than the filling with blood, which is of principal significance to the patient.

Special Types and Diagnosis.—Infarcts of the kidney are typically conical with the apex usually near the cortico-medullary junction and the path of the arcuate arteries. In dogs and pigs, an accompanying chronic valvular endocarditis is frequently demonstrable and may well be the source of the causative embolus. Infarcts of the kidney are rather frequent and typically anemic, may be multiple, and often heal leaving only a narrow, fibrous scar (Fig. 1–11, p. 29).

Infarcts of the spleen are almost always hemorrhagic. Many shallow, subcapsular infarcts, difficult to distinguish from mere subcapsular hematomas, accompany hog cholera (Fig. 10–40B, p. 459). Arterioles are said to be obstructed by extreme proliferation of their endothelium as an effect of the virus.

Infarcts of the myocardium, far rarer in animals than in man and usually of different etiology, are either red or gray at the time they are discovered.

Infarcts of the brain are usually anemic and very quickly reach a state of liquefaction necrosis in accordance with the already mentioned (p. 21) susceptibility of nervous tissue to that termination. The animal may survive, the infarcted area being represented by a sharp gap in the tissue. These are rare in animals.

Intestinal infarctions usually involve a considerable length of the bowel. They are always hemorrhagic and large amounts of blood diffuse into the lumen through the necrotic tissue. They are ordinarily caused by strangulation of the bowel caught in a hernial sac or in a twisted loop of mesentery. In spite of the frequency of thrombosing injury to the anterior mesenteric artery by strongyle worms in the horse (p. 752), emboli of sufficient importance to thwart the rather efficient system of arterial anastomosis are rare. Intestinal infarctions, unless promptly treated by surgical resection, undergo fatal gangrene through invasion of saprophytic bacteria from the intestinal lumen. Obstruction of the lumen of the bowel by some foreign body is frequent in the dog and produces the same hemorrhagic lesion if the obstruction is complete. (Fig. 24–7, p. 1215.)

Infarcts can occur in the lung despite the only moderately effective circulation of the bronchial arteries as a secondary source of supply, but apparently only when that circulation is weakened by abnormally low blood pressure or some other interference. Emboli, single or multiple, brought in via the pulmonary artery are the usual cause. Because of the secondary bronchial circulation, as well as on account of the very extensive capillary network and the pervious nature of lung tissue, pulmonary infarcts are always hemorrhagic, the alveolar spaces being filled with blood.

In animals, infarction of the lung is not common but does occur. It is probable that some areas of lung, filled with blood in a lobular distribution, have been called infarcts without meeting the criterion of necrosis, and certainly without finding the embolus. It is not always easy to distinguish hemorrhagic infarction from simple hemorrhage or from a localized hemorrhagic exudate (p. 160).

True infarcts of the liver are almost nonexistent because of the fact that both the portal vein and the hepatic artery supply large amounts of blood. If an infarct does occur, it is the result of obstruction of a branch of the hepatic artery apparently, for experimental obstruction of the portal vein has failed to have such an effect. Pseudo-infarcts, sometimes called Zahn's infarcts, are reported, but lack the essential feature of necrosis and are really areas of venous and sinusoidal engorgement on a multilobular scale. Except for this greater extent, such pseudo-infarcts might not look very different from the engorgement of sinusoids which accompanies central necrosis (p. 1224). A so-called infarct, in which the circumscribed area of affected hepatic tissue is whitened by degenerative changes (p. 34) and incipient necrosis is stated to be characteristic of infection by Clostridium hemolyticum bovis (p. 573).

Infarction of areas of bovine mammary gland are reported in severe inflammation of that organ. It would seem that the causative emboli would have to be demonstrated in these cases, for such forms of mastitis are usually caused by streptococci of high virulence, and these organisms are entirely capable of killing directly large masses of tissue by their necrotizing toxins.

Indeed the pathologist encounters numerous instances where extensive death of tissue is due to direct bacterial action, chiefly of streptococci, the blackleg organism and other Clostridia. There are occasions where the causative embolus must be found in order to prove that infarction has occurred.

Significance and Effect.—What has been said of the disposition of necrotic tissue in general (p. 24) applies to infarcts. If exposed to the invasion of extraneous saprophytic bacteria, the necrotic area can be expected to become gangrenous. Dead areas lack the resistance of living tissue and afford fertile soil for the development of pyogenic organisms which may chance to be carried to them in the blood. Abscesses (p. 159) then develop and overshadow the infarctive process. However, with the exception of those in the intestine and some in the lungs, infarcts ordinarily are converted into fibrous scars by concurrent slow liquefaction and organization. Many organs survive the injuries of infarction, even repeated, as witness the human heart following the all too frequent myocardial infarcts from coronary thrombosis or coronary sclerosis. Infarcts of the brain result in loss of the functions provided by the particular area involved, which may be fatal or leave the patient with paralysis of certain motor functions or impairment of mental faculties. Infarctions cause one-third and intracranial hemorrhages two-thirds of the paralytic "strokes" suffered by mankind.

General Pathology, The Cell, Necrosis

ABRAHAM, E. P.: "Necrosis, Calcification and Autolysis" in Florey, H. W. (ed.), *General Pathology*, Chapter 15, 4th Ed. Philadelphia, W. B. Saunders Co., 1970.

CRAIG, J. M.: The Etiology of Liver Necrosis in Rats Following Administration of Progesterone Late in Pregnancy. Lab. Invest. *19*:49–54, 1968.

DE DUVE, C.: The Lysosome. Sci. Amer. May, 64–72, 1963.

DE REULK, A. V. S., and KNIGHT, J.: *Ciba Foundation Symposium on Cellular Injury.* Boston, Little Brown & Co., 1964.

ERICSSON, J. L. E., and BIBERFELD, P.: Studies on Aldehyde Fixation. Fixation Rates and Their Relation to Fine Structure and Some Histochemical Reactions in Liver. Lab. Invest. *17*:281–298, 1967.

ESSNER, E.: Endoplasmic Reticulum and the Origin of Microbodies in Fetal Mouse Liver. Lab. Invest. *17*:71–87, 1967.

FAWCETT, D. W.: *The Cell.* Philadelphia, W. B. Saunders Co., 1966.

HARRIS, R. J. C. (ed.): *The Interpretation of Ultrastructure.* New York, Academic Press, 1962.

HERDSON, P. B., KALTENBACK, J. P., and JENNINGS, R. B.: Fine Structural and Biochemical Changes in Dog Myocardium During Autolysis. Amer. J. Path. *57*:539–557, 1969.

HRUBAN, Z., SLESERS, A., and ORLANDO, R.: Structure of Enzymes *In Vitro.* Lab. Invest. *16*:550–564, 1967.

JORGENSEN, F.: Electron Microscopic Studies of Normal Visceral Epithelial Cells. Lab. Invest. *17*:225–242, 1967.

KERR, J. R. F.: An Electron-microscope Study of Liver Cell Necrosis Due to Heliotrine. J. Path. *97*:557–562, 1969.

KING, D. W., *et al.*: Cell Death. I. The Effect of Injury on the Proteins and Deoxyribonucleic Acid of Ehrlich Tumor Cells. II. The Effect of Injury on the Enzymatic Protein of Ehrlich Tumor Cells. III. The Effect of Injury on Water and Electrolytes of Ehrlich Tumor Cells. IV. The Effect of Injury on the Entrance of Vital Dye in Ehrlich Tumor Cells. Amer. J. Path. *35*:369–381, 575–589, 835–849, 1067–1079, 1959.

LITTLEFIELD, J. W., *et al.*: Studies on Cytoplasmic Ribonucleoprotein Particles from the Liver of the Rat. J. Biol. Chem. *217*:111–123, 1955.

MAGEE, P. N.: Toxic Liver Necrosis. Lab. Invest. *15*:111–131, 1966.

MAHLEY, R. W., *et al.*: Lipid Transport in Liver. II. Electron Microscopic and Biochemical Studies of Alterations in Lipoprotein Transport Induced by Cortisone in the Rabbit. Lab. Invest. *19*:358–369, 1968.

MAJNO, G., LaGATTUTA, M., and THOMPSON, T. E.: Cellular Death and Necrosis: Chemical, Physical and Morphologic Changes in Rat Liver. Virch. Arch. Path. Anat. *333*:421–465, 1960.

PALADE, G. E., and PORTER, K. R.: Studies on the Endoplasmic Reticulum. I. Its Identification in Cells *In Situ.* J. Exp. Med. *100*:641–656, 1954.

PALADE, G. E., and SIEKOVITZ, P.: Pancreatic Microsomes. An Integrated Morphological and Biochemical Study. J. Biophys. Biochem. Cytol. *2*:671–691, 1956.

PANABOKKE, R. G.: An Experimental Study of Fat Necrosis. J. Path. Bact. *75*:319–331, 1958.

PEARL, R.: *The Biology of Death.* Philadelphia, J. B. Lippincott Co., 1922.

PRICHARD, R. W.: Descriptions in Pathology. Avoiding Pathological Descriptions. [Editorial, Amer. Med. Ass.] Arch. Path. *59*:612–617, 1955. Reprinted Path. Vet. *3*:169–177, 1966.

RIBELIN, W. E. and DeEDS, F.: Fat Necrosis in Man and Animals. J. Am. Vet. Med. Assn. *136*:135–139, 1960.

SCHLUMBERGER, HANS G.: Origins of Cell Concept in Pathology. Arch. Path. *37*:396–407, 1944.

SMUCKLER, E. A., and TRUMP, B. F.: Alterations in the Structure and Function of the Rough Surfaced Endoplasmic Reticulum During Necrosis *In Vitro*. Amer. J. Path. *53*:315–329, 1968.

TRUMP, B. F., *et al.*: An Electron Microscopic Study of Mouse Liver During Necrosis *In Vivo* (autolysis). Lab. Invest. *11*:986–1016, 1962.

VOGT, M. T., and FARBER, E.: On the Molecular Pathology of Ischemic Renal Cell Death. Reversible and Irreversible Cellular and Mitochondrial Alterations. Amer. J. Path. *53*:1–26, 1968.

WINBORN, W. B., and BOCKMAN, D. E.: Origin of Lysosomes in Parietal Cells. Lab. Invest. *19*:256–264, 1968.

2

Cellular Infiltrations and Degenerations

  More than one hundred years ago, when many changes in diseased cells were first recognized by means of the light microscope, cellular degenerations were recognized by tinctoral characteristics, by the presence or absence of accumulations (fat, pigments, water) and by structural changes in the cells (pyknosis, hypertrophy, etc.). Virchow recognized that these changes must have been based upon chemical phenomena, but only in the past decade or two has sufficient information accumulated on the molecular level to deepen understanding and force change in concepts a hundred years old. The appearance of cells and tissues under the light microscope is still useful for the detection of disease states and to indicate their possible nature and etiology. Precise explanation of the mechanisms involved depends upon the use of sophisticated biochemical methods and the electron microscope. In this chapter, we shall describe those changes recognizable with the naked eye, light or electron microscope (in many of the same words used in early editions) and will attempt to condense some of the concepts which currently seem best to explain them.

FATTY CHANGE

  The intracellular accumulation of lipid (usually as neutral fat) occurs in the liver, kidney and heart under various conditions, most of them pathologic. Since Virchow's time, efforts have been made to distinguish between physiologic and pathologic accumulations of fat in cells and to understand their significance to the function and survival of affected cells. Many terms have been developed over the years, some may be considered synonyms, others based upon concepts now considered invalid, should be abandoned. **Fatty metamorphosis, fatty deposition, intracellular lipid deposition** or **accumulation** are each considered synonymous with **fatty change,** the term currently considered most appropriate. The term **fat phanaerosis,** or **lipophanaerosis,** was based upon the invalid concept that fat was simply "unmasked" in affected cells, that is, the breakdown of lipoprotein membranes and complex lipids resulted in the visible droplets of lipid. This is now known not to be true. The term **fatty degeneration** was used to designate a presumed degenerative change which leads to necrosis of the cell and to distinguish it from **fatty infiltration,** an accumulation of fat that was readily reversible and did not lead to damage to the cell. It now appears that the criteria long considered to distinguish between the two are not supported by present evidence. We shall consider these terms to be less preferred synonyms for fatty change.

Microscopic Appearance.—In ordinary sections, fats and lipoids appear in the cytoplasm as clear, unstained spherical spaces. This shape is due to the well-known fact that oil and water do not mix. The spaces are clear because they are empty, the fat having been dissolved out by the solvents (alcohol, xylene, etc.) used in preparing the tissue for embedding in paraffin or celloidin. If it is desired that the lipids actually be retained, the sections must be cut on the freezing microtome. They can then be handled by techniques which involve a minimal use of fat solvents and stained by special **fat stains.** Sudan III stains fats a yellowish-orange color; Sudan IV, also known as scarlet red or Scharlach red, gives them a redder shade; osmic acid colors them black; Nile blue sulfate imparts a violet color, which is bluish in the case of fatty acids and reddish when neutral fats predominate. Certain techniques have been devised for the differential staining of true fats and lipoids, but the distinction is somewhat more satisfactorily made by means of the polarizing microscope. True fats are isotropic, which means that the light coming through them vibrates in one plane. When viewed with the polarizing microscope, the analyzer can be turned so as to darken these completely. The common lipoidal substances are anisotropic, or birefringent, the light from them vibrating in two or more planes. As a result, these substances are not obliterated as the analyzer is turned. Under the polarizing microscope little points of light in the form of a Maltese cross indicate the lipoid particles, which are especially likely to be esters of cholesterol.

In the liver, the fat appears as droplets in the cytoplasm of the epithelial cells. It is usually in the form of droplets so fine that a large number are contained within the cytoplasm of one cell but at times there is a mixture of large and small

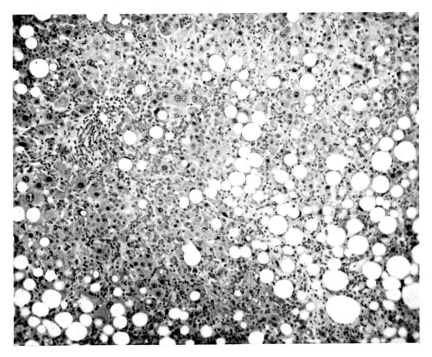

FIG. 2–1. Fatty change of the liver of a rat which received a diet deficient in choline and methionine. H & E, × 115.

droplets. As already explained the fat droplets appear as empty, clear, or almost clear, unstained, round spaces in ordinary tissue sections. The nucleus remains practically unchanged. Usually all parts of the liver are affected almost equally. Within the lobule the distribution is likely to be zonal as explained in the discussion of acute toxic hepatitis (p. 1224). Most, if not all, of the droplets are true neutral fat.

In the kidney, lipids may be deposited in the epithelial cytoplasm of any of the tubules, but as a rule the proximal convoluted tubules or the ascending limbs of Henle's loops, located in the medullary rays, are almost exclusively involved. The droplets are small and indistinct and may easily be overlooked until a fat stain is made. In certain types of glomerular disease, numerous fat droplets may be demonstrated by means of fat stains, in the glomeruli, presumably in the epithelial cells. In cases where the connective tissue surrounding Bowman's capsules has undergone inflammatory increase, fat droplets may be demonstrable in it, fat stains being necessary. Likewise, when the walls of arteries have suffered nephrosclerotic thickening, fat may often be stained in them. Rarely fatty material has been stained in the lumens of the tubules toward the end of the excretory route.

In the heart, fat appears in very fine droplets within the muscle cells. The affected cells are often grouped together in patches which alternate with unaffected areas. Fatty change in the heart is not easily detected without a suitable special stain. It has nothing to do with adipose cells which occur normally in the coronary groove and which may extend a variable distance among the muscle bundles.

Lipids also occur in certain other cells and tissues which will be mentioned in the discussion of causes.

Gross Appearance.—Fat in the liver produces an enlargement of the organ which is limited by a tensely stretched capsule, a slight bulging of the cut surfaces when incised and a less acute angle between its anterior and posterior surfaces where they join each other at the border of the organ. The liver is slightly or markedly lighter in color, approaching a tan or yellow which lacks the greenish tinge that goes with icterus. With rare exceptions all parts of the liver are affected equally. If the fatty change accompanies necrosis, its distribution within the lobule may be limited to a certain zone, which helps to produce the accentuation of lobular architecture characteristic of acute toxic hepatitis (p. 1223). The presence of fat lowers the specific gravity of the tissue; very fatty livers will float in water. Extensive accumulations of lipids make the liver friable, that is, reduce its strength and toughness. It may be possible to force the finger into the hepatic tissue with very little resistance, and in being handled post mortem, a lobe may be fractured unavoidably. Summarizing, the fatty liver is recognized grossly by enlargement, light color, light weight and friability.

Fat in the kidney may bring a slight irregularity in depth of color of the cut surface, but it is only detected with certainty when, as frequently happens in the dog, the ascending loops of Henle contain it. In such a case, the medullary rays stand out as brilliant white streaks radially directed through the cortex but not reaching to the capsule. Diffuse paleness of the renal tissue is seldom, if ever, attributable to fatty changes.

In the heart, fatty degeneration cannot be judged accurately by gross examination (Johnson, 1953).

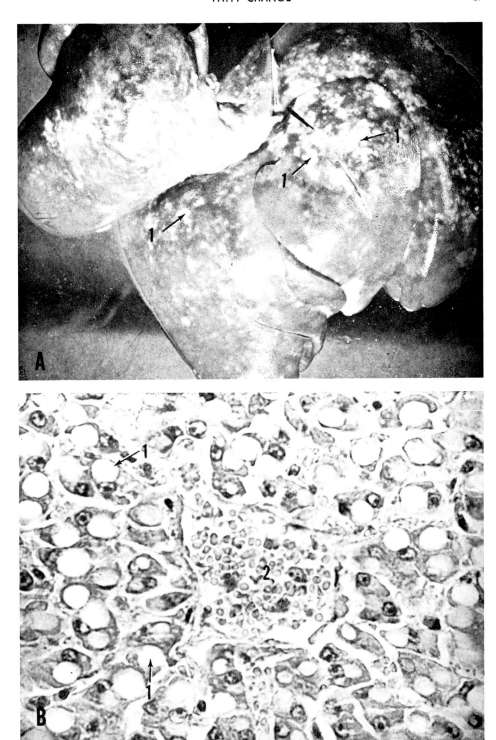

Fig. 2–2. Fatty change, liver of a dog given 200 ml. of olive oil and cream six hours before (unexpected) death. *A*, Deposits of fat (*1*) are seen in all lobes. *B*, Fat droplets (*1*) in liver cells surrounding a central vein. (Courtesy of Armed Forces Institute of Pathology.) Contributor: Dr. Melvin G. Rhoades.

Pathogenesis.—Intracellular accumulation of lipid may occur in any of several situations which interfere with the transport or metabolism of fat, or in special instances, synthesis of protein. These mechanisms are best known in the liver. A short summary of the major means of transport and metabolism of fat by the liver follows: Fat is absorbed from the small intestine and transported via the plasma to the liver in **chylomicra,** tiny lipid particles consisting mostly of triglycerides but also containing small amounts of protein and phospholipid. In the liver, triglycerides are hydrolyzed enzymatically to fatty acids. Protein is synthetized by the endoplasmic reticulum and combined with triglycerides to form low density lipoprotein particles which are released into the plasma. Under the influence of lipoprotein lipase, the lipids are deposited as fatty acids in adipose tissue. Mobilization of fat may return fatty acids to plasma and then to the liver. Also in the liver, esterification of fatty acids to triglyceride, phospholipid or cholesterol ester may occur under enzymatic control.

Some of the mechanisms which may interfere with the transport and metabolism of lipid to result in fatty change, follow:

(1) **Excessive release of free fatty acids** from adipose tissue, resulting in delivery of increased amounts of free fatty acids to the liver (heart or kidney) which may not be able to utilize the increased free fatty acids, thence storing them as neutral fat. This is apparently the process involved in starvation.

(2) **Decreased utilization or oxidation of fatty acids** due to interference with co-factors (*e.g.* carnitine) essential to oxidation of long-chain fatty acids. Bacterial toxins (*e.g.* diphtheria toxin) are considered to produce their effect on fatty change in this manner.

(3) **Lipotrope deficiency** resulting in decreased phospholipid synthesis. Deficiency of methionine or choline decreases phospholipid synthesis and their absence leads to esterification of diglycerides to triglycerides.

(4) **Fatty acids preferentially esterified to triglycerides.** This is believed to explain the fatty change in acute ethanol poisoning.

(5) **Failure of protein synthesis**—thus reducing the protein component available for the lipoprotein particles which are the means of excretion of lipid from the liver. Examples may be found in experimental poisoning by ethionine, carbon tetrachloride, puromycin, yellow phosphorus, etc. Each of these cause dispersion of ribosomes from the endoplasmic reticulum, swelling of the endoplasmic reticulum and accumulation of neutral fat in the cytoplasm.

Fatty change of kidneys, liver and even of the heart commonly accompanies ketosis (p. 1020). Hyperlipemia and hypercholesterolemia are also a part of this syndrome. Ketosis results ordinarily from starvation or from diabetes mellitus. Glycogen and usable carbohydrate are absent in the first instance because they are not available in the food, and in the second because the insulin necessary for their utilization is lacking. Energy has to be obtained from the oxidation of stored fats, and these are imperfectly oxidized. A spectacular example in veterinary practice is the so-called toxemia of pregnant ewes, in which all three organs are heavily laden with fat. The exact reason for this is uncertain. Perhaps there are toxins produced which injure the fat-containing cells in one of the classical ways. Since the level of lipids in the blood is abnormally high, it is possible that the mechanism is the same as that which causes cells to absorb lipids which have accumulated in the local tissue fluids as the result of being released from disintegrating necrotic cells in the vicinity. This latter occurs in leukocytes in many inflamed areas, in phagocytes in such infections as actinomycosis and tuberculosis, in the walls of blood vessels in inflamed areas and elsewhere.

The cells of certain organs and certain tumors contain considerable amounts of lipid deposits. This is true of the adrenal cortex, the corpus luteum, xanthomas, the Sertoli and interstitial cells of the testis and in tumors derived from them. In the normal structures, and probably in the tumors as well, this form of lipidosis should be regarded as a natural characteristic of the particular type of cell. The lipoid substances accumulated in the cells of the adrenal cortex are doubtless there as precursors of the corticosteroid hormones produced by this organ.

The occurrence of lipids in the injured glomerulus may possibly be explained as the absorption of fatty substances released by other dying cells, but this is uncertain. Their rare occurrence in the lumens of the tubules and in the urine can conceivably result from release by disintegrating tubular epithelium. There is no agreement as to the reason for the accumulation of lipids in the renal epithelium in that primarily glomerular affection known as lipoid nephrosis.

Significance.—Fatty change, the intracellular accumulation of lipids, is a process independent of other changes (*e.g.* necrosis) which results from one or more of the five mechanisms described previously (or others not described). These pathogenic mechanisms may be caused by any one of many factors, such as toxins of poisonous plants (Chapter 17), or metabolic disorders (Chapter 18). It may be completely reversible or may lead to rupture and death of the cell. Although independent of necrosis, it may have the same causes, and often occurs in the same organ in association with necrosis. Interpretation of the significance of fatty change, once recognized in a specific case, requires consideration of all of the possible causes and pathogenic mechanisms.

INTERSTITIAL OR STROMAL FATTY INFILTRATION

These terms currently are used to describe the deposition of lipids in the cytoplasm of adipose tissue cells found among the interstitial connective tissue cells throughout the animal body. If the fat is excessive in amounts, obesity is used as a descriptive term. Adipose tissue cells may also replace muscle cells which atrophy for any reason.

EXTRACELLULAR ACCUMULATION OF LIPIDS

Lipid may occur outside of cells in some situations. Necrosis of cells may release lipids into extracellular spaces where pooling may make them visible. Cholesterol is released from cells or pooled from lipoproteins in crystalline form ("clefts," p. 26) as the result of hemorrhage. Fat may be seen in blood vessels also as emboli of adipose tissue or bone marrow (p. 115). Fat droplets in renal tubular epithelium may be shed into the lumen to produce fatty casts (p. 1271).

FATTY DEGENERATION OF MYELIN

This is a condition in which myelin is destroyed with the production of stainable fat as a degeneration product. It will be treated in the study of the nervous system in connection with degenerations of peripheral nerves.

Intracellular Accumulation of Lipids

ABRAHAM, E. P., and ROBB-SMITH, A. H. T.: Degenerative Changes and Some of Their Consequences. Chap. 14 in Florey, H. W., *General Pathology*, 4th Ed. Philadelphia, W. B. Saunders Co., 1970.

ISSELBACHER, K. J., and GREENBERGER, N. J.: Metabolic Effects of Alcohol on the Liver. New Eng. J. Med. *270*:351–371, 1964.

LOMBARDI, B.: Considerations on the Pathogenesis of Fatty Liver. Lab. Invest. *15*:1–20, 1966.

LONGNECKER, D. S., SKINOZUKA, H., and FARBER, E.: Molecular Pathology of *In-Vivo* Inhibition of Protein Synthesis. Amer. J. Path. *52*:891–915, 1968.

MELDOLESI, J., *et al.*: Cytoplasmic Changes in Rat Liver after Prolonged Treatment with Low Doses of Ethionine and Adenine. An Ultrastructural and Biochemical Study. Lab. Invest. *17*:265–275, 1967.

————: Effects of Carbon Tetrachloride on the Synthesis of Liver Endoplasmic Reticulum Membranes. Lab. Invest. *19*:315–323, 1969.

REYNOLDS, E. S., and YEC, A. G.: Liver Parenchymal Cell Injury. VI. Significance of Early Glucose-6-phosphate Suppression and Transient Calcium Influx Following Poisoning. Lab. Invest. *19*:273–281, 1968.

SCHLUNK, F. F., and LOMBARDI, B.: Liver Liposomes. I. Isolation and Chemical Characterization. Lab. Invest. *17*:30–38, 1967.

————: On the Ethionine-induced Fatty Liver in Male and Female Rats. Lab. Invest. *17*:299–307, 1967.

GLYCOGENIC INFILTRATION

Since the visible changes in glycogenic infiltration are somewhat similar to those in lipidosis it is convenient to consider the former at this point. Glycogen is sometimes picturesquely called animal starch since its chemical formula re-

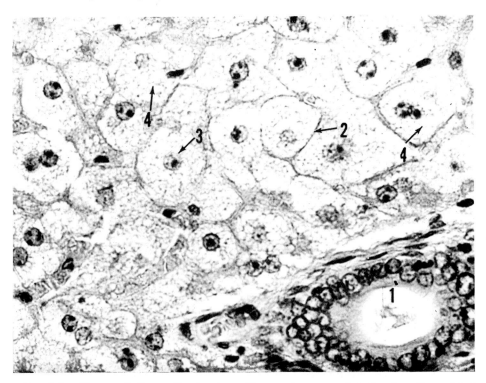

FIG. 2–3.—Glycogen in liver cells of a dog. Glycogen is a normal finding in well nourished animals; it disappears rapidly in many diseased states. Bile duct (*1*) distinct walls of liver cells (*2*), centrally located nuclei (*3*) of hepatic cells and fine droplets of glycogen (*4*) which fill the cytoplasm of these cells. (Courtesy of Armed Forces Institute of Pathology.)   × 500. Contributor: Dr. Lester Barto.

sembles those of the true starches in being multiples of $C_6H_{10}O_5$. Carbohydrates of all kinds are normally carried in the blood as glucose (dextrose) to be stored as glycogen, chiefly in liver and muscle cells. Hence it is normal to find considerable amounts in these tissues.

Occurrence. — Glycogen occurs pathologically in the cytoplasm of epithelial cells lining the straight tubules and Henle's loops of the kidneys, in leukocytes in inflamed and necrotic tissues and, rarely, in cardiac muscle.

Microscopic Appearance. — Whether the glycogen be normally or pathologically deposited, it is to be seen in the cytoplasm of cells as clear spaces or vacuoles. This is because glycogen, being soluble in water, is readily dissolved away in ordinary methods of tissue preparation. The empty spaces are not necessarily round nor do they always have sharp outlines, but they are very clear. All of these facts help one to distinguish glycogenic infiltration from fatty change and from hydropic degeneration. Such vacuoles in the epithelium of Henle's loops are almost surely due to glycogen.

The ultrastructural appearance of glycogen is quite characteristic (Fig. 2–4). The method of fixation influences the appearance of glycogen but usually the electron microscope reveals its smallest unit as roughly isodiametric, slightly irregular particles, 150 to 300 Å in diameter. These, **beta particles,** usually coalesce to form aggregates called **alpha particles** or **rosettes.** The number of particles or rosettes vary a great deal, as is to be expected, and may be present in such numbers to obscure most intracellular organelles.

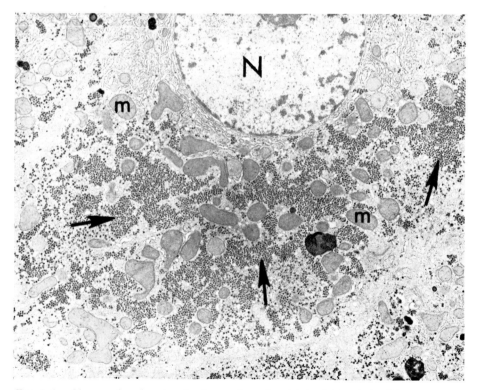

FIG. 2–4.—Glycogen in a hepatocyte of an owl monkey (*Aotus trivirgatus*). Glycogen appears as numerous small electron dense granules (arrows). N = nucleus, m = mitochondria. (Courtesy Dr. Norval W. King.)

The hepatic epithelium of well-nourished animals normally contains considerable glycogen, enough to give the cytoplasm a finely foamy appearance, varying with the amount and recentness of carbohydrate consumption.

Positive identification or differentiation depends upon special technique. The tissue is fixed in alcohol and alcoholic stains are used throughout so that no water comes in contact with it. Best's carmine stain then colors the glycogen a bright pink. Glycogen is also of importance in fungi (pp. 646, 648, 659, 665).

Gross Appearance.—Glycogen is not detected grossly.

The **cause** of glycogenic infiltration is imperfectly understood. Apparently many cells have only to be in contact with it to absorb it. If glycogen is released by dying cells into the intercellular medium, it is absorbed by leukocytes and possibly other cells; in the renal epithelium, its presence ordinarily goes with diabetes and the urinary excretion of glucose.

In people, several specific genetic defects in the enzymes involved in the metabolism and catabolism of glycogen result in the accumulation of glycogen in cells and are grouped as *glycogen storage diseases.*

The **significance** is as implied above. The glycogen is not in itself injurious, but its presence in these situations is indicative of other injury.

CLOUDY SWELLING

Rudolph Virchow, in 1860, proposed the term, *"trübe Schwellung"* to describe a particular swelling and translucency seen microscopically in cells believed to be undergoing degeneration. The translation of the term into the English, "cloudy swelling" was approved by Virchow but over the ensuing years the term has been corrupted by application to other changes, including a grossly recognizable appearance of an organ and therefore no longer has any precise meaning.

ACUTE CELLULAR SWELLING

Possibly equivalent to **cloudy swelling, parenchymatous degeneration, albuminous degeneration** or **granular degeneration,** the term acute cellular swelling is currently preferred as indicating the earliest change manifest by an injured cell. Basically, this concept refers to influx of water into the cell. Numerous changes at the ultrastructural and biochemical level are now known to occur as a result of injury to the cell and may lead to death of the cell, which is eventually detected microscopically by the features of necrosis (p. 10). These changes are assumed to be reversible until a "point of no return" is reached beyond which intracellular events proceed on to death of the cell. This hypothetical point has not been identified by chemical or morphologic criteria.

Acute cellular swelling may be recognized with difficulty in well-preserved specimens under the light microscope in epithelial cells of liver, renal tubules or various glands. The cells are enlarged and the cytoplasm has a homogeneous "ground glass" appearance. Vacuoles may be evident if organelles are sufficiently swollen. Fatty change may accompany it but is now considered to be due to independent factors. Present concepts require definition of this step toward necrosis in ultrastructural and biochemical terms.

Some of the functional and structural events which are now believed to occur in this degenerative process may be summarized briefly as follows:

(1) Injury to the cell (as tested in experimental systems) rapidly leads to the decreased capacity of the cell to carry out oxidative-phosphorylation.

(2) Changes in the cell membrane and energy dependent cation "pumps" lead to increased permeability to water and ions (Na^{++}, Ca^{++}, K^+). These ionic and water fluxes result principally in loss of potassium from the cell and increase in intracellular sodium and calcium. This changes the osmotic situation and results in increased water inside the cell membrane ("cellular edema").

(3) Increased permeability of the cell membrane permits loss of proteins (including soluble enzymes) and coenzymes from the cell. The appearance of these enzymes in the plasma may be used in clinical practice to detect early degenerative changes in cells (especially of liver and heart muscle). Such examples as the transaminases and lactate dehydrogenase are discussed elsewhere in this book (p. 25).

(4) Structural changes such as swelling of organelles which may be detected at the level of light microscopy as vacuoles in the cytoplasm and enlargement of the cell may be more clearly depicted at the ultrastructural level. These include vacuolization at the plasma membrane (probably by accumulation of water), blunting of the microvilli, swelling of the smooth endoplasmic reticulum to form vacuoles and myelin figures. As the process continues, mitochondria become swollen, glycogen and other molecules are lost from the cell. Vacuoles and "myelin" figures (which resemble the laminated multilayer membrane arrays seen in myelin) are formed, possibly as the result of disassociation of lipoproteins and unmasking of hydrophilic groups of phosphatides—thus leading to the uptake of water.

(5) Changes in the ionic environment, decrease in pH due to glycolysis, accumulation of lactate and breakdown of phosphate esters may lead to increased permeability of or rupture of lysosomal membranes (p. 8) releasing their hydrolytic enzymes. These enzymes are believed to be responsible for the self-digestion of the cell—**autolysis** or **necrosis.**

Note: The phenomenon which results in self-digestion of a cell, after the death of the organism (which we prefer to call post-mortem autolysis) (p. 15) is essentially the same as that which occurs in a cell in the living body, except for the response of adjacent, living cells, migration of leukocytes and influx of other materials from the circulation. This antemortem autolysis we prefer to distinguish, primarily for pragmatic reasons, as **necrosis** (p. 17).

HYDROPIC DEGENERATION

Hydropic or vacuolar degeneration, also known as **hydrops,** is a condition in which water in more or less pure form occurs in the cytoplasm of cells. The cells involved are usually epithelial. It occurs, for example, in the epidermis, the epithelium of the amnion at term and a considerable number of epithelial neoplasms. It has no connection with the edematous condition of the fetus known as hydrops amnii, nor with any of the older applications of the term hydrops for extracellular edema. The relationship of hydropic degeneration to acute cellular swelling is not clear except that hydropic degeneration may represent an advanced stage of cellular swelling in which droplets of water are recognizable in cells at the light microscopic level.

The **microscopic appearance** is that of a clear space, frequently surrounding the nucleus, the stainable cytoplasm being pushed back toward the periphery of the cell. The space may be less perfectly clear than is the case with glycogen or fat and its boundaries are hazy and indefinite. It can usually be differentiated by these features, but doubt can be resolved by the application of special stains for fat and glycogen. If these are eliminated, the pale area almost certainly represents water and is properly called hydropic degeneration.

The **gross appearance** is not characteristic. Hydropic degeneration is not likely to be recognized grossly.

The **causes** are (1) lack of nutrition, such as may arise when tumor cells are too far from their blood supply, and (2) old age, perhaps of the individual, as a whole, perhaps of the particular tissue. The amnion and other fetal membranes, at full term, have reached the end of their life span and are showing the changes of senility. Just why the water does not blend with the more normal part of the cytoplasm is not known.

The **significance** of hydropic degeneration is not great. It may be concluded that one of the above causative situations is present.

It will be of assistance to the student to remember that the preceding degenerative changes give a colorless, transparent appearance in ordinary microscopic sections. The several which follow next are pink or red in hematoxylin-eosin sections. The abnormal substances are protein in nature and are sometimes grouped together as **Disturbances of Protein Metabolism.**

HYALINE CHANGES

The adjective "hyaline" is used to refer to any one of several substances which are white, glossy, solid, dense and of smoothly homogeneous texture. The student of anatomy is already familiar with one such substance in hyaline cartilage. A number of substances having these qualities are produced pathologically and have come to be designated by the corresponding noun "hyalin." Quite unrelated to each other, the present-day list includes connective-tissue hyalin, epithelial hyalin and kerato-hyalin. The term "hyaline degeneration" has also been used to refer to these conditions. A form of so-called hyaline degeneration occurs in the cells of the renal tubules. Some think, however, that the hyaline, albuminous granules and droplets seen in these cells represent protein material which the cells have resorbed from the urine-forming glomerular filtrate in the tubules. However this may be, the pathological excretion of protein into the fluid of the tubules is a frequent occurrence. In the microscopic section, the tubular epithelial cells are seen to contain brightly eosinophilic droplets or granules. In the lumina this albuminous material appears as a bright pink precipitate. Sometimes it is very dense, and grossly appears as solid white bodies molded to the form of the tubules. Such bodies are called **albuminous casts** or **hyaline casts.** Under Zenker's Necrosis we have already alluded to the muscle fibers as "hyaline"; some call this also "hyaline degeneration." There has also been a tendency recently to designate as "hyaline degeneration" a partial necrosis and regeneration of voluntary and cardiac muscle encountered in the conditions tentatively and rather primitively called "white muscle disease," a supposed avitaminosis-E (p. 992). It can hardly be said that the muscles fulfill the criteria above outlined.

CONNECTIVE-TISSUE HYALIN

Connective-tissue hyalin is a substance formed in connective tissue and, since it represents a change which has taken place in that tissue, one may refer to the changed connective tissue as "hyaline connective tissue."

Its **occurrence** is, therefore, in structures already formed wholly or partly of connective tissue. These include particularly (1) old scars, (2) the corpus albicans of the ovary, a physiological scarring of the defunct corpus luteum, (3) the walls of arteriosclerotic blood vessels, and (4) other places where connective tissue has been chronically injured or deprived of nutrition.

Microscopic Appearance.—The hyaline area is structureless and smoothly homogeneous under the microscope as well as to the naked eye. It is strongly acidophilic and stains a brilliant pink with the usual stains. When completely hyalinized the connective tissue has no nuclei and no fibrils, but the boundaries of the hyaline area are indefinite, usually with a gradual transition through an outer zone where nuclei are sparse into the surrounding normal fibrous tissue.

Grossly the amount of hyaline material may be too small to be noticeable, but when of greater extent it is seen to be white, shiny, semi-translucent and glassy, but uniformly solid and dense. Old scars are white, even in the skin of dark animals, partly because of the more or less hyaline connective tissue and partly because of the inability of the regenerated epithelium to develop pigmentation.

Causes.—It is probable that the fundamental cause is a lack of nutrition. Large scars are notorious for their poor blood supply. More immediate factors in its production are previous injury as well as advanced age of the individual or tissue. In many species, the placental villi become quite hyaline as the time of parturition approaches. Toxins or injurious substances carried in the circulating blood may be responsible for the change as it occurs in arteriosclerotic blood vessels but this is obscure.

Significance.—While not incompatible with the continued existence of the tissue involved, hyalinization is a degenerative process. The tissue functions less perfectly and connective tissue, so affected, has less than normal strength. It is also inelastic and inflexible, as may be observed in old scars. Once formed, it is relatively permanent. Hyalinization of a blood-vessel wall is by no means conducive to maintaining an even and normal blood pressure, and rupture of the vessel is to be feared.

EPITHELIAL HYALIN

An obsolete synonym for epithelial hyalin is "colloid." The **occurrence** of this change is usually limited to **corpora amylacea** (Latin for "starch-like bodies"), which may be found in (a) the prostate, most commonly of man, and (b) the lung. Also called corpora amylacea by neuropathologists are round, opaque bodies encountered in damaged areas of the white matter of the brain. They are from 5 to 10 microns in diameter and more or less amphoteric (purplish) in their staining. They are considered to be the remains of astrocytes that have disappeared, usually following a stage of gliosis (p. 1387). The term corpus amylaceum should be avoided for granules that are merely calcified, such as those often found in the mammary gland.

Microscopically corpora amylacea are rounded, homogeneous or concentrically laminated bodies, staining pink, perhaps tinged zonally with blue, lying within an alveolus of lung or prostate. They are not detected **grossly.**

Cause and Significance.—Corpora amylacea received their name from the early belief that they were carbohydrate in nature, but it is now known that they are composed of protein. They are considered to result from pressure, dehydration and a prolonged kneading action upon dead cells which have desquamated from the epithelial lining, held together probably by a little fibrin. Thus their presence indicates a previous inflammatory process, although it may have been of subclinical intensity. In the human prostate their presence is so frequent as to be considered almost normal; in animals, with their shorter life-span and less frequent survival from infectious processes, the bodies are rare in either location.

KERATO-HYALIN

Keratin is another name for this substance and the process of its formation may be called either keratinization or **cornification.** It may be normal or it may be pathological because excessive in amount or abnormal in location. It is produced by the slow death of stratified squamous epithelial cells and is normal as the cornified layer, or stratum corneum, of the epidermis and certain other squamous epithelial structures.

Microscopic Appearance.—In a state of complete cornification, this material appears as a solid, homogeneous, pink-staining mass or layer forming the superficial zone of stratified squamous epithelium. It blends gradually with the epithelium of the prickle-cell layer (stratum granulosum), becoming more and more cellular. In locations where it is constantly wet, it occasionally stains bluish.

Its **gross appearance** is that of a hard, colorless, more or less translucent, horny material. In the skin it is likely to be accompanied by much wrinkling.

Occurrence, Causes and Significance.—Abnormal keratinization occurs in the following situations:

(1) In **calluses** such as form on the human hand as the result of prolonged friction and pressure insufficient to cause blistering or erosion. Here it constitutes a physiological and protective hypertrophy but becomes excessive. The same process may result from mild irritation by harness or saddle.

(2) **Corns** on the human foot are essentially similar, but more markedly excessive in extent and irritating because of location. **Corns in the horse's foot** start as a bruise, usually with underlying hemorrhage, and later involve excessive proliferation of the horn. Such lesions as these may also be viewed as excessive proliferative inflammation (p. 165).

(3) In warts, which are focal papillomatoid epithelial proliferations caused by a filterable virus. In addition to the total excess of epithelium, the cornified layer itself is greatly excessive.

(4) In the bovine disease known as specific hyperkeratosis (p. 938) and caused by poisoning by substances containing chlorinated naphthalenes.

(5) In the rare and unexplained disease of man, cattle and dog called **icthyosis,** in which horny scales appear all over the body (Fig. 9–10, p. 339).

(6) In metaplasia (p. 96) of some other kind to stratified squamous epithelium. This occurs in the urinary and other mucous membranes under the influence of

avitaminosis-A, also in chemical irritation of the bronchial lining, where it may be a pre-cancerous condition.

(7) In the "epithelial pearls" of squamous-cell carcinoma, in which the cornified layer finds itself the compressed core of an epithelial mass whose aberrant manner of growth has caused it to be "turned inside out."

Except in the last instance it will be seen that excessive keratinization is caused by continued mild irritation of one kind or another.

While primarily a protective reaction, it is readily seen that excessive keratohyalin can interfere with secretory and absorptive functions and can cause pain when in a tissue which is under mechanical pressure. When the cause is removed the excessive keratin disappears by desquamation.

AMYLOIDOSIS

In this disorder, various organs are infiltrated and to a slight or considerable degree replaced by a firm and solid substance called amyloid. While the name means starch-like, it is now known that amyloid is a protein rather than a starchy substance.

Occurrence.—Being gradually progressive, amyloidosis tends to become generalized and widespread. However, the spleen, liver and kidneys are noteworthy as the sites of its earliest and most extensive formation. Lymph nodes and adrenal glands are rather commonly involved.

In the spleen, the deposits first form immediately around the central arteries of the splenic (Malpighian) corpuscles and gradually spread, replacing these

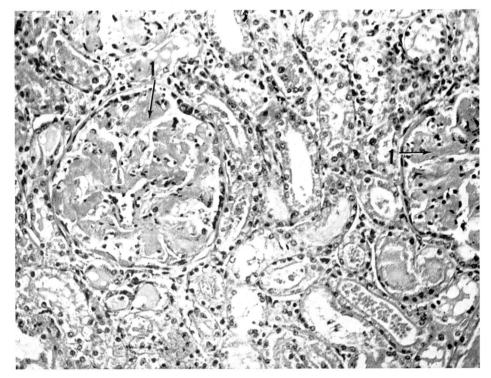

FIG. 2–5.—Amyloidosis, kidney of a dog. Amyloid (1) is deposited in the glomerular tufts. (Courtesy of Armed Forces Institute of Pathology.) × 175. Contributor: Dr. C. L. Davis.

structures and producing what is traditionally called a **sago spleen.** The tiny nodules of white, firm material give the suggestion of a spleen sprinkled with sago or its more modern counterpart, tapioca grains.

In the liver, amyloid accumulates first around the vessels of the hepatic trinities and in advanced cases, it is found spreading along the sinusoids into the lobules. Renal amyloidosis usually appears first in the glomeruli, which it eventually replaces. As the condition progresses the invading substance appears also among the tubules, especially in the outer medulla. It will be seen from the above that amyloid always starts in the immediate vicinity of the smaller blood vessels, if not actually in their walls.

Among the domestic animals, amyloidosis is rare except in the dog and horse but may be induced experimentally in guinea pigs and mice by several means (Barth, *et al.,* 1968).

Microscopic Appearance.—As already implied, amyloid is a dense and nearly homogeneous substance which replaces and obliterates pre-existing cells. The borders of the amyloid are relatively sharp, a fact which assists in distinguishing it from connective-tissue hyalin. By hematoxylin and eosin this substance stains pink, a slightly purplish pink. Reasonably specific staining reactions are obtained with the cresyl violets, which give it a redder or more violet color than the surrounding tissue. Congo red may also be used, imparting a pink color to the amyloid.

On fresh slices of tissue, the application of aqueous solutions of iodine, such as Lugol's, brings out the amyloid as a distinctly brown material. Following the iodine solution with dilute sulfuric acid changes the amyloid from brown to blue, which is possibly more conspicuous.

Gross Appearance.—Small amounts of amyloid are not detected grossly. When accumulations are larger, this substance is white, opaque and somewhat resembles lard but is firmer. The term lardosis (not lordosis) has been used as a synonym in some quarters. As a rule organs other than the spleen show amyloidosis by a slight change in their general appearance rather than in the form of individual deposits. The liver, for instance, when extensively involved is larger, paler and firmer than normal. Microscopic confirmation is essential.

Cause.—Amyloidosis is almost always concomitant to long-standing infections, such as tuberculosis and suppurative processes. It also occurs with frequency in horses which are used for the production of antitoxins. Virchow first described amyloid and postulated that it was formed by certain cells, circulated in the plasma, passed through blood vessel walls under certain circumstances and then was precipitated to form a gel. A recent theory (Teilum, 1966) more nearly fits the known facts concerning natural and experimentally-induced amyloidosis. Teilum's theory on the pathogenesis of amyloidosis postulates a "two-phase cellular theory of local secretion." The first phase involves the proliferation and stimulation of pyroninophilic reticulo-endothelial cells and plasma cells, resulting in elevated levels of gamma globulin in the blood plasma. In the second (amyloid) phase the pyroninophilic cells are suppressed (or exhausted—by persistent stimulation or other means unknown) in their production of gamma globulin (which drops to lower levels in the plasma) and new generations of cells around blood vessels are recognized by material in their cytoplasm which is colored specifically by the periodic acid-Schiff (PAS) method. These PAS-positive cells are believed to produce amyloid *in loco* around blood vessels.

Significance.—Most examples are encountered at autopsy incidental to other diseases, such as those just mentioned. However, if death does not intervene from other causes, amyloidosis progresses to the point where vital functions are destroyed and it is fatal of itself. A cutaneous form of amyloidosis is described in horses (p. 1040).

Amyloidosis

ANDERSSON, A.: On Amyloidosis of the Kidneys in Cattle. Skand. Vet. tidskr. *26*:241–290, 1936.

BARTH, W. F., GORDON, J. K., and WILLERSON, J. T.: Amyloidosis Induced in Mice by *Escherichia coli* Endotoxin. Science *162*:694–695, 1968.

CLARK, L., and SEAWRIGHT, A. A.: Generalized Amyloidosis in Seven Cats. Path. Vet. *6*: 117–134, 1969.

COHEN, A. S.: Preliminary Chemical Analysis of Purified Amyloid Fibrils. Lab. Invest. *15*: 66–83, 1966.

COWAN, D. F.: Avian Amyloidosis. I. General Incidence in Zoo Birds. Path. Vet. *5*:51–58, 1968.

GILMAN, A. L.: Observations on Amyloid Degeneration in Domestic Animals. J. Am. Vet. Med. Assn. *57*:568–578, 1920.

GUEFT, B., and GHIDONI, J. J.: The Site of Formation and Ultrastructure of Amyloid. Amer. J. Path. *43*:837–854, 1963.

GUEFT, B., KIKKAWA, Y., and HIRSCHL, S.: An Electron-microscopic Study of Amyloidosis from Different Species. In *Amyloidosis*, ed. by Mandema, E., Ruinen, L., Schalten, J. H. and Cohen, A. S., Amsterdam, Exerpta Med. Found., 1968.

HADLOW, W. J., and REINHARD, K. R.: Amyloidosis in the Dog. Cornell Vet. *44*:475–489, 1954.

HADLOW, W. J., and JELLISON, W. L.: Amyloidosis in Rocky Mountain Bighorn Sheep. J. Am. Vet. Med. Assn. *141*:243–247, 1962.

HASS, G. M., HUNTINGTON, R., and KRUMDIECK, N.: Amyloid. Properties of Amyloid Deposits Occurring in Several Species under Diverse Conditions. Arch. Path. *35*:226–241, 1943.

JANIGAN, D. T., and DRUET, R. L.: Experimental Murine Amyloidosis in X-irradiated Recipients of Spleen Homogenates or Serum from Sensitized Donors. Amer. J. Path. *52*: 381–390, 1968.

JANIGAN, D. T.: Pathogenetic Mechanisms in Protein-induced Amyloidosis. Amer. J. Path. *55*:379–393, 1969.

KLATSKIN, G.: Non-specific Green Birefringence in Congo Red-stained Tissues. Amer. J. Path. *56*:1–14, 1969.

OSBORNE, C. A., *et al.*: Renal Amyloidosis in the Dog. J. Amer. Vet. Med. Assn. *153*: 669–688, 1968.

SHIRAHAMA, T., and COHEN, A. S.: Ultrastructural Studies on Renal Peritubular Amyloid Experimentally Induced in Guinea Pigs. I. General Aspects. Lab. Invest. *19*:122–131, 1968.

TEILUM, G.: Amyloidosis: Origin from Fixed Periodic Acid-Schiff Positive Reticuloendothelial Cells *In Loco* and Basic Factors in Pathogenesis. Lab. Invest. *15*:98–110, 1966.

TRAUTWEIN, G.: Vergleichende Untersuchungen über das Amyloid und Paramyloid verschiedener Tierarten. I. Histomorphologie und färberische Eugenschaften des amyloids und paramyloids. Path. Vet. *2*:297–327, 1965.

————: Vergleichende untersuchungen über das amyloid und Paramyloid verschiedener Tierarten. II. Histochemie des amyloids und Paramyloids. Path. Vet. *2*:493–513, 1965.

PROTEINS, ALBUMINS AND ALBUMINOUS FLUIDS

It is customary in pathology to refer to nonspecific protein substances by what is almost always their principal constituent, albumin. Pathologically or otherwise, these substances are encountered in the microscopic section in a variety of situations as precipitates from body fluids.

(1) The lumen of a blood vessel may be seen filled with a pink-staining, homogeneous material. This is merely dehydrated blood plasma, with serum-albumin as its visible component, the cells having settled after death to some other part of the vessel.

(2) A similar precipitate is often seen in the renal tubules.   In this case it is albumin (and other protein) precipitated and coagulated from the excreted urine, and the diagnosis is albuminuria or proteinuria (p. 1292).   Sometimes the concentration may be so great that precipitation occurs during life, forming albuminous casts of the tubular lumens, recognizable in the voided urine.   In sections of kidney, these are usually dense and deep-staining.

(3) Most of the various kinds of cysts are filled with albumin-containing fluid. The liquor folliculi, the "colloid" of the thyroid acini and the salivary secretions are physiological examples of similar fluids.

(4) In the case of serous inflammatory exudates (p. 153) or the transudate of edema (p. 134), the only visible substance remaining is the precipitate of albumin and related proteins.   These are seen, for example, filling the alveoli of the lung, as well as in tissue spaces anywhere.

Microscopic Appearance.—Albumin precipitated as outlined above is usually smoothly homogeneous, although occasionally with high magnification, it is in the form of uniformly fine granules.   It stains a bright, clear pink by usual techniques.   This purity of tint helps to distinguish albumin from amyloid, and from fibrin, both of which carry an appearance of opacity because they give impure hues based on a variety of wave-lengths.

The **gross appearance** of all these substances is that of a watery fluid unless, of course, the fluid is mixed with other substances such as blood or pus.

FIBRIN

Fibrin is another proteinaceous substance, physiological or pathological, which the student must learn to recognize.

Occurrence.—Fibrin is seen (1) wherever blood clots, as in internal hemorrhages, intravascular clots, be they ante-mortem (thrombi, p. 108) or post-mortem (2) in the infrequent clotting of lymph, and (3) in fibrinous inflammatory exudates.

Microscopic Appearance.—Fibrin stains pink, but usually it is a "dirty" or smudgy pink.   Ordinarily it is in the form of minute, tangled fibrils readily visible with a magnification of 400 or 500 diameters (high, dry lens), but there are cases where it forms a solid and practically homogeneous mass.   One of the best examples of this is a fibrinous exudate in the pulmonary alveoli, which has to be distinguished from the albumin of a serous exudate, or inflammatory edema. If karyolysis (p. 12) has occurred in its vicinity, fibrin, sponge-like, absorbs the released chromatin, thereby becoming endowed with the blue color characteristic of nuclei.

Gross Appearance.—Fibrin, as seen in clots from which the blood cells have been removed by washing, is a dull white, stringy material, the strands of which form a tangled mass.   In fibrinous exudates, it is likely to be mixed with other exudative components, dead tissue or fecal material (fibrinous enteritis) which modify its form and color.

The **causes** are to be studied in the respective discussions of clotting and exudates.

Significance.—Fibrin is formed by the coagulation of fibrinogen; hence its source is the blood, either directly or through the process of exudation.   Fibrin is not innately a harmful substance; as an exudate upon a mucous or serous surface it forms a valuable protective coating; by closing an opened blood vessel, it

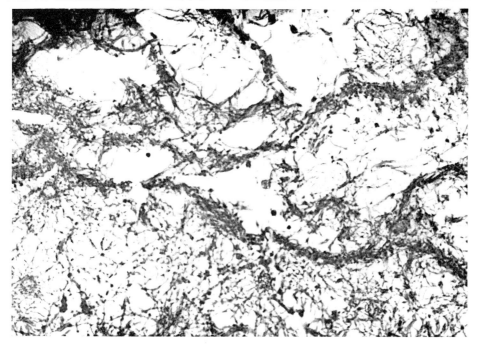

FIG. 2–6.   Microscopic appearance of fibrin in a blood clot in the pulmonary vein of a dog.   Note the thin interlacing fibrils.

terminates the loss of blood which must otherwise be fatal.   But in many situations its ultimate effect is harmful if not disastrous.   Clots, called thrombi (p. 108) all too frequently develop within the blood-vascular system stopping the supply of blood to a certain part with the consequences protrayed under "Necrosis" (p. 17).   In the pulmonary alveoli, it prevents the entrance of air.   While covering and protecting a surface, it interferes more or less with the normal functioning of the surface cells.

As to the ultimate fate of fibrin, there are two possibilities.   The fibrin may be completely liquefied through natural autolysis and the liquefying enzymes of leukocytes.   On the other hand, the mere presence of fibrin appears to act as a stimulus for the proliferation of nearby fibroblasts, with the result that the latter grow into it and in the course of some days the fibrin has disappeared and fibrous connective tissue has taken its place, a process which is called **organization.** Thrombi are thus made permanent, as is also the solidification of the pulmonary alveoli.   On the surfaces which line potential cavities, such as the pleural and peritoneal cavities, there is the strong probability that the two apposed surfaces may be permanently tied together by fibrous **adhesions.**   (See Fibrinous Inflammation, p. 156.)

FIBRINOID DEGENERATION

Fibrinoid degeneration, or merely fibrinoid, is a currently popular name for small areas of nondescript material appearing in connective tissues in various locations.   It is stained by the specific stains for fibrin and is strongly positive to the periodic-acid-Schiff reaction (PAS).   In ordinary hematoxylin-eosin sections it appears as a smudgy, pink material, always in connective tissue, with no distinct boundaries, not exactly necrotic but appearing to lack the numbers of nuclei that would be adequate for normal living tissue. Whether the material is homogenized fibrin from an inflammatory exudate or represents a degenerative change in the collagen or ground substance of connective tissue already present is in dispute. Vasquez and Dixon (1958) have developed evidence by means of fluorescein-coupled antibodies indicating that not all fibrinoid changes are of the same nature. There is general agreement that the change is characteristic of, and doubtless the result of an antigen-antibody reaction going on locally in the connective tissue. It is therefore an outstanding feature of the "collagen diseases" of humans, such as rheumatic fever, periarteritis nodosa (p. 1156) and several others.

MUCUS AND MUCIN

Mucus (the corresponding adjective is "mucous") is a clear, glistening, water-like fluid which is somewhat more viscid than water and which has lubricating properties that give a slimy, slippery impression. It consists of water plus a mucine, a compound containing a nucleoprotein. Due to the nucleic acid in the latter, mucins take the basic stain, which in usual techniques is blue (hematoxylin). (Note that the preceding proteid substances have all taken some shade of red.) On the basis of their origin, two forms of mucin are recognized.

Epithelial Mucin.—A product of epithelial cells, epithelial mucin occurs only upon mucous membranes, coming either from the mucous glands with which most mucous membranes are provided or from those one-celled mucous glands called goblet cells.

A slight amount of mucus is normally secreted by most mucous membranes, especially those of the respiratory and digestive tracts. The "mucus of estrum," which is produced so copiously by the cervical glands at the estrual period, is a physiological phenomenon. Excessive production on other occasions is a response to an irritant and will be treated in detail under Mucous Inflammation (p. 161).

Connective-Tissue Mucin.—Sometimes called **mucoid** to distinguish it from epithelial mucin, this is, potentially at least, one of the intercellular components of connective-tissue matrix. It is abundant in the connective tissue of the embryo and is responsible for the bluish staining of the embryonal type of connective tissue wherever found. Pathologically it occurs in that reversion to embryonal connective tissue which we call mucoid degeneration.

Pseudomucin is a substance related to the true mucins but staining pink instead of blue. It is found in the cystic spaces of ovarian cystadenomas and cystadenocarcinomas of humans. It is not of importance in veterinary medicine.

MUCOID DEGENERATION

Equivalent to this condition are "myxomatous degeneration" and "mucoid atrophy of fat." "Serous atrophy of fat" is also practically synonymous but, owing, probably, to the formation of potassium soaps in the degenerating fat cells, there is a pinkish, rather than a bluish discoloration.

Occurrence.—Mucoid degeneration occurs in tissues which normally contain at least small amounts of fibrous or adipose connective tissue. In this broad territory the more usual locations are (1) around the coronary groove of the heart and extending down between myocardial fibers, (2) in skeletal muscle, between its fibers and bundles, and (3) in the omentum and mesentery.

Microscopic Appearance.—There is a proliferation of connective tissue of embryonal characteristics; its intercellular matrix has the bluish tinge of mucin; its scanty fibrils have a criss-cross arrangement; its hyperchromatic nuclei tend to be stellate, ovoid or spherical. To some extent this connective tissue, which is moderate in amount, is added to the pre-existing elements, but such fibrillar or adipose connective tissue as may have been present tends to decrease in amount, to show pyknotic and pre-necrotic changes and to be replaced by the embryonal tissue.

Gross Appearance.—An appreciable amount of mucoid degeneration produces an area where the tissue is translucent and watery underneath its shiny covering of serosa or other overlying membrane. When mingled with adipose tissue, as is usual, the whole process is obviously an area of degenerated, watery fat. One should watch for it, especially, in the coronary fat of the heart.

Causes.—Certain sorts of blood-borne toxins may possibly play a part, but the principal causative role is to be attributed to lack of proper nutrition. Mucoid degeneration is the most conspicuous alteration accompanying ordinary starvation. Meat inspectors pay much attention to it as pointing to a state of malnutrition which makes mere lack of fat and muscle a case calling for condemnation of the carcass. The condition can occur when the total amount of food is adequate, but when there is some serious short-coming in its quality. It has been noted, for instance, in a lamb which was fed experimentally a diet containing no protein. It is an accompaniment of various wasting and cachectic diseases in their later stages. The possibility that local interference with nutrition may produce mucoid degeneration of a restricted area has to be considered.

Significance.—Mucoid degeneration is important for what it indicates of the general health. It has little effect upon function locally and is a change which is entirely reversible.

References—General

ACHARD, C., VERNE, J., and BARIÉTY, M.: Les graisses du rein chez le chien. Ann. d'anat. path. *9*:780–783, 1932.

ATERMAN, K.: Observations on the Nature of "Watery Vacuolation." The Response of the Liver Cell to the Intravenous Injection of Hypertonic Saline, Evans Blue, Dextran and Heparin. Lab. Investig., *6*:577-605, 1958.

BECKER, J. P.: The Nature of Alcoholic Hyaline (of alcoholic cirrhosis—Mallory). Lab. Invest. *10*:527–534, 1961.

BELL, E. T.: On the Differential Staining of Fats. J. Path. & Bact. *19*:105–113, 1914.

BLOOR, W. R.: II. Fat Absorption and the Blood Lipoids. J. Biol. Chem. *23*:317–326, 1915.

DIBLE, J. H., and HAY, J. D.: The Nature of Fatty Change in the Kidneys. J. Path. & Bact. *51*:1–7, 1940.

FOOTE, J. J., and GRAFFLIN, A. L.: Quantitative Measurements of the Fat-laden and Fat-free Segments of the Proximal Tubule in the Nephron of the Cat and Dog. Anat. Rec. *72*:169–179, 1938.

JENNINGS, R. B., HERDSON, P. B., SOMMERS, H. M.: Structural and Functional Abnormalities in Mitochondria Isolated from Ischemic Dog Myocradium. Lab. Invest. *20*:548–557, 1969.

KING, D. W. (ed.): *Ultrastructural Aspects of Disease.* New York, Harper & Row, 1966.

PEREZ-TAMAYO, R.: *Mechanisms of Disease.* Philadelphia, W. B. Saunders Co., 1961.

PETERS, R. A.: *Biochemical Lesions and Lethal Synthesis.* Oxford, Pergamon Press, 1963.

TRUMP, B. F., and ERICSSON, J. L. E. in *The Inflammatory Process.* Zweifach, B. W., Grant, L. and McClusky, R. T. (eds.). New York, Academic Press, 1965.

VASQUEZ, J. J., and DIXON, F. J.: Immunohistochemical Analysis of Lesions Associated with "Fibrinoid Change. Arch. Path. *66*:504–517, 1958.

3

Mineral Deposits, Pigments

This chapter is concerned with a discussion of pathological deposits of minerals which are encountered in tissues upon gross or microscopic examination; general metabolism of minerals will be treated elsewhere. A number of mineral substances are detected because they are also pigments, *i.e.*, they have an intrinsic color. Also included are pigments of organic origin both endogenous and exogenous which are encountered in tissues as normal components or as pathological deposits.

PATHOLOGIC CALCIFICATION

By pathologic calcification is meant the deposition of calcium salts in tissues other than bone and teeth. The calcium is usually deposited as calcium phosphate and calcium carbonate and may occur in the form of hydroxyapatite similar to that of normal bone. Often the salts are not chemically pure, but may be accompanied by other ions such as iron, which has led some to prefer the noncommittal term of **mineralization.**

Pathologic calcification may be divided into dystrophic calcification, metastatic calcification and calcinosis circumscripta. Calcinosis circumscripta is discussed separately under skin (p. 1032).

DYSTROPHIC CALCIFICATION

Dystrophic calcification is the deposition of calcium salts in dead or degenerating tissues. It is not related to calcium content of blood, which normally is around 10 mg. per 100 ml. It may occur in practically any tissue or organ. While we refer ordinarily to the tissues of the patient, the same may be said of the tissues of metazoon parasites which wander into various regions of the patient's body and perish there, as in trichinosis.

Microscopic Appearance.—The calcium carbonate or phosphate is usually in very irregular granules of microscopic size or a little larger. They usually take a characteristic purplish color from the basic hematoxylin, although occasionally with minor variations in technique the effect of eosin may predominate. The depth of color, in the small particles encountered in microscopic sections, is dependent on the thickness of the particle, and this often shows abrupt variation from point to point as if the mineral were deposited in layers which decrease step by step toward the edge of the calcified granule. Everywhere the form and structure of the granule or clump of granules are entirely irregular and unpredictable, although they may be limited within the confines of a given histologic structure, such as the wall of a small artery.

Calcium salts can be demonstrated to greater advantage with special staining methods such as the von-Kossa and Alizarin-Red-S techniques. However, it should be stressed that certain calcium salts such as calcium oxalate, do not stain with hematoxylin, nor do they react with the usual histochemical stains for calcium salts.

Gross Appearance.—If freed from the surrounding tissue, the calcium particles would be white or gray, irregularly rounded and often honeycombed. The material must be somewhat less dense than ordinary limestone, for small deposits often yield to the microtome knife with about an equal degree of fragmentation of the stone and of the steel.

The most common way of detecting calcification grossly is to slice through the suspected area with a knife in search of a gritty sound and feeling. This is done routinely by meat inspectors examining for tuberculosis and other conditions in which calcification is a more or less constant feature.

Causes.—The presence of dead or dying animal tissue is the fundamental cause of calcium deposition of this type. As indicated, it is not related to an increased amount of calcium in the blood. What local factors initiate the precipitation of calcium are unknown, but it has been suggested that local alkalinity in dead tissue favors the precipitation. There is little evidence to support this hypothesis. Another suggestion is that fatty acids are formed in necrotic tissue which com-

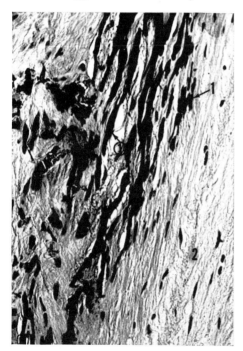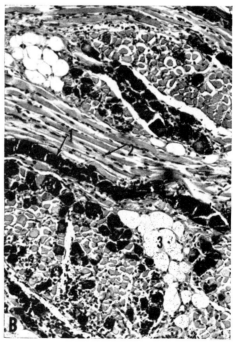

FIG. 3–1.—Calcification. *A*, Deposits of calcium salts (*1*) in the myocardium of a cow. (Courtesy of Armed Forces Institute of Pathology.) × 300. Contributor: Dr. J. F. Ryff. *B*, Calcium deposition in skeletal muscles in the tongue of a foal possibly as a result of vitamin E deficiency. The calcium salt (*1*) replaces the sarcoplasm in many muscle bundles. A few unaffected bundles (*2*) remain. Normal fat cells (*3*) are present. (Courtesy of Armed Forces Institute of Pathology.) × 114. Contributor: Dr. W. O. Reed.

3

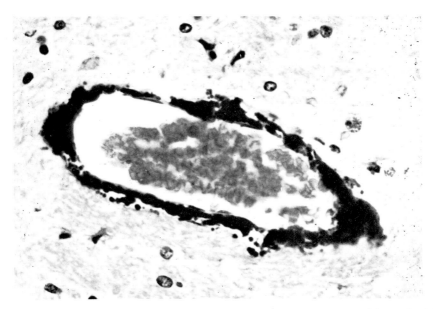

FIG. 3–2.—Cerebrovascular siderosis, marmoset (*Saguinus oedipus*). Iron positive and calcium positive material in the wall of a cerebral arteriole. (Courtesy of New England Regional Primate Research Center, Harvard Medical School.)

bine with calcium forming soaps which are later replaced by phosphates and carbonates. No doubt this is of importance in fat necrosis (p. 22) but again there is little evidence to indicate this mechanism is involved in dystrophic calcification. Increased levels of alkaline phosphatase have been demonstrated within sites of dystrophic calcification but it is not known if this enzyme is involved in the deposition of calcium salts. Also, the enzyme cannot be invariably demonstrated.

Among the situations in which calcification is prone to develop are the caseous centers of tubercles (except avian) and caseous areas in some of the other granulomatous diseases, the rosettes and ensheathed colonies of actinomycosis and staphylococcic granuloma (botryomycosis), old thrombi, degenerating tumors and old areas of scarring, including the injured walls of atheromatous blood vessels. Also included are the remains, more or less encapsulated and scarred, of parasites such as trichinae, flukes, encysted tapeworm larvae and others, which have been unable to complete their life-cycles and have died within the tissues.

Significance.—Calcium deposits are relatively permanent but are harmless unless, by virtue of their location, they interfere mechanically with some function or reduce the strength of a part. It will be recalled that calcification was listed as one of ways by which the body disposes of dead tissue (see Necrosis, p. 17), since calcified material is functionally inert. Occasionally calcification in certain locations may accompany and possibly be causally related to pathological ossification. The latter will receive separate attention presently.

METASTATIC CALCIFICATION

Metastatic calcification is the precipitation of calcium salts as the result of a persistently high concentration of calcium in the blood. The tissues affected need not have been previously damaged. The staining qualities and gross appearance of the calcium salts do not differ from those described for dystrophic calcification.

Causes.—Metastatic calcification can result from (1) primary hyperparathyroidism which is discussed elsewhere (p. 1366), but this condition is exceedingly rare, especially in animals; (2) renal failure in which the excretion of phosphate is reduced, resulting in increased serum inorganic phosphate levels. Secondary hyperparathyroidism may develop in this situation which then accentuates calcium deposition. It becomes difficult to differentiate "dystrophic" from "metastatic" calcification under these circumstances due to the presence of degenerating lesions of uremia (p. 1294). (3) Widespread calcification of the walls of arteries and other tissues can result from a hypercalcemia produced by very large excesses of vitamin-D in the diet. In animals this is most likely to be the result of some scientific experiment, but it may occasionally be encountered in livestock fed too enthusiastically with artificial vitamins. There is evidence that ultrastructural lesions precede renal calcification in hypervitaminosis D in rats. By definition one would have to reassess the use of the term metastatic if similar findings are encountered in other tissues and other forms of metastatic calcification. (4) Widespread disseminated calcification of pulmonary alveolar septa is reported, but in the author's experience this is usually ossification. (5) Evidence has been adduced that deficiency of magnesium and hypomagnesemia may be a cause of widespread calcification. In this deficiency calcification has been noted in the intima of the heart and large vessels of calves, also in the lower nephrons of rats.

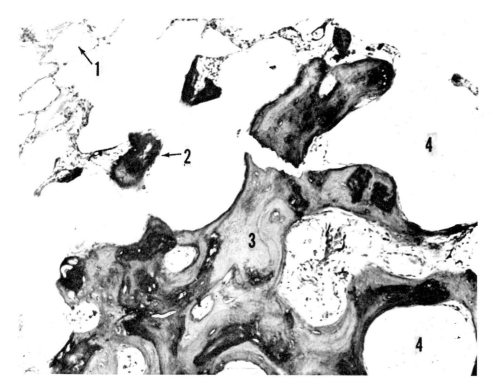

FIG. 3–3.—Pathologic ossification of a bovine lung; cause unknown. Alveoli (*1*), early calcification (*2*), and osteoid (*3*). Dilated alveolar spaces (*4*) are partially surrounded by bone. (Courtesy of Armed Forces Institute of Pathology.) × 250. Contributor: Dr. W. S. Bailey.

(6) Calcification of a variety of tissues, but especially of the lungs, skin, and skeletal muscle is often a feature of hyperadrenalism in the dog (p. 1353). (7) Widespread calcification of the cardiovascular system and lungs are the principal features of Manchester wasting disease (p. 1156).

Occurrence.—Metastatic calcification primarily occurs in the kidneys, lungs, gastric mucosa and media of arteries. A common explanation for the preference of these sites is the local alkaline condition resulting from excretion of acid by the lung, stomach and kidney: precipitation of calcium salts being favored by an alkaline environment. This theory however, remains unproved and does not explain metastatic calcification of other tissues.

PATHOLOGICAL OSSIFICATION

Occurrence.—It is a feature of the normal ontogeny of the turkey that, as the bird approaches maturity, the tendons of its leg muscles turn to bone. In limited and variable degree a similar change is not unknown in other species. **Ossification of the lateral cartilages** (p. 1080) of the horse's foot is an important cause of lameness. It occurs (*a*) in the draft breeds, (*b*) in older individuals, (*c*) in those individuals which have had hard work on hard pavements, and (*d*) in the fore feet, which bear the most weight. Rarely in old horses and old people there is partial ossification of tracheal or laryngeal cartilages, especially if these have been exposed to stresses or have had inflammatory processes nearby. Widespread formation of bony spicules in the interalveolar septa of the lung is not altogether rare. One of us (Smith) has dissected a flat layer of bone measuring 3 by 4 cm. from the wall of the renal pelvis of a bovine animal. He has also encountered a flat plate of bone of larger size between the muscular layers of the belly wall of a pig. Both were in the vicinity of inflammatory processes. Injured muscle is prone to ssification; referred to as myositis ossificans (p. 1054).

Microscopic Appearance.—Small bits of ossified tissue are best distinguished from mere calcification by means of the cells and lacunae which are found in the bone; calcified areas are acellular. Marrow may accompany the bony structures.

Causes.—It appears that ossification is a response to prolonged irritation in older individuals in which there is an hereditary tendency in this directioin Heterotopic bone is also not infrequent at sites of dystrophic and metastatc. calcification. Under these circumstances fibroblasts differentiate to osteoblasts which form osteoid which calcifies to become bone in an identical manner to normal membranous bone formation.

Significance.—The bony structures interfere mechanically with movement; otherwise they appear to do no harm.

GOUT

Gout is a condition in which crystals of uric acid or urates are deposited in the tissues.

Occurrence—The disorder occurs in humans, in birds and, reportedly, in dogs and cats. Parts of the body involved are the articular and periarticular tissues, where the sharp crystals act as irritating foreign bodies, causing intense pain and acute inflammation. Attacks come and recede with poorly understood fluctuations in protein, or purine, metabolism.

In birds two forms are found, the articular, like that just described, and the more frequent visceral form.

Microscopic Appearance.—Inflammatory infiltrations including many macrophages and foreign-body giant cells in conjunction with clusters of sharp acicular crystals, or spaces left after they dissolve, located in an articular surface, joint capsule or adjacent tissues, are indicative of articular gout. In the visceral gout of birds, various serous surfaces are covered with finely crystalline or almost amorphous material which does not stain.

Gross Appearance.—Opportunities for necropsies of cases of this disease are rare except in birds, usually chickens or turkeys. The gross picture of the gouty joint is already obvious. The amount of precipitated material may be so great as to form grossly noticeable white, chalky masses in the tissues. Known as "tophi," these may occur in the subcutaneous tissues elsewhere than in the joints and may ulcerate, but without the severe pain which characterizes involvement of the joints.

In visceral gout, the serous surfaces in the body cavity and especially the outer surface of the pericardial sac are encrusted by a thin grayish layer having a metallic sheen. This appearance is diagnostic.

Causes.—Uric acid and urates are decomposition products of nucleic acid metabolism. Just what happens is not clear, but it is known that in humans the concentration of uric acid in the blood is very considerably increased (from 2.5 mg. per 100 ml. to 4 mg. per 100 ml.). The uric acid in the urine is very low just before an attack, but becomes abnormally high as the attack develops.

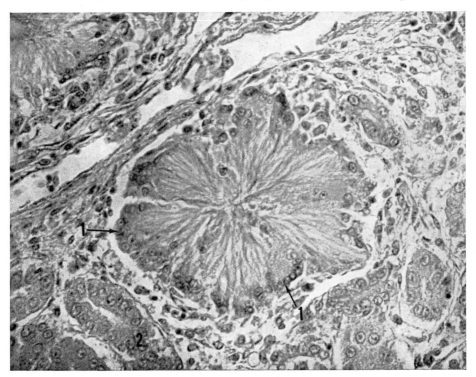

Fig. 3–4.—Gout. Deposit of urate crystals in the kidney of a turkey. The urates are surrounded by multinucleated giant cells (*1*). Renal tubules (*2*). (Courtesy of Armed Forces Institute of Pathology.) × 425. Contributor: Dr. J. F. Olney.

In birds, the kidneys eliminate semisolid urates instead of urine and uric acid. It is known that in deficiency of vitamin-A the elimination of urates is severely impaired, one of the visible lesions being their accumulation in the ureteral ducts. Hence it is now customary to attribute visceral gout to this deficiency. However, the chemical aspects appear not to have been studied sufficiently, and there remains older experimental evidence linking this disorder to diets containing, if not too much protein, at least unusual kinds of protein.

Significance.—The visceral gout of birds is seen only at necropsy. It is difficult to say whether any birds recover, but presumably recovery is possible with a suitable change in diet. Articular gout is stubbornly recurrent in afflicted humans and presumably so in the rare cases in animals.

PIGMENTS

There is nothing logical about considering together the diverse and unrelated substances customarily grouped as pigments except that, in surveying the various abnormalities which one may encounter in cellular pathology, it is convenient to have a look at all those substances which have color of their own instead of being dependent upon artificial staining to make them conspicuous.

A multitudinous number of pigments can be found in animal tissues. The ensuing discussion will make no attempt to cover all pigments, but rather we will

Table 3-1.—Characteristics of Common Pigments as Seen in Tissue Sections

Pigment	Hematoxylin and Eosin	Polaroscopy	Iron Stains	Fat Stains	Acid Fast Stains	Other Distinguishing Characteristics
Carbon	Black	Isotropic	—	—	—	Resistant to all stains and bleaching agents and micro-incineration
Melanin	Yellow:brown to black	Isotropic	—	—	—	Reduce silver; Bleached by $KMnO_4$; Combusted by microincineration
Hemosiderin	Yellow:brown	Isotropic	+	—	—	Non-fluorescent
Acid hematins	Brown	Anisotropic	—	—	—	Removed by saturated alcoholic picric acid
Porphyrin	Usually not visible except in Rodent Harderian Gland	Slightly Anisotropic	—	—	—	Fluorescent at 365 mμ
Bilirubin	Bright Yellow	Anisotropic if crystalline	—	—	—	Gmelin's test positive; Non-fluorescent
Lipofuscins (wear and tear pigments and ceroid)	Yellow to Brown	Isotropic	—	+	+	Fluorescent at 365 mμ

limit ourselves to those pigments that are encountered with frequency or are important components of animal diseases. For our purposes, pigments will be classified as follows:

I. Exogenous Pigments—those formed outside the body.
 A. Carbon
 B. Dusts
 C. Metals
 D. Tattoos
 E. Kaolin
 F. Carotenoids

II. Endogenous Pigments—those formed inside the body.
 A. Phenolic Pigments
  1. Melanin
 B. Hematogenous Pigments
  1. Hemoglobins
  2. Hematins
  3. Parasitic Pigments
  4. Hemosiderins
  5. Bile Pigments
  6. Porphyrins
 C. Lipogenic Pigments
  1. Tissue Lipofuscins
  2. Ceroid
  3. Vitamin E deficiency pigment
 D. Miscellaneous Pigments
  1. Ochronosis Pigment
  2. Dubin-Johnson Pigment
  3. Cloisonné kidney

CARBON—ANTHRACOSIS

Anthracosis is the condition in which carbon particles are found as a black pigment in the tissues. Carbon is foremost among the exogenous pigments.

It **occurs** in the lungs and the lymph nodes which drain them and, rarely, in other organs when carried there in phagocytes. It is common in humans and animals which live in smoky cities, and as pointed out by Hilton Smith in the first edition of this text, universal among men and mules who work in coal mines. The mules have since left the mines but black lungs still plague the miner.

Microscopically carbon appears as minute black granules either between cells or in their cytoplasm. In the lungs, it is in the alveolar walls and in the connective-tissue septa, usually within macrophages. In the lymph nodes, it is chiefly between the lymphoid cells, but large mononuclears frequently phagocytize it and carry it elsewhere. Carbon can be distinguished from other pigments by its black color and histochemically by its resistance to all solvents and bleaching agents.

Grossly moderate or large amounts impart a mottling or speckling with black or gray to the lungs, the ventral portions of the lobes being affected more than the dorsal. Lymph nodes are likewise darkened. One must not confuse with anthracosis the black or brown color which is so common as to be almost the rule

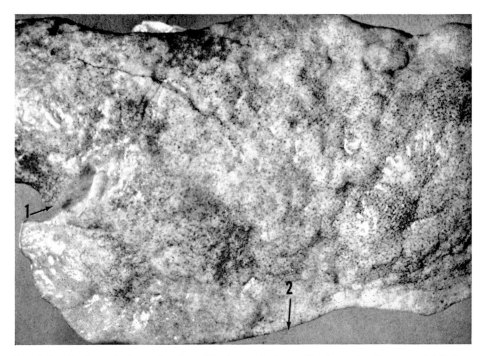

FIG. 3–5.—Anthracosis, lung of a dog. Finely particulate collections of carbon are visible from the pleural surface. Cardiac notch (1) and ventral margin of lung (2).

in the medullary region of bovine lymph nodes. This discoloration is due to a soluble pigment presumed to come from recently hemolyzed blood. Since the pigment is soluble, it is not seen in microscopic preparations. Such lymph nodes do not reflect any form of ill health in the animal.

Causes and Significance.—Anthracosis is due to repeated and continued inhalation of coal smoke, which is the lot of thousands of humans and dogs living in cities, and a few animals of other species. Men (and mules) working in coal mines are markedly afflicted, so that the heavily blackened lung is called a miner's lung. Reasonable amounts of the pigment do little harm and cause no symptoms, but it remains in the tissues throughout life and excessive amounts may cause slight fibrosis and are suspected of predisposing to pulmonary infections.

DUSTS

When dust is inhaled, the organic particles are short-lived owing to defensive mechanisms of the body. Several kinds of mineral dusts, however, leave visible particles in the pulmonary tissues. Collectively, dust retained in the lung is termed pneumoconiosis. Anthracosis discussed above, is a specialized form of **pneumoconiosis** in which the dust particles are carbon. Several other mineral dusts are important causes of pneumoconiosis, some of which induce serious pulmonary disease. The more important ones are:

Silicosis.—**Silicon dioxide** is inhaled in rock quarries and mines or under any other conditions in which rock is being cut or sandblasted. **Microscopically** silicon dioxide occurs in the tissues as fine, anisotropic crystals which can only be visualized with polarized light. The crystals incite collagenous connective tissue proliferation which takes the form of dense sclerotic nodules which may coalesce. A vascular or cellular inflammatory response does not occur. **Grossly** the lungs are nodular and firm and may be pigmented due to concomitant anthracosis.

Siderosis.—Iron dust is inhaled chiefly as hematite or iron oxide from mines. The mineral does not incite fibrosis or an inflammatory reaction and is, therefore, of little significance. However, siderosis is often accompanied by silicosis. **Microscopically** hematite and iron oxide appear as red crystals of varying size. They are anisotropic, appearing orange with polarized light, and iron can be specifically demonstrated with the Prussian blue reaction. The student should note that certain other iron salts and complexes may be black, blue, green, grey or brown, and not all react with the usual Prussian blue stain. In the **gross,** hematite and iron oxide impart a brick red color to the lungs.

Asbestosis.—Asbestos is inhaled from asbestos factories. **Microscopically** asbestos occurs as fine, white anisotropic fibers and as asbestos bodies. Asbestos bodies are long beaded rods with rounded ends, which are yellow due to an iron coating that can be demonstrated with the Prussian blue reaction. Asbestos bodies are isotropic (dark under polarized light). Asbestos incites fibrous scarring of the pleura, around bronchioles and alveolar ducts and within alveolar septae. Discrete nodules as in silicosis do not develop. Foreign body giant cells may form adjacent to the asbestos particles. **Grossly** the pleura is thickened and the lungs are firm.

OTHER METALS AND EXOGENOUS PIGMENTS

Silver.—The disorder known as **argyria** is of academic interest. Formerly a number of infections were commonly treated with various organic silver compounds, of which argyrol is about the only present-day survivor. When large amounts were administered to human patients, silver was sometimes precipitated in the skin in amounts sufficient to impart to it a ghastly gray color. This was a permanent cosmetic injury of considerable importance to the victim. Obviously the same would scarcely be true in animals. **Microscopically** silver occurs as an insoluble albuminate which is brown to black. It is deposited principally extracellularly between connective tissue fibers in the upper corium. Only a small amount may be found within macrophages. In some cases deposits may also occur extracellularly in the liver and kidney. Silver does not produce injury nor incite a cellular reaction.

Lead.—In chronic poisoning due to the prolonged ingestion or assimilation of small amounts of lead compounds a blue-black discoloration is imparted to the gums. Of considerable diagnostic importance, it is most pronounced just above (or proximal to) the teeth and is called the "**lead line.**" Chronic lead poisoning has occurred in animals as the result of eating pasturage contaminated by fumes and smoke from smelters, or drinking water similarly polluted. Chiefly in earlier years, when white lead (lead carbonate) was a more prominent constituent of paints than it is now, animals were sometimes poisoned by gnawing on painted stalls, and painters developed chronic poisoning from absorption of what was spilled on the skin over a period of years (p. 956).

Bismuth.—Occasionally in examining microscopic sections from the edge of a fistulous tract or sinus, such as might have been left by some penetrating foreign body, one sees a faint gray-black pigment in the form of minute granules in and between cells. Investigation reveals that this is a residue from a bismuth-containing paste or powder which was injected into the tract so that it could be visualized by roentgenological examination, bismuth salts being opaque to x-rays. This and similar delicate pigments should be sought by low magnification with a strong light directed down upon the slide and reflected back into the microscope rather than by the usual light transmitted through the section.

Tattoos.—A variety of pigments are used to produce tattoos. These include India ink, China ink, Bismark brown, cinnabar, and kurkuma. These pigments are inert and produce no tissue reaction. They are seen microscopically extra-cellularly between connective tissue fibers of the dermis and within macrophages.

Kaolin.—Also known as china clay or Fuller's earth, kaolin is a kind of clay derived by disintegration of an aluminous material such as feldspar or mica. The essential mineral constituent is hydrated aluminum silicate (kaolinite) but the following elements may also be present: silicon (SiO_2), aluminum (Al_2O_3), iron (Fe_2O_3), titanium (TiO_2), calcium (CaO), magnesium (MgO), potassium (K_2O), sodium (Na_2O), manganese (MnO), copper (CuO), and sulfur (SO_3), with water, carbon, and organic matter. Kaolin has been incriminated as a cause of pneumoconiosis (kaolinosis) in man which leads to dense pulmonary scarring. It has also produced extensive subcutaneous granulomas in the pharyngeal and neck tissues of animals following over-zealous administration of various kaolin contain-ing products for gastrointestinal disease. The kaolin accidentally introduced into the subcutaneous tissue incites a striking influx of macrophages producing dense nodules which displace adjacent tissues. The kaolin is visible as amorphous material and fine anisotropic crystals within macrophages.

CAROTENOID OR LIPOCHROME PIGMENTS

The carotenoid pigments are fat soluble pigments of plant origin. They include carotene-A, carotene-B (the precursor of vitamin A) and xanthophyll, all of which are greenish-yellow. They are classed as lipochrome pigments which are not to be confused with the endogenous lipofuscin pigments discussed shortly (p. 82).

Pigments of this group **occur** normally in the epithelial cells of the adrenal, lutein cells of the corpus luteum, epithelium of the testis and seminal vesicle, Kupffer cells of the liver, ganglion cells, the yolk of eggs, butter fat and the adipose cells of those animals, such as horses and Jersey and Guernsey cattle, which have a markedly yellow body-fat. The amount of carotenoid pigments in tissue varies between species owing to their relative efficiency to convert carotene-B to vita-min A and their efficiency to reject carotenoids in the ingesta which are not re-quired for vitamin A synthesis. The efficiency for these two functions is low in such species as fowl, horses, cattle, humans and non-human primates.

Pathologically the same type of pigment occurs in small tumors of humans known as xanthomas. These tumors are not true neoplasms, but appear to be a disorder of the reticulo-endothelial system.

Lipochrome pigments are seen only grossly, since the material is soluble and the color diffuse and not pronounced.

Hepatic Carotenosis.—Bovine livers are sometimes seen with a brilliant yellow color. perhaps slightly reddish but not with the greenish tinge that is character-istic of jaundice and retention of bile, nor with the pale yellow of fatty change.

It has been shown that the pigment here is carotene, as much as 50 mg. per 100 mg. being demonstrable chemically. This pigment itself is harmless (p. 64) but the affected livers also show toxic changes consisting chiefly of focal or centrilobular necrosis and limited fatty change. These changes progress to varying degrees of portal cirrhosis and even almost complete replacement of the liver tissue by fibrous tissue, mild lymphocytic infiltrations being also present. Feeding such livers experimentally to rats produces similar toxic changes in the livers of the rats but no accumulation of carotene. It is presumed that the carotene remains unconverted and unmetabolized because of the toxic injury to the liver cells but this appears to be a peculiarity of the bovine species only. Investigators, working with material obtained at meat inspection, suspected some unknown toxic plant as the cause.

Livers filled with retained bile pigment in obstructive jaundice, in spite of a usual greenish tinge, may be confusing. The two can be differentiated by extracting a sample of minced liver with ether and water. After thorough shaking, the lighter ether will rise to the top with the yellow color of the carotene if this is present. The water below will be colored yellow by bilirubin, the pigment of icterus, if such is present. The *fatty* liver not only has a lighter yellow color but greater swelling if the condition is pronounced, and a lighter specific gravity, often floating on water.

MELANIN

Passing to the **endogenous** group of pigments, the most important in the **autogenous** sub-group is melanin. Melanin is the pigment which gives color to the skin and hair and to the iris, and provides the black, reflection-proof inner coating of the eyeball.

While the complete chemistry of melanin is not known, it is considered to be formed from the amino acid, tyrosine, which, it will be recalled, differs from phenylalanine (beta-phenyl, alpha-amino propionic acid) by having one hydroxy group attached to the phenyl group, and which is therefore also called hydroxyphenylalanine. Although the oxidative steps necessary to convert tyrosine to melanin are not known, the copper containing enzyme tyrosinase is required. There also exists, by artificial production, the substance dihydroxyphenylalanine, which has one more hydroxy group attached to the phenyl ring. More will be said about this presently.

The mechanisms which control melanin formation are also poorly understood. It has been established in man and some animals that the pituitary produces two melanocyte stimulating factors; α-MSH and β-MSH. Although their function is not clear, they are believed to be of importance in man in the increased pigmentation seen in Addison's disease and in pregnancy. ACTH also has melanocyte stimulating potential but to a significantly lesser degree than MSH. It has also been demonstrated that hydrocortisone decreases MSH release from the pituitary.

Occurrence.—Melanin occurs in several diverse situations. (1) In the epidermis of animals and humans, there is a small amount in light-colored individuals and more in the darker ones. The melanin exists as minute brown or black granules in the cytoplasm of the epithelial cells, chiefly or entirely in the basal layer, the stratum germinativum. In black animals and negroes, some of the pigment extends into cells of the intermediate layers. (2) The hairs partake of the same pigmentation to a degree somewhat proportional to that of the skin. It is reported that the melanin granules are large in dark hairs, smaller in hairs of lighter color. It will be noticed that bay, brown and even sorrel horses have a black skin, as do red and fawn cattle and red swine. In the dog and cat, this may not be the case, depending on the breed. In animals with white spots, both hair and skin are non-pigmented at these places. Gray horses owe their color to a mixture of white and black hairs over a black skin. White rabbits, white rats, white mice and occasional individuals in any of the species, are true **albinos,** having no pigment in hair, skin or elsewhere, except that the retina is not entirely devoid of pigment. (3) In some breeds of cattle, especially Jerseys, and in some breeds of dogs, such as Chows, the mucous membrane of the mouth shares the pigmentation of the adjacent skin. The same is true of hoofs, white hoof tissue growing from white skin, and this is largely true of horns. (4) Melanin gives color to the iris and a thick, black zone of it in a layer of cells where the retina joins the chorioid totally backens the interior of the uveal space. (5) In some people and especially in sheep, among the domestic animals, melanin is found here and there in certain cells of the pia-arachnoid. In sheep this is very frequent over the anterior part of the brain but may be found even over the spinal cord. (6) In some species the substantia nigra of the brain is black because of melanin-containing nerve cells.

The above represent normal physiological deposits of melanin. It occurs **pathologically,** or at least abnormally, in (1) the tumors known as melanomas (p. 267), (2) melanosis, (3) acanthosis nigricans (p. 1035), (4) such abnormalities of the human skin as freckles and (5) hyperpigmentation of the skin associated with hyperadrenalism (p. 1353).

Melanosis is a deposition of melanin in various organs, especially the lungs and aorta, as rather spectacular black or brown spots of irregular shape and often a centimeter or more in greatest diameter. There is no change in the texture, consistency or form of the tissue and no tendency toward neoplasia. The condition is most frequently encountered by meat inspectors, the animals being in normal health.

Albinism represents a pathological absence of melanin. It is thought to result from an inability of the melanocyte to synthesize sufficient functionally active tyrosinase. Melanocytes are present in albinism and are structurally identical to normal melanocytes. Inability to form melanin occurs with the development of *achromotrichia* in copper deficiency in several animal species. As indicated, copper is an essential component of tyrosinase. Focal depigmentation may occur in scars and radiation burns.

Microscopic Appearance.—Melanin takes the form of minute, rounded granules of light or dark brown color, located in the cytoplasm of cells. Ultrastructurally the pigment takes the form of extremely dense, ellipsoidal granules 0.3 by 0.7 microns. In the skin, it is seen to lie in the cytoplasm of the basal and adjoining cells of the epidermis.

It has been shown by certain investigators, using the "dopa reaction" and other special techniques, that the melanin is originally produced in special cells just beneath the epithelium (or within it), which have long dendritic processes interspersed among the epithelial cells. These special cells are **melanoblasts** (or melanocytes). It is postulated that the pigment is transferred from them to the epithelial cells. While in some other locations, to be mentioned shortly, the

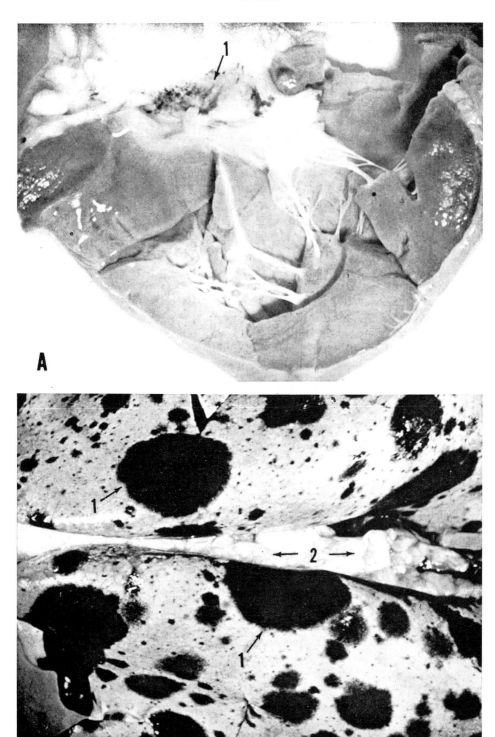

FIG. 3-6.—A, Melanosis, aorta, sheep. Melanin pigment (1) is seen from the intimal surface. B, Melanosis, lung, sheep. Large deposits of melanin (1), mediastinum (2). Photograph courtesy of Dr. C. L. Davis.

presence of melanin may be attributable solely to dendritic cells of more or less similar morphology, it does not appear that all melanin formation can be accredited to cells of this type (for instance in the substantia nigra), and it is difficult to reconcile this view with what one sees in day-to-day observations of skin sections. It is clear, however, that melanin does escape from its intracellular position, is seen extracellularly, is excreted in the urine in cases of great overproduction (malignant melanomas) and is very frequently phagocytized by ordinary reticulo-endothelial macrophages. When laden with melanin these phagocytes receive the special name of **"melanophore"** (or "melanophage"). The melanophores are often seen in the dermis beneath pigmented epithelium and not infrequently migrate in considerable numbers to the regional lymph nodes, where they are recognized as large round cells filled with pigment which is in finer granules than would be the case with hemosiderin, with which it can be confused. The melanophore is not a producer of melanin, as can be shown by the "dopa reaction."

The word "dopa" was coined from the key letters of "dioxyphenylalanine" an older equivalent of dihydroxyphenylalanine which received attention earlier in this section. If a section of fresh tissue is incubated with a suitable solution of this substance, the position of melanin producing cells is indicated by a black granular precipitate. This is pigment which has been formed by the action of the melanin-producing cells upon the dihydroxyphenylalanine. Such cells have the same action on (mono) hydroxyphenylalanine, which is tyrosine, as previously stated. The reaction is considered to be due to an enzyme, called dopa-oxydase (tyrosinase), existing in melanin-forming cells. The dopa reaction, then, is not a test for melanin but for the power of producing melanin. Since it has to be performed upon frozen sections of unfixed, or slightly fixed tissue, precise localization of the enzyme is not easy but, in general, dopaoxydase occurs where melanin occurs except in the case of phagocytized and transported melanin. One may test for the actual melanin granules by Fontana's silver solution, which turns such granules black.

Returning to the question of the exact location of melanin, we may say that in the skin it appears to be produced in specialized dendritic cells called melanoblasts, but that the bulk of it is clearly located in the basal and adjoining layers of the epidermis. In the hairs, the melanin is in their cortical substance, having been derived from the epithelium of the hair follicle. In the eye, there is a layer of "pigment epithelium" at the junction of the retina and choroid and also on the posterior surface of the iris, but there are also dendritic cells comparable to the melanoblasts of the skin scattered through the connective tissue of the choroid and of the iris. In the pia-arachnoid, the pigment is in cells of the dendritic type. These are considered to be of connective-tissue origin, whereas the cutaneous melanoblasts are claimed to be derived from the neural crest, which adds to the perplexity. In the human substantia nigra and certain other small areas of the brain, the pigment is in the cytoplasm of nerve cells and there is no hint as to how it was formed. Melanosis may well be concerned only with melanophores, at least in animals. This seems not to have been determined. In man, there is a "melanosis coli" which may possibly be the result of an abnormal metabolism of tyrosine *in situ*.

The **gross appearance** and **causes** have been implied in the previous discussion.

The color of the skin or hair as seen grossly appears to depend on the concentration of the melanin granules and possibly upon slight differences in molecular structure.

Significance.—The melanin itself is not harmful, although the melanomas, in which it is so conspicuously seen, are major threats to life. Melanosis is not harmful. In the skin, the amount of pigment increases with increased exposure to sunlight (or artificial ultraviolet rays) and it is considered to be of prime importance in protecting the tissues from sunburn. (See also: Photosensitization, p. 77).

HEMATOGENOUS PIGMENTS—HEMOGLOBIN

Hemoglobin, the normal pigment of erythrocytes, is in solution or in a colloidal state within those cells. Hemoglobin consists of a pigment, heme, plus the protein, globin. Heme is divisible into ferrous iron and a porphyrin (protoporphyrin III). The various porphyrins consist principally of four pyrrol rings with various hydrocarbon radicals attached to them. Porphyrins will be discussed shortly. The empirical formula of hemoglobin has been estimated to be approximately $C_{112}H_{1130}N_{214}S_2FeO_{245}$. It is noteworthy, however, that hemoglobin does not respond to the ordinary tests for iron compounds.

Hemoglobin imparts grossly to individual erythrocytes a straw-yellow color, which deepens into crimson red when a thick layer of erythrocytes is viewed in the fresh state. Hemoglobin is ordinarily not seen microscopically, however its presence is responsible for the eosinophilia of erythrocytes. Hemoglobin can be more specifically demonstrated by several histochemical techniques.

The gross tinctorial properties and chemistry of hemoglobin may be slightly altered under certain conditions, such as in some poisonings and due to postmortem changes. In normal hemoglobin the iron is in the ferrous state and is either loosely oxygenated (it is not oxidized) and referred to as **oxyhemoglobin** or has given up its oxygen store and referred to as **reduced hemoglobin.** The bright red of arterial blood is due to the presence of oxyhemoglobin; the dark red of venous blood is caused by reduced hemoglobin.

Methemoglobin is a true oxide of hemoglobin (ferric iron) and is dark red (often called chocolate brown) in contrast to bright red oxyhemoglobin. It is produced by poisonings with nitrites, chlorates, sulphates, and some organic compounds. **Sulfhemoglobin** is a combination of reduced hemoglobin and inorganic sulfide and is a dark brown. It results from the action of nitrites and coal tar preparations (aniline, acetophenetidin, acetanilid) in the presence of excessive amount of sulfur. A **sulfur methemoglobin** can form after death and cause a greenish discoloration to abdominal structures. **Carboxyhemoglobin,** which is a bright cherry-red, is the result of a combination of carbon monoxide with hemoglobin.

When erythrocytes undergo hemolysis, whether it be in the vessels after death, in an external or internal hemorrhage or in a flask of blood withdrawn for some laboratory purpose, the anoxic hemoglobin slowly escapes and carries its dark red color to the surrounding fluids and tissues. Such discolored perivascular tissues after death represent "post-mortem imbibition," which has been discussed (p. 16). As stated above, the color of hemoglobin is not seen microscopically.

HEMATINS

Hematins, or more properly *acid hematins*, are pigments which are formed by the action of acids on hemoglobin. They are not normal breakdown products. The most familiar of the acid hematins is **acid formalin hematin** (formal-precipitated hemoglobin, acid formaldehyde hematin) which is formed when acid aqueous solutions of formaldehyde act on blood rich tissues. It occurs in tissue sections as a dark brown, finely granular, anisotropic pigment that does not stain with iron stains. It may be seen both in vascular spaces and within (or on top of) various cellular elements. Acid formalin hematin is of no pathologic significance, but its presence can be extremely annoying in that it must be differentiated from other pigments. It can be removed from tissue sections with saturated alcoholic picric acid. The use of neutral (pH 7.0) buffered formalin prevents its occurrence. A similar pigment may develop in extremely alkaline (above pH 8.0) formalin solutions. Other acid hematins which closely resemble acid formalin hematin can form from the action of acetic acid and hydrochloric acid. A **hydrochloric acid hematin** is often seen within and adjacent to gastric ulcers. It apparently forms from the action of gastric acid with hemoglobin.

Several parasitic diseases are associated with the deposition of hematin pigments in tissues. In **malaria**, hematins are present in parasitized erythrocytes and in the cytoplasm of reticulo-endothelial cells in the spleen, lymph nodes, liver and bone marrow. In each site the pigment is yellow to dark brown and iron negative. In erythrocytes the pigment is anisotropic whereas in reticulo-endothelial cells it is isotropic. The pigment is formed by the malarial parasites from the host's hemoglobin. Several species of trematodes produce pigments which are believed to be hematins. *Fascioloides magna* (p. 796) in the ruminant liver deposits a grossly visible pigment which accumulates adjacent to the parasite

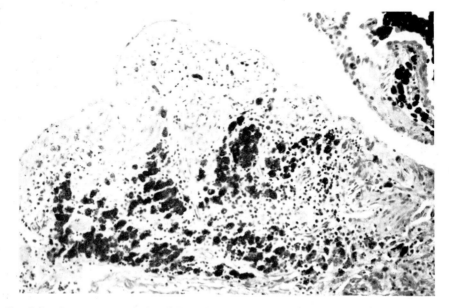

Fig. 3–7.—*Pneumonyssus simicola* infestation of the lung of a rhesus monkey (*Macaca mulatta*). Parasitic hematin pigments within macrophages adjacent to a bronchiole. (Courtesy of New England Regional Primate Research Center, Harvard Medical School.)

within macrophages. Various species of *schistosomes* (p. 802) produce anisotropic, iron negative hematins which accumulate in macrophages of the liver, spleen, bone marrow and lymph nodes.

Pneumonyssus simicola (p. 814) is associated with 2 pigments. One occurs as light brown to colorless, needle-like brightly anisotropic crystals and the other as finely granular brown to black granules which are variably anisotropic. Both pigments are believed to be derived from hemoglobin metabolized by the mite. In contrast to hematins, most of the pigment stains with the usual iron stains although isolated crystals and granules may be negative.

HEMOSIDERIN

Hemosiderin is a shiny, golden yellow or golden brown pigment derived from hemoglobin It is usually seen within macrophages and does respond to the ordinary tests for iron; chemically it is the same as ferritin.

It occurs principally in the red pulp of the spleen and in other places where there has been extensive disintegration of erythrocytes. Such places include the sites of old hemorrhages into the tissues, receding ovarian corpora hemorrhagica and chronically congested lungs. Rarely large amounts are seen within the epithelial cells of the liver, spleen and kidneys, but these cases will be discussed separately under the heading "Hemochromatosis."

Microscopic Appearance.—Hemosiderin commonly takes the form of glittering, golden-colored spherules 2 or 3 microns in diameter packed into oval or rounded phagocytes. These monocyte-like cells are commonly so full of pigment that the nucleus cannot be seen, but it is easy to surmise that the yellow, granular body is a cell because of its size, shape and rounded outline. At times the color tends more toward brown, and the arrangement in spherical granules is less evident. The presence of hemosiderin in the tissues is readily determined by an ordinary chemical test for its component iron the **Prussian-blue reaction.** The application of a solution of potassium ferrocyanide to the microscopic section following treatment with an acid turns hemosiderin a strong greenish blue, the potassium having been replaced by Fe to give ferric ferrocyanide, which, incidentally, is the common pigment of blue paints called "Prussian blue." The same test can also be applied to fresh tissue, the whole area taking a diffuse bluish tinge if large amounts of hemosiderin are present.

Gross Appearance.—Small amounts of hemosiderin are not detected grossly, but large accumulations impart a brownish color to the organ or tissue in which they occur.

Causes and Special Considerations –The cause of the formation of hemosiderin is the destruction, or hemolysis, of erythrocytes to an excessive degree. This happens: (1) locally when there has been a hemorrhage into the tissues; the impounded erythrocytes die because they have no way to replenish their supply of oxygen.

(2) Hemosiderin accumulates in phagocytic cells of the spleen as the result of excessive hemolysis within the circulating blood, as in hemolytic anemia (p. 126). It may also be deposited in the liver in both Kupffer cells and hepatocytes and in the tubular lining cells and interstitium of the kidney.

(3) Hemosiderin gathers in the spleen, lungs and even other organs as the

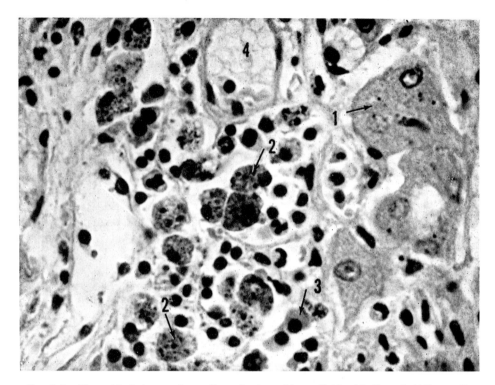

Fig. 3–8.—Hemosiderin in portal area, liver of a dog. Liver cell (*1*) with distended bile canaliculus, macrophages (*2*) with engulfed granules of brown staining hemosiderin, plasma cells (*3*); and branch of portal vein (*4*). (Courtesy of Armed Forces Institute of Pathology.) × 650. Contributor: Dr. D. J. Carren.

result of chronic passive congestion. Chronic congestion of the spleen is most likely to result from cirrhosis, along with congestion of the whole portal circulation.

Chronic passive congestion of the lungs is ordinarily due to disease of the heart, valvular insufficiency or stenosis of the left side. Hence when hemosiderin accumulates here the macrophages of the lung, brilliant with their golden pigment and often lying conspicuously free in the alveolar lumens, are given the nickname of "**heart-failure cells.**" Grossly a brownish tinge is imparted to the lung tissue when the accumulation of hemosiderin is large. As a reaction to the constant pressure of the blood in the distended capillaries, there is a diffuse increase of connective tissue throughout the alveolar walls. This tends to make the whole lung leathery and somewhat hard, or, as we say, indurated. On the basis of these two changes, it is common to refer to the condition as a whole as **brown induration** of the lungs.

The **significance of hemosiderosis** (the deposition of hemosiderin in the tissue) is merely that some one of the above causes has been acting. The pigment in itself is not harmful, nor is it indestructible. The chemistry of its removal is not known, but it apparently can be removed in a period of a few days. In spite of the possibility that chronic passive congestion may be responsible for its presence in the spleen, large amounts almost always mean hemolytic anemia. Such a spleen often also contains numerous **giant-cells** of foreign-body type. Hemosiderosis is related to, but, we believe, separable from hemochromatosis.

HEMOCHROMATOSIS

Under this name, a rare condition is recognized in human beings in which a pigment indistinguishable from hemosiderin is deposited in tremendous amounts in the cytoplasm of the epithelial cells of the liver and pancreas, as well as in kidneys, spleen and various other organs in lesser amounts. It is accompanied by cirrhosis, apparently resultant from irritation by the pigment; by diabetes, probably causally related to the deposited pigment although the islets are not destroyed, and by melanin pigmentation of the skin. On the basis of this triad of lesions, the name of **"bronzed diabetes"** has been in common use clinically. The cause is thought to be an inborn metabolic defect. In view of the fact that the body appears normally to limit its absorption of iron to its very scanty needs and to eliminate the element very slowly or not at all, recent evidence suggests that the trouble may be in excessive absorption of that substance. It is agreed that this iron-containing pigment does not come from hemolysis; hence, it is not related to hemosiderosis. For this reason the name of "cytosiderosis" has been suggested.

In animals the above syndrome has not been reported but there are instances where heavy deposition of what appears to be the same pigment is found in liver and kidney. This is said to occur in equine infectious anemia, without the spleen being similarly involved. It also occurs in anemias due to deficiency of those accessory hemoglobin-forming elements, copper and cobalt (pp. 1011, 1013). It would appear that in those forms of anemia in which the hematopoietic tissue is active but unable to metabolize iron, the latter element accumulates in the tissues and is phagocytized in a form indistinguishable from hemosiderin. In all probability increased amounts of iron are absorbed.

Apparently due to a deficiency of cobalt, Zahawi (1957) has reported a condition in goats grazing the mountains of northern Iraq (inaccessible to other animals) in which 3.6 per cent of 700 goats had brown or blackish kidneys due to heavy deposition of a hemosiderin-like pigment in the epithelium of the proximal convoluted tubules, sometimes with evidence of mild injury to the cells. Lesser amounts of this pigment were found in the Kupffer (rarely the epithelial) cells of the liver and in reticulo-endothelial cells of the spleen and lymph nodes. The testes suffered necrosis of much seminiferous epithelium and gave a Prussian-blue reaction. Other organs were normal. The goats were not clinically ill. The soil here contains as much as 4 per cent copper and 30 per cent iron, but is deficient in cobalt.

BILE PIGMENTS

Since there is a normal destruction each day of a very appreciable number of erythrocytes, a certain amount of hemoglobin is continually being metabolized. The iron and globin are reused by the body, and the porphyrin is changed to a soluble pigment, **bilirubin** by reticulo-endothelial cells in the bone marrow, spleen and elsewhere. In the normal course of events, the bilirubin circulates in the blood until it reaches the liver, where it is excreted in the bile, being responsible for the color of the excreted product. It accumulates pathologically whenever and wherever the disintegration of erythrocytes becomes excessive. Its further history will be related shortly in connection with icterus.

While bilirubin is a soluble substance ordinarily, there is occasionally encountered a brownish pigment, especially at the site of old hemorrhages, which has long been called **hematoidin.** This is now believed to be the same as bilirubin, although it appears as a precipitate, presumably because the solution becomes locally or temporarily supersaturated. Neither bilirubin nor hematoidin are positive to the usual tests for iron. This and the fact that it remains as angular, brown crystals and is seldom phagocytized are the principal features which distingush hematoidin from hemosiderin, for both are formed under the same conditions and have the same significance.

Biliverdin is an intermediary product in the formation of bilirubin; it is of similar chemical structure but it is green rather than yellow. Biliverdin is not ordinarily seen in tissue section but it is responsible in part for the blue-green discoloration of bruises.

In addition to their common presence at sites of hemorrhage, bile pigments are often seen in tissue sections under other circumstances. They may normally be observed in the bile ducts and gallbladder as bright orange yellow amorphous masses. In obstructive jaundice (to be considered shortly) bile pigments may be observed within bile canaliculi, Kupffer cells, hepatocytes, and occasionally in the epithelial cells of proximal convoluted tubules and portions of the loops of Henle in the kidney.

ICTERUS (JAUNDICE)

The formation of bilirubin from the hemoglobin released from destroyed erythrocytes and its normal course to the liver, have been briefly referred to earlier, however prior to considering icterus it is well to examine these events more closely. In the breakdown of hemoglobin in the reticulo-endothelial system, the cyclic structure of the iron-porphyrin compound (heme) is opened and the iron removed and reutilized by the body, as is the globin. The open chained porphyrin is converted to a green pigment called **biliverdin.** Biliverdin is then reduced to **bilirubin,** an orange-yellow pigment. Bound to albumin, bilirubin is then transported from the reticulo-endothelial cell via the blood stream to the liver. In the hepatocyte the pigment is separated from albumin and conjugated with glucuronic acid and excreted in the bile as **bilirubin-diglucuronide.** The conjugated bilirubin in the intestine is reduced by bacteria to **urobilinogen** (mesobilirubinogen and stercobilinogen). Some urobilinogen is reabsorbed into the portal circulation and carried to the liver (enterohepatic circulation) where most of it is converted to a bilirubin-like compound and re-excreted into the bile. A small amount of the absorbed urobilinogen enters the general circulation and is excreted in the urine. The urobilinogen which is not reabsorbed from the intestine, is oxidized in the lower intestine to **urobilin** and **stercobilin** which are normal pigments of feces.

Three pigments in this scheme are of primary importance to the diagnosis of icterus. These are: (1) Bilirubin-diglucuronide which is also called **conjugated bilirubin,** or **direct reacting bilirubin** (direct reaction to the Van den Bergh test) and cholebilirubin; (2) **Non-conjugated bilirubin** which is also called **indirect reacting bilirubin** (indirect reaction to the Van den Bergh test), bilirubin and hemobilirubin; and (3) Urobilinogen.

Icterus is an important clinical and post-mortem disorder in which bilirubin reaches such a high concentration in the circulating blood that the tissues of the whole body are tinged with yellow. Since yellow is a weaker color than red, one must look for it where the tissues normally are white or very pale, such as the sclera of the eye, the omentum and mesentery. In considering the color of adipose tissue as a basis for diagnosis, one must keep in mind the natural color of fat in the particular species and breed. The fat of horses, Jersey and Guernsey cattle, and of certain non-human primates, is normally yellow. Mucous membranes and other tissues normally reddish may still display a yellowish tinge if the icterus is severe. Since the bilirubin is in solution and is not sufficiently concentrated to form a visible precipitate upon dehydration, icterus is seen only *grossly*. However, when the amount of bile pigment (bilirubin) in the circulating blood is large, it is sometimes revealed in microscopic sections of the kidney by a brownish precipitate or bile-stained albumin in the lumens of the tubules and by a brownish tinge in the ordinarily pink-staining (hematoxylin and eosin) cytoplasm of the epithelial lining cells. If the icterus is of the obstructive type, microscopic sections of the liver may also reveal its presence by accumulations of bile pigment in the bile canaliculi and ducts.

Causes.—Depending on the causative mechanism, icterus, or jaundice, is divided into three types, hemolytic icterus, toxic icterus and obstructive icterus.

Hemolytic jaundice is the result of excessive hemolysis of erythrocytes, ordinarily in the circulating blood. The more important diseased conditions in which this type of icterus is pronounced are (1) piroplasmosis, (2) anaplasmosis, (3) leptospirosis (partially hemolytic), and (4) equine infectious anemia. A similar destruction of erythrocytes occurs in infections by (5) hemolytic streptococci, (6) *Clostridium hemolyticum bovis* and (7) *Bacillus anthracis*, but in these cases other aspects of the disease usually overshadow the jaundice. These bacterial infections may, indeed, progress so rapidly that the patient does not survive the two or three days usually necessary for the development of icterus. (8) Ricin, (9) saponin and possibly other plant poisons, (10) potassium or sodium chlorate, (11) pyrogallic acid, (12) nitrobenzene and (13) lead (if chronic) are hemolytic poisons which may or may not produce visible icterus. (14) Most snake venoms owe much of their lethal potency to their hemolytic action, so that icterus is frequent after the lapse of a few days. (15) Massive internal, usually intraperitoneal, hemorrhages result in icterus because of absorption of bilirubin from the disintegrating erythrocytes of the escaped blood. (16) Icterus neonatorum is a form of hemolytic jaundice. It is discussed in connection with hemolytic anemia (p. 126).

Toxic jaundice is caused by toxic substances acting upon the cells of the liver and producing hydropic degeneration, fatty change and necrosis. There are two ways in which jaundice can result from these destructive changes in the liver. First, the hepatic cells may be damaged to such an extent that they cannot perform their excretory function. Hemobilirubin (unconjugated bilirubin) then remains in the blood just as in hemolytic jaundice.

Secondly, the swelling of the hepatic cells may be sufficient to block the bile canaliculi. The bile is excreted from the cells but cannot pursue its course to the gallbladder and intestine. In this case it is bilirubin-diglucuronide, or posthepatic bilirubin, which accumulates in the liver, whence it is reabsorbed into the blood. As a rule both these processes go on simultaneously, so that both kinds of bilirubin accumulate in the blood.

The causes of this hepatic damage are, in general, the things which cause acute toxic hepatitis (p. 1223). They include the hepatic toxins developed in the course of certain infections and a number of extraneous poisons. Outstanding in veterinary medicine are poisonings by lupines and vetches, by plants of the genus *Senecio* ("ragwort," "groundsel"), the genus *Amsinckia* ("tarweed") and others. Several inorganic poisons, as listed under Acute Toxic Hepatitis, are capable of causing more or less jaundice, but chronic copper poisoning is the one most often reported as actually being accompanied by icterus. Numerous infectious diseases are accompanied by severe hepatic injury, but leptospirosis (p. 560) is outstanding in producing toxic (as well as hemolytic) icterus.

Obstructive jaundice results from obstruction to the normal flow of bile. Retained anywhere in the biliary passageways, much of the bile is reabsorbed into the blood. (Some of it becomes dehydrated and is precipitated in the tissue as bile pigment.) The obstruction may be caused by (1) blocking of the bile canaliculi by swollen hepatic cells, (2) obstruction of the ducts, either inside or outside the liver by flukes, fimbriated tapeworms (*Thysanosoma actinioides*) or ascarids, (3) pressure on the intrahepatic ducts by the contracting fibrous tissue of biliary cirrhosis, (4) cholangitis with swelling of the walls of the ducts, (5) gall stones, (6) pressure on any part of the ductal system by neoplasms, granulomas or abscesses, or (7) in duodenitis by pressure of inflammatory swelling on the slanting orifice of the bile duct as it enters the duodenum at the papilla duodeni. The very acute angle at which this duct passes through the duodenal wall subjects it to easy closure by the compression of inflammatory swelling.

Diagnosis of Icterus. — In mild cases the clinical discoloration may not be unequivocal; therefore laboratory tests are often employed to establish the diagnosis of jaundice with certainty. The **"icterus index"** is determined merely by comparing in a colorimeter the color of the blood serum with the yellow tint of a solution of potassium dichromate of standard strength. The **Van den Bergh reaction** depends on the addition of sulfanilic acid and sodium nitrite to the serum and the change in color is a quantitative indication of the presence of bilirubin-diglucuronide. This is the **direct** Van den Bergh reaction. If alcohol is added to the mixture, hemobilirubin also reacts, constituting the **indirect** Van den Bergh reaction. From this it is seen that hemolytic jaundice gives the indirect reaction and obstructive jaundice gives the direct, a valuable aid in differentiation. Toxic jaundice usually gives both direct and indirect reactions since some of the bilirubin accumulates in the blood before being acted upon by the liver (hemobilirubin) and another part afterwards (cholebilirubin, conjugated bilirubin).

As indicated when the bile reaches the intestinal lumen, bacteria change it by chemical reduction into a substance called urobilinogen. A considerable part of the urobilinogen is reabsorbed into the portal blood to be carried to the liver, which normally returns it to the bile, but when the hepatic cells have suffered the types of injury which go with toxic hepatitis, the urobilinogen is very imperfectly removed from the blood and remains to be excreted by the kidneys. Furthermore, the capacity of the liver to eliminate urobilinogen, as has also been pointed out with respect to bilirubin, is by no means unlimited. One can understand, then, that in hemolytic jaundice large amounts of urobilinogen are found in the feces and in the urine, for the amount of cholebilirubin originally excreted is maximal, contributing much urobilinogen to the feces and the very considerable excess above what the liver can decompose goes into the urine. In toxic jaundice, the amount in the urine is considerable, varying with the relative ability of the liver to excrete bilirubin and to decompose the resorbed urobilinogen. In obstructive jaundice, the amount of urobilinogen in the feces and in the urine is diminished, perhaps to zero. The actual test is usually made upon the urine, but the feces can also be tested.

It is also common practice merely to perform certain simple tests for bilirubin (bile) in the urine, the presence of which is called choluria. Since the kidneys are able to excrete bilirubin-diglucuronide but not hemobilirubin, it is obvious that the urine is acholuric in hemolytic icterus, but contains much bilirubin in obstructive jaundice. Because of its dual causative mechanism, toxic jaundice again falls between the two extremes, but some choluria is usually found.

Summarizing, we find that a high icterus index shows the presence of icterus. A positive direct Van den Bergh reaction indicates obstructive jaundice or, at least, the presence of bilirubin-diglucuronide, which may result from toxic jaundice as well as the obstructive type. A positive indirect Van den Bergh test shows the presence of hemobilirubin, which signifies either hemolytic jaundice or toxic jaundice with inability of the hepatic cells to function. With respect to urobilinogen in the urine, a certain amount is normal; smaller amounts or its absence indicate obstructive jaundice (no bile reaching the intestine); large amounts indicate hemolytic icterus with a normal degree of hepatic secretion or, in the absence of hemolytic disease, toxic jaundice with an impairment of the excretory function of the liver. With respect to the mere presence or absence of urinary bilirubin, obstructive icterus is choluric; hemolytic icterus is acholuric.

A number of other laboratory tests are available for determining the degree of icterus, as well as for general hepatic functions. Of course, if hemoglobinuria accompanies the icterus it is practically safe to make a diagnosis of the hemolytic type.

Significance.—From the foregoing it becomes evident that jaundice is an important clue to any one of several different disorders. To profit by its existence the diagnostician needs to have (1) keen observation for its clinical appearance, (2) access to the applicable laboratory tests and (3) a clear understanding of its pathogenetic mechanisms. The bilirubin itself is ordinarily not a seriously harmful substance, although it may well be directly responsible for some of the subjective symptoms which humans feel, such as itching. It possibly contributes to the development of necrosis in the renal epithelium in the poorly understood "hepatorenal" syndrome. The most noteworthy harmful effect of bilirubin *per se* is seen in human infants with kernicterus. In this disorder, most often associated with erythroblastosis fetalis, the hippocampus, basal nuclei, midbrain, medulla and floor of the fourth ventricle are grossly yellow and there is microscopic evidence of neuronal degeneration. Although kernicterus has not been described as a naturally occurring disease in domestic animals, it has been experimentally induced. If the cause can be overcome, the accumulated bilirubin promptly disappears.

PHOTOSENSITIZING PIGMENTS: PHOTOSENSITIZATION

Historically speaking, the condition known as photosensitization or, perhaps better, as photosensitizational dermatitis, has been recognized in farm animals for some time, especially but by no means exclusively in cattle and sheep. The clinical manifestations, appearing a number of hours after exposure to strong sunlight, include burning or itching sensations, erythema, inflammatory edema, which is often extensive—in other words the "rubor et tumor cum calore et dolore" that were recounted as the signs of inflammation nearly two thousand years ago (p. 145). Often the inflammation is so severe that the skin is killed and the necrotic layer sloughs in a few days. These changes are strictly, and often sharply limited to areas of the body surface that are (1) in a position to receive the direct rays of strong light and (2) are unprotected by (*a*) pigmentation of a dark skin or (*b*) a thick coat of hair (or, of course, a blanket or a saddle). In cows the thinly haired and usually unpigmented teats, udder and escutcheon are included. In sheep the head and ears are the most vulnerable areas and the edema is likely to be the most prominent inflammatory change, leading to the colloquial term "bighead," or geeldikkop, which is a South African term meaning thick, yellow head. In New Zealand an equivalent term is **facial eczema**. The ears in these sheep are so swollen that they bend downward; the face is deformed and the mandibular area is so distended and bulging with edematous fluid as to require differentiation from the noninflammatory "bottle-jaw" that is traditional in gastrointestinal helminthiasis (p. 741). The cutaneous lesions usually heal after days or weeks, depending on the degree of severity, but shock and generally disturbed body functions had often been discernible at the beginning, and death is an occasional termination due to infection and gangrenous change in the raw, ulcerated areas where the skin was lost.

This lesion of photosensitization has nothing to do with sunburn, which is less severe. Photosensitization of the tissues is the result of the action of light upon some fluorescent pigment which has accumulated in them. A fluorescent pigment is one that accepts the incoming rays of light and transforms them into light of a

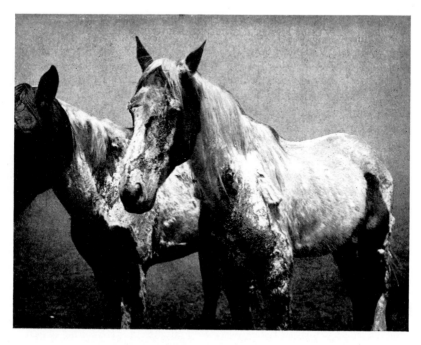

FIG. 3–9.—Photosensitization of skin of horses. Note that the lesions are in the white skin and not in the black areas of these spotted horses. From Bulletin 412 A Colorado State University, Poisonous and Injurious Plants in Colorado, 1950, by L. W. Durrell, Rue Jensen and Bruno Klinger. Photograph courtesy of Dr. Rue Jensen.

longer wavelength (the process of fluorescence). Often the resulting color is red, since this is the color of the longest wavelength; doubtless some of the resulting energy is in the infrared portion of the spectrum. Experimentally, fluorescein, a dye noted for its fluorescent properties, can be injected into the blood and produce a certain photosensitization of the skin. In nature the fluorescent, sensitizing pigments appear under three different and unrelated sets of circumstances, but the pigments, as far as they have been studied chemically, are relatives of hemoglobin and of chlorophyll, being porphyrins or the related phyllocrythrin, a degradation product of chlorophyll. Both chlorophyll and hemoglobin molecules have as their basic components four pyrrole radicals, tied together by methene groups (the basic structure of porphyrin). It is of philosophical interest that these, the principal pigments of the plant and animal kingdoms, are so nearly identical.

The three sets of circumstances which give rise to the presence of photosensitizing pigments in the tissues are (1) **Congenital Porphyria** in which there is a metabolic defect in porphyrin metabolism; (2) **Hepatotoxic photosensitization** in which there is interference with the excretion of phyloerythrin; and (3) **Primary photosensitization** in which preformed photosensitizing pigments are ingested, absorbed and enter the general circulation. In none of these conditions is the pigment seen in usual microscopic preparations. In porphyria the pigment is grossly visible as discussed below. In certain rodents (mice, rats, hamsters) the Harderian gland, an intraorbital lacrimal gland, normally secretes porphyrin which accounts for the red or brown tears seen in these animals. The pigment can be seen in the Harderian gland microscopically as variably sized yellow to reddish granules.

Congenital Porphyria.—Congenital porphyria has been described in cattle, swine, and cats as a metabolic defect in the synthesis of the normal heme pigment ferroprotoporphyrin. This error results in the release of free protoporphyrin, uroporphyrin III and coproporphyrin III which accumulate in serum and tissues. Uroporphyrin III and coproporphyrin III are normally formed in small amounts from precursors of protoporphyrin, but in congenital porphyria the formation of these two pigments greatly exceeds the normal. In cattle the disease is believed to be inherited as a simple Mendelian recessive, whereas in swine and cats it is believed to be inherited as a dominant characteristic (p. 315).

In cattle the accumulation of porphyrins results in the above-described photosensitizational dermatitis when exposed to strong sunlight. Interestingly, photosensitizational dermatitis has not been reported in swine, even when white, or cats with congenital porphyria. The accumulation of porphyrins in dentine and bone, gives rise to a red color which has often gone by the misnomer, "osteohemochromatosis" or by the colorful term "pink tooth." Affected bones and teeth elicit a strong reddish fluorescence with ultraviolet light, a useful aid to clinical and post-mortem diagnosis. Because of increased excretion of porphyrin (porphyrinuria) in the urine, it is reddish brown, or at least tends to develop this color upon standing for a varying period from ten minutes to twenty-four hours. This change must be differentiated from hemoglobinuria and myoglobinuria (p. 1176) and possibly from alkaptonuria (reported in man and one chimpanzee) (p. 321). Fluorescence with ultraviolet light is one distinguishing feature. Discoloration of soft tissues due to the accumulation of porphyrin is less obvious but may be encountered in the lungs or kidneys which also fluoresce. Fluoresence can also be demonstrated in unstained tissue sections as well as in blood smears in which the erythrocytes fluoresce ("fluorocytes").

Except for its photosensitizing effect, this disorder is clinically harmless, as shown by Fourie (1953), who described an ox, imported to South Africa from Switzerland, which reached the ripe old age of eighteen years while excreting 1.6 grams of porphyrin daily, and remaining in good health as long as he was stabled during the day. Exposed to sunlight, he promptly developed the usual lesions of photosensitization. At necropsy the animal's teeth and bones were brown and there was pigment in various internal organs.

Anemia has been reported in cattle and cats with porphyria, apparently resulting from inability to produce normal amounts of hemoglobin and a shortened life span of the erythrocyte.

Other forms of porphyria with varying clinical manifestations occur in humans. The interested student is referred to the chapter by Schmid (1966).

Hepatotoxic Photosensitization.—The great majority of photosensitizations in animals are not of hemoglobinogenous origin but are due to a derivative of the plant kingdom's counterpart of hemoglobin, namely chlorophyll. Furthermore, they are dependent upon toxic injury to the liver. When the chlorophyll of plants passes through the digestive process one of the products is the pigment phylloerythrin. It differs from phylloporphyrin in having a ketone group attached to the sixth carbon atom but for practical purposes can be classed with the porphyrins. Normally this phylloerythrin, with its photosensitizing properties, is eliminated through the liver by the simple expedient of excreting it through the bile (where its brownish color joins that of bilirubin, that not-so-different derivative of the animal kingdom's hemoglobin, p. 69). When the liver or its ductal system is injured in a way that interrupts this excretory function the phylloerythrin, with its photosensitizing properties, reaches the skin via the circulating blood and the results are the same as those outlined above from the presence of (hemoglobinogenous) porphyrin.

As to the liver injury, there is usually no specific morphological pattern although the changes described for acute toxic hepatitis (p. 1223) are usually in evidence. Often, but not invariably, icterus (toxic, p. 75) is an easily recognized part of the general illness and occasionally there are nervous disturbances and other signs of hepatic malfunction (p. 1241). In two forms of hepatotoxic photosensitization, more specific hepatic lesions are seen. In "facial eczema" of sheep and alfalfa associated photosensitization there is a pericholongitis which leads to occlusion of small bile ducts.

The causes of photosensitizing hepatitis are, in general, among those listed for acute toxic hepatitis but it must be emphasized that only a small minority of toxic hepatic illnesses are accompanied by photosensitization. There may be several reasons for this but the outstanding one is that the animal must be on a diet containing liberal amounts of chlorophyll (usually green pasture). Clare (1952) in his admirable monograph on photosensitization, listed the following disorders as being accompanied by photosensitization and by hepatic dysfunction and icterus: (1) Geeldikkop, also known as "thick yellow head," "thick ear," Geelsiekte, etc., caused by *Tribulus terrestris*, plants grown for forage in parts of South Africa; (2) facial eczema of sheep in New Zealand, which is caused by a mycotoxin from the fungus *Pithomyces chartarum* growing on perennial ryegrass and other pastures; (3) poisoning by *Lippia rehmanni*, a South African plant; (4) poisoning by *Lantana camara*, a verbena-like plant which occurs in the United States as well as in South Africa and Ceylon; (5) poisoning by sacahuiste (*Nolina texana*), found in western Texas; (6) poisoning by lechuguilla (*Agave lechugilla*), also a native of western Texas and nearby arid areas; (7) poisoning by second growth from stumps of the Brazilian tree called alecrim (*Holocalyx glaziovii*); (8) poisoning by panick grasses (*Panicum miliaceum et sp.*) in Australia and South Africa; (9) poisoning by leaves of the ngaio tree of New Zealand (*Myosporum laetum*), which affects horses as well as ruminants; (10) poisoning by the Australian grass *Brachiaria brizantha*; (11) poisoning by the American morenita (*Kochia scoparia*); (12) "bighead" from *Tetradymia glabrata*, known as "coal-oil brush" in Utah and as "spring rabbit brush" in Nevada, and *Tetradymia canescens*, the "spineless horse-brush" of Utah. Also included are (13) poisoning by *Microcystis flos-aquae*, a blue-green alga which grows as a scum on lakes; (14) the Norwegian disease of lambs called "alveld," the cause of which is the plant *Northecium ossifragum*; (15) "yellowses," a disease of lambs in Scotland, of uncertain cause; and (16) "black fever," attributed to *Kochia scoparia*. Other plants include the seeds of *Stryphnodendron obovatum*, *Erodium circutorium* and Bermuda grass.

Several of the above plants are discussed as to their general toxic aspects in our Chapter 17 (p. 843). Some other plants, valuable as pasture or cured forage, have also been incriminated or suspected in outbreaks of photosensitizational dermatitis, among them some of the trefoils and bur clovers (*Medicago sp.*), Alsike or Swedish clover (*Trifolium hybridum*), as well as some plants of the cabbage family (rape, *Brassica rapa*, and kale, *Medicago denticulata*) not to mention the common perennial rye grass, which forms so many of our winter pastures. Outbreaks of photosensitization were observed to occur at highly variable periods, often seasonal, and various explanations were offered. Within very recent years investigators in New Zealand have discovered that under certain conditions of growth, temperature and humidity, fields producing these forages became heavily infested with a fungus known either as *Sporodesmium bakeri* or *Pithomyces chartarum*. The fungal growth, when first noticed, was so heavy that mowing machines were blackened by its dark spores. It was demonstrated in these cases that a mycotoxin was really the toxic substance responsible for the photosensitization, rather than the plants themselves. A similar mechanism has been suggested for a photosensitizational dermatitis associated with Bermuda grass in the Southern United States and also for a hepatogenous photosensitivity caused by feeding flood damaged alfalfa. Further investigation is needed to determine to what extent an analogous situation may prevail with other plants.

In addition to these causes there have occurred cases of photosensitization accompanied by toxic hepatic injury and icterus in cattle treated with phenanthridinium, a trypanocidal drug. Carbon tetrachloride poisoning, hepatic fascioliasis (liver flukes) and Rift valley fever can also lead to hepatotoxic photosensitization.

A hereditary defect in the hepatic phyloerythrin excretory mechanisms, which leads to photosensitivity, occurs in Southdown sheep. The disease, which is also associated with hyperbilirubinemia, has been described in New Zealand and the United States. No morphologic lesion is present in the liver. A syndrome has been described in Corriedale sheep similar to the Dubin-Johnson Syndrome in man (p. 85) which is also associated with a failure to excrete phyloerythrin and photosensitivity.

If further evidence is needed of the role of hepatic dysfunction in the production of photosensitization, it is furnished by the experimental work of Quin (1933) in which he produced photosensitization by ligation of the bile duct (obstructive jaundice) provided that fresh green plants were fed.

Primary Photosensitization. — There are several photosensitizational diseases in which neither hepatic injury, icterus nor any form of porphyrinemia has been demonstrated. Two of these have long been known and have received considerable study, namely **fagopyrism,** poisoning by buckwheat (*Fagopyrum esculentum*), and **hypericism,** which is poisoning by *Hypericum perforatum* or closely related species. Common names for the *Hypericum* species include St. John's wort, goatweed, Tipton weed, amber, cammock and Klamath weed. In both fagopyrism and hypericism, a red fluorescent pigment has been obtained from the plant itself and demonstrated in the blood. It would appear that this pigment sensitizes the skin in the same way that phylloerythrin and certain other porphyrins do. The effective wave-lengths of light in this process are near the middle of the visible spectrum, different from that which produces the hepatogenous type of photosensitization just discussed.

The commonly employed anthelmintic **Phenothiazine** is also a cause of primary photosensitizational dermatitis. This drug is oxidized in the intestinal tract to phenothiazine sulfoxide, a photosensitive pigment which is usually metabolized by the liver. However, if it escapes the liver and enters the general circulation, dermatitis will develop upon exposure to sunlight. A damaged liver or the liver of young animals is less efficient in eliminating the sulfoxide. In addition to dermatitis, keratitis is a usual finding, owing to the excretion of phenothiazine sulfoxide in the tears and its entry into the aqueous humor. Photosensitization by this drug occurs most readily in swine but cattle are also susceptible. Sheep are more resistant, apparently due to a greater efficiency of the sheep liver to reduce phenothiazine sulfoxide to phenothiazine sulfate.

A photosensitization of white chickens and ducks has been reported from Uruguay by Cassamagnaghi (1946) due to the seed of an umbelliferous plant, *Ammi visnaga*. Whether this is to be classed with fagopyrism and hypericism or with the hepatogenous photosensitizations has not been determined.

Summarizing, photosensitization as it is ordinarily encountered in veterinary medicine involves a triad of an hepato-toxic plant, fresh green feed in the diet and exposure to direct sunlight. Exceptions exist (1) in the form of plants which supply a sensitizing pigment of their own, apparently involving no hepatic injury, and (2) in certain rare individual animals which form porphyrins in their daily metabolism, only sunlight being required to produce the characteristic dermatitis.

LIPOGENIC PIGMENTS

Lipogenic pigments constitute a group of colored substances that are derived mainly or partly from lipids. They are not the same as the lipochrome or carotenoid pigments (p. 64). Numerous tissue pigments have been classified as lipogenic pigments and the list of names designated to them is exhaustive, despite the fact that their individuality is not established. Included in the list of pigments and synonyms are: ceroid, ceroid-like pigments, abnutzen pigment, wear and tear pigments, pigment of brown atrophy, lipochrome pigment, chromolipoid, hemofuscin, lipofuscin, cytolipochrome, acid fast pigments, and vitamin E deficiency pigments.

Two pigments from the group are encountered with frequency or are of special pathological significance. These are tissue lipofuscins and ceroid.

Tissue Lipofuscins or Pigment of Brown Atrophy.—Synonyms for these terms include "wear-and-tear pigment," the German "abnutzen pigment," "hemofuscin" and "lipochrome." The multiplicity of synonyms suggests the confusion which exists with respect to this pigment. Lipofuscins are believed to represent a homogeneous group of pigments that are derived from the oxidation of unsaturated tissue lipids or lipoproteins. Tissue lipofuscins occur in a variety of tissues and cell types including the heart, skeletal muscle, liver, adrenal, neurons, thyroid, parathyroid, kidney, ovary and testicle, and are referred to by the organ or tissue containing them, *i.e.* cardiac lipofuscin, hepatic lipofuscin, etc. They are resistant to fat solvents and are sudanophilic (*i.e.* stain with fat stains) even after paraffin embedding procedures. They are usually acid fast but are negative to iron stains.

Lipofuscins may occur in great quantity in organs undergoing cachectic or senile atrophy imparting a brown color to them, constituting the pathological entity known as **brown atrophy.** However, lipofuscin may be seen in tissues from animals which are not cachectic, or aged, necessitating caution in interpreting its significance.

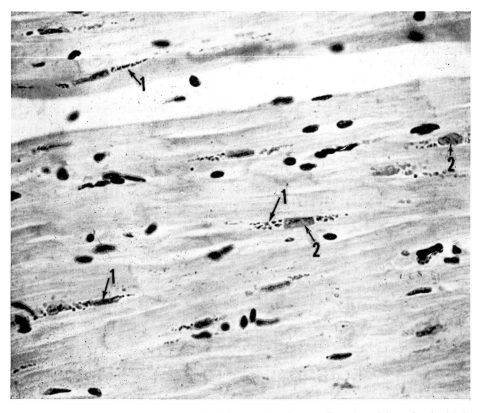

FIG. 3–10.—Pigment of "brown atrophy" in a bovine heart. Granules of hemofuscin (*1*) in cardiac muscle cells at poles of nuclei (*2*). (Courtesy of Armed Forces Institute of Pathology.) × 440. Contributor: Barnes General Hospital.

Microscopically the pigment takes the form of very minute yellowish or darker brown granules. In heart muscle cells it is located chiefly near the poles of the nucleus; in skeletal muscle it is found in any part of the fiber; and in most parenchymatous organs such as the liver or adrenal, it is found distributed throughout the cytoplasm. Ultrastructural studies on lipofuscins are incomplete but in general they appear to consist of irregularly shaped masses composed of varying sized electron-dense bodies embedded in a matrix of lesser density. Each pigment mass is bound by a membrane. **Grossly,** if present in significant quantity, lipofuscin may impart a brownish tinge to cardiac and skeletal muscle. The **significance** of lipofuscin cannot always be established but it often points to some wasting disease, senility or emaciation. The old dairy cows which display the pigment in their skeletal musculature are usually those which go to slaughter when their usefulness as milk-producers is at an end, the condition being found by the veterinary meat inspector. They are always more or less emaciated and the brownish discoloration is one of the grounds for condemning them as cachectic.

A blackish pigment is frequently seen grossly and microscopically in bovine lymph nodes, chiefly but not exclusively in the thoracic, mesenteric and supramammary nodes. Von Wyler (1952) has shown that it is limited to the medulla of the nodes, is minutely granular, intracellular (reticulo-endothelial cells) or extracellular, and has histochemical properties and reactions which appear to place it with the "lipofuscins." While it increases with the age of the animal, being absent in calves, it can hardly be considered pathological since it is very commonly encountered in perfectly healthy cattle at meat inspection.

Apparently limited to certain regions of Australia, there is a diffuse, blackish pigmentation of the livers of sheep which has been called melanosis. Almost 100 per cent of the sheep show the pigment, beginning a few weeks after being brought into the given area. There is a strong suspicion that it results from consumption, perhaps only at certain seasons, of foliage of the Mulga tree (*Acacia aneura*), a widely used forage for sheep in these semi-arid areas, but limited experimentation has not confirmed this. Cattle, which consume the plant less often, develop the pigmentation occasionally. The livers may be slightly darkened or may reach a uniformly distributed dark gray. Microscopic examination shows that the pigment takes the form of minute granules, first in the cytoplasm of the hepatic cells, later in the Kupffer cells, also reaching the portal lymph nodes via macrophages or as free particles. The first particles seen in the cytoplasm of liver cells are yellow; later they become black (oxidation) and look like granules of melanin. Hans Winter (1961, 1963) has shown by extensive histochemical studies that the pigment is not melanin but has the characteristics of a "lipofuscin."

Ceroid.—Ceroid was first described by Lillie (1941) as a pigment which developed in the liver of rats with experimentally-induced cirrhosis. It has since also been produced in the liver of cattle, horses, dogs, pigs, rats, and guinea pigs. Its development is related to choline deficiency, and like other lipofuscins, forms from unsaturated lipids. It occurs principally within macrophages but also within hepatocytes.

An essentially identical pigment occurs in **vitamin E deficiency** in a variety of animal species. This form of ceroid is not restricted to the liver but also occurs within macrophages throughout the body, fat cells, cardiac muscle, smooth muscle

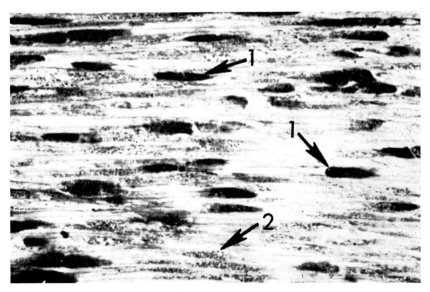

Fig. 3–11.—Vitamin E deficiency pigment (ceroid). Large aggregates (*1*) and fine granules (*2*) of pigment in smooth muscle cells of the small intestine of a dog (PAS stain). (Tissue courtesy Dr. K. C. Hayes.)

of the spleen and intestine (so called "leiomyometaplasts") and ganglion cells. Often the pigment is so abundant that it is visible grossly giving rise to **"yellow fat"** disease or "brown dog gut" (p. 994). **Microscopically** both forms of ceroid are isotropic, granular to homogeneous, and yellow to brown. They are resistant to fat solvents and sudanophilic even after paraffin embedding procedures. They are acid fast and negative to iron stains.

MISCELLANEOUS PIGMENTS

Ochronosis Pigment.—Ochronosis is a feature of a rare hereditary disease of man known as alkaptonuria (urinary excretion of homogentisic acid) in which there is a deficiency of the enzyme homogentisic acid oxidase. Homogentisic acid is a product formed during the metabolism of phenylalanine and tyrosine. The urine in alkaptonuria turns dark upon standing, as the acid is oxidized to a melanin-like product. A pigment is also deposited within tissues, especially in the walls of blood vessels, cartilage, tendons, ligaments and other dense collagenous connective tissues, endocrine glands, kidney and lung. The pigment is believed to be a polymer derived from homogentisic acid and has similarities to melanin. Microscopically it is yellow to brown, isotropic and iron negative. A similar syndrome has been reported in a chimpanzee (p. 321).

Dubin-Johnson Pigment.—The Dubin-Johnson Syndrome, or chronic idiopathic jaundice was first described as a disease in man in 1954. The disorder, which is probably hereditary, is characterized by chronic icterus and an unidentified pigment in the liver cells. The pigment may be a lipofuscin but also shares many properties with melanin. An abnormality in the excretion of conjugated bilirubin is responsible for chronic icterus, but the mechanism of pigment formation is not known. Arias and Cornelius (1964) described a very similar disorder in Corriedale sheep.   In addition to chronic icterus (also due to failure to excrete conjugated bilirubin) and hepatic pigmentation, photosensitivity occurred due to accumulation of phyloerythrin in serum (p. 81).   They suggested that the pigment was melanin and that the disorder appeared to be functionally identical with the Dubin-Johnson syndrome of man.

Cloisonné Kidney.—First described by Al Zahawi (1957), in Cloisonné kidney a dark brown iron negative pigmentation occurs in the basement membranes of proximal convoluted tubules of the kidney, which imparts an appearance, in tissue section, reminiscent of enameled jewelry, Cloisonné.   Al Zahawi described the condition in Angora goats.   It has also been described by Light (1960) in castrated male Angora goats.   Light did not see the condition in female or non-castrated male goats.   The nature and significance of the condition is not known.   The condition is discussed further on p. 1270.

Mineral Deposits, Pigments

ALLISON, A. C., MAGNUS, I. A., and YOUNG, M. R.:   Role of Lysosomes and of Cell Membranes in Photosensitization.   Nature (London) *209*:874–878, 1966.
ARIAS, I., *et al.*:   Black Liver Disease in Corriedale Sheep: A New Mutation Affecting Hepatic Excretory Function.   J. Clin. Invest. *43*:1249–1250, 1964.
BAILEY, J. M., and CARBECK, R. B.:   Porphyria Hepatica with Primary Psychiatric Manifestations.   U.S.A.F. Med. J. *9*:1346–1350, 1958.
BETTY, R. C., and TRIKOJUS, V. M.:   Hypericin and a Non-fluorescent Photosensitive Pigment from St. John's Wort (*Hypericum perforatum*).   Australian J. Exper. Biol. & M. Sc. *21*:175–182, 1943.
BLUM, H. F.:   *Photodynamic Action and Diseases Caused by Light.*   New York, Reinhold Publishing Corporation, 1941.
BROWN, J. M. M.:   Advances in "Geeldikop" (Tribulosis ovis) Research.   J. So. Afr. Vet Med. Assn. *30*:97–111, 1959; *31*:179–193, 1960.
BROWN, J. M. M.:   Biochemical Lesions in the Pathogenesis of Geeldikkop (Tribulosis ovis) and Enzootic Icterus in Sheep in South Africa.   Ann. N. Y. Acad. Sci. *104*:504–538, 1963.
BURGE, W. E., *et al.*:   Mechanism of Pathologic Calcification.   Arch Path. *20*:690–696, 1935.
CAMARGO, W.:   Photosensitization of Cattle by *Stryphnodendron obovatum.*   Biologico *31*:7–11, 1965.
CAMPBELL, W. C.:   Nature and Possible Significance of the Pigment in Fascioloidiasis.   J. Parasitol. *46*:769–775, 1960.
CASSAMAGNAGHI, A.:   Accidentes de Fotosensibilización de orígen alimentico en los animales domésticos.   An. Fac. de vet. Montevideo. *4*:541–549, 1946.
CASSELMAN, W. G. B.:   The *in vitro* Preparation and Histochemical Properties of Substances Resembling Ceroid.   J. Exper. Med. *94*:549–562, 1951.
CLARE, N. T.:   *Photosensitivity in Diseases of Domestic Animals.*   Commonwealth Bureau Animal Health Revue Series *3*, 1952.
————: Photosensitized Keratitis in Young Cattle Following the Use of Phentothiazine as an Anthelmintic. II. The Metabolism of Phentothiazine in Ruminants.   Australian Vet. J. *23*:340–344, 1947.
————: Photosensitization in Animals.   Adv. Vet. Sci. *2*:182–211, 1955.
CLARE, N. T., and STEPHENS, E. H.:   Congenital Porphyria in Pigs.   Nature, London. *153*: 252–253, 1944.
COLLET, P., and HENRY, E.:   Photosensibilisation du dindon par le sarrazin.   Bull. Soc. sci. vét. Lyon. *54* and *55*:437–442, 1952–1953.
CORNELIUS, C. E., and GRONWALL, R. R.:   Congenital Photosensitivity and Hyperbilirubinemia in Southdown Sheep in the United States.   Amer. J. Vet. Res. *29*:291–295, 1968.
CORNELIUS, C. I., ARIAS, I. M., and OSBURN, B. I.:   Hepatic Pigmentation with Photosensitivity: A Syndrome in Corriedale Sheep Resembling Dubin-Johnson Syndrome in Man.   J. Amer. Vet. Med. Assn. *146*:709–713, 1965.
CUNNINGHAM, I. J., and HOPKIRK, C. S. M.:   Experimental Poisoning of Sheep by Ngaio (Myosporum laetum).   N.Z.J. Sci. Tech. Sec. A. *26*:333–339, 1945.
CURTH, H. O., and SLANETZ, C. A.:   Acanthosis Nigricans and Cancer of the Liver in a Dog.   Am. J. Cancer. *37*:216–223, 1939.

DALGAARD-MIKKELSEN, S., KVORNING, S. A., MOMBERG-JORGENSEN, F. H., and SCHAMBYE, P.: Studier over "gult fedt" hos mink. Nord. vet. med. 5:78–97, 1953.

DORMANN, J.: La porphyrine comme pigment de la coquille d'oeufs de la poule. Rec. méd. vét. 120:37–40, 1944.

ENZIE, F. D., and WHITMORE, G. E.: Photosensitization Keratitis in Young Goats Following Treatment with Phenothiazine. J. Am. Vet. Med. Assn. 123:237–238, 1953.

FAWCETT, D. W.: An Atlas of Fine Structure. The Cell, Its Organelles and Inclusions. Philadelphia, W. B. Saunders Co., 1966.

FLESCH, P.: Role of Copper in Mammalian Pigmentation. Proc. Soc. Exper. Biol. & Med. 70:79–83, 1949.

FORD, G. E.: Photosensitivity Due to Erodium spp. Aust. Vet. J. 41:56, 1965.

FOURIE, P. J. J.: The Occurrence of Congenital Porphyrinuria (Pink Tooth) in Cattle in South Africa (Swaziland). Onderstepoort J. Vet. Sci. 7:535–566, 1936.

————: Does Bovine Congenital Porphyrinuria (Pink Tooth) Produce Clinical Disturbances in an Animal which is Protected Against the Sun? Onderstepoort J. Vet. Sci. and Animal Ind. 26:231–233, 1953.

GALLO, G. G.: Dos caso de fotosensibilización en el ganado. [Photosensitization in Two Horses.] Rev. Vet. milit., B. Aires. 2:45–47, 1954.

GJESDAL, F.: Investigations on the Melanin Granules with Special Consideration of the Hair Pigment. Acta Path. Microbiol. Scand. Suppl. No. 133, pp. 112, 1959. Abstr. Vet. Bul. No. 3043, 1960.

GLENN, B. L., PANCIERA, R. J., and MONLUX, A. W.: A Hepatogenous Photosensitivity Disease of Cattle. II. Histopathology and Pathogenesis of the Hepatic Lesions. Path. Vet. 2:49–57, 1965.

GLENN, B. L., MONLUX, A. W., and PANCIERA, R. J.: A Hepatogenous Photosensitivity Disease of Cattle: I. Experimental Production and Clinical Aspects of the Disease. Path. Vet. 1:469–484, 1964.

GLENN, B. L., GLENN, H. G., and OMTVEDT, I. T.: Congenital Porphyria in the Domestic Cat (Felis catus): Preliminary Investigations on Inheritance Pattern. Amer. J. Vet. Res. 29:1653–1657, 1968.

GORDON, H. McL., and GREEN, R. J.: Phenothiazine Photosensitization in Sheep. Australian Vet. J. 27:51–52, 1951.

GROSSMAN, I. W., and ALTMAN, N. H.: Caprine Cloisonné Renal Lesion. Arch. Path. 88: 609–612, 1969.

HANCOCK, J.: Congenital Photosensitivity in Southdown Sheep. Proc. Ruakura N. Z. Farmers Conf. Week. 1949. pp. 85–92. Abstract Vet. Bull. No. 3385, 1951.

HARTLEY, W. J., MULLINS, J., and LAWSON, B. M.: Nutritional Siderosis in the Bovine. N.Z. Vet. J., 7:99–105, 1959.

HEPPLESTON, A. G.: Changes in the Lungs of Rabbits and Ponies Inhaling Coal Dust Underground. J. Path. & Bact. 67:349–359, 1954.

HIGGINSON, J., GERRITSEN, T., and WALKER, A. R. P.: Siderosis in the Bantu of Southern Africa. Am. J. Path. 29:779–815, 1953.

JOERGENSEN, S. K.: Congenital Porphyria in Pigs. Brit. Vet J. 115:160–175, 1959.

KANEKO, J. J.: Erythrokinetics and Iron Metabolism in Bovine Porphyria Erythropoietica. Ann. N.Y. Acad. Sci. 104:689–700, 1963.

KIRKSEN, G., and TAMMEN, C.: Keratitis in Young Cattle Resulting from Photosensitization After Prolonged Medication. Dt. Tierarztl. Wschr. 71:545–548, 1964.

KLECKNER, M. S., BAGGENSTROSS, A. H., and WEIR, J. F.: Iron-Storage Diseases. Am. J. Clin. Path., 25:915–931, 1955.

LAUGHLAND, D. H.: The Nature of a Reddish Pigment Occurring in the Bones of Cattle. Canad. J. Comp. Med. 15:261–267, 1951.

LAZZARO, D. A.: Resus ictericas. [Detection of Jaundice in Animal Carcasses.] Gac. vet. B. Aires 10:242–265, 1948.

LEE, C. S.: Histochemical Studies of the Ceroid Pigments of Rats and Mice and its Relation to Necrosis. J. Nat. Cancer Inst. 11:339–349, 1950.

LEE, H. J.: The Relationship of Copper to Pigmentation in Black-wooled Sheep. M. J. Australia. 2:757, 1948.

LESTER, R., and SCHMID, R.: Bilirubin Metabolism. N. E. J. Med. 270:779–786, 1964.

LIENHART, R.: Remarques à propos de la couleur de la coquille des oeufs des poules domestiques. Compt. rend. Soc. de biol. 140:541–543, 1946.

LIGHT, F. W.: Pigmented Thickening of the Basement Membranes of the Renal Tubules of the G,oat ("Cloissonné Kidney"). Lab. Invest. 9:228–238, 1960.

LILLIE, R. D., DAFT, F. S., and SEBRELL, W. H., JR.: Cirrhosis of the Liver in Rats on a Deficient Diet and the Effect of Alcohol. Public Hlth Rep. 56:1255–1258, 1941.

LORA, R. P.: Fotosensibilización en ovinos merinos por consumo de Hypericum perforatum L. Bol. Zootec., Cordoba. 9:187–190, 1953.

4

LORD, G. H., and WILLSON, J. E.: Foreign Body Granuloma in a Rhesus Monkey. J. Amer. Vet. Med. Assn. *153*:910–913, 1968.

LYNCH, K. M., and McIVER, F. A.: Pneumoconiosis from Exposure to Kaolin Dust: Kaolinosis. Amer. J. Path. *30*:1117–1127, 1954.

MASON, K. E., and HARTSOUGH, G. R.: "Steatitis" or "Yellow Fat" in Mink, and its Relation to Dietary Fats and Inadequacy of Vitamin E. J. Am. Vet. Med. Assn. *119*:72–75, 1951.

MATHEWS, F. P.: Photosensitization and the Photodynamic Diseases of Man and the Lower Animals. Arch. Path. *23*:399–429, 1937.

McFARLANE, D., EVANS, J. V., and REID, C.S.W.: Photosensitivity Diseases in New Zealand. XIV. The Pathogenesis of Facial Eczema. N.Z.J. Agric. Res. *2*:194–200, 1959.

MENKIN, V., and TALMADGE, S. M.: Experimental Siderosis. Arch. Path. *19*:53–65, 1935.

MORTIMER, P. H.: The Experimental Intoxication of Sheep with Sporodesmin, a Metabolic Product of *Pithomyces chartarum*. III. Some Changes in Cellular Components and Coagulation Properties of the Blood, in Serum Proteins and in Liver Function. Res. Vet. Sci. *3*: 269–286, 1962.

MOSES, C.: Photosensitivity as a Cause of Falsely Positive Cephalin-cholesterol Flocculation Tests. J. Lab. & Clin. Med. *30*:267–269, 1945.

NESTEL, B. L.: Bovine Congenital Porphyria (Pink Tooth) with a Note on Five Cases Observed in Jamaica. Cornell Vet., *48*:430–439, 1958.

OPPENHEIMER, B. S., and KLINE, B. S.: Ochronosis. Arch. Int. Med. *29*:732–747, 1922.

OWEN, L. N., STEVENSON, D. E., and KEILIN, J.: Abnormal Pigmentation and Fluorescence in Canine Teeth. Res. Vet. Sci. *3*:139–146, 1962.

PACE, N.: The Etiology of Hypericism, a Photosensitivity Produced by St. Johnswort. Am. J. Physiol. *136*:650–656, 1942.

PLUMMER, P. J. G.: Three Cases of Osteohaemochromatosis in Cattle. Canad. J. Comp. Med. *13*:64–65, 1949.

QUIN, J. I.: The Effect of Surgical Obstruction of the Normal Bile Flow. Onderstepoort J. Vet. Sci. & Animal Ind. *1*:505–526, 1933.

RIMINGTON, C.: Some Cases of Congenital Porphyrinuria in Cattle: Chemical Studies Upon the Living Animals and Post-Mortem Material. Onderstepoort J. Vet. Sci. *7*:567–609, 1936.

————: Pigments of Blood and Bile. Lancet *261*:551–556, 1951.

————: Haems and Porphyrins in Health and Disease. Acta Med. Scandinav. *143*: 161–196, 1952.

ROCHA E. SILVA, M.: En torno da etiologia da doença de fotosensibilização produzida pelo *Holocalyx glaziovii*. Biólogico. São Paulo. *9*:187–194, 1943.

ROUS, P., and OLIVER, J.: Experimental Hemochromatosis. J. Exper. Med. *28*:629–644, 1918.

SALOMON, K., and COWGILL, G. R.: Porphyrinuria in Lead-poisoned Dogs. J. Indust. Hyg. & Toxicol. *30*:114–118, 1948.

SCARPELI, D. G.: Experimental Nephrocalcinosis—A Biochemical and Morphologic Study. Lab. Invest. *14*:123–141, 1965.

SCHLOTTHAUER, C. F., and BOLLMAN, J. L.: Spontaneous Gout in Turkeys. J. Am. Vet. Med. Assn. *85*:98–103, 1934.

SCHLUMBERGER, H. G.: Synovial Gout in the Parakeet. Lab. Investig. *8*:1304–1318, 1959.

SCHMID, R.: The Porphyrias in *The Metabolic Basis of Inherited Disease*. 2nd Edition. McGraw-Hill Book Co., 1966.

SHELDON, J. H.: *Haemochromatosis*. London, Oxford University Press, 1935.

SHIMADA, K., BRICKNELL, K. S., and FINEGOLD, S. M.: Deconjugation of Bile Acids by Intestinal Bacteria: Review of Literature and Additional Studies. J. Infect. Dis. *119*: 273–281, 1969.

SILLER, W. G.: Avian Nephritis and Visceral Gout. Lab. Investig. *8*:1319–1357, 1959.

SLATER, T. F., and RILEY, P. A.: Photosensitization and Lysosomal Damage. Nature (London) *209*:151–154, 1965.

SNELL, A. M.: Fundamentals in the Diagnosis of Jaundice. J. Am. Med. Assn. *138*:274–279, 1948.

SUZUKI, Y., and CHURG, J.: Structure and Development of the Asbestos Body. Amer. J. Path. *55*:79–107, 1969.

SYNGE, R. L. M. and WHITE, E. P.: Photosensitivity Diseases in New Zealand. XXIII. Isolation of Sporodesmin, A Substance Causing Lesions Characteristic of Facial Eczema, from Sporodesmium bakeri, Syd. N. Z. J. Agrig. Res. *3*:907–921, 1960.

TABARELLI NETTO, J. F., RIBEIRO, O. F., and RIBEIRO, I. F.: A propósito do índice ictério e la bilirubinaemia do jejum, em eqüinos. [About the Icteric Index and the Fasting Bilirubinaemia in Equines.] Rev. Fac. vet., São Paulo. *3*:187–194, 1948.

TABUCHI, E., KATADA, M., *et al.*: Haemosiderosis of Spleen and Liver in Equine Infectious Anemia. Nat. Inst. Anim. Hlth. Quart. Tokyo *3*:142–149. (E.)

TAYLOR, F. A.: Pigment of Anthracosis. Proc. Soc. Exper. Biol. & Med. *48*:70–72, 1941.

THORNTON, R. H., and PERCIVAL, J. C.: A Hepatotoxin from *Sporidesmium bakeri* (*Stemphylium botryosum*) Capable of Producing Facial Eczema Diseases in Sheep. Nature. Lond. *183*:63, 1959.

TAYLOR, K. E.: Ham Discoloration Due to Iron Injections. J. Am. Vet. Med. Assn. *145*:470–471, 1964.

TOBIAS, G.: Congenital Porphyria in a Cat. J. Am. Vet. Med. Assn. *145*:462–463, 1964.

TRAUTWEIN, G. W.: The Occurrence of Acid-Fast Lipopigments in Animals. Am. J. Vet. Res. *23*:134–145, 1962.

WALTER, W. G. and BALSWIN, D. E.: Observations on the Parathyroid Glands of Guinea Pigs Affected with Metastatic Calcification. Canad. J. Comp. Med. *27*:140–146, 1963.

WASS, W. M.: *Studies on Bovine Porphyria.* Dissertation, University of Minnesota. pp. 133, 1961.

WASS, W. M., and HOYT, H. H.: Bovine Congenital Porphyria: Studies on Heredity; Hematologic Studies, Including Porphyrin Analyses. Amer. J. Vet. Res. *26*:654–658, 1965.

WENDER, S. H.: Action of Photosensitizing Agents Isolated from Buckwheat. Am. J. Vet. Res. *7*:486–489, 1946.

WHITEHAIR, C. K., SCHAEFER, A. E., and ELVEHJEM, C. A.: Nutritional Deficiencies in Mink with Special Reference to Hemorrhagic Gastroenteritis, "Yellow Fat" and Anemia. J. Am. Vet. Med. Assn. *115*:54–58, 1949.

WHITTEN, L. K.: Photosensitized Keratitis in Calves after Dosing with Phenothiazine. Rep. 15th Internat. Vet. Congress. *2*:56–60, 1952.

WINTER, H.: An Environmental Lipofuscin Pigmentation of Livers. Studies on the Pigmentation Affecting the Sheep and Other Animals in Certain Districts of Australia. Univ. Qd. Pap., Vet. Sci. *1*:1–66, 1961.

————: "Black Kidneys" in Cattle—a Lipofuscinosis. J. Path. Bact. *86*, 253–258, 1963.

WORKER, N. A., and CARRILLO, B. J.: "Enteque seco," Calcification and Wasting in Grazing Animals in the Argentine. Nature (London) *215*:72–74, 1967.

WYLER, R.: Über die Pigmentierung der Rinderlymphknoten. [Pigmentation of Lymph Nodes in Cattle.] Acta anat. *14*:365–382. 1952.

ZAHAWI, S.: Symmetrical Cortical Siderosis of the Kidney in Goats. Amer. J. Vet. Res. *18*:861–867, 1957.

4

Disturbances of Growth

ATROPHY

Atrophy is a shrinking, or wasting away, of an organ or tissue to less than its former, and less than its normal size. This can occur in two ways: (1) Through a decrease in the number of constituent cells, necrosis having eliminated some of those normally present. Atrophy developing by this process is called **numerical atrophy**. The same result is attained (2) by a decrease in the size of each component cell, which constitutes **quantitative atrophy**. Commonly it is parenchymal rather than interstitial cells which undergo this change.

Atrophy may **occur** in any organ or tissue; it may involve the whole organ or a single cell.

Microscopic Appearance.—(1) Cells of certain histological types in an organ or tissue are fewer than normal (numerical atrophy) or smaller than normal (quantitative atrophy). (2) If an organ has a capsule, the wrinkled or undulating capsule may be the most obvious indication that the contents have atrophied. (3) Attention may first be attracted to the condition by the fact that non-atrophying elements appear too large or too numerous. In the spleen, for example, the trabeculæ may appear surprisingly large with too many of them in a given microscopic field, but in reality they have come closer to each other because some of the intervening parenchyma has disappeared. For the same reason, the glomeruli of an atrophic kidney appear too numerous and too close together. Actually the change is in the number of tubules; some of them have been destroyed with a corresponding collapse of the remaining tissue to fill the unoccupied spaces. One should not be misled here by the kidney of a very young animal, which has many small, uniform glomeruli (renal corpuscles), while some of the tubules are yet undeveloped.

In atrophic muscle, the sarcoplasm grows narrower and disappears, leaving for a time the sarcolemma and endomysium, which bear a resemblance to fibrous tissue. In the liver, the hepatic cords may remain intact but become extremely narrow.

Gross Appearance.—The organ or part is smaller than normal as determined by the eye, by measuring or by weight. In our several species and their numerous breeds, varying greatly in weight and stature, it is not easy to say precisely what the size of an organ ought to be. In a few instances, the mean normal weight of an organ has been carefully determined in proportion to the weight of the animal, but even this may be somewhat deceiving. A draft horse weighing 1800 pounds, for instance, is only slightly taller or longer than a racehorse weighing 1000 pounds. As in the case of the spleen, a wrinkled capsule or other distortion may betray the atrophic condition with more certainty than weights and measures. If a paired organ is the subject of scrutiny, it should always be compared with its fellow.

The **causes** of atrophy to some extent duplicate the causes of necrosis, which is not surprising since numerical atrophy involves previous necrosis. (1) **Starvation and malnutrition** cause atrophy of almost the whole body, chiefly quantitative. In starvation the adipose tissue is consumed to produce energy necessary to maintain life. If the oxidation of fat is rapid, ketosis (p. 1020) develops. As the fat becomes exhausted, the muscular and glandular tissues diminish, their protoplasm being catabolized and converted to the production of energy. Practically all organs except the bones and the central nervous system suffer. Malnutrition, caused by some failure of assimilation rather than actual lack of food, has the same effect. (2) **Lack of adequate blood supply** brings deficiency of oxygen and quantitative atrophy of individual cells or numerical atrophy of the organ through necrosis of a certain percentage of the cells. For example, the stagnation of chronic passive congestion causes narrowing of the hepatic cords to half their former width and their ultimate disappearance. (3) **Lack of proper innervation** has already been noted as causing necrosis of muscle cells in "sweeney" of the horse's shoulder. If one considers the whole muscle, supraspinatus or infraspinatus, this is atrophy. In spite of what has been said of the necrosis, some of the muscle cells remain alive, undergoing only quantitative atrophy through loss of their sarcoplasm. It is these cells which regenerate most successfully when recovery supervenes. Progressive atrophy of the muscles of mastication has been observed in a dog as the result of a neurofibroma growing to the root of the trigeminal nerve (mandibular division), an excellent example of this form of pathogenesis. (4) **"Disuse atrophy"** represents a causative mechanism not encountered in the study of necrosis, but one of considerable importance with respect to atrophy. In general, body structures tend to grow larger and more efficient with normal use and activity, a process called hypertrophy (p. 92), and to atrophy if left long unused. This is seen in muscles and even bones. The wasting which occurs in a paralyzed limb is a matter of common observation. In a horse chronically lame from any cause, the foot of the lame leg will be found, by careful measurement, to be slightly smaller than its fellow, a fact which the practical diagnostician takes into account. The lumen of the digestive tract slowly adjusts itself to the load placed upon it; large and bulky meals lead to large stomach and intestines; starvation, or small meals of concentrated foods, leads to atrophy of those organs. If a gland, such as the salivary, has its duct occluded, there is at first an accumulation of dammed-up secretion, then marked atrophy of the gland. (5) Prolonged **pressure** leads to atrophy, at first quantitative and later numerical with necrosis. This is very striking when a neoplasm invades the liver, eventually replacing most of the hepatic tissue. As another illustration, it is possible to tell whether a horse has been working habitually by the slight depression of the healthy tissues where the collar or the saddle rests. (6) Certain **disturbances of endocrine glands** produce atrophy of structures dependent upon their secretions, as, for instance, atrophy of the testes in hypopituitarism. (7) Prolonged **overwork** leads exceptionally to atrophy, as in the thyroid exhaustion following prolonged exophthalmic goiter. (8) **Physiological** atrophy occurs usually as part of the normal aging process. The thymus practically disappears as the individual advances beyond infancy. The stature of a normal man at seventy years may be almost an inch less than it was at thirty years of age.

Classification of Atrophy. — It is sometimes useful to divide atrophy into several classes dependent on special accompanying features. (1) Simple atrophy needs no explanation; the term is used when none of the other classifying adjectives apply. (2) In **fatty atrophy**, the missing cells have been replaced by adipose tissue. This occurs, for instance, in physiological atrophy of the thymus. (3) In **fibrous atrophy**, sometimes called "fibroid" or "scirrhous" atrophy, proliferating fibrous tissue comes in as the pre-existing cells shrink and disappear. The proliferation of new connective tissue really constitutes a chronic inflammatory reaction (p. 165). Quite understandably, then, the irritant which caused the inflammation is either remotely or directly causative of the atrophy. Often this is an infection, as in the case of fibrous atrophy of the testis following orchitis, of the mammary gland following mastitis (shrunken or "lost" quarters of the bovine udder), and of the pancreas following infectious pancreatitis. In cirrhosis, the liver is atrophic as well as fibrotic. The thymus suffers fibrous, instead of fatty, atrophy when it is exposed to roentgen rays, a treatment for persistent hyperplasia of the thymus in human patients. Pressure atrophy is frequently also fibrous atrophy. (4) **Pigment atrophy** is that which is accompanied by deposition of pigment, namely the pigment of brown atrophy (p. 83). (5) **Mucoid atrophy of fat,** also known as **serous atrophy of fat,** has been discussed in connection with connective-tissue mucin and myxomatous degeneration (p. 52).

HYPERTROPHY

In atrophy the affected part is abnormally small, in hypertrophy it is unduly large. When an organ or part enlarges to a size which is disproportionately and abnormally great, the condition is either hypertrophy or hyperplasia. While usage is not always consistent, especially in clinical medicine, hypertrophy can be defined histologically as an increase in size of a part in which each histological component retains its normal proportion and relations to the other components. Some prefer to stipulate that in hypertrophy the functional cells increase in individual size but not in number, while the opposite obtains in hyperplasia. From the physiologic standpoint, hypertrophy can be defined as an increase in size accompanied by an increase in normal functional ability. Actually it is next to impossible to formulate a precise definition which will fit the prevailing usage of hypertrophy as distinguished from hyperplasia in all cases.

The condition occurs in various organs, glands, muscles and tissues. **Microscopically** and **grossly** the appearance is unchanged except that the part in question is abnormally large.

Hypertrophy appears to result as a consequence of increased demand for functional activity of the organ. The fundamental causes and mechanisms involved are essentially unknown.

Pure hypertrophy (without hyperplasia) only occurs in organs whose cells have generally lost the power to undergo mitosis. Synthesis of more cytoplasm in individual cells results in more protein, mitochondria and ribonucleic acid (RNA) (p. 317) per cell but no increase in deoxyribonucleic acid (DNA). Thus it appears that the synthesis of DNA is blocked but that of RNA remains uninhibited. Two types of hypertrophy, not always clearly distinguishable from one another, are usually considered on the basis of their origin and probable cause. These are compensatory and hormonal hypertrophy.

Compensatory Hypertrophy.—This enlargement is believed to result as a consequence of impaired function of a paired organ or part of an organ system. For example, loss of one kidney, for any reason, results in gradual enlargement of the remaining kidney, enabling it to compensate for the loss of function of the paired organ. A paradox here: This hypertrophy reportedly does not occur in the absence of a functional pituitary. Another example of hypertrophy is found in the myocardium, which as a result of back pressure (due to stenosis, hypertension) undergoes remarkable enlargement. Stenosis of the lumen of the pyloris of the stomach leads to hypertrophy of the gastric musculature; similar partial obstruction of the intestinal or urethral lumen leads to hypertrophy of the intestinal or bladder muscle, respectively. The enlargement of skeletal muscles as the result of repeated exercise is well known.

Hormonal Hypertrophy.—This most often is a physiologic phenomenon but in some instance may be pathologic. The enlargement of the mammary gland at the approach of lactation involves hypertrophy (as well as hyperplasia—to be discussed); as does the great increase in size of the testes in birds and some mammals during the mating season.

The **significance** of hypertrophy obviously is that of a protective mechanism and a response to a need for increased function. Occasionally the enlarged organ may constitute a mechanical hindrance to some other function, as when enlargement of the heart muscle may distort the valves from their proper positions or cause the heart to fail due to inadequate blood supply. It should be noted that, while the increase in size occasioned by hypertrophy may be very considerable, there are always definite limits to the maximum size attained.

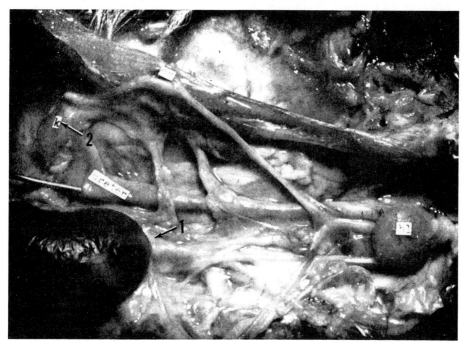

FIG. 4–1.—Compensatory hypertrophy of right kidney (*1*) resulting from congenital hypoplasia of left kidney (*2*). Left ovary (*ov*) and bladder (*bl*). From a five and one-half-month-old female terrier which died of canine distemper.

HYPERPLASIA

In hyperplasia, we see an increase in the size of an organ, tissue or cell, without regard to the maintenance of normal histologic relations. This involves an increase in the number of one kind of cells or another, a feature which some use as the basis of their definition. The epithelium, for example, may increase without

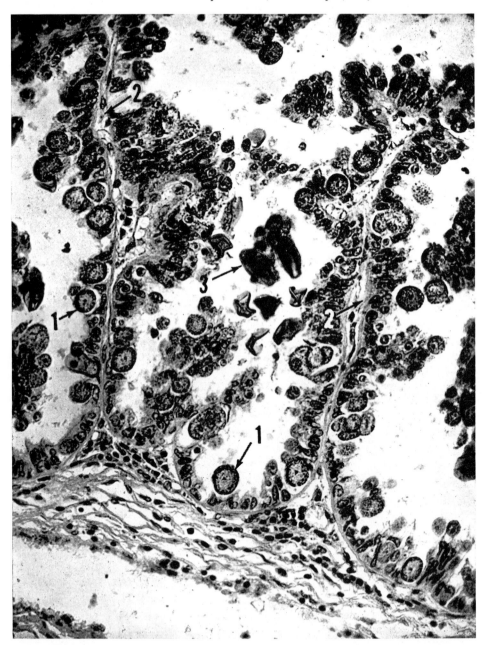

Fig. 4–2.—Hyperplasia of intrahepatic biliary epithelium in liver of a rabbit infected with *Eimeria stiedae.* Gametocytes (*1*) and oocysts (*3*). Note the long fronds of hyperplastic epithelial cells supported by a delicate stroma (*2*). (Courtesy of Armed Forces Institute of Pathology.) × 250. Contributor: Dr. C. L. Davis.

regard to its supporting connective tissue, or the reverse may be true. Normal function based on bodily needs is frequently impaired or distorted.

Gross and microscopic appearances vary. Hyperplasia of a glandular organ usually involves an increase in height of the acinar epithelium and at the same time an increase in the number of its cells. Based on the same principle as the well known fact that one can plant more hills of corn in a crooked row than a straight one, the contours of the acinar lining become crooked, wavy and folded, often to the extent that papillary projections jut into the lumen. Indeed, the acinus may be more or less filled with reduplicated folding of an acinar lining which was originally in the form of a smoothly contoured circle. This is seen especially well in hyperplasia of the thyroid or prostate. In some instances, huge acini are formed at the expense of surrounding structures as in **cystic glandular hyperplasia** of the endometrium or mammary gland. Hyperplastic conditions of the epidermis may take the form of increased thickness of the prickle-cell layer (stratum spinosum), which is known as **acanthosis**, or of the cornified layer, **hyperkeratosis.**

Lymphoid hyperplasia is an increase in the amount of lymphatic tissues of the body, usually as a part of the reaction to a chronic infection. It may be localized in the Peyer's patches and unnamed lymphoid tissue of the intestine, or in the tonsils. Frequently it is generalized, involving all of the lymphoid tissues. In the spleen, it is recognized by an increase in the size and cellular density of the splenic (Malphighian) corpuscles. This condition may be confused grossly with the "sago spleen" (p. 48), but the whiteness and sharpness of the splenic corpuscles is less pronounced in lymphoid hyperplasia. The number of lymphocytes in the red pulp may also be increased, but a heavy concentration of lymphocytes here must be differentiated from malignant lymphoma (p. 208). Affected lymph nodes are enlarged without change in color or consistency. Hyperplasia in these is best detected microscopically by the increased size and prominence of each lymph nodule. The germinal center, with its pale maternal lymphoblasts, is larger than normal and is surrounded by an unusually wide zone of deep-staining lymphocytes, which are very densely packed. The same is true of the lymph nodules of tonsils, Peyer's patches and all tissues which have them. In addition, lymph nodules are increased in number and at times they appear in places where they are not ordinarily found, as in the spleen or thymus. The minute and insignificant collections of lymphocytes which are normal in such organs as the skin, liver and lungs enlarge and may even contain germinal centers.

Lymphoid hyperplasia is often succeeded or accompanied by **lymphoid exhaustion,** in which the pale germinal centers are still larger, but the zone of accumulated lymphocytes around each of them is very much depleted or almost totally absent. The lymphocytes have been sent, like soldiers, into the areas of combat against the causative infection.

Myeloid hyperplasia, or hyperplasia of the bone marrow, is merely a change from the fatty marrow, which is normal in the main marrow cavity of long bones in adults, to normal red marrow with its usual hematopoietic cells. Physiologically it could be called hypertrophy since it is a response to the need for more abundant production of erythrocytes and granulocytes, but there is also an increase of certain particular types of cells, so that the usual designation of hyperplasia is likewise appropriate. It occurs in hemolytic and hemorrhagic anemias, or in infections accompanied by granulocytopenia (Neutropenia. p. 172).

Regenerative hyperplasia is the name given to abnormal enlargement of young cells, or their nuclei, formed in the regeneration (p. 183) of tissues which have been partly destroyed. For instance, many newly regenerated hepatic epithelial cells have huge and hyperchromatic nuclei.

The **causes** of hyperplasia are (1) chronic irritation, as seen in cutaneous hyperplasias, hyperplasia of the bile ducts in coccidiosis of the rabbit and various other disorders, (2) infections, which may possibly owe this effect to irritants produced during the infectious process, (3) imbalances of the endocrine system, as in hyperplasia of the prostate, endometrium and mammary gland, and (4) deficiencies, as exemplified in the hyperplasia of the thyroid which results from deficiency of iodine or the enlargement of bones in rickets (p. 1058) and osteoporosis (p. 1067).

In most respects, the **significance** of hyperplasias seems obvious. It sometimes appears to be but a short step from hyperplasia to the much more serious neoplasia. Still, there are comparatively few conditions where there exists any strong evidence of hyperplasia leading to neoplasia, especially if the hyperplasia is not complicated by metaplasia (below). Chlorinated naphthalene, one of the most potent producers of hyperplasia (bovine specific hyperkeratosis), appears entirely unable to cause neoplasms, even though its hyperplastic effects are demonstrable in many parts of the animal body (p. 938).

METAPLASIA

Change of one variety of tissue into another is called metaplasia. It is always confined to varieties within the limits of the original primary tissue, and, as a matter of fact, only two of the five primary tissues recognized in histology are subject to metaplasia. These are epithelium and connective tissue.

Occurrence.—Metaplasia of columnar or cuboidal epithelium into stratified squamous epithelium, usually cornifying, occurs in the bronchi and bronchioles, in the gallbladder when irritated by gall stones, in the ducts of glands, and in the protruded parts of prolapsed organs such as the cervix. In deficiency of vitamin A, there is a mild metaplasia of the epithelium in a variety of other locations, such as the lining of the renal pelvis.

Connective tissue undergoes metaplasia to cartilage or bone, and cartilage changes to bone in a variety of situations. In cattle, the formation of large numbers of bony spicules in thickened alveolar septa of the lung is not of exceptional rarity. Bony and cartilaginous metaplasia in adenocarcinomas and mixed tumors of the canine mammary gland is frequent and may be so extensive that the major part of the neoplasm consists of bone. The ossification of tendons and cartilage is a form of metaplasia which has already been described (p. 58). Rarely the scars of abdominal wounds develop bony layers. A bony plate of considerable size has been encountered in the submucosa of the bovine renal pelvis.

The fundamental **cause** of metaplasia is a demand for a different kind of function, usually for protection against chronic irritation. The exact mechanisms are essentially unknown.

Significance.—Metaplastic epithelium has a very considerable tendency to go on to neoplasia. Many of the carcinomas of the human lung arise in metaplastic bronchial epithelium.

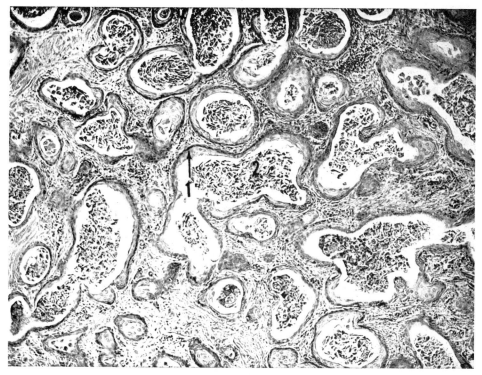

FIG. 4–3.—Squamous metaplasia of prostate of a dog, resulting from estrogen production of a Sertoli cell tumor of the testis. Prostatic acini are lined with squamous epithelium (1) and filled with keratin debris (2). (Courtesy of Armed Forces Institute of Pathology.) × 70. Contributor: Dr. W. H. Riser.

HYPOPLASIA

Hypoplasia is the failure of an organ or part to develop to its normal size. Obviously the disorder occurs during the period of growth, usually before birth. It differs from atrophy in that the atrophic organ has shrunk from a previously normal size; the hypoplastic organ never was any larger. Examples are known of hypoplasia of almost every organ and part. The causes are usually hidden in the obscurity which enshrouds prenatal abnormalities in general. In some cases, a malformation resulting in a restricted blood supply to the hypoplastic structure is demonstrable. Synonyms include agenesis and dysgenesis.

ANAPLASIA

Anaplasia is a reversion of cells to a more primitive and undifferentiated type such as is found in the embryo. More will be heard of it in connection with neoplasia and malignant tumors.

DEVELOPMENTAL ANOMALIES AND MALFORMATIONS

Developmental anomalies ordinarily originate before birth; indeed, in embryonic life, when the development of most body structures has its beginning. But this is not necessarily true; if the epiphyseal cartilages of, let us say, the femur of a child or young animal suffer severe damage, as they may in chronic osteomyelitis, for instance, the bone grows no more and the individual has a shortened and deformed leg, a malformation.

The frequency of pre-natal malformations is surprising; their wide variety is unbelievable. Most of the types have been given names, but these will be omitted here. Reflection on the various forms reveals that they depend upon one of several different errors in the developmental mechanism. Outstanding among these are: (1) Arrest of development in a certain part of the embryo, so that a certain structure is absent or too small (hypoplasia).

(2) Failure of a certain embryonal or fetal structure to disappear when it normally should. There are many examples of this, such as the persistence of the ductus arteriosus, or of the thyro-glossal duct. Atresia ani is a rather common malformation which results from failure of the overlying skin to disappear from the anal opening.

(3) Failure of certain openings, grooves, and fissures to close properly. Many of these are in the mid-line, such as cranioschisis and rachioschisis from lack of closure of the neural groove, but patent foramen ovale in the heart can be included here, as can persistent cloaca, in which the rectal and external genital openings are not separated

(4) Aberrant (ectopic or heterotopic) structures. It is not highly extraordinary to find islands of pancreatic tissue in the wall of the stomach, or of adrenal tissue in the kidney or pelvic tissues. Displacement of cutaneous and mucosal tissues into deeper areas is considered to be the proper explanation of the rather frequent dermoid cysts located near the exterior of the body, as well as of those dentigerous cysts occurring in the head and neck, although just when such malformations become sufficiently complicated to be suspected of resulting from the imperfect duplication now to be discussed it is difficult to say

(5) Duplications. Each cell or group of cells of the early embryo is destined

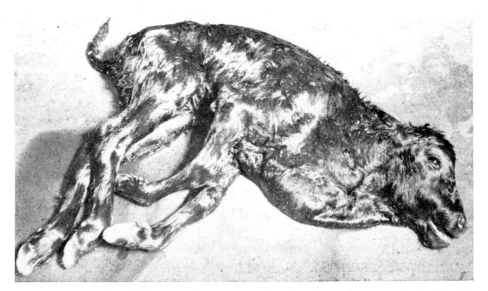

Fig. 4–4.—*Ectopia cordis* in a newborn Angus calf, a full-term twin to a normal calf. The diaphragm was absent; abdominal viscera in the thorax; the heart in the subcutis of the neck. Some calves with this anomaly have lived several months or years.

to produce, as it multiplies, a certain particular structure in the adult. If such a cell were to undergo division without any further specialization or differentiation toward a particular organ or tissue, it is obvious that two cells with identical potentialities would be produced, each destined to form identical body structures, of which there would be two instead of the usual one. If the cell doing this were the recently fertilized ovum, there would be two complete and identical individuals, or twins (of the identical or monozygotic variety). The work of experimental embryologists indicates a slightly different process as actually occurring. The fertilized ovum normally divides into two blastomeres, or primitive daughter cells. In some simple animal species, these two blastomeres have been experimentally separated and each develops into a complete individual, an identical, or uniovular twin. What must be almost complete separation of the two blastomeres has been accomplished by shaking or by inverting the ovum at this two-cell stage with the resulting formation of double monsters, that is, twins like the Siamese twins, almost but not completely separated. In other experiments with certain amphibian species, monsters with two heads or anterior ends have been produced by constricting the developing embryo at a somewhat later stage (during gastrulation). This procedure involves not only the separation of groups of cells, but a division of the supply of a certain chemical hormone called an "organizer." These organizers have been formed in the appropriate region of the embryo and are what supplies the necessary stimulus for the involved cells to differentiate into the peculiar types and structures needed—in this case, to form a head. If the plane of constriction is not exactly median, one of the heads is normal and the other is incomplete and imperfect in one way or another; usually it has only one eye. Double monsters and other radical malformations have also been produced by experimental embryologists in amphibian and similar lower animal species

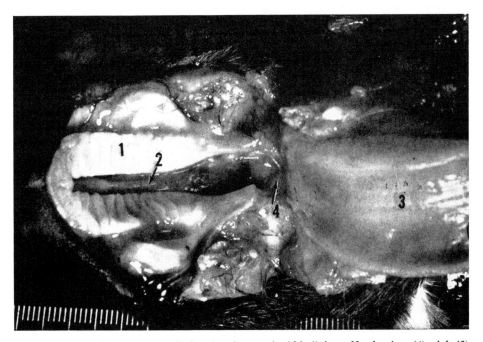

Fig. 4–5.—Congenital anomaly. Cleft palate in a week-old bull dog. Hard palate (1), cleft (2) opening into nasal cavity, deflected tongue (3) and posterior nares (4).

through such means as depriving the very early embryo of sufficient oxygen, by the application of minute amounts of certain toxic chemicals or by lowering the temperature unduly.

There may be all degrees of duplication, such as two separate and perfect twins, two twins which are perfectly formed but joined together by more or less unduplicated tissue, such as belly to belly, back to back, or head to head. In such cases, the vital organs may or may not be duplicated. There may be duplication of almost any part of the animal's body, the muzzle, the head, the cephalo-thorax, the tail, the hind quarters and others. There may be double pairs of fore or hind limbs; the latter are common.

As might be anticipated from the experimental results recorded above, the duplicated parts are not necessarily equal. Especially when the duplication is not a matter of right and left counterparts, the inequality is often such that one set of organs is more or less normal and perhaps functional, while the other recedes to a purely accessory status. We have recently seen a lamb which was born with two mouths, one in the normal place and one, considerably smaller, in the right subparotid region. The accessory mouth chewed when the main mouth chewed, secreted saliva and had three rudimentary teeth, but it did not have an opening into the pharynx. The lamb was raised to well past a year of age (dying of an accident), and in the course of the animal's normal growth the accessory mouth became relatively less and less prominent, since it grew but little.

Supernumerary parts, usually of minor nature, occur in some situations where the conception of duplication is less obvious but probably still applicable, for instance, in the case of supernumerary digits in man or animal. The extra digits are usually bilaterally symmetrical but practically always imperfect and purely accessory. Supernumerary breasts are described in the human female. Supernumerary (and rudimentary) teats are common in the cow. However, in the porcine and even the canine species, a somewhat variable number of pairs of mammæ is considered normal. Likewise, the number of vertebræ and ribs is subject to certain normal variation in some species.

Inequality of duplicated parts attains its logical culmination when the accessory

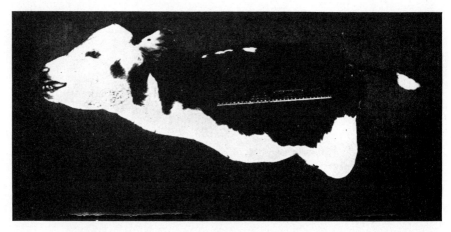

Fig. 4–6.—Congenital anomaly, a calf born alive but without legs lived three days without nourishment and was given euthanasia A similar anomaly in pigs is reported by Hutt to be due to a single recessive gene.

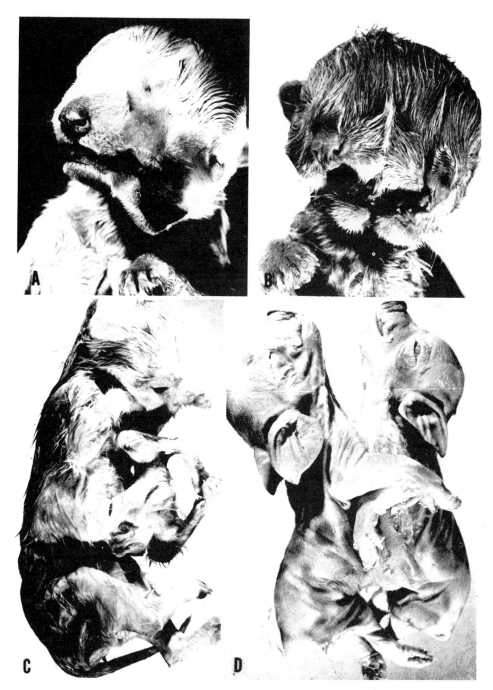

Fig. 4–7.—Congenital anomalies. *A*, Partial duplication of head (diprosopia) in a fox-terrier puppy which lived for two days. *B*, Diprosopia in a kitten. *C*, Twin kittens joined at the abdomen; one of them is only partially developed (heteradelphia). (Courtesy of Armed Forces Institute of Pathology.) Contributor: Major A. C. Girard. *D*, Twin pigs joined at the thorax (thoracopagus).

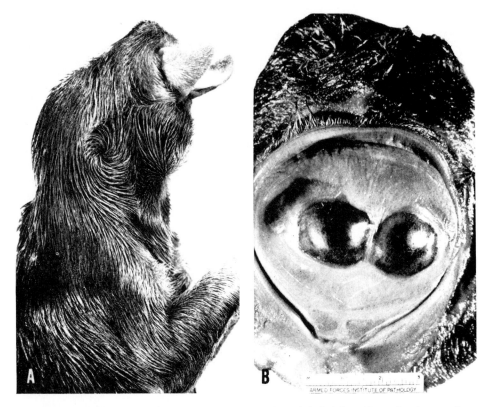

Fig. 4–8.—Congenital anomalies. *A*, Absence of eyes (anophthalmia) and lower jaw in a newborn puppy. *B*, Partially fused eyes (synophthalmia or cyclopegia) in a newborn colt.

structure is no more than a shapeless mass, attached outside or inside the dominant individual and recognizable only as the microscope reveals its histological components. Such a structure constitutes a teratoma. Since teratomas are likely sites for the development of malignant neoplasia, they are discussed in that connection (p. 270).

Etiology.—The causes of many congenital anomalies are essentially unknown. These are to be discussed in the appropriate chapters concerning organ systems. The important known causes are as follows.

(1) Prenatal infection with a virus—for example, panleukopenia (cerebellar hypoplasia) p. 475; Newcastle Disease of chickens (ocular or auditory anomalies) Blattner and Williamson (1951); blue tongue of sheep, p. 466; and Richettsia, p. 536.

(2) Intrauterine effects of poisons ingested by the mother. For example—the plant *Veratrum californicum*, p. 971; thalidomide, p. 974; selenium, p. 901; molybdenum, p. 916; trypan blue and sodium salicylate.

(3) Vitamin deficiencies—for example, Vitamin A, p. 981 and folic acid (B_{12}), p. 984.

(4) Genetic factors—the recombination of mutant genes, inherited from one or (usually) both parents. These are discussed more fully in Chapter 9.

Disturbances of Growth

BARRON, C. N.: Ectopic Pancreas in the Dog. Acta Anat. *36*:344–352, 1959.

BLATTNER, R. J. and WILLIAMSON, A. P.: Developmental Abnormalities in the Chick Embryo Following Infection with Newcastle Disease Virus. Proc. Soc. Exper. Biol. & Med. *77*:619–621, 1951.

DENNIS, S. M., and LEIPOLD, H. W.: Syndactylism in a Neonatal Lamb. Cornell Vet. *60*: 23–27, 1970.

HARRIS, H.: "Cell Growth and Multiplication": Chapter 20 in *General Pathology*, ed. by Florey, H. W. Philadelphia, W. B. Saunders Co., 1970.

KALTER, H., and WARKANY, J.: Experimental Production of Congenital Malformations in Mammals by Metabolic Procedure. Physiol. Rev. *39*:69–115, 1959.

LANDTMAN, B.: Relationship between Maternal Conditions during Pregnancy and Congenital Malformations. Arch. Dis. Childhood. *23*:237–246, 1948.

THOMSON, R. G.: Congenital Bronchial Hypoplasiae in Calvs. Path. Vet. *3*:89–109, 1966.

Chapter

5

Disturbances of Circulation

Coagulation. — When exposed to contact with injured cells, whether tissue cells, leukocytes or even blood platelets, blood coagulates and forms a clot. The non-yielding and tenacious characteristics of the clot are due to a meshwork of fibrils of fibrin coupled with the adhesiveness of the platelets. The process of coagulation can be simply stated as the conversion of the plasma protein **fibrinogen** to **fibrin** by the action of an enzyme **thrombin.** This conversion is accelerated by the presence of **calcium ions** and a **heat labile accelerator.** The fibrin formed by this process, which is soluble, is subsequently converted to an insoluble polymerized fibrin by a specific globulin, **fibrin-stabilizing factor.** The production of thrombin for the conversion of fibrinogen to fibrin cannot be as simply stated. It is the result of a highly complex series of enzymatic events which lead to the conversion of **prothrombin** to thrombin.

In recent years a group of blood clotting factors have been identified. Although a Roman numeral terminology has been suggested by the International Committee on Blood Clotting Factors, these factors are also honored with numerous synonyms. The factors by both number and more important synonyms are:

Factor I   — Fibrinogen

Factor II   — Prothrombin

Factor III   — Thromboplastin, Tissue thromboplastin

Factor IV   — Calcium

Factor V   — Proaccelerin, labile factor

Factor VII   — Proconvertin, precursor of serum prothrombin conversion accelerator, Pro-SPCA

Factor VIII — Antihemophilic factor, Antihemophilic globulin Antihemophilic factor A

Factor IX   — Christmas factor, Plasma thromboplastin component, PTC. Antihemophilic factor C

Factor X   — Stuart-Prower factor

Factor XI   — Plasma thromboplastin antecedent, PTA

Factor XII   — Hagemen Factor

Factor XIII — Fibrin stabilizing factor

The participation of these factors in clot formation can be conveniently divided into an *intrinsic clotting mechanism* and an *extrinsic clotting mechanism*. The two mechanisms share certain factors but are initiated by different means. The factors concerned in each of these systems are as follows:

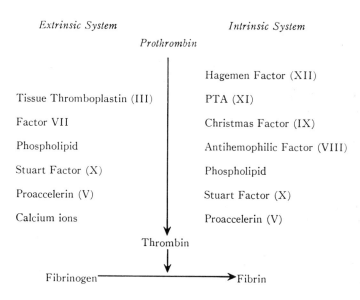

Extrinsic System   *Intrinsic System*

Prothrombin

Hagemen Factor (XII)

Tissue Thromboplastin (III)   PTA (XI)

Factor VII   Christmas Factor (IX)

Phospholipid   Antihemophilic Factor (VIII)

Stuart Factor (X)   Phospholipid

Proaccelerin (V)   Stuart Factor (X)

Calcium ions   Proaccelerin (V)

Thrombin

Fibrinogen ⟶ Fibrin

The interaction of the clotting factors proceeds in an orderly sequential chain of reactions. The intrinsic mechanism, which is independent of tissue damage is initiated by the activation of the Hagemen factor (XII). In a test tube, contact with glass initiates this step. Blood collected into a tube lined with paraffin will not clot owing to the lack of a proper stimulus for the activation of the Hagemen factor. It is not known what mechanism initiates this activation *in vivo*. Activated Hagemen factor then converts thromboplastin antecedent (PTA: XI) to an activated form which in turn activates the Christmas factor (IX). The activation of Christmas factor requires the presence of calcium ions. Activated Christmas factor in the presence of calcium ions and phospholipid activates the antihemophilic factor (VIII) which in turn converts the Stuart factor (X) to an activated form. This conversion also requires calcium ions. Activated Stuart factor in the presence of phospholipid converts proaccelerin (V) to a prothrombin converting principle which then converts prothrombin (II) to thrombin. This sequence of events can be illustrated after the "waterfall sequence" of Davie and Ratnoff (1964) or the "enzyme cascade" of MacFarlane (1964) as follows:

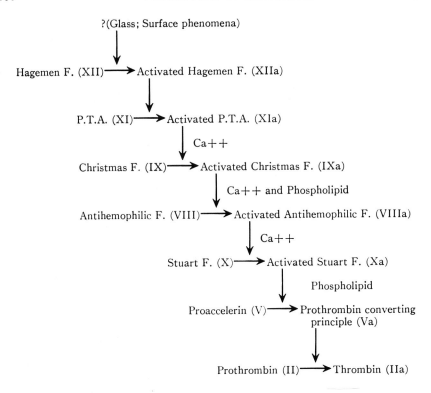

The extrinsic mechanism is dependent upon tissue injury and the release of tissue thromboplastin (III) which in the presence of calcium ions and factor VII activates the Stuart factor (X). The sequence of events then proceeds as in the intrinsic system as follows:

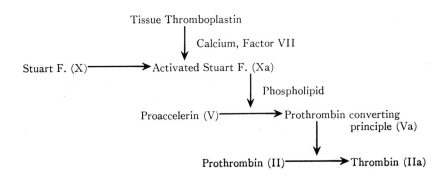

Thrombin formed by either mechanism converts fibrinogen to fibrin as indicated at the beginning of this section. Illustrated this proceeds as follows:

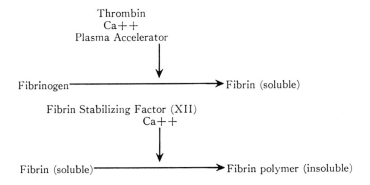

Thrombin
Ca++
Plasma Accelerator

Fibrinogen ⟶ Fibrin (soluble)

Fibrin Stabilizing Factor (XII)
Ca++

Fibrin (soluble) ⟶ Fibrin polymer (insoluble)

Noticeably absent from our discussion to this point is the **platelet.** The presumed role of the platelet in the above described mechanisms of coagulation has lost credence in recent years. Platelets apparently are not a significant source of any of the above clotting factors. They do, however, contribute phospholipids which, as indicated, are necessary for coagulation. The principal role of the platelet in hemostasis is their ability to plug small rents in the vascular integrity. When a vessel wall is injured, platelets aggregate at the site of injury and adhere to the vessel wall and each other, forming a plug and a focus for the deposition of fibrin strands. The stimulus for this aggregation is unknown but it has been suggested that it may be the result of a release of adenosine diphosphate (ADP) by injured endothelial cells. Experimentally, ADP has been shown to cause clumping of platelets.

The *prevention of coagulation* is of equal importance to life as is clot formation. Blood must remain fluid to serve its multiplicity of vital functions. Although not entirely understood, several safeguards prevent coagulation. Normal plasma contains a potent *anti-thrombin substance* which rapidly removes thrombin upon its formation. In addition it is thought that an *anti-thromboplastin* exists. Though not normally present in plasma, *heparin* is an important inhibitor of coagulation. Heparin acts by forming an inactive complex with PTA (factor XI) preventing the activation of the Christmas factor (IX) and also by interfering with the activation of antihemophilic factor (VIII) and the formation of thrombin. The rate of blood flow, blood viscosity, the integrity of the lining endothelium, and the normal separation of formed elements from the vascular endothelium by plasma (laminar flow) are also important factors in maintaining the fluidity of blood. Alteration in these qualities predispose to coagulation and thrombosis.

In addition to factors which prevent clotting, a mechanism exists for clot **dissolution.** A fibrinolytic enzyme **plasmin (fibrinolysin)** is capable of dissolving clots. Plasmin is formed by the activation of a precursor **plasminogen (profibrinolysin)** which is normally present in plasma. Plasminogen activation is stimulated by a tissue activator, **fibrinolysokinase** and also by *streptokinase* and *urokinase.*

Blood clots are of two kinds: (1) Clots formed in the flowing blood stream which necessarily are ante-mortem, and are called thrombi (singular, thrombus). The deposition of the clot in the flowing stream gives it certain identifying characteristics which will be described shortly. (2) Clots not formed in the flowing blood. These include clots formed in the vessels after death, called post-mortem clots, and those formed outside of vessels as the result of hemorrhage. We naturally think of these latter as being formed to close the open vessel, but if the hemorrhage is so located that the blood flows into a body cavity or tissue spaces, the same clotting occurs there.

POST-MORTEM CLOTS

Except when death results from certain septicemias and anoxic conditions, the greater part of the blood is clotted in the venous system soon after life ceases. The arteries contract in rigor mortis so that little blood remains in them. Blood clots formed in this way, as well as those formed outside the vascular channels, whose nature is obvious, have to be distinguished from thrombi by the criteria given in the following paragraphs.

Microscopic Appearance.—The visible components of these clots are the erythrocytes, leukocytes, fibrin and precipitated proteins, chiefly albumin. In post-mortem clots, these elements may be rather uniformly mixed, or the erythrocytes may have settled by force of gravity to the lowest parts of the vessel to be overlain by leukocytes and the precipitated protein of the plasma. Laminations like those in thrombi, however, do not occur. A useful differential feature is the size of the fibrils of fibrin, which in this type of clot are uniformly fine, barely visible individually under the usual low-power magnification of 100 diameters.

Gross Appearance.—The post-mortem clot is (1) dark red in color, (2) smooth and shiny on the outside and moulded to the vessel in which it is formed like jelly in its container, (3) presents a uniform texture to the naked eye and (4) is entirely unattached to the vessel wall. Because of these characteristics it is sometimes called a "currant-jelly clot."

A **chicken fat clot** results from a settling and separation of the red cells from the fluid phase of the blood. This sedimentation is not different from that which occurs in a test tube. This type of post-mortem clot is most likely to be found in the chambers of the heart and when post-mortem clotting is delayed. Such a clot has the smooth and shiny surface of the "currant-jelly," post-mortem clot but has the yellow color of plasma. It is not really attached to the vascular lining but is commonly immobilized through being entangled in the cardiac valves and chordae tendineae.

Cause.—The coagulation mechanisms as discussed above are responsible for post-mortem clotting. The system is probably activated by release of tissue thromboplastin generated from post-mortem autolysis of endothelial cells, leukocytes, and erythrocytes and also the activation of the intrinsic coagulation mechanism.

Significance.—Post-mortem clotting, like post-mortem autolysis, requires only to be distinguished from ante-mortem changes of somewhat similar nature.

ANTE-MORTEM CLOTS, THROMBOSIS

As previously stated, thrombi are clots formed in the flowing blood. This relatively slow process produces a clot of somewhat different qualities from those just described.

Microscopic Appearance.—In addition to the components given for the post-mortem clot, blood platelets, or thrombocytes, accumulate at the site of a thrombus and constitute a significant portion of this type of clot. The platelets tend strongly to adhere to each other, as well as to the vessel wall, forming somewhat amorphous, pink- or gray-staining masses which tend to alternate irregularly with layers or areas where fibrin and leukocytes, fibrin and erythrocytes or fibrin alone predominate. Thus a section through a thrombus tends to be irregularly **laminated.** If the section traverses the right part of the thrombus its area of **attachment** can be seen. On the other hand, a section cut through the trailing end of an obturating thrombus may appear as a lonely island in the middle of the lumen of the vessel. The **fibrils** of fibrin are relatively **thick** and heavy, a feature of prime importance in distinguishing the thrombus from a post-mortem clot.

Gross Appearance.—As seen at the necropsy table a thrombus is friable and has a **dull** and irregularly **roughened** or somewhat stringy surface, in contrast to the shiny, "currant-jelly" aspect of the post-mortem clot. The color is a mixture of red and gray, usually in irregular layers or **laminations.** On at least one side the thrombus will be found **attached** to the wall of the blood vessel. If the thrombus closes the lumen of the vessel entirely, it is an **occluding thrombus.** Rather frequently it occludes the lumen, except that there are one or several small openings which let a certain amount of blood pass through. This is a **canalized** thrombus. The "canals" come to be lined with endothelium continuous with that of the adjacent vessel wall.

Not too infrequently the clotting process continues in the part of the thrombus which is distal to its area of attachment without any further connection to the wall. The free end then trails downstream with the current and may attain surprising length. Such a thrombus is an **obturating** thrombus.

The **causes** of thrombosis are: (1) Injury to the endothelial cells lining the vessel wall. This releases the thromboplastin and possibly adenosine diphosphate (ADP) to start the clotting process and also causes the platelets to adhere to the area, which may be the very first step in thrombosis. The cause of the endothelial damage may be some local injury such as phlebitis of infectious origin or external twisting, ligation or contusion of the vessel. Repeated insertions of the hypodermic needle fall in this category but, fortunately, thrombosis following unskillful intravenous injections is less frequent than might be expected. Thrombosis inside the heart can occur just as readily as in the peripheral vessels and is relatively frequent. Endocarditis due to infection (*Streptococcus, Erysipelothrix*) is causative here. Injury by heartworms, *Dirofilaria immitis*, occasionally but not frequently is sufficient to have a similar effect.

(2) Roughness of the vessel lining which sometimes remains after healing of some earlier injury favors lodgment of platelets. If they are slightly injured in this process, it is thought that they they may release the necessary thromboplastin or ADP. Once started, it is easy to understand how the clotting process can continue by virtue of thromboplastin derived from the disintegration of leukocytes enmeshed in the clot already formed.

(3) Slowing or stasis of the flow of blood may be considered theoretically as a secondary cause but in reality it is of primary importance. Just as a log-jam cannot hold in a swift river, so a thrombus forms with difficulty in a strongly moving stream. Aside from mechanical factors, the current of blood dissipates the thrombin downstream before it can exert its effect. Generalized slowing of the circulation occurs in connection with cardiac insufficiency with its chronic

passive congestion, hence thrombosis is to be feared in this condition. Localized venous congestion and stasis is the rule in extensive inflammations (p. 147). This, with vascular injury due to the infection usually present, accounts for the frequent thrombosis of vessels in extensive areas of inflammation, such as metritis.

(4) Disruption of the laminar flow of blood predisposes to thrombosis by allowing platelets and blood cells to contact the vascular endothelium. Normally these elements are separated from the vascular surface by a zone of plasma. Aneurysms, varices, lodged emboli (p. 113) and extrinsic pressures all produce distortion which results in a turbulence in the flow of blood.

(5) Changes in the composition of blood may also predispose to thrombosis. Thrombosis has been associated with an increase in the number and adhesiveness of platelets which may follow surgical procedures, parturition, accidental trauma and other conditions associated with extensive tissue damage. Thrombosis is frequent in human beings with polycythemia (p. 1170), which produces an increased viscosity of the blood. It has also been demonstrated that increased secretion of catecholamines and epinephrine will hasten coagulation and predispose to thrombosis.

Significance, Effects and Outcome.—Thrombi in arteries completely or partially obstruct the flow of blood to the part supplied by the particular vessel. Depending on the local vascular anatomy, complete occlusion of the artery may be followed by necrosis in accordance with principles already set forth (p. 17), or a **collateral circulation** may fill the breach if there are nearby arteries whose branches anastomose with the terminal network of the occluded artery. If an area of necrosis results, it is called an infarct, as has already been explained (p. 28).

In the horse, severe injury to the **anterior mesenteric artery** (rarely others) caused by invasion of **larvae** of *Strongylus vulgaris* and other worms is so common that every equine autopsy should include examination of this artery. Proliferative arteritis with more or less thrombosis, or perhaps an aneurysm, develops. Thrombi may so restrict the flow of blood to the small intestine that attacks of acute colicky indigestion may become recurrent. This is the "thrombotic colic" described in clinical literature. In many of these cases the artery returns to normal after the parasites leave, as is shown by the much lower incidence of strongyle arteritis in late winter and spring than in the other half of the year.

Thrombosis of the **iliac arteries** is a cause of intermittent lameness of both hind legs in the horse. The obstruction is not complete; if it were, a fatal outcome would soon result; but the flow of blood is typically restricted to the extent that it is sufficient only for the resting animal. Upon vigorous excercise, agonizing and disabling pain arises due to anoxia of the involved muscles, only to disappear when the shortage of oxygen has been relieved by rest. Thrombosis in this location appears to be due also to the ravages of strongyle larvæ, aberrant parasites in this case.

Thrombosis of coronary vessels, so important in human medicine, is rare in the domestic animal.

Despite all that may be said of thrombosis of arteries, the condition is, in general, much more frequent in veins. This is because of the normally slower flow and more easily produced stasis in veins. In humans bedridden from some other cause, thrombosis of the veins of the leg is prone to occur purely because of stagnation of the venous circulation and practical collapse of these almost empty

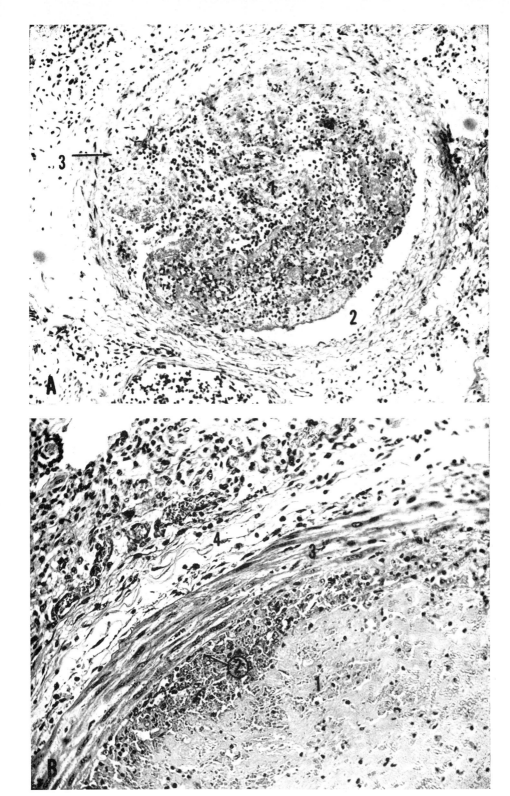

Fig. 5–1.—*A*, Thrombosis of branch of pulmonary artery, lung of a five-year-old Cocker Spaniel with pyometra. Thrombus (*1*), lumen of artery (*2*), attachment of thrombus to intima (*3*). (Courtesy of Armed Forces Institute of Pathology.) × 115. Contributor: Dr. Samuel Pollock.

B, Thrombosis of branch of pulmonary artery in an eleven-year-old Scottish Terrier with chronic valvular endocarditis. Hyaline material in the thrombus (*1*), proliferation of endothelium (*2*), media of distended artery (*3*), and edema in the adventitia (*4*). (Courtesy of Armed Forces Institute of Pathology.) × 185. Contributor: Dr. Elihu Bond.

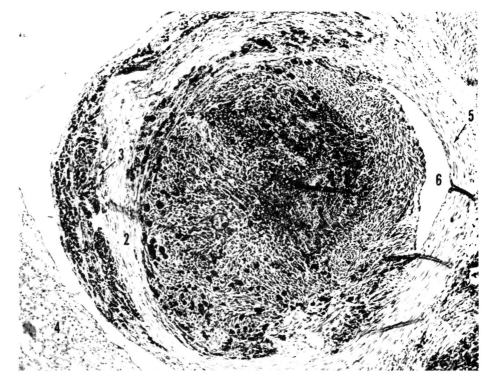

Fig. 5–2.—Thrombosis of renal artery by implantation of a tumor embolus. The neoplasm was a malignant melanoma, primary in the oral mucosa of a nine-year-old dog. Tumor (*1*) attached to artery wall (*2*) which has been penetrated by tumor cells (*3*). Renal tubules (*4*), uninvolved artery wall (*5*) and lumen of the artery (*6*). (Courtesy of Armed Forces Institute of Pathology.) × 70. Contributor: Dr. F. L. Povar.

veins. The same possibility in animals can be added to hypostatic congestion (p. 132), as another reason for frequently turning over a sick animal which is unable to do this for itself. Thrombosis and obstruction of veins tend to cause edema (p. 134) of the part drained because of retarded outflow of fluid.

Ever present in the case of venous thrombosis, wherever it may be located, is the danger of fragments of the clot breaking off to be carried in the blood flow as emboli (p. 113). These continue to float along until stopped at some bifurcation where the lumens become too small to permit their passage. Venous thrombi may release emboli which pass through the heart and are stopped in the smaller vessels of the lungs or brain with fatal results.

Thrombi do not remain as such indefinitely. Many are slowly liquefied by plasmin (p. 107) and possibly by enzymes of leukocytes, the erythrocytes having disappeared by autolysis after two or three days. Others, unfortunately, undergo organization into fibrous connective tissue. Fibrin appears to be an especially fertile field for the multiplication of fibroblasts, which invade it from the surrounding fibrous tissue. The thrombus then becomes a permanent tissue.

The histopathologist needs to be alert in the recognition of such **old, organized thrombi.** The fibrous tissue is usually mature with no special features to make it conspicuous, except that it may take a circular arrangement. Usually, but not invariably, there are some remnants of the encircling smooth muscle. There may be some hemosiderin or hematoidin, the result of hemolysis of erythrocytes caught in the meshes of the developing clot. Occasionally an irregular area of calcification may mark the site of decomposing fibrin and dead blood cells. Sometimes the whole mass is neatly encapsulated by an encircling fibrous wall. If the thrombus has been canalized, it may puzzle the inexperienced with one or more irregular blood passages much too large to be capillaries but having no wall except a single endothelial layer, all buried in fibrous tissue.

EMBOLI AND EMBOLISM

Emboli are foreign bodies floating in the blood stream. Several kinds are recognized. (1) Simple emboli, or **fibrinous emboli** (thrombo-emboli) are pieces of thrombi which have been broken loose by the force of the blood stream. In microscopic and gross appearance, they resemble thrombi. They are almost always found lodged at an arterial bifurcation or other place where the lumen of the artery becomes too small to permit their passage. The cause is obvious.

As can be seen from what has been said on the subject of thrombosis, when an embolus of fibrin becomes arrested in a vessel, it usually brings with it a certain amount of thrombin and the conditions are met for the process of thrombosis to proceed. Hence, if the embolus itself does not entirely obstruct the flow of blood, the thrombus formed around it does so. Thus, the effect of the embolus is to produce obstruction with the same consequences as if it were a thrombus originally.

(2) **Fatty emboli** are drops of the patient's fat, which at normal body temperature has a consistency little beyond that of oil. Since oil and water do not mix readily, the fat remains as separate bodies in the circulating blood. While not detected grossly, they are readily seen microscopically if a fat stain is applied to the section in the usual way. Usually they fill the capillaries or arterioles, being lodged in them.

The cause of fat embolism is the sudden release of body fat from numbers of adipose cells. This may occur when a long bone is fractured with considerable splintering and then subjected to movements which cause jagged ends to jab into the marrow cavity repeatedly. The animal must, of course, have passed the age when the cavity would contain red marrow, Less easily, fatty embolism can occur from severe trauma of subcutaneous fat in obese individuals and from metabolic failure in occasional diabetics (p. 1018).

Fat emboli in the heart, lung or kidney have been known to result from the extreme fatty change of "deficiency hepatitis" brought on by a deficiency of choline, methionine or cystine (p. 38). In these disorders, of experimental animals chiefly, the overloaded hepatic cells in the centers of the lobules sometimes rupture and discharge their accumulated fat so that it coalesces into "fat cysts," whence the fat may find its way into the blood stream. (We must remember, of course, that many body fats are not far from their melting points at the temperature of the living body in a given species.) A similar situation has been known in human alcoholics.

The emboli are usually numerous and are carried back to the heart and into the lungs where they lodge as the blood passages divide and subdivide. Extensive fatty embolism is fatal through interference with the pulmonary circulation and constitutes a cause of unexpected death a short time subsequent to accidents of the nature just outlined. The condition is of some frequency in man and probably is often overlooked in animals, fat stains being necessary to demonstrate it. Nevertheless as much as 10 ml. of melted dog fat has been repeatedly injected into the veins of dogs without any untoward effects by one of the authors (Smith).

(3) **Gas emboli,** usually air emboli, form as bubbles in the blood when there is a sudden and sufficient lowering of the ambient pressure. This occurs when aviators ascend rapidly to great heights, and possibly with more severity when construction workers emerge from underwater compartments in which the air pressure has been raised to several times normal atmospheric pressure. Such a compartment can be placed on the bottom of a river, and if the air pressure is greater than the water pressure the latter is forced out, permitting men to enter and work. These compartments are called by the French name of caissons and the disorder is called **caisson disease.** It is also known as the **bends** because of the severe cramping pain which occurs when the individual is released from pressure. Since the blood has almost unhindered access to pulmonary alveolar air through walls that are quite pervious to gases, the air dissolves in the blood in proportion to the pressure, following ordinary laws of physics. The oxygen dissolved is readily utilized by the tissues but the inert nitrogen, constituting four-fifths of the air, can only remain in solution, the blood being saturated for that particular pressure. If the pressure is suddenly reduced (by ascent of the worker from the caisson), there is nothing for the nitrogen to do but to bubble out. The gas bubbles are capable of stopping the flow in small capillaries and the condition is sometimes fatal. The remedy is to release the pressure very slowly.

Very rarely air embolism may result from air being sucked into the venous circulation through large, gaping wounds so located that respiratory or other move-

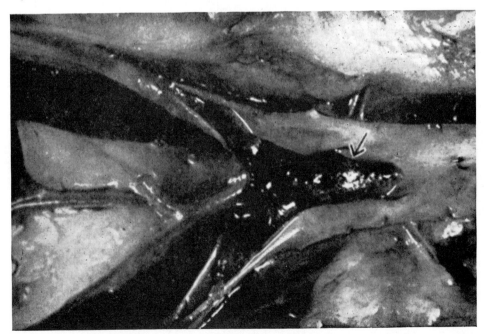

Fig. 5–3.—Saddle embolus (arrow) at bifurcation of the aorta of an eight-year-old spayed female cat. This embolus presumably originated in the left atrium. Courtesy of Angell Memorial Animal Hospital.

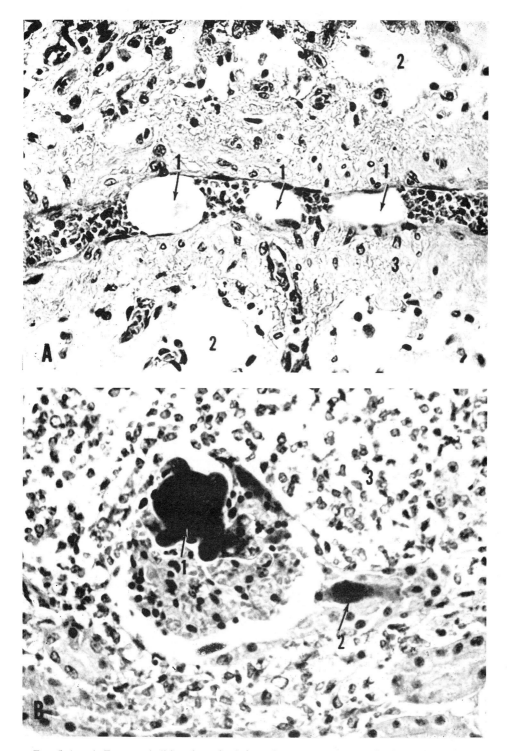

Fig. 5–4.—*A*, Fatty emboli in a branch of the pulmonary artery of a dog hit and killed by an automobile. Globules of fat (*1*) expand the arterial wall and displace blood cells. Pulmonary alveoli (*2*) are present in the section. (Courtesy of Armed Forces Institute of Pathology.) × 395. Contributor: Dr. Elihu Bond.

B, Bacterial emboli in a renal glomerulus of a foal infected with *Shigella equuli*. A bacterial colony is seen in the glomerulus (*1*) and in the efferent tubule (*2*); leukocytes have accumulated around the glomerulus (*3*). (Courtesy of Armed Forces Institute of Pathology.) × 315. Contributor: Army Veterinary Research Laboratory.

ments of the exposed fasciæ and muscles can exert a pumping action. Less un-usual is the pumping of air into surrounding tissues from such wounds, producing merely emphysema (p. 1121), but not involving the blood.

The injection of air into the veins should be mentioned here. In some bio-logical laboratories a routine method of killing experimental rabbits is to inject some 10 ml. of air into the ear vein. This causes almost instant death. However, a comparable amount of air for a man or for most of our domestic animals would be much larger. The accidental inclusion of a little air in making an ordi-nary intravenous injection involves no danger.

(4) **Bacterial Emboli.**—Clumps of bacterial cells are sometimes mechanically detached into the venous flow from tissues heavily infected with pathogenic organisms. Such emboli are often stopped in capillaries to which they are carried after leaving the heart. Interference with the circulation is insignificant, but such groups of bacteria usually multiply at the place where they lodge and are much more likely to set up a new focus, or center, of infection than scattered, single cells would be. Such a transfer of infection is known as **metastasis.** While some organs are not a fertile field for the growth of certain species of bacteria, in general the frequency with which a given organ suffers from such metastases is propor-tional to two things combined, the amount of blood flowing through it in a given time and the extent of fine capillaries through which such blood is filtered. This means that liver, kidneys and lungs are the most frequent recipients of metastatic infections.

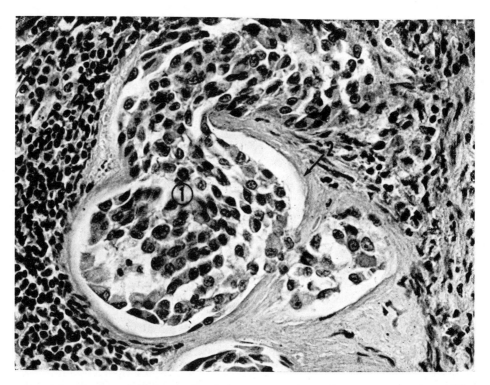

FIG. 5–5.—Tumor embolus in a small splenic artery of a dog. The primary site of this undiffer-entiated carcinoma (1) was not determined. The artery wall is indicated at (2). An infarct resulted from this embolus. (Courtesy of Armed Forces Institute of Pathology.) × 350. Con-tributor: Dr. David E. Lawrence.

(5) **Parasitic emboli** include fragments of adult canine heartworms, *Dirofilaria immitis*, usually in the branches of the pulmonary artery, clumps of blood flukes, *Schistosoma sp.*, and possibly of agglutinated trypanosomes. Embolism of this kind is infrequent.

(6) Emboli of **neoplastic cells** are occasionally seen and must occur with frequency, since it is by clumps of tumor cells carried in the blood that malignant neoplasms are able to colonize in new locations. One may see with some frequency the spot where a growing neoplasm breaks into a vein, and it is easy to understand how clumps of its cells are broken off and carried away to lodge in a new location.

(7) **Spodogenous emboli,** often called spodogenous thrombi, are clumps of blood cells which have been agglutinated (glued together) by immunological processes, or by injection of incompatible types of blood. Also included are masses of precipitated protein which result from certain kinds of irritant chemicals injected into the blood stream. Chloral hydrate, commonly used as an anesthetic, is thought to produce such precipitation rarely, with death sometimes resulting.

(8) Other types of emboli include: red bone marrow emboli following fractures; amniotic fluid emboli; hepatic emboli following trauma to the liver; foreign bodies such as broken needles or hair introduced in venipuncture; trophoblast emboli which occur with frequency in the chinchilla.

FAILURE TO CLOT

Under certain conditions there is partial or total interference with the normal clotting process. Such phenomena are of diagnostic interest to the post-mortem pathologist and are of vital concern during life. The conditions in which the clotting power of the blood is seriously impaired include the following:

(1) In **septicemic diseases,** the expected clotting in the vessels after death may not materialize. This is so much the rule in animals dead of anthrax (p. 570) that failure of the blood to clot is considered an important diagnostic sign. Anoxemia has been blamed for failure of the clotting mechanism but this is not proven.

(2) **Destructive lesions of the liver,** such as occur in severe forms of acute (p. 1223) and chronic hepatitis (cirrhosis, p. 1225), may result in failure of clotting due to deficiency of prothrombin, which is produced by the liver cells. We should be aware, however, of the great reserve capacity of the liver. The damage to hepatic cells must be severe and well-nigh universal if its effect is to be felt in impairment of this function. Fibrinogen, Factor VII, the Stuart factor (factor X) and probably the Christmas factor (factor IX) are also synthesized by the liver.

(3) *Hypocalcemia* can theoretically be included as a cause of failure to clot; however, it is unlikely that this mechanism is of importance *in vivo*. Calcium levels required to prolong coagulation time are well below those which would induce other clinical manifestations of hypocalcemia.

(4) **Deficiency of vitamin K** (2-methyl-1, 4 naphthaquinone) can lower the amount of several clotting factors in the blood with resultant impairment of clotting. Vitamin K is required for the synthesis of prothrombin, Christmas factor (factor IX) Stuart factor (factor X) and factor VII. However, this deficiency is largely limited to the experimental laboratory and is not likely to be

encountered in animals fed any natural or ordinary diet which usually contain ample vitamin K. Also vitamin K is synthesized by bacterial action in the intestine.

(5) **Sweet-clover poisoning** has resulted in uncontrollable and fatal hemorrhage in numerous bovine animals fed for several weeks or longer on sweet-clover hay (*Mellilotus alba et sp.*). The active principle responsible for this action has been found to be *Dicumarol* (3,3'-methylenebis 4-hydroxycoumarin) also known as coumarin and dicoumarin. Dicumarol acts as an antagonist to vitamin K (p. 997). (See Poisoning by Sweet Clover and "Warfarin," p. 906.)

(6) **Thrombocytopenia** or a diminished number of circulating platelets results in an interference with clotting and hemorrhage. The disease occurs as a primary or *idiopathic thrombocytopenia* in which case the cause is not known and as *secondary thrombocytopenia* resulting from certain poisonings, sensitivities and other blood dyscrasias. Both forms are discussed elsewhere (pp. 1173, 1174).

(7) **Hemophilia** is an inherited defect of the coagulation mechanism. Several forms of the disease are known in man, each affecting a specific coagulation factor.

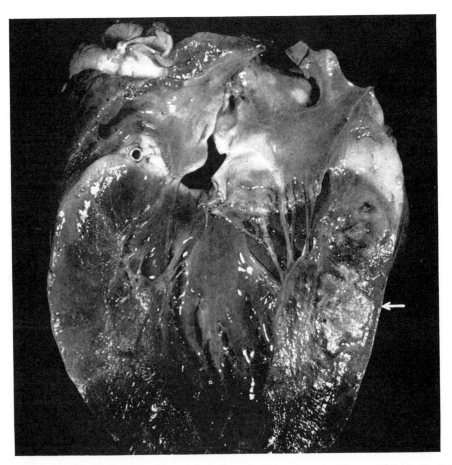

Fig. 5–6.—Infarction of myocardium of left ventricle of heart of an eight-year-old male Airedale dog with malignant lymphoma. The infarction is believed to be the result of occlusion of a branch of the left coronary artery by tumor growth. **Courtesy of Angell Memorial Animal Hospital.**

In dogs, two forms are known to occur: hemophilia A resulting from a deficiency of antihemophilic globulin (factor VIII); and hemophilia B due to a deficiency of the Christmas factor (factor IX). Both are transmitted as recessive sex-linked traits (p. 1175). Sex-linked hereditary hemophilia A also occurs in horses. A disease resembling hemophilia A has been reported in pigs which appears to be transmitted by an autosomal recessive gene (p. 1175). Hereditary factor VII deficiency has also been reported in dogs, but hemophilia is not a usual finding in these animals.

HEMORRHAGE

Hemorrhage is the escape of blood from a vessel, whether it be to the outside of the body, into a body cavity or into adjacent tissues. The ordinary rapid flow of blood through a break or cut in a vessel wall is called **hemorrhage by rhexis** (a bursting)   Considerable amounts of blood may also be lost by a slow oozing of fluid and the escape of blood cells one by one through minute or imperceptible imperfections in the vessel walls. This is called **hemorrhage by diapedesis.**

Tiny hemorrhages which leave dots of blood not much larger than the point of a pin are called **petechiae** (singular, petechia). Somewhat larger hemorrhagic spots on a body surface or in the tissues are called **ecchymoses** (singular, ecchymosis). **Extravasations** refer to hemorrhages in the tissues spread over considerable areas.

When blood escapes into the tissues and produces a tumor-like enlargement, the mass usually goes by the name of **hematoma,** although **hematocyst** is more appropriate. A very simple example is the common "blood blister," familiar to all who have aimed a hammer blow at a nail but somehow had it strike the thumb.

The **causes of hemorrhage** include the following:

(1) Any mechanical **trauma cutting or breaking a blood vessel.**

(2) **Necrosis** or destruction **of a vessel wall,** as when it is invaded by an ulcer or a spreading neoplasm.

(3) **Rupture of a vessel** weakened by aneurysm or atheroma. An **aneurysm** is a sharp bulging of the wall of a blood vessel which occurs when the wall is weakened or partially destroyed. Aneurysms of the anterior mesenteric artery have been mentioned in connection with thrombosis. **Atheromas** are proliferative thickenings which are prone to develop in the walls of larger arteries, including the aorta, from poorly understood causes. They consist of strata of necrotic and semi-necrotic wall, deposits of cholesterol and other lipids, and fibrous tissue proliferated in an attempt at healing. While the vascular wall is thicker, it is by no means stronger.

(4) **Toxic injury to capillary endothelium** culminating in transient openings of punctiform size is chiefly responsible for the petechiæ and ecchymoses seen on serous and mucous membranes, as well as within the depths of the tissues. The causes of this toxic injury are:

(a) Toxins produced by septicemic infections such as hog cholera, pasteurellosis, anthrax, blackleg and the probably allergic purpura hemorrhagica.

(b) Certain plant poisonings, including bracken poisoning, *Crotalaria* poisoning, and sweet-clover poisoning, (p. 906).

(c) Various chemical poisonings including arsenic.

(d) Certain digestive toxemias, especially entero-toxemia of sheep, in which the

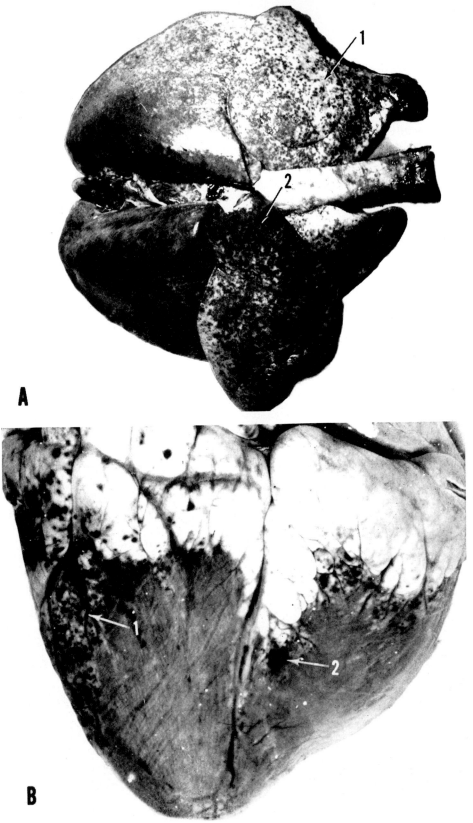

FIG. 5-7.—Hemorrhage. *A*, Petechiae (*1*) and extravasations (*2*) of blood in the pleura of a dog dying of fulminant leptospirosis. *B*, Petechiae (*1*) and ecchymoses (*2*) in epicardium of the heart of a Hereford cow following intravenous injection of formalin solution.

toxin of *Clostridium perfringens* (also known by a variety of other more or less evanescent names) is present, (p. 1211).

(*e*) Vitamin C deficiency, or scurvy (p. 990), results in an increased capillary fragility leading to hemorrhage. Most animals synthesize adequate vitamin C and are not subject to deficiency. However, scurvy is frequently encountered in guinea pigs and non-human primates (monkeys and apes) which require an exogenous source of this vitamin.

(*f*) Last but by no means least, anoxia, whether it results from direct suffocation or from anemia or any other interference with adequate aeration of the blood. It may well be that many of the other causes just listed are fundamentally an interference with oxidative processes.

The fact that the presence of numerous petechiae or ecchymoses is due to some one of the above causes is a very useful aid to the practicing diagnostician. In general they are most commonly found on the epicardial surface but hemorrhages are also frequent in the endocardium. The thymus is an especially frequent site for the development of pin-point hemorrhages.

(5) **Disorders of the clotting mechanism**, such as that due to the action of dicoumarin and other substances listed under "Failure to Clot" (p. 117), can be considered secondary causes of hemorrhage, once a slight weakness of the capillary wall develops. Whether such substances also injure the endothelial lining cells is unsettled.

(6) Rupture of diseased (arteriosclerotic or atherosclerotic) blood vessels or of aneurysms is made more likely by **the increase of blood pressure** which goes with excitement or exercise.

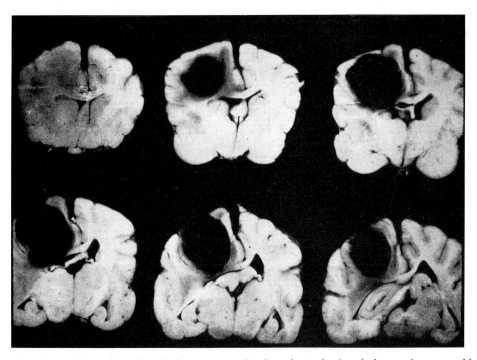

FIG. 5–8.—Hemorrhage into brain as a complication of arteriosclerosis in a twleve-year-old male Spitz dog. The brain has been sectioned at 1 cm intervals. Courtesy of Angell Memorial Animal Hospital.

Significance and Effect.—In reviewing the results of hemorrhage, we have to consider the effects of the escaped blood if it remains in the body cavities or tissues and the effects of the loss of blood from the circulation. Blood which flows into the tissues or cavities of the body soon clots and its subsequent history has been discussed under the heading of "Clots" (p. 108). Its relation to icterus (p. 74) and to hemosiderin (p. 71) have been pointed out.

The location of hemorrhage is of great importance to its significance. Hemorrhage into the brain may result in the loss of vital functions or result in permanent disability. Hemorrhage into the pericardial cavity may mechanically interfere with cardiac function. Hemorrhage into the trachea or bronchi may result in asphyxiation.

Loss of more than one-fourth or one-third of the total blood of the body will be fatal unless some of it is promptly replaced. Before this large amount is lost (25 or 30 pounds, or some 12 liters, in a 1000-pound horse), the arterial blood pressure drops markedly, which facilitates clotting, and tends to reduce further loss, so that only the largest cuts or injuries result fatally.

Following loss of a considerable amount of blood, the volume of fluid is replaced within an hour or two by withdrawal from the intercellular spaces of the tissues, great thirst resulting. Leukocytes are replaced in one or two weeks; replenishment of the full number of erythrocytes is likely to require four to six weeks.

Chronic blood loss does not lead to the serious effects of massive bleeding. Rather the continued loss of blood causes depletion of iron stores, resulting in an iron deficiency anemia (p. 127).

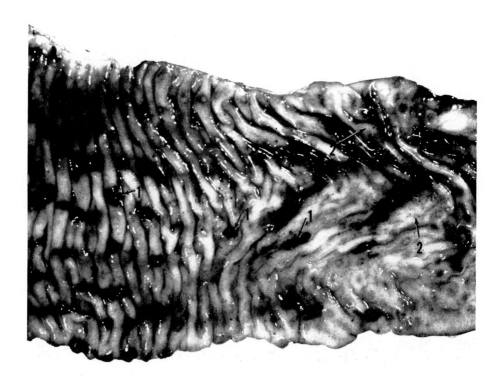

Fig. 5–9.—Hemorrhages in the colon of a dog with rickettsiosis of "salmon poisoning." Ecchymoses (*1*) and petechiae (*2*). Photograph courtesy of Dr. Wm. J. Hadlow.

ANEMIA

Anemia is defined as a reduction below normal of the number of erythrocytes and/or hemoglobin concentration per unit volume of blood. With rare exception, anemia is not a primary disease but rather develops secondary to another disorder. For example, anemia following the rutpure of an aortic aneurysm is secondary to the primary disease of the aorta; and anemia following lead poisoning is secondary to the toxic effects of lead and only represents one facet of the primary disease. Anemia, therefore, is usually a sign of another disorder and as such, the term does not represent a specific diagnosis. Anemia does, however, lead to the development of clinical signs which are secondary to the anemia. In chronic anemia these include pallor of the mucous membranes, cardiac hypertrophy, and dyspnea. Edema (p. 134) may occur secondary to loss of plasma proteins in blood loss anemia. In anemia resulting from acute massive hemorrhage, the clinical signs are referable to those of hemorrhagic shock (p. 140).

Anemias can be classified as to their cause and on the basis of morphologic characteristics of the erythrocytes. Obviously an etiologic classification is more meaningful and useful in that anemia is a secondary lesion, but morphologic characteristics are often extremely helpful in ascertaining the primary disorder.

Morphologic Classification.—Two features of the red blood cell are used to classify an anemia on a morphologic basis—their size and their hemoglobin content. The size is expressed as **mean corpuscular volume (MCV)** which is determined by dividing the packed cell volume (PCV) in per cent by the erythrocyte count in millions per cu. mm. and multiplying by 10. The answer is expressed in cubic microns. For example for a PCV of 42 per cent and an erythrocyte count of 6,000,000/mm.^{3}, the MCV is 70 cubic microns $\left(\dfrac{42}{6} \times 10 = 70 \right)$. The hemoglobin content is expressed as the **mean corpuscular hemoglobin concentration (MCHC)** which is determined by dividing the hemoglobin in grams per 100 ml. of blood by the PCV in per cent and multiplying by 100. The answer is expressed as per cent hemoglobin per cell. For example, for a hemoglobin of 14 gm. per cent and a PCV of 42, the MCHC is 33.3 per cent $\left(\dfrac{14}{42} \times 100 = 33.3 \right)$. Based on MCV and MCHC, anemias can be classified as macrocytic, normocytic, or microcytic and either normochromic or hypochromic. Hyperchromic anemias do not exist in that there is a limit to the percentage of hemoglobin that can exist in an erythrocyte. This is generally accepted as 33.3 per cent (normochromic). However, an abnormally large erythrocyte in a macrocytic anemia may contain more hemoglobin by weight than a cell of normal size, even though both are normochromic. The amount of hemoglobin in micro-micrograms per erythrocyte is termed **mean corpuscular hemoglobin (MCH)** and is calculated by dividing hemoglobin in grams per 100 ml. of blood by erythrocytes in millions per cu. mm. and multiplying by 10. As example, for a 14 gm. per cent hemoglobin and an erythrocyte count of 6,000,000/mm.^{3}, the MCH is 23.3 micro-micrograms $\left(\dfrac{14}{6} \times 10 = 23.3 \right)$. However, in the classification of anemias MCH is not used to determine hypochromasia or normochromasia.

Macrocytic anemias are most frequent following acute blood loss or acute hemolytic anemia. The outpouring of less mature erythrocytes (reticulocytes) in response to the anemia accounts for the increase in MCV. These cells are usually hypochromic. *Macrocytic normochromic anemias* result from deficiency of vitamin B_{12}, folic acid and niacin.

Normocytic normochromic anemias are the most frequently encountered anemias in animals. They result from depression of erythrogenesis and are, therefore, often referred to as *aplastic anemias*. Neoplastic diseases, irradiation and certain toxicities may produce this form of anemia.

Microcytic hypochromic anemia is the classical iron deficiency anemia or "tired blood" to the modern generation. It may follow dietary deficiency of iron or chronic blood loss. Nutritional deficiencies of copper and pyridoxine also produce microcytic hypochromic anemias. Copper is necessary for the utilization of iron in the production of hemoglobin.

Other Features of Anemia.—While the enumeration of erythrocytes, the determination of hemoglobin, and the calculation of MCV and MCHC are the correct and certain way to establish the presence or absence of anemia, certain other signs afford strong presumptive evidence of the disorder. In the blood film, or smear, stained as for making the white-cell differential count, anemic blood is likely to show one or several of the following changes: In **anisocytosis,** the erythrocytes are not of sufficiently uniform size, some are markedly larger than others. One should observe by practice how much variation occurs in normal blood, which is not very much. In **poikilocytosis,** some of the erythrocytes have bizarre and abnormal shapes, being elongated, angular, ovoid or irregularly distorted. The blood film may show occasional **nucleated erythrocytes.** These cells, because of the abnormal demand for replenishment of losses in the circulating blood, were hurried out of the bone marrow before they were completely mature, just as some nations, hard-pressed in war, have sent sixteen-year-olds into battle. By a somewhat similar mechanism **rubriblasts** occasionally are found in the blood smear, although normally they never leave the bone marrow. In **basophilic stippling,** minute dark specks appear in the erythrocyte, usually several

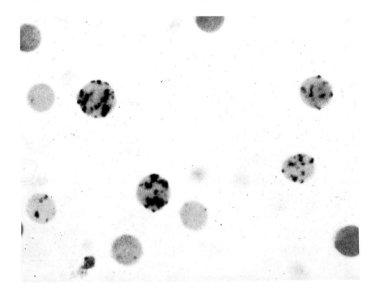

Fig. 5–10.—Reticulocytosis following acute blood loss in a rhesus monkey (*Macaca mulatta*). (Courtesy New England Regional Primate Research Center, Harvard Medical School.)

or many in one cell. This feature is especially common following acute blood loss in cattle and sheep. In **polychromatophilia** the erythrocytes do not stain uniformly, either as one is compared to another or within the boundaries of the same cell. One should be cautious, however, in attaching significance to paleness in cells which take a weak, but uniform stain. *Polychromatophilic erythrocytes* are generally reticulocytes which have entered the peripheral blood in response to blood loss and are evidence of active erythrogenesis.

Other evidences of anemia to be found in the tissues include hyperplasia of the bone marrow (p. 1168), a proliferation of red marrow in places where fatty marrow is normal for a given age. Sections of spleen or liver may rarely show erythropoietic centers in severe and prolonged anemia, these organs regaining some of the hematopoietic functions which they had during embryonic life. Such hematopoietic centers consist of a variety of hyperchromatic cells which are essentially myeloblasts, but which may be confused with foci of inflammatory leukocytes. The finding of nucleated erythrocytes in these collections of dark cells is the needed assurance as to their true nature. Megakaryocytes may also be present in these foci. Extramedullary hematopoiesis is not always indicative of a response to anemia. In most species it is normal for varying periods of time in the liver and spleen and in certain animals such as rodents, hematopoiesis occurs in the spleen throughout life.

In certain hemolytic anemias denaturation and precipitation of hemoglobin results in the occurrence of supravitally stainable, refractile, purplish granules near the erythrocyte membrane known as **Heinz bodies.**

Gross Appearance.—The mucous membranes are unusually pale during life. After death the same is seen to be true of these membranes and the tissues generally. At autopsy the blood may be noticeably pale and watery, but one must not let his enthusiasm run away with his judgment in this observation. Distinct gray dots in the liver may possibly be hematopoietic centers, although they are much more likely to be minute foci of necrosis. The hyperplastic bone marrow is, of course, a gross, as well as a microscopic, observation. With the exception of the last, all these gross indications of anemia are equivocal and have led many observers into error.

Causes.—Like our bank account, the body's store of erythrocytes can be depleted either because of too heavy withdrawals or through failure of replenishment. Anemia can result from loss or destruction of excessive numbers of circulating erythrocytes or from functional failure of the hematopoietic tissue of the bone marrow. On the basis of the causative mechanism, anemias can be classified under five types.

1. **Hemorrhagic** anemia results from severe hemorrhages.

Acute hemorrhagic anemia is that which follows single or multiple severe hemorrhages. The color and cell-volume indices are normal. As stated under the subject of Hemorrhage, regeneration is complete in a month or six weeks. In addition to traumatic causes, acute bleeding may accompany idiopathic thrombocytopenic purpura, sweet clover and warfarin poisoning, bracken fern poisoning and poisoning from trichlorethylene-extracted soybean oil meal.

Chronic hemorrhagic anemia results from continued loss of blood in a series of small hemorrhages. The hemorrhages may be due to unhealed ulcers, such as the human peptic ulcer, but in animals they are much more frequently due to heavy infestations with blood-sucking parasites of which **hookworms, the stomach worm** of ruminants, *Hemonchus contortus,* and the intestinal **strongyles** of the horse are outstanding. This type of anemia tends to be hypochromic and slightly **macro-cytic** or normocytic. Poikilocytosis is prominent, as is hyperplasia of the bone marrow. After some time the iron stores of the body approach exhaustion, and this type of anemia becomes the microcytic anemia of iron deficiency. Hemo-philia and vitamin C deficiency also result in chronic hemorrhagic anemia.

2. **Hemolytic anemia** results from excessive destruction of the circulating erythrocytes, occurring within the blood stream. Accompanying disturbances which assist in identifying this type of anemia are hemolytic icterus, which may be detected by a high bilirubin level in the blood as well as by the physical signs (p. 74), hemoglobinuria in the acute forms and, in more chronic forms, stimula-tion of the bone marrow, shown in the blood picture by nucleated red cells and reticulocytes.

The causes are infectious, toxic and immunologic. They include several infec-tions of the erythrocytes themselves such as (1) piroplasmosis, (2) anaplasmosis, (3) eperythrozoonosis of swine, and cattle, (4) hemobartonellosis of dogs and cats, (5) malaria of humans, monkeys and of birds. Among the piroplasmoses are not only the North American tick fever caused by *Babesia* (*Piroplasma*) *bigemina,* now extinct in the United States, but also similar tick-borne infections caused by other species of *Babesia,* and also piroplasmoses in other species of hosts, particu-larly the dog. (6) The virus of equine infectious anemia is an equally potent destroyer of erythrocytes. (7) The trypanosomiases destroy large numbers of erythrocytes, presumably by the action of toxins; in dourine the red-cell count is said to reach a figure as low as one-tenth of the normal. Several acute bacterial infections, including those due to (8) *Streptococcus "hemolyticus,"* (9) *Clostridium hemolyticum bovis,* (10) *Clostridium welchii* and (11) *Leptospirae* cause rapid destruction of erythrocytes and severe anemia, although this aspect of the disease is likely to be overshadowed by more startling symptoms and lesions. The same may be said about most (12) snake venoms. Certain chemical poisons have a sim-ilar effect, including (13) potassium and sodium chlorate (used to sterilize the soil of weeds and sometimes eaten by cattle), (14) lead, usually as a chronic poisoning, and (15) chronic copper poisoning (p. 866) formerly known as ictero-hemo-globinuria of sheep. (16) Ricin, the toxic principle of castor beans, (17) phenyl-hydrazine and, to a lesser extent, (18) saponin are other strongly hemolytic poisons. (19) The anemia which often accompanies poisoning by kale and rape (p. 925) is believed to be of hemolytic origin.

To this list of causes of hemolytic anemia should be added what is best called **hemolytic disease of the newborn,** also known as **erythroblastosis fetalis, neo-natal isoerythrolysis,** etc. Connected with the red blood cells of most humans, there is an inherited antigen known as the Rh factor which will stimulate in persons not having it (Rh-negative) the formation of antibodies which both agglu-tinate and hemolyze the "Rh-positive" erythrocytes. The process comes to light when an infant inherits the antigen (the Rh factor) from its father and is born of an "Rh-negative" mother. Through placental interchange the mother is exposed to the antigen from the blood of the fetus. To her, being herself without this substance, it is a foreign protein and she develops in her blood the said antibodies against it. Again via placental interchange some of the antibodies enter the blood of the fetus and begin their destructive action on its erythrocytes. When the infant is born, then, it already has a case of hemolytic anemia, and probably of hemolytic jaundice, as well, depending on the severity of the disorder, and it may well be unable to carry on the function of oxygenation as an independent being. It does not appear that the Rh factor exists in animals, but foals, especially mule foals, and pigs and possibly puppies are sometimes born of mothers which have antibodies against the erythrocytes of their newborn offspring. Limited experimental work suggests that the sensitizing antigen is derived somehow from the male parent much as is the case with the inherited Rh factor. There is this difference, however: as is usual in the transmission of antibodies in the species just mentioned, the offspring receives the agglutinating-hemolyzing antibodies, not through the placenta but with its first several nursings of colostrum (which suggests a means of prevention). The resulting jaundice is known as **icterus neonatorum** or **neonatal jaundice.** In non-human primates hemolytic disease of the newborn has been reported in baboons, macaques and marmosets. As in man, antibodies cross the placenta in these species. The diagnosis and/or prediction of this malady in man and animals is aided by the use of the direct or indirect Coombs' test.

Autoimmune hemolytic anemia represents another immunologic hemolytic anemia. Well known for years in man, and more recently in dogs, this disease results from the failure of an individual to recognize "self" with the formation of antibodies against autogenous tissues. Autoimmune disease will be treated in greater detail elsewhere (p. 312).

3. **Deficiency Anemias.**—(a) **Deficiency of Iron.**—Anemia caused by a deficiency of iron compounds in the diet, or rarely perhaps by defective assimilation of that element, is rather common in the human family and is a form easily understood, since hemoglobin cannot be made unless the elementary ingredients are available. It may be for this reason that many of us, when we think of how a case of anemia might be caused, think first of iron.

In reality anemia due to a deficiency of iron is almost never encountered in veterinary medicine, except in nurslings which have no other diet than the mother's milk. The disorder is rather frequent in nursing pigs born in the winter in cold climates, for under those circumstances the sow and her litter often spend the first several weeks in a hog house with a concrete or other type of floor. If pigs can have access to the soil their rooting will, in almost any locality, provide the minute amount of iron which is necessary. Without this or some artificial source of the element, deficiency anemia is likely to develop, for mother's milk, the much heralded "perfect food," does not contain adequate amounts of iron. Other species of animals, and swine, also, when older, almost always have a sufficiently close association with the soil or with plant food that this need is met.

This is the traditional example of hypochromic, microcytic anemia. Poikilocytosis is also prominent.

Anemia reported to result from the (experimental) feeding of certain kinds of raw fish (coal-fish, *Gadus virens*, and raw whiting, *G. merlangus*, and not other kinds) to mink was prevented by cooking the fish and cured by feeding 16 mg. of organic iron per week.

(b) Minute traces of **copper** (p. 1011) are also essential to avoid deficiency anemia. Natural deficiency is not common in that most soils contain an adequate amount of this element. However, usual amounts of copper become insufficient in the presence of excessive molybdenum. Copper is necessary for hematopoiesis by virtue of the fact that it is required for the proper utilization of iron in the production of hemoglobin. As in iron deficiency, the anemia is microcytic hypochromic.

(*c*) **Cobalt** deficiency (p. 1013) is only of concern to ruminant species. Ruminants enjoy the unique position of not requiring a dietary source of B vitamins including vitamin B_{12}. Instead, they depend upon the rumen flora which synthesize these essential metabolites. Synthesis obviously cannot proceed without certain basic raw ingredients. Cobalt being an integral component of vitamin B_{12} (cobalamin) is therefore a dietary requirement for the ruminant and deficiency of this mineral is in essence a vitamin B_{12} deficiency (pp. 984, 1013).

(*d*) *Vitamin B_{12}* deficiency (p. 984) results in a macrocytic normochromic anemia. Deficiency of this vitamin is the basic defect of cobalt deficiency of ruminants. It is required in erythropoiesis for normal development and maturation of erythrocytes, although its exact mechanism of action is not understood. Deficiency is not a commonly encountered clinical problem.

(*e*) **Folic acid** deficiency also results in a macrocytic anemia. Although it is essential for maturation of erythrocytes, an understanding of its exact biochemical function is still incomplete. The actions of vitamin B_{12} and folic acid in erythropoiesis are closely related.

(*f*) Experimentally induced **Pyridoxine deficiency** in dogs, cats, and swine results in a microcytic hypochromic anemia. Pyridoxine is required for hemoglobin synthesis. Deficiency does not appear to occur naturally.

(*g*) Other nutritional deficiencies which may result in anemia include deficiencies of riboflavin, vitamin C and protein.

(*h*) **Pernicious Anemia.** — While this type of anemia may be chiefly of academic importance in veterinary medicine the monumental achievements of Whipple (1935), Peabody (1927), Minot and Murphy (1926) and of Castle (1929) in solving the riddle of human pernicious anemia is worth the attention of anyone in the medical sciences. When one of the authors (Smith) was in college, a needy student could replenish his finances by selling a pint of his blood to be used as a transfusion to keep alive just a little longer some unfortunate person afflicted with **pernicious anemia.** Then came the discovery that the liver (of man or beast) contained a substance, the "erythrocyte-maturing factor," which, if continuously provided, would relieve the patient of all his symptoms. The demand for beef livers became such that liver changed from what was almost a waste-product to one of the more highly priced cuts of meat. Eating two pounds of raw liver a day had its disadvantages but, fortunately, science soon learned how to make concentrated extracts, which could be injected at intervals. It also learned that the mysterious "erythrocyte-maturing factor" in the liver is a storage product made by the action of an unidentified fraction of the gastric juice upon protein (of animal origin) in the food. Vitamin B_{12} is now known to be the essential constituent of the protein, and to become the erythrocyte-maturing factor upon absorption. Pernicious anemia, macrocytic and normochromic, results when this chain is broken. Usually the fault is failure of the stomach to provide its contribution, the "intrinsic factor," in the gastric juice. Many such stomachs have very atrophic glands and secrete almost no gastric juice (achylia gastrica); in others only the hydrochloric acid is demonstrably absent (achlorhydria). While its absence is concomitant with these shortages, the intrinsic factor itself has not been chemically identified. Occasionally the chain is broken through shortage of the "extrinsic factor," apparently through failure of assimilation in certain

chronic diarrheic diseases such as sprue or an actual dietary lack of animal protein, as in pellagra. Rarely the liver is so badly damaged, usually cirrhotic, that
it fails in its part of the process, which is to serve as a storage reservoir for the
finished erythrocyte-maturing substance.

Humans have an anemia of the same macrocytic type when parasitized by the
tapeworm *Diphyllobothrium latum*, apparently because of impaired assimilation
of the extrinsic factor. Perhaps the anemia which dogs show when harboring this
worm represents a parallel condition, although the presence of a hemolytic toxin
has been reported. Beyond this, human pernicious anemia appears to have no
counterpart in animals.

4. **Toxic Aplastic Anemias.**—In aplastic anemia (meaning no growth), the
hematopoietic tissues of the bone marrow are injured in such a way that their
ability to produce erythrocytes is impaired or destroyed. There is nothing remarkable about the size, shape or color of the cells which remain in the circulating
blood. There is an absence of normoblasts, megaloblasts, reticulated erythrocytes
and polychromasia (occasional basophilic staining of the cytoplasm approaching
that of early myeloid cells), all of which are signs of active erythropoiesis in the
marrow. The formation of the granulocytic leukocytes is also depressed, leading
to more or less severe **agranulocytosis.** The bone marrow in aplastic anemia is
predominantly fatty, with scattered islands of hematopoietic cells, or sometimes
it is sclerotic. Myelopoiesis is utterly destroyed in severe cases of feline panleukopenia.

To the extent that they are known, the causes are either toxic radiations or
toxic substances brought to the marrow cells in the circulating blood. These
latter include benzol poisoning, which is the classical example, trinitrotoluene
and, in the case of hypersensitized humans at least, the sulfonamides. A number
of proprietary medicines highly advertized for human self-medication are reported to be almost equally toxic. The **Bracken fern** owes some of its poisonous
effects to production of toxic aplastic anemia, as does poisoning by trichlorethylene-extracted soybean meal. **Irradiation,** whether by x-rays, radium or
the more recently developed radio-active isotopes, is highly destructive of the
hematopoietic tissues and this action is the chief reason that any but very small
dosages are lethal. Anemia from an imperfectly understood disorder of hematopoiesis occurs in association with **nephritis** and uremia, apparently through
direct toxic action of the retained waste products. Interference with the production
in the kidney of a specific enzymic substance called erythropoietin has recently
been reported as the explanation. Anemia develops in various chronic **infections**
apparently because of the effects of toxins upon the mechanism of formation of
hemoglobin. Neoplastic diseases may also result in a selective depression of
erythrogenesis.

5. **Myelophthisic Anemia.**—(*Myelo*, the marrow; *phthisis*, a wasting disease,
usually, but not necessarily tuberculosis.) This type of anemia results from physical destruction of the erythropoietic tissue, usually from its replacement by
metastatic tumor tissues. Various carcinomas are prone to fill the marrow
cavities with neoplastic tissue in their advanced stages, leaving no room for the
normal tissue, which undergoes pressure atrophy and pressure necrosis. This
also applies to the anemia which usually accompanies leukemia and malignant
lymphoma. Osteopetrosis (p. 1070) is similarly destructive to the marrow space.

Significance and Effect of Anemia.—Anoxia of the tissues is the most important product of anemia. This leads to fatty change of the myocardium and other susceptible organs and even necrosis; the heart muscle may be severely damaged. It explains the principal symptoms of rapid and perhaps irregular pulse, shortness of breath and muscular weakness. In hemolytic anemia, the spleen contains much phagocytized hemosiderin. A tendency toward hemorrhage which is characteristic of anemia can presumably be explained on the basis of anoxic damage to capillary endothelium. When edema accompanies anemia, it is conceivably related to increased permeability, but in hemorrhagic anemias protein loss is also contributory and in those cases which go with helminthiasis the continued drain of protein offers ample explanation (p. 138). Removal of the cause cures anemia except in the case of the toxic aplastic anemias, where the changes soon become irreversible.

In perusing the causes of hemolytic anemia, it is noted that they largely duplicate the list given for hemolytic icterus. It is obvious that if erythrocytes are hemolyzed excessively, there tends to be both a shortage of erythrocytes and an accumulation of the products of their destruction. If the rate surpasses the rate at which the liver can eliminate bilirubin, jaundice will result. If the rate of erythrocytic destruction exceeds the capacity of the reticulo-endothelium to convert hemoglobin to bilirubin, hemoglobinemia results, and then hemoglobinuria, as the excess is excreted in the urine.

Sudden severe anemia, otherwise unexplained, usually justifies exploratory laparotomy and search for a site of internal hemorrhage.

HYPEREMIA AND CONGESTION

Both of these terms denote an excess of blood in the vessels of a given part. This can occur in either of two ways, too much blood being brought in by the arteries or too little being drained out by the veins. Some prefer the older term, congestion; some prefer to use the other. In either case, if too much blood is brought in by the arteries, the condition is said to be "active," if the blood simply remains because of impaired venous drainage, it is "passive." Some, therefore, speak of active and passive congestion; others, of active and passive hyperemia. A distinction is also made in that hyperemia, in itself, implies the active condition of too much arterial blood being brought in by dilated arterioles and capillaries, whereas congestion implies that the flow of blood, like the flow of vehicles on a busy street, is impeded because the elements next in front cannot move out fast enough. To make misunderstanding impossible, it is well to speak always of active hyperemia and passive congestion. However, on these pages hyperemia will mean excessive arterial inflow and congestion will signify interference with the venous exit. Synonymous with passive congestion is the term "venous congestion."

ACTIVE HYPEREMIA

This condition may occur in any organ or part of the body.

Microscopic Appearance.—The capillaries are dilated and filled with blood. They also appear to be more numerous than before simply because in the normal state some are empty and collapsed much of the time. Arteries and arterioles are also dilated, but this is seldom apparent after death because post-mortem contraction of their musculature empties and closes their lumens.

Gross Appearance.—To a greater or lesser extent depending on its original color, the part takes on the bright red color of arterial blood. During life the part is also warmer than usual and pulsating arteries may be felt which are not usually perceptible.

Causes.—(1) Active hyperemia is the first stage of inflammation, and the great majority of cases are of this nature. (2) Heat, locally applied, often as a therapeutic measure, promptly brings marked dilatation of the vessels. A person need only expose his bare skin in front of a fireplace to see it redden in a few moments. (3) Increased physiological activity leads to marked increase of arterial blood, which supplies the oxygen and nutrients needed for the functions to be performed. This physiological hyperemia is seen not only in muscles, but also very strikingly in the stomach and intestines during digestion and in the mammary gland at the start of lactation. On a somewhat different basis but still physiological is the hyperemia, followed by congestion, which occurs in the decidual uterus at menstruation (p. 1301). (4) In the human, blushing is a transient hyperemia caused by a psychological disturbance.

The **significance and effect** of active hyperemia are minor when it does not mark the onset of inflammation (p. 145).

PASSIVE CONGESTION

Passive congestion may occur in practically any part of the body and it may be acute or chronic.

Microscopic Appearance.—The capillaries and veins are dilated and full of blood, likewise the sinusoidal blood spaces of the liver and spleen in case those organs are involved. If the congestion is chronic, one looks for a slight or moderate increase of fibrous tissue in the walls of the veins, thickening and strengthening them, a sort of compensatory hypertrophy (p. 93).

Acute passive congestion of the liver is frequently evidenced by sinusoidal capillaries and central veins which are conspicuously dilated but empty. This is because, when a piece of liver is put in the fixative solution preparatory to microscopic sectioning, the blood oozes out into the solution, the blood spaces retaining their dilated shape. There is also a tendency for the more central cells of the hepatic cords to disappear, leaving a central sea of blood, but this will be discussed in the section on Diseases of the Liver, as will also the appearance of chronic congestion in this organ.

Gross Appearance.—The congested part is slightly swollen and tends to have a bluish-red tinge. During life the temperature of the part may be discernibly lower than normal because of the fact that new blood is not being brought in. After death the bluish red darkens as post-mortem hemolysis advances. Considerable amounts of blood can be squeezed from the cut surface. This is an important indication in such organs as the lungs and liver.

Causes.—(1) The most important cause, by far, of acute, generalized congestion is the diminished blood pressure which goes with a failing heart and more or less vasodilation of shock in the terminal stages of many infections and other diseases. The immediate cause of death is spoken of as generalized venous congestion or **congestive heart failure.** When this situation exists, the necropsy shows the vena cava and large veins of the abdominal and thoracic cavities to be large and dark, filled with blood which, quite likely, has clotted. The veins of the mesentery and intestinal walls are prominent and dark. The liver contains much blood, as do, probably, the lungs.

(2) **Chronic passive congestion of the lungs** results from interference with the proper progress of the blood on the left side of the heart, in other words, from hindrance to its free and prompt movement from the pulmonary into the systemic circulation. Such interference occurs through either **insufficiency or stenosis of the mitral valve.** Insufficiency is a leaking back because of failure of the cusps of the valve to seat properly, which usually is the result of irregular thickening of their surfaces with inflammatory granulation tissue (p. 165) or with fibrinous exudate (p. 156). Or, the cusps may have become retracted through the shrinking of fibrous scars so that they do not completely fill the lumen. In either case when the ventricle contracts, some of the blood is forced backward through the leaky valve to impede the incoming flow in the pulmonary vein. Stenosis is a narrowing of the total size of the lumen. It results from the shrinking of fibrous scar tissue when the latter has developed around the base of the cusps. The effect again is to decrease the amount of blood which can pass the valve in a given time. All of these interfering derangements are the result of inflammation, valvular endocarditis, caused by one of a number of infections (p. 1137).

The aortic semilunar valve is subject to the same disorders as the mitral, although attacked less frequently. This does not directly affect the lungs but, in common with other valvular imperfections, leads to "compensatory" hypertrophy (really adaptive as we have classified hypertrophy, p. 93) of the left ventricle. This enlargement of the ventricle sometimes distorts the mitral valve to the extent that insufficiency develops, with the same pulmonary congestion.

(3) **Tricuspid valvular disease** is possibly more frequent in animals than mitral and this valve is subject to the same insufficiency and stenosis. In this case the blood is thrown back into the vena cava and its tributaries, the first appreciably expansible vascular channels being those of the liver. The result is **chronic passive congestion of the liver** (p. 1235). Chronic passive congestion of the liver may also be the result of severe obstruction of the flow of blood through the lungs with retardation of the flow through the right side of the heart and backing up into the liver. Hypertrophy of the right ventricle is usually an accompaniment.

(4) **Cirrhosis** (p. 1225) makes it difficult for blood to get through the liver and causes chronic passive congestion of the portal venous system including the spleen and intestines, usually with ascites (p. 139).

(5) Partial obstruction of any vein of considerable size leads to local congestion of its drainage area, unless collateral drainage is established. Such obstruction may be caused by thrombi or emboli, by stenosis as the result of fibrous scarring following phlebitis (as from repeated puncturing in intravenous administration of medicines) or by external pressure upon the vein from tumors or abscesses.

(6) During the later stages of pregnancy, pressure of the fetus upon the femoral vein as it passes over the anterior border of the pubis causes chronic passive congestion (and consequent edema) of the hind leg. This occurs at least in the equine and bovine species, in which the single fetus reaches relatively large size and in which there is little opportunity for the tensions caused by the fetus to be shifted with changes in the mother's position. The same difficulty occurs in the human species, resulting in so-called **milk-leg.**

(7) Gravity is the cause of **hypostatic congestion.** This is a congestion, often quite noticeable, of the organs and tissues on the lower side of a recumbent ani-

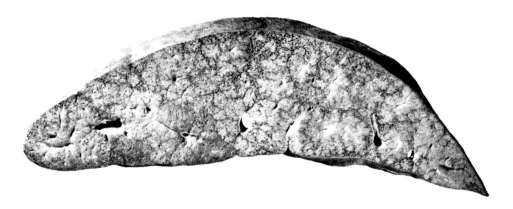

FIG. 5–11.—Chronic passive congestion of the liver of an eight-month-old Hereford steer. The underlying lesions were large firm "vegetative" masses on the leaflets of the tricuspid valve. Photograph courtesy of Dr. W. J. Hadlow.

mal. Especially in large animals, there is a strong tendency for blood to gravitate to the lower side of the body. This may cause the death of an otherwise healthy horse confined for some hours in an unnatural position from which it cannot rise. The gravitational movement continues after death until clotting interferes, so that in many cadavers the condition is interpreted merely as a post-mortem phenomenon. The prosector naturally takes this phenomenon into consideration in his interpretation of the gross lesions.

Significance and Effect.—One of the effects of passive congestion is anoxia, since fresh blood cannot be brought in. Function is impaired; for instance, the congested udder does not secrete milk of normal quantity or quality; the congested intestine does not function properly. In delicate parenchymal cells even necrosis may result. The slow movement of the current predisposes to thrombosis. Edema is a frequent result of either generalized or localized passive congestion which will be discussed presently.

The proliferation of connective tissue in chronic congestion has been mentioned. In the liver this thickens the walls of the central veins, almost nonexistent normally, and of the sinusoidal capillaries, the change being called **central cirrhosis.** Chronic passive congestion of the spleen is characterized by a diffuse fibrosis of the red pulp, with hematoidin and hemosiderin being conspicuous in amount.

Pulmonary chronic passive congestion produces the condition known as **brown induration of the lung.** The lung is indurated (hardened) because of fibrous thickening of the interalveolar septa, that is, of the capillary walls in them. This is visible microscopically and is detected grossly by a certain toughness and lack of resiliency. The brown color is due to hemosiderin. From the congested capillaries, there is a certain amount of hemorrhage by diapedesis into the alveoli. The pigment released from the disintegrating erythrocytes is phagocytized as hemosiderin by reticulo-endothelial cells, which remain to impart collectively their brownish color. Since chronic passive congestion of the lung is ordinarily the result of valvular heart disease, as just explained, the phagocytes filled with hemosiderin (p. 71) are called **heart-failure cells.**

EDEMA

Edema is a disorder characterized by an excessive accumulation of fluid (water) in the intercellular spaces, including the body cavities. Excessive fluid within the cells has already been defined as hydrops, or hydropic degeneration (p. 43), and this definition will be respected here, in spite of a certain looseness in distinguishing between hydrops and edema which is occasionally encountered. The subject of edema has long been a confusing one, and many conflicting theories have been proposed concerning the mechanisms involved. Some of the confusion has come from a certain lack of consistency of ideas regarding edema and inflammation, so that in common medical parlance we formulate certain definitions but fail to abide by them.

May we begin by dispelling one or two fallacies that may have entered the student's mind from older sources or from what may at first have seemed logical assumptions? (1) Edema is *not caused* by a heavy consumption of water. It is possible to fill an animal so full of water that serious disorders result, but edema is not one of them. (2) Edema is *not caused* by a heavy consumption of salt in the diet, notwithstanding the fact that depleting the patient's body of salts already accumulated in the tissues may be markedly beneficial in causing greater elimination of water. Cows have been fed experimentally as much as 2 pounds (Avoir-

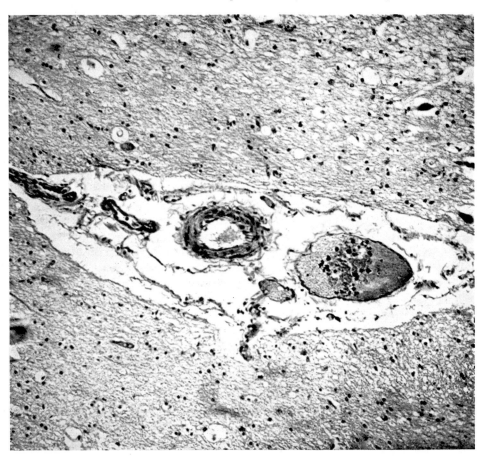

Fig. 5–12.—Perivascular edema, brain of a horse. H & E, × 200.

dupois) of ordinary salt (NaCl) per day over periods of many days without any harmful effects, and certainly without any edema (p. 850). High blood pressure (ordinary arterial pressure) does *not cause* edema. This sometimes fatal disorder is all too common in human beings, but edema is not one of the symptoms.

Edema may be general or local. As the term is freely used it may also be inflammatory or non-inflammatory, but inflammatory edema, being a reaction to an irritant, is, by definition, an inflammation. Strict adherence to this concept in one's inner consciousness, if not in one's common phraseology, should considerably simplify the subject. In this discussion edema means non-inflammatory edema, only.

Occurrence. — Localized edema may occur in most organs and tissues, dependent on local causes. Generalized edema affects the body as a whole but most of the fluid tends to accumulate, because of the force of gravity, in the lowest parts of the body which are capable of stretching to make room for it. In the quadrupeds, such places are along the ventral abdominal and chest wall and in and below the intermandibular space.

Microscopic Appearance. — When tissue is edematous, the spaces between adjacent cells, fibrils or other elemental structures are enlarged. During life they were, of course, filled with fluid; in the microscopic section there may or may not remain a faint, pink-staining residue of precipitated albumin, depending on the amount of albumin (and other protein) in the edema fluid. If the common technical procedure was followed of affixing the section to the glass slide with egg albumin, the beginner will need to guard against mistaking this albumin, which becomes visible when slightly excessive, for the residue from an edema fluid. In case it is the fixative, the pink-staining albumin is seen outside the area of the section as well as in it. Considerable judgment needs to be employed also in interpreting empty intercellular spaces. A certain, but variable amount of space is left between cells by the shrinkage which occurs in the preparation of sections by the paraffin or similar techniques. These artificial shrinkage spaces tend to be less numerous, less uniform in size and less evenly distributed than the spaces which result from edema. Shrinkage follows natural lines of cleavage, which usually lie between one kind of tissue and another, although they do not separate epithelium from its connective-tissue base. A very few erythrocytes, leukocytes or fibrils of fibrin may be present, but any considerable number of the last two indicates inflammation.

Edema of the brain betrays itself first by distention of the perivascular (Fig. 5–12, p. 134) and even the perineuronal spaces, but excessive shrinkage may be deceptive. The sulci are compressed and the convolutions flattened by pressure against the cranial wall, a situation more easily noticed grossly than microscopically. In edema of the lungs, the alveoli are filled with fluid. There is usually enough albuminous residue to render the condition noticeable microscopically.

Gross Appearance. — The edematous part is swollen. Edematous swelling along the ventral belly wall is often of a thickness of several centimeters and rather sharply delimited so that a conspicuous longitudinal ridge marks its boundaries along each side. The swelling commonly diffuses into the preputial region in males and fades out anteriorly in the sternal region. In other cases ("brisket-disease" of cattle), the swelling is most pronounced in the sternal region. Sometimes the edema is conspicuous externally only as a sagging protrusion of the submandibular tissues. This is especially true in sheep suffering from gastro-intestinal parasitism, the condition being called "bottle-jaw" among stockmen.

The swollen tissue is of firm and "doughy" consistency. It "pits on pressure," meaning that if the finger is pressed into the edematous tissue, the fluid is dis-persed into nearby tissue spaces. When the finger is removed, the pit remains for a moment since a certain interval of time is required for the fluid to filter back through the network of tissue cells and fibrils.

The cut surface, in well-marked cases, can be seen to contain a pale yellowish fluid permeating the tissue strands. There may be slight clotting, but usually the fluid drips from the cut surface; if pressure is applied, a much larger amount of fluid can be squeezed from the tissue.

During life the edematous part, if external, is cool, as well as swollen. There is no redness and no sign of pain.

Edema of the lungs is best detected at autopsy by cutting through a lobe, and squeezing the edges. If a watery fluid exudes, perhaps a little tinged with blood, the lung tissue being distended and of firm consistency, the condition is edema. If a definitely bloody fluid is pressed out, the lung is congested; if drops of pus (p. 158) appear, the condition is pneumonia. In edema of the peritoneal, pleural or other serous cavities, the cavity is filled and often distended with a clear watery fluid. Edema of the brain is recognized less, perhaps, by the watery conditions of the tissue than by the flattening of the swollen gyri as they are pressed against the cranium.

The question of whether one is dealing with **inflammatory or non-inflammatory** edema sometimes has to be answered by a study of all accompanying circum-

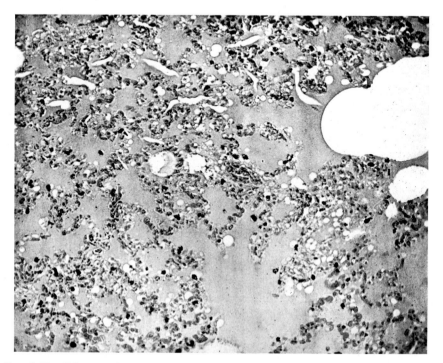

FIG. 5–13.—Edema of the lung of a dog. Note homogeneous protein material fills alveoli. H & E, × 170.

stances. The fluid of non-inflammatory edema is called a **transudate,** because it is conceived as passing from the blood into the tissues purely as the result of deranged physiological mechanisms. The fluid of inflammatory edema is called an **exudate,** being one of the types (serous) of the exudates which characterize acute inflammation. If accessible for physical examination, a transudate can usually be differentiated from a serous exudate by the specific gravity. The specific gravity of a transudate is almost invariably less than 1.017, usually less than 1.015. That of a serous exudate is ordinarily 1.017 or above. The difference is due to the much lower concentration of salts and colloids, especially albumin, in the transudate. Determinations of the total protein usually reveal less than 3 per cent in the transudate of edema; it is likely to be considerably higher in an inflammatory exudate. As would be expected from these figures, the exudate leaves a heavier precipitate of protein, chiefly albumin, in the microscopic section and inflammatory edema can usually be recognized on this basis. The exudate also contains an appreciable, or even considerable number of leukocytes and often some fibrin; the transudate contains no more than traces of these, at most. Grossly the exudate often includes some clotted fibrin and there may be a frank fibrinous inflammation (p. 156) of some of the involved surfaces.

Causes of Edema.—Physiologically the blood enters a capillary with a hydrostatic pressure (blood pressure in the usual sense) of about 45 millimeters of mercury (45 mm. Hg). Since the walls of the capillaries are rather freely permeable to fluids and to the smaller dissolved molecules such as those of crystalloids, this pressure tends to expel those substances into the surrounding intercellular spaces. But this expulsive force is opposed by the (colloidal) osmotic pressure exerted by such molecules as cannot pass through the capillary wall, chiefly the molecules of albumin and globulin, which together, amount to about 6 grams per 100 ml. This force has been computed in the human as from 30 to 35 mm. Hg, leaving an outward force of 10 to 15 mm. Hg. Hence, at the arterial end of the capillary much of the blood serum passes out into nearby intercellular spaces, where it is called lymph. As the blood current travels through the minute lumen of the capillary, its hydrostatic pressure is rapidly dissipated, declining to a figure between 11 and 16 mm. Hg. By this time, the blood passing through the capillary has lost considerable water and has become a more concentrated solution with a higher osmotic pressure than the 30 to 35 mm. given for the arterial end. The fluid already in the tissues has an opposing osmotic pressure of its own, due to the substances dissolved in it. This osmotic attraction tends to draw the water out into the tissues. Toward the lower end of the capillary, this outward attraction is doubtless somewhat diminished because the incoming watery lymph has lowered its concentration of solutes. But this difference appears to be small and is usually disregarded. Conservatively disregarding both these extravascular changes in osmotic pressure, which would lessen the expellant force existing at the terminal end of the capillary, we still have at the venous end of the capillary some 11 to 16 mm. of outward pressure opposed to 30 to 35 mm. of inward osmotic pressure, a balance of 19 mm. tending to draw fluid into the capillary. The result is a normal flow of fluid out of the capillary at its upper end and a return flow into the lumen at its venous end. Edema is the result of some interference with this normal flow.

The fundamental disturbances operating to **cause non-inflammatory edema** can be simplified to (1) decreased plasma colloid osmotic pressure, (2) increased capillary blood pressure, (3) obstruction to lymphatic drainage, and (4) retention of sodium and water.

(1) **Decreased plasma colloid osmotic pressure** is the result of hypoproteinemia. Loss of a large part of the albumin and globulin of the blood occurs in those forms of nephritis (or nephrosis) characterized by severe albuminuria. In the human species, at least, the loss of albumin is much greater than the loss of globulin, causing a "reversed albumin-globulin ratio" of 1 to 3 instead of the normal 3 to 1. In some domestic species (the bovine, especially), the proportion of albumin is normally much lower and the frequency of albuminuria much less and the precise value of the human analogy has not been adequately investigated. The preponderant loss of albumin is especially significant for its molecules are smaller and more numerous than those of globulin, therefore exerting a dominant effect on the osmotic pressure. The above-described mechanism, loss of protein and consequent loss of osmotic pressure, is the cause of the commonly encountered **renal edema.**

Serious deficiencies of blood protein also occur in starvation, protein deficiency and cachexia, the amount assimilated from the diet being just too small to replenish losses. This situation is the cause of **nutritional edema** or **cachectic edema.**

Advanced liver disease, usually in the form of cirrhosis, can also lead to hypoproteinemia due to decreased synthesis of plasma proteins. The liver is the site of production of albumin, fibrinogen and alpha and beta globulins.

Continued daily removal of blood protein can also deplete the available supply and produce hypoproteinemia. This occurs as a result of heavy infestation with bovine and ovine trichostrongyles and some other intestinal parasites whose blood-sucking bites and possibly an anti-coagulant toxin result in repeated minute hemorrhages in large numbers. This daily loss of blood with inadequate replacement accounts for the frequent cases of **parasitic edema,** as well as for the marked anemia.

(2) **Increased capillary blood pressure** usually results from **venous stasis.** This name is given to passive congestion so severe that movement of the blood has all but stopped. Such a severe obstruction of the normal venous flow does two things to the veins and capillaries and the blood in them: it greatly increases the hydrostatic pressure in the veins and the venous ends of the capillaries, and it deprives the capillary endothelium, as well as the other tissue constituents of the area, of their normal supply of oxygen and quite possibly of other nutrients. This certainly does not improve the functional capacity of the capillary walls, and it is believed to weaken them to the point where they permit the passage of albumin and other large molecules. The effect of such a movement of molecules is to lower the osmotic pressure within the capillary and raise it in the surrounding tissue fluid. However this **increased permeability** to large molecules becomes significant only in **inflammatory edema,** as is proven by the fact that the non-inflammatory transudate contains such small amounts of protein.

The effects of (1) the increased intracapillary and venous hydrostatic pressure, (2) the lowered intracapillary osmotic pressure and (3) increased osmotic pressure in the intercellular fluid, combine to neutralize the attractive forces (some 19 mm. Hg) which draw fluid back into the capillary. The result is a marked increase of the fluid which stays in the intercellular spaces, and this constitutes edema.

Since the usual cause of the venous stasis is impaired cardiac function, a weakened and worn-out heart, edema caused in this way is known as **cardiac edema.**

A changed concentration of salts (electrolytes) of course produces a corresponding change in osmotic pressure. While withdrawal of salt (NaCl) from the diet is sometimes sufficient to cause a spectacular cessation of edema, it seems very doubtful that an abnormally high concentration of electrolytes in the intercellular fluids ever occurs to serve as a cause of edema.

For practical purposes the clinician or the pathologist may well ask himself which of the four kinds, renal edema, nutritional edema, parasitic edema or cardiac edema, is present in his patient. The first three exist by virtue of hypoproteinemia; the last results from impaired cardiac action and generalized venous stasis. On the answer to this question depend the first steps to be taken in treatment.

Localized non-inflammatory edema, involving a certain organ or part of the body, is caused by localized **venous stasis** due to some obstruction such as a thrombus or external compression, or it is caused by:

(3) **Obstruction to lymphatic drainage,** which is similar to localized venous stasis, also results in edema. Examples of obstructed lymph drainage are seen in the case of lymph nodes invaded by neoplastic or granulomatous tissue so that the passage of lymph through them is blocked.

In some parts of the world human lymph nodes become obstructed due to the adult filarial worm, *Filaria bancrofti,* whose microfilariae are mosquito-borne and found in the circulating blood. The area drained through such nodes becomes edematous. A special case of obstructed lymph drainage is the accumulation of fluid in the meningeal spaces and ventricles of the brain, communicating and internal **hydrocephalus** respectively. Swelling or fibrous proliferations that would otherwise constitute insignificant anatomical derangements serve to close the minute openings through which the lymph has to drain, with continous increase of fluid and pressure atrophy of the brain parenchyma.

A similar situation exists in the eye; obstruction of the lymph drainage causes increased fluid in the eyeball with destructive intra-ocular pressure and pressure atrophy, a condition known as glaucoma. Edema within the optic papilla, known as papilledema, however, is due to increased intracranial fluid and intracranial pressure projected along the optic nerve within its meningeal covering.

(4) **Retention of sodium and water.** As stated earlier, excess consumption of either salt or water by a normal individual does not cause edema. However, failure to excrete sodium in the urine resulting secondarily in water retention does lead to generalized edema. Reduced urinary excretion of sodium can occur in congestive heart failure and in nephrosis and nephritis. It is important to recall that these diseases also produce edema by other mechanisms as indicated earlier. Increased renal tubular reabsorption is believed to be the cause of renal retention of sodium. However, reduced glomerular filtration may also be of importance in these diseases.

Adrenal cortical hormones may also play a role in congestive heart failure and renal disease. These hormones (particularly aldosterone) cause retention of sodium and increased excretion of potassium. Edema is not infrequently encountered in patients receiving these steroids.

Significance and Effect of Edema.—The fact already noted that edema is almost always of parasitic, nutritional, cardiac or renal origin is of much practical significance to the diagnostician.

Edema fluid remaining for more than a few days tends to become organized with fibrous tissue, perhaps as a chronic inflammatory reaction (p. 165), perhaps through clotting and subsequent organization. This fibrosis is marked in the edema due to lymphatic obstruction in human filariasis (*Filaria*, or *Wuchereria bancrofti*). The human limb becomes permanently and irregularly thickened to the point where it resembles an elephant's leg, the condition being called elephantiasis. In spite of this fibrosing tendency, however, most edemas readily subside if the cause is removed. Surgical drainage, as of the edematous peritoneal cavity, helps but little, for, with the cause unabated, the fluid soon returns.

Accumulation of fluid in the peritoneal cavity is called **ascites**; in the thorax it is **hydrothorax**; in the pericardium, **hydropericardium**; in the scrotal layers, **hydrocele.** In most of these cases, the condition is an inflammatory edema, or serous inflammation, but non-inflammatory ascites is not rare. It may be a part of the picture of generalized edema, or it may result from stasis of the portal circulation caused in most instances by obstruction of the intrahepatic flow by the proliferated connective tissue of cirrhosis (p. 1225). Generalized subcutaneous edema is called **anasarca.** Non-inflammatory hydropericardium occurs rarely in connection with myocardial venous stasis, but in animals, at least, practically all cases are inflammatory. Hydrops amnii is a non-inflammatory edema of the amniotic sac (p. 1322).

Angioneurotic edema is a rare form which will be treated separately because of its rarity and its obscure nature. The term implies a derangement of vasomotor innervation such that there results an increased permeability of capillary endothelium (to large molecules, chiefly albumin and globulin, as has been mentioned with respect to inflammatory edema). The existence of such a mechanism has been postulated to explain certain transient and apparently functional local edemas in humans and, according to some, even the edema of snake-bite (which is obviously inflammatory as we have defined that term). Proof of the existence or nonexistence of a neurovascular mechanism is, of course, much to be desired but it may well be, as Smith and Gault (1948) suggest, that these obscure edemas are "allergic and, therefore, inflammatory in nature." Unexplained edemas also accompany human menstruation, insulin treatment of severe diabetes and the therapeutic or experimental administration of large doses of desoxycorticosterone. Quite recently a practice has developed of feeding estrogenic hormones, such as stilbestrol, to fattening animals for the purpose of producing faster gains in weight. It turns out that edema, variously localized, accounts for at least a part of the increased weight, and this edema has been called angioneurotic. Whether involving nervous or allergic or toxic inflammatory phenomena, it constitutes another example of edema connected with endocrine imbalances. (Angiospastic diseases, such as Buerger's disease in men [chiefly] and Raynaud's disease in women, with somewhat related syndromes in castrated men, may well indicate a relationship between sympathetic vasomotor innervation and imbalance of sex hormones.)

SHOCK

Following immediately or within a few hours after severe traumatic injury to an extensive amount of tissue, or after a major operation, especially one involving considerable exposure and handling of the intestines, or as the result of very severe pain of certain kinds, the baffling and often fatal disorder known as shock is likely to supervene. In humans distressing psychic experiences are often strongly contributory or even principal causes. These latter appear not to apply in the case of animal patients, which is doubtless one reason why shock is less frequently encountered in veterinary practice. The sudden loss of a large amount of blood has practically the same effect, as does also the exudation of a large amount of serum a day or so after a widespread superficial burn.

A patient suffering from shock is in the severest state of functional depression compatible with life and life may cease at any moment. He is conscious but does not show it; humans can answer questions intelligently but do so only with slowness and reluctance. He feels cold and without strength; the body temperature is subnormal and the body surface has no warmth-giving circulation. The fundamental change is a tremendous fall in blood pressure; it is accompanied by the shallow and irregular respirations and the rapid but weak or even irregular pulse of a failing heart.

In spite of extensive studies, all is not yet settled with respect to the etiological mechanisms of shock. It seems to be clear that the volume of circulating blood is too small to fill the space in the vascular system, with the result that the heart has insufficient blood to fill its chambers. In the case of a sudden, severe hemorrhage this is readily understood. Even the copious serous exudate that flows from a large burned area may conceivably reduce the volume of circulating blood sufficiently to produce the situation outlined, although one would suppose that a satisfied thirst would replenish the fluid of the blood as needed. But in the strictly typical cases of shock following operations or injuries, there is no loss of fluid to the exterior. In many instances there is edema of the lungs, and in the case of large muscular bruises, there is considerable exudation of serum into the bruised tissues (inflammatory edema, as it is called). While the loss of some fluid can be explained in these ways, there are many examples of equally extensive edema without the syndrome of shock. It becomes apparent that the real reason for the lack of sufficient blood to fill the vascular channels is that the channels have stretched. To say it a little more precisely, each capillary has expanded until it holds more blood than formerly. This slight expansion becomes the more significant when we realize that it is normal in most, if not all, parts of the body for more than half of the capillaries to be closed at any given moment, especially if the organ or part is resting. The dilatation of capillaries, it may be said, is chiefly in the internal parts of the body, the abdominal area especially; these capillaries are found post mortem to be filled with the blood which should be passing through the heart.

While the type and degree of vasomotor innervation of capillaries is not positively known, there seems little doubt that the dilatation of the capillaries is a nervous phenomenon. The suddenness of the change as well as the circumstances (see above) under which it occurs would strongly indicate this. Another explanation has, however, had its advocates. This is that histamine or a histamine-like substance is liberated from injured tissues and that this substance both paralyzes the capillaries and increases their permeability. Following the theory further we see that the "increased permeability of the capillaries" is the same phenomenon that has already been explained in connection with inflammatory edema (p. 138); increased permeability to large molecules, which escape into the intercellular fluid, raise its osmotic pressure and attract fluid into it. Experimentally the injection of histamine can be shown to have such an action, but there are several objections to attributing to it the condition we have defined as shock. Among the most practical of these are the objections that in some of the causative situations there is little destruction of tissue and little histamine produced, that in many cases of shock there is no edema and that it would seem difficult to explain why a widely diffused substance in the blood would cause dilatation of capillaries in the splanchnic areas, but leave them constricted and empty in the peripheral parts of the body.

From the preceding paragraphs it should be obvious that shock is an entity which has multiple causes, but that many of the causes act through similar mechanisms. Regardless of the original insult, shock is an inequality between blood volume and the capacity of the vascular system which results from blood or fluid loss, or vasodilation of neurogenic origin, and leads to a reduction of blood flow to the tissues. The latter causes anoxia which may sustain and accentuate shock. Based on cause, shock can be classified as *hemorrhagic shock* (blood loss); *neurogenic shock* (trauma, pain, psychic); *traumatic* (or *surgical*) *shock* (probably neurogenic); *burn shock* (fluid loss); and *endotoxic* (septic)*shock* (presumably from bacterial endotoxins).

The **diagnosis** of shock is usually made clinically on the basis of the startling picture already outlined, but a reliably precise diagnosis often is not easy. It is probably for this reason that the exact limitations of the syndrome we call shock are open to doubt. On the one hand it must be distinguished from the fainting which results in some humans from a sudden very severe pain such as may arise from a blow on the testicle or the periosteum. Fainting is a purely nervous reaction involving complete unconsciousness, but is of little more than momentary duration and is unaccompanied by the severe vascular disturbances characteristic of shock. Transient spells of complete unconsciousness are not unknown in animals, at least in the horse, but they appear to have other causes than nervous reflexes. It is doubtful that true fainting occurs in animals. At the other extreme, some have included with shock the premortal coma and near-coma which is often seen in fatal cases of many systemic diseases. If this usage were to be followed, the definition of shock would have to be broad, indeed.

The post-mortem lesions of shock are described as severe congestion of the smaller vessels of the lungs, liver and intestines especially, together with an ischemic state of the peripheral parts of the body. In the lungs the congestion is accompanied not only by the presence of edema fluid in the alveoli, but there is also appreciable hemorrhage into these spaces, a fact which should differentiate the condition from pulmonary congestion and edema from cardiac causes, just as the absence of inflammatory cells should differentiate it from incipient pneumonia. The congestive state of the intestines may also be accompanied by edema and by hemorrhages. There may be small amounts of blood-tinged fluid in the peritoneal, pleural or pericardial cavities. The spleen is empty and bloodless. In patients that live a day or two, degenerative changes and necrosis may be found in the kidneys, liver, heart, adrenal cortex, lymph nodes and spleen. With one or two exceptions the lesions outlined here are very similar to those of poisoning by alpha-naphthyl thiourea. However, the total absence of blood in the fluid in the lungs and elsewhere is an important differentiating feature. The kidneys are markedly congested in the poisoned animals; the peripheral tissues are not strikingly bloodless. In both symptoms and lesions, points of marked similarity between shock and various other diseases could be named. But the essence of our conception of shock is that it is a reflex nervous phenomenon or something closely akin thereto, and not to be explained on the basis of any of the usual causes of disease such as poisons, infections or even trauma in its ordinary aspects. The lesions of the shock-like syndrome which follows severe hemorrhage naturally include little in the nature of congestion; all parts are ischemic. Another important differential feature is the fact that the intravenous administration of blood or isotonic solutions and serum substitutes is promptly beneficial following hemorrhage, but this is not true of shock.

The effects of shock are obvious. If death occurs, it is due largely to cerebral or myocardial ischemia. Fortunately many patients regain their normal circulatory equilibrium almost as mysteriously as they lost it.

Disturbances of Circulation

ARCHER, R. K., and BOWDEN, R. S. T.: A Case of True Haemophilia in A Labrador Dog. Vet. Record 71:560, 1959.

BRENON, H. C.: Further Erythrocyte and Hemoglobin Studies in Thoroughbred Racing Horses. J. Am. Vet. Med. Assn. 133:102–104, 1958.

BRINKHOUSE, K. M., MORRISON, F. C., and MUHRER, M. E.: Comparative Study of Clotting Defects in Human, Canine, and Porcine Hemophilia. Fed. Proc. 11:409, 1952.

BRION, A.: Les phènoménes d'héréto- et d'iso-immunisation chez les animaux. Maroc mèd. 31:597–603, 1952.

————: Réalisation expérimentale de l'ictère du muleton nouveau-né. Compt. rend. Acad. d. sc. 230:1547–1548, 1950.

BROCK, W. E., et al.: Canine Hemophilia. Arch. of Path. 76:464–469, 1963.

BROWN, J. M., KINGREY, B. W., and ROSENQUIST, B. D.: The Hematology of Chronic Bovine Reticuloperitonitis. Am. J. Vet. Res. 20:255–264, 1959.

BRUNER, D. W., HULL, F. E., and DOLL, E. R.: The Relation of Blood Factors to Icterus in Foals. Am. J. Vet. Res. 9:237–242, 1948.

BRUNER, D. W., et al.: Blood Factors and Baby Pig Anemia. J. Am. Vet. Med. Assn. 115:94–96, 1949.

BRYANS, J. T.: Studies on Equine Leptospirosis. Cornell Vet. 45:16–49, 1955.

BUXTON, J. C., and BROOKSBANK, N. H.: Haemolytic Diseases of Newborn Pigs Caused by Iso-immunisation of Pregnancy. Vet. Record. 65:287–288, 1953.

CASTLE, W. B.: Observations on the Etiologic Relationship of Achylia Gastrica to Pernicious Anemia. Am. J. M. Sc. 178:748–764, 1929.

COOK, R.: Frequency at which Blood Can Be Drawn from Farm Animals. J. Anim. Tech. Assn. 10:129–134, 1959. Abstr. Vet. Bull. No. 1658, 1960.

DAVIE, E. W., and RATNOFF, O. D.: Waterfall Sequence for Intrinsic Blood Clotting. Science 145:1310–1312, 1964.

FIELD, R. A., RICHARD, C. G., and HUTT, F. B.: Hemophilia in a Family of Dogs. Cornell Vet. 36:285–300, 1946.

GENGOZIAN, N., et al.: Erythroblastosis Foetalis in the Primate, *Tamarinus Nigricollis*. Nature 209:731–732, 1966.

HELGEBOSTAD, A., and MARTINSONS, E.: Nutritional Anemia in Mink. Nature, Lond. 181:1660–1661, 1958.

HOGAN, A. G., MUHRER, M. E., and BOGART, R.: A Hemophilia Like Disease in Swine. Proc. Soc. Exp. Biol. Med. 48:217–219, 1941.

HOWELL, J. McC., and LAMBERT, P. S.: A Case of Haemophilia A in the Dog. Vet. Record 76:1103–1105, 1964.

HUTYRA, F., and MAREK, J.: *Special Pathology and Therapeutics of the Diseases of Domestic Animals,* 3rd American Edition, translated by J. R. MOHLER, and A. EICHHORN. Chicago, A. Eger, 1926, vol. I, p. 1051.

INTERNATIONAL COMMITTEE FOR THE NOMENCLATURE OF BLOOD CLOTTING FACTORS: The Nomenclature of Blood Clotting Factors. J. Am. Med. Assn. 180:733–735, 1962.

IRVINE, C. H. G.: The Blood Picture in the Race Horse. J. Am. Vet. Med. Assn. 133:97–101, 1958.

KRACKE, R. R., and PLATT, W. R.: Bromide Intoxication from Prolonged Self Medication with B. C. Headache Powder. J. Am. Med. Assn. 125:107–111, 1944.

LIEBERMAN, A. H.: Current Status of Aldosterone in the Etiology of Edema. Arch. Int. Med. *102*:990–997, 1958.

MACFARLANE, R. G.: An Enzyme Cascade in the Blood Clotting Mechanism, and Its Function as a Biochemical Amplifier. Nature *202*:498–499, 1964.

MINOT, G. R., and MURPHY, W. P.: Treatment of Pernicious Anemia by a Special Diet. J. Am. Med. Assn. *87*:470–476, 1926.

MIZUNO, N. S., *et al.*: The Life Span of Thrombocytes and Erythrocytes in Normal and Thrombocytopenic Calves. Blood. *14*:708–719, 1959.

MUHRER, M. E., *et al.*: Antihemophilic Factor Level in Bleeder Swine Following Infusions of Plasma and Serum. Am. J. Physiol. *208*:508–510, 1965.

MUSTARD, J. F., *et al.*: Canine Factor VII Deficiency. Br. J. Haemat. *8*:43–47, 1962.

OSBALDISTON, G. W., COFFMAN, J. R., and STOWE, E. C.: Equine Isoerythrolysis—Clinical Pathological Observations and Transfusion of Dam's Red Blood Cells to Her Foal. Can. J. Comp. Med. *33*:310–315, 1969.

PEABODY, F. W.: Pathology of the Bone Marrow in Pernicious Anemia. Am. J. Path. *3*:179–202, 1927.

POOLE, J. C. F.: Electron Microscopy of Polymorphonuclear Leukocytes. Brit. J. Derm. *81*: 11–18, 1969.

RATOFF, O. D.: Hereditary Defects in Clotting Mechanisms. Adv. Int. Med. *9*:107–179, 1958.

ROWSELL, H. C.: The Hemostatic Mechanisms of Mammals and Birds in Health and Disease. Adv. in Vet. Sci. *12*:337–410, 1968.

ROWSELL, H. C., *et al.*: A Disorder Resembling Hemophilia B (Christmas Disease) in Dogs. J. Am. Vet. Med. Assn. *137*:247–250, 1960.

SANGER, V. L., MAIRS, R. E., and TRAPP, A. L.: Hemophilia in a Foal. J. Am. Vet. Med. Assn. *144*:259–264, 1964.

SHEMANCHUK, J. A., HAUFE, W. O., and THOMPSON, C. O. M.: Anemia in Range Cattle Heavily Infested with the Short-Nosed Sucking Louse, Haematopinus eurysternus (Nitz.) Canad. J. Comp. Med. *24*:158–161, 1960.

SMITH, L. W., and GAULT, E. S.: *Essentials of Pathology*, 3rd ed., Philadelphia, Blakiston Co., 1948.

SZENT IVÁNYI, T., and SZABA, S.: Untersuchungen über die Ursache der haemolitischen Gelsucht der neugeborenen Ferkel. Acta Vet. Hungarie. *3*:75–80, 1953.

THOMPSON, J. E.: Some Observations on the European Broad Fish Tapeworm, *Diphyllobothrium latum*. J. Am. Vet. Med. Assn. *89*:77–86, 1936.

VERBITSKY, M., *et al.*: A Study of Haemolytic Disease of the Foetus and the Newborn Occurring in Hamadryas Baboons under Natural Conditions. Z. Versuchstierk *11*:136–145, 1969.

WATSON, D. F.: Studies on the Hemoglobin Content of Sheep Blood in the Sierra of Peru. Am. J. Vet. Res. *14*:405–407, 195 .

WEIDE, K. D., and TWIEHAUS, M. J.: Hematological Studies of Normal, Ascarid-Infected, and Hog Cholera-Vaccinated Swine. Am. J. Vet. Res. *20*:562–567, 1959.

WHIPPLE, G. H.: Hemoglobin Regeneration as Influenced by Diet and Other Factors, Nobel Prize Lecture. J. Am. Med. Assn. *104*:791–793, 1935.

WIGGERS, C. J.: *Physiology in Health and Disease*, 5th ed., Philadelphia, Lea & Febiger, 1949.

WOLF, S. G., and WOLFF, H. G.: *Human Gastric Function*, 2nd ed., London, Oxford University Press, 1947.

WURZEL, H. A., and LAWRENCE, W. C.: Canine Hemophilia. Thrombosis et Diathesis Haemorrhagica *6*:98–103, 1961.

YOUNG, L. E., *et al.*: Hemolytic Disease in Newborn Dogs. Blood. *6*:291–313, 1951.

Chapter

6
Inflammation and Body Reactions

A pathological phenomenon known and studied from ancient times, inflammation has long been defined as **the reaction of the tissues to an irritant.** Although, owing to its simplicity, this definition is difficult to surpass, two important characteristics which demand emphasis are omitted. First, inflammation is a dynamic process and not a state, and secondly the process depends upon viable tissue. The definition proposed by Ebert (in Zweifach, *et al.*, 1965), though more cumbersome, is more complete: "Inflammation is a process which begins following sublethal injury to tissue and ends with complete healing." This definition also includes the end result of inflammation, *i.e.*, healing, which is a part of the dynamic process and not a distinct entity unto itself. The basic meaning of the verb, "to inflame" is to "set fire to." Many who have suffered the agonies of a severe, acute inflammation in a tender spot will attest to the aptness of the name.

The clinical signs which characterize inflammation are, as stated by Celsus (30 B.C.–38 A.D.) in the first century A.D., and by every medical writer since that time, *rubor et tumor cum calore et dolore*, which, translated, means "redness and swelling with heat and pain." These symptoms are considered of such fundamental importance that they are known as the **cardinal signs** of inflammation, the north, south, east and west of the compass without which no one can proceed! The redness is due to a great increase of blood in the inflamed part. The swelling comes from the increase of blood and the additional presence of substances which, like sap from a tree, have exuded from the blood vessels into the surrounding tissues and are called exudates. The heat, objective but not subjective, also results from the increased flow of blood, carrying warmth to the periphery from the higher interior temperatures of the body. The pain is often attributed to increased pressure upon nerve endings, but it may well be that the irritating effects of toxic products are of greater significance in this, since the degree of pain which accompanies inflammations of apparently equal extent and severity may be highly variable. The Greek physician Galen (A.D. 130–200) later added loss of function as a fifth cardinal sign of inflammation. Pain initiated reflex inhibition of muscle movements, mechanical swelling, and tissue destruction, all contribute to loss of function.

Inflammation is, on the whole, a beneficial phenomenon. It occurs in all the more complex forms of animal life. Without its protection the animal races could not have survived their enemies, facts which appear to have been first perceived by John Hunter (1728–1793) about 200 years ago. The body possesses potent defensive weapons of two quite different forms, its humoral antibodies and its reactive cells, chiefly the leukocytes. The effect of inflammation with its hyperemic changes is to bring these defensive mechanisms into immediate contact with the irritant substance or the cells which have been injured by it. By this means the causative irritant, if still present, can often be destroyed or at least confined, which is the first prerequisite to recovery from the injury.

Although without inflammation survival is not possible, like other vital processes, inflammation may become aberrant and harmful. Just as insulin is necessary for life, its excessive production by a neoplasm of the pancreatic β cells can result in death. Diseases thought to be immunologic in origin (p. 312) such as rheumatic fever, rheumatoid arthritis, glomerulonephritis, and disseminated lupus erythematosus, are associated with inflammatory reactions which provide no obvious benefit, but rather inflict harm upon the host.

Nature and Kinds of Irritants.—These are synonymous with the causes of inflammation and it may be advantageous to review them here, before proceeding to a study of the inflammatory process itself.

The **causes of inflammation** are:

(1) Pathogenic organisms or, more precisely, the toxic and injurious substances produced by them. Included in this group are bacteria, viruses, fungi, protozoa and parasitic metazoa. More will be said later about the effects of each class.

(2) Chemical poisons, which are of endless variety. As explained under the heading of necrosis (which also is produced by many of them), poisons may act either upon the tissues with which they come in immediate contact or upon more distant cells, such as those of the liver, kidney and brain, which are often susceptible to highly diluted poisons in the blood. Some poisons, like cyanides and strychnine, kill without causing either inflammation or necrosis.

(3) Mechanical and thermal injuries. Prominent among these are burns by heat, electricity, light or other radiant energy. Excessive cold, as well as blows and lacerations are also included.

(4) Immune reactions. An inflammatory reaction is associated with antigen-antibody interactions which occur under various circumstances. Included are delayed hypersensitivity (p. 311), the Arthus reaction (p. 310), the Schwartzman reaction, serum sickness (p. 311), and certain of the autoimmune diseases (p. 312).

THE INFLAMMATORY PROCESS

Despite the simple manner in which inflammation has been defined, it is not a simple process, but rather a highly complex series of events whether approached from its morphological, physiological or biochemical characteristics. It is beyond our intentions to cover each of these parameters in depth but rather concentrate on morphological changes and present the more accepted or plausible explanations for their development. The few pages devoted to inflammation in this chapter will hopefully provide a foundation upon which the student of pathology can build. The subject is classically covered with the completeness of current knowledge in 931 pages in *The Inflammatory Process* edited by Zweifach, Grant and McCluskey, and in *Florey's General Pathology*. The inflammatory process, particularly when acute, is primarily a circulatory phenomenon involving changes in the amount and quality of blood reaching the affected area. These changes have already been alluded to in describing the cardinal signs of inflammation (p. 145). Regardless of the nature of the injurious agent or the location of the insult, the basic character of the initial vascular response is remarkably similar. Only as inflammation progresses do features develop which are dependent upon the cause and allow for the morphologic classification of inflammation.

The circulatory events of inflammation were determined with great nicety by Cohnheim (1839–1884) in 1867 and little has been added to our knowledge of the visual sequelae of the vascular events since his original description. Based on Cohnheim's observations the **circulatory** changes are:

(1) **Changes in the blood vessels:**

(a) **Momentary constriction.** Immediately upon application of the irritant the vessels are constricted, apparently by a kind of stimulant action before the full effect of the irritant is felt. Because of its transitory character, this stage is of negligible importance.

(b) **Dilation** of the vessels quickly supervenes, admitting more arterial blood and instituting the stage of hyperemia. This is believed to occur through relaxation of the arteriolar smooth muscle walls and of the pre-capillary sphincters. A noteworthy feature of the dilatation phenomenon is the startling increase in the number of capillaries visible in an inflamed area. This is due to the fact that unfilled capillaries, previously unseen, become distended and conspicuous. As far as acute inflammations are concerned there is no actual proliferation. The cause of the dilation, which is predominantly restricted to arterioles and venules and not capillaries, is probably multiple but as yet not completely understood. In part the **axon reflex** or the so-called anti-dromic reflex is responsible for dilation at the site of injury and the associated dilation beyond the area of immediate injury. The vasomotor nerves are not necessary to the development of dilation or any other aspect of the inflammatory process. Of more importance in causing dilation, and of greater significance in altering vascular permeability are the so-called **chemical mediators** of inflammation which will be discussed shortly. Increase in capillary and venule **blood pressure** is associated with the dilation of vessels.

(c) **Increased permeability** of venules and capillaries develops more slowly, in connection with retardation of the flow, and permits the large molecules of blood protein and a few erythrocytes to leak through into the tissues. Leukocytes also pass through the walls with much greater ease than is normally the case. The exudative stage is thus instituted. Explanations for this increased permeability of the walls differ. Numerous theories have been advanced; some have since been disregarded and others are still in question. The effects of chemical mediators (p. 150) on the venule and capillary wall are probably the principal underlying factors in increasing permeability. Increase in local blood pressure and stretching of vessel walls also contribute to increased permeability. It is uncertain how these mechanisms actually affect the vessel wall and allow large molecules to escape. Undoubtedly the endothelial cells and/or their basement membranes are damaged. Most evidence suggests that materials pass between two adjacent endothelial cells and accumulate between the cell and the basement membrane, eventually leaving through "pores" or rents in the basement membrane. However, there is also evidence to indicate that materials may pass through the endothelial cell in pinocytotic vacuoles.

(2) **Changes in the rate of flow:**

(d) **Acceleration of the rate of flow** naturally accompanies the preliminary dilatation of arterioles but it soon gives way to:

(e) **Retardation of the vascular flow.** Loss of fluid from the blood, to be explained shortly, doubtless increases its viscosity and a certain stickiness of the leukocytes also tends to slow its flow. These factors also account for the increased capillary hydrostatic pressure. The mere dilatation of capillaries and veins, following enlargement of the afferent arterioles, obviously provides space for a more lingering stream. Thus retardation deepens into:

(f) **Stasis** and a well marked passive congestion is established. This situation is much more favorable for the escape of molecular and cellular elements essential to the formation of an exudate.

(3) **Changes in the blood stream:**

(g) **Distribution of the erythrocytes.** Most of us are familiar with the appearance of a flooded river, in which floating debris is drawn to the center of the stream where the flow is fastest. In the normal blood stream, the great majority of the erythrocytes are likewise found in the center of the flow, since this is in accordance with physical laws. But when the stream grows sluggish the heavier, solid elements cease to be drawn to the center and become more evenly distributed. This situation favors the escape of erythrocytes, and the same may well be true of the heavier molecules of globulin and albumin. And globulins are the bearers of the "humoral antibodies" which constitute specific defenses against the most outstanding of all irritants, the micro-organisms of disease.

(h) **Margination of the leukocytes** (sometimes called "pavementing"). The white cells of the blood are naturally influenced by the same physical principles as those which govern the distribution of the erythrocytes, but leukocytes are living, motile individuals, masters, we can almost say, of their own destiny. And what is the behavior of the leukocytes in inflammation? Most of them are found along the walls of the vessels, that is, of the dilated capillaries. They appear to be searching and examining every inlet and bayou of the swollen and roughened capillary lining as if, like houseflies on a screen-door, they were looking for a way to get through. But let us say merely that they have developed some quality of adhesiveness toward the vessel wall, for we do not attribute intelligence to these cells. Or should we say that they are drawn toward the outside by some irresistible force, as a lover is drawn to his lady fair? We can also not exclude that injured endothelium, rather than leukocytes, may be the sticky surface. The adherence of non-motile red blood cells and platelets suggests that the cells may not be acting like houseflies but the vessel wall has become flypaper. However that may be, the leukocytes do stick and succeed in passing through the capillary walls so that the surrounding tissue comes to be filled with them, where, it seems, lies their inevitable destiny. This process of passing into the adjacent tissue is known, by long-standing custom as:

(4) **Emigration of the leukocytes.** They do this by means of their power of ameboid movement. The migration evidently is not accomplished without difficulty for, when studied by means of intravital staining, they are seen to assume a surprising variety of bizarre forms and positions as they squirm through narrow crevices between the cells of the capillaries.

Whatever may be said of other phenomena of inflammation, this emigration of the leukocytes is not a matter of inert and inanimate particles moving in accordance with any law of physics. It is rather the action of living individuals. The force which attracts them into the inflamed tissues is called **chemotaxis,** a chemical attraction. Chemotactic attraction and repulsion are by no means mythical; they have been demonstrated many times in the laboratory, using amebae or other kinds of protozoa as well as leukocytes in a fluid medium to which various attractive or repellant chemicals can be added at one end of the container.

The attracting substance in inflamed tissue may at times be something produced by invading pathogenic organisms. This seems especially likely, since it is known that different infections vary greatly with respect to the kind of leukocyte which enters the zone of inflammation as well as in the extensiveness of the emigration. On the other hand, when the irritant is a burn or any one of the mechanical or thermal injuries listed above, there are no micro-organisms involved. The chemotactic agent is then said to be some substance elaborated by injured cells, and if this is true in noninfectious inflammations, it is argued that it may well be true in all.

A few chemical substances introduced directly into the tissues can cause a marked polymorphonuclear reaction (abscesses from injection of turpentine, etc.) and a few kinds of irritant foreign bodies (lycopodium spores) can cause a very considerable reticulo-endothelial reaction, but there are very few exceptions to the rule that large numbers of leukocytes mean the presence of an infectious agent.

Of the many factors isolated and tested, those which appear most important as chemotactic factors for neutrophils include soluble bacterial factors; a factor derived from complement (C'3); and a complement associated factor (C'(5,6,7)a). Separate factors have been isolated which are chemotactic to mononuclear cells. These include lysates from neutrophils; soluble bacterial factors; and serum derived factors. Although each is clearly chemotactic *in vitro* their precise role *in vivo* is not firmly established (see Ward, 1968).

(5) **Diapedesis of the erythrocytes** is the traditional expression for another phenomenon which needs little explanation. It has already been mentioned that the even distribution of the erythrocytes throughout the more peripheral parts of the slowly moving blood stream favors the escape of an occasional red cell through the permeable capillary wall. The erythrocytes have no power of movement of their own; their passage is hemorrhage by diapedesis (p. 119), a fortuitous result of the changes that have occurred in the capillaries and the stream within them. The erythrocytes are not considered as having any effect on the inflammatory process. In some cases their number becomes very great, leading to the designation of hemorrhagic inflammation (p. 160).

(6) **Exudation of serum.** As would be expected, it is still easier for the fluid part of the blood to exude, or pass through, into the tissues around the capillary than it is for the cells to do so. As was shown in the study of edema, the retention or release of water from the blood vessels depends upon a balance of hydrostatic and osmotic pressures within and without the vessel. It seems safe to say that in inflamed tissue the causative agent has injured cells to the extent that many of their large and complex molecules have been broken into smaller ones and that these enter the intercellular lymph. Thus the osmotic pressure of the extravascular tissue is increased. As indicated above the hydrostatic pressure at the venous end of the capillary is also increased. Both these factors tend to transfer fluid from the vessels into the tissues. The increased permeability of the venules and capillaries (Par. *c*, p. 147) is sufficient to allow the largest molecules of pro-

tein to pass through, which was not the case in edema (non-inflammatory). These molecules also raise the extravascular osmotic pressure.

Thus large amounts of fluid commonly exude into the inflamed area. Contrary to what we find in edema (non-inflammatory), the specific gravity of this exudate approaches that of the blood plasma itself and all of the proteins of the plasma, including fibrinogen, appear in the exudate. This is a most beneficial situation. In the first place, the fluid greatly dilutes toxic substances formed within the body or introduced from without. In such conditions as bee-stings and snake-bites, this dilution process is of primary importance. An even more important benefit in infectious inflammations is the fact that this blood serum brings with it the globulins and antibodies which bring to bear whatever humoral immunity the patient has against the infection in question.

From the fibrinogen of the exudate, fibrin forms. It is believed to afford a supporting framework on which leukocytes can better exercise their ameboid movement. It is difficult to point to the exact mechanism which places much fibrin in one inflammatory exudate and little in another, although the ultimate causes are reasonably well understood and will be discussed with fibrinous inflammation.

The above are the vascular changes of inflammation. The increase of blood is responsible for most of the cardinal signs and other symptoms, but the feature essential to the recovery of the individual animal and which has proved vital to the evolutionary survival of all species of higher animals is the fact that the way is opened for leukocytes and fluid exudates to attack injurious invaders and the deleterious substances produced by injured cells.

CHEMICAL MEDIATORS OF INFLAMMATION

Most of the preceding data describes the early events of the inflammatory process. Why it happens and how it happens bring questions for which we have few answers, although considerable progress has been made in recent years. Some answers were provided in the above discussion, but only brief reference was made to the subject of chemical mediators. It is not our purpose to go far into the field of biochemistry, important though it is, but several chemical substances, participating in the inflammatory reaction, must be mentioned. The constancy of the changes outlined above prompted the search for chemical mediators liberated regardless of the cause of the inflammatory reaction. Such studies are difficult at best, for discovering, and in particular evaluating any given substance is a formidable task in the face of the multitude of events in the inflammatory reaction. Nevertheless several substances have emerged that meet the requirements of chemical mediators constant to the inflammatory process. These include:

Histamine. — Histamine (β-Iminazolylethyamine) was one of the first chemicals associated with inflammatory reactions, and one of the few that is universally accepted as a chemical mediator. Histamine initiates the early vascular responses but only sustains them for thirty to sixty minutes. Histamine is then superseded by other mediators which sustain the vascular reactions or induce what is called the delayed or prolonged vascular reaction. Histamine is widely distributed in tissues in the granules of **basophilic leukocytes** (p. 173) and **mast cells** (p. 180). Following injury of most any nature, histamine is released from the granules, probably by enzymatic action, though details of release are still under investigation, as is its mode of action on the vessel.

Serotonin.—The role of serotonin (5-hydroxytryptamine) in inflammation is less certain than that of histamine. It has vasoactive properties in most species but vascular dilatation and increased permeability have only been clearly documented in the rat and mouse. In most all animals serotonin is widely distributed in the enterochromaffin system with its greatest concentration in the argentaffin cells of the gastrointestinal tract. It is also present in platelets and in the central nervous system. In the rat, mast cells also contain serotonin. Although experimentally serotonin can initiate the vascular phenomena of the inflammatory process, it probably is not of great significance.

Kinins.—The kinins, **bradykinin** and **kallidin** have emerged as the most likely mediators which sustain the vascular reactions after the initial histamine response. Kinins are produced from normal serum precursors by the action of several enzymes in a sequence of events remarkably similar to the coagulation mechanism (p. 104). In fact the systems share at least two factors, the **Hageman factor** (factor XII) and **plasminogen.** The activated forms of these factors, **plasmin** and **activated Hageman factor** act upon serum **kallikreinogen** (prekallikrein) and convert it to an active enzyme **kallikrein.** Kallikrein, which has weak inflammatory properties, in turn releases kinins from α_2-globulins known as kininogens. Schematically the events are as follows:

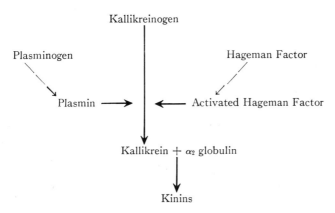

In normal plasma kallikrein is probably a group rather than a single enzyme and the kinins in turn are probably several, though each would appear to be a closely related polypeptide.

No specific antagonistic system to the kinins has been shown to exist, but eosinophils contain a substance capable of inhibiting the effect of bradykinin.

Other Permeability Factors.—Several other compounds have been shown to affect vascular permeability but their role in the inflammatory process or their nature is less certain than that of histamine and the kinins. A *globulin permeability factor* and a *lymph node permeability factor* have been studied in several species, but their exact nature and significance is not clear. *Hyaluronidase, lecithinases* and *nucleosides* have been suggested as permeability factors but their role, if any, is uncertain. By virtue of their abilities to induce vasoconstriction and diminish vascular permeability, *epinephrine* and *norepinephrine* are well established anti-inflammatory agents. Dopa and dopamine, two intermediaries in the formation

Table 6–1. *Summary of Vascular Changes in Inflammation*

1. Transient Vasoconstriction

2. Vasodilation

3. Increased Hydrostatic Pressure

4. Acceleration of Rate of Flow

    Initial Response Mediated by Axon Reflex, Histamine, Kinins and Serotonin (?)

5. Increased Permeability

6. Exudation of Fluid

7. Margination of Leukocytes

8. Emigration of Leukocytes

    Prolonged Response Mediated by Kinins and other factors(?) (lymph node permeability factor?).

9. Diapedesis of Erythrocytes

10. Retardation and Stasis of Flow

of norepinephrine and epinephrine, are similarly anti-inflammatory. When absent, these compounds play a passive role in mediating the inflammatory response, therefore degradation of these compounds is an important step in allowing the inflammatory process to develop. It is suggested that when tissues are damaged, the enzymes monamine oxidase, dopamine β-oxidase and dopa decarboxylase are activated to increase the formation and inactivation of epinephrine, norepinephrine, dopa and dopamine.

Anti-inflammatory Effects of Glucocorticoids. — Mention is made elsewhere of the anti-inflammatory properties of epinephrine and its precursors (p. 151), eosinophils (p. 172), and other agents, but no endogenous or pharmacologic agent possesses anti-inflammatory properties as potent and effective as the glucocorticoids of the adrenal cortex. Indiscriminate "therapeutic" use of these compounds has more than once accentuated rather than cured disease. Corticoids suppress most all aspects of the inflammatory process. They block increased vascular permeability, prevent exudation of inflammatory cells, impair intracellular destruction of bacteria and impede the union of antigen and antibody. The mechanism of these actions is not clear, but probably multiple. One means may be through a stabilizing effect on the membranes of lysosomes and other intracellular granules preventing the release of their contents.

INFLAMMATION CLASSIFIED ACCORDING TO TYPE OF EXUDATE OR OTHER TISSUE REACTION

Following the initial steps discussed up to this point, the inflammatory reaction may subside or continue, depending on the nature of the inciting stimulus. These stimuli, listed above under causes (p. 146), influence the reaction in different manners such that the course of the inflammatory process varies with the cause. What mediates this variance is unknown, but the chemical nature of the agent, the products of tissue necrosis, and in the case of bacteria, exotoxins and endo-toxins, all probably participate. Morphologically the process varies by the character of the exudate. While only a fluid, strictly speaking, can exude, the leukocytes and erythrocytes are inseparable from the fluids and for this reason, it is customary to refer to everything that leaves the blood as part of the exudate. In this sense exudates vary considerably and it is desirable now to divide them, in spite of constant overlapping, into several types. Certain non-exudative mechanisms also enter into some forms of inflammation, which, it will be remembered, was defined as the reaction of the tissues to an irritant.

1. Serous Inflammation

Serous exudative inflammation is characterized by the exudation of blood serum, a clear, albuminous fluid. This is the form which is equivalent to inflammatory edema (p. 149). A common method of more or less humanely killing small domestic or laboratory animals is to inject chloroform into the heart. This brings almost instantaneous death. If the injecting needle misses the heart and the chloroform is placed in the lungs, the animal commonly lives from one to two minutes. Examination of the lungs shows a red and slightly swollen area around the point of injection. Microscopically the alveoli and the septa are filled with a uniformly pink-staining (hematoxylin and eosin) albuminous fluid. Almost any pathologist, examining such a section, will call the condition edema. By the definition of inflammation, it is obviously an inflammatory exudate.

Occurrence.—This type of inflammation is especially frequent in serous cavities, doubtless because of the large areas of well-vascularized surfaces which line these cavities and the thinness of the surface mesothelium. Serous inflammation also occurs in the lungs, as the first stage in certain pneumonias, in response to various inhaled chemical irritants and as the result of at least one irritant which is ingested and presumably eliminated through the lungs, namely, alpha-naphthyl-thiourea (the rat poison, ANTU). Blisters, or vesicles, such as form in the skin when subjected to a bee-sting or a second-degree burn, or in the mucosa in such diseases as aphthous fever, vesicular stomatitis and vesicular exanthema, are examples of localized serous inflammation.

Microscopic Appearance.—Microscopically one sees a homogeneous, pink-staining precipitate like that already described under the title of Albumin (p. 49), natural spaces are distended by it and artificial ones are created, as in the case of vesicles. With the precipitated fluid, there are usually a few scattered leukocytes of various kinds and traces of fibrin. The hyperemic and congested vessels are conspicuous.

Gross Appearance.—There is a watery fluid in the body cavities or tissue spaces which differs little from the plasma of the blood. Neither is it easily distinguished from the fluid of true edema. The presence of small amounts of fibrin clinging to involved surfaces, or of a cloudiness caused by the presence of a few leukocytes indicates an inflammatory origin. A red tinge, coming from small numbers of erythrocytes, also suggests, but does not prove, that the fluid is an inflammatory exudate. The difference in the specific gravity of transudates and exudates has been mentioned (p. 137). If the fluid is within vesicles, it is an exudate. In any case, hyperemia of surrounding tissues indicates that the fluid is of inflammatory origin.

Causes.—This type of inflammation is usually caused by some moderately severe and often transient irritant. In the serous cavities, this is practically always an infection. Joint cavities constitute an exception in that a serous exudate, or excess of synovia, often results from the trauma of tears, sprains and blows. In the peritoneal, pleural and pericardial cavities, colon organisms are frequently responsible, more rarely the actinobacillus and the virus of bovine encephalitis. In the spinal canal and cerebral cavity, an inflammatory increase of fluid accompanies most of the viral and bacterial infections which attack these nervous tissues, with a typical group of symptoms resulting from the increased intracranial pressure.

In the lungs, the usual cause is a bacterial or viral infection, which commonly goes on to produce the more severe purulent or fibrinous reactions some hours later. In fact, most pneumonias begin with a serous exudate, the so-called inflammatory edema. The bacterial causes include *Pasteurella multocida*, the bronchisepticus organism of dogs (currently called *Brucella bronchisepticus*), possibly Hoffman's pseudodiphtheria bacillus (*Corynebacterium pseudodiphthericum*) and others; the viruses include that of psittacosis. The equine and porcine influenza and hog cholera viruses predispose to it, but it is difficult to say just what effects are due to the viruses and what to various bacteria that appear as secondary invaders. Various chemical irritants produce serous exudation in the lungs, chloroform already having been mentioned. Ordinarily they are chemicals that reach the lungs by inhalation and include many irritant gases. The inhalation of chloroform and even of ether tends to have the same effects, an unfavorable feature of their use as anesthetics. Similar to bee-stings, which have been mentioned, are the bites of many venomous creatures ranging from ants to serpents. The usual effect of a bite of the American rattlesnake (*Crotalus sp.*) is a tremendous local inflammatory edema, a serous exudate, even to the extent that the fluid passes through the overlying intact skin. Simple cutaneous abrasions, if of the right depth and severity, induce an exudate of this type. These are abrasions not quite deep enough to cause bleeding. An hour after the injury is inflicted drops of yellowish fluid appear on the surface, where they dry and form a scab.

Significance and Effect.—In politics there is a saying, "If you can't lick them, join them." If a body reaction could be imagined to be concerned with psychology, the massive exudation of serum occurring in such conditions as snake-bite might be considered as designed on a similar philosophy, for in the ordinary nonimmune animal there is slight means of destroying a toxin of this sort but the voluminous exudate dilutes it a thousandfold, greatly weakening its local effectiveness just as all irritants are weakened when diluted. Under conditions where specific antibodies exist, the value of the serous exudate in bringing them to the affected area has already been mentioned.

The pressure of exuded serum produces swelling of the part and interferes with its function, but any pain that is present must usually be attributed to other factors, judging from the sensations of persons who suffer from accumulations of noninflammatory fluids. Indeed, in pleuritis the severe pain disappears when the serous exudate arrives to lubricate and separate the hyperemic and severely irritated surfaces of visceral and parietal pleural membranes. Summarizing, it may be said that as long as an inflammation remains serous, it is comparatively mild. The fluid is promptly resorbed if the cause is overcome.

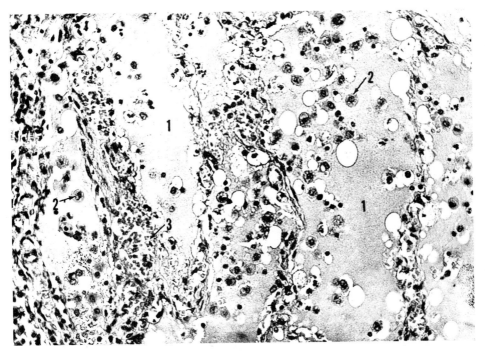

FIG. 6-1.—Inflammatory edema of the lungs of an elephant with pulmonary tuberculosis. Albuminous fluid (1), mononuclear cells (2) and congested capillaries (3). (Courtesy of Armed Forces Institute of Pathology.) × 300. Contributor: National Zoological Park.

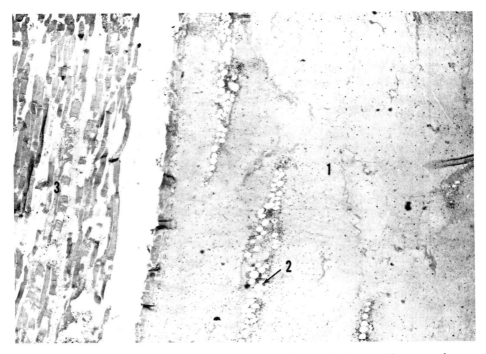

FIG. 6-2.—Inflammatory edema in subcutaneous musculature of a horse with purpura hemorrhagica. Albuminous material (1) containing cells and fibrin; leukocytes accumulated around fat cells (2), and skeletal muscle (3) with fibers separated by edema fluid. (Courtesy of Armed Forces Institute of Pathology.) Contributor: Army Veterinary Research Laboratory.

2. Fibrinous Inflammation

This type of inflammation is characterized by an exudate containing large amounts of fibrinogen, which clots, so that fibrin is the most conspicuous component, although the constituents of the other acute inflammatory exudates are present in some degree.

Fibrinous inflammation **occurs** chiefly on mucous and serous membranes including the alveolar surfaces of the lungs. One of the places where fibrinous exudation is most frequent is the pericardial sac and its surfaces. The respiratory mucous membranes from pharynx to lung alveoli, the pleura and peritoneum, synovial membranes and the lower intestinal mucous membrane are also locations where this type of inflammation is prone to occur.

Microscopic Appearance.—The dirty pink color and general appearance of fibrin have already been described (p. 50). Microscopically the fibrin is seen adherent to the surface which produced it, any detached fibrin seldom remaining as a part of the microscopic section. The fibrils may sometimes be traced into the epithelial or mesothelial cells of the parent surface. These latter, due to the toxic action of the irritant responsible for the fibrin, usually suffer necrosis. Coagulative necrosis is typical, but ultimately the cells pass through the various changes which are characteristic of dead tissue (p. 9). With the fibrin there are small but variable amounts of precipitated serum (protein), leukocytes and even erythrocytes. The underlying living tissue is hyperemic. The amount of exudate may be minute or massive. Not infrequently the exudate is formed in recurrent surges, or waves, so that one zone of exudate may be thin and lacelike, a second dense and deep-staining and a third heavily sprinkled with leukocytes. In the pulmonary alveoli and less commonly in other places, the fibrin may be so densely packed as to form a solid, nonfibrillar mass. Since many leukocytes often accompany the fibrin and die in its vicinity, the already mentioned tendency of fibrin to suffer a blue-staining discoloration from karyolysis and chromatolysis is often pronounced, more so in one area than in another.

Gross Appearance.—In the earliest stages, a dull and cloudy haze on a surface which should be smooth and shiny (serous membranes especially) is all that discloses the presence of a fibrinous exudate, but as the condition advances a conspicuous covering of whitish fuzzy or stringy material develops. This may increase to a thickness of a centimeter with a shaggy outer surface, shreds of fibrin hanging here and there. The fibrin is sometimes reddened with blood, or it may be mingled with the fluid of a serous exudate, which may accompany the fibrinous variety. The layer of fibrin is at times dense and tough and is then very aptly called a **pseudomembrane** (false membrane), for it forms a white or yellowish sheet which is dense and often tough, like a piece of thick paper.

Some fibrinous exudates form a layer which is readily loosened from the underlying parent tissue. Such a layer is called a croupous membrane and the case is said to be one of **croupous inflammation.** The name comes from the "croup" of babies, an infection of the laryngeal and adjacent mucous membranes characterized by a detachable but voluminous and suffocating fibrinous exudate.

A **diphtheritic inflammation,** by contrast, is one in which the fibrinous exudate is so firmly attached to the underlying surface that it cannot be removed except by tearing off with it a superficial layer of bleeding tissue. This diphtheritic membrane is characteristic of human diphtheria, whence the name. Calf diphtheria has an entirely different cause (the necrophorus organism), but the lesion is often much the same as that of human diphtheria.

Croupous exudates, perhaps more than the diphtheritic forms, are sometimes voluminous in amount and retain the shape of the structure in which they were molded, thus forming a **fibrinous cast.** Most astonishing fibrinous casts, several inches long and having the exact form of a bronchus and its branches, are sometimes coughed up by animals, commonly bovines, which may not appear very ill before or after the event. Hollow casts lining an intestine may be several feet in length. When voided with the feces, it may at first seem that the animal has passed a segment of its intestine. These are seen at least in horses and cattle.

Causes.—Fibrinous inflammation usually arises in response to the attack of certain micro-organisms. Prominent among these are the diphtheria bacillus, which attacks humans only, the necrophorus organism (*Sphaeropherus necrophorus* as of the present moment, formerly *Actinomyces necrophorus*), *Salmonella choleraesuis* (*Salmonella suipestifer*), which is thought to be the primary instigator of fibrinous enteritis in the pig, and the virus of avian laryngo-tracheitis. The viruses of feline infectious enteritis (panleukopenia), malignant catarrhal fever and porcine atrophic rhinitis (if it is a virus) are somewhat less notable for the production of fibrinous exudates.

Many fibrinous exudates are mixed with the serous variety and are called serofibrinous; others are combined with purulent inflammation (to be described shortly) constituting a fibrino-purulent type. In these combined forms, we may list many of the causes of serous and purulent inflammations as causes of the fibrinous as well. This applies most frequently to the pyogenic organisms, to which the reaction is usually purulent.

In such cases, the part of the body involved appears to be an important factor in determining whether the exudate is fibrinous. It has been stated that fibrinous inflammation occurs chiefly on mucous and serous surfaces. This is so true that it seems proper to accord to the anatomical location a causative role. For example, any acute inflammation of the pericardium is almost sure to be fibrinous or serofibrinous or fibrino-purulent. The same is likely to be true of inflammations of the pleura, peritoneum and even the meninges.

Burns are at times followed by a fibrinous reaction, apparently without infection.

Significance and Effect.—It is difficult to identify the exact mechanism which is responsible for the outpouring of fibrinogen. We are not aware of any other source than the usual clotting apparatus of the blood. Possibly hydrostatic and osmotic pressures are such that a large amount of blood plasma passes through the abnormally permeable capillaries (see Vascular Changes, p. 147), deposits its fibrin and is then reabsorbed and drained away.

As far as the inflamed area is concerned, the fibrin probably serves a number of useful purposes. We can believe that it prevents loss of blood (erythrocytes) through the dead and unprotected surface which usually underlies it (coagulative necrosis) and that it protects the underlying tissues from further irritation. Certain it is that a "sore throat" coated with a layer of exudate is less painful than it is after the coating has been removed. The strands of fibrin are believed by many to form a framework useful in supporting leukocytes as they migrate through the inflamed zone.

If the inflammation terminates with reasonable promptness, the underlying surface is regenerated and the fibrin is dissolved. On a free mucous surface, it may be sloughed as in the case of the bronchial and intestinal casts previously mentioned. But on the serous surfaces and in the pulmonary alveoli, fibrin remaining there for some days is likely to undergo **organization** by fibrous tissue in much the same way that a thrombus does. The fibroblasts build into the zone of fibrin by proliferation of those in the underlying tissue. Such fibrous tissue is permanent. It is especially unfortunate on serous surfaces such as those of the pleura, pericardium and peritoneum for it tends to build across from one opposing surface to another, forming permanent **adhesions** which tie them together and prevent movement and function. Barring this contingency the organized layer on a surface becomes, as the inflammation subsides, covered with mesothelial cells which form a surface similar to that which existed previously. If fibrin in the alveoli of the lung is organized, that portion of the lung is permanently converted into fibrous tissue, a process known as **carnification** (*carneus*, flesh).

3. Purulent Inflammation

Purulent inflammation and purulent exudates are characterized by pus. **Pus** is typically a liquid of creamy color and consistency, but it may be thin and almost watery or it may be inspissated and semi-solid. Its creamy yellow color is changed to bluish or greenish in case *Pseudomonas aeruginosa* (*Bacillus pyocyaneus*) is

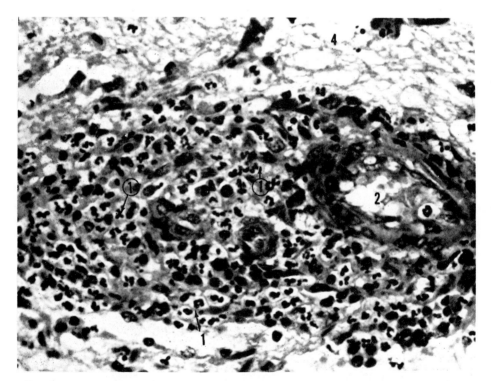

Fig. 6–3.—Purulent inflammation. Polymorphonuclear neutrophilic leukocytes ("neutrophils" or "polymorphs") (*1*) adjacent to an artery (*2*) in the brain of a horse with generalized infection by *Streptococcus pyogenes*. Grossly visible abscesses were found elsewhere in the cerebrum. (Courtesy of Armed Forces Institute of Pathology.) × 600. Contributor: Army Veterinary Research Laboratory.

among the infecting bacteria. It carries a blackish discoloration in case it comes from black hoofs of horses, the color being reportedly due to sulfides. The definitive characteristic of pus is the presence of numerous neutrophilic poly-morphonuclear granulocytes. These "neutrophils," living or necrotic, together with necrotic cells of the pre-existing tissue, more or less liquefied, and minor amounts of the other constituents of inflammatory exudates including serum, constitute the ingredients of pus. When pus is present in major or minor degree, the inflammatory process is said to be purulent. (There is no such adjective as "pussy".)

The term suppurative inflammation or **suppuration** is a variant of the general term and implies that considerable amounts of pus are produced; usually it runs from a surface or fills cavities.

A **phlegmon,** or phlegmonous inflammation, is a condition in which appreciable amounts of pus are diffusely scattered through a tissue, particularly the subcutis. Cellulitis is a more or less synonymous term. A phlegmon tends to spread in-definitely in contrast to an abscess, where the reaction and the causative infection are confined.

An **abscess** is defined as a circumscribed collection of pus. When well devel-oped, it has a wall or capsule of fibrous tissue separating it from the surrounding tissue. In size, abscesses vary from microscopic to almost unlimited dimensions.

Microscopic Appearance.—The appearance of considerable numbers of neutro-philic leukocytes in or on a tissue justifies a diagnosis of purulent inflammation. Usually these are seen in great numbers, but they do not need to be more numerous than accompanying lymphocytes for the purulent designation to be employed. The lymphocyte is looked upon as a sort of accessory, present in various types of inflammation. Many of the neutrophils undergo necrosis and are recognized by their small size, dark and irregularly shaped nuclei and acidophilic cytoplasm. In addition to hyperemia or congestion, a minor amount of fibrin, serum (as a pink-staining precipitate) and various other leukocytes, fixed and wandering cells will be seen in conjunction with the neutrophils.

Gross Appearance.—The purulent exudate consists of pus, the general appear-ance of which has been described as a viscous, cream-colored fluid with possible variations extending from a watery consistency, such as results from some streptococcal infections, to a material which is practically a solid as the result of resorption of water. The red discoloration resulting from hemorrhage, the blue-green color coming from the pigment-forming pyocyaneus bacillus, and the black color from disintegrating hoof material have also been described. Pus may be seen exuding from an infected wound or mucous membrane. It may be con-fined within abscesses or the body cavities. Its presence in the pulmonary alveoli, a phase of pneumonia called gray hepatization, is demonstrated by incising the lung and pressing it out from the cut surfaces. The beginning student is familiar with it, if nowhere else, as the thick yellow and sometimes foul-smelling fluid which he expectorates or blows from his nose in the late stages of a "cold."

Causes.—Purulent or suppurative inflammations are caused by **pyogenic bac-teria.** The word "pyogenic" means "pus-forming." The principal members of this group of bacteria are the pyogenic baciili, *Corynebacterium (Bacterium) pyo-genes,* and its relatives *C. renale* and *C. equi, Pseudomonas aeruginosa,* and rarely *Escherichia (Bacillus) coli.* By pyogenic cocci we mean *Staphylococcus (Micrococcus) aureus* and its relatives *Staph. albus* and *Staph. citreus,* the streptococci, and the human pathogens appearing as diplococci, *Diplococcus pneumoniae*, *Neisseria (Diplococcus) gonorrheae* and *N. meningitidis*. The tubercle bacillus is a pus-former in the very earliest stages of infection, and tuberculous meningitis may be purulent simply because the patient dies before the usual type of tuberculous lesion becomes established. The reaction in several of the infectious granulomas (p. 615) tends to be purulent in the immediate vicinity of the invading organisms. Chief among these granulomas are actinomycosis, actinobacillosis, the form of staphylococcal granuloma formerly called botryomycosis, coccidioidomycosis, blastomycosis, glanders (slightly) and chronic tularemia.

There are a few other pathogens which, under certain circumstances of virulence and resistance, can be pyogenic, but the cocci and corynebacteria far outweigh all others in frequency, importance and pyogenic potency. It is possible to produce a purulent lesion and abscesses by the direct injection into the tissues of various chemical irritants such as turpentine. But in everyday practice the old dictum still holds of, "No infection; no pus," a rule which the budding surgeon may well take to heart. In dealing with tissues surgically removed it is of practical diagnostic importance that a small number of neutrophils may quickly infiltrate a tissue as the result of the slight trauma incident to the living tissue being handled by the surgeon.

Significance and Effect.—The liquefactive necrosis of tissue which is a feature of pus formation is illustrative of the fact that purulent inflammation is a prompt and violent reaction against irritant organisms of high virulence. This does not mean that these diseases necessarily have a high rate of fatality. Along with the vigorous microphagic and other activities of the neutrophils, there is often a very effective production of humoral antibodies (immune bodies) as well as fever, all of which are the body's most potent defenses. These organisms also happen to be among the most vulnerable to available therapeutic agents. However, the mere fact that pus is formed indicates a strong defensive reaction. Without knowing exactly why, physicians of earlier days considered the appearance of pus in a wound a favorable sign, and referred to it as "good laudable pus."

Pus contains large numbers of the causative bacteria, living or dead, and the various toxic products of their metabolism. Confined pus is a source for absorption of toxic substances into the circulation, often with very harmful results including such visible changes as cellular swelling and necrosis of parenchymatous organs. **Toxemia** is the name given to such a state, meaning literally "toxins in the blood." Living organisms also find their entrance into the blood stream facilitated by confinement of the exudate containing them, so that some may be carried by the blood to new locations, where they colonize and multiply, a process called **metastasis**. For these reasons it is of the utmost importance that an abscess or other suppurative lesion have free drainage to the outside, surgical intervention sometimes being necessary.

Abscesses may, however, become sterile, the body defenses having killed all of the causative bacteria. The accumulated pus, with no way to escape, commonly remains for some time before being slowly liquefied and absorbed.

4. Hemorrhagic Inflammation

Hemorrhagic inflammation and hemorrhagic exudates are characterized by large numbers of erythrocytes which leave their normal channels by diapedesis to exude from a body surface or into nearby tissues. With them there are any or all of the components of other types of exudates, serum, leukocytes and especially fibrin, so that the whole exudate bears some resemblance to clotted or unclotted blood.

While this type of inflammation **occurs** within the tissues in such diseases as blackleg, anthrax, pasteurellosis and purpura hemorrhagica, it is especially prone to involve mucous surfaces. The lungs may also suffer this type of inflammation. Hemorrhagic gastritis and enteritis are among the commonest manifestations of this type of exudate.

Microscopic Appearance.—With the components just listed it may be a problem to distinguish hemorrhagic exudate from simple hemorrhage. However, the various components of the blood are present in other than their normal proportions, the constituents of exudates such as fibrin or leukocytes or both always being more plentiful than in normal blood. Also, the exudate is diffuse in distribution, having come from an area, not from one or a few points, as would be the case with a simple hemorrhage.

Gross Appearance.—Blood-colored material, sometimes fluid or semi-fluid, but usually clotted and of gelatinous consistency, appears on a surface or in tissue spaces. It is likely to be somewhat streaked or varying in color and consistency, revealing that the material is not pure clotted blood. The inflamed surface is deep red. It may be confused with the type of catarrhal inflammation in which the principal changes are severe hyperemia and loss of epithelium, but usually in the latter type bloody fluid has not actually escaped from the tissue and the reddening of the surface is not quite so pronounced. Blood, whether as an exudate or as a hemorrhage, coming from any but the most posterior part of the gastro-intestinal tract, colors the feces black. Coming from the lungs it is foamy from admixed air, but when it comes from the respiratory passages this is not the case.

The **causes** of hemorrhagic inflammation are (1) micro-organisms of high virulence and (2) acute poisoning by certain chemicals when in contact in concentrated form with digestive or other mucous membranes, or when such substances are eliminated by way of mucous membranes, especially those of the lower bowel, bladder, or gallbladder. Among these substances are phenol, arsenic, phosphorus and others. The clotted exudate of laryngo-tracheitis of chickens has been mentioned as fibrinous. It is also hemorrhagic with individual cases varying as to which type predominates. The pathogenic leptospiræ and the virus of canine hepatitis are pathogens notable for causing hemorrhagic inflammation, doubtless the direct result of injury to vascular endothelium.

Significance and Effect.—Hemorrhagic inflammation arises quickly and is all too likely to presage an early fatality, although in some instances it subsides with almost equal rapidity upon removal of the cause.

5. Catarrhal or Mucous Inflammation

The characteristic component of this type of inflammatory exudate is mucus, which comes from cells rather than from the blood. Mucus is produced by epithelial cells, either of the more or less complex mucous glands which open upon mucous membranes or of those one-celled mucous glands called goblet cells. For this reason the **occurrence** of mucous or catarrhal inflammation is limited to mucous membranes. The number of goblet cells in a given mucous membrane can vary, increasing under proper stimuli, and it is possible for epithelia not normally equipped with them to develop mucus-secreting cells.

Microscopic Appearance.—Commonly the excessive mucus is readily visible as pale bluish or grayish strands of mucin clinging to the mucous membrane which produced it. The increased number of goblet cells may be conspicuously apparent. In many cases, however, another important feature is loss by necrosis and desquamation of much of the surface epithelium. Rather frequently this becomes the predominant feature of catarrhal inflammation, leaving the affected mucous membrane denuded of its epithelial covering, somewhat hyperemic and containing slight or moderate infiltrations of lymphocytes. Thus, in spite of the fact that the fundamental idea of catarrh is a flowing, we come to speak of a catarrhal inflammation in which there is no flow of mucus. The hyperemia and the presence of reactive cells usually suffice to differentiate this condition from post-mortem desquamation of the epithelium.

Gross Appearance.—The predominantly mucous forms of catarrhal inflammation are recognized by the presence of the clear, slimy mucin-containing fluid which has already been described as mucus (p. 52). This is readily recognized on post-mortem examination. During life it may even drip from the nostrils if the nasal mucosa is the structure involved. Mucous colitis, a fairly common condition, can often be recognized clinically by opaque white shreds or patches of semi-dehydrated mucus adhering to the formed feces or mixed with the excrement if it is softer.

When the inflammation is characterized less by mucus than by hyperemia and loss of epithelium, the inflamed surface shows little but the red color of raw meat with slight swelling. Limited amounts of mucus or of fibrinous or purulent material may or may not be present. Not infrequently there is such an admixture of pus that the term muco-purulent is used. In mucous cholecystitis, the mucus may be seen imperfectly mixed with bile or it may not be discernible.

The increased flow of tears or of saliva which occurs when the respective regions of the body suffer suitable irritation is an entirely comparable reaction to mucous inflammation, although the secretions of the lachrymal and salivary glands differ from mucus.

Causes.—The irritants which cause this type of inflammation are mild in character or of short duration. They include:

(1) Bacterial and viral infections of low virulence or in their early stages. A "cold" as seen most often in humans and poultry forms a good example, in its earlier stages, of catarrhal inflammation. Later the mucous exudate may become purulent.

(2) Mildly or transiently irritating chemicals. Inhaled formalin, chlorine, bromine and chlorpicrin (tear gas) fall in this category, as do many antiseptics used in too great a concentration on delicate mucous membranes. There is considerable difference in what can be endured by the columnar epithelium of the cervix and uterus and by the squamous lining of the mouth.

(3) Irritating foods in the digestive tract have the ability to set up catarrhal inflammation. In some cases it is difficult to say whether a case of transient catarrhal gastro-enteritis is due directly to the food or to micro-organsims in it, but mild forms are often caused by foods of improper quality for the species concerned or consumed excessively, or at a time when the nervous or other status

already been described. It may or may not be well supplied with capillaries depending upon the peculiarities of the causative organism. These also determine whether neutrophils and other leukocytes are present. At its periphery this type of granulation tissue often gives way, sometimes suddenly but more often by imperceptibly gradual changes from rounded to elongated cells, to a fibrous tissue which forms an encircling capsule. (See also Maduromycotic Mycetoma, p. 655, and Cutaneous Habronemiasis, p. 772.)

Epithelial proliferation will be described in connection with the respective causes.

Gross Appearance.—If on an exposed surface, the new tissue is likely to be ulcerated and bloody. If excessive in amount, as it frequently is, the mass bulges grotesquely above the surface. The name, "granulation tissue," is derived from the usual appearance of the new tissue as it proliferates to fill a gaping wound. The growth is not uniform but tends to be in any number of rounded nodules or "granulations" and the wound is said to be "granulating," a sign of satisfactory healing, albeit under a covering of pus.

When incised the tissue is white, tough and hard in the case of mature fibrous granulation tissue; white, smoothly dense and perhaps watery (edematous) if it consists of recently formed fibrous tissue; yellowish, soft and very easily cut when composed of the reticulo-endothelial variety. In the depths of body structures, it is mainly by differences in color and consistency that the presence of a foreign tissue can be distinguished. For example, in a fibrosed liver (see Cirrhosis, p. 1225) the streaks of white criss-crossing through the tissue may be thick enough to reveal themselves readily. A sinus tract, such as results from a penetrating foreign body from the bovine reticulum, is detected by the denseness of its fibrous walls.

Causes.—In general the causes of proliferative inflammation are infectious, toxic, mechanical or rarely radiational irritants which continue to act with

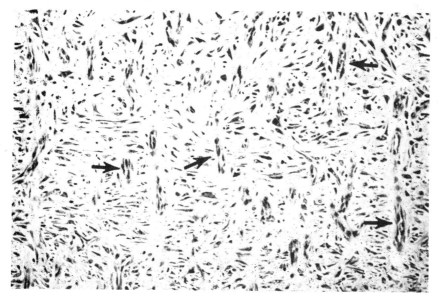

FIG. 6–5.—Fibrous granulation tissue at the base of a healing ulcer of the rectum of a cow. The organization of new blood vessels (arrows) perpendicular to fibroblasts and collagen is typical and allows differentiation from fibroma. (Tissue courtesy Dr. C. L. Davis.)

moderate, or at least non-lethal severity over a considerable period of time. The larval migrations of some metazoan parasites have caused extensive fibrous proliferation, for example, larvæ of the porcine kidney worm (*Stephanurus dentatus*) in the liver and, to a lesser degree, the common ascarid. A proliferative endarteritis is a frequent finding in dirofilariasis ("heart-worm") in the dog. The persistence of other types is dependent upon external factors, but the long duration of infectious inflammations is usually due to the fact that the invading pathogen lacks sufficient virulence to kill the host directly, and the host is unable to provide antibodies, fever or other defensive mechanisms which are able to destroy the invading organisms.

In such a situation, it is usual for the body reaction to consist in the building of granulation tissue around the site of invasion, a sort of defense in depth, as it were. The slow spread of the organisms and their destructive toxins, together with the continual formation of new granulation tissue may go on indefinitely, a fatal outcome perhaps resulting from destruction of vital organs by the mere bulk of the new growths. Allergic hypersensitivity induced by the presence of the invading micro-organisms appears also to play a part in the development of this form of inflammation (See Hypersensitivity, p. 309).

The granulation tissue is chiefly of the reticulo-endothelial variety, but its exact characteristics vary with the disease in question. Among the infections to which these remarks apply are tuberculosis, glanders, syphilis (humans) leprosy (man, rat), Johne's disease, caseous lymphadenitis, actinomycosis, nocardiosis, actinobacillosis, granulomatous staphylococcic infection ("botryomycosis"), coccidioidal granuloma, blastomycosis, histoplasmosis, bovine nasal granuloma, chronic aspergillosis, chronic tularemia (at least in man) and Hjarre's coli-granuloma of birds. Toxoplasmosis essentially belongs in the group, especially as it involves muscle and the human eye.

Small foreign bodies accidentally buried in the tissues can initiate a similar granulomatous reaction which is likely to be both reticulo-endothelial and fibrous. Bits of certain kinds of surgical sutures, minute splinters of wood and metals, fragments of plant tissue and lycopodium spores (formerly used as a powder for surgeons' gloves) have had this effect.

Epithelial proliferation, reserved for discussion in this section, results in limited extent from continued local pressure, the cornified layer (keratin) being thickened especially. The best example is a "corn" on the human foot, but similar proliferations of the epidermis form over the elbows and other bony prominences of animals due to repeated pressure when lying down. Chemical irritants produce overgrowth of epithelium in the case of highly chlorinated naphthalenes, which, through external or internal contact, produce proliferation of the epidermis and of various internal epithelia (the specific bovine "hyperkeratosis"). An appreciable amount of lymphocytic and other inflammatory infiltration is present in these tissues. The irritants (smoke?) which cause bronchial carcinoma start their work merely with overproduction of epithelium. The most spectacular example of epithelial proliferation is that which results from the invasion of the coccidium, *Eimeria stiedae*, in the bile ducts of the rabbit. Retaining its simple columnar type, the overgrowth of epithelium, with the necessary underlying stroma, produces a multitude of papillary projections which simulate an adenoma (although neoplasia never occurs). Since it is clearly caused by the presence of an extrinsic irritating object, the justification for considering the process inflammatory seems ample. The gastritis associated with *Gongylonema neoplasticum* in rodents is another example of epithelial proliferation in inflammation.

Significance and Effect.—As the reader has probably already inferred, the changes described for proliferative inflammation frequently fulfill the definition of hyperplasia (p. 92). Indeed the term **hyperplastic inflammation** is in common use for those forms in which the mere overgrowth of a pre-existing tissue is prominent. The tendency already noted for hyperplastic tissues to progress to metaplasia and neoplasia has to be considered here. A possible example in the bronchi has just been noted. In the ordinary pyogenic or reticulo-endothelial granulomas, there is no reason either in the histological appearances or in the clinical course for one to think of neoplasia. However, there are cases in which it is most difficult to distinguish histologically between fibrous granulation tissue and a fibrous neoplasm. Ordinary fibrous granulation tissue regularly makes a second (or continued) growth following anything but very complete removal, and there are plenty of cases in equine practice where the impossibility of perfect separation of granulating from normal tissue leads to repeated recurrence and eventual euthanasia. Indeed, some of these border-line growths have come to be called **equine sarcoids**. **Hodgkin's disease** is a fatal proliferative disease of humans thought to belong with the lymphoma-myeloma group of neoplasms but which has never been certainly separated from the inflammatory reactions.

THE LEUKOCYTES IN INFLAMMATION

It is desirable to consider briefly the functions and capabilities of the various reactive cells in inflammatory processes. Reticulo-endothelial cells having received attention in preceding paragraphs, the cells to be considered are, with one exception, the leukocytes of the blood.

NEUTROPHIL LEUKOCYTES

These cells, sometimes known as polymorphs, polymorphonuclear cells and granulocytes, but for which the most popular designation is neutrophil(e)s, are the characteristic component of the purulent exudate and probably the most potent of the leukocytes in the inflammatory battle. In professional slang, reference is sometimes made to them as "pus cells." The term **heterophil(e)** is used to describe the functional counterpart of the neutrophil in certain species such as the rabbit and guinea pig in which the granules of the cells are eosinophilic. The less desirable term pseudoeosinophil has also been applied to the neutrophil of these species.

Formed in the bone marrow from primitive cells, the mature neutrophil when released into the circulation, has a bizarre multilobed nucleus and numerous cytoplasmic granules which resemble lysosomes. When observed by electron microscopy, the nuclear lobes often appear disconnected due to ultrathin sectioning. The chromatin is concentrated near the nuclear membrane. The granules are surrounded by a membrane, relatively uniform in size, round to elongate and have a homogeneous, moderately electron-dense matrix. There is a paucity of organized cytoplasmic structures other than the granules. Mitochondria are generally few and little or no endoplasmic reticulum is present. A Golgi apparatus is usually evident. The granules contain a host of hydrolytic, oxidative, and

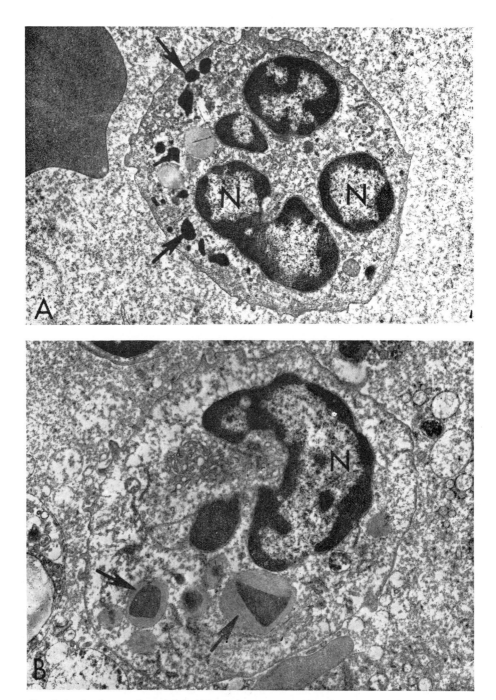

FIG. 6-6.—Leukocytes in peripheral blood of a marmoset (*Saguinus nigricollis*). *A*, Neutrophil. The lobes of the nucleus (*N*) appear separate due to thin sectioning. The granules (arrows) resemble lysosomes. *B*, Eosinophil. The granules (arrows) contain dense crystalline bodies. (Courtesy Dr. N. W. King, Jr.)

proteolytic enzymes as well as two antibacterial substances **lysozyme** and **phago-cytin.**

The half life of neutrophils is approximately six hours, requiring their continual replenishment both to the circulation and to inflammatory exudates, as neutrophils are end cells, incapable of division. It is not certain what constitutes the graveyard for dying neutrophils, but probably most leave the body to the outside world via the intestines, skin and lungs.

The neutrophils leave the blood in large numbers in response to invasion and injury by pyogenic bacteria to enter the zone of inflammation as explained in the description of the purulent exudate. They reach the scene quickly, within a few hours, utilizing their marked ability of ameboid movement.

Their function of engulfing small particles is so readily observable that they are called the **microphages** of the body, a term coined by Metchnikoff in 1905. This phenomenon known as **phagocytosis** is probably the principal function of neutrophils. They may ingest foreign matter such as carbon, pigments, cellular debris and most importantly, bacteria. To phagocytize bacteria, certain serum proteins called **opsonins** are required. Opsonins generally represent specific antibodies directed against the bacterium, although normal serum from non-immunized or previously exposed individuals also contain proteins (which may in fact be specific antibodies) which coat bacteria and bind complement. Once engulfed "digestible" materials are disposed of by "digestive" enzymes held by the neutrophil's granules. If perchance the material is "nondigestible" like carbon particles, it is released upon the death of the short-lived neutrophil to be engulfed by another neutrophil or possibly a macrophage (p. 176). Most bacteria are killed following phagocytosis, but not by usual enzymes such as proteases, for these living objects are resistant to most enzymes. Two substances, lysozyme and phagocytin, are held responsible for this ability. Other functions ascribed to neutrophils include secretion of lytic substances to degrade dead bacteria and dead body cells, secretion of substances which augment the inflammatory reaction, secretion of chemotactic chemicals, and secretion of a pyrogen (fever producing substance) to initiate and maintain fever.

As indicated, neutrophils, unlike some of the reactive cells, have no ability to multiply by mitosis or otherwise. Replacements for the large numbers killed on the inflammatory battleground have to come from their original source, the myeloid tissue in the red bone marrow. It is not surprising then that as an acute suppurative inflammation develops the number of neutrophils in the circulating blood is perceptibly, often markedly increased. Moderate increases in the numbers of these cells may also accompany certain toxemias such as uremia, severe loss of blood, and pregnancy.

Practical use is made of this fact by determining the **total** and **differential white-cell counts** of the blood in the diagnosis of suspected pyogenic infections. The percentage of neutrophils among all leukocytes is markedly increased in acute pyogenic infections, in the human, dog and horse from a normal of 60 to 70 per cent up to 75 to 90 per cent. In cattle, sheep and swine the normal of around 50 per cent shows a similar tendency. The total leukocyte count of 6,000 to 10,000 per cubic millimeter in the human, with a somewhat higher normal in the domestic mammals, rises commonly to 12,000 to 15,000 and less often to 20,000, 30,000 or even higher in these infections although in cattle the first twenty-four or forty-eight hours of an acute pyogenic process may actually be marked by a decrease. This inflammatory change is known as (neutrophilic) **leuko-cytosis.** It has to be distinguished from **leukemia,** (p. 208), a neoplastic increase in the numbers of one kind or another of white cells in the blood, sometimes to much higher levels. On the other hand, in some other infections, chiefly viral, there is a marked decrease in the white-cell count known as **leukopenia** or if the change is only in the neutrophils, as **neutropenia.**

Something can also be learned concerning the diagnosis and prognosis from the "**Schilling count.**" This consists in determining how many of the neutrophils are young ("juvenile," or "stab" from the German) cells. These should not exceed 6 per cent of the total white cells. If their number is higher, it indicates an active but possibly losing battle against a pyogenic invader, since larger numbers of juvenile forms appear only when production by the myeloblastic tissue is inadequate. A high neutrophil count consisting of mature types (horseshoe or multi-lobed nucleus) is a favorable sign. The term "shift to the left," based on a common way of writing the figures for the different types, is a frequent method of expressing an increase in the count of juvenile neutrophils.

EOSINOPHIL LEUKOCYTES

The functions of the eosinophil leukocyte in the battle against disease have long been a matter of speculation and study, but still remain mysterious. It is well recognized that eosinophils are increased in numbers and must play an important part in allergic reactions such as asthma, the invasions by many (but not all) parasitic helminths and arthropods (where again allergy may be the fundamental excitant) and diseases of the skin.

The mature circulating eosinophil, produced in the bone marrow, varies in appearance between species. In most, the nucleus is slightly lobed but rarely to the extent of a mature neutrophil. As seen in man, dogs, and horses, the nucleus consists of two tear drop lobes connected by a thin strand, whereas in the rat the nucleus is usually an annular ring without distinct lobation. The cytoplasmic granules also vary in the different species, unusually large in the horse, rod-like in the cat, ovoid in sheep, round in the cow and pig, and round but variable in size in the dog. The ultrastructure of the eosinophil nucleus is similar to that of neutrophils with condensation of chromatin at the periphery. The granules are membrane-bound structures with a moderately dense matrix in which is embedded a very dense structure of crystalline appearance. This crystalloid varies in shape from round (dog) to square (man) to rectangular (cat, rat). Other cytoplasmic organelles are not numerous; mitochondria are few and the endoplasmic reticulum is sparse. Eosinophils contain a complement of enzymes similar to those of the neutrophil but lack detectable lysozyme and phagocytin. They have an unusually high concentration of peroxidase.

Like neutrophils, eosinophils have a short life span (a few days) and are end cells incapable of reproduction. Although the normal number in the circulating blood in most species is small, vast reserves are present in the marrow and in the walls of the intestines, lungs, skin and vagina. These sites represent a pool of eosinophils, which can contribute to the circulation. Rapid changes can occur in the circulating number apparently from interchanges with the tissue pool. Adrenal cortical steroids induce a swift reduction or disappearance in eosinophils (eosinopenia) which accounts for the eosinopenia in shock or the "alarm" reaction. Experimental injection of histamine also induces eosinopenia.

As indicated, their function is obscure. They are motile and phagocytic and therefore presumed to play a role in engulfing and destroying particulate matter such as dead cells, bacteria, parasites and very likely **antigen-antibody precipitates.** A most probable role of the eosinophil is an antagonist to the inflammatory response. Recent evidence has shown that eosinophil extracts are antagonistic to histamine (p. 150), serotonin (p. 151) and bradykinin (p. 151), all of which are mediators of the inflammatory response. This may also explain the close association of eosinophils to mast cells (p. 180) in tissues which has led some to regard the eosinophil as a physiological opposite of the mast cell. Eosinophils are also thought to play a role in the immune response, possibly accepting antigen or "information" from macrophages which have engulfed antigen.

In the tissues, eosinophils, with or without other leukocytes, congregate at the site of allergic reactions (lungs in asthma), in the vicinity of animal parasites (intestinal worms, trichinae [p. 762], recent acute sarcosporidiosis) (p. 694). The reason for their presence in huge numbers in eosinophilic myositis (p. 1052) has never been discovered. They are numerous in the sinuses of lymph nodes that drain other tissues containing eosinophils and also under other circumstances not understood. In the tissues and even on a glass slide they are attracted by histamine, while they at the same time antagonize its action. This attraction is presumed to be the reason why they are drawn to the types of injury just mentioned but it does not explain the selective attraction to these types of injury and not others.

BASOPHIL LEUKOCYTES

Basophils are found in very low numbers in the circulating blood. They have a lobed nucleus and the cytoplasm contains deeply basophilic and metachromatic granules. Their function and their role in the inflammatory process is unknown. Like mast cells, the granules are thought to contain histamine and heparin and therefore the function of these two cells may be analogous, but must wait confirmation. The ultrastructural characteristics of basophils is similar to that of neutrophils, but the granules are larger and have a lamellated or whorled matrix rather than homogeneous.

LYMPHOCYTES

The lymphocytes have received considerable discussion under the heading of Lymphocytic Inflammation. They appear in a great variety of acute and chronic inflammatory processes but only in limited numbers. Probably because they have only limited powers of ameboid movement, they remain at some distance from the center of active acute inflammation. Frequently many of them only succeed in getting just outside the blood vessel which brought them, constituting **perivascular lymphocytic infiltration.** They usually appear rather late in the course of an infection, some days after its beginning. They are not phagocytic.

Lymphocytes are produced by the lymphoid tissues of the body where they comprise the major cellular constituent of these organs. The normal development of the lymphoid organs requires that the thymus provide either an original stock

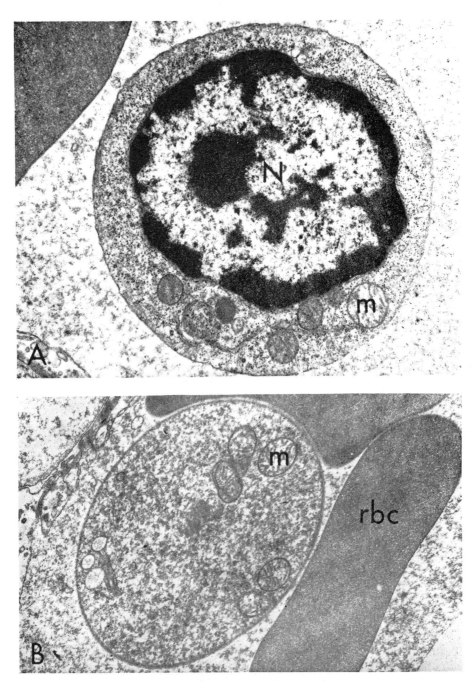

FIG. 6–7.—*A*, Lymphocyte in peripheral blood of a marmoset (*Saguinus oedipus*). *N* = nucleus, *m* = mitochondria. *B*, Thrombocyte, *m* = mitochondria. (Courtesy Dr. N. W. King, Jr.)

of cells or provide a humoral factor. Without the thymus (thymectomy) lymphoid tissues fail to develop normally. Antigenic stimulation is also required for the development of the non-thymic lymphoid organs. The lymphoid organs of animals reared under "germ-free" conditions fail to develop normally. This is undoubtedly related to the role of the lymphocyte in the immune mechanisms which will be discussed later. Once formed, lymphocytes are released via the major lymph channels to the blood stream where they comprise a large percentage of the circulating leukocytes. Most are small cells containing a round nucleus and a narrow rim of cytoplasm. A smaller number of lymphocytes have larger nuclei with more prominent nucleoli, a greater amount of a more basophilic cytoplasm, and are called large lymphocytes. The cytoplasm of small lymphocytes contains only mitochondria and a few small vesicles whereas large lymphocytes contain, in addition, a prominent Golgi apparatus and endoplasmic reticulum. Lymphocytes are not end cells, large lymphocytes are capable of division into small lymphocytes and small lymphocytes of differentiation to a large cell which in turn is capable of division into small lymphocytes. Thus it is not appropriate to assign a life span to lymphocytes. However, assuming the cell does not divide or differentiate, small lymphocytes are known to remain alive *in vivo* for at least ninety days.

In contrast to granulocytes which remain within the circulation until death or unless "called forth," lymphocytes do not normally remain in the blood stream continuously but recirculate from the blood back to the lymph. They enter lymph by passing through endothelial cells of post capillary venules located in the cortex of lymph nodes. This unique ability of lymphocytes to pass through another cell is not shared by any other leukocyte. Lymphocytes also find their way from the blood to the lymphocytic follicles of the spleen and other lymphoid organs such as Peyer's patches. The route in these cases is not clear. From the node or spleen, the lymphocytes then either directly re-enter the blood or travel via lymphatics to regain the blood circulation.

Several functions have been ascribed to lymphocytes. These include (1) that lymphocytes can differentiate into other cell types to include macrophages, fibroblasts, plasma cells and multipotential stem cells. However, with the exception of differentiation into plasma cells, there is no direct evidence that any of these transformations can or do occur; (2) that lymphocytes serve as "trephocytes," *i.e.*, cells which supply nutrients to other cells. Direct evidence for this function is also lacking; (3) that lymphocytes participate in the immune response. It is now relatively certain that lymphocytes do, in fact, participate in the immune mechanisms, however their exact role remains elucidation.

In addition to immunological responses mediated by humoral antibody, lymphocytes are also necessary for cell mediated immunological responses such as homograph rejection and delayed type hypersensitivity. In both cases it is the small lymphocyte that is necessary for these responses. It is now known that there are two populations of small lymphocytes, one dependent upon the thymus for development, called T-lymphocytes, and one independent on the thymus, called B-lymphocytes. In birds development of B-lymphocytes is dependent upon the bursa of Fabricius, but no single organ or tissue has been identified in mammals which serves this function. Most circulating small lymphocytes are T-lymphocytes while B-lymphocytes are largely restricted to lymphoid tissue. B-lymphocytes are concerned with immunoglobulin synthesis by differentiating into plasma cells (p. 178). In contrast the T-lymphocytes are responsible for cell mediated immunological reactions; they do not form immunoglobulins. Recent evidence suggests that T-lymphocytes are necessary to stimulate B-lymphocytes to antibody production; thus there is a dependence of the humoral antibody system on the thymus dependent T-lymphocytes.

In man there is a long list of disorders characterized by immunological deficiencies centering around both B-lymphocytes and T-lymphocytes. Undoubtedly future research will reveal many similar disorders in animals.

MONOCYTES, LARGE MONONUCLEAR, RETICULO-ENDOTHELIAL CELLS

These are closely related cells of mesenchymal origin which have been discussed in connection with proliferative inflammation. Responding to stimuli initiated by the infections and other irritants listed under that heading, they become numerous in the inflamed areas some days after the beginning of the inflammatory process, which may well have been purulent at its very outset. They have marked capability of ameboid movement.

The blood monocyte characteristically has an indented nucleus with condensation of the nucleoplasm near its membrane. The cytoplasm is similar in many ways to that of the lymphocyte but is more abundant. It contains mitochondria, a well formed Golgi apparatus, and rough and smooth endoplasmic reticulum which usually appears as "vesicles." Lysosomes or other "granules" are absent. The tissue macrophage and reticulo-endothelial cells have a similar structure to

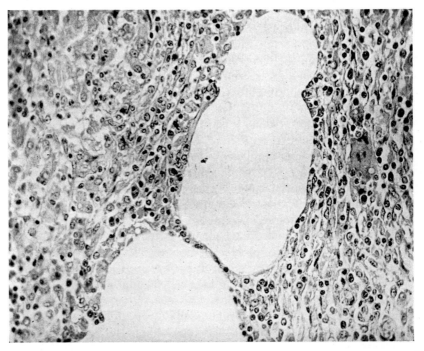

FIG. 6–8.—Reticulo-endothelial cells surrounding lipid foreign material (spaces) injected subcutaneously as an adjuvant in a tissue vaccine. Subcutis of a cow. H & E × 300. Contributor: Col. Fred D. Maurer, V.C.

the monocyte, but also contain many membrane-bound granules. These granules are reminiscent of lysosomes and presumably contain a packet of enzymes including lysozyme and acid-phosphatase.

Their functions include the phagocytosis of the microscopically larger particles, animate or inanimate, including the pathogenic bacteria responsible for their presence. This faculty gives them the name of **macrophages,** as contrasted with the microphages, which are polymorphonuclear neutrophils. The macrophages frequently fuse together to form giant cells, which are able to phagocytize still larger particles such as pathogenic yeast cells and fungi, of which the *Cryptococcus* (*Torula*) and the *Coccidioides* are among the largest. A **Langhans' giant cell** is of irregular shape and some 50 or 60 microns in diameter. Its cytoplasm is fused into a homogeneous mass, but it has many spherical nuclei arranged in a more or less complete wreath just inside its hazy and indefinite periphery. A **foreign-body giant cell** is similar except that its somewhat larger nuclei are piled up in a jumbled mass at the center of the cell.

Functions of the mononuclear cells other than phagocytosis are thought to include the secretion of various enzymes and neutralizing substances. They may also play a role in the immune processes by altering antigen or transferring antigen or "information" to an immunologically competent cell. Their function of providing a physical barrier in the form of a frequently wide zone of granulation tissue between the infected and healthy areas has been described in connection with proliferative inflammation.

The first of these cells may be brought to the inflamed area by the blood in

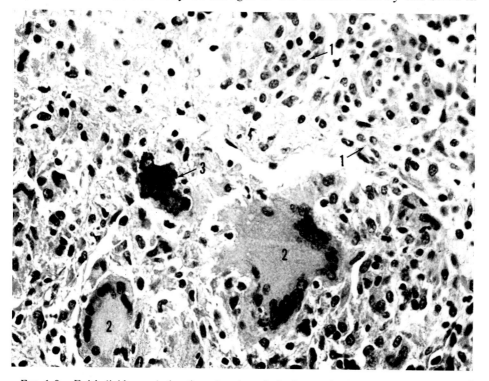

FIG. 6–9.—Epithelioid granulation tissue in tuberculosis of an equine lung. Epithelioid cells (*1*), Langhans' giant cells (*2*) and calcareous debris (*3*). (Courtesy of Armed Forces Institute of Pathology.) × 435. Contributor: Dr. J. R. M. Innes.

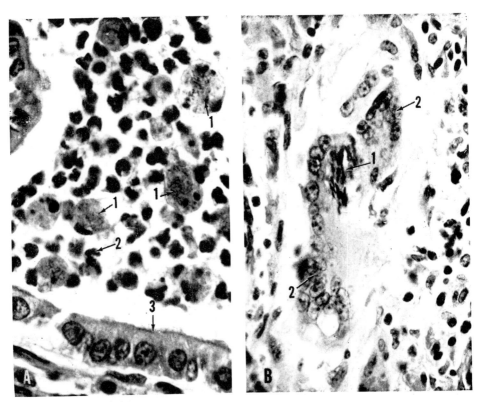

FIG. 6–10.—*A*, Macrophages in a bronchiole of a foal infected with *Corynebacterium pyogenes*. Organisms in macrophages (*1*), neutrophils (*2*), bronchiolar epithelium (*3*). (Courtesy of Armed Forces Institute of Pathology.) × 1000. Contributor: Army Veterinary School. *B*, Foreign body type giant cells in spermatic granuloma in a ram. Phagocytized spermatozoa (*1*), nuclei of giant cell (*2*). (Courtesy of Armed Forces Institute of Pathology.) × 648. Contributor: Dr. K. McEntee.

many instances, but the great majority are attributable to mitotic reproduction at the site of the activity. Numbers in the circulating blood may be increased slightly but seldom enough to be of diagnostic utility.

PLASMA CELLS

Plasma cells are not found in the blood but are an important constituent of many inflammatory reactions. These cells are smoothly spherical or elliptical with much more cytoplasm and therefore somewhat larger than a lymphocyte. The nucleus resembles that of a lymphocyte in being spherical and having a "clock-face" peripheral arrangement of chromatin granules. An important aid in recognition is the fact that the nucleus is almost always eccentrically placed in the cell. The cytoplasm appears homogeneous and as a rule, but not invariably, is a little more basophilic in its staining reaction than most cytoplasm, taking a nearly magenta shade of purplish red. Often the cytoplasm contains a distinct hyaline sphere called a **Russell body.** The electron microscopic features of the nucleus are not distinctive, however, the cytoplasm in addition to distinct Golgi bodies and mitochondria is filled with an abundant amount of endoplasmic reticulum. Within the cisternae of the endoplasmic reticulum, homogeneous material (gamma globulin) is found which as it increases in amount, dilates the cisterna and gives the Russell body its characteristic microscopic appearance.

Plasma cells do not undergo mitosis, they originate from small lymphocytes. Once formed they live a short life; about twelve hours. It is assumed the plasma cell then dies, but it has not been proved that death is the fate, it is possible they change in morphology to remain in the tissues as "memory" cells for immunologic mechanisms.

The function of the plasma cell is the production of antibodies (immunoglobulins). Plasma cells are known to produce all recognized types of humoral antibodies. The homogeneous material described above which lies in the cisternae of the endoplasmic reticulum represents accumulation of gamma-globulins produced by the cell.

Their occurrence seems to be influenced both by the type of injurious agent and the part of the body involved. With regard to the latter, the female reproductive tract is an outstanding location for plasma-cell reactions. Almost all inflammations here involve small or large numbers of plasma cells. They are also seen with some frequency in intestinal inflammations and in those of the male reproductive organs. The infections which bring them out are chronic in nature and include some of the granulomas (p. 615). Plasma cells have been found to increase in the spleen and lymph nodes of rats affected with experimentally induced tumors.

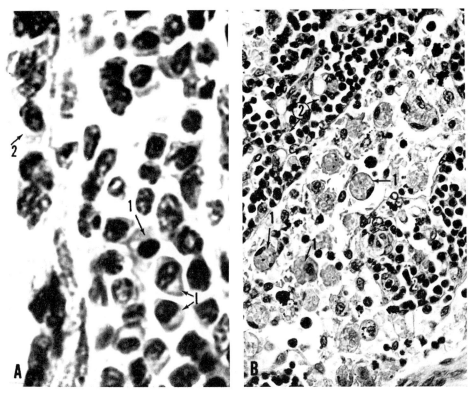

FIG. 6–11.—A, Plasma cells in an intestinal villus of a dog. Plasma cells (1), intestinal epithelium (2). (Courtesy of Armed Forces Institute of Pathology.) × 1000. Contributor: Dr. Samuel Pollock. B, Erythrophagocytosis, lymph node of a dog with acute leptospirosis. Erythrocytes in macrophages (1), lymphocytes (2). (Courtesy of Armed Forces Institute of Pathology.) × 440. Contributor: Division of Veterinary Medicine, Walter Reed Army Institute of Research.

MAST CELLS

Although mast cells are not usually looked upon as a cellular component of the inflammatory exudate, their probable relationship to the inflammatory process demands their consideration here. Mast cells arise from undifferentiated mesenchymal cells, and by mitosis from other mast cells. They are found in loose connective tissue throughout the body and in organs rich in connective tissue such as the mammary gland. Generally they are few in number in parenchymatous organs which contain little connective tissue such as the kidney and liver. However, in certain species even in these tissues they may be numerous. For example, the dog liver contains an appreciable number of mast cells.

Mast cells vary in shape and size within and between species. The nucleus is round or oval and contains a prominent nucleolus. The cytoplasm is distinctive, containing many spherical basophilic and metachromatic granules. The ultrastructure of the granule varies from finely granular to concentric lamellae of filaments presenting a whorled or scrolled pattern not dissimilar from the granules of the basophil (p. 173). Mitochondria, Golgi and endoplasmic reticulum are also found in the cytoplasm although often obscured by the multitude of granules.

The granules contain, in addition to a variety of enzymes, heparin (p. 107), histamine (p. 150), and at least in the rat and mouse, serotonin (p. 151). It is these compounds which relate the function of the mast cell to the inflammatory process. Each has been discussed earlier. Upon proper stimulation, which includes mechanical trauma, venoms, bacterial toxins, heat, cold, irradiation, etc., mast cells degranulate and release their vasoactive amines. Indeed in an acute inflammatory response there is a reduction in stainable mast cells. In contrast mast cells increase in number in chronic inflammatory processes.

Of greater concern to the diagnostic pathologist is the neoplastic transformation of mast cells to produce the mast cell tumor. This is discussed in Chapter 7.

THE DURATION OF INFLAMMATION

Of absorbing interest to a patient or its owner in case of illness is an answer to the question, "How long will it last?" Since many of our infectious and inflammatory diseases have more or less characteristic periods of duration, the diagnostician is almost equally anxious to know, "How long has it lasted?" As a rule the descriptive diagnosis of a disease or a lesion is incomplete without an indication of whether the disorder shows evidence of long or short duration. As the reader has doubtless already surmised, the characteristic clinical and pathological changes are usually quite different in diseases of long standing from those in sudden severe illness. The term **acute** and **chronic** designate the two types, with **subacute** in an intermediate position.

Clinically an acute disease is one that arises suddenly, often within a few hours and progresses rather promptly within a matter of some days or, at most, a few weeks to recovery or death, as the case may be. A chronic disease begins slowly and insidiously, it often being impossible to say just when the patient passed from a state of health. The disease then continues indefinitely or for a long time.

Pathologically speaking, the distinction in the case of inflammatory diseases is made on the basis of changes demonstrable in the affected tissues. Acute inflammation is characterized by any of the exudative or alterative changes mentioned in preceding pages but there is no proliferation. Any proliferation of new tissue whatsoever renders the inflammation chronic or **subacute**. The latter is an intermediate grade detected by the presence of immature proliferated tissue, which is a reparative process that has been started but not completed. Inflammation is chronic if any mature proliferated tissue is present as the result of it. This ordinarily means mature fibrous connective tissue. Reticulo-endothelial, bony or epithelial proliferations are also regularly chronic but enough mature fibrous tissue, not a part of pre-existing histological structures, can usually be found to fulfill the above criteria. **Mononuclears, plasma cells and even lymphocytes are characteristic of subacute or chronic inflammations but are not, in themselves definitive.**

It should be understood that some of the exudative, hyperemic or alterative changes characteristic of acute inflammation are also present in subacute and chronic inflammations. Indeed, if one encounters only mature proliferated fibrous tissue this is a **scar**, a completed repair or healed inflammation. On the other hand, if, in addition to the signs of subacute or chronic inflammation, the acute exudative changes occupy a prominent place in the picture, it is well to call attention to that fact by diagnosing "chronic (or subacute) inflammation, still active." Summarizing, acute inflammation is characterized by hyperemia and exudative (or alterative) changes. Subacute is the same plus immature fibrous tissue. Chronic inflammation has all the preceding plus mature fibrous tissue.

THE DEGREE OF INFLAMMATORY REACTION

While inflammation serves as a protective reaction assisting in the defense of the body against its enemies, the process is governed by physical and chemical laws rather than by intelligence, and is capable of destroying by its severity the life it ordinarily would protect. Estimation of the degree of reaction is of prime importance in formulating suitable treatment. From this standpoint inflammation may be adequate, inadequate or excessive.

(1) An **adequate inflammatory reaction** is one which is sufficient to bring about prompt destruction of the irritant and repair of the injury and no more. Its successful and satisfactory termination is often called **resolution**. Some examples are the uncomplicated rhinitis of the common "cold" in humans and birds, the uncomplicated case of equine strangles, the healing of a simple cut, accidental or surgical, the amount of granulation tissue which replaces an extracted tooth.

(2) **Inadequate Inflammatory Reaction.**—In this type there is a reaction, but it is not sufficient to destroy or overcome the irritant or produce recovery. Examples include such exostoses as the spavin on the horse's hock. This is caused by mechanical strains and concussion which all too often act continuously or repeatedly. The chronic proliferation of bony and fibrous tissue goes on indefinitely. Cirrhosis, to be studied with diseases of the liver, is of this type. Not only does the chronic fibrous proliferative reaction fail to overcome the irritant toxic substance, but the proliferated fibrous tissue acts as an irritant to cause further injury. Among the infections, bovine brucellosis is a good example. The immediate damage attendant upon abortion, if it occurs, is usually healed within a reasonable time, but the animal is not able to free herself completely of the causative bacteria, which survive in her body to repeat the acute exacerbation when susceptible embryonic tissue is again available by virtue of another preg-

nancy. The animal becomes a **carrier** of the organisms for a long time. Many protozoan diseases fall into this category, such as dourine or human malaria, the patient developing a sort of tolerance for the pathogen. The reaction against ringworm fungi is similarly slow and insufficient to produce decisive results. While most viral infections are quite the opposite, that of equine infectious anemia belongs here. The horse may live for years with repeated inflammatory and febrile exacerbations but probably never becomes free from the infection.

(3) **Excessive inflammatory reaction** is the opposite. While in many cases capable of destroying the injurious irritant, the reaction, either because of its great violence or on account of special anatomical and physiological considerations, threatens or destroys the patient before the former outcome is achieved. There are various examples. In many of the acute febrile infections, the body temperature (see Fever, p. 184) reaches such heights that experience promises a better chance for survival if it is artificially reduced. Heat prostration, the common overheating of draft horses and swine, is essentially of this nature. It is not the immediate exposure to excessive heat that kills but, rather, the maladjustment of body mechanisms, hyperemic or congestive, if not really inflammatory. In severe pneumonias, death is occasionally due to suffocation because too many of the pulmonary alveoli have been rendered temporarily useless when filled with exudate. Comparatively mild inflammation of the mucosa of the esophagus, brought on by mechanical trauma or by chemical irritant, like lye, accidentally swallowed, may have fatal results because the healing process so narrows the lumen that swallowing is impossible due to stricture of the esophagus. Laminitis of the horse is another instance where a process, comparatively trivial elsewhere, has dire results on account of its particular location. Commencing as a hyperemia which usually is only incidental to a transient generalized vasodilation, the capillaries of the sensitive laminæ, enclosed in the unyielding hoof, become so involved in swelling that blood can neither leave nor enter, with destruction of the hoof, and perhaps of life.

Treatment is not within our scope but it is obvious that, in addition to attacking the cause in any way possible, the clinician will wish to treat an excessive reaction by measures which subdue it, such as cold applications if the site is accessible. Inadequate reactions he will often decide to stimulate by counterirritants, and in the adequate reactions he will, perhaps, be on guard lest he do too much.

It remains to acquaint the student with certain qualifying adjectives applied to inflammation which are somewhat, but not quite self-explanatory.

Hyperplastic inflammation is accompanied by the proliferation of certain histological structures without others, so that the definition of hyperplasia (p. 94) is fulfilled. It is naturally also proliferative and also chronic. Johne's disease (p. 637) furnishes an example of hyperplastic enteritis.

Hypertrophic inflammation is a justifiable term if proliferation results in increased function as well as increased size of the part (p. 92). We often hear of hypertrophic gastritis, for increased secretion and acidity accompany the thickening of the mucous membrane.

Fibrosing, or fibrous inflammation is a term emphasizing the production of large amounts of fibrous granulation tissue. It is also chronic, proliferative and hyperplastic, but it may at the same time be atrophic if the functional tissue is compressed or diminished, as is frequently the case. Chronic mastitis is usually fibrous, as well as atrophic (p. 1327).

Atrophic inflammation results in atrophy (p. 90) of the pre-existing organ or part, usually through necrosis of the parenchymal cells. The lost cells are often replaced by fibrous tissue and then it is also fibrosing and hyperplastic inflammation if one chooses to use those designations. In atrophic cirrhosis (p. 1225) the hepatic lobules are abbreviated. In atrophic rhinitis of swine (p. 1094) the turbinate bones and eventually the nasal septum are completely obliterated.

Obliterative inflammation involves obliteration through slow necrosis of certain structures in the inflamed area. Atrophic rhinitis could be called obliterative. In obliterative glomerulonephritis (p. 1263), many glomeruli are changed into hyaline scars or disappear entirely. In obliterative orchitis (p. 1336), the seminiferous tubules disappear.

Adhesive inflammation is characterized by extensive fibrous adhesions due to the organization of a fibrinous exudate (p. 156). It is, of course, chronic and may be called proliferative, if it is thought that some of the increase of fibrous tissue resulted directly from the irritation without the area in question being first occupied by fibrin, a difficult thing to decide.

HEALING AND REGENERATION

Healing is the process which, after an injurious agent has been overcome, restores the injured part as nearly as possible to its previous normal condition. The task commonly involves three phases.

(1) **Removal** of the products of inflammation such as exudates and dead cells. This is usually accomplished by liquefaction, the fluid being readily absorbed into the lymph and blood. The fact that dead tissue tends to be liquefied by its own autolytic enzymes (autolysis) and by enzymes derived from inflammatory leukocytes (heterolysis) has already been reported (p. 21). Several kinds of leukocytes are thought to produce substances aiding this process as explained in immediately preceding pages. If the dead tissue is on a surface the main mass desquamates or sloughs as soon as preliminary liquefaction has loosened its attachment. Everyone is familiar with the lossening of a scab, which is simply dried and hardened exudate.

(2) **Repair** of damaged or disjoined parts is accomplished by proliferation of fibrous tissue, the building of a scar (p. 181). Much more to be desired, however, is the healing by regeneration now to be discussed.

(3) **Regeneration** is the process by which lost cells and tissues are replaced by others of the same kind. Some tissues regenerate readily; others do not, a situation which often determines what extent of recovery is possible from a given injury.

Epithelium can, in general, regenerate with considerable facility. That of the digestive, respiratory and similar **mucous membranes**, of the lung alveoli following pneumonia, of the endometrium after menstruation, all such epithelium is readily replaced by multiplication of some few cells which remain, albeit in glands or ducts opening on the surfaces destroyed. Secretory epithelium of badly damaged **glands,** however, is commonly not replaced. This is true of the gastric glands, mammary gland, seminiferous tubules, etc. In the **liver,** the epithelial cells regenerate readily provided the framework of the lobule is intact; otherwise, there is often an unsuccessful attempt in the form of proliferation of large numbers of bile ducts. But these scarcely produce functioning hepatic tissue. In the **kidney,** individual cells of the tubular lining are replaced, but no new nephrons

7

are formed. The **epidermis** readily regenerates from the edges of a wound, but accessory skin structures are not reproduced. Papillation and often pigmentation remain absent.

Muscle.—Severed muscles are usually reunited by a fibrous scar which restores them to normal functional ability. Smooth and cardiac muscles never regenerate. A certain amount of regeneration sometimes occurs in voluntary striated muscle, with buds of muscle cells building out into the tissue of the fibrous union. Often these appear as multinucleated "giant-cells" which might be mistaken for foreign-body giant cells, since they have many nuclei and little sarcoplasm. If the sarcolemma remains intact, as in atrophy of a muscle, the sarcoplasm can be replaced.

Nerve.—If a peripheral nerve is severed, the distal portion dies but is slowly regenerated by new growth from the proximal end. Rarely perhaps there is union of the proximal and the original distal ends. If a nerve cell body dies, the whole neuron dies and is not replaced, the peripheral process undergoing what is called "wallerian degeneration." Sometimes, after a time, more or less perfect function is restored by training (for particular acts, etc.) by virtue of a new route being found to carry the impluse around the destroyed portion of the brain or cord. Neuroglia proliferates readily.

Blood.—Restoration of blood has been treated under Hemorrhage (p. 119).

Connective Tissue.—It has already been seen that fibrous tissue proliferates readily, replacing its own kind or other tissues which are not able to regenerate. When young it is areolar in arrangement, often rich in young capillaries. It becomes denser and less vascular with age, until finally old scars may be very dense and even hyaline with a very poor blood supply. (See Granulation Tissue.)

Cartilage and bone are regenerated first as fibrous tissue by multiplication of the undifferentiated connective-tissue cells of the perichondrium or periosteum, and, to a lesser extent, of the endosteum. In the healing of a fracture the sequence is (1) hemorrhage, (2) clotting, the formation of fibrin, (3) organization of the fibrin by fibroblasts, as is prone to occur in fibrin anywhere, (4) calcification and ossification of the fibrous tissue into imperfect bone (the provisional callus), which is then slowly destroyed and replaced by more perfect bone (the true callus).

Tendons and ligaments regenerate slowly but perfectly as a rule.

Blood vessels are easily replaced by newly formed capillaries. These may become much larger than capillaries normally are, but a muscular coat (characteristic of arteries and veins) is seldom, if ever, developed.

Mesothelium of the serous surfaces is quickly regenerated.

FEVER

Fever is a characteristic accompaniment of most infectious diseases, the principal exceptions being those which are localized to a small area of the body or those of a very chronic, slowly progressing nature. The word may be used in a strict sense to mean merely hyperthermia, an increase of the body temperature above the normal, or its meaning may include other phenomena which are concomitant with elevated temperature in these infectious diseases, particularly the increased pulse rate and cardiac output and the more rapid respiration.

While fever is ordinarily almost synonymous with infection and presumably due to toxins from the invading pathogen, it may also result from the presence of decomposition products of proteins, as when parts of large tumors are undergoing necrosis or burned tissue is being lysed, or in the course of anaphylactic reaction of antibodies upon the antigens of foreign proteins. Local injury to the thermo-taxic (heat-regulating) center in the hypothalamus can also produce fever. This, plus the fact that experimental severance of the nervous connections of this center with the rest of the body prevents the induction of fever, shows that the basic mechanism of hyperthermia is in the nervous center, although the rise in tempera-ture naturally must depend either upon increased production or diminished dissipation of heat. During fever, regulation of body temperature involves the normal mechanisms, but at a higher baseline level. It appears that the setting of the "thermostat" in the thermoregulatory center in the hypothalamus has been simply set too high. Possibly bacterial toxins, or tissue decomposition products act directly on the center to change its setting, or they may act by causing the formation and release of a common endogenous pyrogen which mimics the effect of cold on the hypothalamic center.

Since, in the earlier and maximal stages of a fever, sweating ceases in spite of the abnormally high body temperature, it is easy to understand how, in those species possessed of sweating mechanisms, one important outlet for the escape of heat is closed. Dogs, likewise, do not pant and are thus deprived of their most effective mechanism for the elimination of surplus heat. It is well known from human experience that during the early stages of severe fevers the patient feels cold, he "has a chill," and in both man and animals there may actually be shiver-ing, a form of muscular exertion which generates heat. Swine, affected by a febrile disease, have no perspiratory function to be arrested, but they tend to burrow into the bedding and to lie closely one against another, their natural methods of keeping warm. Undoubtedly such pigs feel chilled; probably this aspect of fever is more prolonged and possibly more pronounced in swine than it is in the human. Concerned in the development of fever are other mechanisms, such as temporary vasoconstriction at the body surface (during the chill), less efficient heat radiation by a too concentrated blood and others not well under-stood, but all are directed toward the retention of body heat. Once the higher temperature is attained, its maintenance can be explained simply by van't Hoff's law that the speed of a chemical reaction increases as the ambient temperature rises (usually two to four times for each 10° C.), for the heat of the body is, of course, generated by the various oxidative reactions taking place within it.

While the above centrally controlled mechanisms operate in most examples of fever and all of those associated with infections or extensive tissue damage, body temperature can be elevated without disturbance of central nervous regulation. For example increased heat production in hyperthyroidism or reduced heat loss with pheochromocytoma may cause fever. Also, increased heat production re-sulting from vigorous muscular exercise can elevate body temperature; but we do not call this fever.

We may conclude that fever most often arises principally because of reduced dissipation of heat through functional changes controlled by the heat-regulating center in the brain, and that this center is influenced by blood-borne toxins from pathogenic micro-organisms or from protein decomposition or possibly by a common endogenous pyrogen.

Whether the phenomenon of fever was developed through a long evolutionary survival of the most resistant, was arbitrarily decreed by the omniscient Creator, or whether it just happened, it is a response possessed by all homiothermic species. This fact has led us to believe that fever is ordinarily beneficial, however there is still no direct *in vivo* evidence that fever is beneficial. It is known that the processes of phagocytosis (p. 165) and antibody-antigen reactions are more rapid in its presence (logically by the same van't Hoff's law just mentioned), and it can be shown bacteriologically that many of the pathogenic organisms grow only slowly and with difficulty at the temperatures corresponding to febrile levels in the host. For example, the anthrax organism loses much of its virulence at such temperatures, a fact of which advantage is taken in making immunizing vaccines. Conversely, it has often been shown that lowering an animal's temperature below the normal level is one of the most potent methods of lowering its resistance to many infections. Using anthrax again as an example, the chicken (normal body temperature about 107° F.) is ordinarily not susceptible to anthrax, but can be infected after its temperature is lowered by exposure to refrigerator temperatures.

Nevertheless, extremely high body temperatures cause cellular swelling and necrosis of delicate parenchymatous cells as has been pointed out (p. 42). This fact has received confirmation from the experimental production of "artificial fever." Hyperthermias occasionally reach levels which are in themselves incompatible with life.

STRESS

An animal learns that a certain thing or situation is harmless or dangerous, agreeable or disagreeable, and is content to approach it or avoid it without making any great effort to understand it. Fortunately for human progress, man is more curious and wishes to understand the various phenomena which he encounters. If this proves currently impossible, man has at least one last recourse: He gives the object or the phenomenon a name, and then he feels considerably more tranquil. Whole populations, indeed, are often quite content to talk glibly about a certain subject which they do not understand but for which they do have a name. Such names come and go and are widely used, often with a very poor conception of what it is to which the name applies. Such a name, in much of the lighter medical thinking of the day, is "stress." We are tempted to infer that whatever illness or abnormality an animal (or person) may have, "stress" is the cause of it and "stress" must be treated by a proposed medicament (which the proponent often has for sale at a very reasonable or unreasonable price). There is perhaps no better place than this to have a look at so popular a term and to try to see what it properly connotes.

Nearly a generation ago, Cannon (1929) pointed out that the observable signs and symptoms of fright, rage or pain are entirely comparable to those that result from a suitable dose of epinephrine and are just what would be expected if a considerable amount of that substance were suddenly released into the circulation from the adrenal gland. If a cat is held at bay by a dog, the hair of the cat stands erect, its pupils dilate and its eyes bulge, its muscles are tense, its heart beats faster. Investigation shows that the level of blood sugar rises, making it immediately available for the production of energy, more blood flows into the musculature and less into the digestive organs, whose activities are held in relative abeyance. The bronchioles dilate, increasing the animal's capacity for rapid oxidation of sugar; the spleen empties its reserve erythrocytes into the circulation; even the clotting power of the blood is enhanced, as if in preparation for a wound. If the cat then decides to run, it is capable of extreme speed and unbelievably long jumps; its claws dig with unerring accuracy into the bark of an unfamiliar tree, up whose trunk it runs as if on level ground. This is the "alarm reaction" of Cannon and his school and, while not proven, it is widely accepted that these uncanny powers are due to an increased supply of epinephrine from the adrenal medulla, the hormone acting through the medium of the sympathetic nerves.

Selye (1950) carried this idea further and has postulated an increase of various adrenal and pituitary hormones as one of the protective agencies operating against the "stress" of infections, cold, muscular fatigue, nervous strain and even of heat and ionizing radiations. Following upon the epinephric reaction of Cannon, Selye theorized that increased adrenocorticotrophic hormone, ACTH, from the pituitary stimulated the adrenal cortex to greater release of various of its steroid hormones, which are sometimes known as "corticoids." The supply of all these hormones is held to be subject to exhaustion in the case of the prolonged "stress" of the disorders mentioned. The theory then goes on to propose that a number of stubborn and poorly understood diseases of man are due to an imbalance of the cortical hormones so produced. These diseases include rheumatoid arthritis and similar disorders characterized by excessive production of collagen, hypertension and its etiological relatives, nephrosclerosis and glomerulonephritis, and even the apparently very dissimilar ulcerative colitis. The basis for this theory was that the administration of certain of these cortical hormones (the mineralocorticoids) to experimental animals produced lesions similar to those found in most of these human diseases. Furthermore, these lesions are relieved or prevented by another group of cortical hormones (the glucocorticoids) of which cortisone is now a well-known example. If this theory be correct, we can say that the diseases listed have as their original cause the "stress" occasioned by environmental attacks of the kinds outlined, infections, cold, mental and nervous tribulations and the like. For diseases such as rheumatoid arthritis and glomerulonephritis, other causes and mechanisms have been advanced which seem far more plausible, but how is stress to be eliminated as an underlying factor?

While proof in either direction is very difficult to obtain and, so far, not available, there have been many arguments for and against the theory. Nothing would be gained by recounting them here, especially since these human diseases are practically nonexistent in the domestic animals. Indeed, the fact that animals rarely suffer, apparently, from some of the strains under consideration (the nervous ones) might be an argument in favor of the theory as it applies to humans. At any rate, there is no evidence that "stress" as above described is of importance in veterinary medicine. Admittedly the word "stress" is at times used with much broader and less definite implication but such vagueness is not characteristic of the precision of thought which scientific persons are expected to display. Even a stone wall is subject to "stress" as any architect will explain.

STATUS THYMICO-LYMPHATICUS

In human medicine there have long been recognized cases of sudden death which were unexplained and unexplainable. As an apparently precipitating circumstance, there has commonly been some trivial injury or disturbance, the extraction of a tooth or other minor operation, sudden excitement, anesthesia under circumstances ordinarily quite safe, or even a cold bath. At necropsy the only lesions to be found have been pronounced hyperplasia of the thymus with generalized increase of lymphoid tissue in many lymph nodes, the Peyer's patches, tonsils and elsewhere. No abnormalities in structure were noted beyond the unusual, hyperplastic development in size. Further investigation has shown that the adrenals in these cases are decidely smaller than normal. The heart and aorta tend to be hypoplastic also. Differences of opinion are still unsettled as to whether these abnormalities are responsible for the sudden deaths, but numerous careful investigators have found in the affirmative. Current beliefs in endocrinology suggest the hypoplastic adrenals may well explain the overgrowth of lymphoid tissue as well as the lack of normal tenacity of the spark of life. There are authorities, however, who attach no importance to the above changes and believe that some other cause of death was overlooked in each case.

It is not for us to say which opinion is correct, but we do say with considerable certainty that what appears to be an identical syndrome has been found in the dog with a fair degree of frequency. The last case seen by one of the authors (Smith) occurred during the excitement of feeding time in the kennel of an experienced dog-raiser. Another was in a pup that died inexplicably following routine manipulation preparatory to a distemper "shot." A third was an entirely unexpected death during ether anesthesia given by thoroughly competent individuals of long experience. In all cases the only lesions discoverable were those described above, the persistent hyperplastic thymus, the widespread increase of lymphoid tissue, the small adrenals. Estimation of the size of the heart and aorta was a matter of judgment and not unequivocal. We are inclined to attribute death in such cases to the so-called status thymico-lymphaticus, with awareness that the state may not be a single entity.

Inflammation and Body Reactions

ABRAMSON, H. A.: The Electrical Charge of the Blood Cells of the Horse and Its Relation to the Inflammatory Process. Cold Spring Harbor Symposia on Quantitative Biology. *1*:92–106, 1933.

ACKERMAN, G. A.: Ultrastructure and Cytochemistry of the Developing Neutrophil. Lab. Invest. *19*:290–302, 1968.

ADAMI, J. G.: *Inflammation: Introduction to the Study of Pathology.* London, Macmillan & Company, Ltd., 1909.

ANDERSON, V., and BRO-RASMUSSEN, F.: Autoradiographic Studies of the Kinetics of Eosinophils. Ser. Haemat. *4*:33–44, 1968.

ARCHER, R. K.: *The Eosinophil Leucocytes.* Philadelphia. F. A. Davis Co. 1963.

ARCHER, R. K., and BROOME, J.: Bradykinin and Eosinophils. Nature *198*:893–894, 1963.

ARCHER, R. K.: The Eosinophil Leucocytes. Ser. Haemat. *1*:3–32, 1968.

ARCHER, R. K., and BOWDEN, R. S. T.: True Haemophilia (Hemophilia A) in a Thoroughbred Foal. Vet. Rec. *73*:338–340, 1961.

ARCHER, R. K.: Eosinophil Leucocytes and Their Reactions to Histamine and 5-Hydroxytryptamine. J. Path. Bact. *78*:95–103, 1959.

BOYD, WM.: *Text-book of Pathology.* 6th ed. Philadelphia, Lea & Febiger, p. 294 ,1953.

CANNON, W. B.: *Bodily Changes in Pain, Hunger, Fear and Rage.* 2nd ed. New York, D. Appleton Co., 1929.

————: Organization for Physiological Homeostasis. Physiol. Rev. *9*:399–431, 1929.

CRANSTON, W. I.: Temperature Regulation. Br. Med. J. *2*:69–75, 1966.

DURAN-REYNALS, F.: Tissue Permeability and the Spreading Factors in Infection. Bact. Rev. *6*:197–252, 1942.

FLOREY, H. W. (Editor): *General Pathology.* 4th Ed., Philadelphia, W. B. Saunders Co., 1970.

FORBUS, W. D.: *Reaction to Injury.* Baltimore, The Williams & Wilkins Co., 1943.

EISEN, V., and GLANVILLE, K. L. A.: Separation of Kinin-Forming Factors in Human Plasma. Br. J. Exp. Path. *50*:427–437, 1969.

GELLHORN, E., and DUNN, J. O.: Undernutrition. Starvation and Phagocytosis. J. Nutrition. *14*:145–153, 1937.

HAYTHORN, S. R.: Multinucleated Giant Cells with Particular Reference to the Foreign Body Giant Cell. Arch. Path. *7*:651–713, 1929.

KRUMBHAAR, E. B.: The Stigmata of St. Francis of Assisi. Ann. Med. Histroy. *9*:111–119, 1927.

MALLERY, O. T., JR., and McCUTCHEON, M.: Motility and Chemotaxis of Leukocytes in Health and Disease. Am. J. Med. Sci. *200*:394–399, 1940.

MANN, P. R.: An Electron-Microscope Study of the Relations Between Mast Cells and Eosinophil Leucocytes (Plates LXVIII and LXIX). J. Path. *98*:183–186, 1969.

McCUTCHEON, M., and DIXON, H. M.: Chemotropic Reactions of Polymorphonuclear Leukocytes to Various Micro-organisms. Arch. Path. *21*:749–755, 1936.

MENKIN, V.: *Dynamics of Inflammation.* New York, Macmillan Co., 1940.

————: Chemical Basis of Injury in Inflammation. Arch. Path. *36*:269–288, 1943.

MILNE, F. J.: "Thoughts and Observations on Counter Irritation in the Horse" (TT) Translated Title. Zbl. Vet Med. *8*:1095–1140, 1961.

MOON, V. H.: The Vascular and Cellular Dynamics of Shock. Am. J. Med. Sci. *203*:1–18, 1942.

————: Pathology of Secondary Shock. Am. J. Path. *24*:235–274, 1948.

MOVAT, H. Z. *et al.*: Allergic Inflammation. III. The Fine Structure of Collagen Fibrils at Sites of Antigen-Antibody Interaction in Arthus-type Lesions. J. Exp. Med. *118*:557–564, 1963.

OPIE, E. L.: Experimental Pleurisy—Resolution of a Fibrinous Exudate. J. Exper. Med. *9*:391–413, 1907.

————: Inflammation. Arch. Int. Med. *5*:541–568, 1910.

————: Inflammation and Immunity. J. Immunol. *17*:329–342, 1929.

POOLE, J. C. F.: Electron Microscopy of Polymorphonuclear Leukocytes. Brit. J. Derm. *81*:(Suppl. 3): 11–18, 1969.

REBUCK, J. W.: The Modification of Leukocytic Function in Human Windows by ACTH. Gastroenterol. *19*:644–657, 1951.

ROUS, P., and GILDING, H. P.: Is the Local Vasodilatation after Different Tissue Injuries Referable to a Single Cause? J. Exper. Med. *51*:27–39, 1930.

SCOTT, R. E., and HORN, R. G.: Ultrastructural Aspects of Neutrophil Granulocyte Development in Humans. Lab. Invest. *23*:202–215, 1970.

SELYE, H.: *The Physiology and Pathology of Exposure to Stress.* Montreal, Canada, Acta, Inc. Abstr. Vet. Bul. No. 3115–1951. 1950.

SHIVLEY, J., FELDT, C., and DAVIS, D.: Fine Structure of Formed Elements in Canine Blood. Amer. J. Vet. Res. *3*:893–906, 1969.

SPECTOR, W. G. (Editor): The Acute Inflammatory Response. Ann. of N.Y. Acad. Sci. *116*:747–1084, 1964.

SPICER, S. S., and HARDIN, J. H.: Ultrastructure, Cytochemistry, and Function of Neutrophil Leukocyte Granules. Lab. Invest. *20*:488–497, 1969.

WARD, P. A.: Chemotaxis of Mononuclear Cells. J. Exp. Med. *128*:1201–1221, 1968.

WETZEL, B. K., HORN, R. G., and SPICER, S. S.: Fine Structure Studies on the Development of Heterophil, Eosinophil, and Basophil in Rabbits. Lab. Invest. *16*:349–382, 1967.

WELSH, R. A.: Light and Electron Microscopic Correlation of the Periodic Acid-Schiff Reaction in the Human Plasma Cell. Am. J. Path. *40*:285–296, 1962.

WOLF-JURGENSEN, P.: The Basophil Leukocyte. Ser. Haemat. *1*:45–68, 1968.

ZWEIFACH, B. W., GRANT, L., and McCLUSKEY, R. I. (Editors): *The Inflammatory Process.* New York, Academic Press, 1965.

7

Neoplasia

A neoplasm is a new growth of cells which (1) proliferate continuously without control, (2) bear a considerable resemblance to the healthy cells from which they arose, (3) have no orderly structural arrangement, (4) serve no useful function and (5) for the present, at least, have no clearly understood cause. There have been many definitions of a neoplasm but the above, changed but little from that offered by Mallory more than a generation ago, possibly comes as near as any to enlightening the novice on what the general public calls a "cancer." "Tumor" is a less precise but commonly used synonym which originally meant a swelling, but which now is almost exclusively reserved for enlargements of neoplastic nature.

Manner of Growth.—It is the **continuous proliferation,** the uncontrolled growth, which makes neoplasia the formidable and destructive process that it is. Rates of growth vary, and naturally the tumor of rapid growth is most to be feared. But there is also a difference in type of growth; neoplasms may grow by expansion or by infiltration. In the tumor endowed with the power of infiltrative growth, the outermost cells multiply actively and unevenly and, as more room is required for the growing population, individual cells or small groups force themselves in amongst the cells and structures of the surrounding tissues. Since the infiltrating tumor cells are usually possessed of great vitality, they can endure more pressure and more successfully compete for oxygen and nutrient substances, with the result that the pre-existing tissues are crowded out and disappear through necrosis of one cell after another.

It is thus obvious that the tumor able to grow by infiltration destroys whatever is in its path, even bones, and this continues until life itself is destroyed. Because of this great destructiveness, neoplasms of this nature are classed as **malignant,** while those which grow only expansively, much less dangerous to their host, are said to be **benign.** (Details of the differentiation between benign and malignant neoplasms are discussed on page 272.) There is one other feature of malignant neoplasms, which, indeed, reinforces their malignancy, the capacity for **metastasis.** It is obvious that an infiltrative growth will sooner or later make its way into blood vessels and lymph vessels. As the neoplastic cells reach the lumen, they are in contact with the flowing stream and, as might be expected, it is not unusual for single cells or small groups of them to be detached and carried away as emboli in the blood stream or lymph, as the case may be. They travel until their progress is stopped by lodgment in the fine meshes of the next lymph node or in small, terminal arterioles or capillaries. More often than not lodgment occurs in the lungs, liver, spleen or kidneys, whose capillary networks provide fine and extensive filters.

The malignant neoplastic cells may multiply and continue their uncontrolled and disorderly growth at the point where they lodge, setting up a new colony, a **metastatic neoplasm.**

While malignant neoplasms have the sinister powers of both infiltrative and metastatic growth, the **benign neoplasm** is limited to the expansive type of growth. The tumor is able to grow outward if on a body surface or to exert expansive pressure against surrounding tissues, but the neoplastic and normal cells remain segregated along a fairly sharp line. Because of its inability to infiltrate, the benign growth is not likely to penetrate a blood vessel, but if some of its cells do chance to be carried about by blood or lymph they are usually not able to survive in a new location.

We do not know why these differences exist nor, indeed, just how neoplastic cells of any sort differ from the normal. It can be said that in proportion to their malignancy, tumor cells resemble less and less the histological tissue from which they arose, even to the point that the tissue of origin cannot be guessed. This quality of not conforming to any histological prototype in structure, arrangement and staining qualities is called **anaplasia.** Such cells are **anaplastic,** or **undifferentiated.** That the "non-conformist attitude" is not restricted to their physical appearance but extends to their whole behavior and manner of living is freely attested by their uncontrollably rapid rate and undisciplined manner of reproduction. It may be supposed that such cells are equally unorthodox in many of their metabolic processes, indeed, that there must be certain basic metabolic aberrations which permit them to flout so successfully what, for other cells, are basic laws. Chemists have found a few differences, the most important of which appears to be the much greater ability of neoplastic tissues to obtain energy by splitting glucose into lactic acid (called glycolysis). This apparently makes them more or less independent of an extensive supply of oxygen, which, to ordinary adult tissues, is essential. This property of relative anaerobiosis, the rapid rate of multiplication and, to a certain extent, the lack of accepted histological patterns are characteristic of embryonic tissues. In some tumors, such as the chordoma, the microscopic picture is unlike anything existing in the adult, but does resemble rather closely the embryonal structure from which it is doubtless derived. For these reasons malignant neoplastic tissue is sometimes said to be of embryonal type. However, no embryo ever possessed the uncontrolled invasive power which exists in the malignant neoplasm and the resemblance is not fundamental.

The **resemblance** which tumor cells bear **to the healthy cells** from which they arose is the basis for our system of classification and nomenclature of neoplasms. There are many different kinds of neoplasms, depending on the histological type of tissue which furnished them genesis, and to which they bear a likeness. Classification of neoplasms according to the different histological types is of more than academic importance for the various types differ markedly in their clinical course and effect on the patient, as well as in their possibilities for successful treatment by the diverse methods currently available. It will be seen when a classification is presented shortly that there is at least one type of tumor for almost every histological prototype and that no part of the body escapes the threat of neoplasia.

The **lack of orderly structural arrangement** will be appreciated by the student after a few tumors have been examined. He will find that microscopically the fibrous strands of a fibroblastic tumor run harum-scarum in all directions: the epithelium of an epidermal tumor finds itself surrounded by connective tissue **stroma,** whereas the opposite is the normal arrangement.

As to **function,** most neoplasms have none at all. Exceptions to this are to be found among the benign neoplasms of some of the ductless glands and hormone-producing organs. Such tumors, being benign, have diverged but slightly from the normal ancestral tissue, either morphologically or functionally. As an example, we see occasionally a tumor (adenoma) of the pancreatic islets. While its cells proliferate in a disorganized manner, they individually have an appearance very similar to that of normal cells of the same kind. As islet cells should do, they secrete insulin, producing an excess of this substance with a resultant hypoglycemia, which may be fatal. In man and dogs (p. 251), surgical removal of the tumor has cured the hypoglycemia. Certain interstitial-cell tumors of the testis have produced hypermasculinity and prostatic hyperplasia. Arrhenoblastomas of the ovary have brought masculinity to the female (human), as do also many adrenocortical tumors (man, bovines, p. 252). The Sertoli-cell tumor of the dog's testis often has a marked feminizing effect (p. 260). Adenomas of the thyroid may or may not cause hyperthyroidism (toxic goiter, p. 255), depending on the individual case. Several tumors of the hypophysis bring disorders of growth, depending on the particular hormone produced. Adenomas of the parathyroid cause decalcification of bones, hypercalcemia and even renal calculi, through their excessive secretion. Since none of these functions are useful, but often quite the contrary, the original definition of a neoplasm is not violated.

In man some neoplasms that are not related to endocrine glands secrete hormones. For example, certain carcinomas of the lung have been found to secrete adrenocorticotropic hormone and anti-diuretic hormone and some adenocarcinomas of the colon secrete a substance with parathyroid hormone activity. Comparable tumors have not been reported in animals. In general the more anaplastic the neoplasm the less its cells retain their original function. Functional abilities which are not detrimental are also evident in well differentiated non-hormone secreting neoplasms. For example squamous cell carcinomas may produce keratin, osteosarcomas, bone; chondromas, cartilaginous matrix; adenocarcinomas, mucin; and hepatomas, bile.

A discussion of the causes is perhaps best deferred until the student has formed a closer acquaintance with the nature of neoplasms. To gain the aid of realistic visualization, it is well that the student become better acquainted with the discernible features of neoplasia.

Gross Appearance.—The microscopic appearances of tumors have already received incidental notice. More will be said as each kind of neoplasm is discussed. The gross appearances of neoplasms are seldom as informative as one would wish, but a few points will possibly be of assistance. The general conception of a neoplasm as an enlargement is ordinarily applicable, but there are exceptions. Some of the more malignant carcinomas and melanomas may never reach conspicuous size before they kill the patient through the effects of their metastases or by virtue of interfering with some vital function, such as the passage of food through the intestine. This remark refers to the primary, or original tumor. The metastatic tumors arising by transfer of cells from the primary are often called secondary tumors.

Cases are not rare where the patient dies of a metastatic tumor without the primary being discovered even in a reasonably thorough autopsy. For instance, if a rather spherical, circumscribed tumor (these being gross characteristics of a metastatic rather than a primary growth) consisting of mucus-forming glandular epithelium (an adenocarcinoma) is found in the spleen, this is a metastatic tumor because there is no mucus-forming glandular epithelium in the normal spleen. We must look for the primary where such epithelium normally occurs, for instance in the gastro-intestinal mucosa. Adenocarcinomas of the intestine often consist of little more than a short stretch of annular thickening and if there is no constriction of the lumen and no ulceration, it is quite possible for the inexperienced prosector to overlook such a tumor. A nicety of expression should be noted here: in this hypothetical case, the neoplasm is a tumor *of* the intestine but the growth in the spleen is not a tumor *of* the spleen; it is still an adenocarcinoma of the intestine, metastatic *in* the spleen. "Of" refers to the site of the primary tumor, always.

In contrast, some neoplasms may reach very large size. Before the days of surgical removal, instances were known where human tumors weighed more than the patient. The same could occur in an animal if its life were conserved with equal care, but usually the daily struggle for food and with enemies terminates such a case at an earlier stage. Such tumors must obviously be of the benign variety; a malignant tumor would bring death before any such tremendous size was attained.

Tumors of any considerable size cause a bulging of the organ or part involved. This is especially noticeable in tumors arising in or just beneath the skin. Such protruding masses lead eventually to pressure necrosis of the overlying skin or mucous membrane with ulceration and bleeding.

Some malignant neoplasms (carcinomas) of the skin or mucous membranes ulcerate before they reach any very noticeable gross proportions. In such cases the ulcer may be the presenting symptom. Benign epithelial tumors (papillomas) protrude in simple or complicated branching forms.

The cut cross-section usually reveals the tumor as a mass of foreign tissue of different color and consistency from that which surrounds it. The color is likely to be white or nearly so. Melanomas are typically black, although some are "amelanotic" and white. A few, such as the interstitial-cell tumor of the testis, are yellow. The consistency may be harder or softer than that of the surrounding tissue; one learns to recognize the tissue of lymphomas by its rather soft, very homogeneous, white character. Incision not infrequently reveals hemorrhages, cysts or other special structures, also areas of necrotic tissue.

Neoplastic tissue, bulging, ulcerated or otherwise, has to be distinguished from inflammatory granulomatous tissues, including those of actinomycosis, tuberculosis and the excessive granulation tissue of wound healing. Sometimes this can be done by the clinical history, the location, or the presence of abscesses, "sulfur granules" or other special structures. In most instances, the decision must await microscopic examination.

CLASSIFICATION OF NEOPLASMS

The fundamental plan for the nomenclature of neoplasms has long been to name each type according to the tissue from which it arose, and which, of course, it resembled more or less closely. It was found that there was a neoplasm to correspond to almost every type of cell recognized in histology, the latter being called the "type cell" for the particular variety of neoplasm. We now recognize several additional tumors which are traceable, not to any tissue found in normal histology, but to a type of tissue occurring only at a certain stage of embryonal

development.   From the fibroblast of fibrous connective tissue originally came
the fibroblastoma, the suffix "oma" meaning a tumor.   Fibroblastomas were of
two kinds, fibromas if benign and fibrosarcomas if malignant.   However, present-
day usage reserves the suffix "-blastoma" for tumors derived from a stage encountered in embryonal development and not in the histology of mature tissues,
so that "fibroblastoma" in the above sense is better avoided.   The suffix "-sar-
coma" is used to indicate malignancy for all tumors of "supporting-tissue" origin,
that is, for those arising from the following three of the five primary tissues:
connective tissue, muscle, blood and lymph tissue.   We may list the following
tumors as belonging to the "supporting-tissue" class:

Fibroma; Fibrosarcoma.—These tumors arise from fibrous connective tissue
in its ubiquitous locations and resemble it in appearance.   The cells with their
collagenous fibrils run aimlessly in a variety of directions.   Fasciculi of cells lying
in the same plane are often seen (Fig. 7–2B) and are of value in distinguishing the
fibrosarcoma from the hemangiopericytoma, in which this is not a feature.   If the
fibrous material predominates at the expense of the nuclei and plump cell bodies,
the tumor is hard grossly and is called a **fibroma durum.**   If cell bodies and nuclei
predominate, with fewer fibrils, the tumor is softer and is called a **fibroma molle.**
All degrees of malignancy exist.   Among the criteria of malignancy in general, a
high degree of cellularity, hyperchromatic staining of the nuclei and a tendency
for the nuclei to be plump, rounded or even stellate are especially significant in
the fibrosarcoma.   Virus-caused fibropapillomas are discussed on page 511.

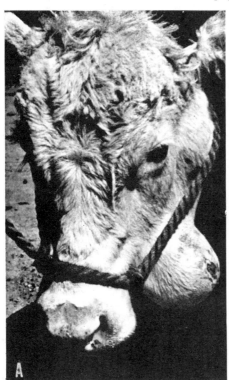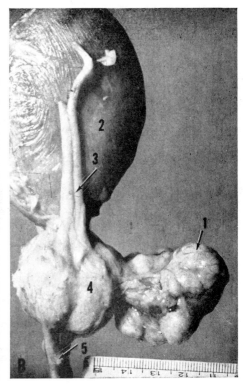

Fig. 7–1.—*A,* Fibrosarcoma involving mandible of a Hereford steer.   This neoplasm could
easily be confused clinically with actinomycosis.

B, Leiomyoma of the prostate of a dog.   Tumor (*1*), urinary bladder (*2*), ductus deferens (*3*),
prostate (*4*) and urethra (*5*).

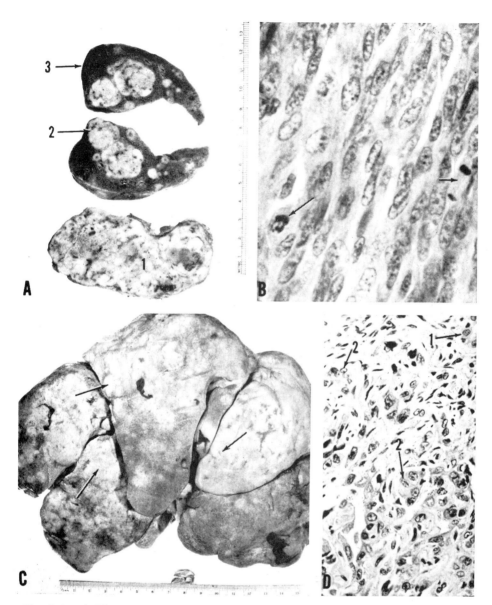

FIG. 7–2.—A, Fibrosarcoma, primary (1), in cheek of a 12-year-old male Scottish terrier, with metastases (2) to lung (3). B, Photomicrograph of same tumor (× 700). Note spindle-shaped cells with ovoid nuclei and mitotic figures (arrows). (Courtesy of Armed Forces Institute of Pathology.) Contributor: Dr. John E. Craige. C, Adenocarcinoma of intrahepatic bile ducts, liver of a fifteen-year-old male beagle. Masses of tumor (arrows) enlarge the liver and elevate the capsule. D, Photomicrograph of the neoplasm in C (× 300). The neoplastic cells form structures resembling bile ducts (1) in some places, but in others they are undifferentiated (2). (Courtesy of Armed Forces Institute of Pathology.) Contributor: Dr. D. N. Bader.

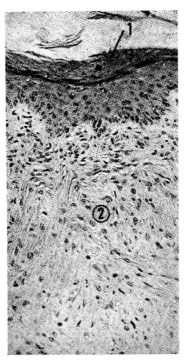

FIG. 7–3.—Equine sarcoid, skin of the ear of a mule (× 160). Hyperkeratotic epidermis
(1) covers the mass in this section. Note hyperplastic cells of dermis.

Equine Sarcoid.—A cutaneous growth peculiar to equines was first recognized
by Jackson (1936) who named it equine sarcoid because, despite contrary clinical
behavior, its histological appearance is certainly that of a sarcoma of moderate
malignancy. The lesion, often multiple, is most frequently found on the lower
legs, head and prepuce. It occurs perhaps even more frequently in mules and
donkeys than in the horse. The growths may reach the size of a man's fist,
variable in shape and in extent of the base, and bulging under the skin, which is
thickened and roughened (acanthotic), and which sooner or later becomes ulcerated and infected. The growing mass may extend into the dermis, especially
when it recurs after incomplete removal, but the underlying muscle is not invaded.

Microscopically the new growth is made up principally of interlacing bundles of
spindle-shaped cells which may form whorls and bundles suggestive of those of a
neurofibroma. It is not surprising that most pathologists, confronted with the
lesion for the first time, consider it a neurofibroma, neurofibrosarcoma, fibroma
or fibrosarcoma. The proportion of collagen fibrils to nuclei varies but it is not
high enough that the sarcoid is likely to be mistaken for a keloid. Inflammatory
infiltration is of course present near an ulcerated surface; a few lymphocytes and
eosinophils may appear anywhere among the fibroblastic cells but these are so
few that there is no likelihood of mistaking the lesion for inflammatory granulation tissue. Neither is the number of capillaries great enough to favor such an
error. The real difficulty is in distinguishing the sarcoid from a sarcoma. Usually
there is less anaplasia of nuclei and fewer mitoses than in a sarcoma but in
borderline cases differentiation may not be possible on histological grounds alone.
Indeed, when the day comes that everything is known about neoplasia it may be

found that there is no real distinction. The overlying epidermis often sends long fronds deep into the mass, a feature which to Jackson was more or less confirmatory of his opinion that the epithelium participated in the neoplastic process. However, it must be remembered that this bizarre epithelial proliferation is not unusual in any epidermis which is struggling under difficulties to cover a stubborn subcutaneous enlargement of any sort.

Anything less than complete removal is invariably followed by a recurrent growth that tends to be more richly cellular, the spindle-shaped cells being increased in size, with large, hyperchromatic nuclei and more frequent mitotic figures. Metastasis, however, does not occur, the situation being reminiscent of the diagnosis of "sarcoma of local malignancy only." The apparently viral etiology of this growth is discussed with the tumor-forming viruses (p. 507).

Chondroma; Chondrosarcoma.—These tumors differ from the fibroma and fibrosarcoma in that in certain parts they consist of cartilage, of the hyaline variety. Cartilage normally grows by proliferation of the perichondrium, which is a specialized layer of connective tissue. The same is true of the formation of cartilage in neoplasms; the cartilage cells in their lacunæ are not in a position to proliferate. It is the connective tissue cells which do this; certain of them differentiate into chondroblasts to form more cartilage, but the latter is always surrounded by fibroblasts. The malignant cells of a chondrosarcoma are anaplastic fibroblasts, and malignancy is judged by the same histological characteristics as in a fibrosarcoma, any tumor being as malignant as its most malignant part (Fig. 7–4).

Osteoma; Osteosarcoma.—The same may be said of these as has been said of the cartilage tumors, substituting bone for cartilage. The bone appears as irregular islands or spicules always surrounded by proliferating connective tissue. The degree of malignancy is that represented by the connective tissue in its most anaplastic areas. Osteomas have to be distinguished from inflammatory exostoses, which are bony enlargements resulting from mechanical trauma. The latter are simpler and more orderly in their architecture, each individual cell conforming well to the form and appearance of a normal histological fibroblast or osteoblast, as the case may be. The neoplasm consists of less well differentiated cells, more indiscriminate in form and structure but still betraying an identifying resemblance to the cells from which they arose. (See Anaplasia, p. 191.) The bones of the lower parts of the horse's limbs are especially subject to exostoses.

Osteosarcoma, Osteogenic Sarcoma, or Periosteal Sarcoma.—Some tumors arising from the periosteum, are capable of forming bone but do so only to a minimal extent. They continue to proliferate as a rather distinctive type of fibrous tissue. This tissue is rich in nuclei which, however, are not hyperchromatic. The majority tend to have the shape of short spindles with pointed ends or they may appear somewhat triangular. They are oriented to point in various directions with no tendency for groups to lie parallel (to which the technical term parallelism is applied).

The critical, identifying characteristic of cells of an osteosarcoma is their ability to produce **osteoid,** the ground substance of bone. The osteoid may or may not become calcified to produce irregular spicules of bone (Fig. 7–5C). Radiographically (Fig. 7–5A), this tumor is usually found at the extremity of a long bone and produces a radiolucent enlargement which erodes the pre-existing calcified bone. Multinucleated cells are frequent.

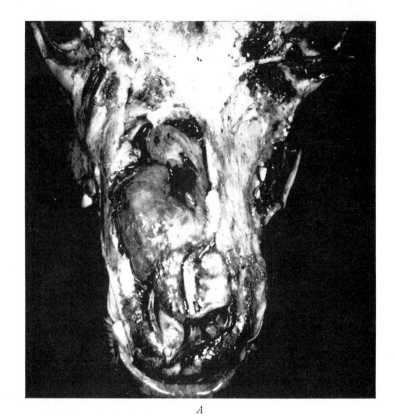

A

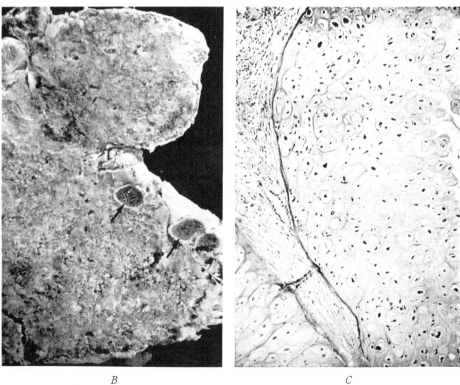

B   C

FIG. 7–4.—*A*, Chondrosarcoma of nasal septum of a seven-year-old male pointer. (Courtesy of Angell Memorial Animal Hospital.) *B*, Chondrosarcoma of the ribs of a five-year-old ewe. The tumor metastasized to the lung. Contributor: Dr. C. L. Davis. *C*, Chondrosarcoma (× 120) of the ribs of an aged ewe. Note cells with irregular polarity and variable size in cartilaginous matrix. Metastasis to lungs also occurred in this case. (Courtesy of Armed Forces Institute of Pathology.) Contributor: Dr. C. L. Davis

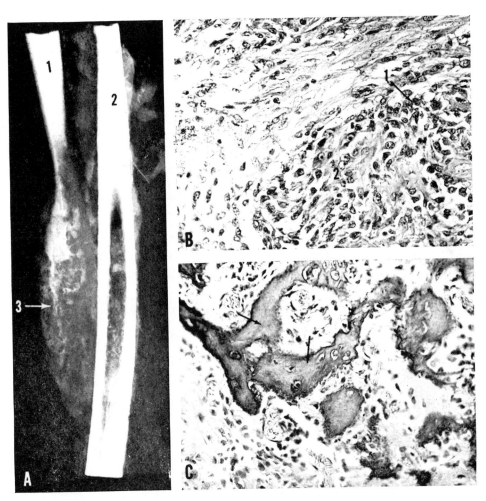

FIG. 7–5.—Osteosarcoma of the ulna of a ten-year-old female golden retriever. *A*, Radiograph of the neoplasm (*3*) in the distal third of the ulna (*1*). The radius (*2*) is not directly involved. *B*, Photomicrograph (× 250) in an area of the neoplasm made up of densely packed cells (*1*) which form osteoid (*2*). *C*, Photomicrograph (× 250) of the same tumor from an area with irregular spicules of new bone (arrows). (Courtesy of Armed Forces Institute of Pathology.) Contributor: Fourth Medical Field Laboratory, U.S. Army.

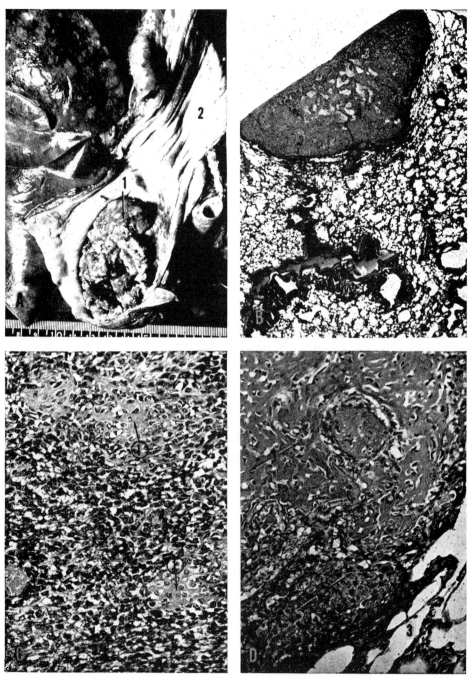

FIG. 7–6.—Osteosarcoma, primary, in the esophagus of a seven-year-old male hound. The neoplasm was associated with long-standing infection of the esophagus by *Spirocerca lupi*. *A*, The tumor (*1*) involves the terminal esophagus (*2*). The lung is identified at (*3*). *B*, Metastasis (*1*) of osteosarcoma to lung (× 12). *C*, An area of the tumor (× 150) in which osteoid (*1*) is formed by the densely packed hyperchromatic cells (*2*). *D*, Higher magnification (× 150) of *B*, showing osteoid (*1*) and spindle-shaped cells. Bone was formed in other parts of this tumor. (Courtesy of Armed Forces Institute of Pathology.) Contributor: Dr. H. R. Seibold.

Osteosarcoma may originate in tissues other than bone in some circumstances. Two such circumstances are noteworthy in animals. One such extra-osseous origin is the esophagus of the dog, adjacent to a long standing lesion produced by the spirurid worm, *Spirocerca lupi* (p. 755). A second such site is the mammary gland as a part of a mixed tumor (p. 244).

These tumors are highly malignant and metastasize early. They are more frequent in dogs than in the other domestic species, especially the large breeds, and the epiphyses of long bones are sites of predilection.

Giant-cell Tumor of Bone, or **Osteoclastoma. Epulis.**—Not too infrequently there occurs on the end of one of the long bones of the human limbs a tumor of very bizarre microscopic structure consisting chiefly of large, dark-staining, fusiform nuclei in a moderately fibrous stroma. With these are large multinucleated giant-cells in great numbers. The histologic picture is highly bizarre and suggestive of malignancy, but clinical experience shows the tumor to be practically always benign. A growth of very similar histological structure occurs on the gums and is called an epulis. Epulides have been reported occasionally in the dog.

In general, this tumor is rarely encountered in animals although multinucleated osteoclasts in an osteosarcoma may cause this diagnosis to be considered. The epulis in the gums of the dog must be differentiated from the much more common non-neoplastic lesion called "fibrous hyperplasia of the gum," "fibrous epulis" or "gingival hypertrophy" (p. 1192).

Myxoma; Myxosarcoma.—These tumors are composed of connective tissue which forms mucin, in other words, connective tissue of embryonal type. The nuclei tend to be round or stellate; the intercellular fibrils are bluish (hematoxylin and eosin) and show little parallelism. These tumors are always more or less malignant, but the term myxoma is generally used in spite of that fact. They are encountered with some frequency in veterinary medicine. Some effort must be made to distinguish this neoplasm from a fibrosarcoma with myxomatous degeneration.

Lipoma; Liposarcoma.—Lipomas, often multiple, occur in a great variety of locations as masses of adipose tissue of various sizes and shapes. The fat may be yellowish in color. These benign tumors are distinguished grossly from the excessive fat of obesity, which they frequently accompany, by the fact that they form discrete lumps or masses in contrast to the diffuse distribution of ordinary adipose tissue. Microscopically, close comparison will show a greater variation in the size and shape of the fat cells than occurs in normal adipose tissue. The liposarcoma, which is rare, is characterized by areas of anaplastic fibrous tissue in company with adipose tissue and an intermediate tissue in which only rudimentary fat cells with very small vacuoles exist.

A particular type of fatty tumor occurs in the subcutis in the midline of the back over the thorax or in the axilla. This is called a **"tumor of brown fat"** or **"hibernoma."** It forms solid masses of cells which resemble those of the "brown fat" or "hibernating gland" of many animals. This fat is brownish grossly and the lipid in the cytoplasm is in the form of tiny droplets uniformly distributed throughout the rather dark brownish cytoplasm. These fat cells contain much more potential energy than do ordinary fat cells. The tumors may reach large size but are usually benign. Dogs, rats and wild animals have been found with **these tumors.**

Chordoma.—In humans, a rare neoplasm arises at the upper (spheno-occipital) or lower (sacro-coccygeal) extremities of the vertebral column from "ecchordoses," which are remnants persisting from the fetal notochord. With a rather variable histologic appearance and frequently a superficial resemblance to cartilage, the chordoma consists of large rounded cells with central nuclei and clear, mucoid-appearing cytoplasm. These cells are seen in areas or clumps which are ordinarily connected to fibroblastic tissue but which sometimes appear surrounded by a non-cellular mucinous matrix, probably a distintegration product of other similar cells. Both the cytoplasmic and the extra-cellular material usually contain numerous vacuoles. As one might guess, the chordoma consists grossly of a gelatinous, semi-transparent tissue. The tumor infiltrates surrounding tissues and may reach considerable size. There appear to be few reports of chordomas in animals.

Neurofibroma; Neurofibrosarcoma; Neurogenic Sarcoma.—Arising from the fibrous connective tissue of nerve sheaths, the perineurium, the neurofibroma is distinguished microscopically from the ordinary fibroma by the fact that some of the fibrous tissue is arranged in tight, circular whorls. Malignant tumors of this class occur rarely and are usually known by the name of neurogenic sarcoma although neurofibrosarcoma is not improper. However, these are not clearly distinguishable from malignant tumors thought to arise from the neurilemma or from the ordinary type of fibrosarcoma. Microscopically, the neurogenic sarcoma resembles a fibrosarcoma, but the cells tend to have the form of plump spindles and have a whorled or at least a curly arrangement. Grossly, the neurofibromas

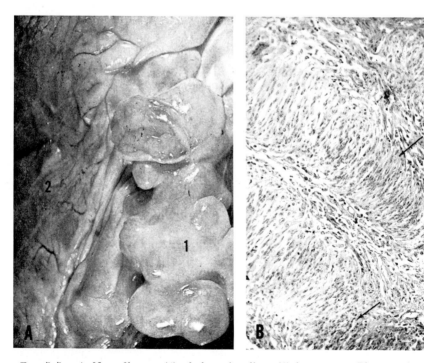

FIG. 7–7.—*A*, Neurofibroma (*1*) of the epicardium (*2*) in a steer. Photograph courtesy of Dr. C. L. Davis. *B*, Neurofibromatosis involving brachial plexus, myocardium and intercostal nerves of an eight-year-old cow. Section (× 150) is from the tumor in the brachial plexus. (Courtesy of Armed Forces Institute of Pathology.) Contributor: Dr. C. L. Davis.

form rounded masses, usually subcutaneous, sometimes located more deeply. They occur at least in bovines and chickens. In cattle they are fairly frequent in the myocardium, sometimes with more than one in a single heart. The tendency to form whorls is sometimes recognizable grossly in the moist, slightly bulging cut surface. In man, large numbers of cutaneous neurofibromas occur in the same patient in what is known as von Recklinghausen's neurofibromatosis. A tumorous condition having similar characteristics has been reported in the dog (Antin, 1957). A neurofibroma or a very close relative of it occurs at the origin of the acoustic nerve in man and is known as the acoustic-nerve tumor. We have no reports, as yet, of this tumor in animals.

Neurilemmoma; Schwann-Cell Tumor.—Either of these terms describes a neoplasm, usually benign, which is considered to arise from the neurilemmal cells surrounding the axones of peripheral nerves. There is considerable difference of opinion as to whether this tumor is distinguishable from the neurofibroma, which arises from the perineurial connective tissue, a question which we shall leave to others. The neurilemmoma ("Schwannoma") resembles the fibroma in its general microscopic structure, but here and there areas are found in which the elongated, spindle-shaped nuclei are gathered together in windrows. The nuclei lie practically parallel in a direction crosswise of the windrow. This feature is the principal distinctive characteristic of the tumor. As would be expected the growths are located along the course of a nerve or at a plexus or ganglion. While the number of cases reported in animals is not adequate for final conclusions, it appears that the common sites are in the deeper somatic structures (brachial plexus, intercostal nerves) or internal organs. In respect to size, the tumors seldom exceed a few centimeters in diameter. Their growth is not rapid and, if accessible, complete removal should be curative.

Meningioma. — These tumors arise from the cranial or spinal meninges, presumably from their mesothelial (older histologists called them endothelial) cells which form the surface of these membranes. (Some say they arise from "arachnoid cells.") In most meningiomas, the cells are more plump and the nuclei more rounded than in the neurofibroma, but there is the same tendency toward a whorled arrangement. Occasionally meningiomas form areas of bone. Rather commonly at the center of many of the whorls, there is a compressed hyaline or calcified body suggestive grossly of a grain of sand. This form of meningioma is sometimes called a **psammoma** (from *psammos*, meaning sand), and the little granules are known as brain sand. Grossly the meningioma forms a more or less spherical subdural mass. It compresses the underlying brain or cord and may extend deep into sulci. Meningiomas have been found somewhat frequently in the horse and are the most common intracranial neoplasm in the cat (Fig. 7–50).

Mesothelioma is a term, its usefulness denied by some, which designates a tumor arising from the mesothelial (formerly called endothelial) lining cells of serous membranes, particularly the pleura and peritoneum. These growths usually take the form of diffusely disseminated nodular growths covering extensive areas of the membrane concerned. Microscopically, the majority have the structures of rounded or papillary projections consisting of a fibrous core covered by large mesothelial cells which bear a close resemblance to epithelium. It appears that either of these constituents can become dominant and develop into a neoplasm which (1) has a structure resembling a fibroma or (2) consists of carcinoma-like masses of large epithelioid cells. Grossly, these neoplasms must

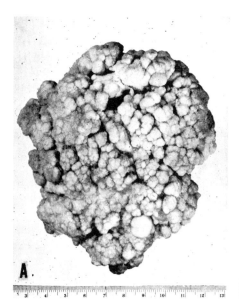
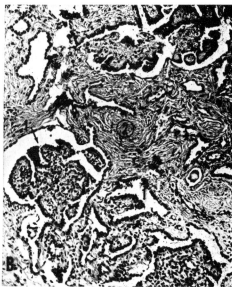

FIG. 7–8.—Mesothelioma of the pleura of a six-year-old cow. *A*, Gross appearance of the nodular pleura. *B*, Photomicrograph (× 105) showing papillary growth of mesothelium (*1*) and supporting stroma (*2*). (Courtesy of Armed Forces Institute of Pathology.) Contributor: Dr. C. L. Davis.

be differentiated from actinobacillosis, tuberculosis ("pearly disease") and probably other granulomatous infections, which sometimes cover the peritoneum or pleura with masses of closely placed nodular proliferations.

Synovioma denotes a neoplasm derived from the mesothelium (formerly called endothelium) lining synovial cavities. Like the mesothelioma, these tumors may be composed of cells resembling those of a somewhat pleomorphic fibroma or of epithelioid cells arranged to form continuous sheets, or papillary or cystic structures. They are difficult to recognize without knowledge of their site of origin (Fig. 7–9).

Hemangioma; Hemangioendothelioma.—These tumors arise from the endothelial cells which line blood vessels. The tumor consists of a mixture of cellular areas, the endothelial cells resembling short, plump fibroblasts, and of endothelium-lined blood spaces filled with normal, circulating blood. The hemangioma having medium-sized blood spaces and no great amount of cellular tissue is designated **hemangioma simplex,** the one with very large blood spaces, **hemangioma cavernosum,** and the opposite type, with a large amount of cellular tissue and minimal blood spaces is an **hemangioma hypertrophicum.** The great majority are benign. In fact an area of tumor sufficiently anaplastic to be malignant would be unlikely to have any features distinguishing it from other sarcomas, although other areas of the same tumor may be sufficiently well differentiated to betray its origin. Logically or not, those forms considered malignant are usually called **hemangioendotheliomas, malignant hemangiomas,** or **hemangiosarcomas.**

In the dog, hemangioendotheliomas with malignant potentialities are encountered arising from the spleen, right atrium and occasionally from the subcutis. These neoplasms consist of ovoid cells with hyperchromatic nuclei and scanty cytoplasm. The cells form or tend to form many small capillaries, the distin-

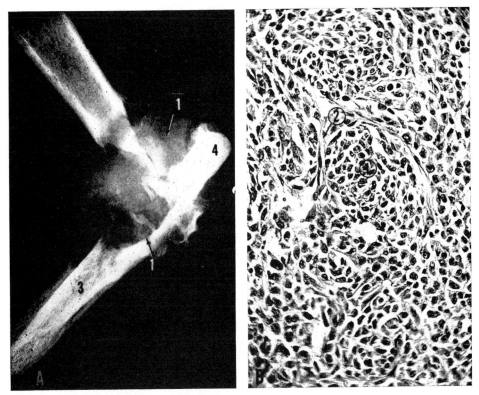

FIG. 7–9.—Malignant synovioma involving elbow joint, humerus, radius and ulna of an eleven-year-old female spitz dog. *A*, Radiograph of the tumor (*1*) which replaces the joint and destroys the distal part of the humerus (*2*), proximal part of the radius (*3*) and ulna (not shown). The olecranon (*4*) is partially invaded. *B*, Photomicrograph (× 330) of the highly cellular neoplasm (*1*) with indistinct stroma (*2*). (Courtesy of Armed Forces Institute of Pathology.) Contributor: Dr. Leo L. Lieberman.

guishing feature of the growth. The term **capillary hemangioma** has been used for this variety. Cutaneous hemangiomas have been produced in ducks by the application of methyl-cholanthrene (Rigdon, 1952). In man, the familiar fiery red birthmarks have the structure of superficially placed hemangiomas, although they do not grow and are usually rich in blood.

Hemangiopericytoma.—A related type of neoplasm recently described as a separate entity is the hemangiopericytoma (Mulligan, 1955, Stout and Murray, 1942, Yost and Jones, 1958). It consists in general of spindle-shaped cells with ovoid or elongated nuclei and considerable cytoplasm which frequently becomes fibrillar. The tumor thus bears a superficial resemblance to "spindle-celled sarcomas," neurofibromas and hemangioendotheliomas, with which, in the past, many specimens of this type have doubtless been classed. The distinguishing characteristic, however, is the presence of numerous small capillaries, open or collapsed, which are lined by endothelium but closely encircled by the more or less anaplastic and pleomorphic "spindle" cells, which are considered to be pericytes. In some specimens, encircling cells are flattened and extended in a circumferential direction; in others, their relationship to the vessel wall is less obvious but the cells tend to form whorls or clusters around a capillary space. By suitable

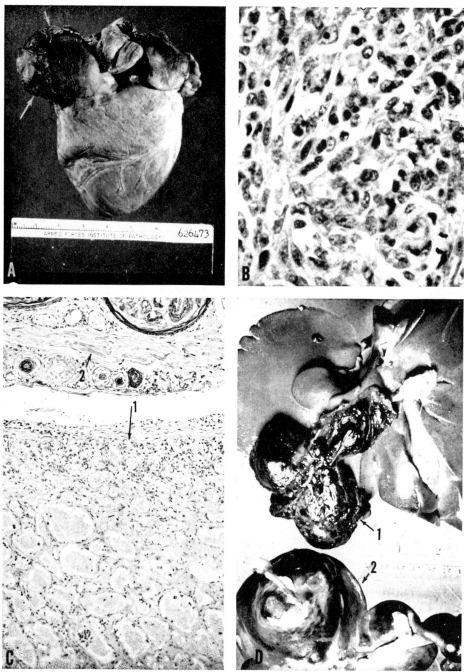

FIG. 7–10.—*A*, Hemangioendothelioma (arrows), primary in the myocardium of the right auricle of a seven-year-old female beagle dog. Contributor: Dr. Leo L. Lieberman. *B*, Hemangio-endothelioma (× 300), primary in spleen of a dog. The tumor cells have elongated nuclei and frequently form vascular channels. *C*, Hemangioma (× 75) in the subcutis of tarsal region of a two and a half-year-old wire-haired fox terrier. The new growth is encapsulated (*1*) and sep-arated from the dermis (*2*). (Courtesy of Armed Forces Institute of Pathology.) Contributor: Dr. Leo L. Lieberman. *D*, Hemangioendothelioma involving liver (*1*) and spleen (*2*) of a dog.

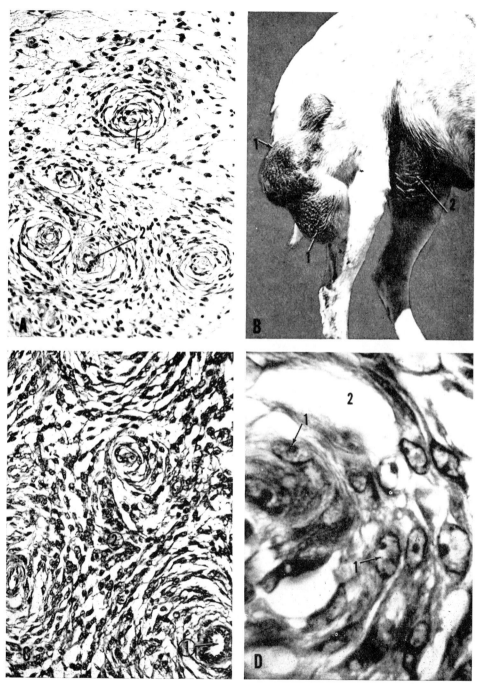

FIG. 7–11.—Hemangiopericytoma of the subcutis of the dog. *A*, Photomicrograph (× 160) showing whorl arrangement of tumor cells around occult (*1*) and overt capillaries (*2*). Contributor: Dr. S. W. Stiles. *B*, Large subcutaneous hemangiopericytoma (*1*) in a fifteen-year-old terrier dog. Note metastasis to inguinal region (*2*). Contributor: Dr. W. J. Zontine. *C*, Section (× 210) in a densely cellular area with capillaries (*1*) and spindle-shaped cells (*2*) concentrically arranged around them. Contributor: Dr. W. H. Riser. *D*, Higher magnification (× 1080) of another tumor. Note ovoid nuclei (*1*) which are often vesicular and contain a single nucleolus. Clear, empty spaces (*2*) are common. (Courtesy of Armed Forces Institute of Pathology.) Contributor: Phillips Veterinary Hospital.

reticulum stains (Lillie, 1947) large and numerous reticular fibers can be demonstrated in concentric layers around the vessels. The tumor is always subcutaneous. It recurs after many months and in the course of several years has been shown to metastasize. This, in our experience, is one of the most common neoplasms encountered in surgically removed specimens from dogs.

The term **perithelioma** has been applied to this tumor, or one very similar, by European writers.

Histologists are poorly agreed on just what constitutes a pericyte. Just how widely the conception of this neoplastic type will be accepted, only time will tell. It must be admitted that the designation of whorl-forming tumors as of perineural origin (neurofibromas) has often been grounded more on habit than on proof.

Lymphangioma; Lymphangioendothelioma.—These tumors are entirely comparable to the hemangiomas, except that the vascular spaces are connected to the lymphatic system and contain lymph instead of blood. They are much less frequent than their blood-containing counterparts.

Leiomyomas and **Leiomyosarcomas** are smooth-muscle tumors. It is not always easy to distinguish the neoplastic smooth muscle from connective tissue, especially since the muscle is often so poorly differentiated that it does not respond typically to special stains such as Van Gieson's. One relies largely on the fact that the muscle nuclei, while long and slender, have well rounded ends. They, with their fibers, have a strong tendency to lie parallel with each other, although the composite band of cells and fibers may curve freely. Malignancy is betrayed by the usual signs, especially by lack of differentiation into typical smooth muscle, bizarre nuclei, hyperchromatic nuclei and numerous mitotic figures (the name given to nuclei in the process of mitosis). Leiomyomas are relatively frequent in the digestive and other organs whose structure includes much smooth muscle (intestine, uterus).

Rhabdomyoma and **Rhabdomyosarcoma** are the names given respectively to benign and malignant neoplasms arising from striated muscle, either skeletal or cardiac. These tumors, including cardiac examples, are known in most of the domesticated species but are rare. In a few, the resemblance to striated muscle is obvious, but the majority have to be differentiated from fibrous or smooth-muscle tumors by the recognition of an occasional fiber which contains cross striations.

Malignant Lymphoma.—Among the neoplasms of the blood-forming tissues, those consisting of lymphoid cells are by far the most prominent. Indeed this is the most frequently encountered tumor in American veterinary practice, none of the usual domestic species being exempt. Jackson (1936), however, found lymphoid tumors uncommon in South Africa. Goats appear to be rarely affected.

The tumors are usually multiple, causing pronounced enlargement of a number of lymph nodes in various parts of the body and, in about half of the cases similarly involving the spleen, which may reach a most astonishing size. These lymphoid organs are not invaded by discrete metastases, as would be the case with other tumors, but are remade and transformed into neoplastic tissue which differs from the previously existing normal organ in having none of the characteristic histological structures, such as germinal centers and splenic (malpighian) corpuscles. The evidence justifies the prevalent view that this neoplasm is multicentric in origin and arises through a more or less generalized proliferation of normal lymphocytes of an uncontrollable neoplastic type.

In addition to involving many or perhaps all of the lymphoid organs, the malignant lymphoma, which is never benign, invades, in what we may call a metastatic manner, practically any organ of the body. These invasions may take the form of discrete metastatic masses or they may display themselves as insidious infiltrations of neoplastic cells among the normal histological structures. The latter is common in the kidney, where lymphoid cells may be interspersed through certain areas of intertubular stroma, and in the bovine heart, where they

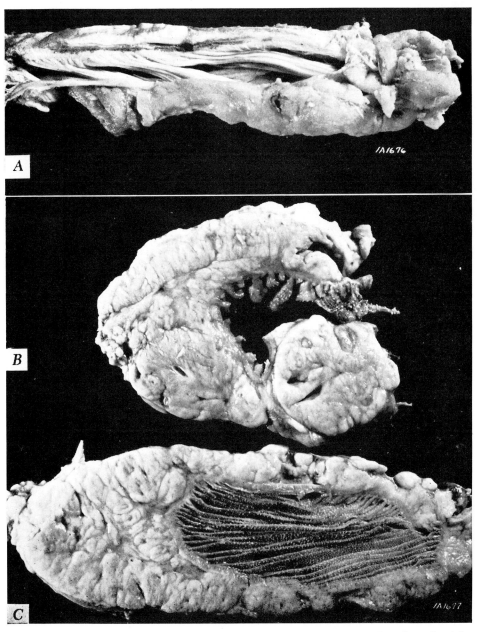

FIG. 7–12.—Bovine malignant lymphoma, illustrating neoplastic invasion of cauda equina (*A*), reticulum (*B*) and omasum (*C*). Photograph courtesy of Dr. M. J. Twiehaus, Kansas State University.

may infiltrate among the muscle fibers. Other organs in which metastatic tumor tissue is encountered with some degree of frequency in cattle include the liver, the walls of the reticulum, abomasum, uterus and ureter, the retrobulbar area, where it produces extreme exophthalmos, and the meninges of the cauda equina, where it causes paralysis of the posterior limbs (Fig. 7–12). In the dog, involvement is more likely to be limited to the lymphoid and parenchymatous organs, although Peyer's patches and tonsillar areas are not exempt. In one case, the roof of the dog's mouth was extensively invaded between the mucosa and the palatine bones. Discrete nodules occur in the kidney, as well as the diffuse infiltrations mentioned.

The nomenclature of tumors of the lymphoid group has varied through the years. In accordance with an early plan of classification (Mallory, 1914), a malignant lymphoid tumor was properly called a **lymphosarcoma.** While not necessarily incorrect in this sense, the term today usually connotes a special subvariety, one showing a mild degree of histological anaplasia according to some and one having cells which approach a fibroblastic type according to others. Somewhat later the term **lymphoblastoma** was in vogue, based on the concept that any neoplasm is a "blastoma." By another group the obviously logical term of **lymphocytoma** was preferred. Each of these is best avoided as a general term, partly because of lack of agreement on them but more because each now has a special significance, designating a class or subvariety of the group. Malignant lymphoma is the preferred name for the lymphoid tumors in general.

It is now customary to subdivide malignant lymphomas into several classes or types. The classification of Gall and Mallory (1942) is usually followed with slight modifications. The principal classes now commonly recognized are briefly as follows:

1. Malignant lymphoma, lymphocytic type, often subdivided into well differentiated and poorly differentiated subgroups. In these the cells are close replicates of normal lymphocytes although in the poorly differentiated subgroup they have lost some uniformity in this respect. One sees a monotony of lymphocytic cells which have replaced all architectural features of lymph node or spleen and, of course, invade other organs as mentioned above. Mitotic figures are practically non-existent.

(2) Malignant lymphoma, histiocytic (formerly clasmatocytic) type, and (3) malignant lymphoma, stem-cell type, together correspond to what some have called the reticulum-cell type and the most atypical specimens have been called reticulum-cell sarcomas in some quarters. Here also belong most examples of Gall and Mallory's earlier lymphoblastic type. In (2) the histiocytic type the cells resemble histiocytes (reticulo-endothelial cells) in having considerable to large amounts of cytoplasm, its outer contour indistinct. The nuclei are vesicular (pale and empty-appearing), often indented, reniform or folded, sometimes almost triangular. A prominent nucleolus appears in some of the cells. Mitotic figures occur with some frequency and are often atypical. There is considerable pleomorphism, no two cells being exactly alike. In some examples the cytoplasm tends to form stringy, attenuated strands of eosinophilic material (reticulin, collagen) approaching the appearance of connective tissue. Rarely there may be large binucleate cells resulting from incompleted cell division and resembling but not duplicating the Reed-Sternberg cells of Hodgkin's disease.

3. The stem-cell type of malignant lymphoma is the most anaplastic. The cytoplasm is minimal. The nuclei are very large, round and hyperchromatic

(dark-staining). Indentation of the nucleus is exceptional. Mitoses are numerous and frequently abnormal in form. Nucleoli are exceptional.

4. Malignant lymphoma, Hodgkin's type, is equivalent to that clinically variable and morphologically heterogeneous group of human lymphadenopathies known as **Hodgkin's disease,** itself divisible into three subtypes which we shall overlook. The true nature of this obscure disease has never been entirely settled. Evidence has been brought forth linking it with the infectious granulomas (p. 615) but present opinion classes it with the lymphomas. Its course, while often slow, is relentlessly fatal, a fact tending strongly to support the neoplastic concept of its etiology. There probably have been no true examples of Hodgkin's disease in the domestic animals but cases are reported from time to time bearing such strong similarity to it that the veterinary pathologist needs to be aware of the exact criteria that would justify such a diagnosis. Characterized by slowly enlarging lymph nodes, especially in the thoracic and cervical regions, the disease involves continuous proliferation of four kinds of cells in varying proportions: lymphoid cells, histiocytes, fibroblasts and eosinophils. If the embryological precursors of these cells are traced back far enough they all have the same parent cell, hence it may be that Hodgkin's disease should be viewed as a disorder arising in prelymphoid and premyeloid stem cells. The histologic picture may be difficult to distinguish from that of a lymphoma (histiocytic type especially) or from that of inflammatory granuloma, depending on the predominant cell types in a given case. In this dilemma we fall back, for diagnostic purposes, upon what is known as the Reed-Sternberg cell, which can be found after more or less searching in all cases. This giant cell, which is fundamentally a syncytium of at least two, and usually more, incompletely divided histiocytes, has a multilobed, or at least bilobed, nucleus or a piled-up, overlapping group of single vesicular nuclei. Each nucleus or nuclear lobe has a single prominent, acidophilic (reddish) nucleolus near its center. At least one or two of these nucleoli must be visible in the plane of the microscopic section under study. Less than these specifications does not permit interpretation of a giant cell as a Reed-Sternberg cell and without Reed-Sternberg cells Hodgkin's disease can not be diagnosed with certainty.

As to the practical value of these rather meticulous classifications and subdivisions of malignant lymphomas and their relatives it may be answered that in human medicine it has become possible to predict with considerable accuracy the clinical course of the disease and thus adjust the treatment to a slow or rapid progress. In the less anaplastic types a reasonably satisfactory state of health may be maintained for months or years; the more malignant ones have an early fatal termination in spite of any known treatment. It is not possible on the basis of cellular morphology to say whether actual leukemia will be manifested. In animals the same general tenets as to the clinical course doubtless hold true, although for economic or humane reasons the course has not been followed to its natural end in most cases. We do know of some animals, especially cattle, which have lived for a considerable part of their natural life-span with obvious lesions of malignant lymphoma.

Since it is normal for a considerable number of lymphocytes to enter the blood stream and be carried away as circulating lymphocytes, it is not surprising that in some cases the same thing happens with neoplastic lymphoid cells. In some patients with malignant lymphoma, the total leukocyte count may rise to many thousands per cubic millimeter, for instance to a point between 30,000 and 200,000.

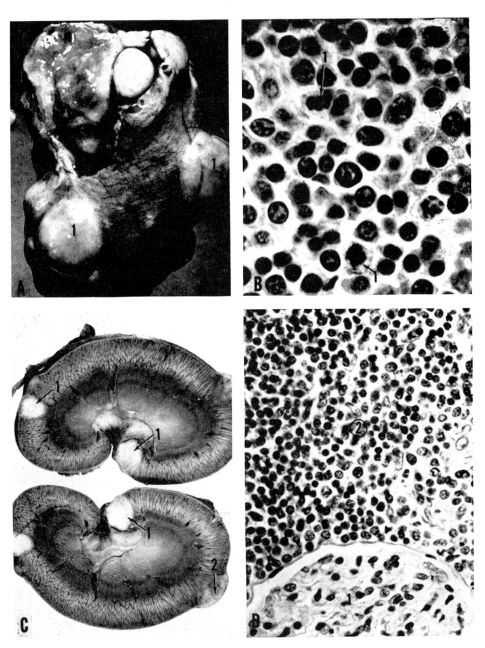

Fig. 7–13.—Malignant lymphoma. *A*, Metastatic lesions (*1*) in the kidney of a dog. *B*, Photo-micrograph (× 1190). Note individually discrete tumor cells and mitotic figures (*1*). *C*, Gross appearance of tumors (*1*) and (*2*) shown in *B* and *D*, from the kidney of a five-year-old male shepherd. *D*, Infiltration of the renal cortex (× 500), the renal corpuscle (*1*) is not yet replaced by the tumor (*2*). (Courtesy of Armed Forces Institute of Pathology.)   Contributor: Dr. Leo L. Lieberman.

The increase represents an increased number of lymphocytes only, their percentage of the total white-cell count rising to a very high figure. This condition is called **lymphatic, lymphocytic,** or **lymphoid leukemia.** It must be differentiated from the increased leukocyte count of an inflammatory leukocytosis (p. 172). This can be done by noting morphological differences in the neoplastic cells seen in the blood and usually, also, by the fact that the white-cell count of leukemia is likely to be far higher than that of leukocytosis, the latter commonly being below 20,000 per cubic millimeter, and rarely exceeding 30,000. The malignant lymphoma accompanied by leukemia is said to be **leukemic;** without leukemia it is an **aleukemic** malignant lymphoma (or lymphocytoma, lymphoblastoma, lymphosarcoma). The evidence indicates that a malignant lymphoma may be at one time leukemic; at another, aleukemic.

In some patients, the first and perhaps the only manifestations of disease are those of **leukemia,** this being, of course, substantiated by the leukocyte count. This fact led to the conception of leukemia as a separate disease entity, and there was formerly considerable difference of opinion as to its cause. It is generally accepted nowadays that lymphatic leukemia is a phase of malignant lymphoma even though, as rarely happens, no discrete neoplastic formations can be found. Leukemia may be regarded as a circulating neoplasm, the supply of new cells, however, being still derived from the usual lymphoblastic tissues.

A tendency is evident among many workers to call all neoplasms of blood-forming organs "leukemia." In this usage, malignant lymphoma would be included, even in cases without malignant cells in the circulation. This tendency is decried by some (Payne, 1969) and certainly indicates a lack of precision.

The **diagnosis** of malignant lymphoma in lymph nodes is not as simple as might be assumed. Neither generalized enlargement of lymph nodes nor, microscopically, the presence of primitive or immature (in other words, undifferentiated or anaplastic) lymphoid cells is proof of the presence of neoplasia. Such undifferentiated and embryologically immature cells are recognized by their larger and paler nuclei and more hazily bounded cytoplasm. The nuclei, usually round but occasionally indented, reniform or folded, have sharply outlined nuclear membranes but the dark-staining chromatin is not concentrated at those peripheral membranes as it is in the lymphocyte with its "clock-faced" nucleus, nor are the internal chromatin granules darkly stained. The nucleus, thus, is of the "vesicular" type and much lighter in color than that of the lymphocyte. The cell as a whole has a diameter two or three times that of the lymphocyte—a large pale cell in contrast to the small, dark lymphocytes which often surround it.

Now cells of this type can be found scattered here and there in a normal lymph node, where they are interpreted as histiocytes, a form of reticulo-endothelial cell. How much do they differ from the "maternal lymphoblasts" of the "germinal" centers? One prominent school of thought says, "Very little", and that the relationship is close. As to the germinal centers, it is well accepted that proliferative increase in their size and number is the essence of classical lymphoid hyperplasia (p. 95), a frequent lesion of many chronic infections such as brucellosis and canine distemper. If the cells of the germinal center proliferate in response to such chronic irritants why should not the scattered histiocytes do likewise? At any rate, lymph nodes are not infrequently encountered as part of a localized or generalized process in which the population of undifferentiated histiocytic cells of this kind is markedly or even tremendously increased, with consequent enlargement of the nodes, sometimes to astonishing size. If the causative infection or irritant is discernible the reactive nature of the process is readily apparent but when no causative agent is in evidence many of these examples of reactive hyperplasia are easily confused with malignant lymphoma.

The principal criteria for differential diagnosis include, pointing toward reactive hyperplasia, the persistence of any of the architectural components of normal lymph node, whether they be follicles, sinuses, including the subcapsular sinus, recognizable lymph cords with normal lymphocytes or the recognition of cortex and medulla. Variety rather than uniformity of cell types, some approaching the characteristics of normal lymphocytes, also argues for hyperplasia. One should search carefully for other signs of inflammatory reaction, such as albuminous or fibrinous precipitate from an exudate. Unsuspected micro-organisms can occasionally be demonstrated by the application of special techniques. Pointing toward malignant neoplasia are uniformly large size of cells, the presence of really large numbers of mitotic figures, atypical mitotic figures, and the presence of cells which are so undifferentiated or abnormal as to be difinitely outside the range of any but neoplastic proliferation. Extensive infiltration of the capsule of the lymph node by lymphoid cells is an oblique indication of considerable but not decisive importance that a malignant lymphoma is present. Of course, if a clinical history is available this may be such as to dispel all doubts. Neoplastic invasion of such non-lymphoid organs as the heart, stomach, kidney or uterus may be present to settle the question.

A lymphoma can arise in the thymus; in fact in laboratory mice this is a common occurrence. Its characteristics, either grossly or microscopically, need not differ from those of a lymphoma located elsewhere. The term **thymoma** is then sometimes used but, according to most authorities, a true thymoma must contain more than purely lymphoid elements, namely structures traceable to the Hassall's corpuscles of the normal thymus. We need not enter into the controversy whether the cells of Hassall's corpuscles or even the "thymocytes" themselves are epithelial or mesenchymal in nature but as seen in sections they are identified because of their similarity to epithelial cells. Occasionally they form laminated whorls resembling Hassall's corpuscles; rarely, they line spaces of cystic appearance. The lymphoid-appearing cells are ordinarily in the great majority, however. One sees no fibrous stroma except along the course of blood vessels.

Malignant Myeloma.—Practically everything that has been said about the malignant lymphoma is true of the malignant myeloma except with respect to the cell of origin, which for the myeloma is the myelocyte of the bone marrow or its progenitor, the myeloblast. The comparable synonyms, **myelocytoma, myeloblastoma** and **myelosarcoma,** have been used but in present-day terminology the usually preferred names for this tumor are either (1) **multiple myeloma,** which is based upon the fact that with few exceptions the tumors arise at a number of separate sites in the bone marrow, or (2) **plasma-cell myeloma,** based upon the histological appearance of the most frequently encountered type-cell. Some even go so far as to prefer the term **plasmacytoma** but to others this name is reserved for a tumor consisting of what appear to be plasma cells occurring in nonosseous sites (respiratory passages of head, etc., in human beings) without any detectable involvement of bone marrow. The myeloma is always malignant and may be leukemic or non-leukemic. While **myelogenous leukemia** is not inappropriate, this form of leukemia is commonly designated **granulocytic leukemia,** a term more expressive of the types of cell usually encountered and at the same time permitting differentiation from the much rarer forms such as plasmacytic leukemia, monocytic leukemia and erythroid leukemia.

Grossly, some myelomas have a greenish hue, which is due to a high prevalence of eosinophilic granulocytes and their precursors. This greenish color, if faded, can be temporarily restored by oxidation with hydrogen peroxide. Because of their color, these have been designated **chloromas** in the older literature. Most myelomas in animals have involved lymph nodes but few generalizations are possible until more cases have been studied.

Myelomas are very rare in domesticated mammals but do occur in laboratory mice and the equine, bovine, canine and feline species. Since these are tumors of bone-marrow cells, their anatomical location is naturally the bone marrow, specifically in those bones having red marrow. While solitary myelomas are not unknown, it is usual to find the marrow involved at a number of spots within the same or different bones. But neoplasms of this general nature are also encountered outside the bone marrow, especially in the spleen, lymph nodes and liver. Presumably these should invariably be metastases from primary tumors of bone marrow but the frequency with which such primaries were not discovered forces us to an opposite conclusion. Furthermore, a prevalent opinion among histologists points to a "common lymphoid stem cell" as the original precursor of myeloid cells, which ultimately differentiate into erythrocytes or any of the granulocytes (neutrophilic, eosinophilic, basophilic). If this concept is correct it serves to explain the occasional myelomas which seem to be primary in the spleen or lymph nodes, the mast-cell tumor probably and those "plasmacytomas" seen in human nasal and pharyngeal regions and elsewhere.

The diagnosis of myeloma depends upon recognition of cells of the myelocytic series. These vary in morphology and staining characteristics in accordance with the stage of differentiation from the large "stem-cell" with its extensive cytoplasm and pale vesicular nucleus, all the way to the mature granulocytes and erythrocytes. The cytoplasm of these myeloid cells is described by hematologists as basophilic but for the tissue pathologist working with sections stained by hematoxylin and eosin this merely means that the cytoplasm is less pink than that of most cells, a lavender or somewhat purplish hue. This difference in color, if present, is of considerable value in diagnosis. In some specimens these cells not only have a darker cytoplasm but their nucleus is definitely eccentric in position, rounded, with peripheral chromatin granules, and perhaps partially surrounded by a pale halo in the cytoplasm. These, then, are the "plasma cells" responsible for the frequently used name, plasma-cell myeloma.

As usually seen in tissue sections, cells of general myeloid type are to be recognized as individually discrete, rounded cells with considerable cytoplasm and a central nucleus which is large, round and vesicular if the cell is at an early stage of differentiation, smaller, possibly indented, and with prominent chromatin granules if at a later stage. While many of these cells are granulocytes or the precursors of granulocytes, the only cytoplasmic granules that can ordinarily be seen in hematoxylin-eosin sections are those of the eosinophils. When these cells are numerous and of immature type they constitute strong diagnostic evidence that the cells of the whole group are of myeloid nature. The immature eosinophilic granulocytes, which are known as eosinophilic myelocytes, are distinguished from the mature ones by the fact that the former have large round nuclei with only a limited amount of granular chromatin, whereas the mature eosinophil has a lobed nucleus (most frequently two lobes), with darker, denser chromatin.

Outside the bone marrow any appreciable numbers of eosinophilic myelocytes mean the presence of either (1) this neoplastic condition, perhaps as granulocytic leukemia, or (2) extramedullary hematopoiesis (myeloid metaplasia) such as occurs as compensatory mechanism in some severe and prolonged anemias (p. 123). As differential clues between these two we have the facts that in compensatory hematopoiesis (1) a certain proportion of the granulocytes become mature forms, (2) the differentiation tends strongly toward erythropoiesis rather than granulocytopoiesis, nucleated erythrocytes being recognizable, and (3) with this erythropoiesis there appears a larger number of megakaryocytes, than with granulocytic leukemia. Summarizing, it may be said that if the appropriate cell types can be recognized and if compensatory hematopoiesis can be excluded, a diagnosis of some variety of malignant myeloma is in order.

Xanthoma.—This term refers to tiny yellowish nodules which form on the skin of the eyelids and on tendons and tendon sheaths in man. They consist of collections of large, pale "foam cells," doubtless of reticulo-endothelial origin, whose extensive cytoplasm is made granular by many minute droplets of cholesterol and other lipoids. With them are fibroblasts and other phagocytes. This is not truly a neoplasm, but a reactive lesion. It possibly bears some significant relation to cholesterol metabolism.

Within very recent years rather wide-based, sessile proliferations called xanthomas have been encountered subcutaneously in chickens. They consist mostly of connective tissue and "foamy", cholesterol-containing phagocytes similar to those in human xanthomas. The proliferations are quite irregular in contour but do not grow to extensive heights. They are not true neoplasms. A typical xanthoma also occurs with some frequency in subcutis of the shell parakeet (budgerigar) (Petrak and Gilmore, 1969).

Granular Cell Myoblastoma.—This is a microscopically startling growth consisting principally of large, or even huge, polyhedral and spherical cells of epithelioid appearance which have a comparatively small central nucleus and an extensive, pale, granular cytoplasm. There is more or less collagen-bearing stroma. In the human tongue, especially, these cells appear related to, and derived from striated muscle and this conception is responsible for the name applied to the tumor. However, these growths have also been described in structures, such as the human mammary gland and hypophysis, where there is no striated muscle. One school of thought places the origin of the peculiar cells in nervous tissue; another considers them as altered fibroblasts. Whatever their nature, the tumor constitutes a readily recognizable entity and its metastasis is known to be highly unlikely. Hyperplastic changes (acanthosis) of the overlying epidermis are likely to accompany it. There are those who believe the large cells to be degenerative or possibly regenerative and not truly neoplastic. Such a tumor has been recorded in the subcutaneous tissue of a dog (Troy, 1955). Some foreign material of plant origin was found embedded in the overlying dermis, which may or may not be significant. The tumor was excised with an apparent cure. Additional cases have been reported in the horse (Misdorp and Nauta-van Gelder, 1968), dog and mouse.

EPITHELIAL NEOPLASMS

A different system of nomenclature prevails with respect to the epithelial, or "covering tissues." Epithelium is, first of all, considered as being divided into two kinds, gland-forming and non-gland-forming. A moment's reflection on the histology of glands reminds us that their epithelium is, or is derived from columnar or cuboidal epithelium and that it is this kind of epithelium which forms glands. The non-glandular epithelium is a surface-covering epithelium, chiefly stratified squamous (transitional in the urinary tract). New growths of surface epithelium can grow downward into the tissues only if malignant; benign growths must project from the surface. These often very complicated, branching projections are called papillomas. The basic classification for epithelial neoplasms thus becomes:

Papilloma, a benign epithelial neoplasm growing from a surface, usually, but not necessarily stratified squamous in type.

Carcinoma, a malignant epithelial neoplasm. Those coming from stratified squamous epithelium are designated squamous-cell carcinomas.

Adenoma, a benign gland-forming tumor. Usually the parent tissue, and the tumor as well, form glandular acini but the non-acinar sebaceous glands and the ductless glands are included here.

Adenocarcinoma, a malignant gland-forming neoplasm.

The term "epithelioma" is used in some quarters, usually with the implication of malignancy, but the older "carcinoma" and its variants are the names commonly employed. A number of special types of epithelial tumors will be described shortly.

Papilloma.—The term papilla denotes a small projection; a papilloma is a tumor consisting of papillary projections, usually a large number of them. As already stated, it is a benign epithelial neoplasm but, since epithelium always rests upon a connective tissue base, which provides the blood vessels supplying necessary nutrients, the epithelial tumor always has a core of fibrous connective tissue. As the epithelial cells grow and multiply, their excess population finds room by bulging and folding outward from the surface. As these bulges grow into more and more complicated papillary projections, the underlying connective tissue grows with them. It is believed that the true neoplastic process resides in the epithelium, however. The type of epithelium is that which belongs to the surface which gave origin to the tumor. Non-squamous epithelium, however, not infrequently undergoes squamous metaplasia previous to the development of neoplasia. Papilloma of known viral etiology are discussed on page 508.

Common sites of papillomas include the skin, where they are covered with stratified squamous epithelium, cornified but usually unpigmented and always without accessory skin structures and rete pegs. Also productive of squamous papillomas are the esophagus and the bovine rumen. The latter rather frequently bears multiple, simple papillary formations up to 2 cm. in height, which are not truly neoplastic but are believed to represent an excessive healing reaction as a result of the superficial ulcerations frequently seen in the rumens of fattening cattle (Smith, 1944). Long, slender papillary growths, of horny hardness and measuring typically perhaps 2 or 3 mm. in diameter and 2 or 3 cm. in height, occur in the region of the esophageal groove and, likewise, are not true neoplasms.

Papillomas covered with simple cuboidal or columnar epithelium occur in the intestine. Papillomas of complicated architecture resembling the petals of a

dahlia are not altogether rare in the bladder. Smaller but similarly formed papillomas near the corneo-scleral junction constitute an early stage of squamous-cell
carcinoma of the bovine eye. Whether the malignant change is to be attributed
to the original or to some further carcinogenic stimulus is not known. Papillomas
may also occur within the ducts of glands, but the papillary growths found frequently in the lactiferous sinus of cows are not truly neoplastic. Their growth is
always limited. While they are infrequent in other parts of the world, Plowright
(1955) has reported a remarkably high incidence of papillomas and papillary
carcinomas of the rumen and esophagus in a more or less inbred strain of indigenous Zebu cattle in a remote African valley.

Polyps (*polypus*; plural, *polypi*) are inflammatory tumor-like growths which
are rather frequent in the nasal passages (horse, etc.) and in the lower bowel.
They may reach a size that more than fills the nostril but are not neoplasms.
Histologically, they consist of loosely arranged fibrous or myxomatous tissue
covered by epithelium and liberally infiltrated with leukocytes of various kinds

Adenomas are benign epithelial neoplasms which form glands. Lying in a
small or large amount of fibrous stroma, the glands may be large or small, tubular
or somewhat spherical. Their epithelium, in reality, extends to form an unseen
connection with that from which it originated. The lining epithelium is typically
simple cuboidal or simple columnar. Any tendency for the epithelial cells to
"pile up" in more than one layer or to invade the underlying stroma is a strong
suggestion of malignancy (adenocarcinoma). The lining may be smoothly
circular in contour or may form rounded bulges or long papillary projections into
the lumen. When these latter are extensive with a tendency to branch and subdivide, malignancy should be suspected. The glandular acini may or may not
contain secretion, manifested by a pink-staining precipitate.

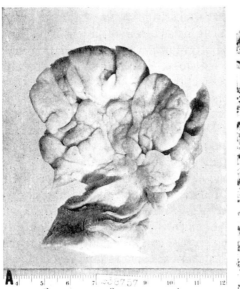 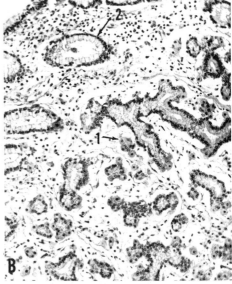

Fig. 7–14.—Adenomatous polyp or adenoma in the gallbladder of a seven-year-old cow. *A*, The
gross specimen, attached by its sessile stalk (bottom of photograph) in the neck of a gallbladder.
B, Photomicrograph ($\times$ 160) of a tumor. Note "parietal" (*1*) and "chief" (*2*) cells resembling
those of the gastric mucosa. These cells are normally present in the neck of the bovine gallbladder.
(Courtesy of Armed Forces Institute of Pathology.) Contributor: Dr. C. L. Davis.

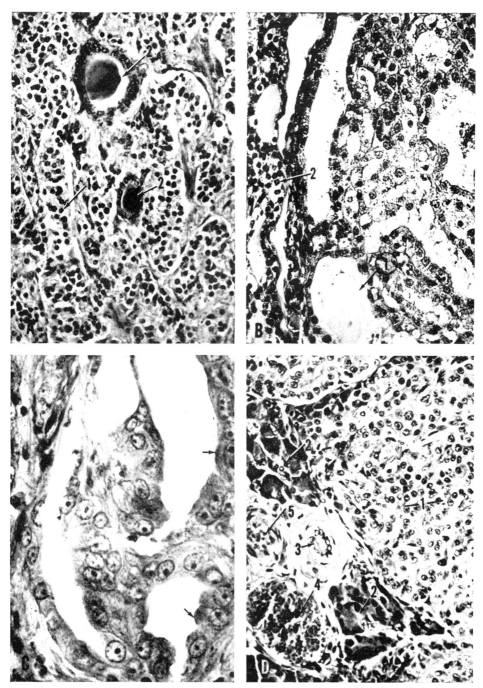

FIG. 7–15.—Adenocarcinoma of the thyroid of an eight-year-old cow. Solid nests of cells (*1*) and acini containing colloid (*2*) are present. Contributor: Dr. C. L. Davis. *B*, Adenoma of the thyroid of a ten-year-old male cat. The tumor ($\times$ 335) is forming large acini (*1*) and compresses the adjacent normal thyroid tissue (*2*). Contributor: Dr. Leo L. Lieberman. *C*, Adenoma of ceruminous gland ($\times$ 545), ear of an eight-year-old mongrel dog. Tumor contains large columnar cells with granular cytoplasm (arrows). Contributor: Dr. S. W. Stiles. *D*, Adenoma of islet cells, pancreas of a ten-year-old female Persian cat ($\times$ 575). Tumor (*1*) is compressing normal pancreatic acini (*2*). Pancreatic duct (*3*), vein (*4*) and artery (*5*). (Courtesy of Armed Forces Institute of Pathology.) Contributor: Dr. M. A. Troy.

In some adenomas, the acini become very large, in addition to being filled with fluid. These are called **cystadenomas.** If there are papillary projections jutting into the glandular lumens the term **papilliferous cystadenoma** is applied. In one kind of tumor, seen especially in the mammary gland, both the glandular epithelium and the extensive fibrous stroma appear to share equally in the neoplastic proliferation. These are called **fibroadenomas.** They differ from the mixed mammary tumors (p. 244) in that their connective-tissue elements are much less anaplastic.

Grossly, adenomas commonly lie wholly or partly in the gland from which they arose. There is usually a rather sharp demarcation between the adenomatous and the healthy tissue, with perhaps a thin fibrous capsule, and as a rule the two tissues have a visibly different appearance or consistency.

Adenomas may be encountered in any of the glandular organs, at least theoretically. They are relatively frequent in the mammary gland (dog) and thyroid (horse).

Benign tumors of the non-acinar ductless glands are also included with the adenomas. These will be discussed individually, as will adenomas of the various cutaneous glands.

Adenomas, like papillomas, may develop the invasive and metastatic powers characteristic of malignancy, becoming adenocarcinomas.

Adenocarcinomas show the same general pattern as adenomas, consisting of epithelial-lined acini lying in a fibrous stroma. In reality, the epithelial acini of adenomas and adenocarcinomas are extensions from some pre-existing epithelial surface which furnished them genesis. Only occasionally is the section of tissue cut in such a way that this is readily apparent.

Adenocarcinomas differ from adenomas in that the epithelium is less well differentiated, less like the normal. This may be shown by excessive proliferation

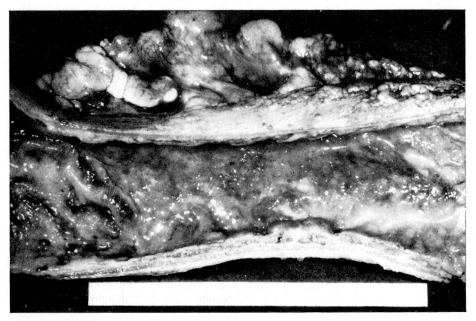

Fig. 7–16.—Adenocarcinoma of the colon of a seven-year-old male German shepherd. Note that the mucosa is eroded and the lumen is partially stenotic due to the invasion of the wall by the tumor. (Courtesy of Angell Memorial Animal Hospital.)

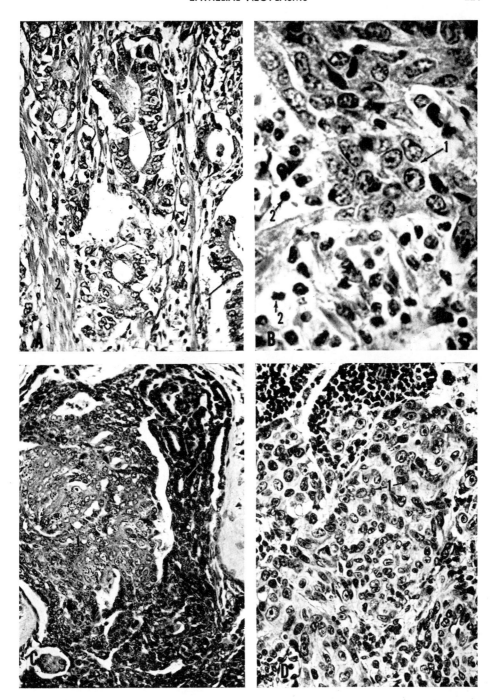

Fig. 7–17.—Differences in the microscopic appearance of adenocarcinomas. *A*, Adenocarcinoma arising in the gastric mucosa and invading the stomach wall in an eight-year-old female Boston terrier. Neoplastic cells (*1*) form irregular acini as they invade the muscularis (*2*). Contributor: Dr. A. E. Rappoport. *B*, Undifferentiated cells (*1*) and lymphocytes (*2*) in an adenocarcinoma (× 750) in the mammary gland of a twenty-five-year-old mare. Contributor: Dr. C. L. Davis. *C*, Squamous cells (*1*), solid nests (*2*) and acini (*3*) in an adenocanthoma of the mammary gland of a six-year-old female English setter. Contributor: Angell Memorial Animal Hospital. *D*, Solid nests of carcinoma cells (*1*) (medullary carcinoma) in a lymph node (*2*) metastasis of a primary adenocarcinoma of bile ducts of a fifteen-year-old beagle. (Courtesy of Armed Forces Institute of Pathology.) Contributor: Dr. D. N. Bader.

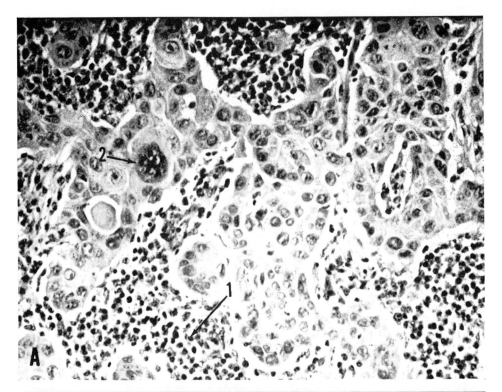

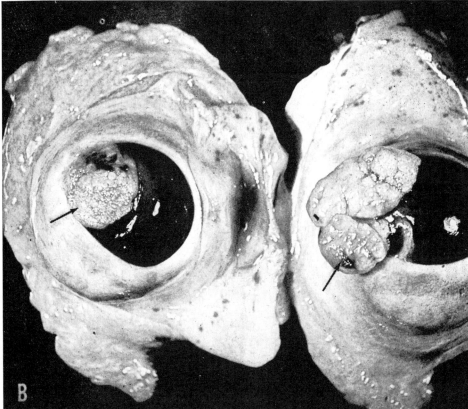

Fig. 7–18.—Squamous cell carcinoma ($\times$ 224) arising in corneal epithelium, eye of an eleven-year-old Hereford cow. The infiltrating tumor cells are surrounded by leukocytes (*1*) and have a bizarre giant nuclei (*2*). (Courtesy of Armed Forces Institute of Pathology.) Contributor: Drs. C. N. Barron and G. T. Easley. *B*, Squamous cell carcinomas in both eyes of a Jersey cow. Note that each is attached at the limbus but extends over the cornea. Photograph courtesy of Dr. C. L. Davis.

of epithelium into the acini, either in several layers or in numerous papillary projections or both. But the essential difference is the power of the epithelium to invade. At some place or other the epithelial cells are seen breaking through their basement membrane, real or assumed, and infiltrating into the connective tissue. It is by this means that pre-existing tissues and organs are destroyed. In the more malignant examples, this invasiveness is carried to the point where the cells fail, in certain areas, to form glands at all, and appear as solid masses of epithelial cells. Malignancy is also shown, as in other neoplasms, by the anaplasia, or lack of differentiation, of the individual cells. They tend to be larger, rounder, and more hyperchromatic, with large, dark-staining nuclei. Nuclei in various stages of mitosis may be seen. As is true of squamous-cell carcinomas, adenocarcinomas are sometimes graded from grade 1 to grade 4 as their degree of malignancy increases.

Cystadenocarcinomas are those in which certain of the acini become large, cyst-like spaces, usually filled with pink-staining proteinaceous secretion. **Papil-**

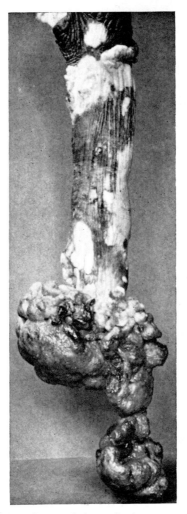

Fig. 7–19.—Squamous cell carcinoma of the penis of a twenty-five-year-old horse. The lower mass was a transplant of the tumor to the prepuce.

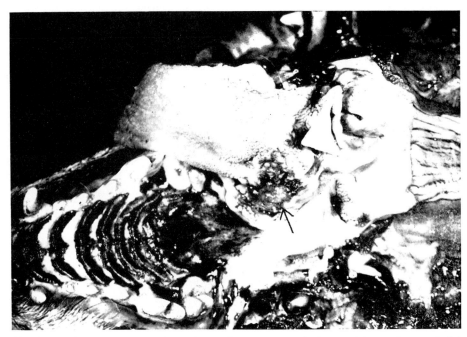

Fig. 7–20.—Squamous-cell carcinoma in tonsilar crypt (arrow) of a spaniel-type dog, aged eight years, spayed female. Note that lesion is eroded and depressed. The left retropharyngeal lymph node was infiltrated by the tumor. (Courtesy of Angell Memorial Animal Hospital.)

liferous **adenocarcinomas** or papilliferous cystadenocarcinomas are those which have extensive papillary projections into the lumens.

Squamous Cell Carcinoma.—This, the commonest form of carcinoma, is characterized by, and derived from stratified squamous epithelium. Its epithelium cornifies or not, in accordance with the epithelium from which it was derived. Pigmentation and papillation (formation of rete pegs), however, are not carried over into the neoplasm. In a reasonably well-differentiated tumor of this type, the usual succession of layers is preserved from the underlying connective-tissue stroma, the dark, basal stratum germinativum, the larger and paler cells of the stratum spinosum, or prickle-cell layer, gradually flattening out to join the stratum corneum, or cornified (keratinized) layer, if this is present. However, this epithelium is by no means restricted to the outer surface of the neoplasm as would be the case in a papilloma. On the contrary, epithelial masses and columns extend promiscuously into and through the neoplastic mass. Cross sections of these masses present themselves as islands of epithelium surrounded by stroma. The basal layer of epithelial cells thus comes to lie at the periphery of such an island, with what would normally be the most superficial epithelium occupying the center of the mass. In the case of a cornifying tumor, the red-staining keratohyalin (p. 46) of the stratum corneum comes to lie at the center of the epithelial mass, becomes quite dense from the pressure of growing cells and forms a rounded, laminated structure known as an **epithelial pearl.**

The term **epidermoid carcinoma** is sometimes used to designate these tumors, inasmuch as they are derived from the epidermis. (Tongue, esophagus, rumen, ocular surfaces and vagina also bear cornifying squamous-cell carcinomas.)

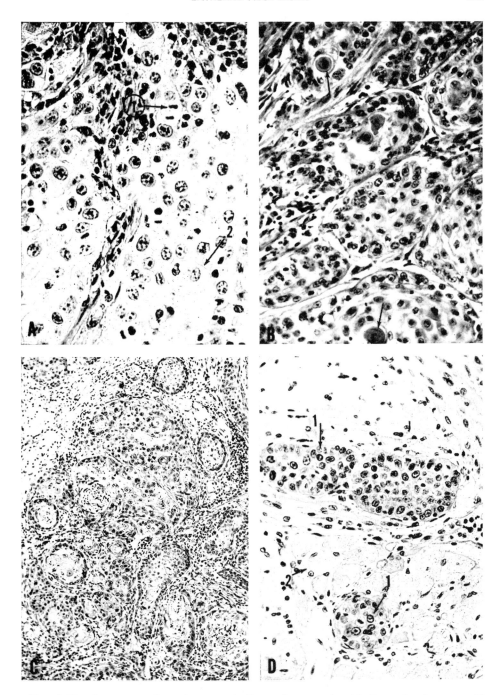

Fig. 7–21.—Squamous-cell carcinoma. *A*, From the corneal epithelium of a four-year-old Hereford cow. Mitotic figures (*1*) are frequent and cell borders (*2*) are prominent (× 335). Contributor: Drs. C. N. Barron and G. T. Easley. *B*, Primary tumor in the vulva of a six-year-old Hereford cow (× 224). Keratinized centers of epithelial "pearls" are indicated by arrows. Contributor: Dr. C. L. Davis. *C*, Primary tumor (× 90) from epithelium of tongue of a thirteen-year-old male cat. Note inflammation surrounding irregular nests of tumor cells. *D*, Extension of tumor (*1*) deep into the musculature (*2*) of the tongue. These are probably tumor emboli in lymphatics (× 235). (Courtesy of Armed Forces Institute of Pathology.) Contributor: Dr. Edward Baker.

The more anaplastic squamous-cell carcinomas lack differentiation into layers and the epithelial masses consist of cells which are all more nearly uniform, with dark, hyperplastic nuclei, sometimes in the process of mitosis. Occasionally, the epithelial cells of a highly anaplastic carcinoma, squamous-cell or adenocarcinoma, may assume a fusiform or spindle shape, so that it becomes very difficult even to make the primary determination whether the tumor is a carcinoma or sarcoma. Of some assistance is the fact that the cells of a sarcoma, being relatives of endothelium, can and usually do form the walls of the blood vessels in the tumor. Epithelial cells cannot do this but must be provided with at least enough interstitial tissue to form an endothelium for the blood vessels. These endothelial cells almost always have a different appearance from the neoplastic cells. Also, among the cells of an anaplastic sarcoma, there almost always run minute fibrils of stroma; carcinoma cells are merely in juxtaposition. Of course, carcinoma cells must always rest upon a fibrous stroma somewhere, and in all but the most anaplastic the difference between the tumor cells and their stroma is readily perceived.

Squamous-cell carcinomas arise from the skin and from the stratified squamous epithelium of all body openings and are rather frequent in all domestic species. These, like other carcinomas, are especially liable to metastasize to the regional lymph nodes, thence to visceral organs.

Keratoacanthoma.—In recent years an increasingly frequent lesion in the human skin has been recognized under various names including "non-metastasizing squamous-cell carcinoma" and "keratoacanthoma," the latter being most favored. What appears to be a corresponding entity in the dog has gone unreported or has been considered to be a neoplastic cyst or tumor of follicular, adnexal or basal-cell origin. The numerous lesions studied by one of us (Jones) have all been reasonably small, confined to the dermis and initiated by downward growth of epidermis consequent to proliferation of all epidermal layers. In spite of the fact that later appearances may suggest altered hair follicles or adnexa, it can be seen in all early cases that the process starts *between* hair follicles. The thickened,

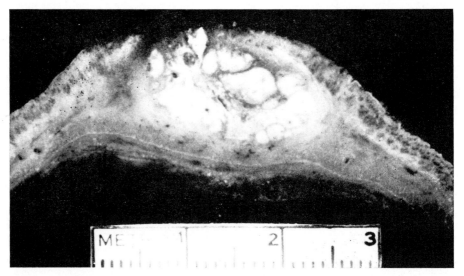

Fig. 7–22.—Keratoacanthoma, skin of a four-year-old male German shepherd. Note ulceration of the epidermis and the multilobulated masses in the dermis and subcutis. (Courtesy of Angell Memorial Animal Hospital.)

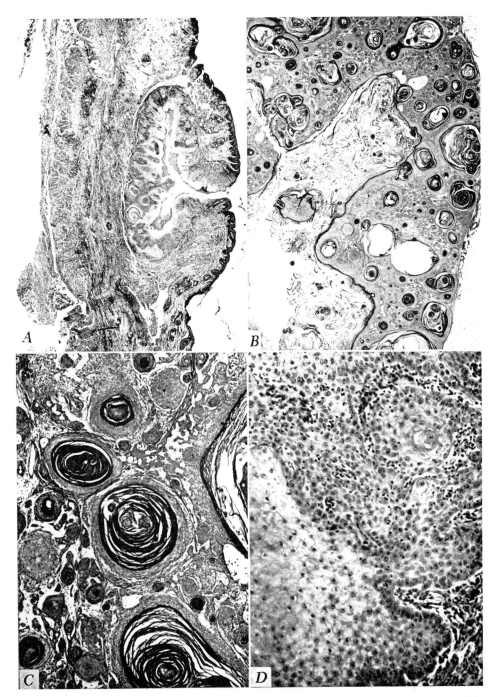

Fig. 7–23.—Keratoacanthoma (canine). *A*, Early lesion (× 9) arising from epidermis which is thickened and forced downward into the dermis. *B*, A more fully developed lesion (× 9) with multiple keratin nests and a cystic center. *C*, Another lesion with many epithelial nests filled with keratin and cords of cells between them (× 50). *D*, Solid zones of epithelium in the early development of the lesion. H & E (× 150). (Courtesy of Angell Memorial Animal Hospital.)

downward-growing epidermis forms a crypt which eventually becomes a multi-loculated cyst crowded with persistent keratin. Continued folding of this epi-thelium produces few or many concentrically laminated masses of keratin sur-rounded by a uniform layer of squamous epithelium whose cells maintain their usual polarity and orderly arrangement. As the epithelial mass continues to ex-pand the central collections of keratin may become very conspicuous. In most, but not all cases, columns of cuboidal cells grow out from the basal surface of the epithelium into the dermal stroma and in some instances join one another to form interlacing cords or columns (Fig. 7–23). This feature sometimes suggests an abortive attempt to form sweat glands but such an interpretation is by no means established. Inflammation may become a prominent feature in the surrounding dermis, especially if any keratin or other detritus escapes through a rupture in the epidermis.

All available evidence indicates that the keratoacanthoma in the dog, as in man, is a self-limiting disease, although multiple tumors and recurrent lesions are common.

Basal-cell Tumor.—The adjective, "basal-cell," is applied to this clinically homogeneous group of epithelial neoplasms in the belief that they arise from the basal, or germinal layer (stratum germinativum) of the epidermis. The classical name for these tumors is **"basal cell carcinoma"** but their proclivity to remain

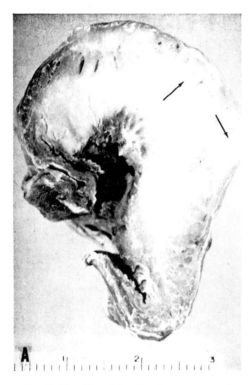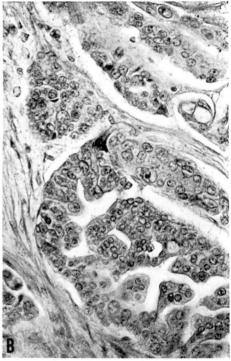

Fig. 7–24.—Transitional and squamous-cell carcinoma of the epithelium of the urinary bladder of an eleven-year-old male collie-shepherd dog. *A*, The tumor invades and replaces the mucosa as well as the muscular coat and elevates the serosa (arrows). *B*, Photomicrograph (× 305) of a part of the neoplasm in which transitional epithelium is simulated. In other areas squamous cells predominate. (Courtesy of Armed Forces Institute of Pathology.) Contributor: Dr. Leo L. Lieberman.

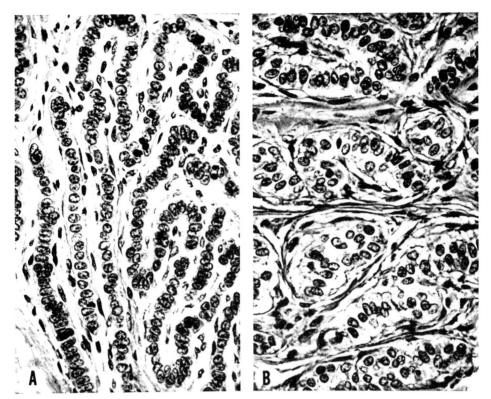

FIG. 7–25.—Basal-cell tumor, skin of nose of a four-year-old male, mongrel dog. *A*, Characteristic long, tortuous cord of cells with elongated nuclei perpendicular to length of cord (× 400). *B*, Another area in same tumor (× 400) with tumor cells forming nests. (Courtesy of Armed Forces Institute of Pathology.) Contributor: Dr W. H. Cowan.

localized seems to make it inconsistent to call them carcinomas. Other terms used to indicate the character of this tumor include: **"basal cell epithelioma"** and **"basiloma."** While some pathologists make certain distinctions and subdivisions, it may be said in general that the basal layer in question may be that of the epidermis proper, of the hair follicles, of the sebaceous glands or of the sweat glands (which have only one epithelial layer).

Clinically, basal-cell tumors in man are locally and persistently invasive but rarely metastasize. They are also highly sensitive to roentgen rays. Sufficient numbers have scarcely received careful study to justify conclusions on all phases of their clinical behavior in animals, but indications are that this is about the same in animals as in man. In the dog, as in man, various regions about the face are favorite sites of localization. Grossly, the tumors are likely to remain small but, with the exception of the trichoepithelioma (p. 230), tend to ulcerate early.

The arrangement of the tumor cells varies in different cases, but the cells themselves are rather constantly of small or medium size, ovoid and closely packed. The nuclei are small, round and darkly stained, like those of the normal stratum germinativum. The cytoplasm is scanty and pale. Projecting spines, prickles, or intercellular bridges, as they are variously designated, are absent, which again relates the neoplasm to the germinal rather than the more superficial layers of epidermis. Mitoses are usually scarce.

In most basal-cell tumors, the cells form solid masses, rounded and sharply contoured, which lie just beneath the epidermis but separated from it by a zone of dermal connective tissue. Occasionally, a place may be found where the two epithelia join; such a spot is considered one of the points of origin of the neoplastic process. Like the basal layer in normal skin, the outermost layer of cells of the mass is often unusually dark (hyperchromatic) with its individual cells elongated in a direction perpendicular to the base line. These tumors are differentiated from squamous-cell carcinomas by the lack of any gradation or transition from basal cells to larger and paler "prickle cells," and by the absence of any semblance of the cornification which characterizes cutaneous and some other squamous-cell carcinomas. (Very exceptionally intermediate types are reported with limited formation of cornified foci and with a clinical behavior which is also intermediate between that of the basal-cell and the more malignant squamous-cell carcinomas.) These tumors may, on occasion, contain melanin.

Some basal-cell tumors form small or large cystic spaces. These often resemble glands and possibly should be so considered, although the cells lining the glands are usually not different in appearance from their neighbors at some distance from the gland-like space. This situation has led to the belief that such tumors arise in sweat glands, justifying a separate classification of sweat-gland carcinoma or adenoma, or such special terms as syringocarcinoma, syringadenoma, and others. Some authorities also ascribe a sweat-gland origin to a type in which the basal cells insinuate themselves into the stroma in long, twisting lines composed of just one or two rows of transversely elongated cells, thus resembling the single layer of cells which lines a normal sudoriferous gland. However, this type and the first-described solid type both occur in the same tumor.

Some pay considerable attention to the epithelium of the hair follicles as a site of origin for tumors of the general group. Most pathologists agree that basal-cell carcinomas can probably arise from the basal layer of hair follicles as well as from basal cells elsewhere. One type of benign subepidermal growth thought to arise from the hair follicle as a whole, or rather from cells sufficiently well differentiated to simulate parts of such structures, is recognized under such names as **trichoepithelioma**. The growth consists of a stroma in which lie numerous gland-like structures resembling hair follicles, but often with a lumen that is cystic or with an epithelial wall of excessive thickness or thinness, and, of course, without any hairs. A rather uniform type consistent with the concept of trichoepithelioma occurs in the dog. It forms areas and islands with typical basal cells peripherally but with a precipitous change to larger, vacuolated and indistinctly staining cells which fill the central areas. The tendency of these tumors to form a structure which histologically resemble parts of the hair follicle is the critical point used to classify them.

A special kind of tumor related to basal cells is the **hair matrix tumor** or **benign calcifying epithelioma** (of Malherbe) which occurs in the skin of man and the dog. This neoplasm is made up of lobules of epithelial tissue (Fig. 7–26), the outer rim of which contain groups of cells which resemble the hair matrix. The interior of these lobules is usually made up of masses of cells resembling those at the periphery but which are necrotic, as evidenced by their failure to take the usual hematoxylin stain. The outlines of the cells may be seen, however, causing some to call them "ghost cells"—an apt description. Calcification often starts in the center of the tumor lobules and may involve much of the necrotic tumor.

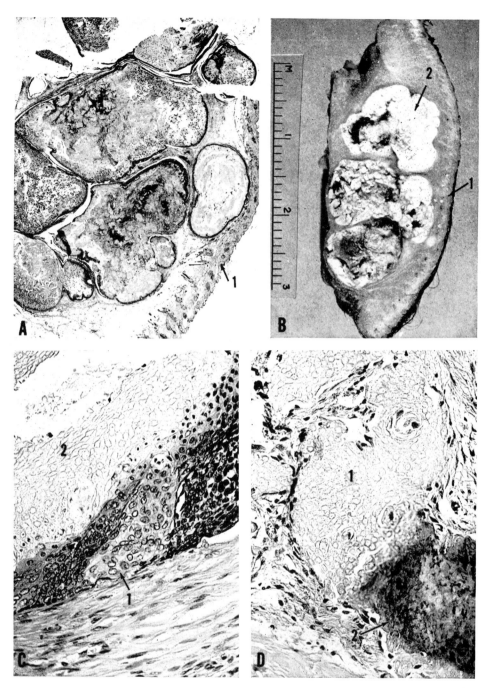

Fig. 7–26.—Benign calcifying epithelioma (hair matrix tumor). *A*, Tumor (× 4) in dermis and subcutis of right prescapular region of a three-year-old female French poodle. Note the lobulated nature of the new growth. Epidermis (*1*). *B*, Gross appearance of the same tumor. Epidermis (*1*) chalky, granular and lobulated tumor (*2*). Contributor: Dr. M. G. Rhoades. *C*, A similar tumor from the dermis of a two-year-old Kerry blue terrier (× 250). Epithelial cells (*1*) simulating hair matrix, and cells (*2*) in center of lesion which stain poorly but maintain their outline ("shadow" or "ghost" cells). *D*, Another area of same tumor as C (× 200). Outlines of cells (*1*) in center of lesion; calcification is present (*2*). (Courtesy of Armed Forces Institute of Pathology.) Contributor: Dr. G. A. Goode.

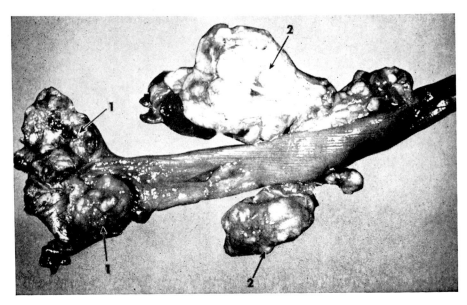

A

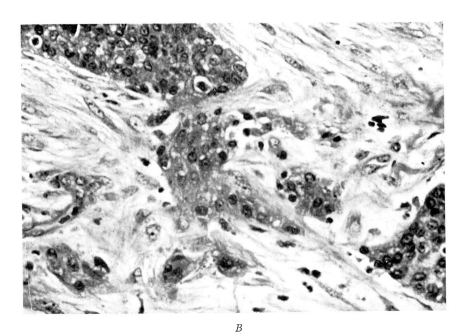

B

FIG. 7–27.—Adenocarcinoma of perianal gland of a ten-year-old spayed female cocker. *A*, Two tumor masses (*1*) near anus and metastatic tumors in iliac lymph nodes (*2*) adherent to the rectum. (Courtesy of Angell Memorial Animal Hospital.)

B, Microscopic appearance of malignant cells of adenocarcinoma of perianal gland. Note irregular bizarre shape of the cells and their isolation into small groups in the cellular stroma.

These tumors are benign but may be multiple, may ulcerate the overlying skin and if their necrotic contents escape into the dermis, incite much inflammatory reaction.

The confusion which exists in the classification and nomenclature of the basal-cell group is illustrated by the fact that for one form which constitutes a rather definite entity in human medicine the following synonyms exist: turban tumor, cylindroma, multiple sarcoma, nevoepithelioma adenoides, sweat-gland carcinoma epithelioma adenoides cysticum, syringoma, syringocystadenoma, plexiform sarcoma, angiosarcoma, endothelioma capitis and tomato tumors (Cooper, 1946). Various authors attribute the origin of this tumor to sweat glands, sebaceous glands and basal cells. It is probable that all are correct, depending on the variety encountered in the individual case.

Adenomas and Adenocarcinomas of Sebaceous Glands.—A rather common benign tumor closely simulating the normal sebaceous glands histologically is readily recognized in dogs. Often there is little but its size to distinguish it from the normal glands and the question of a mere hyperplasia arises. The adenomas tend to be sharply localized in the dermis but not encapsulated. Hyperplasia is more apt to be a diffuse process with many enlarged, hypercellular sebaceous glands over a larger part of the dermis.

Adenocarcinomas, which occur in the dog, are much more anaplastic, with many undifferentiated cells and few cells with vacuolated cytoplasm resembling sebaceous cells. They often extend haphazardly into the dermis, are not sharply circumscribed or encapsulated and may metastasize.

Adenomas and Adenocarcinomas of the Ceruminous Glands.—These tumors of the external ear are occasionally encountered in the dog and cat. They are usually benign, nodular growths, 1 or 2 cm. in diameter, which bulge into the auditory canal, but may become locally invasive or metastasize to the regional lymph nodes. Microscopically, they consist of rather ordinary glandular acini with lumens of generous size and linings of simple columnar or cuboidal epithelium (Black, 1949). This tumor is distinguished by a golden brown, crystalline pigment in the cytoplasm of the epithelial cells.

Adenomas and Adenocarcinomas of Perianal Glands.—The perianal or circum-anal glands in the dogs are paired, modified sebaceous glands located in the sub-cutis on each side of the anus. Their excretion is discharged into two epithelial-lined sacs, lateral to the anus, which communicate with the anus through a small opening near the mucocutaneous junction. The glands are made up of irregular columns of large, closely packed polyhedral cells with eosinophilic cytoplasm rich in finely particulate lipid. The cells extrude their holocrine secretion through ducts lined by modified perianal gland cells, emptying into perianal sacs.

Benign tumors (adenomas) are quite common, particularly in male dogs and are usually sharply circumscribed, thinly encapsulated, spherical masses of varying size. Their cut surface is usually orange-tinted and greasy in texture, sometimes altered by dark hemorrhage or ulceration of the overlying skin. Histologically the adenoma closely resembles the normal gland except that the glands are usually larger and more closely packed; the epithelial cells hyperplastic and hypertrophic and ducts irregular in numbers and location. Ulceration and hemorrhages due to external trauma are frequent. The modified sebaceous cells cling together and usually have an orderly relationship to their scant stroma (Fig. 7–28).

Adenocarcinomas are much less frequent but surprisingly, are apt to arise in

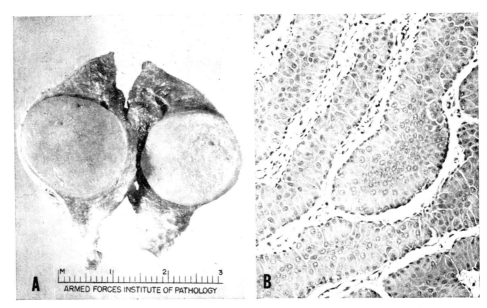

FIG. 7–28.—Adenoma of perianal gland of a six-year-old male beagle. *A*, Gross specimen with its spherical outline and orange-tinted, greasy cut surface. *B*, Photomicrograph ($\times$ 150) of the new growth. Irregular columns of large polyhedral cells supported by delicate stroma. (Courtesy of Armed Forces Institute of Pathology.) Contributor: Major C. N. Barron.

aged spayed females in which the benign form is quite rare. This malignant form may metastasize to the iliac lymph nodes (Fig. 7–27) and thence to sublumbar and other intraabdominal lymph nodes and eventually reach the general circulation. The identifying feature of this malignant variety is the isolation of individual tumor cells and small irregular groups of these cells in the stroma which is apparently invaded. This is the only reliable histologic criterion for malignancy in this tumor. To the uninitiated who has not studied and followed the biologic behavior of the neoplasm, many adenomas may appear to be malignant from their histologic appearance.

The Mast-cell Tumor of the Dog's Skin.—The mast-cell has been considered synonymous with the basophilic granulocyte of the blood. However, the mast-cells seen in canine pathology, with their rounded, primitive-appearing nuclei, have little save the basophilic granules in the cytoplasm to tie them to the basophils of the blood, which are never numerous in the dog. Similar cells occur here and there among the varied mesodermal types found in the cutaneous tissues, omentum and mesentery.

The term "mastocytoma" often appears in the literature in reference to tumors made up largely of tissue mast cells. The word "mast" in this context comes from the German, meaning fattened or stuffed and the "cyte" comes from the Greek, *kytos*—a hollow cell. The combining form "mast" from the Greek *mastos* (breast) has quite a different meaning. In deference to the sensitivities of our classical, scholarly, colleagues, we chose not to use this incorrect combination of two languages.

A neoplasm arises with some frequency in the cutis of the dog and rarely of the cat, and still less frequently in the skin and omentum of bovines which is considered to be derived from these mast cells. Its cells are of the large round type,

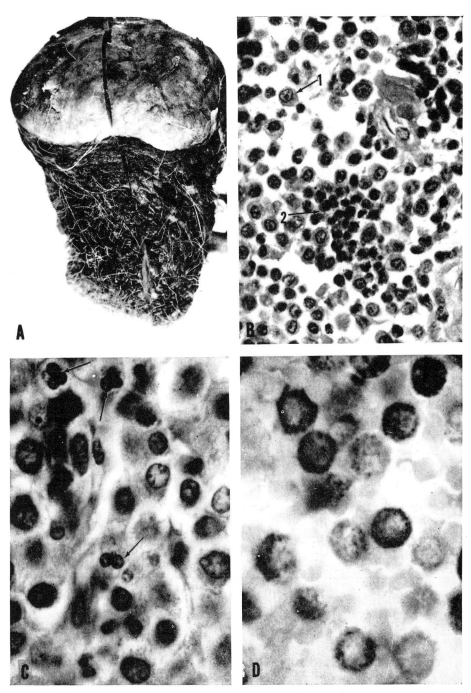

FIG. 7–29.—Mast-cell tumor. *A*, Ulcerated tumor involving the skin of the scrotum of a thirteen-year-old male spitz dog. Contributor: Dr. S. W. Stiles. *B*, Photomicrograph (× 545) of a mast-cell tumor from the cheek of a ten-year-old male cocker spaniel. Hematoxylin and eosin stain. Mast cells (*1*) and nests of eosinophils (*2*) are present. Contributor: Dr. W. H. Riser. *C*, Higher magnification (× 650) of a mast-cell tumor from the skin of the leg of a twelve-year-old male Boston terrier. H & E stain. A few mast cells contain cytoplasmic granules. Eosinophils (arrows) are common. Contributor: Army Veterinary School. *D*, Section with Giemsa stain (× 1200) to demonstrate metachromatic granules in the cytoplasm of the neoplastic mast cells. (Courtesy of Armed Forces Institute of Pathology.) Contributor: **Dr. C. L. Davis.**

rather loosely put together, forming shapeless masses beneath the bulging epidermis. They infiltrate among the coarse collagen fibers of the region, the fibers often persisting for some time, so that a marginal area of the tumor might be mistaken for an inflammatory infiltration. From the standpoint of diagnosis, the cells of the mast-cell tumor differ from those of a malignant lymphoma in that the nuclei of the former are more dense and dark-staining with less tendency to show individual chromatin granules. The mast cells have more cytoplasm than is the case with, at least, the lymphocytic type of malignant lymphoma. The mast-cell tumor, for unknown reasons, usually contains a few scattered collections of cells resembling neutrophilic and eosinophilic granulocytes. Its individually discrete cells are less uniform in size and shape, while the nuclei are more deeply staining than those of the transmissible veneral tumor, with which it may be confused. It also lacks the rather frequent mitotic figures (nuclei in various stages of mitosis) which are seen in the transmissible tumor. The proof of the diagnosis of mast-cell tumor lies in the demonstration of the dark cytoplasmic granules. In some examples of the tumor, these are so numerous that the nucleus is obscured in a black smudge around it. More frequently, the granules are hard to find. They are much more evident by the Giemsa or a similar metachromatic stain than when hematoxylin and eosin are used, and it is commonly necessary to resort to such a procedure for diagnosis.

The mast-cell tumor is most likely to be located on the posterior part of the animal's body. It produces a bulging cutaneous tumor commonly reaching a diameter of 2 to 5 cm. and a height of 1 to 3 cm. Ulceration is common.

Metastases are rare but the tumor has definite local malignancy, so that wide excision is imperative. This neoplasm has only a rare counterpart in the human species, although urticaria pigmentosa presents somewhat similar aggregations of mast cells.

In the cat neoplastic mast cells sometimes proliferate in the spleen, nearly replacing most of its normal structure. The spleen is usually very much enlarged with a characteristic deep mahogany color and fleshy consistency. Mast cells are usually found in small numbers in the peripheral circulation in such cases. These circulating cells are morphologically identical to tissue mast cells rather than basophils. An interesting concomitant feature is the presence of small, sharply demarcated ulcers in the mucosa of the pylorus or duodenum. These ulcers are probably the result of excess histamine (or possibly serotonin) produced by the mast cells.

The Canine Transmissible Venereal Tumor. — Known by a variety of names, such as Sticker tumor, venereal granuloma, transmissible sarcoma, and transmissible lymphosarcoma, this tumor occupies a unique place among neoplastic conditions in that it is rather readily transmitted through transplantation of cells by contact, is likely eventually to disappear spontaneously and, having disappeared following either natural or experimental occurrence, leaves the patient in a state of appreciable immunity. Nevertheless it appears to fulfill the criteria of malignancy in its histological appearance and in the fact that metastases are not rare.

Historically, this neoplasm is of interest as the first frank neoplasm to be transmitted experimentally from one animal to another. A Russian veterinarian, M. A. Novinsky, is credited with accomplishing this feat (p. 525) (Stewart, et al., 1957).

Like the mast-cell tumor, the transmissible tumor consists of large round cells (polyhedral when subjected to pressure) which bear some resemblance to lymph-oid cells. Both in total volume and in size of nucleus these cells are larger than lymphocytes, being more comparable to the maternal lymphoblasts of lymph nodes. However, their nuclei, rounded or slightly indented, stain more strongly than those of lymphoblasts, both in their chromatin granules and in their nuclear membranes. In spite of these general statements, a characteristic of some value in diagnosis is a rather pronounced variation in size of individual cells and nuclei. Mitotic figures are numerous, quite out of proportion to what one would expect from the comparatively low infiltrative and metastatic powers of the tumor.

Diagnosis is made by these characteristics after eliminating the mast-cell tumor, and by location of the (primary) tumor in close relation to the genital mucous membranes. Without a knowledge of the location, the transmissible tumor could be confused with a number of others, including the aortic-body tumor and the seminoma.

Clinically, the majority of these tumors are found on or in close proximity to the external genitalia, being transmitted by coition. They also occur, however, on the face, shoulders and in other locations. The same dog may have a growth in two widely separated parts of the body. Commonly sessile, ulcerated and a few centimeters in diameter, they may attain formidable size, for instance distending and protruding from the vagina. While metastasis has been frequent enough to convince numerous experimenters of the neoplastic malignancy of this type of

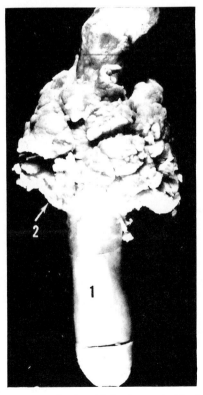

FIG. 7–30.—Canine venereal tumor. Lesion (2) in the penis (1) of a dog. (Courtesy of Armed Forces Institute of Pathology.)

growth, that is not the usual clinical experience. Unmolested, it attains its very considerable size in the course of several months, then remains stationary or ultimately shrinks and disappears. Probably because of its behavior as a transmissible disease, this tumor is much more common in some parts of the country than in others, and in some places where formerly frequent it is now seldom seen. On the whole, it is the paradox among neoplasms.

It has been shown by Machino, 1963, and confirmed by Weber *et al.*, 1964, that the cells of the transmissible venereal tumor have chromosome configurations quite different from that of normal canine cells. (See Chapter 9.) Normal cells of the dog at metaphase contain 76 autosomal chromosomes, all of them acrocentric. The sex pair are metacentric; the X is the largest of the complement and the Y near the smallest in size. The cells of the venereal tumor, on the other hand, contain only 59 chromosomes, 17 of them metacentric and 42 acrocentric. M. Reiter, in our laboratory (T.C.J.), has demonstrated that cells of the "canine cutaneous histiocytoma" contain morphologically normal canine chromsosomes in normal numbers.

Canine Cutaneous Histiocytoma.—This lesion of the dermis of the dog has been known for many years as one of the commonest "tumors" of the skin of that species. It has borne a number of names over the years, each indicating lack of solid knowledge about the exact nature of the lesion. Such names as "round cell tumor," benign lymphoma, "extragenital venereal tumor" and "histiocytoma" have been applied, the last of the list by Mulligan who believed it was identical to the venereal tumor described previously. This lesion bears no resemblance to

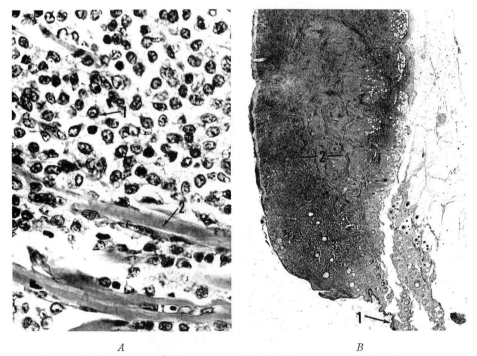

A   *B*

Fig. 7–31.—Canine cutaneous histiocytoma. *A*, Cells of the new growth (*1*) infiltrating collagen bundles (*2*) of the dermis (× 440). *B*, Low power of the cutaneous nodule (× 8). The epidermis (*1*) is elevated by the mass (*2*) which also infiltrates the subcutis. (Courtesy of Armed Forces Institute of Pathology.) Contributor: Dr. Elihu Bond.

the human lesion which is usually called histiocytoma and some evidence indicates it may not be a neoplasm at all. Nevertheless, for want of a better label, we shall use this appellation, "canine cutaneous histiocytoma" to label a specific entity. We now feel that it is not identical to the canine venereal tumor (p. 236).

This lesion occurs for the most part in young dogs. It appears within a week or two as an elevated mass, movable in the dermis, 1 to 3 cm. in diameter. It apparently irritates the canine patient, who licks and rubs it until it may become ulcerated. Simple excision usually results in complete cure although no interference at all also usually is followed by disappearance of the lesion. Apparently, no recurrence or further lesions appear once the initial lesion is healed. Transmission attempts have uniformly failed. This cutaneous lesion apparently still occurs in regions in the United States where the canine venereal tumor has not been encountered for many years.

The canine cutaneous histiocytoma is seen with the light microscope to be made up of rather large, individually discrete cells which are closely packed in the dermis, separating fibers of dermal collagen and elevating the epidermis. These cells may extend into the subcutis, infiltrating fat and connective tissue (Fig. 7–31). The typical cells have round or ovoid, finely stippled to vesicular nuclei and distinct, non-granular cytoplasm. They are not phagocytic. Mitoses may be found and the cells appear to be actively invasive. The benign course of the lesion is in contrast to its "malignant" histologic appearance.

Subtle differences in cell morphology and the normal karyotype of these cells, differentiate the lesion from the venereal tumor. Epizootiologic data and failure of transmission are also different. It is quite possible that this lesion is not a "neoplasm" at all but more data will be required to settle this point. It is a common lesion which the veterinary pathologist or clinician must be able to recognize.

The Adamantinoma.—Also known as **ameloblastoma** and **enameloblastoma,** this tumor arises from the enamel-organ, the embryological predecessor of a tooth. The name adamantinoma is based upon the exceeding hardness of the dental enamel, hence adamant. However, the tumor remains as a soft tissue, forming no enamel. (Obviously a tissue which had already differentiated into enamel would be as unable to proliferate as is the bone of an osteosarcoma or the cartilage of a chondrosarcoma (p. 197). It will be recalled that in the development of a tooth the gingival epithelium forms an invagination into the underlying connective tissue which later loses its connection with the surface and remains as an epithelial cavity whose superficial wall contains several layers of rather tall, pale epithelium and whose deeper wall consists of a single layer of lower, darker cells. This constitutes the enamel organ. Directly beneath, the connective tissue forms the bulb of the tooth which pushes into the enamel organ, distorting it into a horseshoe shape whose convex side is gradually pushed to the surface as the tooth erupts.

The adamantinoma forms epithelial masses which tend, in a bizarre fashion, to retain this horseshoe shape, a very useful diagnostic feature if present. Internally the epithelial structures vary from a single layer of small dark cells like those of the deeper side of the enamel organ to a many-layered epithelial island of larger, more typically epithelial-appearing cells, in the midst of which pale, angular "star-cells" resembling embryonal connective tissue may or may not be present, representing the original central cavity of the developing enamel organ. It is typical for the nuclei of the outer, or basal layer of epithelium to be at the opposite end of the cell from the connective tissue base. There is, however, much deviation from this more or less ideal structure. The epithelium may have an arrangement characteristic of squamous-cell carcinoma in many areas, of basal-cell carcinoma in others, all in the same tumor. The star-cells corresponding to the central structure of the enamel organ are often replaced by small or large cysts. The connective tissue may exceed the epithelium in amount.

The neoplastic mass, consisting of these epithelial structures permeating fibrous connective tissue, grows from a dental primordium in either, usually the lower, jaw to form a locally destructive tumor of considerable size. While locally malignant, metastasis seldom occurs. Adamantinomas are among the rarer tumors in man; among animals they have been reported rarely in several species. While some authorities describe several subvarieties, the adamantinomas with the fibrous epulides (p. 1192) and the odontomas, which are tooth-like structures derived from dental residues, essentially comprise the special tumors of the jaw.

The **craniopharyngioma** is a rare tumor occurring in the roof of the nasopharynx, between the latter and the cranial cavity in the region of the sella turcica. It originates from remnants of Rathke's pouch, a fetal tube or stalk of pharyngeal epithelium which extends upward toward the brain to form all but the pars nervosa of the pituitary. This tumor is rather variable in histological structure ranging from that of a squamous-cell carcinoma to a basal-cell type, often with degenerative cysts. The tumor often produces adiposity (Fröhlich's syndrome) and diabetes insipidus through pressure on the hypothalamus. Craniopharyngiomas have been reported in the dog (Saunders and Rickard, 1952; White, 1938).

Mixed salivary-gland tumors, containing what appear to be epithelium, cartilage, myxomatous and endothelial tissue, constitute a well-known entity in

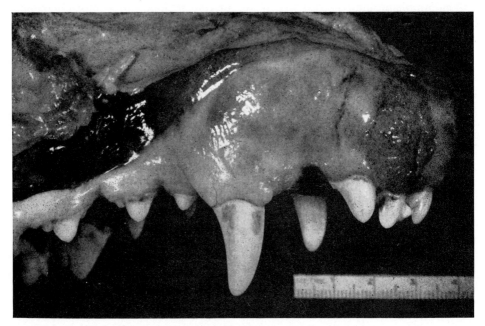

FIG. 7–32.—Adamantinoma of maxilla of a fourteen-month-old standard poodle.
(Courtesy of Angell Memorial Animal Hospital.)

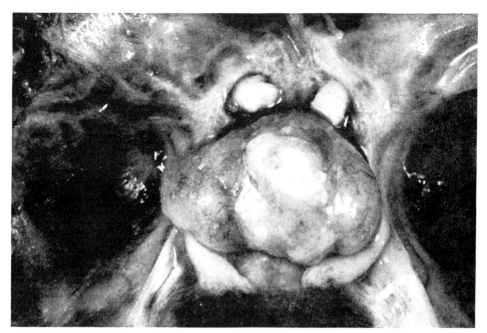

Fig. 7–33.—Craniopharyngioma involving the pituitary of a ten-year-old female boxer. (Courtesy of Angell Memorial Animal Hospital.)

man. In general, they have not been recognized in veterinary patients. However, there is one rather incomplete reference to their occurrence in dogs (Harvey, Dawson and Innes, 1939) and one has recently been seen in a slaughtered cow. (Contributed to the Armed Forces Institute of Pathology by Dr. M. J. Eggert.) It formed a mass of considerable size, not grossly separable from the parotid itself. Microscopically both glandular and supporting tissues were neoplastic but the most conspicuous feature was a startlingly extensive ossification within the connective-tissue elements. A morphological similarity to the canine mixed mammary tumor thus was obvious.

Primary Carcinoma of the Lung.—Carcinoma arising in the lung tends to differentiate toward any of four types: adenocarcinoma, squamous-cell carcinoma, small-round-cell carcinoma and an infrequent spindle-cell form. The squamous-cell type arises from bronchial epithelium which has previously undergone metaplasia to the stratified squamous variety. The other types come from normal histological elements, including, probably, the mucous glands. The types are not inflexibly separate but are useful histopathological entities. True adenomas also occur, which may or may not be antecedent to adenocarcinoma.

The term **bronchogenic carcinoma** is applied to those primary tumors of man which presumably originate from bronchial epithelium. These tumors most often arise near the hilus of the lung and have doubled in frequency during recent years (Goldberg, et al., 1956). This class of pulmonary neoplasms has generally been associated with cigarette smoking, is most frequent in men and makes up 90 per cent of all primary pulmonary neoplasms. Most (about 70 per cent) of bronchogenic carcinomas are squamous cell carcinomas histologically; about 10 per cent are adenocarcinomas and 20 per cent are undifferentiated carcinomas (Robbins, 1967).

The more frequent type of pulmonary neoplasm in animals is the **bronchiolar-alveolar cell carcinoma** (terminal bronchiolar carcinoma, or adenocarcinoma of the lung) which, as in man, appears first in the periphery of the lung and is believed to arise from alveolar or bronchiolar epithelium. These tumors characteristically are made up of tall columnar epithelium (Fig. 7–34) supported by a thin stroma, arranged in a complex papillary structure. Sometimes these tumors appear to grow into and use the alveoli as a lattice for their growth. Some of these tumor cells produce large amounts of mucus.

The so-called adenomatosis of sheep and cattle, which reaches its culminative form in the South African **jaagsiekte** (p. 1113) is an extreme example of hyperplastic inflammation. There are all gradations up to a picture including areas of complicated, gland-like alveoli with folded linings of large cuboidal cells. Less pronounced examples of a similar nature occur in Marsh's **ovine chronic progressive pneumonia** (p. 1112). As a milder manifestation of the same tendency, the cells lining pulmonary alveoli have often been noticed to undergo considerable enlargement, with hyperchromaticity of their nuclei, in many cases of chronic pneumonitis, attracting such attention that they formerly received a special designation, "cells of Tripier," "fetalization" of the cells being synonymous.

Metastatic neoplasms are encountered with much greater frequency, but primary carcinomas are not exactly rare in the lungs of cattle and dogs and are known in the horse (Monlux, 1952).

Hepatoma.—The liver is subject to ordinary adenoma and adenocarcinoma, which arise from the lining of intra- and extra-hepatic bile ducts. A special type of neoplasm is the hepatoma, or **liver cell adenoma or carcinoma.** In histologic structure, it may differ little from the healthy liver tissue which adjoins it. The lobular architecture, however, is disarranged and bizarre; normal portal triads do not occur; and its cells usually show a staining reaction differing in one direction or another from that of the healthy tissue. Fatty change may be pronounced. Grossly the tumorous tissue, often considerable in extent, is likely to show greenish or yellowish discoloration from bile which has been secreted by the neoplastic cells but which cannot escape because of the lack of outlet to normal ductal connections. At the other extreme, some hepatomas consist of highly anaplastic cells with no resemblance to normal liver either in form or arrangement of the cells. Bizarre giant-cell forms occur in some specimens.

This must be considered one of the rarer tumors in animals, in spite of the fact that hepatomas have been recorded in all the common domestic species. Very little can be contributed with respect to causes. In man, a statistical relationship appears to exist between hepatomas and hemochromatosis (p. 73) and cirrhosis (p. 1225), but data are too scanty to afford any information in connection with these conditions in domestic animals. Experimentally, azo dyes and some other substances have been shown to have a specific carcinogenic action on the liver. Since the advent of poisoning by chlorinated naphthalenes (p. 938), an associated "adenomatosis" of bile ducts has been seen, but no true neoplasia has resulted from this type of substance. Fascioliasis (the usual liver fluke being *Fasciola hepatica*) commonly causes hyperplastic proliferation but does not lead to neoplasia. Neither, as far as known, do the other parasites which invade the liver, such as the larvæ of ascarids and of the porcine kidney worm, *Stephanurus dentatus*. The adenomatoid hyperplasia of bile ducts resulting from biliary coccidiosis (*Eimeria stiedæ, Coccidium oviforme*) in the rabbit has not been observed

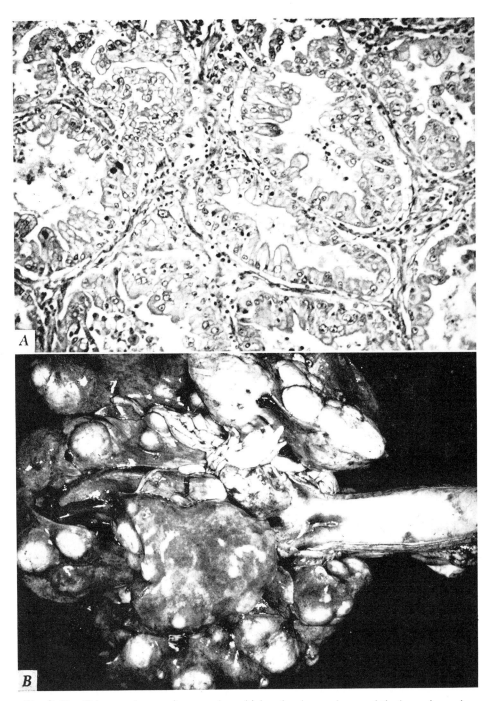

FIG. 7–34.—Primary adenocarcinoma or bronchiolar-alveolar carcinoma of the lung of a cocker-dachshund, male, nine years old. *A*, Section of one of the tumor nodules. H & E ($\times$ 200). *B*, The gross lung. (Courtesy of Angell Memorial Animal Hospital.)

to develop into neoplasia. Aflatoxin (p. 888) has been shown to be associated with hepatomas in experimental animals.

Mucoid, or Signet-ring Carcinoma.—This is a type which deserves mention because, when encountered even in metastatic form, the type of cell points to probable origin somewhere in the gastro-intestinal tract. While in some of these are acini whose cells secrete a mucinous fluid into the lumen, the form which attracts most attention is characterized by cells containing a single large vacuole in the center, the nucleus being pushed to one side. The cell thus has the appearance of a signet ring. The vacuole might well contain fat, judging by its appearance, but appropriate stains show the content to be mucinous. Only a certain portion of the cells show this appearance, others being merely ordinary epithelial cells, often in masses without the formation of acini. Some human mammary adenocarcinomas show this type of cell, the same appears to be true in some canine mammary tumors.

Mammary Tumors.—Of considerable interest in the general study of neoplasia is the fact that in the bovine, where anatomical development and functional activity of the mammary gland are greater by far than in any other species, mammary neoplasms are practically unknown. While they have been reported in equines, the only domestic species in which they are common is the canine. They are, of course, frequent in laboratory mice and are not uncommon in rats.

As would be expected, adenocarcinomas of varying degrees of anaplasia occupy a prominent place among canine mammary neoplasms. Many begin as intraductal tumors; that is, they arise from the epithelium lining the ducts and grow for a time within their lumens. In this location they grow as papillary projections, often of very complicated pattern. As they invade the surrounding parenchyma or metastasize to other organs they commonly continue this architectural pattern by producing acini which are more or less filled with papillary projections, all being covered by a layer of columnar or cuboidal epithelium. A neoplasm of this structure, whether of mammary origin or not, is known as a **papilliferous cyst-adenocarcinoma** which usually exhibit low grade malignancy. Other adenocarcinomas arise by malignant transformation of acinar cells, then grow by proliferation of these cells. Some of these lack the essentials of malignancy; hence, are adenomas. Rarely the above forms occur in the mammary gland of the male; ordinarily they are in females.

Almost as frequent in the dog as the pure adenocarcinoma is the **mixed mammary tumor.** Any epithelial neoplasm has its fibrous stroma, which scarcely differs from the connective tissue upon which any normal epithelium must always rest. But in the mammary mixed tumor both the glandular epithelial elements and the fibrous stroma assume the neoplastic characteristics of anaplasia, hyperchromatism, hypercellularity and the other features of malignancy. Very commonly the fibrous elements may in places undergo metaplasia to cartilage or bone. Any one of these tissues may constitute the major part of the primary tumor or of its metastases. Thus tumors consisting principally of bone are not rare as the culmination of this metaplastic and neoplastic process, a situation all but limited to the canine mammary gland. While ordinarily restricted to females, this tumor has been seen rarely in males.

Whether pure sarcomas occur in the mammary gland or whether the supposed fibro-, chondro-, and osteosarcomas represent mixed tumors whose epithelial elements have been overlooked we are not prepared to say. According to one school

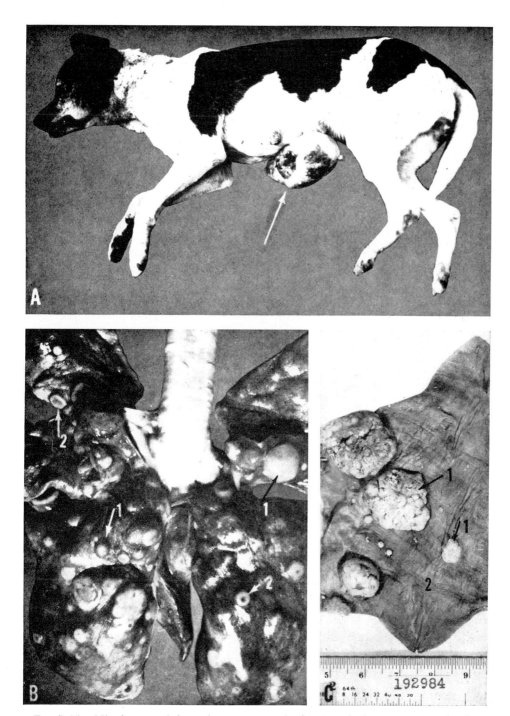

FIG. 7–35.—Mixed tumor of the canine mammary gland. *A*, A single tumor of bony hardness in a five-year-old fox terrier. *B*, Metastatic nodules of a malignant mixed tumor from the mammary gland of a thirteen-year-old female chow. *C*, Metastatic mixed tumor (*1*) on the diaphragm of a thirteen-year-old female dachshund. (Courtesy of Armed Forces Institute of Pathology.) Contributor: Dr. A. M. Berkelhammer.

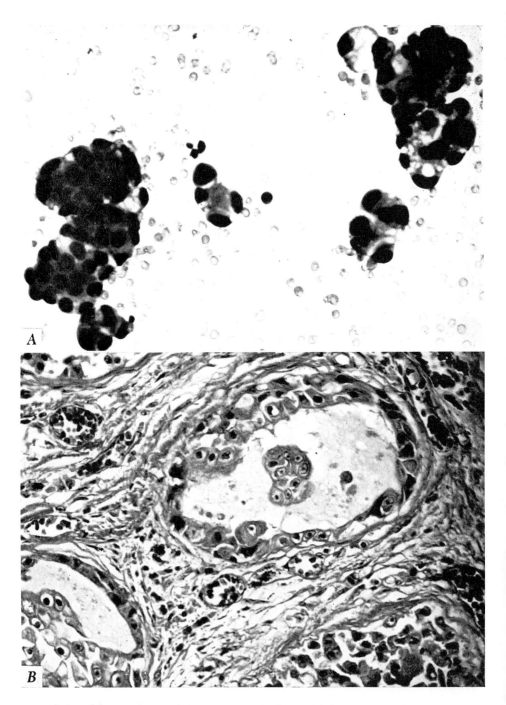

Fig. 7–36.—Adenocarcinoma of the mammary gland of a thirteen-year-old spitz. Metastases had occurred to the lungs, pleura and liver. *A*, Smear of fluid aspirated from the pleural cavity. Wright-Giemsa's stain (× 400). *B*, Section of the primary tumor in the mammary gland. H & E (× 400). (Courtesy of Angell Memorial Animal Hospital.)

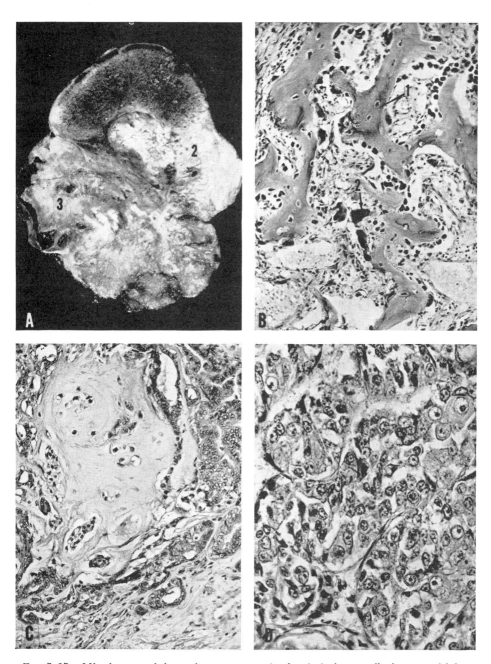

Fig. 7–37.—Mixed tumor of the canine mammary gland. *A*, A circumscribed tumor with bone (*1*) glandular tissue (*2*) and fibrous areas (*3*) recognizable grossly. *B*, Section of the osseous part in *A* (× 130). Spicules of bone (*1*) surrounded by osteoblasts and some osteoclasts (*2*). Contributor: Major Randall J. J. Foley. *C*, Cartilage (× 145) surrounded by epithelial cells in a malignant mixed tumor (see Fig. 7–35C). *D*, Undifferentiated epithelial cells (×350) in the same tumor as *C*. (Courtesy of Armed Forces Institute of Pathology.) Contributor: Dr. A. N. Berkelhammer.

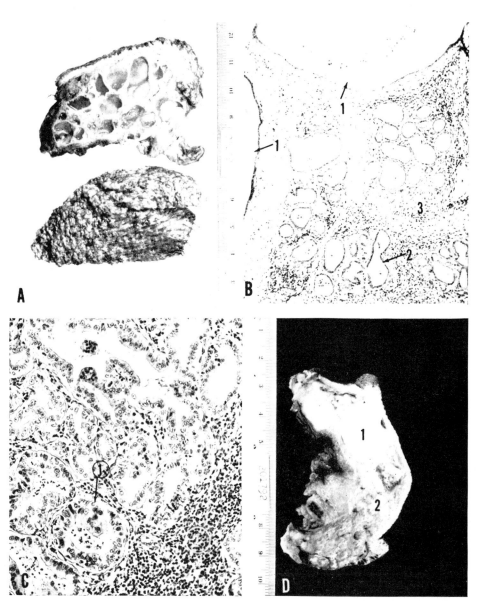

Fig. 7–38.—*A*, Cystic hyperplasia of the mammary gland of a seven-year-old coonhound. *B*, Higher magnification (× 80) of the same lesion. Cystic (*1*) and hyperplastic acini (*2*) and dense stroma (*3*) containing leukocytes. Contributor: Dr. R. F. Vigue. *C*, Adenocarcinoma (× 150) of the mammary gland of a nine-year-old female cocker spaniel. *D*, The gross specimen with solid areas of tumor (*1*) and diffuse neoplastic infiltration (*2*). (Courtesy of Armed Forces Institute of Pathology.) Contributor: Angell Memorial Animal Hospital.

of thought, it is possible for epithelial cells to undergo a "dysembryogenetic" transformation into cartilage or bone. Another derives the connective tissue from the "myoepithelial" cells which invest the acinar epithelium.

Chorion-epithelioma, also known as **chorio-carcinoma** and **syncytioma.**—This neoplasm occurs uncommonly in man and very rarely in animals, only two clearly identifiable cases, one in an armadillo (Marin-Padilla and Benirschke, 1963) and a rhesus monkey (*Macaca mulatta* [Lindsay, *et al.*, 1969]), have been reported. In the human female, it arises in the endometrium from chorionic villi that have remained attached to the maternal tissue following parturition (or abortion) and expulsion of the bulk of the fetal membranes. The bits of chorionic tissue remain alive through absorption of nutrient materials from surrounding fluids and frequently proliferate slowly to form a botryoid, cystic structure known as a **hydatidiform mole.** Chorionic epithelial cells, so retained, with or without the formation of a distinct "mole," occasionally acquire neoplastic properties from unknown causes and grow to form a highly malignant neoplasm. It is characterized histologically by masses or strands of epithelial cells with very lightly staining cytoplasm characteristic of the Langhans layer of the chorionic villi. (This is less well differentiated in the domestic animals.) Mingled indiscriminately with these Langhans cells are syncytial masses of large, darkly staining epithelium corresponding to the outer, syncytial layer of chorionic epithelium. Having the same invasive power as the normal hemochorial placenta (p. 1305), the tumor elements tend to penetrate blood vessels and to lie in the areas of hemorrhage so produced. Like the normal chorionic tissue, these tumors secrete gonadotropic hormones, with a positive Aschheim-Zondek test the same as in pregnancy. Cystic corpora lutea also result. Chorion-epithelioma is occasionally found in the testis as part of a teratoma (p. 270). Whatever the origin, early blood-borne pulmonary metastases are much to be feared.

Nephroblastoma, also known as **Embryonal Nephroma** and **Wilms' Tumor.**— This tumor arises in the kidney or occasionally outside but near it. It is now known to arise from the renal blastema, from which the kidney is formed but which, in early embryonic stages, is not greatly differentiated from the primitive mesenchyme. The latter is pluripotent in its capacity for differentiation into several types of mature tissue, a fact which explains how this embryonal tumor contains more than one kind of tissue. An old name, of little value histogenetically but very suggestive of the usual microscopic picture, is **adenosarcoma.** It consists typically of what appears to be highly cellular fibroblastic tissue with, here and there, an inexplicable, epithelial-lined glandular acinus in its midst. In some examples the glands are scarce and hard to find; at the other extreme are occasional tumors in which many areas consist chiefly of gland-like epithelial structures suggestive of an adeno-carcinoma. In man, it is common for the growth to include smooth muscle, doubtless as a result of aberrant differentiation of certain mesenchymal cells, but this is seldom seen in the nephroblastomas of animals. While still rare, this is one of the relatively frequent tumors of swine; it has been reported in cattle and sheep, as well as in chickens, rabbits and other small mammalian species, becoming evident usually at an early age.

Sullivan and Anderson (1959) studied embryonal nephromas collected from meat-inspection sources, all but two being in swine. Seventy-seven per cent of these occurred in pigs less than one year of age but, since the great majority of pigs encountered in meat inspection are of this age, it may be more significant that one

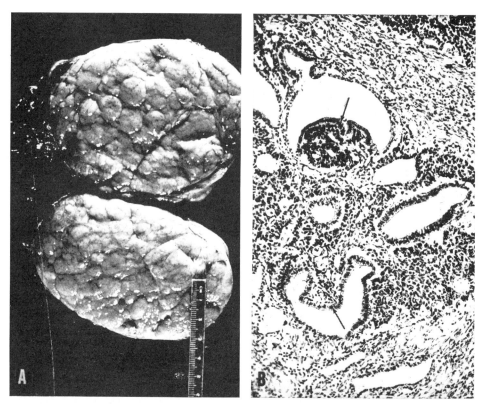

FIG. 7–39.—Embryonal nephroma, kidney of a six-month-old male fox terrier. *A*, The gross specimen. *B*, Photomicrograph (× 100). Note structures simulating renal corpuscles. (Courtesy of Armed Forces Institute of Pathology.) Contributor: Dr. H. R. Seibold.

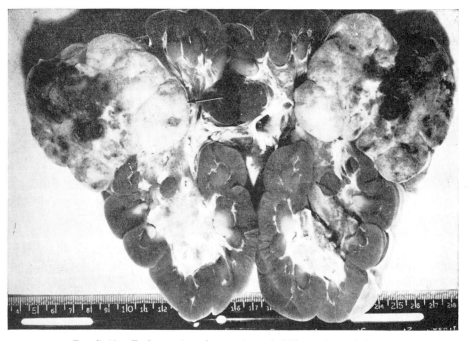

FIG. 7–40.—Embryonal nephroma (arrow), kidney of an adult cow.

occurred in a sow six years old. There were twice as many in females as in males for some unknown reason. The tumors were multiple in 30 per cent, usually bilateral. Most often, but by no means invariably, arising at one pole of the kidney, they ranged from very small up to a diameter of 80 cm. and a weight of 27 kg. These authors described the typical tumor as a "firm, lobulated, light-colored growth" having a "distinct capsule and numerous trabeculae of dense, mature connective tissue." While growth was described as rapid, metastases were exceptional, being chiefly to the lungs or liver. Partially calcified bone was demonstrated in one of the tumors and striated (not smooth, as in human patients) muscle was definitely recognized in five.

Hypernephroma.—This name has long been used to designate a neoplasm arising usually near one end of a kidney and characterized by columns of large cells with a clear, lipoid-containing cytoplasm. These were conceived to be misplaced adrenocortical cells, thus accounting for the name. The prevalent view today is that they arise from the epithelium of renal tubules. They appear to blend by imperceptible gradations with "clear-celled adenocarcinomas" and more ordinary adenocarcinomas and adenomas which are known to originate from the renal tubules. Benign or malignant tumors of this general class have been found in the dog, horse, monkey and laboratory rodents.

Islet-cell Adenoma.—The pancreas is subject to adenocarcinomas derived from the acinar epithelium and to a tumor, usually benign, arising from the epithelial cells of the pancreatic islets (islands of Langerhans). The former presents no unusual architectural features. Cells of acinar origin ordinarily contain zymogen granules demonstrable by azure-eosin techniques (Lillie, 1947), a fact which can be utilized in the rare event that difficulty is experienced in differentiating the two tumors.

The islet-cell adenoma (rarely carcinoma) is characterized by masses of round polyhedral epithelial cells with round nuclei centrally placed in a considerable

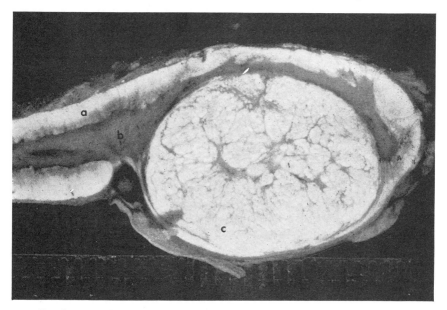

FIG. 7–41.—Adenoma of the adrenal cortex of an eight-year-old male hound.
Adrenal cortex (*a*), medulla (*b*), tumor (*c*).

amount of pale pink, and possibly granular cytoplasm. The nuclei vary considerably in size and rarely have nucleoli. Thin trabeculae divide the tumor into lobules. The neoplasm usually appears as an indistinctly nodular mass of pinkish tissue imbedded in the pancreas. Most of these tumors attract attention, however, because of hyperinsulinism and hypoglycemia resulting from their functional activity.

Adreno-cortical Adenomas and Carcinomas.—The benign tumors of the adrenal cortex are adenomas whose histologic structure closely simulates that of the normal adrenal cortex, including the zona glomerulosa; the malignant forms consist of highly anaplastic epithelial cells held in place by fibrous trabeculæ. Grossly the carcinomas may reach large size and spread extensively to nearby organs. While always rare, these tumors have been reported in dogs and horses and quite a number are on record in cattle and sheep. Richter (1957) reported what were considered to be adenomas in the adrenal cortex of goats. Among castrated males there were 169 adenomas in 770 adrenal glands, among uncastrated males the findings were 0 out of 244; in females, 2 out of 273. Most tumors were less than 5 mm. in diameter; the largest was 11 mm. Nodular hyperplasia was considered to have been excluded.

A masculinizing functional effect is characteristic but not universal in tumors of the adrenal cortex. This has been noted in some of the bovine cases, the cow's voice becoming more like that of the bull and a crest developing over the neck. In humans, an excess of adrenogenic hormones is demonstrable in the urine of patients having a masculinizing adreno-cortical tumor. These hormones belong to the 17-ketosteroid group (steroids with a ketone group on the 17th carbon atom) and a test of the urine for these steroids can be performed as an aid to diagnosis. In a few human cases these tumors are feminizing (Cushing's syndrome)

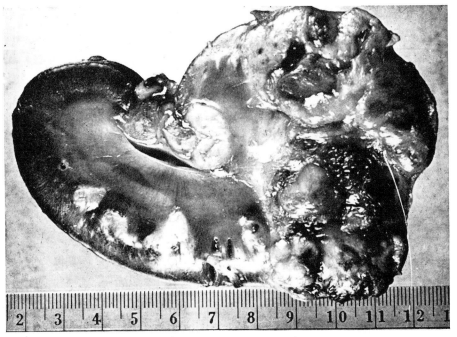

Fig. 7–42.—Papillary adenocarcinoma of the kidney of an eight-year-old male springer spaniel.

and an excess of estrogenic hormone has been demonstrated in the urine. Feminizing cases have not been reported in animals; they would not be expected to present recognizable symptoms in other than entire males. We are also told that the cells of masculinizing adrenocortical tumors show fuchsinophilic and siderophilic cytoplasmic granules (Goormaghtigh, 1940).

Pheochromocytoma.—The adrenal medulla, as modified nervous tissue connected with the sympathetic nervous system, gives rise to neoplasms of poorly

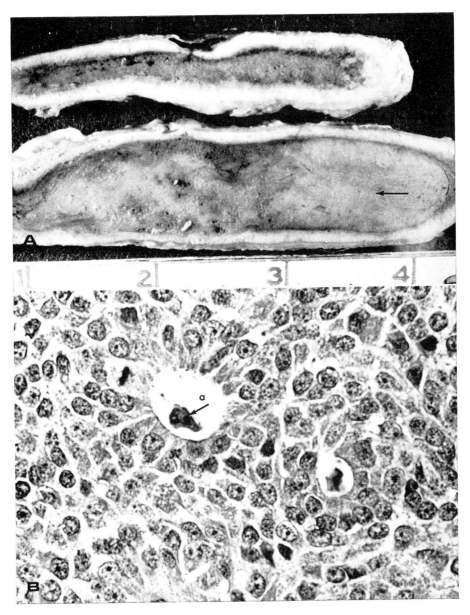

FIG. 7–43.—*A*, Pheochromocytoma (arrow), medulla of the adrenal of an eight-year-old male dalmatian dog. *B*, Same tumor (× 1000) H & E stain. Note intimate relationship of tumor cells to small capillaries (*a*), forming "pseudo rosettes" around them. The empty space around the capillary is due to shrinkage artefact. (Courtesy of Angell Memorial Animal Hospital.)

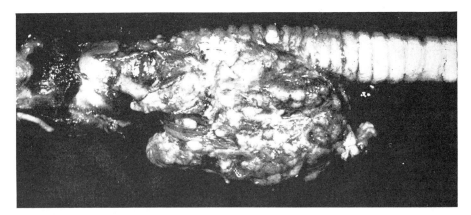

Fig. 7–44.—Adenocarcinoma of the left thyroid, of a 12-year-old male cocker spaniel. Note the relation of the tumor mass to the larynx and trachea. (Courtesy of Angell Memorial Animal Hospital.)

or well differentiated nerve cells, neuroblastomas and ganglioneuromas respectively. These will be discussed with neoplasms of nervous tissue. Also arising from the cells of the adrenal medulla is the pheochromocytoma (meaning a dark-celled tumor). Other names are **chromaffinoma** (having an affinity for chromium fixatives) and **paraganglioma** (coming from the "paraganglia" of the abdominal area). These tumors are commonly brown upon gross examination because of a pigment in them, hence the first name. Whether this is the case or not, if the tissue is fixed in chromium salts (Mueller's fluid), the cells commonly develop a brown color which is seen in the microscopic section (a feature characteristic of the chromaffine tissue of normal histology). Another method is to place the fresh tissue in a 5 to 10 per cent solution of potassium dichromate and a yellow or brown color should develop in the solution within a half-hour. But failure of the typical color to develop does not necessarily exclude the diagnosis of pheochromocytoma. The cells have the appearance of large epithelioid cells with central nuclei and abundant cytoplasm. Their outlines tend to be indefinite and fuzzy, as is true in the normal adrenal medulla. They are usually held in groups by thin fibrous strands. Blood spaces are likely to be numerous. Pheochromocytomas of the adrenal medulla have been recorded in the horse, cow and dog, but they are very infrequent. In man, they usually liberate adrenalin and produce vascular hypertension; this feature has not been studied in animals.

Aortic Body Tumor.—The term *paraganglioma* is best reserved for chromaffin tumors occurring outside the adrenal. At least related to the general group, but with an equivocal chromaffinity, are the carotid-body tumor in man and the similar and probably corresponding aortic-body tumor in dogs. These two "bodies" are considered to be nervous receptors activated by the amounts of oxygen and carbon dioxide in the blood, thereby influencing respiration; there is dispute as to whether the tumors truly belong in the chromaffinoma or paraganglioma groups. Some refer to this group of tumors as **non-chromaffin paragangliomas.**

Sometimes called the **heart base tumor,** the **aortic body tumor** is located at the base of the heart, usually intimately related to both the aorta and pulmonary artery. This anatomic relationship corresponds to that described by Bloom (1943)

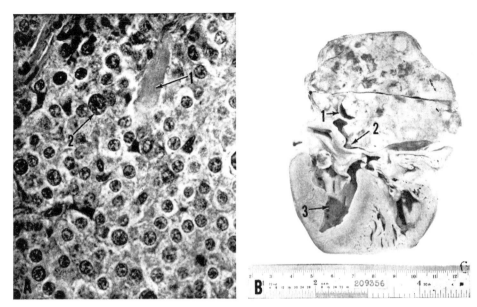

Fig. 7–45.—Aortic body tumor. *A*, Photomicrograph (× 500). Collagen-rich supporting stroma (*1*) and polyhedral cells with spherical nuclei, some large and hyperchromatic (*2*). *B*, The gross tumor at the base of the heart of a ten-year-old male English bulldog. Tumor invades the aorta (*1*), compresses the atrium (*2*). Left ventricle (*3*). (Courtesy of Armed Forces Institute of Pathology.) Contributor: Dr. W. H. Riser.

for the normal aortic body of the dog. The media of both the pulmonary artery and aorta is often infiltrated by tumor cells, occasionally with encroachment upon the lumen. The anatomic site is of importance because the morphology of the tumor cells could be confused with that seen in a number of other tumors. The tumor cells are usually polyhedral in shape with vacuolated or granular cytoplasm and spherical, finely stippled nuclei. Very large hyperchromatic nuclei are often scattered through the neoplasm. It is divided into lobules of irregular size by fine strands of connective tissue; blood vessels are in close proximity to the tumor cells. Apparently without any endocrine function, aortic body tumors have ordinarily been found only in the dog, most frequently in brachiocephalic breeds (Bulldog, Boston Terrier, Boxer). However, one of the authors (Smith) encountered an aortic-body tumor in a 12-month-old heifer. It formed a mass 20 cm. in diameter, encircling the base of the heart, attached to it and to nothing else. Death resulted from cardiac failure and edema. A few **carotid body tumors** of dogs have been seen in the experience of the authors. Scott (1958) reported one which was successfully removed by the surgeon. Others have been reported in a cow (Nordstoga, 1966) and in a cat (Buergelt and Das, 1968).

Thyroid Adenomas and Adenocarcinomas.—These tumors are among the commoner neoplasms of dogs and adenomas, at least, frequently affect the horse. Both types of tumor are more frequent in geographical areas where goiter is frequent. (See Thyroid, p. 1357.) Adenomas of the thyroid may present a picture closely resembling normal thyroid, but they consist of rounded, lightly encapsulated nodules, often more than one, in which the adenomatous thyroid tissue can be seen to differ from healthy thyroid tissue in one way or another when the two are compared. Commonly the acini of the adenoma are smaller and the lining cells more highly chromatic than is the case with the nearby healthy thyroid, but almost the reverse may be true. A sharp difference of one kind or another is almost sure to betray the adenomatous character of one area as compared to the other. Many thyroid adenomas are **toxic,** meaning that they secrete thyroxin and cause hyperthyroidism.

In bovine animals, Jubb and McEntee (1959) have proposed that some thyroid tumors arise from remnants of the **ultimobranchial bodies** from which the thyroids originate during embryologic development. The ultimobranchial bodies are found in sections of the lateral lobes of the thyroid as tubular or cystic structures lined by squamous or columnar epithelium which may undergo metaplasia and hyperkeratinization (in poisoning due to hexachloronaphthaline, vitamin A deficiency, or hyperestrogenism). This epithelium contributes to the formation of thyroid acini in fetal life and apparently retains some of this potential. Origin of thyroid tumors from this body is offered as an explanation of the multiple types which are found in tumors of bovine thyroid.

While most follow the pattern of the parent tissue, carcinomas of the thyroid are likely to be highly anaplastic and to bear no resemblances that would apprise the uninitiated of their origin. A few take the form of a papilliferous adenocarcinoma with papillary projections extending into the glandular acini. A larger proportion consist of solid masses of epithelial cells put together in pavement-like fashion. The cells have central nuclei, which may be small or large, pale or dark, round or more bizarre, depending on the milder or more marked degree of malignancy of the neoplasm. Some even approach a spindle-cell form.

These tumors invade the nearby organs and tissues and metastasize to various organs, most frequently the lungs. The primary tumor is not likely to be large, although some exert enough pressure on the trachea and larynx to interfere with breathing (Fig. 7–46).

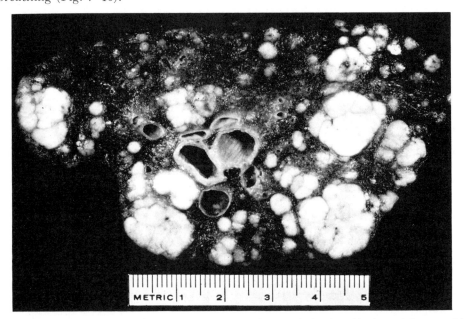

Fig. 7–46.—Metastases in the lung from adenocarcinoma of the thyroid of an eight-year-old male Irish setter. Note that the single and confluent nodules are not all the same size. (Courtesy of Angell Memorial Animal Hospital.)

Parathyroid Adenoma.—Clear-cut examples of this tumor have not been reported in animals, but such growths are not entirely unknown and documented reports may be expected as the volume of veterinary observations grows. Parathyroid adenomas in man are usually brownish or grayish and small in size. The microscopic structure is similar to that of the normal parathyroid, consisting of areas of epithelial cells with central nuclei and a liberal amount of rather dark-staining cytoplasm mingled with other areas where the cytoplasm stains scarcely at all (light cells). Slender trabeculæ, pseudo-acini and blood spaces complete the picture. Most parathyroid adenomas have the important functional effect of removing calcium from the bones, placing it in the blood, whence it is excreted by the kidneys as far as they are able to do so. Results of this process are osteitis fibrosa cystica (von Recklinghausen's disease), hypophosphatemia and often urinary calculi consisting of calcium phosphate. This condition is not to be confused with the parathyroid hyperplasia which results from long-continued drainage of blood calcium when nephritic kidneys are unable adequately to excrete phosphates. This parathyroid hyperplasia also deprives the bones of calcium resulting in their softening ("rubber jaw"). This condition does occur in animals, chiefly in the dog (p. 1064).

Pituitary Adenomas.—There are three kinds of adenomas which arise from the pars glandularis of the anterior lobe of the pituitary gland. The **acidophil adenoma** consists chiefly of cells with eosinophilic cytoplasm which are derived from the acidophilic chromophiles of the normal organ. This tumor in man usually produces an excess of the growth hormone which results in gigantism, or acromegaly. Among the five acidophil adenomas reported in animals, all have been in dogs, none of these exhibited signs of acromegaly. Capen, Martin and Koestner (1967), studied the ultrastructure of acidophil adenoma from a dog in which clinical signs of a space occupying lesion of the hypophysis were evident. These authors found two types of acidophils among the cells making up the adenoma. In the first and predominating type cell the cytoplasm was densely packed with secretory granules and the endoplasmic reticulum, and golgi apparatus were poorly developed. These cells were considered to be in the storage phase. The second type of cell had well developed endoplasmic reticulum and golgi but few secretory granules, therefore were believed to be actively synthesizing the product which eventually makes up the acidophil granules.

Chromophobe adenomas are made up of chromophobe cells which in the past have been believed to be functionally inactive or in a "resting" stage. In the dog, however, tumors made up of what appeared to be chromophobe cells have been associated with severe clinical manifestations. Capen, Martin and Koestner (1967), carefully studied twenty-six tumors of the adenohypophysis of dogs, twenty were classified as chromophobe adenomas and six as **adenomas of the pars intermedia.** Fourteen of the adenomas of chromophobe cells and two of the pars intermedia were functionally active and were manifest clinically by diabetes insipidus (p. 1020) and hyperadrenocorticism (p. 1353). Evidence that these functional tumors produced adrenocorticotrophic hormone (ACTH) was seen in the clinical manifestations following adrenal cortical hyperplasia: muscular weakness and wasting; bilateral symmetrical loss of hair; calcification in dermis and other tissues; neutrophilia, eosinopenia and lymphopenia; increased corticosteroid in serum and increased 17-hydroxycorticosteroids in urine.

Ultrastructural study of functionally active chromophobe adenomas in the dog

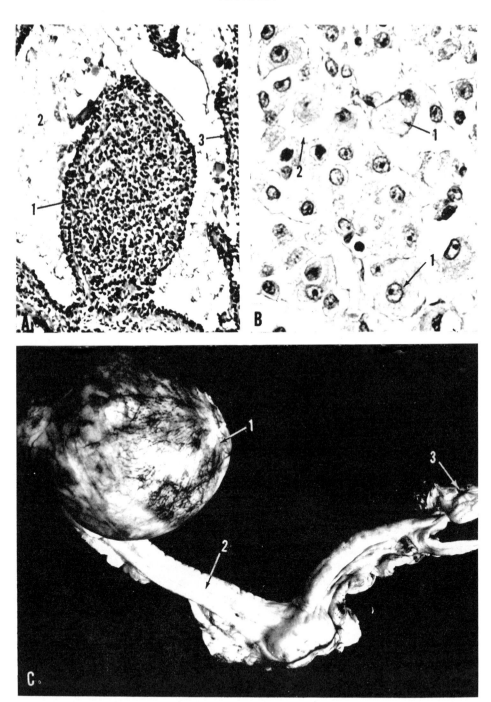

FIG. 7–47.—Granulosa cell tumor. *A*, Photomicrograph ($\times$ 136) of a tumor of a mare's ovary showing cells in a nodule (*1*) with a cystic space (*2*) suggesting Graafian follicle lined by granulosa cells (*3*). Contributor: Dr. F. A. Howard. *B*, Large polyhedral cells (*1*) and lipid (*2*) in a granulosa cell tumor ($\times$ 540) in ovary of a twelve-year-old wire-haired terrier. *C*, Gross tumor in left ovary (*1*), left cornu of uterus (*2*) and right ovary (*3*). This animal exhibited estrus for six months until the tumor was removed. (Courtesy of Armed Forces Institute of Pathology.) Contributor: Major Howard Kester.

pituitary by Capen and Koestner (1967) led them to conclude that the cells making up these adenomas were actually pituitary corticotrophs, the cells now believed responsible for the secretion of ACTH. This supports the other evidence of functional activity which we have alluded to.

Granulosa-cell Tumor, Theca-cell and Luteal-cell Tumors.—The granulosa-cell tumor arises from the stratum granulosum of the ovarian follicle, or the cells capable of forming that structure. The embryologic origin of these structures is not a matter of universal agreement, but it is commonly considered that the stratum granulosum is derived from the theca folliculi and that the luteal cells of the corpus luteum may be formed from either of these. The usual granulosa-cell tumor consists of masses of cells of epithelial appearance with round central nuclei and considerable cytoplasm. In some, there are fluid-filled, rounded open spaces here and there which bear a suggestive resemblance to Graafian follicles. In others, there are places where a dozen or fewer cells cluster radially around a tiny open space, producing a formation called a rosette. (Rosettes are also found in ependymomas, medulloblastomas, retinoblastomas and neuroblastomas.) In still others, the cells are diffusely distributed in no particular pattern except that they are held in elongated or cylindrical lobules by thin fibrous trabeculæ. Grossly, the granulosa-cell tumor is usually rounded and smoothly encapsulated and may reach a weight of several pounds, being attached to the ovary rather than included in it. The cut surface is usually yellowish.

The theca-cell tumor differentiates to form spindle-shaped cells, thus resembling the theca interna and theca externa of the follicle.

The luteal-cell tumor is similar to the usual type of granulosa-cell tumor but is even more yellow grossly, the cells containing numerous lipoidal droplets, microscopically suggestive of a corpus luteum.

The tumors of this group secrete a feminizing hormone, an estrogen. In the cow, this has brought relaxation of the sacro-sciatic ligaments, suggestive of late pregnancy and, more spectacularly, nymphomania. The granulosa-cell tumor has also been seen in mares, ewes, cats and bitches. In the latter, it tends to cause cystic glandular hyperplasia of the endometrium, as in women.

The arrhenoblastoma is a rare masculinizing tumor arising in connection with the rete ovarii, which is considered to be the female counterpart of the testis. Its cells may be highly anaplastic but when well differentiated, they form structures closely resembling the seminiferous tubules or the Sertoli-cell tumors (see below) of the testis. Dacorso (1947) has described an anaplastic arrhenoblastoma from a bovine ovary in which the cells varied from polyhedral to fusiform types.

The dysgerminoma arises from undifferentiated primitive cells of the ovary. Its histological picture resembles that of the seminoma (below). It has no hormonal effect. The dysgerminoma has been found in the cow and in dogs.

Still more rare are the Brenner tumor and the Berger tumor, the latter arising from ovarian cells considered to be counterparts of the interstitial (Leydig) cells of the testis. Neither of these appears to have been recognized in animals.

Seminoma.—One of the three neoplasms peculiar to the testicle, the seminoma is believed to arise from the germinal epithelium of the seminiferous tubules. Its large polyhedral cells with prominent round nuclei, centrally located, are not unlike spermatogonia and spermatocytes. Their nuclei contain conspicuous chromatin bodies, a feature which aids in distinguishing this tumor from some of the larger-celled malignant lymphomas and from the transmissible venereal tumors

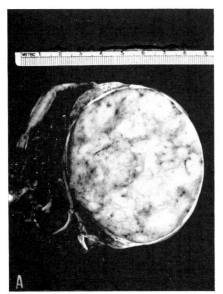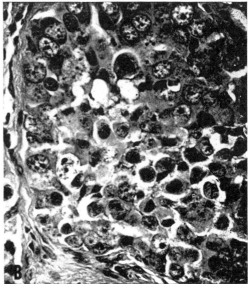

Fig. 7–48.—Seminoma. *A*, Spherical mass in the testicle of a seventeen-year-old chow dog. Contributor: Dr. Edward Records. *B*, Seminoma ($\times$ 355) testicle of an eight-year-old Pomeranian. Large spherical cells with hyperchromatic nuclei. (Courtesy of Armed Forces Institute of Pathology.) Contributor: Angell Memorial Animal Hospital.

in cases where a diagnosis is to be made without knowledge of the source of the tissue. Mitotic figures are likely to be frequent in all these tumors. Fine trabeculae divide the masses of cells into compartments. The seminoma occurs most frequently in the dog, although its rarity in other domestic species may well be due merely to the castration of most males among other species. While this tumor is often deadly in men, in the dog it is much less to be feared. It tends to spread slowly along the spermatic cord (where the surgeon should seek it), but reasonably early removal is usually curative.

A unique feature of some value in distinguishing the seminoma from other tumors encountered in the canine testicle is the rather frequent occurrence of small collections of cells which are apparently lymphocytes in the midst of the neoplastic cells.

Sertoli-cell, or Sustentacular-cell Tumor.—As its name implies, this tumor arises from the sustentacular, or Sertoli cells of the seminiferous tubules. While a few may develop areas so anaplastic as to consist of solid masses of round or polyhedral cells with central nuclei, the majority of these tumors contain some areas in which continuity can be traced to seminiferous tubules of normal size and shape but with their lining devoid of germinal cells, one or two irregular layers of tall Sertoli cells remaining. An intermediate type of structure consists in solidly filled tubules, the cells being radially elongated, angular and with a cytoplasm which is more or less clear because of high lipoid content. The common synonym of **tubular adenoma** aptly describes this, the usual appearance of the Sertoli-cell tumor.

Grossly, the Sertoli-cell tumor is likely to consist of one or more nodules which may greatly distend the tunica albuginea, reaching several times the size of the normal testis. The cut surface bulges and is gray or light yellow in color. The rare anaplastic forms of this tumor spread into the surrounding structures and up the spermatic cord, and may metastasize to the sublumbar lymph nodes.

The Sertoli-cell tumor occurs almost exclusively in the dog, the human counterpart being exceedingly rare. It commonly produces a feminizing hormone with the result that the mammae enlarge, the hair of the belly is thinned and the dog becomes sexually attractive to other males. Squamous metaplasia of the prostate and urinary epithelium also results. This is comparable to the metaplasia noted

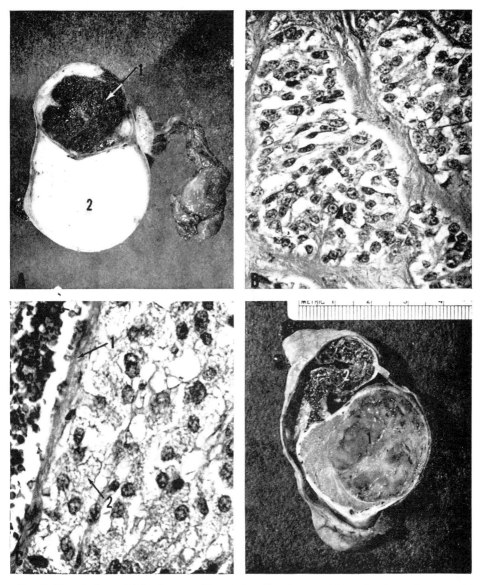

Fig. 7–49.—*A*, Interstitial cell tumor (*1*) and Sertoli cell tumor (*2*), testis of a twelve-year-old dachshund. Contributor: Dr. Robert Ferber. *B*, Sertoli cell tumor (× 355), testicle of a nine-year-old Boston terrier. Elongated, lipid-containing Sertoli cells in irregular nests. Contributor: Angell Memorial Animal Hospital. *C*, Interstitial cell tumor (× 435) testis of an eight-year-old beagle. Blood vessels (*1*) intimately related to lipid-bearing interstitial cells (*2*). *D*, Interstitial cell tumor (*1*) displacing testicular parenchyma. Epididymis (*2*). Same case as *C*. (Courtesy of Armed Forces Institute of Pathology.) Contributor: Angell Memorial Animal Hospital.

following the feeding of stilbestrol to fattening sheep. The metaplasia has also been produced experimentally in dogs (Fig. 4–3).

Interstitial, or Leydig-cell Tumor.—This neoplasm arises from the interstitial, androgen-secreting cells of the testis. Its cells are larger and have more eosinophilic cytoplasm than the two previous testicular tumors. The cytoplasm contains large amounts of lipids, which accounts for the foamy character of its cytoplasm and for a distinctly yellow color grossly. Much of the fat is anisotropic under the polarizing microscope. The cells form masses divided into compartments by fibrous trabeculae. Mitotic figures are seldom found. This tumor is not infrequent in the dog and, like the other testicular tumors, would probably be seen more frequently in other species, if the males were not castrated at an early age. It has been reported in a cryptorchid equine testicle (Smith, 1954) and in a six-year-old bovine which had been castrated by inversion of both testes within the scrotum and torsion of their spermatic cords. Secretion of excess androgen by the tumor can sometimes be demonstrated in early life, but at a later period the opposite hormonal effect may be demonstrable. Usually in the dog no hormonal effects are observed clinically.

An interesting compilation from the Angell Memorial Animal Hospital shows that, of 520 canine testicular tumors, 38 per cent were interstitial-cell tumors, 32 per cent seminomas and 30 per cent Sertoli-cell tumors. In a surprisingly high number of cases the same patient had two different testicular tumors and in four patients all three types were present. Among 42 cryptorchid testicles 12 were tumorous.

TUMORS OF NERVOUS TISSUE

Neoplasms arising in nervous tissue, ordinarily in the brain, come chiefly from the neuroglia, and those having this source are known as **gliomas.** Gliomas can be subdivided into a great many groups or varieties, but the classes commonly recognized are (1) astrocytoma, (2) glioblastoma multiforme, (3) medulloblastoma, all of which arise from astrocytes or early, undifferentiated forms of neuroglial tissue, (4) ependymoma, which arises from the ependymal lining cells, and (5) oligodendroglioma. These represent the recognized types of neuroglial tissue except the microglia, which does not form tumors. The above classes are not sharply demarcated and some gliomas partake of the characteristics of two different classes. The several classes of gliomas are characterized by different rates of growth, so that the terms benign and malignant are used to refer to them but no glioma metastasizes to locations outside the cranial cavity (or spinal canal). Infiltration to adjoining areas of the brain is, however, marked in the case of the more malignant ones, so that grossly and even microscopically it may be very difficult to discern the limits of the tumor. In man the usual location, biological history, operability and outcome are well known with respect to each class of tumor. Judging by the comparatively few cases of glioma reported in animals, it appears that this information has only a very limited application to veterinary surgical problems. As more case-records accumulate, our knowledge of these aspects of the gliomas found in animals can be expected to increase. If diagnosable, it would seem that surgical treatment of such tumors need not be more forbidding than it is in the human being.

The **astrocytoma** varies considerably in histological appearance, for a thorough study of which special techniques are necessary. Several different types are recognized, whose description would be beyond the scope of this work. In general, the cells have round or somewhat elongated nuclei which are relatively pale although chromatin granules can be seen. The nuclei, which are rather sparsely distributed, may or may not be accompanied by a poorly outlined cytoplasm, but

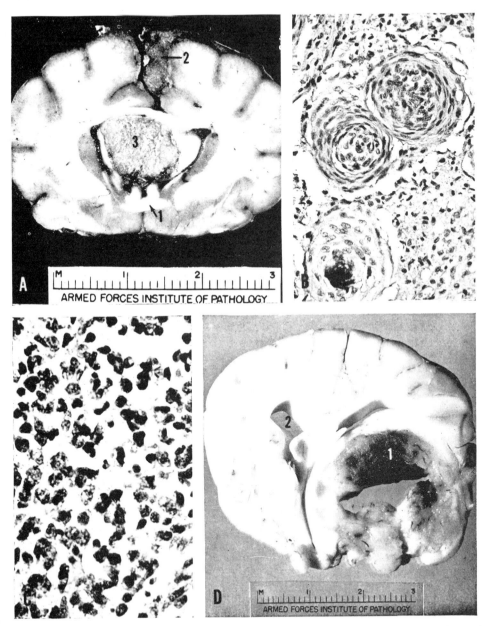

FIG. 7–50.—*A*, Meningioma, brain of a fourteen-year-old castrated male cat. Section of brain through the anterior commissure (**1**) with tumor in pia (**2**) and in midline (**3**). *B*, Same tumor as *A* (× 210); note concentrically laminated structures. Contributor: Dr. J. Holzworth. *C*, Oligo-dendroglioma, brain of an eight-year-old female boxer. *D*, Gross specimen of same tumor. The tumor (*1*) displaces the midline. Slight hydrocephalus, lateral ventricle (*2*). (Courtesy of Armed Forces Institute of Pathology.) Contributor: Dr. L. N. Loomis.

the bulk of the internuclear space is occupied by pink-staining fibrils which criss-cross in various directions. This tumor occurs in almost any part of the brain and is among those of lesser malignancy.

The **glioblastoma multiforme** differs histologically from the astrocytoma in that its nuclei are more numerous, more deeply stained, and very irregular and pleomorphic in size, shape and position. In man, this tumor is the most frequent of the gliomas, as well as the most malignant and is usually located in the cerebral hemispheres.

The **medulloblastoma,** arising from embryonal glial tissue, consists of masses of round cells with deeply staining, round nuclei. It thus resembles a malignant lymphoma in its microscopic appearance. At times there is formed a kind of "rosette" consisting of a flower-like circle of radially arranged nuclei around a tiny pale central spot which may contain a capillary. This tumor occurs in young individuals and is located ordinarily just dorsal to the fourth ventricle, where it appears as a more or less spherical, discrete reddish-gray mass.

The **ependymoma** consists of cells of medium size with irregularly rounded or polyhedral nuclei, centrally placed. The nuclei are moderately deep-staining; the cytoplasm, pink. The cells are put together in solid masses, broken here and there by a thin trabecula. Occasionally they reveal their innate tendency to line cavities by forming a tiny open space around which a single zone of cells is radially arranged. Such a structure is called a "rosette." Ependymomas form well-demarcated masses in the region of the fourth or the third ventricles, from whose lining they conceivably arise.

The **oligodendroglioma,** not altogether rare in the dog, consists of polyhedral cells separated into compartments by thin trabeculae. The cytoplasm of the cells takes practically no stain by ordinary methods. This gives the tumor the appearance of rather small, round nuclei arranged alongside of, but separated from the trabeculæ. Calcified granules equal to the size of several cells are often scattered through the tissue.

Pinealoma.—This tumor, also known as pineal adenoma, is a very rare neoplasm derived from the pineal body, or epiphysis cerebri. Its histologic appearance is distinctive in that it consists of an indiscriminate mingling of groups of large epithelioid cells with groups of small (neuroglial) cells with small round nuclei suggestive of lymphocytes. Sexual or other forms of precocity have accompanied some pinealomas in children, but these are suspected of being due to disturbance of nearby structures rather than to the direct effect of the tumors. A pinealoma has been reported in a silver fox, a horse, and a rat.

Cholesteatoma.—This term relates to a tumor-like formation consisting of layers of epithelial-appearing cells containing so much cholesterol and other lipids that the gross tumor resembles a cluster of pearls. Some are in the brain tissue. In the horse, this term has been applied to a lesion in the choroid plexus which more appropriately should be called cholesterinic granuloma (Fig. 28–9). These are considered to result from degenerative processes and have been related to the granulomas. Those in the brain tissue of man are said to be the result of epidermal or even dermal (dermoid cyst) remnants left there during embryonal development.

Psammoma.—This is an old term used to designate intracranial tumors containing numerous calcified granules. Most of these were meningiomas (p. 203) but some may have been overgrowths related to the "cholesteatomas."

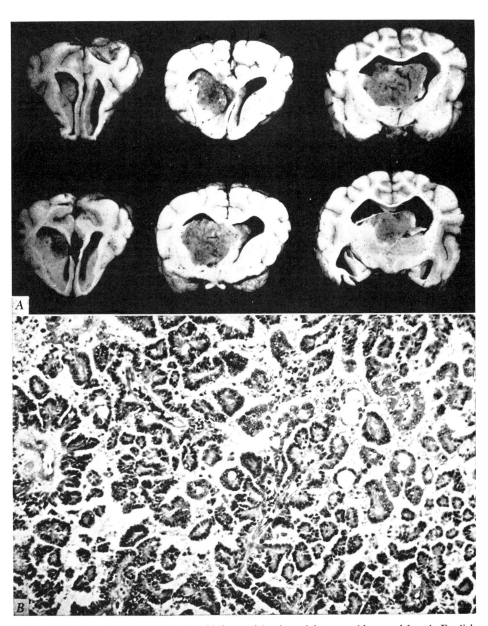

FIG. 7–51.—Ependymoma, arising in third ventricle of an eight-year-old spayed female English bulldog. *A*, The gross brain cut at 1 cm. intervals. Note the deviation of the midline and the hydrocephalus of the lateral ventricles. *B*, Section of the tumor, H & E × 200. (Courtesy of Angell Memorial Animal Hospital.)

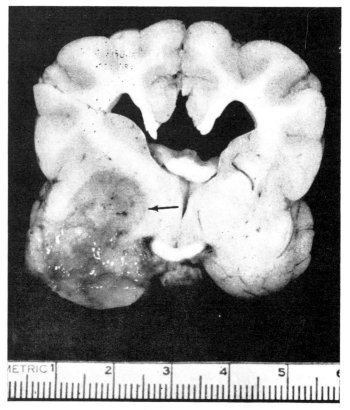

Fig. 7–52.—Astrocytoma, right pyriform lobe of cerebrum of a nine-year-old castrated male boxer. (Courtesy of Angell Memorial Animal Hospital.)

Neuroblastoma.—These are tumors consisting of small, round cells of undifferentiated embryonal aspect. The microscopic appearance is similar to that of the medulloblastoma (above) to which the neuroblastoma is embryologically related, since both arise from nervous tissue at a very early stage of embryonal development. Like the medulloblastoma, this tumor also typically forms "rosettes," which, if present, are a prime aid in the microscopic diagnosis. In the case of the neuroblastoma, the cells of the rosette are arranged around a small tuft of fibrils of nervous origin.

The neuroblastoma can originate in the central nervous system, but the majority occur in the adrenal medulla; a few arise from sympathetic nervous tissue elsewhere in the abdominal cavity. In the adrenal medulla the tumor sometimes receives the name of **sympathoblastoma.** Wherever located, it occurs in the young and is highly malignant.

Retinoblastoma, or Neuroepithelioma.—This tumor arises in the eye from the precursors of the neuro-epithelial receptor cells of the retina. Like the medulloblastoma and the neuroblastoma it consists of small cells with nuclei suggestive of lymphocytes. It also tends to form rosettes. It is malignant, metastasizing to the regional lymph nodes. It occurs in the very young and has a startlingly high incidence in some human families. These tumors appear to be very rare in animals.

Ganglioneuroma.—Arising from nervous tissue capable of forming neurons, this tumor is related to the neuroblastoma. But where the neuroblastoma is undifferentiated, or anaplastic, the ganglioma is well differentiated into "ganglion cells" looking much like multipolar and other nerve cells and a supporting tissue suggestive of normal neuroglia. These very rare tumors may occur in the brain but, like the neuroblastomas, are more likely to arise in the adrenal medulla or occasionally in sympathetic ganglia.

MELANOMAS

Melanomas arise from melanin-forming cells. They are malignant or, at least only temporarily, benign. Cells which have the ability to produce melanin (melanocytes) arise embryologically in the neural crest which originates from the neuroectoderm. Early in embryonic life, these cells migrate to other positions in the body, particularly the skin, where they eventually produce melanin. This

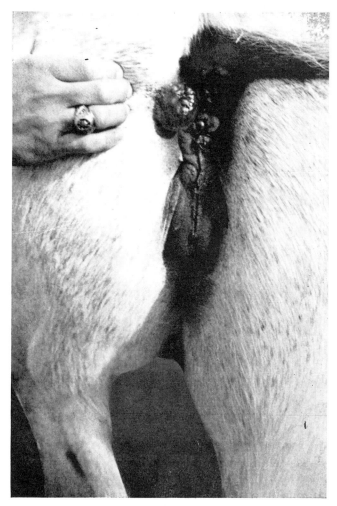

Fig. 7–53.—Melanoma in the perineum of an aged gray mule.
(Photograph, courtesy of Dr. Thomas Hardy.)

pigment enters into other tissue cells (dermis, epidermis, choroid, retina, ciliary processes, meninges, etc.) adjacent to the melanocyte. It is not surprising therefore that tumors of melanin-producing cells are most common in the skin but may originate elsewhere. Their nature and chemistry have been discussed in connection with melanin (p. 65). Since some melanomas consist of cells formed and arranged like epithelium and others equally resemble undifferentiated fibrous or supporting tissue, they have been called melanocarcinomas and melanosarcomas respectively. Present usage employs neither of those terms.

Melanomas of the skin are common tumors in most species, even in fishes. Their mode of origin has been the subject of much speculation and study. In humans, most cutaneous melanomas arise in the small, raised, brown spots present somewhere on almost everyone's skin, known as pigmented moles, or nevi (singular: nevus). These may be merely islands of detached epithelium according to one belief. The extensive work of Masson (1926) which has been rather widely accepted, indicates that they are derived from or, at least, connected with cutaneous nerves, thus constituting aberrant nerve-endings. An intriguing but unsubstantiated theory is that nevi are phylogenetic vestiges of a pigmented sensory organ, which exists in amphibia and may possibly have been present in the ancestors of the human race at the amphibian stage of evolution. Whatever may be the truth about nevi, they do not explain the origin of melanomas in animals nor of those human melanomas not located in the skin.

The histologic appearance of melanomas varies considerably. The cells may be so filled with the brown pigment that little else can be seen or, at the other extreme, there may be no melanin at all, an **amelanotic melanoma.** The shape of the cells varies in different tumors, or sometimes within the same tumor, from round or polyhedral forms resembling epithelium to elongated, fusiform cells which one would take for fibroblasts. Typically the latter type predominates and the spindle-shaped cells fit together somewhat like the segments of an orange, to fill compartments clearly or vaguely marked off by thin fibrous trabeculæ. The cytoplasm tends to be basophilic and typically, when stained with the milder hematoxylin preparations (Mayer's hemalum), the nuclei have a distinctive violet hue which is not seen in other than melanoma cells. In most cases the large amounts of melanin in the cytoplasm of the tumor cells, as well as that phagocytized by melanophores in the vicinity leave no doubt as to the diagnosis, but some melanomas are so amelanotic that the diagnosis must be made on the morphological features of the cells.

While we incline to the view that all melanomas are potentially malignant, a very considerable number follow a course which can be considered benign for months or even years, the patient perhaps dying meanwhile of some other cause. Attempts to separate the malignant from the benign by histological examination depend on the general criteria of malignancy already given. These include large, hyperchromatic nuclei, bizarre forms and mitotic figures. An underlying lymphocytic infiltration is considered a sign of malignancy, as is also invasion of lymphatics.

Grossly, the melanoma is ordinarily recognized by its deep black color and by the inky pigment which diffuses from it into any watery medium with which the cut surface may come in contact. The true nature of an amelanotic melanoma may be discoverable only by microscopic examination.

Melanomas occur in so many forms and locations that generalization is difficult.

In the horse, quiescent or actively malignant melanomas are especially frequent in old gray horses, although they are by no means non-existent in horses of other colors. Their location is especially likely to be in the perianal and perineal region (Fig. 7–53), whence they spread to perirectal and other pelvic lymph nodes. One case is recalled in a brown mare in which the first symptom was complete inability to use one hind leg. Investigation showed that an intrapelvic melanoma had spread along the femoral canal and had enveloped the sciatic nerve. A number of

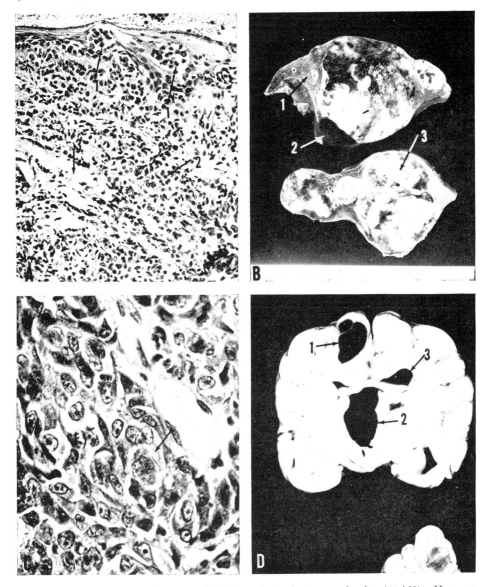

FIG. 7–54.—Malignant melanoma. A, Primary lesion in tongue of a dog (× 160). Note neoplastic cells in epidermis (1) and dermis (2) displacing collagen fibers (3). B, Metastatic malignant melanoma in lung (1) of a dog. Note melanotic (2) and amelanotic (3) areas. Contributor: Dr. M. L. Povar. C, Higher magnification (× 574) of tumor in A. Large cells laden with melanin (arrow). Contributor: Dr. Leo L. Lieberman. D, Metastatic malignant melanoma (1) and (2) in brain of a dog. Note slight internal hydrocephalus (3). (Courtesy of Armed Forces Institute of Pathology.) Contributor: Dr. C. L. Davis.

equine cases have been seen in which death resulted from metastases to the spleen, lungs or other internal organs without the primary having been found. One case is recalled in which a mare's mammary gland was half replaced by melanoma, probably by direct extension from a tumor of the overlying skin.

In cattle, melanomas arise in the skin at various locations. In swine, cutaneous melanomas varying in diameter from a few millimeters to several centimeters and usually somewhat elevated are common. The smaller ones usually remain until the pig is slaughtered; larger ones are often removed surgically, a perfect cure usually resulting. In the meat-producing animals, there is little opportunity to observe the ultimate outcome of these tumors. In the dog, cutaneous melanomas arise in various parts of the body and not a few occur in the mouth in those breeds having pigmented oral mucosa.

As to non-cutaneous melanomas, we are acquainted with one or two in the canine eye, which is rare. Melanomas occur from time to time in the spinal meninges, where they are apparently primary, arising from the pigmented cells previously mentioned.

Teratomas.—Teratomas require separate consideration. These are neoplasms containing tissues derived from more than one of the three primary germ layers, ectoderm, mesoderm and entoderm. The great majority of them occur in either the ovary or the testicle but a few are found in the retroperitoneal region, anterior mediastinum and other places close to the midline of the body. They usually are first discovered while the patient is still young and all evidence points to their having existed since fetal life. Growth may be slow or rapid at the time of discovery but in most cases has been very gradual over a long pre-symptomatic period.

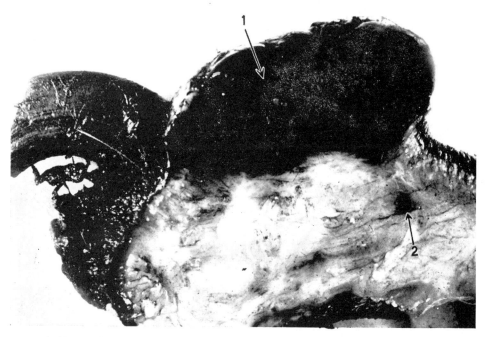

Fig. 7–55.—Malignant melanoma arising at base of toe nail of a sixteen-year-old male dachshund-collie crossbred dog. The tumor mass (*1*) is not encapsulated and a small mass is separated from it (*2*). (Courtesy of Angell Memorial Animal Hospital.)

The different tissues are in a jumbled mass and of various kinds. Most frequently encountered are connective tissue, cartilage and bone, epithelial structures of ectodermal or entodermal type, skin, hair and neuroglia. In one relatively common form, there is a cystic cavity lined with skin and filled with an increasing amount of hair which grows from the skin. This is commonly called a **dermoid cyst**. Some of the cysts have one or more teeth protruding into them and are called **dentigerous cysts**. To qualify as true teratomas, there must be active growth. In many instances, teratomas continue slow and benign growth over a long period, the various histological components apparently changing but little in their relative proportions. In other cases, one component or another assumes malignant qualities with rapid growth, infiltration and metastasis, thus constituting in effect a carcinoma or a sarcoma, as the case may be.

There have been a number of theories on the causation of teratomas. In view of the fact that many teratomas are discovered when the patient is at an age comparable to childhood, or even at birth, it is well agreed that teratomas are initiated early in fetal or, more likely, embryonic life. Also, since so many histological types of tissue make up a teratoma, tissues derived from each of the three primary layers usually being present, it must be concluded that the parent cell or cells are set apart at an extremely early stage of embryonal development. The fact that teratomas are practically restricted in location to tissues which, in the embryo, lie close to the median axis is construed to mean that their origin is related to abnormal development in the primitive streak. Beyond this there diverge two principal theories. One is that the teratoma develops from one ancestral cell which is the product of an abnormal mitosis at this very early stage. Such a parent cell would have the ability, as it subsequently underwent repeated subdivision, of producing practically any kind of tissue that the ovum could produce. The product of its growth would constitute essentially a twin, included within the body of the more normal descendant of the ovum itself. It would differ from ordinary enzygotic (identical) twins, or from Siamese twins, only in that the twin included within the body of the other was prevented from attaining any degree of normal development, presumably because of the limitations of its environment. Such a mode of origin would be in accord with the frequently observed twinning or duplication of various parts and segments of the animal body, as exemplified by two-headed calves and similar well-known malformations.

The second theory, also prominent, is that certain cells in the region of the primitive streak escape, by some developmental accident, from the control of certain chemical "organizers," substances which many embryologists believe exist in the normal embryo and regulate the relative development of its component structures in such a way as to develop a normal body.

The theory that teratomas represent parthenogenetic development of male or female reproductive cells has also been advanced. Certain experimenters have induced parthenogenetic development of ova in lower animal forms by means of physical and chemical stimuli and such ova, implanted in the maternal body, have grown into jumbled masses of tissue not unlike teratoid growths in higher animals. The misplacement of primordial ova during embryonic life to any of the locations where teratomas occur is, of course, conceivable, as well as their parthenogenetic development.

In any case, it appears that if all the tissues of the teratoma are well differentiated into their respective histological types, the teratoma remains a slowly enlarging mass with benign effects. If the tissues, on the other hand, retain embryonal characteristics, morphologic and otherwise, they can be expected, sooner or later, to be guilty of rapid and malignant growth, stimulated by some unknown factor, possibly no different from one of the carcinogenic stimuli which incite neoplasia in other tissues.

DIFFERENTIATION BETWEEN
BENIGN AND MALIGNANT NEOPLASMS

From what has been said of the respective effects of benign and malignant neoplasms, it is obvious that one of the first questions to be settled when neoplastic disease is encountered is that of whether the tumor is benign or malignant. Since this is commonly impossible by clinical examination alone, the task ordinarily falls to the pathologist.

It should be emphasized, however, that the benign and malignant classes are not set apart by an iron-clad boundary. Benignity is a relative quality and certainly there are all degrees of malignancy. Still, it is possible in more than 90 per cent of cases to predict the clinical behavior of a tumor from its histological structure and other characteristics. The clinician will learn some things from the gross appearance of the tumor; the pathologist will determine more by applying the microscopic criteria of malignancy; but our most effective aid at times is a personal acquaintance with the characteristic life-history of each tumor entity. For instance, it is well known that the usual carcinoma of the bovine orbit, histologically of grade 1 or grade 2 malignancy, is prone to cause great destruction by direct infiltration into surrounding tissues but seldom metastasizes. This encourages the surgeon to hope for a complete cure in cases where complete removal is possible. On the other hand, a similarly well-differentiated adenocarcinoma of the canine mammary gland offers a much poorer prognosis. As another example, a seminoma in the dog has about the same histological appearance as its human counterpart, but metastasis is much less likely than it is reputed to be in the human. It is to be hoped that more and better recorded observations on the outcome of tumors will bring a more accurate knowledge of many of them.

Microscopically, there are several accepted criteria to be considered in estimating the degree of malignancy of a neoplasm. (1) The fundamental measure of malignancy is the **degree of anaplasia,** meaning the extent to which the neoplastic tissue diverges from the normal histological pattern for the kind of tissue in question. Some tumors resemble the normal histology closely in the shape, size and staining reactions of the cells and their nuclei, and are put together in a way which simulates closely the architecture of the parent tissue. These are usually benign. Proportionately as these characteristics deviate from the normal and as the neoplastic cells cease to resemble the normal or as they come to resemble the embryonal stages of such cells, so the degree of malignancy rises. Such growths are said to be anaplastic, or undifferentiated.

(2) The mode of growth is of prime importance. If metastases are known to have occurred, the question of malignancy is obviously settled. If any extensive infiltration can be demonstrated, the tumor is malignant. This criterion is useful especially in the early stages of epithelial tumors; if it can be shown that the neoplastic epithelial cells have infiltrated below the basement membrane, or the basal line where a theoretical basement membrane separates epithelium from

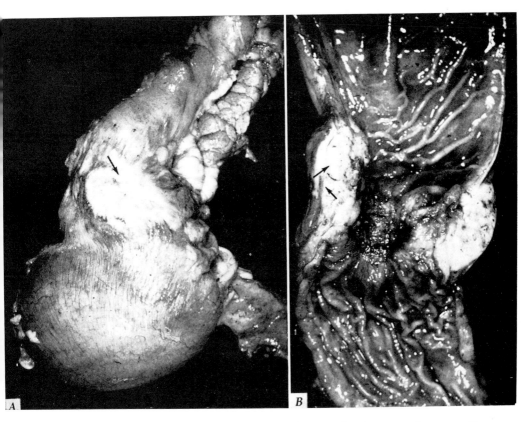

FIG. 7–56.—*A*, Adenocarcinoma of stomach of an Irish setter, female, age twelve years. Note white scar (arrow) on serosal surface. A large ulcer was found on the opposing mucosal surface. *B*, Adenocarcinoma (arrow) of the rectum of an eight-year-old male springer spaniel. The tumor encircled the rectal wall, causing partial obstruction. (Courtesy of Angell Memorial Animal Hospital.)

connective tissue stroma, the tumor is malignant, a carcinoma. Some epithelial growths are characterized by very extensive projections with crowded folds and many subdivisions. These may project into the lumina of glands (prostate, mammary) or ducts, or into cystic structures, presenting a startling and bizarre appearance. If it can be shown that the epithelium always remains above the line corresponding to a basement membrane and does not infiltrate, the neoplasm is to be classed as benign. Indeed the condition may be only hyperplasia, as in the hyperplastic thyroid of cretinism.

(3) The degree of cellularity is important in fibrous and similar neoplasms. If the nuclei are closely spaced, indicating a large number of cells per unit of area, this is an indication of malignancy.

(4) If the nuclei tend to be hyperchromatic, taking a stronger nuclear stain (such as hematoxylin) than usual, they are thus more like what is seen in an embryo, hence probably malignant. Nuclei of unusually large size are also significant.

(5) Numerous mitotic figures (nuclei in some stage of mitosis) mean rapid growth and the tumor is probably malignant. The kind of tumor is important

here; some characteristically show many mitoses; others do not, even though malignant.

(6) Abnormal mitotic figures, such as a division into three daughter nuclei instead of two, occur in some malignant tumors and are very significant if recognized.

Gross criteria afford some assistance in determining whether a tumor is benign or malignant. If it is growing on a surface and is pedunculated (attached only by a narrow neck), it is in all probability benign. Sessile tumors (relatively flat and having a broad base) are much more likely to be malignant. Ulceration is somewhat suggestive of malignancy, but may occur in either kind. Within the tissues, the tumor may have a distinct fibrous capsule. Such a tumor is probably benign. In the process of removal, the well-encapsulated, benign tumor may "shell out," like peas from the pod, leaving the smooth inner lining of the capsule. The physical examination should, of course, include careful examination for metastases in the regional lymph nodes and other accessible sites.

When tumors are encountered in such organs as lungs, liver, kidney and spleen, the question arises whether they are **primary or metastatic.** The form of the growth is usually very significant. Primary neoplasms are seldom regular in shape or smooth in outline. Metastatic growths, though obviously malignant, grow largely by expansion and produce a more or less spherical tumor. If more than one are present, one recalls the extreme improbability of several similar primary tumors developing in the same organ at the same time. If more than one organ is involved some, perhaps all, of the growths are metastatic.

Grading.—As a means of facilitating the conveyance to the clinician of the pathologist's estimate of the degree of malignancy of a given tumor, a system of grading has come into common use for neoplasms of certain kinds, particularly squamous-cell carcinomas and adenocarcinomas. Grade 1 applies to a squamous-cell tumor whose epithelium is well differentiated into the layers characteristic of normal epithelium; germinal layer, spinous-cell layer, and cornified layer, if the tumor is the cornifying kind. In the case of an adenocarcinoma, the glandular acini are well formed and rather uniform in size and shape, although their epithelial lining may have several reduplicated layers. Grades 2 and 3 resemble the normal tissue of origin less and less, with grade 4 representing an adenocarcinoma which scarcely forms any recognizable glandular structures at all, or a carcinoma whose large, round cells have become so undifferentiated and embryonal in morphology that it may be difficult to decide even whether the tumor is a carcinoma or a sarcoma.

Carcinomas of grade 1 obviously have the lowest malignancy, grow rather slowly and metastasize late or perhaps not at all. The other grades increase successively in malignancy, rapidity of growth, invasiveness and tendency to metastasize. The chances of complete, surgical removal of tumors of grade 4, even when taken early, are far from favorable. The more anaplastic cells of grades 3 and 4 are, however, highly susceptible to the destructive effects of roentgen rays or other forms of irradiation, so that the hope of improvement or cure by these means is much better than it is for grades 2 and 1. Against the latter, irradiation is of little effect for the tumor cells are scarcely more vulnerable than the normal tissues.

While grading is useful as a scale or code of measurement, it has decided limitations because of the variations that frequently exist in different parts of the same tumor. No hard and fast rule can be formulated for treatment on the basis of grade; each case must be handled as an individual problem and the use of modifying adjectives or grades are of value only when they convey some information between the pathologist and clinician.

CAUSES OF NEOPLASMS

Although much has been learned about the nature of neoplasms, no unifying theory has yet been established to explain the exact etiology of all neoplastic diseases in man or animals. Mechanisms at the molecular level which control the growth and multiplication of cells are now in some respects defined but not yet thoroughly understood. These will be referred to later. We shall review some historical concepts of the causes and nature of "cancer" and take up present-day theories after the older ideas are considered.

The earlier students of neoplasia noticed that in their microscopic appearance most neoplastic cells were remarkably similar to their embryonal predecessors, and were inclined to view this feature in a causative light. They found on rare occasions neoplasms developing from islands of unmatured and undifferentiated tissues or even what appeared to be tissues which should have formed one organ but were entrapped within another. The best example was the supposed inclusion within the kidney of tissue which, on the basis of similarity, should have been a part of the adrenal, the tumor being the well-known hypernephroma. From such as these, they postulated fetal misplacements, fetal rests and fetal inclusions as causes of neoplasms, **Cohnheim's theory of fetal residues.** A pronounced form of such misplacement of embryonal tissues is the teratoma (p. 270), a slowly enlarging mass containing several histological types of tissue. Such disorders of embryonal and fetal development do occur, areas of persistent embryonal tissue not being altogether rare in the young. The incidence of active neoplasia in such areas appears to be high, but it is by no means universal and direct causal relationship is no longer credited.

Chronic Irritation.—This came to occupy a prominent place in theories which were prevalent for many years, Virchow being one of its leading proponents. It was early observed that severe burns were likely to be superseded years later by squamous-cell carcinoma. Such burns heal very slowly and with difficulty. It is easy to reason that the earlier attempts at healing are frustrated by inability of newly proliferated epithelial cells to survive under conditions of poor blood supply and external trauma, and that the process is successful only after a race of extremely prolific cells has been developed by natural selection and survival of the fittest through many generations. Such a race of cells might well be conceived as having acquired in this way the faculty of rapid and uncontrolled growth which is characteristic of neoplasia. It was, however, difficult to explain the delay of years which often intervened between apparently successful healing of the burn and the appearance of the neoplasm. A comparable lesion occurs in cattle which have been branded by application of a burning-hot iron to the skin. A proliferative epithelial growth occasionally develops at the site and rarely becomes carcinomatous, the so-called brand-cancer.

It was observed that among the people of Khurdistan, India, carcinoma of the skin of the anterior abdominal wall is frequent, although almost unknown in other races and nationalities. These people have a custom of carrying a pot filled with live coals or hot stones resting on the anterior belly wall. A causative relationship seemed obvious, apparently in terms of heat and pressure.

A generation ago, when pipe-smoking was much commoner among men than it is in the present "cigarette age" and when smoking among women was incompatible with respectability and almost unknown, carcinoma of the lip, known as "pipe-smoker's cancer," was many times more frequent in men than in women. The man usually had a favorite position in which the pipe was held, the carcinoma developing where the stem rested against the lip. Chronic irritation from heat and pressure were strongly suspected of having a causative effect.

When large chimneys used to be cleaned by men descending into them while heat and smoke were still rising from a smouldering fire, these "chimney-sweeps" had a high incidence of carcinoma of the scrotal skin, which is almost unknown in other men. Irritation from the rising heat and fumes was considered responsible. We know nowadays that specific carcinogens, such as will presently be described, were present in the smoke.

The incidence of cutaneous neoplasms on the feet and legs appears to be much higher among bare-foot peoples than in the races whose feet usually are clad. At least such were the findings of Vos (1936) who reported 33.4 per cent of all cutaneous carcinomas and 82.5 per cent of malignant melanomas were on the feet or legs of Javanese natives, the corresponding figures in Holland being 0.7 per cent and 22.5 respectively. Whether the feet and legs were exposed to any other irritant than physical trauma would be a matter for speculation.

No corresponding observations on animals have been compiled, but against the theory that ordinary mechanical injury, even though persistently repeated, is a cause of neoplasia is the experience with millions of horses that have been used as draft animals. Injury and chronic ulcerated areas from pressure of the collar were unfortunately everyday occurrences in the days of horse-drawn implements and vehicles, but neoplasia at that site remained practically unknown.

The present tendency is to eliminate ordinary physical injury as a cause of neoplasia, but the same may not be said of certain other factors in the local environment.

Actinic Light Rays.—These may be considered among the environmental irritants. It is generally accepted that exposure to sunlight is responsible for the fact that as many as 90 per cent of human cutaneous tumors are on the unclothed parts of the body. The backs of the hands of many outdoor workers show areas of hyperkeratosis and hyperpigmentation which, in a certain number of instances, go on to carcinogenesis; statistics also show such neoplasms to be noticeably more frequent in the sun-drenched Southwest than in the more somber parts of the United States. Statistically a similar situation exists in cattle with respect to carcinomas of the ocular and periocular tissues; they are much more prevalent in the Southwest. There is little doubt that the brilliant sunlight bears some responsibility for this, although some place importance on a possible hereditary tendency in the breeds and families prevalent in the area. There is no reason to suppose that photosensitization (p. 77) is concerned in this situation.

In humans there is a rare disease, hereditarily recessive, called xeroderma pigmentosum (a pigmented, dry skin), in which, due to a great sensitivity to light, a dermatitis terminating in fatal carcinomatosis is inescapable before more than a few years of life have passed.

Experimental confirmation of the carcinogenic effects of light, particularly of ultraviolet light, is rather extensive.

Irradiation.—Roentgen rays are notorious for their carcinogenic effect when total exposure to them is excessive over an extended period of time, as in x-ray technicians, who, in the early history of roentgenology, worked without protective clothing or other safety devices. Ample experimental studies have confirmed these clinical observations. There is a chronic dermatitis, then ulceration and finally some of the ulcers develop into carcinomas, the whole process usually requiring several years.

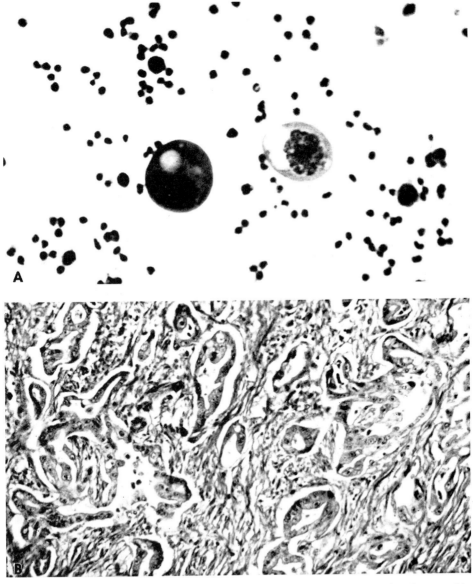

Fig. 7–57.—Adenocarcinoma of the cecum of a fourteen-year-old castrated male cat, with metastases to diaphragm, abdominal wall, liver and spleen. *A*, Smear of ascitic fluid containing large malignant cells, Giemsa's stain (× 400). *B*, Section of metastatic tumor in diaphragm. H & E (× 250). (Courtesy of Angell Memorial Animal Hospital.)

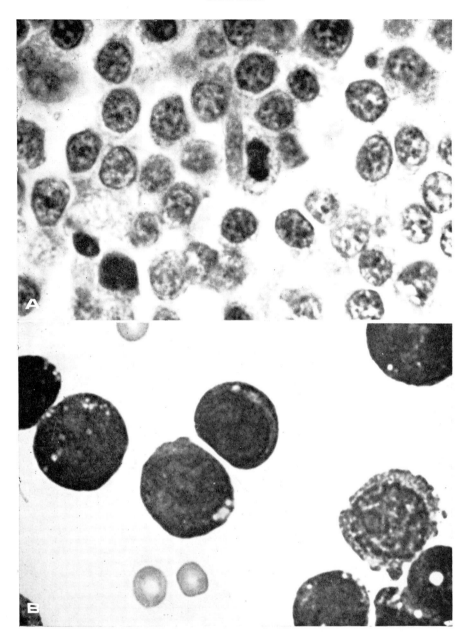

Fig. 7–58.—Malignant lymphoma involving pleura of a cat. *A*, Section of pleura, H & E (× 1600). *B*, Smear of fluid aspirated from pleural cavity. Wright-Giemsa's stain (× 1600). Note the apparent difference in the size of the tumor cells prepared by sectioning and smear techniques.

Radium and thorium, when accidentally or experimentally introduced into the body, localize in the bone and produce a chronic osteitis in which osteosarcoma supervenes. The first knowledge of this fact came when it was found, as reported by Martland (1931), that persons engaged in painting a radioactive preparation on watch dials to make them luminous, died of osteogenic sarcoma a few years later. The effects of the newer radio-active substances (uranium, cobalt, etc.) may prove to be similar. A number of years is always necessary before the carcino-genic effects of these various forms of energy become apparent.

Parasites.—As agents setting up irritation which may lead to neoplasia, para-sites deserve some attention. Bilharziasis, better known as schistosomiasis (*Schistosoma hematobium*), has been considered a cause of carcinoma of the human bladder, especially since the two conditions occur together and the incidence of carcinoma of the bladder is high in those populations (Egypt) which are heavily parasitized. The blood flukes produce considerable cystitis of a chronic nature, but they are not universally accepted as causing the neoplasms.

The small nematode *Gongylonema* (*Spiroptera*) *neoplasticum*, parasitizing the wall of the rat's stomach, occasions the development of carcinoma or a carcinoma-like proliferation of the gastric mucosa. The tumors were produced experimen-tally by Fibiger (1914) and what he considered pulmonary metastases occurred in some cases. More recently some other plausible explanations have been offered for the pulmonary growths, causing some doubt that the gastric tumors were really no more than inflammatory hyperplasia similar to that occurring in coccidiosis of the rabbit's gallbladder. There is also evidence that deficiency of vitamin A may have been an important factor in production of these hyperplasias (Hitchcock and Bell, 1952).

Cysticercus fasciolaris, the cystic, or larval, stage of the tapeworm of the cat, *Tænia crassicolis* (*tæniæformis*), developing in the liver of rats, either naturally or experimentally, results in what some consider true sarcomatous proliferation of the connective tissue which surrounds the parasitic cysts (Bullock and Curtis, 1920; Dunning and Curtis, 1939, 1946).

In the dog, a nematode which is rather common in warm countries, *Spirocerca lupi*, invades the wall of the lower esophagus. One or more worms are often found at the center of a spheroidal fibrous tumor 1 or 2 cm. in diameter. These tumors, obviously resulting from the worm's presence, usually have the histologic structure of fibrosarcomas or osteosarcomas (metaplasia of fibrous tissue to bone). They commonly form a large mass extending into the mediastinal tissue and ul-cerating on the esophageal surface. A number of them have been reported as metastasizing to the lungs (Seibold, *et al.*, 1955) and other viscera. The evidence that the embedded worms have a causal relationship appears incontrovertible.

The occurrence of true neoplasia in connection with metazoan parasites is thus an apparent fact at present. If true carcinogenic effect is present we do not know whether it is physical or chemical.

Chemical Carcinogens.—While the chimney-sweep's cancer mentioned pre-viously was described as early as 1775, the carcinogenic nature of soot and gaseous products of combustion was at that time unknown. As tars and oils found more uses in our industrial age, the suspicion arose that neoplasms might result from contact with them. A number of persons attempted to demonstrate this experi-mentally. Two Japanese, Yamagiwa and Ichikawa, finally succeeded in produc-ing cutaneous papillomas and carcinomas in the ears of rabbits after repeated applications of tar throughout a period of many months. Many similar experi-ments by various researchers brought out the fact that mice are readily suscep-tible to "tar cancer," rabbits somewhat less so, the other common laboratory animals being refractory. Chemists naturally set out to discover the exact com-pounds or radicals which exert the carcinogenic effect. A very considerable num-ber of such substances are now known. Nearly all of them are hydrocarbons, not necessarily obtainable from tar but not altogether unrelated to some of its components. The first chemically pure hydrocarbons found to be carcinogenic were derivatives of 1:2-benzanthracene, such as 1:2:5:6-dibenzanthracene, the most powerful being 9:10-dimethyl-1:2-benzanthracene:

Another outstanding carcinogenic derivative is methylcholanthrene:

This substance has been directly synthesized and has also been prepared from cholic and desoxycholic acids of bile. This and the fact that desoxycholic acid itself has shown some carcinogenic effect have led to the suspicion that carcinogenic substances of similar composition may possibly be formed in animal tissues.

In general, chemical carcinogens produce carcinomas when applied externally to the epidermis, sarcomas when introduced into the connective tissues and, not infrequently, their introduction into an internal organ results in a special type of neoplasm derived from certain tissues of that organ. However, the relative susceptibility or resistance of the various tissues is a factor, and under some circumstances a carcinogenic substance causes neoplasia of a certain organ regardless of where or how it is introduced into the body. This is illustrated by the work of Orr (1943), who regularly produced carcinomas of the mammary glands of suitably susceptible mice by applying the carcinogen to the nasal mucosa. A few types of carcinogen appear to have a positive predilection for a particular organ or tissue, as, for instance, o-aminoazotoluene (used for dying leather) and other azo-compounds, which produce epithelial tumors of the liver when introduced in a variety of ways. On the other hand, the type of tumor produced sometimes appears to vary with the species of experimental animal, as in the work of Rigdon (1952), who produced cutaneous hemangiomas by the local application of methyl-cholanthrene to the skin of ducks, but obtained carcinomas when chickens were given the same treatment. All these differences are probably dependent on variations in susceptibility, which will be discussed shortly.

Hormones.—Some investigators have been impressed by the similarity of the structural formulas of the carcinogenic hydrocarbons, such as benzanthracene and cholanthrene, to those of certain hormones produced in the body, particularly ovarian follicular estrogens, progesterone of the corpus luteum, testosterone of the testis and the corticosterones of the adrenal, and have theorized that disordered metabolism of these hormones may result in their transformation into carcinogenic compounds. There is no real evidence that this happens, however, and the similarity of the formulas would appear to be no greater than that which exists between various carcinogenic and noncarcinogenic members of the anthracene or benzpyrene groups themselves.

The chemical relationship between the carcinogenic hydrocarbons and the bile acids has been mentioned. Here, again, any spontaneous transformation into carcinogenic substances remains hypothetical.

Limited experimentation has been reported on the production of neoplasms by the administration of massive doses of the estrogenic hormones. It appears that such hormones are able to induce hyperplastic and even neoplastic growth of the interstitial cells of the testes of mice. There are reports of similar effects in other organs normally under hormonal control, such as the prostate and the uterus, but these are not unequivocal. It is only in the mammary gland that estrogen-induced neoplasms, usually adenocarcinomas, are well established. These have been shown to occur in mice of susceptible strains, usually preceded by cystic glandular hyperplasia comparable to the "chronic cystic mastitis" thought to predispose the human gland to neoplasia.

Heredity.—The vast amount of experimentation on this aspect of neoplasia, chiefly in mice, has shown that whether one of the recognized carcinogens actually produces a tumor depends on the relative susceptibility not only of the individual, but of the organ or tissue in question. The susceptibility or the lack of it is transmitted from one generation to the next. For instance, certain strains of mice are highly susceptible to carcinoma of the skin, but resistant to other types. Other strains have been bred which have a high susceptibility to mammary adeno-carcinoma. Some families have a high resistance to all forms. These characteristics are thus to be considered hereditary although neoplasms, themselves, are not inherited.

Practically no data are available on the possible inheritance of susceptibility or resistance in the domestic animals, although there is evidence which leads some to believe in an inherited susceptibility to ocular (corneal or conjunctival) carcinoma in certain families of the Hereford breed. Human pedigrees are too short and medical histories too fragmentary to offer any general assistance on this point. There are, however, a few striking instances where a given tumor has reappeared in members of the same family with the most extraordinary frequency. There are also cases where both monozygous twins, although living under entirely different environments, have developed the same malignant tumor at almost the same age. It has also been shown that a person or animal with one tumor has a considerably more than average likelihood of acquiring some other of different type. This fact is obviously susceptible of more than one interpretation.

It has proved possible to breed a strain of mice 80 per cent of whose members develop carcinoma of the mammary gland. But if the newborn mice are placed on foster mothers of a resistant strain and not allowed to suckle their own mothers very few mammary tumors develop in them. Thus it was shown that high incidence of mammary cancer is, at least partly, due to some substance in the milk. This substance (so-called milk factor), be it hormone, virus or some more ordinary chemical component, is found also in the neoplastic tissue.

Oncogenic Viruses.—It has been known since 1908 that extracts of animal tumors, filtered to be free of cells and bacteria, were capable of inducing new tumors upon injection into a suitable host. The first such demonstration of a tumor-inducing (oncogenic) virus in avian leukosis, was the work of two Danish veterinarians, Ellermann and Bang. Rous, in 1910, produced similar results with the fowl (Rous) sarcoma. These demonstrations of viral-associated neoplasms have been followed over the years by many others, as outlined in Table 7-1. The evidence is overwhelming therefore that certain viruses can cause tumors in birds, invertebrates and mammals. Incontrovertible proof is only lacking in man because of the difficulties and proscriptions in experimenting with the human species.

The reluctance to accept the role of viruses as predominant in the etiology of neoplasms has in part been caused by the lack of a unifying theory which would explain the occurrence of tumors as the result of trauma, ultraviolet or x-irradiation, chemical carcinogens, etc., in the absence of a demonstrable virus. During the past few years, great strides have been made toward understanding the intracellular events leading to neoplasia but the exact mechanisms, at this writing, are still unknown.

Fundamental to the understanding of virus and cell interactions is the fact that genetic control of all cell processes and transmission of information to successive generations is determined by the deoxyribonucleic acid (DNA) and ribonucleic acid (RNA) in the cell (p. 318). Viruses are now known to contain a "core" of DNA or RNA, usually coated by a protein. Viral DNA or RNA may differ from cellular DNA or RNA only by the sequence of the nucleotides (base pairs) along the length of the molecule, or perhaps the acutal length of the viral molecule may be different (p. 507). It appears likely that viral DNA or RNA may become incorporated in the DNA or RNA of cells and may influence the processes controlled by the cellular genome. (The genome includes all the genetic material in the cell.) The incorporation of viral DNA into the genome of a cell may be the means of transforming a normal to a neoplastic cell and may explain why viruses

Table 7-1.—Viral-Induced Neoplasms

Year	Species	Type of Neoplasms	Author	Page
1908	Chicken	Fowl leukosis	Ellermann & Bang	517
1910	Chicken	Fowl sarcoma	Rous	520
1920	Cow	Bovine papilloma	Magalhaes	508
1932	Dog	Oral papilloma	DeMonbreun & Goodpasture	512
1932	Rabbit	Fibroma	Shope	516
1933	Rabbit	Cutaneous papilloma	Shope	513
1933	Chicken	Lymphomatosis, myelomatosis	Furth	518
1936	Rabbit	Oral papilloma	Parsons & Kidd	514
1936	Mouse	Mammary adenocarcinoma	Bittner	523
1938	Frog	Renal adenocarcinoma	Lucké	524
1951	Horse	Cutaneous papilloma	Cook & Olson	512
1951	Mouse	Malignant lymphoma	Gross	523
1953	Mouse	Tumor of parotid gland	Gross	283
1953	Squirrel	Fibroma	Kilham, Herman & Fisher	283
1954	Goat	Cutaneous papilloma	Moulton	283
1955	Deer	Fibroma	Shope, et al.	284
1956	Mouse	Leukemia	Friend	283
1957	Mouse, hamster	Polyoma	Stewart & Eddy	524
1964	Cat	Malignant lymphoma	Jarrett, et al.	521
1966	Mouse	Osteosarcoma	Finkel, Biskis & Jinkins	283
1967	Guinea pig	Malignant lymphoma	Opler	523
1969	Simian primates	Malignant lymphoma	Melendez, Hunt, et al.	523

which apparently initiate neoplastic growth are at times later "masked" and cannot be recovered from the tumor cell.

One of the *in vitro* demonstrations of the effect of oncogenic viruses is accomplished by introducing them into certain cultures of tissues. Two general effects are produced by these viruses—one is to cause dissolution of the cells and replication of the virus, the other is to transform the growth pattern of the cells. This **transformation** results in more luxuriant and less controlled growth of the cells in tissue cultures. This phenomenon resembles malignant transformation (neoplasia).

The details of this fascinating field of viral oncogenesis and the control of intracellular activities are outside the scope of this book. Additional reading may start with the references to follow.

Viral-Induced Neoplasms

BITTNER, J. J.: Some Possible Effects of Nursing on the Mammary Gland Tumor Incidence in Mice. Science *84*:162, 1936.
COOK, R. H., and OLSON, C., JR.: Experimental Transmission of Cutaneous Papilloma of the Horse. Amer. J. Path. *27*:1087–1097, 1951.
DEMONBREUN, W. A., and GOODPASTURE, E. W.: Infectious Oral Papillomatosis of Dogs. Amer. J. Path. *8*:43–56, 1932.
DULBECCO, R.: Viruses in Carcinogenesis. Ann. Intern Med. *70*:1019–1029, 1969.
DULBECCO, R.: Cell Transformation by Viruses. Science *166*:962–968, 1969.
ELLERMANN, V., and BANG, O.: Experimentelle leukäemie bei Hühnern. Centralbl. f. Bakt. *46*:595–609, 1908.
FINKEL, M. P., BISKIS, B. O., and JINKINS, P. B.: "Virus Inducton of Osteosarcomas in Mice." Science *151*:689–701, 1966.
FRIEND, C.: Cell-free Transmission in Adult Swiss Mice of a Disease Having the Character of a Leukemia. J. Exper. Med. *105*:307–318, 1967.
FURTH, J.: Observations with a New Transmissible Strain of the Leucosis (Leucemia) of Fowls. J. Exp. Med. *53*:243–267, 1931.
————: Lymphomatosis, Myelomatosis and Endothelioma of Chickens Caused by a Filterable Agent. 1. Transmission Experiments. J. Exp. Med. *58*:253–275, 1933.
GROSS, L.: "Spontaneous" Leukemia Developing in C3H Mice Following Inoculation, in Infancy, with AK-leukemic Extracts, or AK-embryos. Proc. Soc. Exp. Biol. & Med. *76*: 27–32, 1951.
————: A Filterable Agent Recovered from AK-leukemic Extracts Causing Salivary Gland Carcinomas in C3H Mice. Proc. Soc. Exp. Biol. & Med. *83*:414–421, 1953.
————: Viral Etiology of "Spontaneous" Mouse Leukemia: A Review. Cancer Res. *18*:371–381, 1958.
HABEL, K.: Tumor Viruses. Yale J. Biol. & Med. *37*:473–486, 1965.
HUEBNER, R. J., and TODARO, G. G.: Oncogenes of RNA Tumor Viruses as Determinants of Cancer. Proc. Nat. Acad. Sci. *64*:1087–1094, 1969.
JARRETT, W. F. H., *et al.*: Leukemia in the Cat. Transmission Experiments with Leukemia (Lymphosarcoma). Nature *202*:566–568, 1964.
KILHAM, L., HERMAN, C. M., and FISHER, E. R.: Naturally Occurring Fibromas of Grey Squirrels Related to Shope's Rabbit Fibroma. Proc. Exp. Biol. & Med. *82*:298–301, 1953.
LUCKÉ, B.: Carcinoma in the Leopard Frog. Its Probable Causation by a Virus. J. Exp. Med. *68*:457–468, 1938.
MAGALHAES, O.: Warts in Cattle. Brazil-Med. *34*:430, 1920.
MELENDEZ, L. V., *et al.*: Herpesvirus Saimiri. II. Experimentally Induced Malignant Lymphoma in Primates. Lab. Anim. Care *19*:378–386, 1969.
MOULTON, J. E.: Cutaneous Papillomas on the Udders of Milk Goats. North Amer. Vet. *35*:29–33, 1954.
OPLER, S. R.: Observations on a New Virus Associated with Guinea Pig Leukemia: Preliminary Note. J. Nat. Cancer Inst. *38*:797–800, 1967.
PARSONS, R. J., and KIDD, J. G.: Oral Papillomatosis of Rabbits. A Virus Disease. J. Exp. Med. *77*:233–250, 1943.
ROUS, P.: A Transmissible Avian Neoplasm (Sarcoma of the Common Fowl). J. Exp. Med. *12*:697–705, 1910.

Shope, R. E.:   Infectious Papillomatosis of Rabbits.   J. Exp. Med. *58*:607–624, 1933.
————————:   A Transmissible Tumor-like Condition in Rabbits.   J. Exp. Med. *56*:793-802, 1932.
————————:   An Infectious Fibroma of Deer.   Proc. Soc. Exp. Biol. & Med. *88*:533–535, 1955.
Stewart, S. E., *et al.*:   The Induction of Neoplasms with a Substance Released from Mouse Tumors by Tissue Culture.   Virology *3*:380–400, 1957.
Syverton, J. T.:   Present Status of Studies on Tumor-producing Viruses.   Nat. Cancer Inst. Mono. No. 4, 345–353, 1959.

Summarizing, it seems safe to say that some neoplasms arise in cells whose embryonal life was in some way distorted, as by displacement or by ill-timed mitosis, but that, wherever they originate, all neoplasms depend upon some stimulus to initiate the change from normal to uncontrolled reproduction. A number of chemical and physical agents are able to instigate this reproductive change but a pre-existing, and often dormant, susceptibility is an important, and probably decisive, prerequisite to their effective action. This susceptibility is a characteristic of species and of families, as well as of individuals; hence, it must be presumed to have been passed from parents to offspring. This transmission is assumed to be by the ordinary processes of heredity, dependent on some change in those rather ephemeral constituents of nuclear material called genes. The assumption of ordinary heredity is, however, placed in serious jeopardy by the discovery that, in one instance, at least, the transmission occurs only through the mother's milk or through the intimate association incident to nursing.

Furthermore, while neoplasia represents a single pathological phenomenon, the susceptibility essential for a neoplasm to develop is not universal either with respect to all the different kinds of neoplasms or with regard to all the different tissues or parts of the body which might be involved. If neoplasms can be judged by the experimentally demonstrable susceptibility or resistance to them, can we not almost borrow the terminology of the bacteriologists and virologists and say that various neoplasms are, at least to a considerable extent, "immunologically distinct"? Indeed, it becomes more and more apparent that, while neoplasia, like inflammation, is a unique phenomenon, we possibly have, on an etiological basis, almost as many kinds of neoplastic disease as we have inflammatory.

Since susceptibility, or the lack of it, is a characteristic of each tissue or part of the body, is it not fair to conclude that susceptibility or resistance resides in the cell, a situation analogous to cellular immunity and cellular hypersensitivity? Perhaps this brings us back to some change in the genes, previously mentioned. Genes are said to consist of desoxyribonucleic acid and to have close chemical relationship to nucleoproteins constituting both enzymes and viruses. Perhaps when we know more about the chemical nature of viruses, enzymes and genes, all of which are self-perpetuating living substances, it will be easy to understand how a virus-like living substance gains entrance to body cells, becomes a part of their hereditary make-up and, with or without the aid of a suitable external stimulus, introduces a change in the enzymatic functions of the cell which permits continuous and uninhibited growth and reproduction!

An aspect of neoplasia that is attracting more and more attention is that of the delay commonly involved between the patient's first contact with a carcinogenic environment and the appearance of the tumor. As stated above, rabbits and mice develop carcinomas following the application of carcinogenic substances, but only after the lapse of an interval of time which constitutes a considerable portion of their life-span. In most experiments the carcinogen has been repeatedly applied through all or much of this interval. It is unusual, although not unknown, for a neoplasm to follow a single exposure to a carcinogenic agent. This is the opposite of the outcome of a single exposure to an ordinary pathogenic virus or bacterium, although in the case of tuberculosis and some other chronic granulomatous infections there is evidence suggesting that the disease develops most readily after there has been a previous sensitizing exposure. The roentgenologist develops carcinoma—or lymphoma—but only years after his first exposure, during which time he has usually continued to suffer further exposure.

We could continue with other illustrations of the principle that the action of carcinogenic agents is not immediate. Several explanations of this observed fact have been enunciated. One, not currently stressed but by no means disproved, is that the appearance of the neoplasm awaits the arrival of the "cancer age" of the individual, say the fifth decade in humans. At that age some change in the situation of the body cells, possibly a degeneration or weakening of normal biological control of cell multiplication, would presumably permit those watching, waiting tumorously inclined inhabitants to arise and have their way. Certainly the concept of a bodily resistance to uncontrolled reproductive processes, which might wax and wane, needs to be kept always in our consciousness as we ponder over this, the greatest biological problem of mankind. That a resistance or defense mechanism, which probably resides in the gamma-globulin, is indeed a reality is indicated, for instance, by the work of Reyniers and Sacksteder (1959). They were able to transmit an artificially induced tumor from one germ-free (raised without access of any microorganisms) chicken to another but not from an ordinary germ-infected one to another. However, the ("conventional") germ-infected chickens could be made susceptible by feeding antibiotics.

A second explanation offered for the delay in development of neoplasia following an inciting exposure is that this disease, like infectious diseases, has an "incubation period," in the case of neoplasia a very long one. It is easy to accept this proposal since we are already accustomed to it in connection with infections, but proof is lacking.

A third theory, which is receiving serious consideration at the present time, is that of a neoplastic "threshold" which must be crossed. Just as a very definite threshold of toleration in the blood must be crossed in diabetes before sugar appears in the urine, so it may be that a certain level of carcinogenic power must be built up before the process actually appears. Whether this would be essentially different from a weakening of resistance as mentioned above we are hardly able to speculate at this time. Certainly it would seem that the threshold to be crossed must reside in the individual cell for it is fundamental that the phenomenon of neoplastic change is highly localized. At any rate, the idea is, for example, that you might have received a certain amount of carcinogenic activity, say quantity X, from an endocrine imbalance. Then you get quantity Y from a certain mild radioactivity to which you are exposed. X and Y are additive but you are all right until you get quantity Z of some known or unknown carcinogenic substance, say from eating pesticide-treated cranberries or inhaling irritant gases. If X plus Y plus Z add up to a figure above the threshold, neoplasia develops in the least resistant or most susceptible group of cells. But, cheer up, tobacco-loving friends; Whatever may be the exact truth about cigarettes and lung cancer, you may have a chance. Perhaps your fate is not already prematurely sealed. Perhaps you have not crossed the threshold. It is upon such premises that much is presently being done toward the elimination of suspected carcinogenic substances. The results will bear watching.

Resistance to Neoplasia.—Why does one patient develop a neoplasm and another similar patient escape that fate? Preceding paragraphs have carried the implication, at least, of susceptibility to neoplasms or to the carcinogens that cause them (p. 275). In the light of everyday experience it is difficult not to conclude that different individuals vary in susceptibility either to particular forms of neoplasms or to the phenomenon in general. Certainly some animal species are susceptible to neoplasms of given types, while others are not. If, indeed, neoplasia is inherited, it is the state of susceptibility that is inherited, not the neoplasm itself.

What is the difference between susceptibility and lack of resistance? Or what is the difference between resistance and lack of susceptibility? In general, the answers are largely unknown. But we do know that the body is able to offer resistance to a neoplasm. How much unseen resistance of humoral or intracellular nature there may be is largely speculative but, to a variable extent, there are demonstrable cellular reactions to a developing neoplasm. The most frequently recognized reaction is fibrous encapsulation (p. 165) which is attempted with many of the benign growths. This reaction is essentially similar to that which helps confine many of the infectious granulomas.

Infiltrations of lymphocytes occur in and around many tumors, and statistical studies have shown longer survival time when these occur. Regional lymph nodes may be hyperplastic with increased lymphoid tissue and more than the usual complement of germinal (now often called "reactive") centers, or their lymph sinuses may be distended with lymph and extensive accumulations of large (reticuloendothelial) histiocytes. Black, Opler and Speer (1954) have made extensive studies of histiocytic and hyperplastic reactions in lymph nodes regional to both mammary and gastric carcinomas in humans and have found the destructive action of both these forms of cancer to be strongly retarded or inhibited when these reactions were pronounced. In many instances the tumors themselves were also markedly infiltrated with lymphocytes.

THE FREQUENCY OF NEOPLASMS

A knowledge of "what kind of tumor occurs where and how often" not only satisfies a natural scientific curiosity, but is essential to studies of many sorts dealing with etiology and possible prevention. Unfortunately precise information of this kind is not easy to obtain. Some of our best works on animal neoplasms have dealt with frequency of occurrence in a general way without giving figures susceptible of precise tabulation and analysis. Certain variations in terminology and interpretation have been in vogue over the years and in some instances have rendered one author's report scarcely comparable with another's, not to mention the doubts that have existed in all our minds concerning some of the more difficult classifications.

Although it is interesting to know which histologic types are found in a large series of neoplasms collected over the years at a clinic or hospital, this does not lead to data which are useful to study the frequency of particular tumors. In order to have information of value to determine rate of occurrence, the population from which the neoplasms came must be carefully and thoroughly defined. Only such data are of value in comparing trends under varying conditions. A few studies have been made of animals in which adequate laboratory identification of the neoplasms were combined with sound epidemiologic methods. Examples of studies which consider the epizootiologic aspects of neoplasia are found in the reports of Dorn, *et al.*, 1966 and 1968; Anderson, *et al.*, 1969 and Zaldivar, 1967. The kinds of tumors and their order of frequency in a specific organ or system are discussed further in Chapters 19 through 29.

Neoplasia—General References

ANDERSON, L. J., and SANDISON, A. T.: Tumours of Connective Tissues in Cattle, Sheep and Pigs. J. Path. *98*:253–263, 1969.

ANDERSON, L. J., SANDISON, A. T., and JARRETT, W. F. H.: A British Abattoir Survey of Tumours in Cattle, Sheep and Pigs. Vet. Rec. *84*:547–551, 1969.

ANDERVONT, H. B., and DUNN, T. B.: Occurrence of Tumors in Wild House Mice. J. Nat. Cancer Inst. *28*:1153–1163, 1962.

BLOCK, M. M., OPLER, S. R., and SPEER, F. D.: Microscopic Structure of Gastric Carcinomas and their Regional Lymph Nodes in Relation to Survival. Surg., Gyn., & Obstet. *98*: 725–734, 1954.

BULLOCK, F. D., and CURTIS, M. R.: Experimental Production of Sarcoma of the Liver of the Rat. Proc. N. Y. Path. Soc. N.S. *20*:149–175, 1920.

CHAPMAN, W. L., JR., and ALLEN, J. R.: Multiple Neoplasia in a Rhesus Monkey, *Macaca mulatta*. Path. Vet. *5*:342–352, 1968.

CHESTERMAN, F. C., and POMERANCE, A.: Spontaneous Neoplasms in Ferrets and Polecats. J. Path. Bact. *89*:529–533, 1965.

DAVIS, C. L., LEEPER, R. B., and SHELTON, J. E.: Neoplasms Encountered in Federally Inspected Establishments in Denver, Colorado. J. Amer. Vet. Med. Assn. *83*:229–237, 1933.

DORN, C. R., *et al.*: The Prevalence of Spontaneous Neoplasms in a Defined Canine Population. Amer. J. Pub. Hlth. *56*:254–265, 1966.

DORN, C. R., *et al.*: Survey of Animal Neoplasms in Alameda and Contra Costa Counties, California. I. Methodology and Description of Cases. J. Nat. Cancer. Inst. *40*:295–305, 1968.

DORN, C. R., *et al.*: Survey of Animal Neoplasms in Alameda and Contra Costa Counties, California. II. Cancer Morbidity in Dogs and Cats from Alameda County. J. Nat. Cancer Inst. *40*:307–318, 1968.

FELDMAN, W. H.: *Neoplasms of Domesticated Animals* Philadelphia, W. B. Saunders Co., 1932.

FIBIGER, J.: Weitere Untersuchungen uber das Spiropteracarcinom der Ratte. Ztschr. f. Krebsforsch. *14*:295–326, 1914.

HARVEY, W. F., DAWSON, E. K., and INNES, J. R. M.: Debatable Tumors in Human and Animal Pathology. Edinburgh M. J. *45*:275–284, 1938, and *46*:256–266, 1939.

JACKSON, C.: Incidence and Pathology of Tumors of Domesticated Animals in South Africa. Onderstepoort. J. Vet. Sci. *6*:3–460, 1936.

LILLIE, R. D.: *Histopathologic Technique.* Philadelphia, Blakiston Co., 1947.

KENT, S. P.: Spontaneous and Induced Malignant Neoplasms in Monkeys. Ann. New York Acad. Sci. *85*:819–827, 1960.

KOVACS, A. B., and SOMOGYVÁRI, K.: (Incidence of Tumours in Domestic Animals): Data from the Budapest Veterinary School for the Past 50 Years. Magy. Allatorv. Lap. *23*: 460–463, 1968. V.B. *39*:2132, 1969.

KROOK, L.: A Statistical Investigation of Carcinoma in the Dog. Acta Path. et Microbiol. Skand. *45*:407–422, 1954.

LOEB, W. F.: Leucyl Aminopeptidase Activity in Canine Neoplasia. Lab. Invest. *15*:1118–1119, 1966.

MAWDESLEY-THOMAS, L. B.: Neoplasia in Fish—a Bibliography. J. Fish Biol. *1*:187–207, 1969.

MEIER, H., *et al.*: Epizootiology of Cancer in Animals. Ann. New York Acad. Sci. *108*: 617–1326, 1963.

MISDORP, W.: Tumors in Newborn Animals. Path. Vet. *2*:328–343, 1965.

MONLUX, A. W., ANDERSON, W. A., and DAVIS, C. L.: A Survey of Tumors Occurring in Cattle, Sheep and Swine. Amer. J. Vet. Res. *17*:646–677, 1956.

MUGERA, G. M.: Canine and Feline Neoplasms in Kenya. Bull. Epizoot. Dis. Afr. *16*: 367–370, 1968. V.B. *39*:2610, 1969.

MURRAY, M.: Neoplasms of Domestic Animals in East Africa. Brit. Vet. J. *124*:514–524, 1968.

PAMUKCU, A. M.: An Annotation on the Occurrence of Tumours in Sheep. Brit. Vet. J. *112*:499–506, 1956.

PLUMMER, P. J. G.: A Survey of Six Hundred and Thirty-six Tumours from Domesticated Animals. Canad. J. Comp. Med. *20*:239–251, 1956.

RATCLIFFE, H. L.: Incidence and Nature of Tumors of Captive Wild Animals and Birds. Amer. J. Cancer. *17*:116–135, 1933.

REYNIERS, J. A., and SACKSTEDER, M. R.: Tumorigenesis and the Germfree Chicken. Ann. N.Y. Acad. Sci. *78*:328–353, 1959.

ROUS, P.: A Transmissible Avian Neoplasm (Sarcoma of the Common Fowl). J. Exper. Med. *12*:697–705, 1910.

————: The Virus Tumors and the Tumor Problem. Amer. J. Cancer *28*:233–272, 1936.

SCHARDEIN, J. L., FITZGERALD, J. E., and KAUMP, D. H.: Spontaneous Tumors in Holtzman Source Rats of Various Ages. Path. Vet. *5*:238–252, 1968.

WEBSTER, W. M.: Neoplasia in Food Animals with Special Reference to the High Incidence in Sheep. N. Z. Vet. J. *14*:203–214, 1966.

ZALDIVAR, R.: Incidence of Spontaneous Neoplasms in Beagles. J. Amer. Vet. Med. Assn. *151*:1319–1321, 1967.

Skin and Appendages

ADAMS, E. W., MOORE, E. G., and CARTER, L. P.: Canine Venereal Tumor: Biologically Active Deoxyribonucleic Acid from Canine Venereal Tumor. Amer. J. Vet. Res. *29*:1241–1244, 1968.

ALLEN, A. C.: So-called Mixed Tumors of the Mammary Gland of Dog and Man. Arch. Path. *29*:589–624, 1940.

BIGGS, R.: Comparison of Mixed Tumors of Human Breast and Mammary Gland of the Bitch. J. Path. & Bact. *59*:437–444, 1947.

BITTNER, J. J.: Possible Relationship of the Estrogenic Hormones, Genetic Susceptibility and Milk Influence in the Production of Mammary Cancer in Mice. Cancer Res. *2*:710–721, 1942.

BLOOM, F.: Spontaneous Solitary and Multiple Mast-cell Tumors in Dogs. Arch. Path. *33*:661–676, 1942.

BORLAND, R., and WEBBER, A. J.: An Electron Microscope Study of Squamous Cell Carcinoma in Merino Sheep Associated with Keratin-filled Cysts of the Skin. Cancer Res. *26*:172–182, 1966.

BURDIN, M. L.: Squamous-cell Carcinoma of the Vulva of Cattle in Kenya. Res. Vet. Sci. *5*:497–505, 1964.

COOPER, D. L.: Cylindroma; Report of an Unusually Extensive Case. J. Amer. Med. Assn. *132*:575–577, 1946.

COTCHIN, E.: Further Observations on Neoplasms in Dogs, with Particular Reference to Site of Origin and Malignancy. I. Cutaneous, Female Genital and Alimentary Systems. Brit. Vet. J. *110*:218–232, 1954.

————: Melanotic Tumours of Dogs. J. Comp. Path. *65*:115–129, 1955.

DAHME, E., and WEISS, E.: Zur systematik der mammatumoren des Hundes. Dtsch. tierarztl. Wschr. *65*:458–461, 1958.

DODD, D. C.: Mastocytoma of the Tongue of a Calf. Path. Vet. *1*:69–72, 1964.

DROMMER, W.: Submikroskopische untersuchungen am Basaliom des Hundes. Path. Vet. *5*:174–185, 1968.

DROMMER, W., and SCHULTZ, L.-CL.: Vergleichende licht-und electromen-mikroskopische Untersuchungen am übertragbaren venerischen Sarkom und Histiozytom des Hundes. Path. Vet. *6*:273–286, 1969.

FIDLER, I. J., and BRODEY, R. S.: A Necropsy Study of Canine Malignant Mammary Neoplasms. J. Am. Vet. Med. Assn. *151*:710–715, 1967.

————: The Biological Behavior of Canine Mammary Neoplasms. J. Am. Vet. Med. Assn. *151*:1311–1318, 1967.

FLATT, R. E., et al.: Pathogenesis of Benign Cutaneous Melanomas in Miniature Swine. J. Am. Vet. Med. Assn. *153*:936–941, 1968.

FOWLER, E. H., KASZA, L., and KOESTNER, A.: Enzyme Histochemical Comparison of the Canine Mastocytoma Cell *In Vivo* and *In Vitro*. Am. J. Vet. Res. *29*:853–862, 1968.

FUJIMOTO, Y., and OLSON, C.: The Fine Structure of the Bovine Wart. Path. Vet. *3*: 659–684, 1966.

GREENE, H. S. N.:   Familial Mammary Tumors in the Rabbit.   J. Exper. Med. 70:147–184, 1939.

GREVE, J. H., and MOSES, H. E.:   Histopathologic Changes in Xanthomatosis in Chickens. J. Am. Vet. Med. Assn. 139:1106–1110, 1961.

HOTTENDORF, G. H., and NIELSEN, S. W.:   Collagen Necrosis in Canine Mastocytomas. Amer. J. Path. 49:501–513, 1966.

HOTTENDORF, G. H., NIELSEN, S. W., and KENYON, A. J.:   Canine Mastocytoma.   I. Blood Coagulation Time in Dogs with Mastocytoma.   Path. Vet. 2:129–141, 1965.

HOTTENDORF, G. H., and NIELSEN, S. W.:   Pathologic Report of 29 Necropsies on Dogs with Mastocytoma.   Path. Vet. 5:102–121, 1968.

HOTTENDORF, G. H., NIELSEN, S. W., and KENYON, A. J.:   Ribonucleic Acid in Canine Mast Cell Granules and the Possible Interrelationships of Mast Cells and Plasma Cells.   Path. Vet. 3:178–189, 1966.

HOWARD, E. B., et al.:   Mastocytoma and Gastroduodenal Ulceration.   Gastric and Duodenal Ulcers in Dogs with Mastocytoma.   Path. Vet. 6:146–158, 1969.

JABARA, A. G.:   Canine Mixed Tumors (Mammary).   Aust. Vet. J. 36:212–221, 1960.

—————:   Two Cases of Mammary Neoplasms Arising in Male Dogs.   Aust. Vet. J. 45: 476–480, 1969.

JOHNSON, R. M., and SANGER, V. L.:   Lipids in Avian Xanthomatous Lesions.   Am. J. Vet. Res. 24:1280–1282, 1963.

JONES, T. C.:   Tumors of Specialized Sebaceous Glands of Dogs.   Bull. Internat. Assn. Med. Museums (now Lab. Investigation) 28:66-72, 1948.

LIU, S K., and HOHN, R. B.:   Squamous Cell Carcinoma of the Digit of the Dog.   J. Am. Vet. Med. Assn. 153:411–424, 1968.

LOMBARD, L. S., and MOLONEY, J. B.:   Experimental Transmission of Mast Cell Sarcoma in Dogs.   Fed. Proc. 18:490, 1959.

MASSON, P.:   Les naevi pigmentaires, tumeurs nerveuses.   Ann. d. Anat. Path. 3:417–453, and 656–696, 1926.

MAWDESLEY-THOMAS, L. E., and BUCKE, D.:   Squamous Cell Carcinoma in a Gudgeon (Gobio golio, L).   Path. Vet. 4:484–489, 1967.

McCLELLAND, R. B.:   Benign Neoplasms of the Skin Glands of Dogs.   Cornell Vet. 30:67–72, 1940.

MOULTON, J. E.:   Histological Classification of Canine Mammary Tumors.   Cornell Vet. 44:168–180, 1954.

MULLIGAN, R. M.:   Neoplastic Diseases of Dogs: Mast Cell Sarcoma, Lymphosarcoma, Histiocytoma.   Arch. Path. 46:477–492, 1948.

—————:   Hemangiopericytoma in the Dog.   Amer. J. Path. 31:773–789, 1955.

MUSTAFA, I. E., CERNA, J., and CERNY, L.:   Melanoma in Goats.   Sudan Med. J. 4:113–118, 1966.   V.B. 37:2244, 1967.

NEILSEN, S. W., and AFTOSMIS, J.:   Canine Perianal Gland Tumors.   J. Am. Vet. Med. Assn. 144:127–135, 1964.

NIELSEN, S. W., and COLE, C. R.:   Canine Mastocytoma—A Report of One Hundred Cases. Am. J. Vet. Res. 19:417–432, 1958.

—————:   Cutaneous Epithelial Neoplasms of the Dog.   A Report of 153 Cases.   Am. J. Vet. Res. 21:931–948, 1960.

OLSON, C., JR.:   Equine Sarcoid, a Cutaneous Neoplasm.   Am. J. Vet. Res. 9:333–341, 1948.

OLSON, C., JR., and COOK, R. H.:   Cutaneous Sarcoma-like Lesions of the Horse Caused by the Agent of Bovine Papilloma.   Proc. Soc. Exper. Biol. & Med. 77:281–284, 1951.

ORKIN, M., and SCHWARTZMAN, R. M.:   A Comparative Study of Canine and Human Dermatology.   II. Cutaneous Tumors, the Mast Cell and Canine Mastocytoma.   J. Invest. Derm. 32:451–466, 1959.

PECKHAM, M. C.:   Xanthomatosis in Chickens.   Am. J. Vet. Res. 16:580–583, 1955.

PETERS, J. A.:   Canine Mastocytoma: Excess Risk as Related to Ancestry.   J. Nat. Cancer Inst. 42:435–443, 1969.

PETRAK, M. L., and GILMORE, C. E.:   In Petrak, M. L. (ed.) Diseases of Cage and Aviary Birds.   Philadelphia, Lea & Febiger, 1969, pp. 459–489.

POWERS, R. D.:   Immunologic Properties of Canine Transmissible Venereal Sarcoma. Amer. J. Vet. Res. 29:1637–1645, 1968.

PRIER, J. E., and JOHNSON, J. H.:   Malignancy in a Canine Transmissible Venereal Tumour. J. Amer. Vet. Med. Assn. 145:1092–1094, 1964.

RAGLAND, W. L., KEOWN, G. H., and GORHAM, J. R.:   An Epizootic of Equine Sarcoid. Nature (Lond.) 210:1399, 1966.

ROSENBERG, J. C., et al.:   The Malignant Melanoma of Hamsters.   I. Pathologic Characteristics of a Transplanted Melanotic and Amelanotic Tumor.   Cancer Res. 21:627–631, and 632–635, 1961.

SAKURAI, Y.: Adenoid Cystic Epithelioma ("Brooke's Tumor") in a Dog. J. Jap. Vet. Med. Assn. *13*:206–208, 1960.

SCHULZ, K. C. A., and SCHUTTE, J. A.: Multiple Acanthoma in the Skin of Swine. J. S. Afr. Vet. Med. Assn. *31*:437–442, 1960.

SHOPE, R. E., *et al.*: An Infectious Cutaneous Fibroma of the Virginia White-Tailed Deer (*Odocoileus virginianus*). J. Exp. Med. *108*:797–802, 1958.

SMIT, J. D.: Skin Lesions in South African Domestic Animals with Special Reference to the Incidence and Prognosis of Various Skin Tumors. J. S. Afr. Vet. Med. Assn. *33*:363–376, 1962.

STOUT, A. P., and MURRAY, M. R.: Hemangiopericytoma: A Vascular Tumor Featuring Zimmermann's Pericytes. Ann. Surg. *116*:26–33, 1942.

STRAFUSS, A. C., *et al.*: Cutaneous Melanoma in Miniature Swine. Lab. Anim. Care *18*: 165–169, 1968.

TRAUTWEIN, G., and STOBER, M.: (Leucaemic Mast Cell Reticulosis in a Cow; a Contribution to Non-Lymphatic Leucosis in Cattle). Zentbl. Vet. Med. *12A*:211–231, 1965. V.B. *35*: 3088, 1965.

UBERREITER, O.: (Mammary Tumours in Dogs and Cats.) Wien. Tierarztl. Mschr. *55*: 415–442, 1968 and 481–503, 1968 V.B. *39*:2141, 1969.

WEISS, E.: Intranukleäre und intrazytoplasmatische Glycogenablagerungen in Mastzellentumoren des Hundes. Path. Vet. *2*:514–519, 1965.

WEISS, E., RUDOLPH, R., and DEUTSCHLANDER, N.: Untersuchungen zur Ultrastruktur und Atiologie der mastzellentumoren des Hundes. Path. Vet. *5*:199–211, 1968.

WEISS, E., and FEZER, G.: Histologische Klassifizierung der Schweissdrusentumoren von Hund und Katze. Berl. Münch. Tierarztl. Wschr. *81*:249–254, 1968.

WEST, G. B.: Pharmacology of the Tissue Mast Cell. Brit. J. Derm. *70*:409–417, 1958

YOST, D. H., and JONES, T. C.: Hemangiopericytoma in the Dog. Amer. J. Vet. Res. *19*: 159-163, 1958.

Musculoskeletal System

HEMMING, R. B., and SEAWRIGHT, A. A.: Multiple Osteogenic Sarcoma in the Skin of a Dog. Aust. Vet. J. *41*:182–185, 1965.

HOWARD, E. B., and KENYON, A. J.: Malignant Osteoclastoma (Giant Cell Tumor) in the Cat with Associated Mast Cell Response. Cornell Vet. *57*:398–409, 1967.

SALM, R., and FIELD, J.: Osteosarcoma in a Rabbit. J. Path. Bact. *89*:400–402, 1965.

SULLIVAN, D. J.: Cartilaginous Tumors (Chondroma and Chondrosarcoma) in Animals Amer. J. Vet. Res. *21*:531–535, 1960.

TJALMA, R. A.: Canine Bone Sarcoma: Estimation of Relative Risk as a Function of Body Size. J. Nat. Cancer Inst. *36*:1137–1150, 1966.

QUIGLEY, P. J., *et al.*: Two Cases of Haemangiosarcoma of the Radius in the Dog. Vet. Rec. *77*:1207–1209, 1965.

WOLKE, R. E., and NIELSEN, S. W.: Site Incidence of Canine Osteosarcoma. J. Small Anim. Pract. *7*:489–492, 1966.

Respiratory System

AMARAL-MENDES, J. J.: Histopathology of Primary Lung Tumours in the Mouse. J. Path. *97*:415–427, 1969.

COTCHIN, E.: Spontaneous Neoplasms of the Upper Respiratory Tract in Animals. In *Cancer of the Nasopharynx* edited by C. S. Muir and K. Shanmugaratnam. 203–259. Copenhagen, Munksgaard. 1967.

DUNCAN, J. R., *et al.*: Enzootic Nasal Adenocarcinoma in Sheep. J. Amer. Vet. Med. Assn. *151*:732–734, 1967.

FERRI, A. G., and TAUSK, EVA: Primary Pulmonary Carcinomas of the Dog. J. Comp. Path. & Therap. *65*:159–167, 1955.

GUSTAFSON, P. O., and WOLFE, D.: Bone-Metastasizing Lung Carcinomas in a Cat. Cornell Vet. *58*:425–430, 1968.

HÄNICHEN, T., and SCHIEFER, B.: Zur morphologie und Häufigkeit primärer Geschwülste der Nasenhöhlen und Nasennebenhöhlen bei Hund und Katze. Z. Krebsforsch. *71*: 255–266, 1968.

JONAS, A. M., and CARRINGTON, C. B.: Vascular Patterns in Primary and Secondary Pulmonary Tumors in the Dog. Amer. J. Path. *56*:79–95, 1969.

LOMBARD, C.: (Lung Cancer in Comparative Pathology). Le Cancer Pulmonaire en Pathologie Comparée. Econ. Med. Anim. *5*:305–325, 1964.

MISDORP, W. and NAUTA-VAN GELDER, H. L.: "Granular Cell Myoblastoma" in the Horse. Path. Vet. *5*:385–394, 1968.

MONLUX, W. S.: Primary Pulmonary Neoplasm in Domestic Animals. Southwestern Vet. 6:131–133, 1952.

NIELSEN, S. W., and HORAVA, A.: Primary Pulmonary Tumors of the Dog. A Report of Sixteen Cases. Am. J. Vet. Res. 21:813–830, 1960.

ROBBINS, S. L.: Pathology, 3rd Ed. Philadelphia, W. B. Saunders Co., 1967.

SEFFNER, W., and FRITZSCH, R.: (Multiple Occurrence of Pleural Mesothelioma in Pigs.) Arch. Exp. Vet. Med. 18:1395–1405, 1964. V.B. 35: 2679, 1965.

SEIBOLD, H. R.: An Embryonal Mixed Tumor in the Lungs of a Calf. J. Am. Vet. Med. Assn. 108:157–160, 1946.

SNYDER, R. L., and RATCLIFFE, H. L.: Primary lung cancers in birds and mammals of the Philadelphia Zoo. Cancer Res. 26:514–518, 1866.

SWOBODA, R.: Über das Lungenkarzinom bei Tieren mit besonderer Berücksichtigung des Rindes. Path. Vet. 1:409–422, 1964.

Cardiovascular System

DIAMANDOPOULOS, G. TH.: Histopathology of Sarcomas Induced in Hamsters by Clones of In Vitro SV-40 Transformed Homologous Heart Cells. Amer. J. Path. 53:753–767, 1968.

GEIB, L. W.: Primary Angiomatous Tumors of the Heart and Great Vessels. A Report of Two Cases in the Dog. Cornell Vet. 57:292–296, 1967.

GRICE, H. C., SAY, R. R., and McKINLEY, W. P.: Rhabdomyosarcoma in the Heart of a Chicken. J. Am. Vet. Med. Assn. 130:530–532, 1957.

HIYEDA, K., and FAUST, E. C.: Aortic Lesions in Dogs Caused by Infection with Spirocerca sanguinolenta. Arch. Path. 7:253–272, 1929.

KAST, A., and HÄNICHEN, T.: Rhabdomyome in Schweineherzen. Zbl. Vet. Med. 15: 140–150, 1968.

MAGNUSSON, G.: Primartumoren im Herzen des Rindes. Dtsch. tierarztl. Wschr. 68: 405–409, 1961.

McCONNELL, R. F., and EDIGER, R. D.: Benign Mesenchymoma of the Heart in the Guinea Pig. A Report of Four Cases. Path. Vet. 5:97–101, 1968.

OMAR, A. R.: Congenital Cardiac Rhabdomyoma in a Pig. Path. Vet. 6: 469–474, 1969.

ROBERTS, S. R.: Myxoma of the Heart in a Dog. J. Amer. Vet. Med. Assn. 134:185–188, 1959.

SYVRUD, R.: Rhabdomyoma in the Cat. Western Vet. (Washington State University, Pullman, Wash.) 6:49–50, 1959.

WALLER, T., and RUBARTH, S.: Haemangioendothelioma in Domestic Animals. Acta Vet. Scand. 8:234–261, 1967.

Hemic and Lymphatic System

BEDERKE, G., and TOLLE, A.: (Transmissibility of Bovine Leucosis to Calves by Blood and by Contact.) Zbl. Vet. Med. 11B:433–445, 1964.

BENJAMIN, S. A., and NORONHA, F.: Cytogenetic Studies in Canine Lymphosarcoma. Cornell Vet. 57:526–542, 1967.

BLOOM, F.: Intramedullary Plasma-cell Myeloma in a Dog. J. Cancer Res. 6:718–722, 1946.

CLAGUE, D. C., and GRANZIEN, C. K.: Enzootic Bovine Leucosis in South East Queensland. Aust. Vet. J. 42:177–182, 1966.

CONNER, G. H., et al.: Studies on the Epidemiology of Bovine Leukemia. J. Nat. Cancer Inst. 36:383–388, 1966.

CORDY, D. R.: Plasma Cell Myeloma in a Dog. Cornell Vet. 47:498–502, 1957.

CORNELIUS, C. E., GOODBARY, R. F., and KENNEDY, P. C.: Plasma Cell Myelomatosis in a Horse. Cornell Vet. 49:478–493, 1959.

DIGIACOMO, R. F.: Burkitt's Lymphoma in a White-handed Gibbon (Hylobates lar). Cancer Res. 27:1178–1179, 1967.

DORN, C. R., TAYLOR, D. O., and HIBBARD, H. H.: Epizootiologic Characteristics of Canine and Feline Leukemia and Lymphoma. Amer. J. Vet. Res. 28:993–1001, 1967.

DUNGWORTH, D. L., THEILEN, G. H., and LENGYEL, J.: Bovine Lymphosarcoma in California. II. The Thymic Form. Path. Vet. 1:323–350, 1964.

DUTCHER, R. M.: Bovine Leukemia: Growth 29:1–5, 1965.

FRANK, W., and SCHEPKY, A.: Metastasierendes Lymphosarkom bei einer Riesenschlange, Eunectes murinus (Linnaeus, 1758). Path. Vet. 6:437–443, 1969.

FUJIMOTO, Y., MILLER, J., and OLSON, C.: The Fine Structure of Lymphosarcoma in Cattle. Path. Vet. 6:15–29, 1969.

GALL, E. A., and MALLORY, T. B.: Malignant Lymphomas. Amer. J. Path. 18:381–429, 1942.

GARD, S.: The Pathogenesis of Bovine Lymphomatosis. Path. Microbiol. *28*:638–690, 1965.

GILMORE, C. E., GILMORE, V. H., and JONES, T. C.: Reticuloendotheliosis, a Myeloproliferative Disorder of Cats: A Comparison with Lymphocytic Leukemia. Path. Vet. *1*: 161–183, 1964.

HARE, W. C. C., YANG, T. J., and MCFEELY, R. A.: A Survey of Chromosome Findings in 47 Cases of Bovine Lymphosarcoma (Leukemia). J. Nat. Cancer Inst. *38*:383–392, 1967.

HATZIOLOS, B. C., *et al.*: Bovine Lympho-sarcoma: The Effect of Inoculations on Newborn Calves and Mice—First Year of Observation. J. Vet. Res. *27*:489–502, 1966.

HAYDEN, D. W.: Generalized Lymphosarcoma in a Juvenile Rabbit. A Case Report. Cornell Vet. *60*:73–82, 1970.

HOLZWORTH, J.: Leukemia and Related Neoplasms in the Cat. II. Malignancies other Than Lymphoid. J. Amer. Vet. Med. Assn. *136*:107–121, 1960.

HOWARD, E. B., NIELSEN, S. W., and KENYON, A. J.: Cutaneous Lymphomatosis in a Boxer Dog. Pathologic and Biochemical Observations. Path. Vet. *6*:76–85, 1969.

HUGOSON, G.: A Case of Congenital Skin Leukosis in a Calf. Zentbl. Vet. Med. *13B*: 748–757, 1966. V.B. *37*:2749, 1967.

HUNT, R. D., *et al.*: Morphology of a Disease with Features of Malignant Lymphoma in Marmosets and Owl Monkeys Inoculated with *Herpesvirus saimiri*. J. Nat. Cancer Inst. *44*: 447–465, 1970.

JÄRPLID, B.: Studies on the Site of Leukotic and Preleukotic Changes in the Bovine Heart. Path. Vet. *1*:366–408, 1964.

JARRET, W. F. H., *et al.*: A Virus-like Particle Associated with Leukaemia (Lymphosarcoma). Nature *202*:567, 1964.

————: Experimental Studies of Feline and Bovine Leukeamia. Proc. Roy. Soc. Med. *59*:661–662, 1966.

JARRETT, W. F. H., CRIGHTON, G. W., and DALTON, R. G.: Lymphosarcoma or Leukaemia in the Domestic Animals. Vet. Rec. *79*:693–699, 1966.

KRÜGER, K. E., and RABL, R.: (Pathology of Leucosis in Cattle Having a Leucosis-positive Blood Picture.) Zentbl. Vet. Med. *12A*:161–170, 1965. V.B. *35*:2675, 1965.

LaBELLE, J. A., and CONNER, G. H.: Hemolymph Node Involvement in Bovine Leukemia. J. Am. Vet. Med. Assn. *145*:1107–1111, 1964.

LÖLIGER, H. C.: Leucosis in Rabbits. Berl. Münch. Tierarztl. Wschr. *79*:192–194, 1966. V.B. *36*:4417, 1966.

LOMBARD, L. S., *et al.*: Myelolipomas of the Liver in Captive Wild Felidae. Path. Vet. *5*: 127–134, 1968.

LUKES, R. J., *et al.*: Canine Lymphomas Histologically Indistinguishable from Burkitt's Lymphoma. Lancet, 13th August, 389–390, 1966.

MARSHAK, R. R., *et al.*: Observations on a Heifer with Cutaneous Lymphosarcoma. Cancer *19*:724–734, 1966.

MIURA, S., and OHSHIMA, K.: Monocytic Leukemia in Cattle. I. Cytological Observation of Two Cases. Jap J. Vet. Sci. *29*:141–150, 1967.

MOLDOVANU, G., *et al.*: Cellular Transmission of Lymphosarcoma in Dogs. Nature (Lond.) *210*:1342–1343, 1966.

OHSHIMA, K., and MIURA, S.: Mast-cell Leukosis in Cats—A Report of Two Cases. Jap. J. Vet. Sci. *27*:233–238, 1965.

OSBORNE, C. A., *et al.*: Multiple Myeloma in the Dog. J. Am. Vet. Med. Assn. *153*: 1300–1319, 1968.

PARKER, J. W., WAKASA, H., and LUKES, R. J.: Canine and Burkitt's Lymphomas. Lancet 28th Jan., 214–215, 1967.

PAYNE, B. J.: Editorial on Leukemia. Path. Vet. *6*:89–93, 1969.

POST, J. E.: Experimental Transmission of Two Canine Neoplasms: Lymphosarcoma and Mast Cell Leukemia. Diss. Abstr. *29B*:259–260, 1968. V.B. *39*:1223, 1969.

PRASAD, M. C., and CHANDRASEKHARAN, K. P.: Generalised Lymphosarcoma in a Bovine Foetus. Indian J. Path. Bact. *11*:131–134, 1968. V.B *39*:1215, 1969.

PRICE, R. A., and POWERS, R. D.: Reticulum Cell Sarcoma in a Sykes Monkey (*Cercopithecus albogularis*). Path. Vet. *6*:369–374, 1969.

REID, J. S., and MARCUS, L. C.: Granulocytic Leukemia in a Cat. J. Small Anim. Pract. *7*:421–425, 1966.

RICKARD, C. G., *et al.*: C-type Virus Particles in Spontaneous Lymphocytic Leukemia in a Cat. Cornell Vet. *57*:302–307, 1967.

SCHAPPERT, H. R., and GEIB, L. W.: Reticuloendothelial Neoplasms Involving the Spinal Canal of Cats. J. Am. Vet. Med. Assn. *150*:753–757, 1967.

SCHNEIDER, R., *et al.*: A Household Cluster of Feline Malignant Lymphoma. Cancer Res. *27*:1316–1322, 1967.

SCHULZE, P., WITTMANN, W., and GRALHEER, H.: Electron Microscope Studies on the

Specificity of Virus-like Particles Contained in the Colostrum in Bovine Leukosis. Acta Virol., Prague *10*:467–470, 1966. V.B. *37*:1755, 1967.

SIMON, N., and HOLZWORTH, J.: Eosinophilia Leukemia in a Cat. Cornell Vet. *57*:579–597, 1967.

SIRBU, Z., *et al.*: Cytochemical and Ultrastructural Studies on Bovine Lymphoid Leucosis. Archiva Vet. *5*:27–34, 1968. V.B. *39*:4707, 1969.

SMITH, H. A.: Leukemic Neoplasia in the Dog. Ann. New York Acad. Sci. *108*:633–641, 1963.

————: Malignant Lymphoma in Animals. A Survey of Present Knowledge. Amer. J. Clin. Path. *38*:75–87, 1962.

————: The Pathology of Malignant Lymphoma of Cattle. Path. Vet. *2*:68–94, 1965.

SQUIRE, R. A.: A Cytologic Study of Malignant Lymphoma in Cattle. Amer. J. Vet. Res. *26*:97–107, 1965

STOVER, M.: (Cytochemistry of Leucocytes in Bovine Leucosis). Zentbl. Vet. Med. *13A*:320–328, 1966. V.B. *37*:294, 1967.

SWIERENGA, S. H., and BASRUR, P. K.: DNA Synthesis in Normal and Neoplastic Lymphocytes of Domestic Animals. Cornell Vet. *58*:292–304, 1968.

THEILEN, G. H., and DUNGWORTH, D. L.: Bovine Lymphosarcoma in California. III. The Calf Form. Am. J. Vet. Res. *26*:696–709, 1965.

VAN KAMPEN, K. R.: Lymphosarcoma in the Rabbit. A Case Report and General Review. Cornell Vet. *58*:121–128, 1968.

VAN PELT, R. W., and CONNER, G. H.: Clinicopathologic Survey of Malignant Lymphoma in the Dog. J. Am. Vet. Med. Assn. *152*:976–989, 1968.

WEIPERS, W. L., *et al.*: Leukaemia in the Domestic Animals. Ann. Rep. Br. Emp. Cancer Campaign *44*:Part II, 417–420, 1966. V.B. *38*:1041, 1968.

WEISS, E.: Formale genese der leukosen und RH.S-Neoblastome von Rind. Zbl. Vet. Med. *15*:151–155, 1968.

ZALUSKY, R., *et al.*: Leukemia in the Rhesus Monkey (*Macaca mulatta*) Exposed to Whole-body Neutron Irradiation. Radiat. Res. *25*:410–416, 1965.

Digestive System

ANDERSON, N. V., and JOHNSON, K. H.: Pancreatic Carcinoma in the Dog. J. Am. Vet. Med. Assn. *150*:286–295, 1967.

ANDERSON, W. A., MONLUX, A. W., and DAVIS, C. L.: Epithelial Tumors of the Bovine Gallbladder.—A Report of Eighteen Cases. Am. J. Vet. Res. *19*:58–65, 1958.

BASKERVILLE, A.: Mesothelioma in the Calf. Path. Vet. *4*:149–156, 1967.

BENJAMIN, S. A., and LANG, C. M.: An Ameloblastic Odontoma in a Cebus Monkey (*Cebus albifrons.*) J. Am. Vet. Med. Assn. *155*:1236–1240, 1969.

BRODEY, R. S., and COHEN, D.: An Epizootiologic and Clinicopathologic Study of 95 Cases of Gastrointestinal Neoplasms in the Dog. Proc. 101st A. Meet. Am. Vet. Med. Assn. 167–179, 1964.

BRODEY, R. S.: Alimentary Tract Neoplasms in the Cat: A Clinciopathologic Survey of 46 Cases. Am. J. Vet. Res. *27*:74–80, 1966.

BULLOCK, F. D., and CURTIS, M. R.: Experimental Production of Sarcoma of the Liver of the Rat. Proc. New York Path. Soc. N.S. *20*:149–175, 1920.

DAVIS, C. L., and NAYLOR, J. R.: Carcinoma in the Stomach of a Dog. J. Am. Vet. Med. Assn. *102*:286–288, 1943.

DOS SANTOS, J. A.: (Enzootic Hepatoma in Rabbits: Second Series of Observations.) Pesquisa Agropec. Bras. *1*:97–100, 1966. V.B. *38*:1049, 1968.

DUNNING, W. F., and CURTIS, M. R.: Malignancy Induced by *Cysticercus fasciolaris:* Its Independence of Age of the Host when Infested. Amer. J. Cancer *37*:312–328, 1939.

————: Multiple Peritoneal Sarcoma in Rats from Intraperitoneal Injection of Washed Ground, *Taenia* Larvae. Cancer Res. *6*:668–670, 1946.

FELDMAN, W. H.: Metastasizing Hepatoma in a Hog (*Sus scrofa*). Amer. J. Cancer *27*: 111–114, 1936.

HITCHCOCK, C. R., and BELL, E. T.: Studies on the Nematode Parasite, *Gongylonema neoplasticum*, and Avitaminosis A in the Forestomach of Rats: Comparison with Fibiger' Results. J. Nat. Cancer Inst. *12*:1345–1387, 1952.

HIYEDA, K., and FAUST, E. C.: Aortic Lesions in Dogs Caused by Infection with *Spirocerca sanguinolenta*. Arch. Path. *7*:253–272, 1929.

HUEPER, W. G., and PAYNE, W. W.: Observations on the Occurrence of Hepatomas in Rainbow Trout. J. Nat. Cancer Inst. *27*:1123–1142, 1961.

JEFFCOTT, L. B.: Primary Liver-cell Carcinoma in a Young Thoroughbred Horse. J. Path. *97*:394–397, 1969.

KARBE, E., and SCHIEFER, B.: Primary Salivary Gland Tumors in Carnivores. Canad. Vet. J. *8*:212–215, 1967.

KOESTNER, A., and BUERGER, L.: Primary Neoplasms of the Salivary Glands in Animals Compared to Similar Tumors in Man. Path. Vet. *2*:201–226, 1965.

KROOK, L.: On Gastrointestinal Carcinoma in the Dog. Acta Path. Microbiol. Scand. *38*:43–57, 1956.

LANGHAM, R. F., et al.: Oral Adamantinomas in the Dog. J. Am. Vet. Med. Assn. *146*: 474–480, 1965.

MANKTELOW, B. W.: Hepatoblastomas in Sheep. J. Path. Bact. *89*:711–714, 1965.

McDONALD, J. W., and LEAVER, D. D.: Adenocarcinoma of the Small Intestine of Merino Sheep. Aust. Vet. J. *41*:269–271, 1965.

PARSONS, R. J., and KIDD, J. G.: Oral Papillomatosis of Rabbits: A Virus Disease. J. Exp. Med. *77*:233–250, 1943.

PLOWRIGHT, W.: Malignant Neoplasia of the Esophagus and Rumen of Cattle in Kenya. J. Comp. Path. & Therap. *65*:108–114, 1955.

RAGLAND, W. L., and GORHAM, J. R.: Tonsillar Carcinoma in Rural Dogs. Nature, Lond. *214*:925–926, 1967.

RIBELIN, W. E., and BAILEY, W. S.: Esophageal Sarcomas Associated with *Spirocerca lupi* Infection in the Dog. Cancer *2*:1242–1246, 1958.

ROWLATT, U.: Spontaneous Epithelial Tumours of the Pancreas of Mammals. Brit. J. Cancer *21*:82–107, 1967.

SALMON, W. D., and NEWBERNE, P. M.: Occurrence of Hepatomas in Rats Fed Diets Containing Peanut Meal as a Major Source of Protein. Cancer Res. *23*:571–575, 1963.

SCHÄFFER, E., and SCHIEFER, B.: Incidence and Types of Canine Rectal Carcinomas. J. Small Anim. Pract. *9*:491–496, 1968.

SCHMIDT, J., and GEMMER, H.: "Squamous-cell Carcinoma of the Stomach of a Horse with Anemia" (Trans. Title). Dtsch. Tierarztl. Wschr. *67*:494–496, 1960.

SCHUTTE, K. H.: Esophageal Tumors in Sheep: Some Ecological Observations. J. Nat. Cancer Inst. *41*:821–824, 1968.

SEIBOLD, H. R., et al.: Observations on the Possible Relations of Malignant Esophageal Tumors and *Spirocerca lupi* Lesions in the Dog. Am. J. Vet. Res. *16*:5–14, 1955.

WERLE, E., HAENDLE, H., and SCHMAL, A.: Ein fall von Carcinoid bei einem Elefonten. Path. Vet. *5*:81–83, 1968.

WETTIMUNY, S. G. DE S.: Primary Liver Tumors of Cattle in Ceylon. J. Comp. Path. *79*: 355–362, 1969.

WOODRUFF, J. M., and JOHNSON, D. K.: Hepatic Hemangioendothelioma in a Rhesus Monkey. Path. Vet. *5*:327–332, 1968.

YOSHIDA, S.: Contribution to the Study on *Gnathostoma spinigerum* Owen 1836, Cause of Esophageal Tumor in the Japanese Mink, with Especial Reference to its Life History. Tr. 9th Congress, Far East Assn. Trop. Med., Nanking, China *1*:625–630, 1934.

Urinary System

COTCHIN, E.: Spontaneous Carcinoma of the Urinary Bladder of the Dog. Brit. Vet. J. *115*:431–434, 1959.

FELDMAN, W. H.: Embryonal Nephroma in a Sheep. Amer. J. Cancer *17*:734–747, 1933.

FERGUSON, A. R.: Associated Bilharziosis and Primary Malignant Disease of the Urinary Bladder, with Observations on a Series of Forty Cases. J. Path. & Bact. *16*:76–94, 1911.

FIBIGER, J.: Weitere Untersuchungen uber das Spiropteracarcinom der ratte. Ztschr. f. Krebsforsch. *14*:295–326, 1914.

HARBUTT, P. R., and LEAVER, D. D.: Carcinoma of the Bladder of Sheep. Aust. Vet. J. *45*:473–475, 1969.

HATAYA, M., USUI, K., and SHIRASU, Y.: Studies on the Treatment of Transmissible Venereal Tumor of Dogs by X-ray and Gamma-ray Irradiation. Proc. XVIth Internat. Vet. Congr. Madrid. *2*:287–288, 1959.

HEAD, K. W.: Cutaneous Mast-cell Tumors in the Dog, Cat and Ox. Brit. J. Dermatol. *70*:389–408, 1958.

JABARA, A. G.: Three Cases of Primary Malignant Neoplasms Arising in the Canine Urinary System. J. Comp. Path. *78*:335–339, 1968.

JONES, T. C., and FRIEDMAN, N. B.: Pathologic and Clinical Features of Canine Testicular Tumors. Bull. Internat. Assn. Med. Museums (now Lab. Investigation). *31*:36–53, 1950.

MUGERA, G. M., NDERITO, P., and SORHEIM, A. O.: The Pathology of Urinary Bladder Tumours in Kenya Zebu Cattle. J. Comp. Path. *79*:251–254, 1969.

OLSON, C., et al.: A Urinary Bladder Tumor Induced by a Bovine Cutaneous Papilloma Agent. Cancer Res. *19*:779–782, 1959.

OSBORNE, C. A., *et al.*: Neoplasms of Canine and Feline Urinary Bladder: Incidence, Etiologic Factors, Occurrence and Pathologic Features. Amer. J. Vet. Res. *29*:2041–2055, 1968.

PAMUKCU, A. M., GÖKSOY, S. K., and PRICE, J. M.: Urinary Bladder Neoplasms Induced by Feeding Bracken Fern (*Pteris aquilina*) to Cows. Cancer Res. *27*:917–924, 1967.

PRICE, J. M., and PAMUKCU, A. M.: The Induction of Neoplasms of the Urinary Bladder of the Cow and the Small Intestine of the Rat by Feeding Bracken Fern (*Pteris aquilina*). Cancer Res. *28*:2247–2251, 1968.

SULLIVAN, D. J., and ANDERSON, W. A.: Embryonal Nephroma in Swine. Amer. J. Vet. Res. *20*:324–332, 1959.

WALTER, W. G., BURMESTER, B. R., and CUNNINGHAM, C. H.: Studies on the Transmission and Pathology of a Viral-induced Avian Nephroblastoma (Embryonal Nephroma). Avian Diseases *6*:455–477, 1962.

Genital System

ADAMS, E. W., and CHINEME, C. N.: Canine Venereal Tumor. Serum Protein Electrophoresis, Transaminase, and Lactic Dehydrogenase Activity. Cornell Vet. *57*:572–579, 1967.

ADAMS, E. W., CARTER, L. P., and SAPP, W. J.: Growth and Maintenance of the Canine Venereal Tumor in Continuous Culture. Cancer Res. *28*:753–757, 1968.

ANDERSON, L. J., and SANDISON, A. T.: Tumours of the Female Genitalia in Cattle, Sheep and Pigs Found in a British Abattoir Survey. J. Comp. Path. *79*:53–63, 1969.

BELTER, L. F., CRAWFORD, E. M., and BATES, H. R.: Endometrial Adenocarcinoma in a Cat. Path. Vet. *5*:429–431, 1968.

CORDES, D. O.: Equine Granulosa Tumours. Vet. Rec. *85*:186–188, 1969.

COTCHIN, E.: Spontaneous Uterine Cancer in Animals. Brit. J. Cancer *18*:209–227, 1964.

GUARDA, F.: Contributo allo studio dei tumori ovarici. L'arrhenoblastoma nella varieta di adenoma tubulare nel suino. Ann. Fac. Med. Vet. Torino *8*:9–21, 1958.

HISAW, F. L., and HISAW, F. L., JR.: Spontaneous Carcinoma of the Cervix Uteri in a Monkey (*Macaca mulatta*). Cancer *11*:810–816, 1958.

INNES, J. R. M.: Neoplastic Diseases of the Testis in Animals. J. Path. and Bact. *54*:485–498, 1942.

KARLSON, A. G., and MANN, F. C.: The Transmissible Venereal Tumor of Dogs; Observations of Forty Generations of Experimental Transfers. Ann. New York Acad. Sci. *54*:1197–1213, 1952.

KURTZE, H.: (An Infectious Venereal Disease in Dogs in Nigeria.) Dt. tierarztl. Wschr. *72*:203–204, 1965. V.B. *35*:3930, 1965.

LEAV, I., and LING, G. V.: Adenocarcinoma of the Canine Prostate. Cancer *22*:1329–1345, 1968.

LINDSAY, J. R., *et al.*: Intrauterine Choriocarcinoma in a Rhesus Monkey. Path. Vet. *6*:378–384, 1969.

MAKINO, S.: Some Epidemiological Aspects of Venereal Tumors of Dogs as Revealed by Chromosome and DNA Studies. Ann. New York Acad. Sci. *108*:1106–1122, 1963.

MARIN-PADILLA, M., and BENIRSCHKE, K.: Thalidomide-induced Alterations in the Blastocyst and Placenta of the Armadillo, *Dasypus novemcinctus Mexicanus*, Including a Choriocarcinoma. Amer. J. Path. *43*:999–1016, 1963.

McENTEE, K, and ZEPP, C. P., JR.: Canine and Bovine Ovarian Tumors. Proc. First World Congress on Fertil. & Sterility, N.Y., 1953.

MONLUX, A. W., *et al.*: Adenocarcinoma of the Uterus of the Cow—Differentiation of its Pulmonary Metastases from Primary Lung Tumors. Am. J. Vet. Res. *17*:45–73, 1956.

MULLIGAN, R. M.: Feminization in Male Dogs, a Syndrome Associated with Carcinoma of the Testis and Mimicked by the Administration of Estrogens. Amer. J. Path. *20*:865–873, 1944.

MURRAY, M., JAMES, Z. H., and MARTIN, W. B.: A Study of the Cytology and Karyotype of the Canine Transmissible Venereal Tumour. Res. Vet. Sci. *10*:565–568, 1969.

NORRIS, H. J., TAYLOR, H. B., and GARNER, F. M.: Equine Ovarian Granulosa Tumours. Vet. Rec. *82*:419–420, 1968.

————: Comparative Pathology of Ovarian Neoplasms. II. Gonadal Stromal Tumors of Bovine Species. Path. Vet. *6*:45–58, 1969.

PAMUKCU, A. M.: Seminoma of the Testicles in an Ankara Goat. Vet. Facültesi dergisi *1*:42–43, 1954 (In Engl.)

PLOWRIGHT, W.: Malignant Neoplasia of the Esophagus and Rumen of Cattle in Kenya. J. Comp. Path. & Therap. *65*:108–114, 1955.

PREISER, H.: Endometrial Adenocarcinoma in a Cat. Path. Vet. *1*:485–490, 1964.

PRIER, J. E.: Chromosome Pattern of Canine Transmissible Sarcoma Cells in Culture. Nature Lond. *212*:724–726, 1966.

RANGEL, N. M., and MACHADO, A. V.: Leidigocitoma (Tumor de celulas interstitiasis) em testiculo de bovino. Arq. Esc. Sup. Vet. Minas Gerais, Brazil 5:22–33, 1952.

RUST, J. H.: Transmissible Lymphosarcoma in the Dog. J. Am. Vet. Med. Assn. 114: 10–14, 1949.

SCHLOTTHAUER, C. F., McDONALD, J. R., and BOLLMAN, J. L.: Testicular Tumors in Dogs. J. Urology 40:539–550, 1938.

STREETT, C. S.: Sertoli Cell Carcinoma and Multiple Metastasis in a Dog. Cornell Vet. 57:597–619, 1967.

SMITH, G. B., and WASHBOURN, J. W.: Infective Venereal Tumours in Dogs. J. Path. & Bact. 5:99–110, 1898.

SMITH, H. A.: Interstitial Cell Tumor of the Equine Testis. J. Am. Vet. Med. Assn. 124: 356–359, 1954.

STUBBS, E. L., and FURTH, J.: Experimental Studies on Venereal Sarcoma of the Dog. Amer. J. Path. 10:275–286, 1934.

TAKAYAMA, S., et al.: Cytological Studies of Tumors. XXV. A Study of Chromosomes in Venereal Tumors of the Dog. Z. Krebsforsch. Bd. 64:253–261, 1961.

TERLECKI, S., and WATSON, W. A.: Adenocarcinoma of the Uterus of a Ewe. Vet. Rec. 80: 516–518, 1967.

THORNBURN, M. J., et al.: Pathological and Cytogenetic Observations on the Naturally Occurring Canine Venereal Tumour in Jamacia (Sticker's Tumour). Brit. J. Cancer 22: 720–727, 1968.

Endocrine System

ASDRUBALI, F., LATINI, A., and PATRIZI, R.: (Functional B Cell Insuloma in Cattle.) Arch. Vet. Ital. 15:191–203, 1964. V.B. 35:674, 1965.

BECK, A. M., and KROOK, L.: Canine Insuloma. Two Surgical Cases with Relapses. Cornell Vet. 55:330–339, 1965.

BLOOM, F.: Structure and Histogenesis of Tumors of the Aortic Bodies in Dogs. Arch. Path. 36:1–12, 1943.

BRODEY, R. S., and KELLY, D. F.: Thyroid Neoplasms in the Dog. A Clinicopathologic Study of Fifty-seven Cases. Cancer 22:406–416, 1968.

BUERGELT, C. D., and DAS, K. M.: Aortic Body Tumor in a Cat. A Case Report. Path. Vet. 5:84–90, 1968.

CAPEN, C. C., MARTIN, S. L., and KOESTNER, A.: Neoplasms in the Adenohypophysis of Dogs. A Clinical and Pathologic Study. Path. Vet. 4:301–325, 1967.

CAPEN, C. C., and KOESTNER, A.: Functional Chronophobe Adenomas of the Canine Adenohypophysis. An Ultrastructural Evaluation of a Neoplasm of Pituitary Corticotrophs. Path, Vet. 4:326–347, 1967.

CAPEN, C. C., MARTIN, S. L., and KOESTNER, A.: The Ultrastructure and Histopathology of an Acidophil Adenoma of the Canine Adenohypophysis. Path. Vet. 4:348–365, 1967.

CAPEN, C. C., and MARTIN, S. L.: Hyperinsulinism in Dogs with Neoplasia of the Pancreatic Islets. A Clinical, Pathologic and Ultrastructural Study. Path. Vet. 6:309–341, 1969.

CELLO, R. M., and KENNEDY, P. C.: Hyperinsulinism in Dogs Due to Pancreatic Islet Cell Carcinoma. Cornell Vet. 47:538–557, 1957.

CLARKSON, T. B., NETSKY, M. G., and DeLa TORRE, E.: Chromophobe Adenoma in a Dog; Angiographic and Anatomic Study. J. Neuropath. 18:559–562, 1959.

COHEN, A. H., et al.: Histologic and Physiologic Characteristics of Hormone-secreting Transplantable Adrenal Tumors in Mice and Rats. Amer. J. Path. 33:631–652, 1957.

GOORMAGHTIGH, N.: Cytology and Functioning of Adrenal Cortex Tumors. Amer. J. Cancer 38:32–40, 1940.

GRAUBMANN, H. D.: (Thyroid Carcinoma in Pigs.) Mh. Vet. Med. 20:574–576, 1965. V.B. 36:258, 1966.

HARE, T.: Chromophobe-cell Adenoma of the Pituitary Gland, Associated with Dystrophia Adiposo-genitalis in a Maiden Bitch. Proc. Royal Soc. Med. 25:1493–1495, 1932.

JOHNSON, K. H.: Aortic Body Tumors in the Dog. J. Am. Vet. Med. Assn. 152:154–160, 1968.

JUBB, K. V., and KENNEDY, P. C.: Tumors of the Non-chromaffin Paraganglia in Dogs. Cancer 10:89–99, 1957.

LOEB, W. F., CAPEN, C. C., and JOHNSON, L. E.: Adenomas of the Pars Intermedia Associated with Hyperglycemia and Glycosuria in Two Horses. Cornell Vet. 56:623–639, 1966.

MARCUS, L. C., BUCCI, T. J., and KRAMER, K. L.: Pancreatic Islet Cell Tumor in a Dog. J. Am. Vet. Med. Assn. 145:1198–1203, 1964.

NORDSTOGA, K.: Carotid Body Tumor in a Cow. Path. Vet. 3:412–420, 1966.

RAHKO, T.:   The Ultrastructure of Beta Cell Islet Tumour in a Dog.   Acta Path. Microbiol. Scand. *77*:405–413, 1969.

RICHARDS, M. A., and MAWDESLEY-THOMAS, L. E.:   Aortic Body Tumours in a Boxer Dog with a Review of the Literature.   J. Path. *98*:283–288, 1969.

ROUSE, B. T., and WILSON, M. R.:   A Case of Hypoglycaemia in a Dog Associated with Neoplasia of the Pancreas.   Vet. Rec. *79*:454–456, 1966.

SANDISON, A. T., and ANDERSON, L. J.:   Tumours of the Endocrine Glands in Cattle, Sheep and Pigs Found in a British Abattoir Survey.   J. Comp. Path. *78*:435–444, 1968.

SIEGEL, E. T., *et al.*:   Functional Adrenocortical Carcinoma in a Dog.   J. Am. Vet. Med. Assn. *150*:760–766, 1967.

Nervous System

ANTIN, I. P.:   Neurofibromatosis or von Recklinghausen's Disease in a Dog.   J. Am. Vet. Med. Assn. *130*:352, 1957.

BARONTI, A. C., and RHODES, D. A.:   Meningioma in a Dog.   J. Am. Vet. Med. Assn. *130*: 520, 1957.

BEEZLEY, D. N.:   A Trigeminal Ganglioneuroma in a Dog.   Cornell Vet. *59*:585–594, 1969.

BOTS, G. T. L. A. M., KROES, R., and FERON, V. J.:   Spontaneous Tumors of the Brain in Rats.   Path. Vet. *5*:290–296, 1968.

DAVIES, H. W.:   Tumors of the Brain in the Dog.   Vet. Rec. *10*:717–719, 1930.

DUNCAN, T. E., and HARKIN, J. C.:   Electron Microscopic Studies of Goldfish Tumors Previously Termed Neurofibromas and Schwannomas.   Amer. J. Path. *55*:191–202, 1969.

FERRELL, J. F., HUNT, R. D., and NIMS, R. M.:   Cervical Ganglioneuroma in a Dog. J. Am. Vet. Med. Assn. *144*:508–512, 1964.

FERRI, A. G., and MATERA, E. A.:   Glomus Tumor in a Dog.   J. Comp. Path. *70*:373–379, 1960.

GEIB, L. W.:   Ossifying Meningioma with Extracranial Metastasis in a Dog.   Path. Vet. *3*: 247–254, 1966.

HAYES, K. C., and SCHIEFER, B.:   Primary Tumors in the CNS of Carnivores.   Path. Vet. *6*:94–116, 1969.

JACOB, K.:   Grosshirnmeningom beim Hund.   Berl. Münch. tierarztl. Wschr. *72*:226–228, 1959.

JOHNSON, D. F., and BROWN, D. G.:   Intradural Spinal Lipoma in an Experimental Swine. Path. Vet. *6*:342–347, 1969.

JOLLY, R. D., and ALLEY, M. R.:   Medulloblastoma in Calves. A Report of Three Cases. Path. Vet. *6*:463–468, 1969.

JOSHUA, J. O., and OTTAWAY, C. W.:   A Case of Cranial Nerve Tumor with Acquired Hydrocephalus in the Dog.   Vet. Rec. *59*:649, 1947.

KOESTNER, A., and ZEMAN, W.:   Primary Reticuloses of the Central Nervous System in Dogs.   Amer. J. Vet. Res. *23*:381–393, 1962.

LUGINBUHL, H.:   Comparative Aspects of Tumors of the Nervous System.   Ann. New York Acad. Sci. *108*:702–721, 1963.

————— –:   Meningiomas in Cats.   Review of the Literature and Report of Eight Cases. Am. J. Vet. Res. *2*:1030–1040, 1961.

—————:   Zur vergleichenden pathologie der tumoren des nervensystems. I. Teil. Schweiz. Arch. Tierheik *104*:305–322, 1962.   V.B. *32*:3853, 1962.

—————:   Spontaneous Neoplasms of the Nervous System in Animals.   Prog. Neurol. Surg. *2*:85–164, 1968.

MILKS, H. J., and OLAFSON, P.:   Primary Brain Tumors in Small Animals.   Cornell Vet. *26*:159–170, 1936.

MISDORP, W., and NAUTA-VAN GELDER, H. L.:   "Granular Cell Myoblastoma" in the Horse.   A Report of Four Cases.   Path. Vet. *5*:385–394, 1968.

MONLUX, A. W., and DAVIS, C. L.:   Multiple Schwannomas of Cattle.   Am. J. Vet. Res. *14*:499–509, 1953.

PILLERI, G.:   Hirnlipom beim Buckelwal, *Megaptera novaeangliae*.   Path. Vet. *3*:341–349, 1966.

—————:   Cerebrale neurofibrome beim Finwal, *Balaenoptera physalus*.   Path. Vet. *5*: 35–40, 1968.

SAVAGE, A., ISA, J. M., and FISCHER, W: Malignant Ependymoma in a Dog.   Cornell Vet. *52*:68–70, 1962.

SCHLOTTHAUER, C. F., and KERNOHAN, J. W.:   Glioma in a Dog and Pinealoma in a Silver Fox (*Vulpes fulvus*).   Amer. J. Cancer *24*:350–356, 1935.

SIMON, J., and BREWER, R. L.:   Multiple Neurofibromatosis in Cow and Calf.   J. Am. Vet. Med. Assn. *142*:1102–1104, 1963.

TETERNIK, D. M., *et al.*: Neurogenous Neoplasms in Cattle. (Trans. title.) Veterinariya, Moscow *37*:[No. 5 pp.] 56–60, 1960.

TROY, M. A.: Granular-cell Myoblastoma in a Dog. J. Am. Vet. Med. Assn. *126*:397, 1955.

Special Sense

ANDERSON, D. E.: Effects of Pigment on Bovine Ocular Squamous Carcinoma. Ann. New York Acad. Sci. *100*:436–446, 1963.

BARRON, C. N.: The Comparative Pathology of Neoplasms of the Eyelids and Conjunctiva with Special Reference to Those of Epithelial Origin. Dissertation, University of Michigan, 1962. Pub. by Acta Dermato-venereologica 42, Suppl. 51, Hakan Ohlsson Boktryckeri, Lund, 1962. Stockholm.

BARRON, C. N., *et al.*: Intra-ocular Tumors in Animals. V. Transmissible Venereal Tumor of Dogs. Amer. J. Vet. Res. *24*:1263–1270, 1963.

BECKWITH, J. B., and PERRIN, E. V.: *In Situ* Neuroblastomas: A Contribution of the Natural History of Neural Crest Tumors. Amer. J. Path. *43*:1089–1104, 1963.

BELLHORN, R. W., and HENKIND, P.: Adenocarcinoma of the Ciliary Body. A Report of Two Cases in Dogs. Path. Vet. *5*:122–126, 1968.

BLACK, M. B.: Adenoma of Ceruminous Gland in the Dog. Arch. Path. *48*:85–88, 1949.

DMOCHOWSKI, L., *et al.*: Electron Microscope Studies of the Replication of a Virus Isolated from Bovine Cancer-eye Lesions. Proc. Amer. Assn. Cancer Res. *8*:14, 1967.

FRENCH, G. T.: A Clinical and Genetic Study of Eye Cancer in Hereford Cattle. Austr. Vet. J. *35*:474–481, 1959.

MAGRANE, W. G.: Tumors of the Eye and Orbit in the Dog. J. Small Anim. Pract. *6*: 165–169, 1965.

MOHIYUDDEEN, S.: A Study of the Eye Cancer among Bovines in Mysore State with Special Reference to its Histopathological Features, Biological Behavior and Some Factors Associated with its Causation. Indian Vet. J. *36*:125–132, 1959.

RICHTER, W. R.: Tubular Adenomata of the Adrenal of the Goat. Cornell Vet. *47*:558–577, 1957.

————: Adrenal Cortical Adenomata in the Goat. Amer. J. Vet. Res. *19*:895–901, 1958.

RUSSELL, W. O., WYNNE, E. S., and LOQUVAM, G. S.: Studies on Bovine Ocular Squamous Carcinoma ("Cancer Eye"). I. Pathological Anatomy and Historical Review. Cancer N.Y.), *9*:1–52, 1956.

SAUNDERS, L. Z., STEPHENSON, H. C., and McENTEE, K.: Diabetes Insipidus and Adiposo-genital Syndrome in a Dog Due to an Infundibuloma. Cornell Vet. *41*:445–458, 1951.

SAUNDERS, L. Z., and RICKARD, C. G.: Craniopharyngioma in a Dog with Apparent Adiposogenital Syndrome and Diabetes Insipidus. Cornell Vet. *42*:490–494, 1952.

SCOTTI, T. M.: The Carotid Body Tumor in Dogs. J. Am. Vet. Med. Assn. *132*:413–419, 1958.

SYKES, J. A., *et al.*: Bovine Ocular Squamous-cell Carcinoma. IV. Tissue-culture Studies of Bovine Ocular Squamous-cell Carcinoma and its Benign Precursor Lesions. J. Nat. Cancer Inst. *26*:445–471, 1961.

TOKARNIA, C. H.: Islet-cell Tumor of the Bovine Pancreas. J. Am. Vet. Med. Assn. *138*: 541–547, 1961.

ÜBERREITER, O., and KÖHLER, H.: (Primary Corneal Tumors in Horses, Dogs and Cats.) Wien. tierarztl. Wschr. *50*:70–86, 1963.

WHITE, E. G.: A Suprasellar Tumour in a Dog. J. Path. & Bact. *47*:323–326, 1938.

ZEDLER, W., and MÜLLER, E.: (Eye Tumours in Cattle.) Berl. Münch. Tierarztl. Wschr. *79*:222–226, 1966. V.B. *36*:4411, 1966.

8

The Cause and Nature of Disease

In subsequent chapters, we propose to consider the pathological changes characteristic of individual diseases, grouping the latter in accordance with their causes. It will be worthwhile, then, to pause long enough to see what things cause diseases in our animal patients and to examine the nature of those causes. Any disease involves the effects of some detrimental situation in the environment and the reactive activities by which the body tissues more or less successfully protect themselves from those effects.

An apparent exception to the preceding statement might seem to exist in those diseases which we view as hereditary, and those which, like diabetes mellitus, are attributed to some **intrinsic flaw** in the machinery of the body. But the question naturally arises, why is there a flaw in the machinery or how did a given family or strain come in the first place to have a genetic peculiarity transmissible by one defective individual to its descendants? As is explained briefly under the subject of heredity (p. 315), there are grounds for the tenet that even the **"hereditary"** and **congenital** diseases have their basis in injured germ plasm, if not, indeed, in unperceived injury to the developing embryonic individual itself (which makes the disease "congenital"). If this view proves to be correct, we shall eventually know more about the various injuries which can affect germ plasm, producing imperfections that are to be transmitted from generation to generation. Chapter 9 is devoted to this complex subject of **heredity** and cytogenetics.

Leaving this group, we find that diseases may be caused by the lack of some necessary ingredient or of some accessory substance essential to the animal mechanism. This is not difficult for most of us to believe; a motor does not run without fuel, neither will it do so without oil. The particular lesions and malfunctions which result from such **deficiencies** have, however, availed themselves of many hiding places and to discover them has required long and perspicacious search. These are given attention under the heading of Deficiency Diseases (p. 980).

A third group of causes of disease can be brought together under the caption of **mechanical and thermal injuries.** This has already been done, since such injurious agents—blows, cuts, heat, irradiations and the like—cause disease by producing necrosis or related changes (p. 17). It should be noted that injuries of this kind usually are not continuous but of short duration. The tissues are promptly free to accomplish whatever repair is possible. Unless the injury is repeated, the bodily reaction is relatively acute and normally subsides when repair and regeneration have been completed.

A fourth group of causes are **poisons,** substances which, by the direct and immediate chemical unions which they consummate and the abnormal chemical processes which they are able to institute, upset metabolic and functional activities and produce disease. Somewhat paralleling mechanical and thermal injuries, the effects of poisons are proportional to, and limited by the size of the dose or doses received; poisons do not perpetuate themselves. A considerable number of poisons in concentrated form are sufficiently injurious to bring immediate death (necrosis) to the cells with which they come in contact. However, in the case of most poisons the nature of the chemical malfeasance is not known; sometimes it is interference with oxidative processes in the tissue cells or in the blood; frequently it is a particular action on some part of the nervous system. A few poisons, such as ricin from the castor bean, have the same faculty as bacterial toxins and viruses to cause the production of neutralizing antibodies on the part of the body cells. Presumably such poisons have a similar ability to alter or combine with certain special cellular components which form the antibodies. (See below.) Also to be considered as poisonous are certain of the essential nutrients which, when fed in excess, result in disease. The fat soluble vitamins A and D are examples (p. 999).

The fifth and last group of causes of disease comprises the living organisms which invade the body and produce injuries of various kinds. Most of the living pathogens are host-specific, that is, a given pathogen only attacks hosts of a particular species. This becomes less true among the simpler forms; for instance, the virus of rabies is able, as far as known, to attack all warm-blooded species. But many of these simple bits of living protoplasm are so finely attuned to their environment that they react to differences in the tissues and fluids of host species so subtle as to be undetectable by our most exquisite chemical analyses. It is desirable to subdivide the living organisms according to their biological classification, especially since the injuries that they inflict, as well as the types of body reaction against them, can, to a certain extent, be grouped in corresponding categories. The subdivisions or classes to be considered are (a) metazoan parasites, (b) protozoa, (c) fungi, (d) higher bacteria, (e) lower bacteria and (f) viruses.

The **metazoan parasites,** of which the intestinal worms are the outstanding but by no means exclusive representatives, injure the host mechanically if they are actually within the tissues. The kidney worm of swine, the lungworms and the cystic intermediate stages of *Trichinella spiralis*, *Hypoderma bovis*, a number of tapeworms and many other types and species are examples of this form of injury, which, on the whole, is mild and of less significance than might be expected. There are exceptions to this, however, as, for example, the lesions resulting from invasion by *Spirocerca lupi* (p. 755) in the dog's esophagus and aorta. If the metazoan parasite is in the alimentary canal, its main detrimental effect is commonly to rob the host of nutriment. Some, however, are blood-suckers (hookworms, trichostrongyles) and the resulting anemia becomes the predominant injury. Mechanical obstruction of the lumen of the gut or of the bile-duct is a comparatively rare manner of injury. Hypersensitivity (p. 309) represents another manner in which parasites may initiate harmful effects.

It is probable that some of the metazoan parasites liberate toxic substances more or less similar to those produced by pathogenic bacteria, although positive information on this point is limited at the present time. Such toxic products have been suspected in the case of the common ascarid worm. Certain it is that hookworms, leeches and possibly other blood-sucking parasites release an anti-coagulant substance which prevents prompt cessation of hemorrhage from the wounds left by their bites. A single tick of certain species (*Dermacentor andersoni*, *Ixodes holocyclus*, *I. pilosus*) liberates a substance which causes paralysis in the parasitized animal or human, but which is usually terminated by early detachment of the tick (see p. 813).

The pathogenic **protozoa** seldom do violent damage to their host, protozoan diseases being almost always slow in progress with fatalities occurring only after an extended period, if at all. Some species invade individual cells, which they ultimately destroy. Whether this destruction is entirely a mechanical disintegration, it is difficult to say. The seriousness of the destructive effects depends upon the kind of cells involved, as well as their number. Destruction of erythrocytes by the organisms of piroplasmosis (babesiosis) or anaplasmosis generally produces a more dangerous disease than does destruction of intestinal epithelium by coccidia, because of the relative functional importance of the two kinds of cells. A characteristic of many protozoan diseases, rarely seen elsewhere, is the frequent ability of the host animal and the parasitic organism to acquire a toleration for each other so that they live in an almost symbiotic relationship, neither able to injure the other very seriously. This is noted in many piroplasmoses, plasmodioses (malarias) and trypanosomiases as well as in intestinal protozoan infections. It is interesting that nearly all protozoan diseases are infections of the intestinal tract or of the blood.

Passing to the **fungi**—microscopic plants lacking the green pigment chlorophyll and multiplying by methods more complicated than simple fission—we find that their ability to produce disease is limited. With a few exceptions, fungous diseases involve the skin or the mucous surfaces including the lungs, probably because the ability of fungi to invade tissues and their adaptability to a completely internal environment are not great. The vast majority of fungi are not parasitic at all, but this, of course, can be said likewise of the bacteria, as well as the protozoa and metazoa. The pathogenetic qualities of a few fungi, however, must not be minimized. A number are able to grow successfully, though perhaps slowly, within the tissues and produce some of our most formidable diseases (histoplasmosis, coccidioidomycosis, blastomycosis and others). Pathogenicity is doubtless due to toxic products of the organisms which diffuse into the surrounding tissues and injure or kill the nearby cells. Of the chemical nature of these toxic substances very little is known.

The pathogenic **"higher bacteria"** (bacteria other than the order *Eubacteriales*) produce diseases of slowly progressive and chronic nature as a rule. In several of the most important diseases (tuberculosis, glanders, necrobacillosis, etc.), an important and conspicuous feature is massive and progressive necrosis in the vicinity of the colonies of organisms. Necrotizing toxins are evidently at work. In other diseases of this group (Johne's disease, actinomycosis and others), the injury falls short of producing necrosis but, as will be seen shortly, causes a cellular reaction which is entirely comparable to the reaction against the necrotizing diseases. A minority of the pathogens of this group are capable of causing acute, reactive disease. In all these, the destructive and often lethal actions are due to toxic substances elaborated by the bacteria.

The pathogenic **simple bacteria** (*Eubacteriales*) regularly cause acute disease, which is often severe. This is evidently accomplished through the action of powerful toxins, although little is known about their chemistry or their exact mode of action. Certain types of toxic substances, it is true, are recognized and named according to their particular effects, as, for example, hemolysins, which hemolyze erythrocytes, leukocidins, which kill leukocytes, and aggressins which drive away the leukocytes and other protective substances, but these designations tell us nothing about how those effects are produced. Many of the bacterial pathogens prefer to localize in a particular organ or tissue; certain others grow and multiply in practically all the tissues of the body. Examples of the former are *Corynebacterium renale*, which regularly attacks the bovine kidney, the swine-erysipelas organism, which has a predilection for joint surfaces or the endocardium, the streptococcus of equine strangles, which only rarely localizes elsewhere than in the upper respiratory mucous membranes, or the Salmonellæ which limit their activities to the intestines.

Viruses, the least discernible and supposedly the most primitive of living things, constitute, from the standpoint of injuries inflicted, the most formidable and the most important of the several groups of disease-producers. It is not certain even that they are living organisms, especially since Stanley, in 1935, reduced the virus which causes mosaic disease of the tobacco plant to a crystalline form. Other plant viruses, as well as animal viruses, such as the virus of poliomyelitis have also been crystallized. The idea had been advanced at a much earlier date that viruses may be organic catalyzers differing from the ordinary enzymes in that they not only induce abnormal (and pathological) metabolic processes in body cells, but also affect the chemical activities in those cells in such a way that a new and larger supply of the virus is continually produced. More recently, the possibility has been studied that they differ but little from the genes which compose the chromosomes and govern heredity. These hypotheses now appear correct for most viruses. The DNA or RNA of the virus carries all the information needed for the hereditary transmission of its specific characteristics. Upon infecting a cell the viral genome assumes command of the cellular machinery and redirects its activities to reproduce new viral particles. Thus a virus does not, and cannot, reproduce in a manner comparable to an animal or plant cell, but rather must borrow the synthesizing machinery of a cell in order to be reproduced. Viruses are therefore, obligate intracellular parasites.

Viruses are particles of rather definite and constant size and shape, as has been shown by their passage or retention by various filters, by ultracentrifugation and by the electron microscope. Animal viruses consist of a central core of nucleic acid (DNA or RNA, but not both) surrounded by a protein shell called a capsid. The capsid together with the nucleic acid form the nucleocapsid of the virus which is divided into basic subunits called capsomeres. Surrounding the nucleocapsid some viruses have an envelope or membrane which is believed to be derived from cytoplasmic or nuclear membranes of the infected cell. A single complete viral particle is referred to as a virion. Viruses are rather easily killed (or "inactivated" if they were never really alive) by the same disinfectants that kill bacteria, as well as by the same degree of heat (55 to 60° C.), but some are very resistant to drying. If the degree of heating or disinfectant action is suitable, they retain the power to induce the formation of antibodies of the same kinds and in the same way as do bacteria. Similarly, their pathogenicity but not their antigenicity is easily destroyed by ultraviolet rays. With the exception of a few which approach the bacteria in the size of their particles, they are not affected by sulfonamides and antibiotics as are many bacteria. Viruses can only be propagated in, or in the presence of the living body cells of a host (the chick embryo serving as a very useful artificial host for many). They cannot be seen or detected by any ordinary laboratory means. Hence, their presence is established only by their effects, the disease produced. As Hagan (1960) cleverly expresses it, viruses are better known by what they do than by what they are.

The type of disease produced by viruses may be either destructive or proliferative. Tissue destructive viruses or cytocidal viruses produce necrotizing diseases which in general are comparable to those produced by the simple bacteria; acute and often severe infections. The proliferative lesions may vary from simple hyperplasia to neoplasia. We can do little more than speculate on the mechanisms by which viruses produce injury, but the cytolytic effects are probably directly related to altered cellular metabolism induced by the virus resulting in a disturbance of one or more vital cellular processes. Proliferation and neoplasia appear to result from the incorporation of the viral genome into the cell without causing death but rather causing unrestricted growth. Viral infection need not invariably result in visible lesions as many viruses are capable of invading a cell and remaining dormant. Such viruses are said to be *latent* and the "disease" *sub-clinical*. Under proper circumstances, which are not understood, latent viruses may be activated to produce disease. This relationship is best illustrated with *Herpesvirus simplex* in man which is usually latent, but if the host is stressed, as for example by fever, the virus is activated and a characteristic lesion develops; in this case a "fever blister." Latent infections are to be differentiated from *virus persistence* which is characterized by the presence of the virus in the body after recovery, or during a period without clinical signs as is the case with the virus of equine infectious anemia. A third relationship, not leading to lesions, is *virus symbiosis* which is an association of a non-pathogenic virus and host tissue which is of mutual benefit.

It is notable that a given virus regularly (but, in the case of some, not invariably) attacks a certain body tissue or structure and, to a considerable degree, localizes in the same tissue or structure where it produces lesions. For instance, the virus of equine encephalomyelitis is found in the nervous tissues (which are the ones injured) and only very transiently elsewhere. On the basis of the kind of tissue usually attacked, viruses have been divided into epitheliotropic (attracted to epithelium), neutrotropic, pneumotropic and pantropic (attracted to all tissues) types. However, these divisions are not highly precise. The classification of viruses is discussed further in Chapter 10.

In many of the viral diseases, peculiar structures known as **inclusion bodies** or **cell inclusions** (Plate I, p. 348) appear regularly and have come to possess great and often decisive importance in diagnosis. These inclusions vary considerably in appearance, although most of them are acidophilic in their staining reactions. In some diseases, the characteristic inclusions are found in the nucleus, while in others they are in the cytoplasm. The first discovered and the best known of these inclusions are the intracytoplasmic Negri bodies of rabies, named for the Italian pathologist who discovered them.

The nature of viral inclusion bodies has prompted considerable discussion and argument. Some considered them to be aggregates of virions and others believed them to be artefacts. Both views appear to be correct; depending on the stage of the inclusion body's development and the virus inducing their formation. Electron microscopic studies have demonstrated that most viral inclusion bodies do in fact represent virions in various stages of development embedded in a protein matrix of uncertain significance. Certain viruses can apparently vacate the inclusion body, leaving behind the protein matrix. Whether or not virus is present at a given time, it seems reasonably certain that inclusion bodies are, or had been, sites of viral synthesis and accumulation. It is not known why some viral diseases are invariably associated with inclusion bodies whereas in other viral diseases inclusion bodies are never observed. Regardless of their exact significance, inclusion bodies represent a result of virus-host cell interaction of great diagnostic importance.

The Reactions of Disease.—Thus far we have considered the various pathogenic agents and what they do to the patient. Let us now see what the patient can do to the pathogen. The reaction of the body tissues is in many diseases directly responsible for more of the symptoms and lesions than are the discernible alteration of, and damage to the tissues. The story of bodily reaction is largely the story of inflammation and that has already been told (Chapter 4). It is reinforced by the various processes of regeneration and repair. Hyperplasia has been discussed and shown to be usually a reaction to injury or irritation (p. 94). The same is true of the neoplasms caused by chemical carcinogens. The question whether all forms of neoplasia may not be manifestations of reactions to irritants is most intriguing and one that may be answered in the not too distant future. Fever, a generalized bodily reaction, has been discussed and its benefits enumerated. (p. 184) Such physiological mechanisms as increased rates of respiration and heart-beat are of the same nature as are also polydipsia and polyuria in cases of mild renal injury. The elaboration of immunizing antibodies is in the same category and will require discussion presently.

Reviewing the several types of causes of disease as outlined earlier in this chapter, we find that there is little, if any, reaction to those diseases and abnormalities resulting from some **innate flaw** in the germ plasm or body mechanisms. Compensatory and adaptive hypertrophy (p. 92) is a process able to amend the situation in the case of some of these defects. Examples include not only the hypertrophy of one kidney, when the other is missing or non-functional, or hypertrophy of the cardiac musculature to compensate for a patent foramen ovale, but also such phenomena as hypertrophy of the bone marrow in cases of anemia. Hyperplasias arise in reaction to some of the deficiency diseases, for instance the enlarged thyroid in iodine deficiency or the enlargement of bones and joints in rickets.

To **mechanical and thermal injuries** the reaction is regularly inflammatory. Acute serous inflammation (p. 153) followed by proliferative inflammation and repair is the rule here. There is also an inflammatory reaction against the necrotic tissue that may have resulted from the injury; it is usually sero-purulent and lymphocytic. An outstanding example is the inflammatory line of demarcation that separates the living from a gangrenous area.

Against **poisons**, in general, the animal body is unable to offer marked resistance or reaction. Most poisons, when taken into the digestive tract, are sufficiently irritant that they cause nausea, thereby dissuading the animal from partaking further of the offending substance, vomiting (depending on the species of patient) which gets rid of much of the poisonous material, and diarrhea, which quickly expels the poisonous ingesta that may have reached the intestine. The local reaction on the part of whatever areas of the gastro-intestinal mucosa come in contact with the poison is the prompt appearance of acute catarrhal or hemorrhagic inflammation. Pronounced edema (serous exudate) of the deeper layers of the gastric or intestinal wall and even of the mesentery occurs in many of these poisonings, which is in contrast with what is seen in infectious inflammations.

Probably the most spectacular reaction against a poison is seen when most venoms of animal origin and a few plant poisons enter the cutaneous and subcutaneous tissues. An outpouring of serum into the surrounding tissue occurs in unbelievable amount and with unbelievable rapidity. This is carelessly called edema, but is by definition a serous inflammatory exudate. In some individuals, reactions of this type become extreme, apparently on the basis of allergic hypersensitivity (bee stings, etc.). The serous exudation is highly beneficial at least in diluting the poison; a similar but miniature accumulation of serum occurs when certain inorganic poisons are injected subcutaneously, but this reaction depends purely on local irritation. The injection of a fatal dose of a solution of strychnine, for instance, would not provoke it.

In the case of the frequently encountered hepatotoxic and nephrotoxic poisons, it is difficult to say that there is any reaction to the poison except in so far as an alterative inflammation (p. 164) can be considered a reaction. Hyperplasia of the liver cells, for instance, is regenerative and consequent upon the death of the original cellular inhabitants. Similarly the fibrous proliferations, whether cirrhotic or nephritic, are reactions and reparative attempts which would follow toxic necrosis of the previously existing hepatic or renal epithelium whatever its cause.

Against the **metazoan parasites,** there are only very limited bodily reactions, at least as viewed from the standpoint of what may occur in response to bacterial infections. In general, when we think of parasitism we think of eosinophilia, but in reality this applies only to certain parasitisms. In trichinosis (acute stage), ascariasis and a number of other intestinal helminthiases, the esoinophil count of the blood may rise to several times the small normal percentage, that is, to 6 or possibly 10 per cent of the total white cells. However, this is highly variable, being possibly on an allergic basis. In some common intestinal helminthiases, eosinophilia is minor or absent. Eosinophils are usually prominent in the exudates which surround parasitic larvæ or adults which have invaded the tissues, but here also there are exceptions, as for instance infection by *Spirocerca lupi.*

Local reactions to migrating parasites, usually larvæ, vary from practically nothing to the extensive granulomatous lesions, heavily infiltrated with eosinophils, lymphocytes and reticulo-endothelial cells, which form the "summer sores" characteristic of cutaneous habronemiasis (p. 772) of the horse. The nodules of intestinal "nodular disease" (oesophagostomiasis, p. 743) are examples of small granulomatous encapsulations of a parasite, the central part of the nodule usually becoming necrotic. Encysted parasites, such as cysticerci (p. 787) and trichinae (p. 762) eventually die and then undergo hyaline degeneration or calcification. As contrasting examples, we may cite the hookworms (p. 738) which in limited numbers inflict their blood-sucking bites and occasion almost no reaction. When their numbers are great enough to produce gross mechanical injury to the mucous membrane, a diffuse catarrhal or hemorrhagic enteritis results, but probably has secondary bacterial infection of the injured tissue as an important immediate cause.

Humoral antibodies (p. 307), in the usual sense, are not formed in response to attack by metazoan parasites. Complement-fixing bodies do develop against certain genera or classes of parasites. The best known of these occur in echinococcosis, the complement-fixation test being of use in the diagnosis of suspected hydatid cysts.

In spite of the absence of demonstrable immunizing antibodies and despite the comparative lack of inflammatory reaction, there is an undeniable resistance to most metazoan parasites which accompanies maturity of age and, in the case of some parasites, at least, a state of superior nutrition and vigor. An example of the latter is readily available in pediculosis; in the same herd of cattle, horses or pigs, individuals that are already unthrifty or are very young or very old become lousy in late winter, while their more robust companions have practically no lice. Whether the well-known resistance of older animals to intestinal helminths is the result of previous infestation has not been proved. The fundamental nature of this resistance, which is strong but not perfect, has baffled investigators.

The **pathogenic protozoa** are notable for doing serious and often fatal injury to the host while inciting practically no inflammatory reaction. A more meaningful statement would be that the animal body has almost no weapons with which to fight protozoa. A successful defense appears to depend considerably upon regenerating the victimized cells (erythrocytes, intestinal epithelium) faster than they are destroyed. There is, however, a gradually developing resistance against protozoa which, like that against metazoa, appears not to be related to any form of humoral antibody. In toxoplasmosis (a protozoan infection), there is a very limited reaction of mononuclear and other leukocytes and giant cells. Rarely a coeval invasion by large numbers of sarcosporidia appears to be met by a transient neutrophilic and lymphocytic infiltration of the affected muscles.

The invasive **fungi** and **higher bacteria** can be grouped together in considering body reactions. As is readily seen by contemplating such well-known diseases as tuberculosis, glanders, Johne's disease, actinomycosis, blastomycosis, syphilis and leprosy (the last two belonging to the human family), the defensive reactions, cellular and humoral, are not sufficient in most cases to destroy the pathogen, once it is established. The humoral antibodies (p. 307) are especially ineffective, although their presence can sometimes be shown by careful tests and a certain relative degree of increased resistance is demonstrable against tuberculosis following certain immunizing procedures (B.C.G., etc.). In several diseases, complement-fixing bodies exist and can be used diagnostically. The cellular reaction against pathogens of these groups is more conspicuous and possibly more potent. In some of the diseases it is purulent, in others it is not, but in all cases it involves reticulo-endothelial cells, lymphocytes and fibroblasts, which together form an encapsulating, granulomatous mass of tissue which, with more or less success, separates the infected from the healthy areas. The infected foci are, as it were, placed in quarantine and the spread of the infection is prevented or, at least, delayed. While this is the average and typical picture in this group, there should be mentioned at the mildest extreme the dermatophytes, or ringworm fungi, which elicit only a mild infiltration of inflammatory cells, and, at the severest extreme, a few acute infections comparable to those produced by the simple bacteria.

It is against the bacteria and viruses that the reactive forces of the animal (or human) body are most active and vigorous or, at least, most in evidence. This is not to say that the battle is more likely to have a favorable ending, for it will be recalled these invaders were described on an earlier page as producing **severe and formidable infections.** Still, it can be said to the credit of modern medical science that by taking advantage of the host's potentialities for vigorous reaction and supplementing them with artificial devices (vaccines, antibiotics), it has been possible to remove much of the sting from most of the diseases in this group.

Of the diseases caused by higher bacteria, the preceding statement is less true than of those caused by the **simple bacteria** and **viruses**. The latter may be grouped together, since the body reactions against them are similar. Except in the case of infections which are strictly localized, fever is usually a prominent aspect of the body reaction. The cellular reactions are those of acute exudative (p. 152) inflammation typically, but there are important exceptions. In many viral diseases, the cellular exudate is minimal or practically absent (rabies); in a majority of these, lymphocytic infiltrations predominate; in some (equine encephalomyelitis) lymphocytic and neutrophilic infiltrations are combined. Brucellosis may be mentioned as an infection which is exudative during acute exacerbations (abortions) and in restricted localizations but is reticulo-endothelial and even granulomatous during remissions.

Antibodies.—It is against the simple bacteria and viruses that the **humoral antibodies** assume prime importance. Details must be left to works on immunology, but certain features of antibodies and their formation will be reviewed here. The adjective "humoral" is a vestige of the Hippocratic teachings. It will be remembered that in the conception of the renowned Greek physician the body contained four humors, or fluids (blood, phlegm, black bile and yellow bile), and that diseases represented disorders of those humors (fluids). Humoral antibodies therefore are the substances (chemical, but not concrete bodies) which work against (*anti*) disease and are found in the body fluids, chief of which is the blood serum. The antibodies are the basis of humoral immunity, immunity being defined as a marked and unusual resistance to disease. It is principally through their effects that an animal is immune to further attack after having recovered from, or after having been successfully vaccinated against an infectious disease. Antibodies are formed in the body as the result of exposure to, and attack by pathogens, usually microorganisms and their toxic products, rarely proteins from some other organic source. They are specific, meaning that a given antibody has immunizing effect only against the particular microorganism or protein which brought it into being. That antibodies are of cellular origin is not in doubt, but considerable confusion has existed as to what cell or cells are responsible for their formation, *i.e.*, what cells are *immunologically competent*. Most evidence indicates that plasma cells (p. 178) produce antibody, and that lymphocytes (p. 173) are an integral component of the immunological mechanisms. The relationship of lymphocytes to plasma cells; the transformation of lymphocytes into immunologically competent cells; and whether lymphocytes can produce antibody are questions of prime importance but still unanswered. Also yet to be solved is the relationship (if any) of reticulum cells and macrophages to antibody production. To date the plasma cell remains the only cell known to produce antibody. Plasma cells are derived from B-lymphocytes (p. 175).

How a foreign protein induces the production of a specific antibody has been the subject of extensive investigation and debate but remains a mystery. Two theories have been set forth and although to date both are hypothetical, they deserve brief consideration prior to our later discussion of hypersensitivity and autoimmunity. The **instructive theory** postulates that antigen upon entering the body comes into contact with **immunologically competent cells** and acts as a templet to instruct the cell to produce a specific gamma globulin. This theory implies that any immunologically competent cell can be instructed to produce any specific antibody, a difficult task in view of the potential number of antibodies. Other major obstacles to the theory are (1) the templet (antigen) would have to persist for the duration of the immunity, (2) it does not account for the anamnestic response, and (3) it does not allow for an adequate explanation of the body's ability to recognize "self," or how an individual can be tricked into recognizing "non-self" as self. It is well known that except under unusual circumstances, antibodies are not produced against one's own tissues. Yet for a period of time while the immune system is "immature," foreign proteins can be introduced which in later life will be recognized as self and not as foreign. This is well illustrated in free-martin cattle who share placental circulation resulting in a transfer of cellular (and humoral) components. As adults these dizygotic twins are chimerics (p. 327) which share blood groups and which are immunologically tolerant of each other's tissues. Other experimentally induced forms of immunological tolerance also support this phenomenon.

To explain recognition of self and non-self as well as to meet other objections to the instructive theory, Burnet advanced the **selective theory,** or **clonal theory** of antibody production. This theory proposes that clones of cells exist which have the inherent capacity to produce antibody upon stimulation by the proper antigen; and that this clone is stimulated to reproduce more cells with the same capacity. The theory indicates that for every possible antigen (including self), a cell or clone of cells exists which have the genetically endowed ability to produce a specific antibody to that specific antigen, and that the antigen must find (select) the proper cell or cells with which to interact. To explain self recognition and immunological tolerance before birth, it is then theorized that body antigens or self, interact with the proper cells, or clones, before birth and before these cells have the ability to proliferate upon antigenic stimulus and that this interaction results in the destruction of these clones.

The antibodies known to exist in the blood serum are (1) antitoxins, which chemically and quantitatively neutralize specific bacterial exotoxins (tetanus, diphtheria, botulism); (2) agglutinins, which agglutinate bacterial cells, sticking them together in such large masses that they spread to other areas of the body only with difficulty; (3) precipitins, which precipitate dissolved proteins, thus inhibiting their dissemination and chemical activity; (4) lysins, which dissolve cells, including pathogenic bacterial cells; and (5) opsonins, which facilitate and stimulate phagocytosis of bacterial cells (cocci and certain bacilli) by the microphages (neutrophils) or even by the macrophages (p. 178).

The antitoxins, as stated, enter into chemical combination with certain toxic substances produced by the parent species of bacterial pathogen, thereby nullifying their disease-producing power. The agglutinins are thought to act by neutralizing or nullifying the electric charge which is normally carried by bacteria in suspension. With this charge, normally negative, the cells repel each other in accordance with the well-known electrical law that like charges repel and unlike attract. Once the charges have been eliminated, the cells clump together pursuant to Newton's first law of motion (gravity), and the same can probably be said of molecules when they are precipitated by precipitins. To accomplish this change of electrical potential, a chemical reaction has doubtless occurred. Similarly there must be chemical reactions between each of the other humoral antibodies and appropriate molecules in or on the bacterial cell or virus but little is known definitely. It is quite possible that there are other "antibodies" in the body fluids of which we have no knowledge because we cannot identify their effects. At any rate, it is by the various actions just described and probably by others, as yet unrecognized, that the body fluids play their part, often a decisive one, in combatting the microörganisms which cause disease.

There is also **cellular mediated immunity** (and hypersensitivity, p. 309) which is independent of humoral antibodies. Cellular immunity accounts for resistance to tuberculosis and certain other infections, all forms of delayed hypersensitivity such as transplant rejection (p. 311), and possibly prevention of endogenous tumor formation. Cellular immunity is mediated through T-lymphocytes (p. 175) which are sensitized by appropriate antigens to proliferate and release cytotoxic factors to neutralize antigen. This process is further discussed under hypersensitivity (p. 309) and tuberculosis (p. 635).

A form of cellular immunity which is better understood is the production of **interferon** by cells infected with a virus. Interferon is probably of greater importance in limiting a viral infection in non-immune animals than are humoral antibodies. It has been long recognized that an animal or tissue, infected with virus, was resistant to infection with a second virus, a phenomenon labeled *viral interference*. It is now known that most viruses, upon infecting a cell, stimulate the production and release of a protein called interferon, which prevents or interferes with the action of the same virus, or of another virus, on new cells. The mechanism of this interference is not known, but it is believed to hinder the formation of complete and infective virus. Thus, in the presence of interferon a virus is capable of infecting a cell and even altering its metabolism which may destroy the cell, but new infective virus is not duplicated. Virus which may be formed is incomplete and not capable of reinfecting new cells. Interferon is not virus specific but it is species, or host specific.

The degree of the reaction to these bacterial and viral pathogens depends upon the immunological state of the individual patient. The normal, susceptible individual, upon exposure to infection contracts the disease and suffers the acute inflammatory and febrile reaction outlined as usual for pathogens of the simple bacterial and viral groups. But there are two other states possible: he may be immune or he may be hypersensitive. If he is immune, it is, of course, because of a plentiful supply of humoral or cellular antibodies ("species immunity" excepted). If he is hypersensitive to the particular pathogen or its products, a severe reaction results from slight contact with the pathogenic products in a way which ordinarily would have insignificant effects.

Hypersensitivity.—Hypersensitivity is a reactive status which is very imperfectly understood. It represents an accelerated or accentuated immune response to the degree that it is often detrimental rather than beneficial. This is especially true when violent reactions, which may lead to death, develop in response to exposure to ordinarily innocuous substances. Hypersensitivity reactions are divided into *immediate-type* and *delayed-type*. The immediate reactions include *Anaphylaxis*, the *Arthus reaction*, and *serum sickness*. Delayed reactions are classically illustrated by *tuberculin sensitivity*, *transplant rejection*, and *allergies* such as contact dermatitis and certain drug allergies. **Anaphylaxis** can be experimentally demonstrated when an animal is given parenterally a minute dose usually of a protein-containing substance, such as white of egg or the blood serum of another species of animal. After an "incubation" period of about ten days or two weeks, it is then given a larger dose of the same substance in the same way. The dose and the material are such as would be harmless to a normal animal, but in this "sensitized" animal a state of "anaphylactic shock" supervenes within a matter of minutes. The fundamental reaction here is contraction of smooth muscle, which produces varied symptoms according to the anatomical characteristics of the species involved. In the guinea pig, contraction of the smooth muscle of the bronchioles is the outstanding effect with dyspnea and partial or fatal suffocation. In the dog, contraction of venous passages is the salient manifestation with severe congestion of the liver and other splanchnic organs. In some species, such as the rabbit, the effects are less clearly defined but areas of ischemic necrosis result from the same or a similar mechanism. Anaphylaxis (and other immediate-type but not delayed-type hypersensitivities) is dependent on circulating serum antibodies which can be transferred to another individual. For reasons poorly understood, the interaction of antigen and antibody induces the release of chemical mediators from cells and tissues which in turn act upon smooth muscle cells resulting in the anaphylactic symptom complex. Four substances have been incriminated as mediators, though variation exists between species as to which of the four assume importance. These are (1) *histamine* (p. 150) which is released from mast cells and platelets, (2) *serotonin* (p. 151) which is released from enterochromaffin tissue, mast cells (rats only) and platelets, (3) *kinins* (p. 151) produced from plasma precursors and (4) *slow reacting substance* which is a substance of unknown composition and origin. Each of these in the appropriate host causes contraction of smooth muscle.

As is widely recognized, certain individual human beings suffer from hypersensitivity to organic substances of great variety. If the offending substance is a particular food, such as strawberries in one instance or lobsters in another, the hypersensitivity is shown by digestive disturbances or cutaneous rashes. If the object of the hypersensitivity is an inhaled substance, the result is either "hay fever," a seromucous inflammation of the upper air passages, or asthma, a spasmodic and hypertrophic narrowing of the bronchioles. Immediate hypersensitivity of these types is known as **allergy** or **atopy.** It is presumed to depend on a previous sensitization although in the case of hypersensitivity to such substances as sulfonamides, it is not always evident how the hypersensitive state arose. Comparable disorders, while infrequent, are known to occur in domestic animals and appear to be very similar to those of man. They are less rare in those species whose life spans are longer, perhaps because long life affords greater opportunity for previous sensitization.

The Arthus reaction represents another expression of hypersensitivity which is probably of importance in disease processes characterized by vascular injury and necrosis of ill defined pathogenesis (as in some cases of glomerulonephritis). The Arthus reaction consists of a focal area of inflammation and necrosis at the site of antigen injection in a previously sensitized animal. As in anaphylaxis, it is dependent upon circulating antibody. The injected antigen combines and precipitates with antibody (and complement) in vessel walls; a reaction which results in damage to the vessel, though the mechanism leading to damage is not understood. The antigen-antibody complex attracts large numbers of polymorphonuclear leukocytes which infiltrate and surround the vessel and by some means contribute to further damage; leading to necrosis, edema, hemorrhage and thrombosis. If polymorphonuclear cell infiltration is blocked, the Arthus reaction does not develop. In brief, the Arthus reaction is an antigen-antibody mediated acute vasculitis dependent upon polymorphonuclear leukocytes.

Serum sickness is in some respects similar to the Arthus reaction, but classically serum sickness develops in individuals not previously sensitized to the responsible antigen. Instead, when a large amount of antigen such as horse serum is injected, some remains in circulation as an antibody response becomes evident, which is generally six to twelve days. The resulting circulating antigen-antibody complex leads to the development of serum sickness. Although most of this complex is removed from circulation by the reticuloendothelial system, some is deposited in vessel walls which leads to a necrotizing vasculitis. Many vessels may be affected, but in particular, lesions are seen in the major arteries, the endocardium and the renal glomeruli.

Delayed Hypersensitivity.—Probably the most important form of hypersensitivity in the domestic animals is that which accompanies the presence of a number of well-known chronic diseases. Histologically these diseases are characterized by granulomatous proliferation and there is reason to believe that the granulomatous reaction (p. 166) is dependent upon a state of hypersensitivity. Tuberculosis is the outstanding example, together with the familiar tuberculin reaction. Other diseases in which the same phenomena are of importance are Johne's disease, glanders, coccidioidomycosis, and histoplasmosis. Diagnostic use is made of the hypersensitivity existing in these diseases and also in the case of hydatid disease (echinococcosis) and to some extent in brucellosis. If the metabolic products of one of these pathogenic species is introduced in minute amount into the tissues of an animal harboring infection with the same species, a reaction of totally inordinate severity results, whereas in a noninfected animal no appreciable change occurs. The usual method is to inject intradermally about 1 or two drops of a bacteria-free filtrate of the broth medium in which the pathogen in question has been grown in laboratory culture. This is the intradermal tuberculin (or johnin, mallein, etc.) test. After an incubation period which is usual in antigen-antibody reactions, a localized inflammatory swelling develops. It is composed of the usual ingredients of acute, non-purulent inflammatory exudates—serum (inflammatory edema), a little fibrin, lymphocytes, mononuclears of the reticuloendothelial group and a scattering of other inflammatory cells. The swelling subsides after several days. The tuberculin is sometimes instilled into the conjunctival sac, a mucopurulent exudate resulting after a few hours. If the same filtrate is injected into the subcutaneous tissue, so that absorption occurs, there is fever and general malaise, beginning after a few hours and lasting perhaps twenty-four hours. It is possible experimentally to give a normal animal a dose of overwhelming size and perhaps produce a reaction and lesions resembling those of the disease itself, but from doses such as are used in diagnostic tests no effects can be discerned in the healthy animal. The diagnostic tests used in humans to detect a state of allergy consist in the cutaneous injection of minute amounts of the suspected protein, plant pollen or animal product and sensitivity is revealed by the same type of hyperemic inflammatory swelling.

The delayed-type reaction is not dependent on circulating antibodies but rather cellular mediated immunity. The sensitivity cannot be transferred by injecting

11

serum into another individual but can be transferred with whole cells (lymph node or circulating leukocytes).

Autoimmunity.—In the discussion of hypersensitivity we saw how a normal process can become aberrant or over-reactive and become more harmful than the noxious stimuli initiating the reaction. Autoimmunity represents another aberrant reaction on the part of the immunological mechanisms which harm the host and for which no advantage can be found. As defined by Burnet (1969), autoimmunity is *"a condition in which structural or functional damage is produced by the reaction of immunocytes or antibodies with normal components of the body."* How can antibodies form against one's own tissues? What happens to self-recognition (p. 308)? Using Burnet's clonal theory of antibody formation several conceivable mechanisms can be set forth to explain autoimmunity.

(1) *Anatomic segregation of antigen:* If during maturation of the immune system a particular antigen is anatomically segregated, or not formed until later in life, this antigen will not be recognized as self as it will never have had the opportunity to inactivate immunologically competent clones capable of reacting to it. For all practical purposes the antigen is foreign. Thyroglobulin which never leaves the lumens of the follicles to gain entrance into the circulation is an example of such an antigen. If for any reason thyroglobulin does enter the circulation, antibodies are formed which react with the thyroid. Hashimoto's disease of man and similar forms of lymphocytic thyroiditis in the dog are believed to represent this form of an autoimmune disease. Spermatozoa and the lens of the eye are other examples of isolated antigens.

(2) *Alteration of antigens:* If tissues are altered such that new and foreign reactive antigenic sites are present, they will stimulate antibody formation. It is postulated that radiation, mutations, infections, and certain chemicals might produce antigenic alteration of tissue proteins.

(3) *Cross reactions between antigens:* If foreign antigens possess reactive sites in common with tissue proteins, the antibodies to the foreign antigen might react with tissue proteins. Rheumatic fever and glomerulonephritis in man are believed to be the result of this type of cross reaction between tissue proteins and certain strains of streptococci.

(4) *Forbidden clones:* It is postulated that autoimmunity might be caused by alteration of immunocytes with the appearance of new clones or a failure of the normal suppression mechanisms allowing clones to persist or reappear. These forbidden clones, as termed by Burnet, would then be capable of producing antibodies to tissue proteins. It is in this category which most autoimmune diseases in man are placed. It is not known why new, forbidden, or abnormal clones appear, but it is believed that in certain individuals a genetic predisposition exists.

Whatever the mechanism, autoimmunity represents a failure to recognize self, and the development of serious and often fatal disease for which no satisfactory treatment exists.

In man, many diseases are believed to be autoimmune in origin, whereas in animals examples are few. Autoimmune hemolytic anemia has been described in dogs (p. 1174). A disease resembling systemic lupus erythematosus has been reported in dogs (p. 1262). Lymphocytic thyroiditis (p. 1363) has already been mentioned. Autoimmunity is believed to play an important role in the pathogenesis of the lesions of Aleutian disease, a viral disease of mink (p. 501). Autoimmunity probably participates in other diseases such as *Brucella ovis* epididymitis in rams (p. 594). Undoubtedly the list of autoimmune diseases in animals will grow as this mechanism of disease is studied further.

The Cause and Nature of Disease

ATKINS, E.: Pathogenesis of Fever. Physiol. Rev. *40*:580–646, 1960.

BAGDONAS, V., and OLSON, C., JR.: Observations on Immunity in Cutaneous Bovine Papillomatosis. Am. J. Vet. Research. *15*:240–245, 1954.

BERGSTRAND, H.: On the Pathological Anatomy of the Allergic Reaction. Odontologisk tidskr. *4*:339–343, 1945.

BEVERIDGE, W. I. B.: Immunity to Viruses; General Discussion with Special Reference to Role of Allergy. Lancet. *2*:299–304, 1952.

BORRELL, A.: Sur les inclusions de l'épithélioma contagieux des oiseaux (molluscum contagiosum). Comp. rend. Soc. de biol. *57*:642, 1904.

BURNET, MACFARLANE: *Cellular Immunology* (Books One and Two). Melbourne University Press, 1969, pp. 1–726.

BURNS, P. W.: Allergic Reactions in Dogs. J. Am. Vet. Med. Assn. *83*:627–634, 1933.

CHURG, J., and STRAUSS, L.: Allergic Granulomatosis, Allergic Angiitis and Periarteritis Nodosa. Am. J. Path. *27*:277–302, 1951. [The patients had asthma, therefore allergic.]

COFFIN, D. L., COONS, A. H., and CABASSO, V. J.: Histological Study of Infectious Canine Hepatitis by Means of Fluorescent Antibody. J. Exper. Med. *98*:13–20, 1953.

COONS, A. H., LEDUC, E. H., and CONNOLLY, J. M.: A Method for the Histochemical Demonstration of Specific Antibody and Its Application to a Study of the Hyperimmune Rabbit. J. Exper. Med. *102*:49–60, 1955.

FENNER, F., and MARSHALL, I. D.: Passive Immunity in Myxomatosis of the European Rabbit. J. Hyg. *52*:321–336, 1954.

GOLDGRABER, M. B., and KIRSNER, J. B.: Granulomatous Lesions—An Expression of a Hypersensitive State. An Experimental Study. Arch. Path. *66*:618–634, 1958.

HAGAN, W. A., and BRUNER, D. W.: *Infectious Diseases of Domesitc Animals*. 4th ed. Ithaca, Comstock Publishing Co., 1960.

HOWARD, F. A., and CRONIN, M. T. I.: Colostral Transfer of Anti-erythrocyte Agglutinins from Mare to Foal. J. Am. Vet. Med. Assn. *126*:93–94, 1955.

HULLAND, T. J.: Arteriosclerotic Changes in the Visceral Arteries of Sheep. Canad. Vet. J. *1*:195–205, 1960.

IZSOF, Z.: Anafylaxia u ošípanych. [Anaphylaxis in Pigs.] Čas. československ. Vet. *5*:200–201, 1950. Also (Abstr.) Vet. Bull. No. 1031, 1951.

KEUNING, F. J., and VAN DER SLIKKE, L. B.: Role of Immature Plasma Cells, Lymphoblasts and Lymphocytes in the Formation of Antibodies as Established in Tissue Cultures. J. Lab. & Clin. Med. *36*:167–182, 1950.

ROCHA LAGÔA, F.: Imunidade e permeabilidade celular. Mem. Inst. Oswaldo Cruz. *43*:431–456, 1945.

LAMBERT, H. P., and RICHLEY, J.: Action of Mucin in Promoting Infections: Anticomplementary Eff-ct of Mucin Extracts and Certain Other Substances. Brit. J. Exper. Path. *33*:327–339, 1952.

LURIA, S. E., and DARNELL, J. E., JR.: *General Virology*. 2nd ed. New York, John Wiley & Sons, 1967, pp. 1–512.

MAPLESDEN, D. C., COTE, J. F., and MITCHELL, D.: Allergy in a Horse. J. Am. Vet. Med. Assn. *128*:152, 1956.

MELLORS, R. C., SIEGEL, M., and PRESSMAN, D.: Histochemical Demonstration of Antibody Localization in Tissues. Lab. Investigation. *4*:69–89, 1955.

MOULTON, J. E., and BROWN, C. H.: Antigenicity of Canine Distemper Inclusion Bodies as Demonstrated by Fluorescent Antibody Technic. Proc. Soc. Exper. Biol. & Med. *86*:99–102, 1954.

PAPPENHEIMER, A. M., and MAECHLING, E. H.: Inclusions in Renal Epithelial Cells Following the Use of Certain Bismuth Preparations. Am. J. Path. *10*:577–588, 1934.

PATTERSON, R.: Ragweed Allergy in the Dog. J. Am. Vet. Med. Assn. *135*:178–180, 1959.

RIVASSEAU, D., and RIVASSEAU, P.: Injection d'extraits d'*Ascaris* et choc anaphylactique chez le cheval. Rev. méd. vet. *105*:15–17, 1954.

ROCHA E SILVA, M.: The Histamine Theory of Anaphylactic Shock. Arch. Path. *33*:387–408, 1942.

SMITH, H.: The Virulence-enhancing Factor of Mucins. II. Fractionation Studies on Hog Gastric Mucin. Biochem. J. *46*:356–363, 1951.

SMITH, W. (Ed.): *Mechanisms of Virus Infection*. New York, Academic Press, 1963. pp. 1–368.

STANLEY, W. M.: Isolation of a Crystalline Protein Possessing the Properties of Tobacco-Mosaic Virus. Science. *81*:644–645, 1935.

STROBLE, C. P., and GLENN, M. W.: A Fatal Case of Bovine Anaphylaxis. J. Am. Vet. Med. Assn. *126*:227–232, 1955.

STROCKBINE, J. K.: Anaphylaxis and the Ox Warble. J. Am. Vet. Med. Assn. *77*:106–107, 1930.

VILČEK, J.: *Virology Monographs 6, Interferon.* New York, Springer-Verlag, 1969, pp. 3–141.

TYRRELL, D. A.: The Role of Interferon in the Response to Infection. Proc. Roy. Soc. Med. *62*:13–14, 1969.

9

Genetically Determined Disease; Cytogenetics

INTRODUCTION

During recent years, many significant discoveries have been made in the field of genetics, particularly in application to genetically determined disease in the human subject. The fundamental nature of much of the new knowledge has inspired and challenged investigation in many disciplines; many of the new techniques are being used to explore disease problems. Much of the work is being done in relation to human disease but most principles undoubtedly apply to animals. The search for models and the probe for underlying causes of genetically influenced disease in animals is challenging to the veterinary pathologist. It is now clear that genetic mechanisms are not only involved in transmitting characteristics from one generation to the next, but also are important in controlling the activities of cells in the body, particularly as they change from one cell generation to another.

The veterinary pathologist needs to understand the principles of genetics in order to judge the quality and significance of genetic evidence in the cause and pathogenesis of disease. He also needs to know enough about the field in order to communicate effectively with scientific colleagues who are geneticists. Complete discussion of this field is outside the scope of this book, but some of the principles will be recounted briefly, particularly those which appear at this time to be fundamental in disease processes.

The student is strongly advised to read further in the literature; some of the most pertinent information is found in the references listed at the end of this chapter. *Animal Genetics* by F. D. Hutt should be a delightful book with which to start. This book is precise and readable with Hutt's spritely style, and genetic principles are beautifully illustrated by examples in animals.

The founder of genetics was undoubtedly the Austrian monk and teacher, Gregor Johann Mendel, whose careful studies of a few characteristics of garden peas led to the discovery of some basic principles which influence heredity in all living things. In *simple mendelian inheritance*, characteristics inherited from one generation by the next are controlled by unit characters called genes. Two of these units of inheritance occur in each of the cells of living creatures which reproduce sexually, one gene derived from each parent. In the gametes (ova, sperm) produced by the parents, these paired genes segregate from one another, each gamete acquiring half the number found in somatic cells. When two gametes unite at random to form a zygote, their genes recombine. By studying the characters resulting from these recombinations, Mendel discovered the principle of **independent assortment.** It is now known, of course, that genes are carried in the chromosomes of cells and segregate independently if carried on different chromosomes, but if close together ("linked") on the same chromosome are more apt to remain together. Genes which occupy the same site (*locus*) on a chromosome, can only be alternates for one another and are called **alleles.**

When the genes at one locus are the same from both parents (homozygous), only one characteristic controlled at this locus will be conveyed to the next generation, but when these genes are different (heterozygous) the sex cells (gametes) will contain alternate alleles in approximately equal numbers. In the heterozygous state, the characteristic manifest in the phenotype of the progeny may be controlled by only one gene, which in this case is considered **dominant,** the unexpressed gene is called **recessive.** In matings between heterozygotes, recombinations at random will result in homozygous dominant, heterozygous, and homozygous recessive zygotes in the approximate ratio of 1:2:1. Since the dominant gene will be expressed whenever present, the recessive gene will be expressed only when homozygous, thus giving a 3:1 ratio in the phenotype. This principle, reported by Mendel in 1865, is useful today in the study of genetically controlled disease conditions in man and animals. As an example, brachycephalic dwarf ("snorter") calves; if it is controlled by a single recessive gene, the defect should appear in about one-quarter of the progeny of matings between bulls and cows which are both heterozygous (carriers) for that gene. Some evidence indicates that the situation is somewhat more complicated in this condition (Julian, 1959).

The preceding paragraph illustrates the ratios which can be expected in progeny in animals heterozygous for a single gene which controls a hereditary defect. This is the simplest ratio which is useful as genetic evidence but is only applicable to a few disease conditions and only when all parents are heterozygous. Other ratios occur in progeny, depending upon the frequency of the controlling gene in the population.

Mendelian Genetics

ALTMAN, P. L., and DITTMER, D. S. (ed.): Growth—Including Reproduction and Morphological Development. Table I, pp. 1–7. *Biological Handbook*, Fed. Amer. Soc. Exp. Biol. Wash., D.C., 1962.

EMERY, ALAN, E. H.: *Heredity, Disease and Man.* Berkeley, Univ. Calif. Press, 1968.

GRÜNEBERG, H.: *The Genetics of the Mouse.* 3rd Ed., The Hague, Bibliographia Genetica, 1963.

HADORN, E.: *Developmental Genetics and Lethal Factors.* New York, John Wiley & Sons, 1961.

HUTT, F. B.: Inherited Lethal Characters in Domestic Animals. Cornell Vet. *24*:1–25, 1934.

————: *Genetic Resistance to Disease in Domestic Animals.* Ithaca, Comstock Publishing Co., 1958.

————: *Animal Genetics.* New York, Ronald Press Co., 1964.

INNES, J. R. M., and SAUNDERS, L. Z.: *Comparative Neuropathology.* New York, Academic Press, 1962.

MONTAGUE, F. A.: *Genetic Mechanisms in Human Disease.* Springfield, Charles C Thomas, 1961.

PAULING, L.: Molecular Disease and Evolution. Bull. New York Acad. Med. *40*:334–342, 1964.

ROBINSON, R.: Genetics of the Domestic Cat. Bibliographia Genetica *18*:271–362, 1959.

SRB, A. M., and OWEN, R. D.: *General Genetics.* San Francisco, W. H. Freeman and Co., 1952.

DNA, RNA, AND THE GENETIC CODE

For a long time, nucleic acids have been known to occur in the nuclei of cells and, as indicated on page 322, genetic information is transmitted in the chromosomes. A particular nucleic acid, deoxyribonucleic acid (DNA) is now believed to be the molecular substance with the characteristics needed to be genetic material—namely, it is self-replicating and it is able to control all chemical processes which are specific to the organism. In microbial systems, DNA has been shown to be the sole carrier of genetic information. Although perhaps best viewed as a theory at the present, strong evidence exists that DNA is the fundamental genetic material in all living things. The presumption of the truth of this hypothesis has led to great research efforts and many fundamental facts are emerging as a result.

The **structure of the DNA** molecule was first demonstrated in 1953 by Watson and Crick, whose findings (now amply confirmed) won them a Nobel Prize. The DNA molecule was shown by Watson and Crick to be made up of three types of "building blocks," *viz.*, phosphate (which gives it acid properties), deoxyribose (a sugar) and four bases (two purines: adenine and guanine and two pyrimidines: cytosine and thymine). The molecule consists of elongated chains in which the sugar and phosphate form a double helix around a central axis; these paired helical bands are linked together at regular intervals by pairs of bases (Fig. 9–2). These bases are joined in very specific ways: one purine is held to one pyrimidine by hydrogen bonds—*i.e.*, adenine (A) is always paired with thymine (T) and guanine (G) with cytosine (C). Each single group, consisting of base pair, sugar and phosphate, is sometimes referred to as a **nucleotide** and the DNA molecule as a polynucleotide chain.

Replication of DNA is visualized by Watson and Crick as based upon the specific base-pairing of adenine-thymine and guanine-cytosine along the length of the molecule. As illustrated in Figure 9–3, this results in a pair of templates when the two chains of the DNA molecule separate. Bases, sugar and phosphate that are free in the cell are combined and the base pairs are joined at their specific sites to form a new polynucleotide chain. The specific sequential arrangement of the base-pairs along the molecule is therefore replicated as new double-stranded chains are formed which exactly duplicate the parent DNA. This is an over-

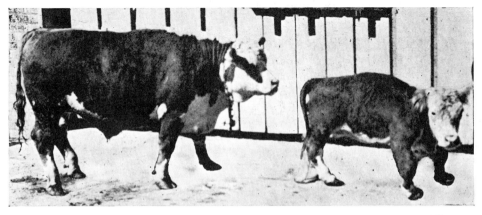

FIG. 9–1.—Dwarfism 'C' in a Hereford calf. Note small size, large head, and distorted limbs in affected calf. Normal calf of same age and breed on left.

simplified explanation of a very complicated process, but outlines the basic concept which now seems to be amply confirmed.

The Control of Function by DNA.—The synthesis of specific proteins has been shown to be controlled by genetic factors, suggesting that at least some, if not all, of the genetic information carried by DNA concerns the sequence of amino acids in proteins. The sugar-phosphate part of the double helix is perfectly regular, but the sequence of the four base pairs along the length of the DNA molecule is variable and therefore must be the component which in some way determines the sequence of amino-acids in proteins. The **coding problem** involves the manner in which a sequence of nucleotides in the DNA molecule can, without ambiguity, determine the sequence of amino acids in a polypeptide chain (protein).

The view of Crick *et al.* (1957) of the *coding problem* involves the concept of non-overlapping triplet codes. These are explained as follows: By designating each of the nucleotides by a letter, an arbitrary sequence along the chain may be designated as: AGTAGCTGC. If the code is a triple one, a sequence of three

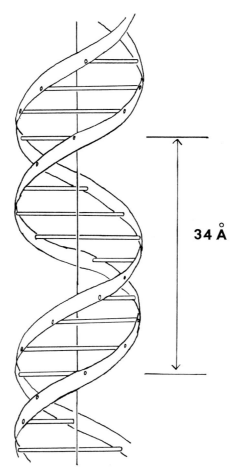

34 Å

Fig. 9–2.—The deoxyribonucleic acid (DNA) model of Watson and Crick. The coiled double helix, made up of sugar (deoxyribose) and phosphate, form paired "backbones" which are held equal distances apart by base pairs (purines and pyrimidines) represented by the horizontal lines. (After Symonds, N. D., *Chromosomes in Medicine*, 1961, Wm. Heineman.)

adjacent nucleotides is necessary to code for one amino acid. Assuming that AGC is such a sequence, and the code is non-overlapping, then none of these three nucleotides, AGC, can be part of any adjacent triplet. The next triplet to the left, AGT, and the next to the right, TGC, would be codes for different amino acids. This triplet code therefore could be AGT AGC TGC; other combinations would be meaningless. It was shown by Crick *et al.* that it is theoretically possible to construct a number of codes of this type in which, of the 64 possible triplets, 20 could provide codes for individual amino acids. As 20 amino acids commonly make up proteins, these codes adequately satisfy the requirements of the coding problem.

In the period between our third and fourth editions, the coding problem has been essentially solved. The nucleotide triplet code for each amino acid has been demonstrated by experimental methods. Although specific for each amino acid, more than one code is effective for several of them. This is summarized succinctly by Jukes (1966).

The simplest explanation of protein synthesis, assuming that its specificity is determined by some such coding mechanism as described in the preceding paragraph, would be that it was assembled directly on the DNA. However, the site of protein synthesis has been shown experimentally to be in the cytoplasm of the cell; specifically in tiny particles called ribosomes which contain a large quantity of **ribonucleic acid** (RNA). The molecule of RNA is very similar to DNA, except that one of its bases, **thymine,** is replaced by a similar pyrimidine, **uracil,** and the sugar, deoxyribose, becomes ribose. It appears that RNA molecules are involved in the transfer of genetic information from the DNA of the nucleus to the cytoplasm; and within the ribosomes, act as templates for the synthesis of protein. This process as now visualized (Sutton 1963) requires three types of RNA: **Messenger RNA** (mRNA, template RNA) which is unstable in most systems, and contains 1500 nucleotides; **ribosomal RNA** which is stable, has 1650 and 3300 nucleotides; and **transfer RNA** (soluble RNA, sRNA, adapter RNA) which is stable and contains only 70 nucleotides. Twenty amino acids are necessarily present in the cell, plus 20 enzymes, each capable of attaching a specific amino acid to one of 20 specific **transfer RNA**'s. Each molecule of sRNA is believed to attach to its specific amino acid and, recognizing the sequence (code) of base pairs in the **messenger RNA** in the ribosomes, attaches the amino acids in the proper sequence for the specific protein. After alignment in the proper order, condensation occurs between adjacent peptides to form the specific protein which then separates from the sRNA which in turn becomes available for further synthesis of protein.

The Gene and DNA.—Each of the non-overlapping regions of DNA which contains a particular sequence of nucleotides and which indirectly controls the synthesis of one specific protein can be called a gene. In this sense, it is a unit of function and can be subdivided into smaller units or **mutational sites.** The number of amino acids in a typical protein is in the order of 1000, and as three nucleotides are necessary to code for each amino acid, a gene contains about 3000 nucleotide pairs. A small organism, such as a virus, may contain sufficient DNA to include 100 genes of this size, while higher organisms may have enough DNA to provide as many as 1 million genes.

The student can visualize by the use of the foregoing schemata, that a change or defect in one or more base pairs in DNA may lead to the formation of an

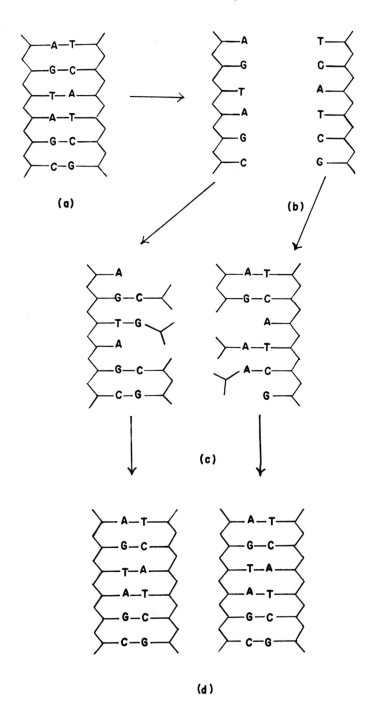

Fig. 9–3.—Replications of DNA. In (a) the base pairs (adenine-thymine and guanine-cytosine) are represented by letters (A–T, G–C) separating the "backbone" of sugar-phosphate. In (b) the base pairs separate, leaving two single strands of DNA with bases in linear sequence. Enzymes and a source of energy cause binding of free bases with their sugar-phosphates to specific sites (c) resulting in two double strands of DNA (d) with exactly the same base sequence as the original (a). (After Symonds, *Chromosomes in Medicine*, 1961, Wm. Heineman.)

abnormal protein or may preclude its production entirely. At the molecular level, such a change in base pairs is believed to be one underlying mechanism in **mutation.** It is known that major errors can occur in DNA replication, sometimes involving chromosomal segments or whole chromosomes. These may have very significant effect upon the resultant phenotype. The recognition of abnormal phenotypes in the language of the geneticist, represents pathologic diagnosis to the pathologist and is the point of interest in much of this book.

The first disease clearly shown to be the result of genetic influences at the molecular level is sickle cell anemia of man. Pauling, Itano *et al.*, in 1949, found that the essential defect underlying the loss of erythrocytes involved the hemoglobin molecule. Amazing as it may seem, the concept of such genetic defects was thoroughly considered and expanded by Garrod in 1909. The introduction of biochemical techniques and philosophy into genetics resulted in development of an important modern area of research, sometimes called **Molecular Genetics.** Some genetic defects of man now recognized at the molecular level are: phenylketonuria, alkaptonuria, cystinuria, cystinosis, glycinuria, galactosemia, and various glycogen storage diseases. For the most part, these defects are each controlled by a single recessive gene. The concept of the gene is still valid but can now be considered in biochemical terms on the molecular level.

Studies with microbial organisms, particularly *Neurospora*, have disclosed that single enzymes control the synthesis of specific proteins and each enzyme is determined by a specific gene. Organisms which are normally able to produce all of their nutritional needs from simple substances can be caused, by radiation-induced mutation, to lose the ability to synthesize one or more of these essential nutrients. Mutation of one gene results in the loss of one enzyme. These facts have led some (Pauling, 1949) to state that vitamin deficiency states are actually genetically determined diseases which are the result of the loss during evolution of the ability to synthesize the necessary vitamin. As an example, man and the guinea pig have each lost the ability to synthesize ascorbic acid and therefore are subject to scurvy when this vitamin is absent from the diet. Most other animals still retain the capacity to synthesize ascorbic acid—presumably because they still have the gene which controls this function.

DNA, RNA and The Genetic Code

JUKES, THOMAS H.: *Molecules and Evolution.* New York, Columbia University Press, 1966.
KORNBERG, A.: Biologic Synthesis of Deoxyribonucleic Acid. Science *131*:1503–1508, 1960.
SUTTON, H. E.: Genes and Protein Synthesis. In *Second International Conference on Congenintal Malformations*, New York, International Medical Congress, Ltd., 1963.
SYMONDS, N. D.: DNA, Genes and Chromosomes. pp. 7–16 in Hamerton, J. L. *Chromosomes in Medicine.* London, Wm. Heineman (Medical Books) Ltd., 1963.
WATSON, J. D., and CRICK, F. H. C.: Molecular Structure of Nucleic Acids. A Structure for Deoxyribose Nucleic Acid. Nature *171*:737–738, 1953.

CHROMOSOMES

Shortly after the beginning of the 20th century, geneticists were enthusiastically testing the principles of Mendel in plants and animals. One of them (Sutton, 1902) observed that the multiplication and reduction-division of chromosomes in meiosis preceding the formation of germ cells, could provide mechanisms for the segregation of genes, with recombinations occurring at fertilization in accord with mendelian principles. Thus, observations in genetics were combined with others in cytology to establish that genes are carried in chromosomes. This was the beginning of **cytogenetics.** The techniques of cytogenetics have long been used in the study of plants, but have only recently been shown to be applicable to animals. Phenomenal progress has been achieved in applying cytogenetic methods to the elucidation of those human diseases in which abnormalities occur in the chromosomes. Only the beginning has been made in the study of chromosomes of other animals. However, enough has been learned to indicate that detectable abnormalities do occur in the chromosomes of animals, as well as man, and many of these abnormalities underlie the occurrence of genetically determined disease. Chromosomes are therefore of great interest to the veterinary pathologist.

Number and Morphology.— Chromosomes are most readily studied at metaphase at which time individual chromosomes are separately distinct and can be counted and studied morphologically. Appropriate techniques usually involve the culture of cells of the animal under study in order to obtain adequate numbers undergoing mitosis. Rapidly multiplying cells in tissue culture are treated with colchicine (or a related compound) in order to arrest many cells in the metaphase stage of mitosis. The cells are then expanded with hypotonic saline solution, forcing the chromosomes apart, permitting their fixation on a glass slide individually separated from one another. After proper staining, the chromosomes may

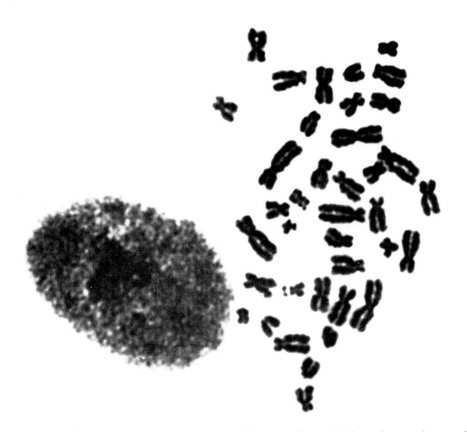

Fig. 9–4.—Chromosomes of the cat (*Felis catus*) in metaphase. An interphase nucleus at the left. Smear prepared from cultures of lung treated with colchicine *in vitro*.

be studied under the light microscope or, better, photographed. Photographic enlargements of the chromosomes (Fig. 9–4) are used to count their number, align them in homologous pairs in a systematic arrangement (called a karyotype) (Fig. 9–5) and to study their morphologic features.

The number of chromosomes is characteristic for each species; each somatic cell in the body contains the same number of homologous pairs (diploid, $2n$), one derived from each parent. Following meiosis, the germ cells each contain half the diploid number, therefore are haploid (n). Fertilization of the ovum restores the diploid number to the zygote. The determinors of sex are found in the **sex chromosomes** which are individually distinguishable in most species. In most normal mammals, females have a pair of X chromosomes (XX) and males have one X and one much smaller Y chromosome (XY). In *Lepidoptera*, birds, reptiles and some other animals, males are the homogametic sex, with two chromosomes (usually designated ZZ); females have one Z and a smaller chromosome designated W (ZW). Birds have many tiny chromosomes, called microchromosomes, which present difficulties in counting and tend to obscure the small W chromosome. Drones of honey-bees are of particular interest because they have a haploid (n) number of chromosomes, all originating by parthenogenesis from unfertilized eggs.

The remaining chromosomes are called **autosomes** and contain most of the genetic material. Genes which are carried in these chromosomes are called **autosomal,** in contrast to those carried on the X chromosome (the Y apparently determines only the male sex, does not carry other genes) which are called **sex-linked.** The pattern of inheritance differs between autosomal and sex-linked

Table 9–1.—*Chromosomes of Some Common Species*

Common Name	Scientific Name	Chromosomes 2n	Female	Male
Ass	*Equus asinus*	62	XX	XY
Mule	*Equus mulus*	63	XX	XY
Horse	*Equus caballus*	64	XX	XY
Przewalsky horse	*Equus caballus prezewalskii*	66	XX	XY
Mrs. Hartmann's Mountain Zebra	*Equus zebra hartmannae*	32	XX	XY
Man	*Homo sapiens*	46	XX	XY
Mouse	*Mus musculus*	40	XX	XY
Dog	*Canis familiaris*	78	XX	XY
Cat	*Felis catus*	38	XX	XY
Rabbit	*Oryctolagus cuniculus*	44	XX	XY
Guinea pig	*Cavia cobaya*	64	XX	XY
Goat	*Capra hircus*	60	XX	XY
Sheep	*Ovis aries*	54	XX	XY
Cattle	*Bos taurus*	60	XX	XY
Zebu	*Bos indicus*	60	XX	XY
Pig	*Sus scrofa*	38(?)40	XX	XY
Fox	*Vulpes fulva*	38	XX	XY
Mink	*Mustela vision*	30	XX	XY
Parakeet	*Melopsittacus undulatus*	58	ZW	ZZ
Turkey	*Meleagris gallopavo*	81–82	ZW	ZZ
Duck	*Anas platyrhyncha domestica*	79–80	ZW	ZZ
Fowl	*Gallus gallus*	77–78	ZW	ZZ
Honey Bee	*Apis Mellifera*	32 (16-drone)	ZW	ZZ

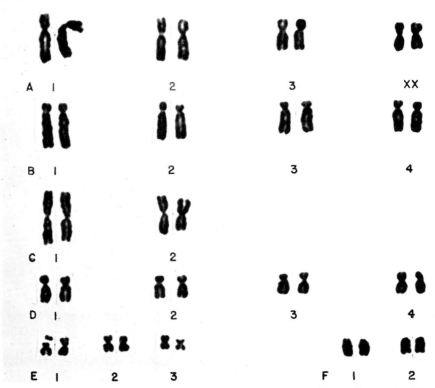

Fig. 9–5.—Karyotype of the domestic cat, *Felis catus*, prepared according to the "San Juan System" (agreed upon by a group of scientists in San Juan, Puerto Rico, November, 1964). *A*, Female, from a cell cultured from the spleen. (Continued on page 325)

genes and lesions in the autosomal *vs.* the sex chromosomes have different effects, making their distinction of importance. Identification of the sex chromosomes may be facilitated by the use of autoradiography. Cultures of multiplying cells are exposed to tritiated thymidine which has been made radioactive. This substance is utilized by the replicating DNA and can be identified later in the metaphase chromosomes by means of an autoradiograph which is prepared from a photographic film placed over the cell preparation on the slide. After prolonged exposure, the film is developed in place over the chromosome spreads and the radioactivity is identified as blackened spots of silver grains. One or more of the sex chromosomes replicate out of phase with the autosomes and are heavily labelled by the radioactive thymidine.

The number of chromosomes currently believed to occur in several common species is indicated in Table 9–1. The correct number of human chromosomes was not settled until new techniques were introduced in 1958. Revisions in this table may be necessary as each species is studied more adequately with the newest techniques.

Chromosomes—General Aspects

BENIRSCHKE, K., BROWNHILL, L. E., and BEATH, M. M.: Somatic Chromosomes of the Horse, the Donkey and their Hybrids, the Mule and the Hinny. J. Reprod. Fertil. *4*:319–326, 1962.

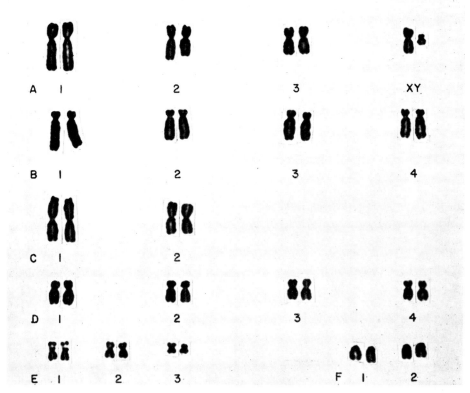

FIG. 9–5.—(*Continued*)

B, Male, cell cultured from the kidney. Note that in this system the groups can be readily described—viz: Group A, large submetacentric chromosomes; Group B, large subtelocentrics; Group C, large metacentrics; Group D, small metacentrics or submetacentrics; Group E, small metacentrics (the first pair satellited); and Group F, small acrocentric chromosomes.

BENIRSCHKE, K., LOW, R. J., SULLIVAN, M. M., and CARTER, R. M.: Chromosomes Study of an Alleged Fertile Mare Mule. J. Hered. *55*:31–38, 1964.

BORLAND, R.: The Chromosomes of Domestic Sheep. J. Hered. *55*:61–64, 1964.

CHU, E. H. Y., and BENDER, M. A.: Chromosome Cytology and Evolution in Primates. Science *133*, 1399–1405, 1961.

DEROBERTIS, E.: Advances in the Ultrastructure of the Nucleus and Chromosomes. J. Nat. Cancer Inst. Mono. No. 14, May, 1964.

EBERLE, P.: Comparative Studies on Sex Chromosomes in Different Species. Genetica *35*: 34–46, 1964.

GUSTAVSSON, I.: The Chromosomes of the Dog. Hereditas *51*:187, 1964.

HAMERTON, J. L. (ed.): *Chromosomes in Medicine.* London, Wm. Heinemann (Medical Books) Ltd., 1961.

HARE, W. C. D., *et al.*: Cytogenetics in the Dog and Cat. J. Small Anim. Pract. *7*:575–592, 1966.

HSU, T. C., and BENIRSCHKE, K.: *Atlas of Mammalian Chromosomes.* Vol. 1–5. New York, Springer-Verlag, 1967–71.

LEHMAN, J. M., MACPHERSON, I., and MOORHEAD, P. S.: Karyotype of the Syrian Hamster. J. Nat. Cancer Inst., *31*:639–649, 1963.

MAKINO, S.: *An Atlas of the Chromosome Numbers in Animals.* Ames, Iowa, Iowa State University Press, 1951.

MOORE, W., JR., and LAMBERT, P. D.: The Chromosomes of the Beagle Dog. J. Hered. *54*: 273–276, 1963.

MUKHERJEE, B. B., and SINHA, A. K.: Cytological Evidence for Random Inactivation of X-chromosomes in a Female Mule Complement. Proc. Nat. Acad. Sci. *51*:252–254, 1964.

Rothfels, K., Aspden, M., and Mollison, M.: The W-chromosome of the Budgerigar, *Melopsittacus undulatus.* Chromosoma *14*:459–467, 1963.

Weitkamp, L. R., *et al.*: Inherited Pericentric Inversion of Chromosome Number Two: A Linkage Study. Ann. Hum. Genet. (Lond.) *33*:53–59, 1969.

Wurster, D. H., and Benirschke, K.: Comparative Cytogenetic Studies in the Order *Carnivora.* Chromosoma (Berl) *24*:336–382, 1968.

————————: Indian Muntjac, *Muntiacus muntjak:* A Deer with a Low Diploid Chromosome Number. Science, *168*:1364–1366, 1970.

Aberrations of Chromosomes.—Surprisingly, abnormalities are not infrequent in chromosomes of animals, notwithstanding the admittedly preconceived idea that chromosomal material must be inviolate in order for the species to survive. It is now known that a large variety of lesions occur in chromosomes with alarming frequency but subsequent death of the gamete or zygote has a species-cleansing effect, permitting only a few abnormal chromosomes to persist in the embryo through birth or into adult life. In spite of this "cleansing" mechanism, some chromosomal aberrations do persist and have significant effect upon the adult phenotype. Several such abnormal chromosomes are now known to underlie important disease syndromes in man and an increasing number are being found in animals as the search is continued.

Aberrations in Number (Heteroploidy).—Possession of chromosome numbers (Table 9–1, p. 323) other than the haploid (n) set in the gametes, or the diploid ($2n$) complement after fertilization, is called **heteroploidy.** If the abnormal number involves exact multiples of the haploid set, the resulting cells are called **euploid** and the condition **euploidy** or **euploid heteroploidy.** Examples of this condition have been found in mammalian embryos, particularly mice, although most of the affected animals die within the first few days of embryonic life. The usual explanation for this abnormality is that the error occurs during meiosis, particularly in the ovum, and that distribution of the chromosome sets to the gametes is erroneous. For example, the polar body may fail to be extruded from the ovum, leaving the diploid set ($2n$) to be fertilized by a haploid sperm (n) resulting in a $3n$ **(triploid)** zygote. Various possibilities and their theoretical explanation are summarized by Russell (1962).

Aberrations in the number of chromosomes which do not involve exact multiples of the haploid (n) number are termed **aneuploid heteroploidy.** This may involve specific chromosomes in triple number **(trisomy)** or single number **(monosomy)** rather than the normal double dose. Errors of this type are more apt to persist into adulthood and result in significant abnormalities. Several of these are now known in man, involving either autosomes or sex chromosomes, and a few have been found in animals. These will be described later.

Duplications and deficiencies of a section of a chromosome may also occur, leaving the total number intact. Long known to occur in *Drosophila* and plants, these defects have now been observed in chromosomes of man and mouse. Deletion or duplication of a part of a chromosome may not necessarily be lethal, and may result in an abnormal phenotype. **Translocation** involves the rearrangement of genetic material of at least two non-homologous chromosomes. This translocation may be reciprocal or non-reciprocal between the two chromosomes. If the zygote survives, and some (with this defect) do survive, genetic effects are usually evident in the resulting phenotype and the translocations may be detected by cytologic study of the chromosomes.

Two more definitions are indicated before we consider some of the specific chromosomal abnormalities that have been discovered so far.

Mosaicism may refer to genes or to whole chromosomes and usually means that more than one population of cells is present in the body, each population differing in some respect in their chromosomes or genes. Usual usage implies that the differing cell populations are inlaid by some error within the individual during its development. Chromosomal mosaicism, for example, could result from a defect (*i.e.*, non-disjunction) in certain cells in the embryo, giving rise to two populations of cells, one with an extra X chromosome (XXY in a male) the rest of the cells could be normal (XY).

Chimerism, in this context, implies mosaicism in which one cell type is acquired *in utero* from a twin. For example, Owen (1945) demonstrated that fraternal bovine twins, one male and one female, with placental anastomoses permitting exchange of hematopoietic cells during fetal life, could be shown later to have red blood cells of two types, one acquired *in utero* from its twin. Germ cells may also circulate in embryonic life and could give rise to germ cell chimerism.

Anomalies in Sex Chromosomes.—In most mammals, male sex is determined by the presence of the Y chromosome which is received by the zygote from the male parent. Somatic cells resulting from union of an X- and a Y-bearing gamete each contain one Y chromosome derived from the male and one X from the female parent (XY). The female zygote receives one X-bearing gamete from each parent and therefore each somatic cell normally contains two X chromosomes (XX). Female cells during anaphase were discovered by Barr (in neurons of *Felis catus*) to differ from male cells in that a small heteropyknotic body was often demonstrable along the nuclear membrane in female cells only. This body (Fig. 9-6) is now called the Barr Body or **sex chromatin.** According to the concept first proposed by Lyon (1962), this sex chromatin body consists of one of the X chromosomes which is genetically inactivated. Presumably, inactivation of this X chromosome occurs early in embryonic life. This inactivated, heteropyknotic X chromosome could be either maternal or paternal in origin in different

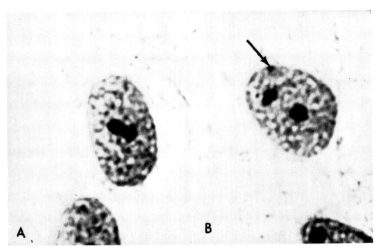

Fig. 9-6.—Sex chromatin in interphase nuclei, H. & E. × 1600. *A*, Cell from buccal smear of normal male (XY) cat. Sex chromatin absent (negative).

B, Nucleus from buccal smear of a tortoiseshell male cat (XXY). Barr Body (arrow) at nuclear membrane—one fewer than the number of X chromosomes in the cell.

cells of the same animal. Apparently, only one X chromosome is needed in the activity of the cell because if more X chromosomes are present in the cell, all but one will be inactivated and appear as sex chromatin. The number of sex chromatin bodies in a cell will therefore be one fewer than the number of X chromosomes present. An XX cell will contain one, and XXX cell two and an XXXX cell, three sex chromatin bodies. In the absence of sex chromatin, as in a male (XY) cell or an XO female cell, the cell is sometimes depicted as "sex chromatin negative." The sex chromatin is easily demonstrated with simple techniques and is therefore useful in studies of animals with heteroploidy involving the X chromosome.

Klinefelter's syndrome in the human subject is recognized in adolescence by small testes, and sometimes eunuchoid features, gynecomastia, low urinary excretion of 17-ketosteroids and high excretion of gonadotropins. A slender, tall body build is most common and frequently sexual hair is sparse. Many affected individuals are intellectually subnormal and many later prove to be infertile. Most males with this syndrome are sex chromatin positive and therefore have more than one X chromosome in their somatic cells. The usual karyotypes are shown to be XXY, with most cells containing the extra X chromosome. The modal chromosome count is 47, one more than the normal number. In some cases of this syndrome, some cells (10 to 50 per cent) contain a different number of X chromosomes. Therefore, these are called XX/XXY mosaics. In some cases XXYY and in others XXXY chromosomal configuration have been described. The cause of this abnormality is not known but one theory ascribes it to non-disjunction of the X chromosome during gametogenesis. Non-disjunction may be further described as the failure of two chromosomes of a pair to migrate to opposite poles of the cells in meiosis. One gamete may receive both chromosomes and the next none. The exact cause of this phenomenon is unknown.

The Tortoiseshell Male Cat.—In the domestic cat, *Felis catus*, orange coat color and its alternative, black, are determined by genes which are within the X chromosome, therefore are sex-linked. The orange gene (σ) is co-dominant with its allele for black (σ^+) and both characteristics are expressed in the heterozygote. Modifying genes may result in a panoply of patterns and intensity of color, but the essential feature of the heterozygote is occurrence of both black and orange hair. The black hair may be diluted to blue and the orange hair to cream by the recessive gene for Maltese dilution (d) but the σ/σ^+ genotype still can be detected in the phenotype. This heterozygote is commonly called the tortoiseshell or "tortie." Cats in which the orange and black are mixed with white (due to a dominant gene, S, for piebald) are called "calico" or "tricolor."

Tortoiseshell cats are therefore heterozygous for two sex-linked alleles and therefore must have two X chromosomes and consequently must be females. Most tortoiseshells are females, but exceptional male torties sometimes occur. Most tortie males have been reported to be sterile but a few were said to be fertile. Recently, Thuline and Norby (1961) demonstrated that blood cells of two tortoiseshell male cats contained one more than the normal number of chromosomes ($2n-39$). In our laboratory, we were able to identify the additional chromosome to be an X chromosome in two cats (Fig. 9–7). Further, in one case, XX/XY/XXY mosaicism was demonstrated. Both of these male cats had small testicles and lacked libido. A third male calico studied by Malouf and Benirschke (1965) has an XX/XY mosaic karyotype with a normal ($2n-38$) number of chromosomes.

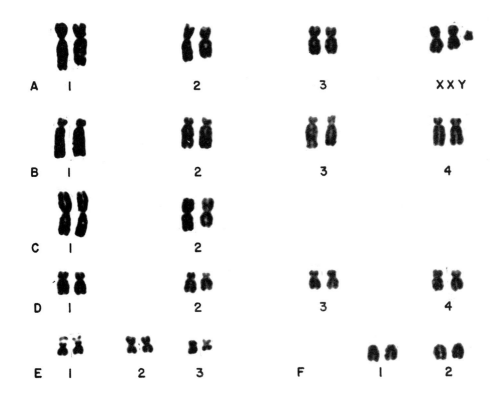

A   1   2   3   X X Y

B   1   2   3   4

C   1   2

D   1   2   3   4

E   1   2   3   F   1   2

FIG. 9–7.—Karyotype of a male tortoiseshell cat. Note the diploid (*2n*)
number is 39 and the sex chromosomes are XXY.

Chu, Thuline and Norby (1964) described triploid-diploid chimerism in a male
tortoiseshell cat which was reportedly sterile and whose testicles histologically
contained Sertolic cells and spermatogonia but no spermatids or spermatozoa.
Cell cultures from the skin of the ear of this cat were shown to contain about
55 per cent triploid cells (*3n*–57) with XXY sex chromosomes. Most of the
remainder of the cells in these tissue cultures contained normal (XX *2n*–38)
chromosomes. The two X chromosomes were believed to carry both alternative
genes for yellow and black coat color; the Y chromosome was the male sex determi-
nant. This syndrome in the cat appears to mimic Klinefelter's syndrome in man
in many respects and may provide a useful model for studies on its pathogenesis
and etiology.

Anomalies of sex chromosomes which are similar to those described in Klinefelter's syndrome in man and in the tortoiseshell male cat have been reported in
sheep (Bruere, Marshall and Ward, 1969), cattle (Rieck, Höhn and Herzog, 1969)
and horses (Basrur, Kanagawa and Gilman, 1969).

Turner's Syndrome.—A clinical syndrome in women described originally by
Turner (1938) consisted of sexual infantilism, webbing of the neck and cubitus
valgus. Similar findings were reported by Ullrich (1930) in children, but sexual
deficiency was not recognized in his patients. Oftentimes the syndrome is not
recognized until puberty when menstruation does not begin when expected.
These patients are usually short in stature and of slightly lower than average

intelligence. It is now known that most of the patients with this syndrome do not have sex chromatin in their somatic cells and have only 47 chromosomes, one less than the normal number of 46. The missing chromosome is the X, therefore the karyotype can be designated as XO. The lack of this one X chromosome appears to underly the clinical syndrome, but neither is the cause of the chromosomal abnormality known, nor is the mode of action of the missing X understood. Females of XO karotype have been described in mice which were fertile and presumably otherwise normal but this situation has not yet been uncovered in any other species. Mice with XXY karyotype have also been reported, but no adequate comparison has been made with XXY individuals in man or cat (Russell, 1962).

Intersexes.—An intersex or gynandromorph is defined as an animal or person with some ambiguity in genitalia or secondary sexual characteristics suggesting both male and female. Hermaphroditism (p. 1340) includes those animals or persons with both male and female genitalia, external and internal. A pseudo-hermaphrodite has the external genitalia of one sex and the gonads of the opposite sex, the gonadal sex usually added as an adjective in its name. Thus, a male pseudohermaphrodite has female external genitalia and male gonads (testes). It is not unusual for both an ovary and testis, or a fused ovotestis to be present in some intersexes.

Study of the chromosomes of such intersex animals has added new dimensions to this problem presented by such anomalies and has led to new theories concerning the factors controlling determination of sexual characteristics. Intersexes have been described in many species and increasing numbers are now being studied from the genetic and cytogenetic points of view. No completely consistent chromosomal pattern has yet emerged but most affected animals appear to be chimeric as far as their sex chromosomes are concerned. This aspect has been reviewed in admirable detail in all species by Benirschke (1970).

A problem of continued interest is the hypogonadism and sterility of female bovines which are carried *in utero* with a male twin. These particular heifers have been recognized for many years and are usually designated by a name of obscure origin: **Freemartin.** The phenomenon of freemartinism is not thoroughly explained but appears to be associated with several situations. First, the male and female co-twins share a common placental circulation *in utero* which allows them to exchange hematopoietic and germ cells early in embryonic life. Second, the cells from one embryo establish themselves in the co-twin, producing chimerism which can be demonstrated in sex chromosomes and erythrocyte antigens. The presence of XX cells in gonads and other tissues of male calves which are twins of females, appears to reduce fertility and the XY cells in the female co-twin is associated with sterility. However, in twin marmosets, germ cell chimerism is not associated with sterility, hence a direct causal effect of the heterosexual germ cells is not established.

The earlier theory concerning the etiology of freemartinism induced the postulate that androgenic hormones produced by the testicles of the male twin, had a deleterious effect upon the development of the female gonad. This theory still remains viable although definitive evidence to support it has not yet been forthcoming.

Testicular Feminization.—This is another anomaly which affects the phenotypic expression of sexuality, is reported in human patients and appears to have a counterpart in animals. The patient has female secondary sexual characteristics including female external and internal genitalia except for the presence of testes in place of ovaries. The karyotype in all cells is XY. This situation is explained on the basis of an inherited, single gene defect which makes all tissues unresponsive to androgenic hormones, particularly testosterone. Thus, in spite of the presence of a functioning testis, male genitalia and secondary sex characteristics do not develop.

Ohno and Lyon (1970) have described a sex-linked genetic characteristic in mice which has these features of testicular feminization. These workers demonstrated that cells of mice homozygous for the defective gene are unable to respond to testosterone or dihydrotestosterone. This is demonstrated in renal tubular cells in which alcohol dehydrogenase is produced in normal mice by stimulation with androgens but no alcohol dehydrogenase is developed in mice homozygous for the defective gene. Similar cases have been described in sheep (Bruere, McDonald and Marshall, 1969) and cattle (Short, 1967).

Anomalies of Sex Chromosomes

ARMSTRONG, C. N., and MARSHALL, A. J.: *Intersexuality in Vertebrates Including Man.* London, Academic Press, 1964.

BASRUR, P. K., KANAGAWA, H., and GILMAN, J. P. W.: An Equine Intersex with Unilateral Gonadal Agenesis. Canad. J. Comp. Med. *33*:297–306, 1969.

BASRUR, P. K., KOSAKA, S., and KANAGAWA, N.: Blood Cell Chimerism and Freemartinism in Heterosexual Bovine Quadruplets. J. Hered. *61*:15–18, 1970.

BENIRSCHKE, K.: Spontaneous Chimerism in Mammals. A Critical Review. Curr. Topics. Path. *51*:1–61, 1970.

BENIRSCHKE, K., and BROWNHILL, L. E.: Further Observations on Marrow Chimerism in Marmosets. Cytogenetics *1*:245–257, 1962.

BENIRSCHKE, K., et al.: Chromosomes Study of an Alleged Fertile Mare Mule. J. Hered. *55*:31–38, 1964.

BIGGERS, J. D., and McFEELY, R. A.: Intersexuality in Domestic Mammals. In A. McLaren (ed.) *Advances in Reproductive Physiology*, Logos Press, London, 1966.

BRUERE, A. N.: Male Sterility and an Autosomal Translocation in Romney Sheep. Cytogenetics *8*:209–218, 1969.

BRUERE, A. N., MARSHALL, R. B., and WARD, D. P. J.: Testicular Hypoplasia and XXY Sex Chromosome Complement in Two Rams: The Ovine Counterpart of Klinefelter's Syndrome in Man. J. Reprod. Fert. *19*:103–108, 1969.

BRUERE, A. N., McDONALD, M. F., and MARSHALL, R. B.: Cytogenetical Analysis of an Ovine Male Pseudohermaphrodite and the Possible Role of the Y Chromosome in Cryptorchidism of Sheep. Cytogenetics *8*:148–157, 1969.

CATTANACH, B. M.: XXY Mice. Genet. Res. *2*:156–160, 1961.

————: XO Mice. Genet. Res. *3*:487–490, 1962.

CARR, D. H.: Chromosome Studies on Abortuses and Stillborn Infants. Lancet *2*:603–606, 1963.

CHU, E. H. Y., THULINE, H. C., and NORBY, D. E.: Triploid-diploid Chimerism in a Male Tortoiseshell Cat. Cytogenetics *3*:1–18, 1964.

CLENDENIN, T. M., and BENIRSCHKE, K.: Chromosome Studies on Spontaneous Abortions. Lab. Invest. *12*:1281–1292, 1963.

CLOUGH, E., et al.: An XXY Sex Chromosome Constitution in a Dog with Testicular Hypoplasia and Congenital Heart Disease. Cytogenetics *9*:71–77, 1970.

DUNN, H. O., McENTEE, K., and HANSEL, W.: Diploid-triploid Chimerism in a Bovine True Hermaphrodite. Cytogenetics *9*:245–259, 1970.

HARD, W. L.: The Anatomy and Cytogenetics of Male Pseudohermaphroditism in Swine. Anat. Rec. *157*:255–256, 1967.

JONES, T. C.: Anomalies of Sex Chromosomes in Male Tortoiseshell Cats. In *Comparative Mammalian Cytogenetics.* Ed. by K. Benirschke, Springer, Berlin-Heidelberg, 1969.

KANAGAWA, H., and BASRUR, P. K.: The Leukocyte Culture Method in the Diagnosis of Freemartinism. Canad. J. Comp. Med. *32*:583–586, 1968.

KOSAKA, S., et al.: Abnormal Blood Type and Female Type of Chromsome in a Male of Heterosexual Bovine Twins. Jap. J. Zootech. Sci. *40*:238–242, 1969.

LOUGHMAN, W. D., FRYE, F. L., and CONDON, T. B.:   XY/XXY Bone Marrow Mosaicism in Three Male Tricolor Cats.   Amer. J. Vet. Res. 31:307–314, 1970.
LUBS, H. A., and RUDDLE, F. H.:   Chromosomal Abnormalities in the Human Population: Estimation of Rates Based on New Haven Newborn Study.   Science 169:495–497, 1970.
LYON, M. F.:   Sex Chromatin and Gene Action in the Mammalian X Chromosome.   Amer. J. Human Genetics 14:135–148, 1962.
McFEELY, R. A., HARE, W. C. D., and BIGGERS, J. D.:   Chromosome Studies in 14 Cases of Intersex in Domestic Animals.   Cytogenetics 6:242–253, 1967.
McKUSICK, V. A.:   On the X Chromosome of Man.   Washington, D.C., Amer. Inst. Biol. Sci., 1964.
MILLER, O. J.:   The Sex Chromosome Anomalies.   Amer. J. Obstet. Gynec. 90:1078–1139, 1961.
MUKHERJEE, B. B., and SINHA, A. K.:   Cytological Evidence for Random Inactivation of X-chromosomes in a Female Mule Complement.   Proc. Nat. Acad. Sci. 51:252–254, 1964.
OWEN, R. D.:   Immunogenetic Consequences of Vascular Anastomoses Between Bovine Twins.   Science 102:400–401, 1945.
PAYNE, H. W., WILLSWORTH, K. and DeGROTT, A.:   Aneuploidy in an infertile mare.   J. Amer. Vet. Med. Ass. 153: 1293–1299, 1968.
RIECK, G. W., HÖHN, H., and HERZOG, A.:   Hypogonadismus, Intermittierender Kryptorchidismus und segmentäre Aplasia der Ductus Wolffii bei einem männlichen Rind mit XXY—Konstellation bsw. XXY/XX/XY—Gonosomen-Mosaik.   Deutsch. Tierarztl. Wschr. 76: 133–138, 1969.
RIGDON, R. H., and MOTT, C.:   Testis in the Sterile Hybrid Duck. A Histologic and Histochemical Study.   Path. Vet. 2:553–565, 1965.
RUSSELL, L. B.:   Chromosome Aberrations in Experimental Mammals, Chapter 7 in Progress in Medical Genetics, Vol. II by Steinberg, A. G. and Bearn, A. G.   New York, Grune & Stratton, 1962.
SAMPATH KUMARAN, J. D., and IYA, K. K.:   Sex Chromatin in Bovines.   Indian Vet. J. 42: 377–383, 1965.
THULINE, H. C., and NORBY, D. E.:   Spontaneous Occurrence of Chromosome Abnormalities in Cat.   Science 134:554–555, 1961.

Anomalies in Autosomal Chromosomes.—Autosomes would appear at first examination to be more frequently involved in defects than the sex chromosomes, simply because there are more of them.   Clinical deviations related to abnormal sex chromosomes are, on the contrary, much more frequent in the human subject. The explanation may be that abnormal autosomes may be more apt to lead to death of the zygote, therefore leaving fewer abnormal living phenotypes.   It does appear that lesions in autosomes do have a more serious effect on the individual than similar defects in sex chromosomes.   **Down's syndrome** or **mongolism** in children, although described over one hundred years ago (Down, 1866), was only recently shown to be associated with one of two anomalies of autosomal chromosomes.   Affected children are mentally retarded and have other physical features which characterize the syndrome.   The cells of patients with this syndrome are usually aneuploid with a chromosome number of 47.   The extra chromosome is usually found to be one of the small acrocentric chromosomes defined as number 21.   This trisomy was the first discovered, apparently is the most frequent, and currently is called the "regular mongol."   Some mongols were subsequently found to have the normal number (2n–46) of chromosomes, but karyotype analysis revealed evidence of a translocation involving chromosome number 21.   These latter cases are referred to as "translocation mongols."

Trisomy of a small acrocentric autosomal chromosome in a young female chimpanzee (Pan troglodytes) has been reported by McClure, et al. (1969).   This chimpanzee was born in the Yerkes Regional Primate Research Center from parents with normal karyotypes and phenotypes.   The sire was twenty-one years old and the dam fourteen at the time of birth of the trisomic offspring.   The dam

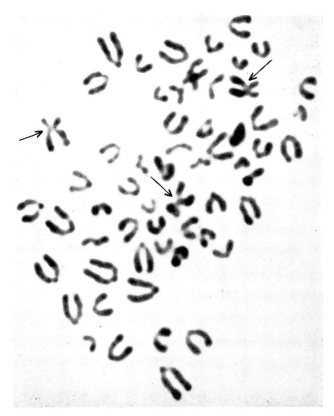

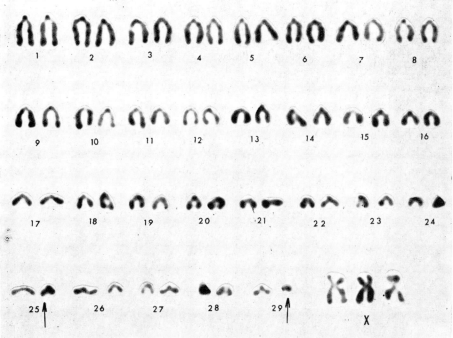

FIG. 9–8.—Metaphase spread (top) and karyotype of a cell from a cow with malignant lymphoma (lymphosarcoma). Note the two large extra metacentric chromosomes and the total number ($2n$–61). (Courtesy of Dr. Parvathi K. Basrur, Ontario Veterinary College.)

had delivered a premature stillborn infant twenty-eight months prior to this parturition. At birth, this chimp was in the low normal range of weight in comparison with other chimps born in this laboratory. She grew significantly slower than normal chimps. Several congenital anomalies were noted: bilateral partial syndactyly of the toes with clinodactyly, prominent epicanthus, hyperflexibility of the joints and a short neck with excess skin folds. Several neurologic abnormalities were present, including absence of the Moro reflex, marked hypotonia, abnormal traction and suspension responses and general inactivity. Several deficiencies in postural behavior were evident in comparison to other chimpanzees at the same age.

Each of these features in this trisomic chimpanzee are similar to those observed in human infants with Down's syndrome. This raises interesting speculation about the possible homology of the small acrocentric chromosomes of man and chimpanzee.

Another defect of autosomes has been established as occurring repeatedly in man and involves trisomy of chromosome 17 or 18. This defect has been associated with odd-shaped skull, low-set and malformed ears, micrognathia, webbing of the neck, probable mental retardation and a congenital heart defect. A third autosomal abnormality, trisomy of the group 13–15 of large acrocentric chromosomes, has been found in children with multiple congenital anomalies such as harelip, cleft palate and bilateral coloboma. Other abnormal chromosomes have been reported but the above serve to illustrate aberrations in autosomes which result in viable but seriously altered phenotypes.

It is also of interest that in human cases of chronic granulocytic leukemia, cells have been found with a small isologous chromosome, presumably number 21 which has lost $\frac{1}{4}$ of its long arm. This "marker" chromosome is called the "Philadelphia" or Ph[1] chromosome after the city in which it was first described (Nowell & Hungerford, 1961). The consistent occurrence of an extra and a marker chromosome in granulocytic leukemia of the mouse has been reported by Wald et al. (1963).

In cases of bovine lymphosarcoma (malignant lymphoma), interesting chromosomal alterations have been found. Basrur and associates (1964) described the occurrence of three large submetacentric chromosomes, resembling the X chromosome in this species, in a complement of 61 ($2n$) chromosomes (Fig. 9–8). In other cells cultured from the circulating blood of cattle affected with lymphosarcoma, Hare et al. (1964) have found several chromosomal abnormalities. Although some inconsistency between individuals was evident, in several cases modal chromosome numbers were heteroploid due to the presence of large extra telocentric and metacentric chromosomes and the loss of one X chromosome.

Dr. P. K. Basrur graciously permitted me to study karyotypes of cells cultured from five dogs with lymphosarcoma (malignant lymphoma). Two of these were males; three females. All had more than the normal number of metacentrics— two females with normal diploid complement ($2n$–78) had three (one more than normal) large submetacentric chromosomes and one female with $2n$–77, had two large and two smaller metacentric chromosomes. One male dog had a normal complement ($2n$–78) but an extra large metacentric chromosome was present. The second male dog with lymphosarcoma also had two large metacentrics and $2n$–77. Further details may be found in the publication by Dr. Basrur (1966).

Malignant Lymphoma in Cats.—This disease is accompanied by a panoply of chromosomal abnormalities in affected cells (Jones, 1969). Four groups of anomalies have been identified: I.—Due to loss of a single chromosome in group E (see normal karyotype, p. 324) resulting in a modal chromosome number of 37. II.—A single chromosome was lost from group D, causing the modal number of chromosomes to be 37. III.—An additional acrocentric chromosome in group F resulted in a total number of chromosomes of 39. IV.—Additional chromosomes in groups C, D, E and F of the feline karyotype, resulted in 2-n numbers of 40 and 41. In a final category (V) no abnormalities were detected in the lymphomatous cells. This severe aneuploidy in malignant cells may be the effect of the feline lymphoma virus. Any possible effect of these changes in chromosome number on the malignant behavior of the cells is yet to be demonstrated.

Sterility in Hybrids.—The mule, our best known hybrid, has been described as "without pride of ancestry or hope of posterity." The underlying reason for the mule's sterility is of much scientific interest and is still clouded with mystery. In spite of published descriptions of allegedly fertile mules, doubt has been expressed by Benirschke (1963) that reportedly fertile mules were actually mules. In his view, in fact, they may have been donkeys. Karyotype analysis now offers one approach to this problem but is yet to be done on such allegedly fertile mules. The domestic horse (*Equus caballus*) is now known to have a *2n* number of 64 chromosomes, the ass (*Equus asinus*) 62 chromosomes and the mule, not unexpectedly, has the sum of the haploid number of each of his parents—namely, 63. Benirschke (1964) has demonstrated an intriguing panoply of chromosome numbers in many varieties of wild equines (Table 9–1). Variation in chromosome number and arrangement may provide an important mechanism which affects evolution. The sterile hybrid, on the other hand, presents a dead end in the development of new varieties or species. The cause of sterility in hybrids such as the mule is unknown. One of the possibilities is that unequal numbers of chromosomes are unable to pair off ("synapse") during that specific phase of meiosis. The problem has many aspects needing more adequate study.

Spontaneous Human Abortions.—Studies by several investigators, particularly Benirschke (1963), Clendenin (1963), and Carr (1963) have uncovered chromosomal abnormalities in human aborted and stillborn fetuses. It appears likely that the chromosomal defects were causally related to the intrauterine death of these fetuses. Among the defects in the chromosomes of these abortuses or fetuses were the following: Translocation on chromosome A (*2n*–46); Trisomy of Group E (pair 16) (*2n*–47); Anencephaly, XO sex chromosomes (*2n*–45); Triploidy and XXY sex chromosomes (*2n*–69); Trisomy of group D (*2n*–47) and Tetraploid cultures. It has been estimated that about one chromosomal abnormality occurs in 200 live births. These aberrations are much more frequent in aborted and stillborn fetuses; one estimate puts this frequency at about 30 per cent of all spontaneously interrupted pregnancies (Benirschke, 1963).

The significance of the finding of defective chromosomes in these human patients is yet to be fully determined, but it appears that such defects may well contribute significantly to the non-viable state of many human embryos.

The chromosomes of aborted animals of any species are yet to be studied Such studies may prove to be quite revealing.

Anomalies of Autosomal Chromosomes

BASRUR, P. K., GILMAN, J. P. W., and McSHERRY, B. J.: Cytological Observations on a Bovine Lymphosarcoma. Nature (Lond.) *201*:368–371, 1964.

BASRUR, P. K. and GILMAN, J. P. W.: Chromosome Studies in Canine Lymphosarcoma. Cornell Vet. *56*:451–469, 1966.

BENIRSCHKE, K., BROWNHILL, L. E., and BEATH, M. M.: Somatic Chromosomes of the Horse, the Donkey, and their Hybrids, the Mule and the Hinny. J. Reprod. Fertil. *4*:319–326, 1962.

BENIRSCHKE, K.: Chromosomal Studies on Abortuses. Trans. New Eng. Obstet. and Gyn. Soc. *17*:171–183, 1963.

BENJAMIN, S. A. and NORONHA, F.: Cytogenic Studies in Canine Lymphosarcoma. Cornell Vet. *57*:526–542, 1967.

HARE, W. C. D., *et al.*: Chromosomal Studies in Bovine Lymphosarcoma. J. Nat. Cancer Inst. *33*:105–118, 1964.

—————: Cytogenetics in the Dog and Cat. J. Small Anim. Pract. *7*:575–592, 1966.

JONES, T. C.: Chromosomal Analyses of Feline Lymphomas. Nat. Cancer Inst. Monograph No. 32, p. 95, 1965.

McCLURE, H. M., *et al.*: Autosomal Trisomy in a Chimpanzee: Resemblance to Down's Syndrome. Science *165*:1010–1012, 1969.

NOWELL, P. C. and HUNGERFORD, D. A.: Chromosome Studies in Human Leukemia. II. Chronic Granulocytic Leukemia. J. Nat. Cancer Inst. *27*:1013–1035, 1961.

RICH, M. A., TSUCHIDA, R., and SIEGLER, R.: Chromosome Aberrations: Their Role in the Etiology of Murine Leukemia. Science *146*:252–253, 1964.

RUSSELL, L. B.: Chromosome Aberrations in Experimental Mammals, Chapter 7 in *Progress in Medical Genetics*. Vol. II by Steinberg, A. G. and Bearn, A. G. New York, Grune & Stratton, 1962.

TSUCHIDA, R. and RICH, M. A.: Chromosomal Aberrations in Viral Leukemogenesis. I. Friend and Rauscher Leukemia. J. Nat. Cancer Inst. *33*:33–47, 1964.

WALD, N., *et al.*: The Consistent Occurrence of an Extra and a Marker Chromosome in Mouse Granulocytic Leukemia. Mamm. Cyto. Confer. Vergennes, Vermont, 1963.

WEBER, W. T., NOWELL, P. C., and HARE, W. C. D.: Chromosome Studies of a Transplanted and a Primary Canine Venereal Sarcoma. J. Nat. Cancer Inst. *35*:537–547, 1965.

Pathologic States Determined by Single Genes

In conformity with our policy of considering pathologic entities in relation to their specific etiology when known, in the following section will be described some such entities which have been characterized adequately and for which convincing evidence of their genetic basis is available. The numbers of such diseases is increasing rapidly and it will not be possible to include all which should be so categorized. Some will be listed in Table 9–2, may be found only in the references, or are described in the chapter directed toward the anatomic system involved (Chapters 19 through 29).

Lethal Genes.—One should not be surprised, after consideration of even a few aspects of genetic mechanisms, to learn that some defective genes result in death of the zygote. This lethal effect may be expressed at any time after fertilization —in the embryo, fetus, newborn or adult animal. Many other (sublethal) genes result in defects which lower vitality or produce other undesirable characteristics, but do not result in death. Most completely lethal genes are recessive and are only recognized by their full expression in the homozygous animal. In most instances, one normal gene is sufficient to overcome the presence of the homologous abnormal gene.

An example to demonstrate present concepts concerning the pathogenesis of a characteristic controlled by a single lethal gene is found in hemophilia A, which occurs in nearly identical form in man and the dog. This gene is sex-linked— *i.e.*, carried in the X chromosome. The female, with her two X chromosomes, can be either homozygous or heterozygous for this gene. The male, with only one X can only be hemizygous. If his single X chromosome contains the abnormal gene, he will be affected with hemophilia. The affected male produces no anti-hemophilic globulin (AHG) which is needed to protect him against uncontrolled bleeding. The homozygous normal and the heterozygous female usually produce normal amounts of AHG but in some instances (Graham *et al.*, 1963) the hetero-zygote (carrier) woman produces somewhat reduced amounts of AHG. No

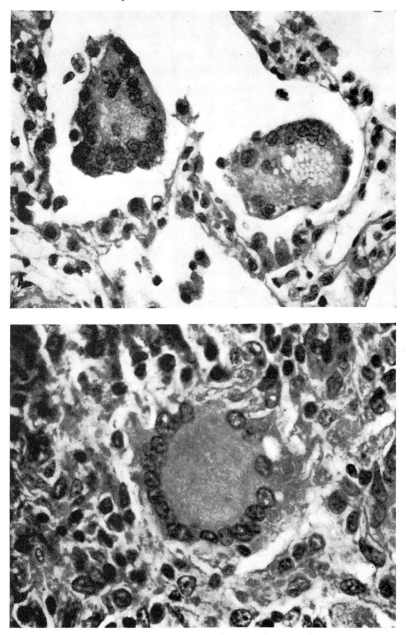

Fig. 9–9.—Vegetative dermatosis of swine. *A*, Multinucleated giant cells with vacuolated cytoplasm in alveoli of lung. *B*, Langhan's type of multinucleated giant cell in bronchial lymph node. (Courtesy of Drs. Dean H. Percy, Thomas J. Hulland and *Pathologia Veterinaria.*)

matter which of several explanations now current for this phenomenon are most accurate, it can be seen that quantitative analysis of the specific protein or specific enzyme may provide a means of detecting the carrier heterozygote. This is a matter of potential importance in control of genetically determined diseases in animals.

One important and practical problem should be considered in the study of the effect of lethal or sublethal genes in animals. This involves what the pathologist would call specific pathologic diagnosis and the geneticist might call "identification of the phenotype." In some cases, simple clinical inspection may be adequate, but in most instances, careful study by chemical and pathologic methods is necessary. For example, clinically manifest cerebellar ataxia in young kittens may be found at necropsy to result from grossly recognizable hypoplasia of the cerebellum; from absence of Purkinje cells in the cerebellum; or from microscopically detectable encephalitic lesions in the cerebellum. These three lesions may each have different causes, only one, or none of them due to genetic factors. Much needs to be done in the elucidation of the character of the lesions in animals as well as in underlying genetic mechanisms.

Mendelian ratios in progeny, study of pedigrees, test matings, coupled with adequate studies using clinical and pathological technics, are helpful in gaining presumptive evidence to decide whether a disease is merely congenital (acquired *in utero* and usually evident at birth) or whether it is also actually genetically controlled (*i.e.* inborn or inherited from the parents and the result of the recombination of genetic factors). Much more must be learned about the mechanisms involved at the molecular level before an adequate understanding is reached. The interactions of environmental factors (*i .e.* viruses, toxic chemicals, X-radiation, nutritional factors) must be more carefully studied to uncover all possible modes of action upon animal cells and particularly upon their genetic mechanisms (especially DNA and RNA).

Vegetative Dermatosis (Dermatosis Vegetans) in Swine.—Hjärre (1953) has described in young swine in Sweden a syndrome involving vegetating dermatosis of unknown etiology associated with a specific type of pneumonia. The cutaneous lesions usually appeared in newborn animals which occasionally survived for as long as a year but usually were dead by the seventh week. Usually only one pig in a litter was involved, and no abnormalities were evident in the parents or siblings of the same litter, but subsequent litters frequently contained an affected piglet.

The lesions usually appeared first on the distal parts of the extremities, but frequently spread to the rest of the body, particularly the inner surfaces of the legs and the abdomen. The lesions appeared as elevated, roughened, hairless plaques which sometimes assumed a papillomatous character. Involvement of the growing hoof often resulted in some deformity.

Microscopically, the cutaneous lesions in the early stages consisted principally of acanthosis and hyperkeratosis in the epidermis with elongation of the rete pegs. Microabscesses occurred in the elongated dermal papillae and in the epidermis. Older lesions consisted of severe acanthosis involving broad areas of the epidermis, often with moderate to severe hyperkeratosis. In some instances, the dermis was thrown up into papillary folds. In some, the sweat glands were cystic, presumably as a result of occlusion of their ducts by the acanthotic epidermis.

The lungs were often consolidated by the presence of many mononuclear cells and multinucleated giant cells in the alveoli. Fetalization of the alveolar lining was also recognized.

The inheritance as an autosomal recessive of the underlying factors in this disease was originally reported by Larsson (1953) in Sweden and confirmed by Percy and Hulland (1967) in Canada. The gene appears to be carried only by swine of the Landrace breed and common ancestors in Sweden appear to be responsible for the gene demonstrated in swine in Norway, England and Canada.

Vegetative Dermatosis of Swine

HJÄRRE, A.: Vegetierende Dermatosen mit Riesenzellem-pneumonien bei Schwein. Deutsch. tierarztl. Wschr. *60*:105–110, 1953.
LARSSON, E. L.: Klumpfotgrisar. Svenska Svinavelsför Tidskr. *1*:1–15, 1953.
PERCY, D. H., and HULLAND, T. J.: Dermatosis Vegetans (Vegetative Dermatosis) in Canadian Swine. Canad. Vet. J. *8*:3–9, 1967.
————: Evolution of Multinucleate Giant Cells in Dermatosis Vegetans in Swine. Path. Vet. *5*:419–428, 1968.
————: The Histopathological Changes in the Skin of Pigs with Dermatosis Vegetans. Canad. J. Comp. Med. *33*:48–54, 1969.

Congenital Ichthyosis.—A rare congenital disease of newborn infants, ichthyosis is sometimes encountered in calves. The name ichthyosis was suggested by the scaly epidermis which resembles the skin of fish. The severe form, *ichthyosis congenita fetalis* (Harlequin fetus, from the grotesque garb of Harlequin clown), astounding in appearance, was first described more than one and one-half centuries ago, and still is incompletely explained. The animal counterpart is infre-

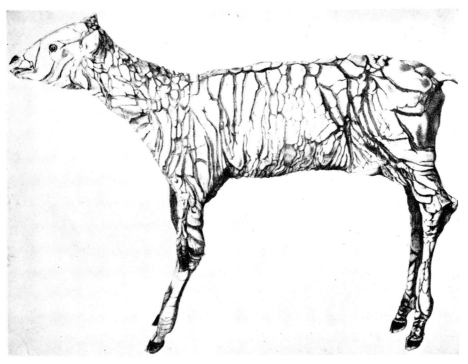

FIG. 9–10.—Congenital ichthyosis, skin of a newborn calf. (Courtesy of Armed Forces Institute of Pathology.)

quently recorded in the literature, although accounts are found in the old literature, and most veterinary museums in Europe have at least one skin from an
affected calf. One of the writers (Jones) has studied pathologic material from
calves in a herd in which several cases reportedly occurred. Hutt (1934) considers this condition in cattle to be due to a simple autosomal recessive gene,
homozygous in the affected calf.

The skin of the affected newborn infant and calf are strikingly similar; neither
survive more than a few hours or days. The entire skin is hairless and is covered
with thick, scaly, horny epidermis which is divided into plates by deep fissures.
These fissures are often wide, with a red, raw-appearing base, and follow a pattern
that corresponds to the cleavage planes of the skin. The skin is everted around
the lips, eyes and other body orifices, giving the impression of being too small for
the body which it encases. One explanation offered for the appearance of the
skin is that a defect in keratinization inhibits the proper expansive growth of the
epidermis, preventing it from keeping pace with growth of the rest of the body.

Microscopic sections reveal the epidermis to be covered by an extremely thick,
dense and tightly adherent layer of keratin. The rete pegs are elongated; the

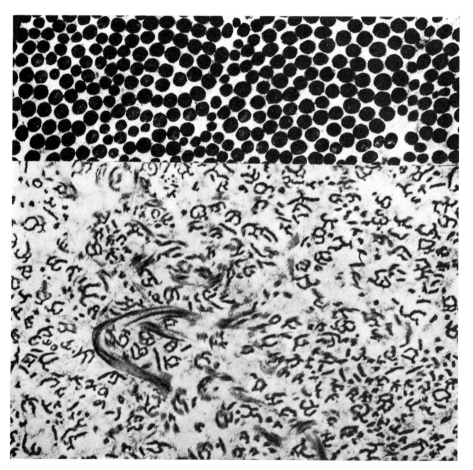

Fig. 9–11.—Bovine dermal collagen. × 49,400. *Top*—Normal collagen fibers in cross section.
Bottom—Collagen of calf affected with dermatosparaxis. (Courtesy of Dr. W. Kay Read and
Laboratory Investigation.)

dermis is moderately thickened and contains congested capillaries, particularly in areas underlying the fissures. The fissures extend through the hyperkeratotic stratum corneum and separate the upper layers of the stratum germinativum, but the basal layer is usually intact.

Other types of congenital and adult ichthyosis are known in man but apparently have not been recognized in animals.

Congenital Ichthyosis

EDMONDS, H. W. and DOLAN, W. D.: Ichthyosis Congenita Fetalis, Severe Type (Harlequin Fetus). Bull. Internat. Assn. Med. Mus. *32*:1–21, 1951.

JULIAN, R. J.: Ichthyosis Congenita in Cattle. Vet. Med. *55*:35–41, 1960.

TUFF, P. and GLEDISH, L. A.: Ichthyosis congenita hos Kalveren arvelig letal defekt. Nord vet. med. *1*:619–627, 1949.

Congenital Dermal Asthenia.—Collagenous tissue dysplasias which result in cutaneous asthenia, hyperelasticity and fragility of the skin and hypermobility of joints have been reported in man, dog, mink and cattle. It is not certain at this writing whether these are identical pathologic processes in each species although the evidence now points toward their similarities. The bovine entity has been called "dermatosparaxis" and has distinctive morphologic characteristics. Light microscopy indicates deficiency in the amount of collagen of the skin and its fine fibrillar nature. Ultrastructural studies (Fig. 9–11) indicate that the collagen fibrils in the dermis are inadequately packed and fail to form the orderly, uniform, fibers characteristic of normal collagen. This bovine disease appears to be inherited as an autosomal recessive characteristic. The canine disease seems to resemble closely *cutis hyperelastica* (Ehlers-Danlos syndrome) of man.

The human skin affected with this disease is reported to contain excessive numbers of compact masses of elastic fibers distributed throughout the dermis. These are demonstrable in microscopic sections treated with special stains for elastic fibers (Weigert's or van Gieson's elastica stains).

Congenital Dermal Asthenia

ANSAY, M., GILLET, A., and HANSET, R.: (Hereditary Dermatosparaxia [Fragility of the Skin] in Cattle. I. Biochemical Constitution of the Skin. II. Additional Observations on Collagen and Acid Mucopolysaccharides.) Ann. Med. Vet. *112*:449–464 and 465–478, 1968. V.B. *39*:2636, 1969.

HANSET, R., and ANSAY, M.: (Dermatosparaxia [Fragility of the Skin]—A New Hereditary Defect of Connective Tissue in Cattle.) Ann. Med. Vet. *111*:451–470, 1967. V.B. *38*:2079, 1968.

HEGREBERG, G. A., and PADGETT, G. A.: Ehlers-Danlos Syndrome in Animals . Bull. Path. *8*:247, 1967.

HEGREBERG, G. A., et al.: A Connective Tissue Disease of Dogs and Mink Resembling the Ehlers-Danlos-Syndrome of Man. J. Hered. *60*:249–254, 1969.

HEGREBERG, G. A., PADGETT, C. A., and HENSON, J. B.: Connective Tissue Disease of Dogs and Mink Resembling Ehlers-Danlos Syndrome of Man. III. Histopathologic Changes of the Skin. Arch. Path. *90*:159–166, 1970.

In Table 9–2 are listed several examples of lethal or semilethal congenital diseases in domestic animals. These examples were selected on the basis that presumptive evidence indicates that they are controlled by genetic factors and the lesions have been described in adequate detail. In most cases a single recessive gene is involved (a few dominant ones are indicated by D) and some are sex-linked. A very large number of lethal genes have been studied (see Hutt, 1964,

Stormont, 1958; and Wiesner, 1960) but many have not been adequately characterized pathologically. Analysis of chromosomes in these conditions is also yet to be done. The list will give some conception of the complexity of the problem of genetically determined disease in animals and will provide some clues to the great effort still needed to arrive at adequate understanding of these conditions.

Table 9-2.—Examples of Genetically Controlled Diseases

Diseases in which (1) evidence indicates genetic determination and (2) pathologic manifestations have been described. A = autosomal, S = sex-linked, D = dominant, r = recessive, gene symbol (if established) = ( ).

Scientific and Common Names	Genetic Designation and Gene Symbol	Clinical and Pathologic Features	Reference
CATTLE: Achondroplasia, recessive, ("Bull-dog calves")	A, r, ( )	Dexter breed heterozygous for gene; occurs also in other breeds; fetus aborted 4th to 6th months of gestation; anasarca, phocomelus, prognathia, domed skull, protruding tongue, achondroplasia.	Hutt, 1964; Stormont, 1958; Innes and Saunders, 1962.
Hypotrichosis congenita ("hairless")	"Hairless" A, r, ( )	Guernsey and Holstein; viable and non-viable forms—may be different genes; complete atrichia.	Hutt and Saunders, 1963: Schleger, 1967.
Hereditary congenital ataxia; Hypomyelinogenesis congenita	"Jittery" A, r, ( )	Jersey; Shorthorn; Angus; (may occur in many breeds), calves 2–3 weeks of age—incoordination, micro: leucodysplasia of cerebellum, midbrain and medulla w/loss of neurons and myelin.	Saunders et al. 1952; Innes and Saunders, 1962; Young, 1962.
Ichthyosis faetalis "fish skin"	A, r, ( )	Norwegian red poll cattle, probably other breeds (similar to "Harlequin fetus" in man), alopecia, scaly fissured skin, hyperkeratosis, acanthosis (p. 1026) deep fissures.	Tuff and Gledish, 1949.
Epitheliogenesis imperfecta (epithelial defects, skinless)	"Skinless" A, r, (ep)	Ayrshire, Holstein, and Jersey breeds, calves born alive, absence of skin in patches over fettocks and knees, sometimes ears and over muzzle.	Hutt and Frost, 1948; Hutt, 1964.
Hydrocephalus internus	Hydrocephalus A, r, ( )	Hereford and Holstein-Friesian; congenital hydrocephalus interna in newborn calves, symmetrical distention of lateral ventricles.	Baker et al., 1961; Innes and Saunders, 1962; Urman and Grace, 1964.
Hairlessness, streaked	"Streaked hairlessness" S, D, ( )	Holstein-Friesian breed, vertical streaks of atrichia over hips in heterozygous females, hemizygous males presumed dead in utero.	Eldridge and Atkeson, 1953; Hutt, 1964.
Aphakia, microphakia, cataract, ectopia-lentis, iridermia; multiple eye defects.	Hereditary eye defects A, r, ( )	Jersey breed, newborn calves blind due to congenital cataract, with iridermia, microphakia, and ectopia-lentis.	Saunders and Fincher, 1951.

Table 9–2.—Examples of Genetically Controlled Diseases (Continued)

Scientific and Common Names	Genetic Designation and Gene Symbol	Clinical and Pathologic Features	Reference
Dwarfism "snorter dwarfs"	Dwarfism, A, r, ( ) (may be more complex)	Hereford, Angus, calves are short in stature, fail to grow, short bulging foreheads, malocclusion, nasal obstruction may cause dyspnea.	Julian *et al.*, 1959; Hutt, 1964; Pahnish *et al.*, 1955.
Acroteriasis congenita (adactyly) "amputated"	A, r, ( ) Amputations	Holstein-Friesians; forelegs terminate at elbow, hindlegs at hock; cleft palate, adentia; prognathism and maxillar distortion; death near time of birth.	Stormont, 1958; Wiesner, 1960.
Bovine Porphyria	A, r, ( )	Porphyrins stain teeth and bones; fluoresce in ultraviolet light.	Kaneko and Mills, 1970; Wass and Hoyt 1965.
Dermatosparaxia; Fragility of skin; Ehlers-Danlos syndrome	A, r, ( )	Skin fragile, stretches and tears easily (also dog and man).	Ansay, Gillet and Hanset, 1968; Hanset and Ansay, 1967; O'Hara, *et al.*, 1970.
Chediak-Higashi syndrome	A, r, ( )	Partial albinism, abnormal cytoplasmic granules in leukocytes, increased susceptibility to infection; also in man and mink.	Padgett, *et al.*, 1970.
Dog: Hemophilia A	S, r (h)	Aberdeen terrier, greyhound, Irish setter, Scotch terrier; hemizygous males affected—homozygous females also; deficiency of antihemophilic factor or Factor VIII, results in failure of blood to clot; hemorrhages into joints, subcutis, etc. may result in death.	Hutt *et al.*, 1948; Brinkhous, 1959.
Hemophilia B; Christmas Disease	S, r, ( )	Cairn terriers; deficiency of Factor IX results in deficiency of plasma thromboplastin.	Rowsell *et al.*, 1960.
Atrichia; Hairlessness	A, D, ( )	Hairless breeds heterozygous for this gene, homozygotes usually born dead, lack pinnae; may have stenotic esophagus.	Hutt, 1934.
Hereditary blindness and deafness	A, r, ( ) "dappling"	Merle or harlequin hair coat in heterozygotes; homozygotes white hair coat, microphthalmia, coloboma, often deaf. Collies, Norwegian dunker hounds, Great Danes, bull terriers.	Stormont, 1958.

12

Table 9–2.—*Examples of Genetically Controlled Diseases (Continued)*

Scientific and Common Names	Genetic Designation and Gene Symbol	Clinical and Pathologic Features	Reference
Ehlers-Danlos syndrome; cutaneous asthenia	A, r, ( )	Lack of tensile strength in connective tissue; skin easily torn, also in man, cattle and mink.	Hegreberg and Padgett, 1967; Hegreberg, et al., 1969; Hegreberg, Padgett and Henson, 1970.
Cyclic neutropenia "Gray Collie syndrome"	A, r, ( )	Collie dogs; associated with gray coat color; intermittent neutropenia results lowered resistance to infection; intestinal malabsorption.	Lund, Padgett, and Gorham, 1970; Windhorst, et al., 1967.
Subluxation of carpus	S, r, ( )	Closely linked with hemophilia A, carpus easily over-flexed and subluxated.	Pick, et al., 1967.
Cystinuria: cystine urolithiasis	S, r, ( )	Amino acid, cystine, in urine in increased amounts, possibly transport mechanism defective; uroliths may obstruct urethra; also in man.	Cornelius, Bishop and Shaffer, 1967.
Congenital, hereditary lymphedema	A, D, ( )	Lymphatic obstruction at regional lymph nodes—distal lymphatics distended; also in man, swine, cattle.	Patterson, et al., 1967; Luginbuhl, et al., 1967.
DOMESTIC FOWL: Achondroplasia (Creeper)	Creeper A, D, (*Cp*)	Scots dumpies, Japanese bantams, heterozygous breeds; assume crouching stance due to shortened extremities; achondroplasia; homozygotes usually die during first week of incubation.	Hamburger, 1942; Hutt, 1949.
Short limbs; Cornish lethal	Cornish lethal A, D, (*Cl*)	Shortened extremities in heterozygotes; homozygotes die during last week of incubation. Note similarity to "creeper."	Stormont, 1958; Hutt, 1949.
Featherless chicks; (naked)	Naked S, r (*n*)	Many homozygous chicks die few days before hatching; other featherless chicks die after hatching; more survivors if kept warm; almost complete absence of feathers at hatching, but grow some plumage after 4 months of age; females hemizygous and affected.	Hutt, 1949.
CAT: Manx, tailless	A, D(?) (*M*)	Manx cats heterozygous dominance incompletely expressed, homozygotes die *in utero*, some presumed heterozygotes have imperforate anus, and defects in pelvic bones.	Todd, 1964.

Table 9–2.—Examples of Genetically Controlled Diseases (Continued)

Scientific and Common Names	Genetic Designation and Gene Symbol	Clinical and Pathologic Features	Reference
Deaf, white	A, r (de)	Deafness in dominant white (W) cats with blue or yellow eyes; due to agenesis of organ of Corti, spiral ganglia and cochlear nuclei.	Innes and Saunders, 1962.
Polydactyly	A, D, (P)	Extra toes on front feet, sometimes hind feet affected also, but not without involvement of front feet; one to three extra digits.	Robinson, 1959.
MOUSE: Yellow coat color	A, D, (A^y)	All yellow mice heterozygous; first lethal gene demonstrated (by Cuenot) in mammals. *Note:* A very large number of lethal and semilethal genes are known in the mouse. The reader is referred to Grüneberg for details.	Grüneberg, 1956.
SWINE: Amelia, congenital	Amputated A, r, ( )	All appendages missing; piglets are born alive.	Johnson, 1940; Hutt, 1964.
Cerebrospinal lipodystrophy; (Tay-Sachs)	A, r(?) ( )	Lipodystrophy of neurons in central nervous system. Ultrastructure: membranous inclusions— resembles Tay-Sachs disease of man.	Read and Bridges, 1968.
Renal hypoplasia (bilateral)	A, r (?) ( )	Kidneys in newborn swine very much smaller than normal.	Cordes and Dodd, 1965.
Cerebral meningocele	A, r, ( )	Meningocele vary in size usually midline over dorsal aspect cerebrum.	Myer and Trautwein, 1966; Trautwein and Myer, 1966.

Pathologic States Determined by Single Genes

BAKER, M. L., PAYNE, L. C., and BAKER, G. N.: The Inheritance of Hydrocephalus in Cattle. J. Hered. 52:134–138, 1961.

BARDIN, C. W., *et al.*: Pseudohermaphroditic Rat: End Organ Insensitivity to Testosterone. Science 167:1136–1137, 1970.

BLUMBERG, B. S.: *Proceedings of Conference on Genetic Polymorphisms and Geographic Variations in Disease.* New York, Grüne & Stratton, 1963.

BRINKHOUS, K. M. and GRAHAM, J. B.: Hemophilia in the Female Dog. Science 111:723–724, 1959.

BROWN, R. C., SWARTON, M. C. and BRINKHOUS, K. M.: Canine Hemophilia and Male Pseudohermaphroditism; Cytogenetic Studies. Lab. Invest. 12:961–967, 1963.

CORDES, D. O., and DODD, D. C.: Bilateral Renal Hypoplasia of the Pig. Path. Vet. 2:37–48, 1965.

CORNELIUS, C. E., BISHOP, J. A., and SCHAFFER, M. H.: A Quantitative Study of Amino Aciduria in Dachshunds with a History of Cystine Urolithiasis. Cornell Vet. 57:177–183, 1967.

ELDRIDGE, F. E. and ATKESON, F. W.: Streaked Hairlessness in Holstein-Friesian Cattle. J. Hered. 44:265–271, 1953.

FISHBEIN, M. (ed.): *Second International Conference on Congenital Malformations.* New York, Internat. Med. Congress, Ltd., 1964.

FRYE, F. L., McFARLAND, L. Z., and ENRIGHT, J. B.:   Sacrococcygeal Agenesis in Swiss Mice. Cornell Vet. 54:487–495, 1964.

GARROD, A. E.:   *Inborn Errors of Metabolism*, 1909.   Reprinted, London Oxford University. Press, 1963.

GLUECKSOHN-WAELSCH, S.:   Mammalian Genetics in Medicine.   Chapter 8 in *Progress in Medical Genetics*, Vol. II, Steinberg, A. G. and Bearn, A. G., New York, Grune & Stratton, 1962.

GRAHAM, J. B., McLENDON, W. W., and BRINKHOUS, K. M.:   Mild Hemophilia; an Allelic Form of the Disease.   Am. J. Med. Sci. 225:46–53, 1953.

HUTT, F. B.:   Inherited Lethal Characters in Domestic Animals.   Cornell Vet. 24:1–25, 1934.

HUTT, F. B. and FROST, J. N.:   Hereditary Epithelial Defects in Ayrshire Cattle.   J. Hered. 39:131–137, 1948.

HUTT, F. B., RICKARD, C. G., and FIELD, R. A.:   Sex-linked Hemophilia in Dogs.   J. Hered. 39:2–9, 1948.

HUTT, F. B. and SAUNDERS, L. Z.:   Viable Genetic Hypotrichosis in Guernsey Cattle. J. Hered. 44:97–103, 1953.

JULIAN, L. M., TYLER, W. S., and GREGORY, P. W.:   The Current Status of Bovine Dwarfism. J. Am. Vet. M. A. 135:104–109, 1959.

KANEKO, J. J., and MILLS, R.:   Hematological and Blood Chemical Observations on Neonatal Normal and Porphyric Calves in Early Life.   Cornell Vet. 60:52–60, 1970.

LUND, J. E., PADGETT, G. A., and GORHAM, J. R.:   Additional Evidence on the Inheritance of Cyclic Neutropenia in the Dog.   J. Hered. 61:47–49, 1970.

LUNGINBUHL, H., *et al.*:   Congenital Hereditary Lymphoedema in the Dog.   II. Pathological Studies.   J. Med. Genet. 4:153–165, 1967.

MYER, H., and TRAUTWEIN, G.:   Experimentalle Untersuchungen uber erbliche Meningocele cerebralis beim Schwein.   I. Zuchtversuche and genetische analyse.   Path. Vet. 3:529–542, 1966.

O'HARA, P. J., *et al.*:   A Collagenous Tissue Dysplasia of Calves.   Lab. Invest. 23:307–314, 1970.

OHNO, S., STENIUS, C., and CHRISTIAN, L. C.:   Sex Differences in Alcohol Metabolism; Androgenic Steroid as an Inducer of Kidney Alcohol Dehydrogenase.   Clin. Genetics 1:35–44, 1970.

OHNO, S., and LYON, M. F.:   X-linked Testicular Feminization in the Mouse as a Non-inducible Regulatory Mutation of the Jacob-Monod Type.   Clin. Genet. 1:121–127, 1970.

PADGETT, G. A., *et al.*:   The Chediak-Higashi Syndrome: A Comparative Review.   Curr. Topics Path. 51:175–194, 1970.

PAHNISH, O. F., STANLEY, E. B., SAFFLEY, C. E., and ROUBICEK, C. B.:   Dwarfism in Beef Cattle.   Ariz. Agric. Exper. Sta. Bull. 268, 1955.

PATTERSON, D. F., *et al.*:   Congenital Hereditary Lymphoedema in the Dog.   I. Clinical and Genetic Studies.   J. Med. Genet. 4:145–152, 1967.

PAULING, L. ITANO, H. A., SINGER, S. J., and WELLS, I. C.:   Sickle Cell Anemia, a Molecular Disease.   Science 110:543–548, 1949.

PICK, J. R., *et al.*:   Subluxation of the Carpus in Dogs.   An X-chromosomal Defect Closely Linked with the Locus for Hemophilia A.   Lab. Invest. 17:243–248, 1967.

READ, W. K., and BRIDGES, C. H.:   Cerebrospinal Lipodystrophy in Swine.   A New Disease Model in Comparative Pathology.   Path. Vet. 5:67–74, 1968.

ROWSELL, H. C., DOWNIE, H. G., MUSTARD, J. F., LEESON, J. E., and ARCHIBALD, J. A.: A Disorder Resembling Hemophilia B (Christman Disease) in Dogs.   J. Am. Vet. M. A. 137:247–250, 1960.

SABOURDY, M.:   Hereditary Disease of Laboratory Animals, their Interest for Research. Proc. 18th World Vet. Congr., Paris 2:675–678, 1966.

SAUNDERS, L. Z.:   A Check List of Hereditary and Familial Diseases of the Central Nervous System in Domestic Animals.   Cornell Vet. 42:592–600. 1952.

SAUNDERS, L. Z. and FINCHER, M. G.:   Hereditary Multiple Eye Defects in Grade Jersey Calves.   Cornell Vet. 41:351–366, 1951.

SAUNDERS, L. Z., SWEET, J. G., MARTIN, S. M., FOX, F. H., and FINCHER, M. G.:   Hereditary Congenital Ataxia in Jersey Calves.   Cornell Vet. 42:559–591, 1952.

SHORT, R. V.:   Reproduction.   Ann. Rev. Physiol. 29:373–400, 1967.

STANBURY, J. B., WYNGAARDEN, J. B., and FREDRICKSON, D. S.:   *The Metabolic Basis of Inherited Disease*, New York, McGraw-Hill Book Co., 1964.

STORMONT, C.:   Genetics and Disease.   Vet. Sci. 4:137–162, 1958.

TODD, N. B.:   The Manx Factor in Domestic Cats.   J. Hered. 55:225–230, 1964.

TRAUTWEIN, G., and MYER, H.:   Experimentelle Untersuchungen über erbliche Meningocele Cerebralis beim Schwein.   Path. Vet. 3:543–555, 1966.

The student will soon observe that viral diseases in this chapter are taken up in approximate relation to the tissue affected by the virus. This present arrangement is still the most satisfactory to the pathologist but may be changed in future editions when more complete knowledge of the interaction of viruses and cells give a more fundamental or useful basis upon which to study viral disease.

The definition of viruses (Lwoff, 1957) is of interest: "Viruses are infectious, potentially pathogenic nucleoprotein entities possessing only one type of nucleic acid, which reproduce from their genetic material; are unable to grow and to undergo binary fission, and are devoid of metabolic enzymes." Thus, viruses so defined may contain deoxyribonucleic acid (DNA) or ribonucleic acid (RNA), but not both. Agents which contain both DNA and RNA, such as those of the psittacosis-lymphogranuloma venereum-trachoma group, are excluded by this definition. The perceptive student will quickly recognize the importance of the discovery of DNA in viruses, this being the same self-replicating molecule which is the genetic material of the cell (p. 317). In fact, DNA may control all the activities of the cell. The fact that the same chemical substance occurs in viruses and in self-replicating cells also provides a clue to the means by which viruses are reproduced and interact with the cell (p. 319).

The effects of some viruses are characterized by the formation of tumors (pp. 281, 507). Of particular importance in this group are avian lymphomatosis, papillomatosis of various species and the Shope fibroma of rabbits. Some malignant tumors have been associated with a virus, *i.e.*, the squamous cell carcinoma that develops in the Shope papilloma of the skin of rabbits. The "milk factor" which occurs in mouse mammary carcinoma is also of interest in this connection. This factor, now known to be a virus, has been shown to be transmitted to suckling mice by their mothers' milk, and a high incidence of mammary carcinoma is observed in the progeny as they mature. Delivery of mice by cesarean section and raising them on foster mothers not excreting the "milk factor" result in a much lower incidence of mammary carcinoma. In recent years, it has been increasingly evident that other neoplastic diseases of animals, for example "polyoma virus" of rodents, mouse leukemia and feline lymphoma are caused by viral agents.

Many viruses produce leukopenia in the earliest stages of infection. This is particularly severe and persistent in feline panleukopenia and rinderpest; in both, leukopenia is a direct result of destruction of leukocytes and their precursors. In other diseases, such as hog cholera, equine influenza, and canine distemper, leukopenia is less pronounced and transitory, and may be the result of mobilization of leukocytes in certain parts of the body, temporarily removing them from the blood stream.

NEUROTROPIC VIRAL DISEASES

Rabies

(Hydrophobia, Lyssa, Rage, Tollwut)

Rabies is a viral encephalitis to which almost all mammals, including man, are susceptible. The virus is usually present in the saliva of infected animals and is transmitted by their bite; therefore the disease is most common in carnivores such as dogs, wolves and foxes. As a rule rabies in man results from the bite of a rabid dog, wolf, fox, or skunk. These animals also transmit the disease to cattle, horses, and sheep, which, however, seldom spread it further. Insectivorous and frugivorous bats have in recent years been shown to harbor the virus, often without clinical signs of disease. These animals may have an important role in the dissemination of the virus and its survival in nature during inter-epizootic periods of time. In some parts of the world, vampire bats are important in the spread of the disease to other animals and man. Bats are the only animals which can become infected with, and excrete, rabies virus without developing clinical disease leading to death. In domestic animals rabies is most frequent in cattle, dogs, and cats. Wildlife rabies is most prevalent in skunks, foxes, raccoons and bats.

Signs.—Following the bite of a rabid animal, or penetration of the virus through the skin by some other means, the virus invades the central nervous system via peripheral nerve pathways. Centrifugal passage from the brain, also via peripheral nerves, results in salivary gland infection. The incubation period varies from a few days to several months. The clinical symptoms usually appear in one of two forms: the "dumb" and the "furious." In the "dumb" form of rabies, the animal falls into a stupor and has the peculiar staring expression associated with paralysis of the muscles of mastication. In the "furious" form, the animal goes into rages, biting and slashing at any moving object or even inanimate objects, such as sticks and trees. The furious champing of the jaws is accompanied by excessive salivation; the saliva streams from the mouth or is

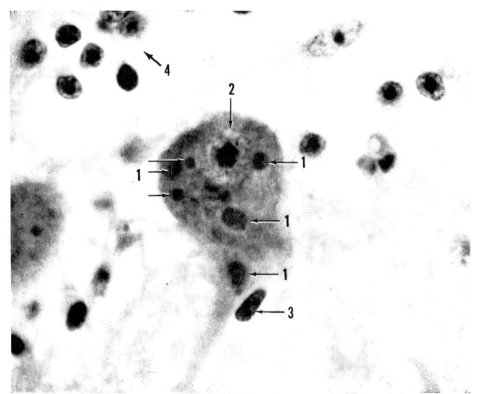

Fig. 10–2.—Rabies, cerebellum of a cow (× 1350). An unusual number of Negri bodies (*1*) are present in a Purkinje cell. Nucleus of the Purkinje cell (*2*), nucleus of a microglial cell (*3*), and cells of a granular layer (*4*). Schleifstein modification of the Wilhite stain. (Courtesy of Armed Forces Institute of Pathology.) Contributor: Lt. Col. F. D. Maurer.

PLATE I

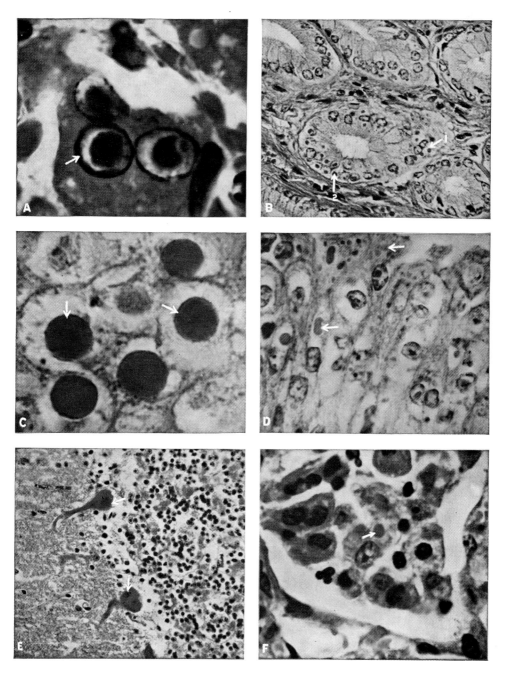

CELLULAR INCLUSIONS OF VIRAL INFECTIONS

A, Infectious canine hepatitis, intranuclear inclusions in liver cells. × 1850, H & E stain. Note margination of nuclear chromatin (arrow) surrounding a clear halo around the inclusion body.

B, Canine distemper, cytoplasmic (1) and intranuclear (2) inclusion bodies in gastric epithelium. × 470. H & E stain.

C, Fowl pox, Bollinger bodies (arrows) in cytoplasm of epidermal cells. × 1300, H & E stain.

D, Canine distemper, cytoplasmic inclusions (arrows) in epithelial cells of urinary bladder. × 525. Shorr's S–3 stain.

E, Rabies, cytoplasmic inclusions (arrows) in Purkinje cells, cerebellum of cow. × 350, Schleifstein modification of Wilhite stain.

F, Canine distemper, cytoplasmic inclusion (arrow) in cells from pulmonary alveolar wall. × 825. H & E stain.

churned into foam which may adhere to the lips and face. A radical change in temperament occurs; wild animals which normally shun man will venture into the open and attack human subjects. The rabid dog, fox or wolf tends particularly to attack a moving person or animal. Paralysis may follow either the "furious" or "dumb" stage of the disease. Death occurs within ten days of the first symptoms. Recovery is unknown.

Lesions.—The lesions of rabies are microscopic, limited to the central nervous system, and extremely variable in extent. They may be very subtle and indiscernible except for early necrosis of neurons with specific cytoplasmic inclusion bodies in the affected nerve cells. In some cases, diffuse encephalitis is demonstrated by perivascular cuffing, neuronophagic nodules, and other indications of destruction of neurons throughout the brain. These changes tend to be particularly prominent in the brain stem, the hippocampus, and tne gasserian ganglia. According to Lapi, Davis and Anderson (1952) specific lesions develop earlier and more constantly in the gasserian ganglia than elsewhere in the nervous system, and may be present even before specific inclusion bodies can be demonstrated. These lesions consist of focal proliferation of the capsule cells surrounding the ganglion cells, mild infiltration of lymphocytes and plasma cells, and encroachment of proliferating glial cells upon the neurons. These collections of prolifer-

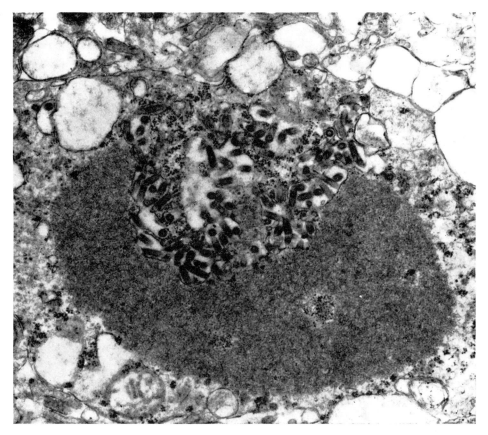

Fig. 10–3.—Rabies, hippocampus, fox. A neuronal inclusion containing bullet shaped and rod shaped virus particles. (× 30,000). (Courtesy Dr. R. E. Dierks and American Journal of Pathology.) (Electronmicrograph taken by Dr. F. A. Murphy.)

ating glial cells replacing neurons are known as **Babes nodules.** They may be seen in association with inclusion bodies in the cytoplasm of nearby ganglion cells.

In 1903, spherical cytoplasmic inclusion bodies with specific tinctorial characteristics were described by Negri in neurons of dogs, cats and rabbits experimentally infected with rabies virus. These inclusion bodies have subsequently been called **Negri bodies** and are accepted as specific indications of infection with rabies virus. This wide acceptance of Negri bodies as proof of rabies has developed in spite of a prolonged controversy as to the exact nature of these inclusions. Negri's idea that they were protozoan is not generally held today. Electron microscopic observations indicate that Negri bodies represent well-defined electron dense masses, which may or may not contain, or be associated with rabies virions. The nature and significance of the matrix is not understood but may represent a necessary component for viral replication or a reaction on the part of the infected neuron. Negri bodies are not always present in rabies and certain strains of rabies virus do not produce inclusion bodies, indicating that Negri bodies are not necessary for viral replication. Negri bodies are always intracytoplasmic; in the rabid dog they are found most readily in the hippocampus, but in cattle they are more numerous in the Purkinje cells of the cerebellum. It is possible for all neurons, even those of the ganglia, to contain these inclusions. Negri bodies have a distinct limiting membrane and may be encircled by a narrow, clear halo. In tissue sections, they usually measure from 2 to 8 microns in diameter. One or several may be present in an affected nerve cell. These inclusions may be entirely within the cell body or they may occur in dendrites where they are likely to be elongated, conforming to the shape of these processes. A granular, slightly basophilic internal structure can be demonstrated in preparations with Mann's stain.

The staining characteristics of the Negri body are of considerable interest. The hematoxylin and eosin method does not differentiate Negri bodies well. They become only a slightly darker shade of the color of the surrounding cytoplasm, but the clear halo may serve to delimit them. The Schleifstein modification of the Wilhite stain is particularly successful with tissue fixed in Zenker's solution. When stained by this method, Negri bodies are bright magenta, contrasting with the purplish cytoplasm of the neuron; red blood cells are somewhat yellowish or copper colored. The Williams modification of the van Gieson stain gives a similar effect. In impression smears, Seller's stain is effective; the inclusion body is bright red or magenta against the pale blue background of the neuronal cytoplasm. Mann's and Giemsa's stains are also useful, particularly in impression smears. No matter which stain is used, it is important that the person who examines material to confirm the diagnosis be thoroughly familiar with the characteristics of the stain and the appearance of Negri bodies. The final recognition of Negri bodies should not be left to the novice.

Moulton (1954) who has studied the histochemical characteristics of the Negri body, has found that it gives positive reactions to stains for protein, arginine, tyrosine, and alpha-amino acids. The inner granules are positive for desoxyribonucleic acid and organic iron. The periodic acid-Schiff reaction is inconclusive. Negative reactions are obtained in tests for ribonucleic acid, glycogen, hyaluronic acid, mucopolysaccharides, ascorbic acid, neutral fats, phospholipids, cholesterol, inorganic iron, calcium, alkaline phosphatase, dehydrogenase and cytochrome oxidase.

When the virus centrifugally invades the salivary gland, degenerative changes leading to necrosis may be encountered in the acinar epithelium, principally affecting mucogenic cells of the mandibular salivary gland. Virus can readily be demonstrated by fluorescent antibody techniques and electron microscopy within these cells. A moderate infiltration of lymphocytes and plasma cells accompanies the degenerative changes.

Diagnosis.—The diagnosis of rabies can be based upon the symptoms if they are typical, but should be confirmed by laboratory examination. Demonstration of typical Negri bodies is considered diagnostic; however, the brains of as many as 30 per cent of infected animals may not contain demonstrable Negri bodies. In cases in which Negri bodies cannot be demonstrated, animal (mouse) inoculations should be done. Mice injected intracerebrally with a 10 per cent suspension of infected brain tissue will die within six to twenty-one days. Identification of infection in mice is accomplished by demonstration of Negri bodies or by neutralization tests with immune serum. The former is the more common practice. Microscopic lesions in the gasserian ganglia may also be useful in diagnosis, but this method is not widely used at present.

The fluorescent antibody technique is very useful in specific identification of rabies inclusion bodies. In this method, specific anti-rabic serum is conjugated with a fluorescent dye and used to treat suspected impressions or other cell preparations. The Negri body absorbs the labeled antibody in the anti-rabic serum which clings to and identifies the Negri body as it fluoresces typically under ultraviolet light. With suitable controls, this method is quite specific in identification of Negri bodies or more specifically, antigens of rabies virus, even when Negri bodies cannot be demonstrated by conventional staining techniques.

The mouse inoculation test and the fluorescent antibody technique which are almost equally sensitive are much more sensitive than the examination for Negri bodies. It should be stressed, however, that no test is completely reliable.

In those animals in which rabies is suspected but cannot be demonstrated, an attempt should be made to determine the cause of death or cause of encephalitis. Diseases to consider are canine hepatitis, toxoplasmosis, distemper in dogs, *Oestrus ovis* infestation in sheep, and listeriosis in sheep and cattle. The brain, spinal cord or meninges may also be involved by diseases of unknown etiology. Differentiation of canine hepatitis and canine distemper are of considerable importance, since inclusion bodies may occur in both of these diseases. Both are also much more common in dogs than is rabies. In canine hepatitis involving the brain, intranuclear inclusions are found in endothelial cells in association with rupture of capillary walls and microscopic hemorrhages. The inclusions of canine distemper, further described on page 441, are most readily demonstrable in glial cells, particularly in the nuclei of gemistocytic astrocytes and microglia. Fluorescence antibody techniques show that distemper inclusions occur in neurons but they are less readily demonstrable with other methods. Cytoplasmic inclusions are less frequently found in the brain in canine distemper (p. 445).

Groups of tiny spherical bodies without a definite limiting membrane are encountered in the cytoplasm of neurons of nonrabid animals. Since at one time these were thought to be associated with rabies, they were given the name "Lyssa bodies." It now seems clear that they are not specific for rabies. They have been described in the dog, cat, skunk, fox, and laboratory white mouse. Although they can be easily confused with Negri bodies they lack an internal structure, are more acidophilic and are highly refractile. In the brains of normal cats, other cytoplasmic inclusions with tinctorial characteristics essentially the same as those of Negri bodies have been described. These feline inclusions cannot be differentiated morphologically from Negri bodies; therefore, it may be necessary to resort to animal inoculation or fluorescent antibody techniques when rabies is suspected in the cat.

Rabies

BEAUREGARD, M., BOULANGER, P., and WEBSTER, W. A.: The Use of Fluorescent Antibody Staining in the Diagnosis of Rabies. Can. J. Comp. Med. 29:141–147, 1965.
BURNS, K. F., SHELTON, D. F., and GROGAN, E. W.: Bat Rabies: Experimental Host Transmission. Ann. New York Acad. Sci. 70:452–466, 1958.
COVELL, W. P., and DANKS, W. B. C.: Studies on the Nature of the Negri Body. Am. J. Path. 8:557–571, 1932.
DIERKS, R. E., MURPHY, F. A., and HARRISON, A. K.: Extraneural Rabies Virus Infection. Virus Development in Fox Salivary Gland. Am. J. Path. 54:251–273, 1969.
DUPLESSIS, J. L.: The Topographical Distribution of Negri Bodies in the Brain. J. S. Afr. Vet. Med. Assn. 36:203–207, 1965.
ENRIGHT, J. B.: Bats and Their Relation to Rabies. Ann. Rev. Microbiol. 10:369–392, 1956.
GOODPASTURE, E. W.: Studies of Rabies with Reference to Neural Transmission of Virus in Rabbits and Structure and Significance of Negri Bodies. Am. J. Path. 1:547–582, 1925.
HERZOG, E.: Histologic Diagnosis of Rabies. Arch. Path. 39:279–280, 1945.
HOTTLE, G. A., et al.: Electron Microscopy of Rabies Inclusion (Negri) Bodies. Proc. Soc. Exp. Biol., N.Y. 77:721–723, 1951.
JENSON, A. B., et al.: A Comparative Light and Electron Microscopic Study of Rabies and Hart Park Virus Encephalitis. Expl. Molec. Path. 7:1–10, 1967.
LAPI, A., DAVIS, C. L., and ANDERSON, W. A.: The Gasserian Ganglion in Animals Dead of Rabies. J. Am. Vet. Med. Assn. 120:379–384, 1952.
MATSUMOTO, S.: Electron Microscope Studies of Rabies Virus in Mouse Brain. J. Cell. Biol. 19:565–591, 1963.
McQUEEN, J. L.: Rabies Diagnosis. Special Application of Fluorescent Antibody Techniques. Proc. 63rd Meet. U.S. Livestock Sanit. Assn. San Francisco. 1959. pp. 356–373.
MITCHELL, F. E., and MONLUX, W. S.: Diagnosis and Incidence of Rabies in a Selected Group of Domestic Cats. Am. J. Vet. Res. 23:435–442, 1962.
MOULTON, J. E.: A Histochemical Study of the Negri Bodies of Rabies. Am. J. Path. 30:533–543, 1954.
NEGRI, A.: Beitrag zum Studium der Aetiologie der Tollwuth. Ztschr. f. Hyg. u. Infektionskr. 43:507–528, 1903.
NINOMIYA, S.: Histopathologic Studies on Salivary Glands of Rabid Dogs with Special Reference to Parotid and Mandibular Glands. Appendix: On Cervical Lymph Nodes. Gumma J. Med. Sci. Japan 4:117–127, 1955.
SCHINDLER, R.: Studies on the Pathogenesis of Rabies. Bul. World Health Org. 25:119–126, 1961. V.B. 1091–62.
SZLOCHTA, H. L., and HABEL, R. E.: Inclusions Resembling Negri Bodies in the Brains of Nonrabid Cats. Cornell Vet. 43:207–212, 1953.
THOMPSON, S. W., et al.: The Protein Nature of the Matrices of Negri Bodies. Am. J. Vet. Res. 21:636–643, 1960.
TIERKEL, E. S.: Rabies. Adv. Vet. Sci. 5:183–226, 1959.
VONMICKWITZ, C. V.: Einschlusskorperchen in den Ganglienzellen des Ammonshornes und des Thalamus von Hausund Zookatzen. Path. Vet. 3:569–587, 1966.
WEBSTER, L. T.: *Rabies*. New York, The Macmillan Co., 1942.

Equine Encephalomyelitis

A widespread disease of the central nervous system of horses was recognized in the United States as early as 1912 and was known to be the cause of serious losses, particularly in the central part of the country, during the 1920's and 1930's. The disease was variously known as "forage poisoning," "cerebral spinal meningitis," "staggers," "Borna disease," botulism, and "Kansas horse plague."

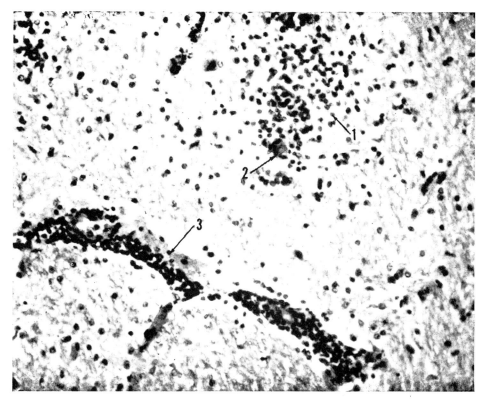

Fig. 10–4.—Equine encephalomyelitis (western strain) cerebrum of a horse (× 280). A nodule of lymphoid cells (*1*) adjacent to a neuron undergoing phagocytosis (*2*). Lymphocytes (*3*) in the wall of a blood vessel and the Robin-Virchow space. (Courtesy of Armed Forces Institute of Pathology.) Contributor: Dr. L. T. Giltner.

During the summer of 1930 a virus was isolated from a horse with symptoms indicating involvement of the central nervous system by Meyer, Haring and Howitt (1931), who suggested adoption of the name "equine encephalomyelitis" originally proposed by Stange (1948). This important discovery was the fore-runner of many significant advances in the understanding and control of viral encephalitis in many species, including man. The virus isolated by Meyer and colleagues is now known as the "western" strain of equine encephalomyelitis virus to distinguish it from an antigenically different virus isolated from horses in the eastern part of the United States, the "eastern" strain. A third strain of virus producing similar symptoms and lesions was isolated by Kubes and Rios (1939), Beck and Wyckoff (1938) from animals in Venezuela and is known as the "Venezuelan" strain. The Western strain occurs throughout most of the United States west of the Mississippi but also has been recognized in several states along the Eastern Seaboard and in Central and South America. In contrast, the Eastern strain is principally limited to the Eastern Seaboard. The Venezuelan strain occurs in several South American countries, Panama, Trinidad and Mexico. It also exists in Florida and in 1971 a serious epizootic occurred in Mexico and Texas.

The demonstration by Kelser, in 1933, that mosquitoes may serve as vectors of the virus of equine encephalomyelitis provided an explanation for many of its epizoötiologic features and was followed by the discovery that the equine encephalomyelitis viruses are infective for large numbers of animals, including man. It is now apparent that birds and reptiles serve as the main reservoirs for the virus and that mosquitoes are the principal vectors. The prime vectors for the Western and Eastern strains are *Culex tarsalis* and *Culiseta melanura* respectively; however other mosquitoes may also transmit the disease. *Aedes taeniorhynchus* is known to be an important vector of the Venezuelan strain. The infection in most avian species is asymptomatic, however in certain birds such as the ring-neck pheasant, clinical disease with high mortality can occur. Owing to mosquito transmission, the disease is seasonal with its greatest incidence in summer and fall, ending abruptly with the first killing frost.

Even though equine encephalomyelitis is an important disease in horses and man, infection of these species is rather incidental to the perpetuation of the virus in that viremia is generally not adequate to infect mosquitoes. Since the symptoms and lesions caused by the three strains of virus are essentially the same, they will be considered together.

Signs.—The symptoms, referable to derangement of the central nervous system, usually appear suddenly after an incubation period of one to three weeks. Affected animals lose awareness of their surroundings and wander about aimlessly, walk continuously in circles, are unresponsive to commands, and may collide with objects or crash through fences. High fever often occurs at the outset, but in some cases the body temperature has returned to normal by the time nervous symptoms appear. As the disease advances, stupor is evident and paralysis of various groups of muscles sets in. This flaccid paralysis increases rapidly, the animal lies down, is unable to regain its footing and soon succumbs. It is estimated approximately 50 per cent of horses infected with the western strain of virus die; with the eastern strain, this figure reaches 90 per cent.

Lesions.—There is no gross lesion that may be considered characteristic of this disease. The viruses of equine encephalomyelitis attack neurons, hence the lesions are principally referable to damage of these cells. Affected neurons undergo various degenerative changes, culminating in necrosis. These changes are manifest by dissolution and loss of tigroid substance (tigrolysis) and chromatin (chromatolysis), fragmentation of the cell and its removal by phagocytes (neuronophagia). This process attracts leukocytes and glial cells, which form small nodules around the injured neuron; such nodules may persist after all traces of the nerve cell are gone. The gray matter around affected neurons may also become edematous and diffusely infiltrated with lymphocytes, neutrophils and small numbers of erythrocytes. Lymphocytes escaping from nearby arterioles are often trapped in the Virchow-Robin space (p. 357) to form a wide collar of densely packed cells around the blood vessel. This "perivascular cuffing" may extend into the white matter where it is the only significant change. Perivascular cuffing is a striking microscopic finding, but it is not specific for equine encephalomyelitis; it occurs in numerous inflammatory lesions of the central nervous system.

Small intranuclear acidophilic inclusion bodies in neurons have been described by Hurst (1934) in western equine encephalomyelitis of horses and laboratory animals, but because similar bodies have been demonstrated to occur in other viral diseases, it is doubted that they can be considered pathognomonic.

The distribution of the lesions in the central nervous system varies, depending somewhat on the strain of virus. With the eastern strain, the gray masses are diffusely involved, the lesions are numerous and neutrophils are often a prominent component of the exudate. The presence of these neutrophils appears to be the result of the severity of the infection and the short fatal course of the disease, thus is not absolutely diagnostic of the eastern type. Infection with any strain of virus may result in lesions in the gray matter of the cerebral or cerebellar cortex, but they are most numerous in the olfactory bulbs, thalamus, hypothalamus, brain stem and in both dorsal and ventral gray columns of the spinal cord. The gasserian and other ganglia may contain increased numbers of mononuclear cells.

In certain laboratory animals (rabbits, guinea pigs, mice) which have been experimentally infected, there is a tendency toward massive necrosis of certain olfactory centers (rhinencephalic cortex ventral to *fissura rhinica* and *cornu Ammonis*); however, other viruses may also affect these species in a like manner. A fatal encephalitis is produced by these viruses in man with lesions comparable to those of the equine disease. Neutrophils are a much less prominent component of the exudate when the western rather than the eastern strain of virus is the etiologic agent involved. Western equine encephalomyelitis in man produces widely disseminated lesions which are especially numerous in the putamen and caudate nuclei; fewer are found in the cerebral cortex and spinal cord.

Diagnosis.—A presumptive diagnosis may be made upon the finding of the above described microscopic lesions diffusely distributed through the gray matter of the central nervous system. A confirmed diagnosis can be made only on the basis of isolation and identification of the virus.

Equine Encephalomyelitis

ANONYMOUS: Editorial note. J. Am. Vet. Med. Assn. *113*:464, 1948.

BAKER, A. B., and NORAN, H. H.: Western Variety of Equine Encephalitis in Man. Arch. Neurol. & Psychiat. *47*:565–587, 1942.

BECK, C. E., and WYCKOFF, R. W. G.: Antigenic Stability of Western Equine Encephalomyelitis Virus. Science *88*:264, 1938.

CHAMBERLAIN, R. W.: Vector Relationships of the Arthropod Borne Encephalitides in North America. Ann. New York Acad. Sci. *70*:312–319, 1958.

EHRENKRANZ, N. J., *et al.*: The Natural Occurrence of Venezuelan Equine Encephalitis in the United States. New Eng. J. Med. *282*:298–302, 1970.

FOTHERGILL, L. D., DINGLE, J. H., FARBER, S., and CONNERLEY, M. L.: Human Encephalitis Caused by Virus of Eastern Variety of Equine Encephalomyelitis. New England J. Med. *291*:411, 1938.

GLEISER, C. A. *et al.*: The Comparative Pathology of Experimental Venezuelan Equine Encephalomyelitis Infection in Different Animal Hosts. J. Infect. Dis. *110*:80–97, 1962. VB 2271–62.

HARING, C. M., HOWARTH, J. A., and MEYER, K. F.: Infectious Brain Disease of Horses and Mules. North Am. Vet. *12*:29–36, 1931.

HESS, A. D, and HOLDEN, P.: The Natural History of the Arthropod-Borne Encephalitides in the United States. Ann. New York Acad. Sci. *70*:294–311, 1958.

HURST, E. W.: The Histology of Equine Encephalomyelitis. J. Exper. Med. *59*:529–542, 1934.

JENNINGS, W. L., ALLEN, R. H., and LEWIS, A. L.: Western Equine Encephalomyelitis in a Florida Horse. Am. J. Trop. Med. *15*:96–97, 1966.

KELSER, R. A.: Mosquitoes as Vectors of the Virus of Equine Encephalomyelitis. J. Am. Vet. Med. Assn. *82*:767–771, 1933.

KING, L. S.: Studies on Eastern Encephalomyelitis; Histopathology in the Mouse. J. Exper. Med. *71*:107–112, 1940.

KISSLING, R. E.: Host Relationship of the Arthropod-Borne Encephalitides. Ann. New York Acad. Sci. *70*:320–326, 1958.

KUBES, V., and RIOS, F. A.: Causative Agent of Infectious Equine Encephalomyelitis in Venezuela. Science *90*:20–21, 1939.

MEYER, K. F., HARING, C. M., and HOWITT, B.: The Etiology of Epizoötic Encephalo-myelitis of Horses in the San Joaquin Valley, 1930. Science *74*:227–228, 1931.

MEYER, K. F.: Summary of Recent Studies in Equine Encephalomyelitis. Ann. Int. Med. *6*:645–654, 1932.

PEERS, J. H.: Equine Encephalomyelitis (Western) in Man. Arch. Path. *34*:1050–1064, 1942.

TEN BROECK, C., and MERRILL, M. H.: Serological Differences Between Eastern and West-ern Equine Encephalomyelitis Virus. Proc. Soc. Exper. Biol. & Med. *31*:217–220, 1933.

WEIL, A., and BRESLICH, P. J.: Histopathology of the Central Nervous System in the North Dakota Epidemic Encephalitis. J. Neuropath. and Exper. Neurol. *1*:49–58, 1942.

WOLF, A., and ORTON, S. T.: The Occurrence of Intranuclear Inclusions in Human Nerve Cells in a Variety of Diseases. Bull. Neurol. Inst., New York, *2*:194–209, 1932.

Encephalomyelitides of Swine

Certain viral agents have an affinity for the central nervous system of swine and cause diseases of some importance in this species. The virus of hog cholera (p. 455) for example, may upon occasion attack the cells of the central nervous system. The lesions resulting from the presence of hog cholera virus may be distinguished with reasonable certainty by histologic methods utilizing that virus' affinity for the vasculature. *Herpesvirus suis* (Pseudorabies, p. 369) is highly neurotropic producing encephalitis in piglets and other domestic animals. The lesions in pseudorabies are distinguished by the presence of intranuclear inclusion bodies. Japanese B encephalitis (p. 379) also affects pigs. Other viruses which have an even more selective affinity for the nervous system of swine have been recognized during the past few years. The first of these is called Teschen Disease, so named from the province of Czechoslovakia where the first outbreak was identified. Several outbreaks of porcine diseases with similar clinical features and histo-pathologic effects upon the central nervous system have been described subse-quently from widely scattered parts of the world. These diseases have received various local names and have been studied with some intensity. Of particular importance is the development of evidence that similar viral agents are involved in each of these diseases. New techniques which have been utilized to study these viral agents and to compare one with another indicate that each is caused by a variant strain of Teschen disease virus. Each of these disease conditions will be described briefly, comparisons made and the present evidence outlined concerning their probable relationship to one another. Another encephalitis of piglets has been described in Canada and Japan which is caused by a hemagglutinating virus that is not related to the Teschen group. This is also briefly described.

Teschen Disease

Teschen disease is also known as encephalomyelitis or poliomyelitis of swine, Bohemian pest and meningo-encephalomyelitis suum. This disease occurs in many countries of central and western Europe, but is not clearly recognized in the Western Hemisphere. It is caused by a filtrable virus approximately 25 to 30 mμ in diameter and classified in the picornavirus group. This virus is found in the central nervous system of infected pigs, at times in feces, transiently in the blood, and rarely in other tissues or excretions. The disease is limited to swine and morbidity and mortality are both high in this species. This disease is similar to poliomyelitis of man in that the virus may be isolated from the intestinal tract, and the ventral columns of gray matter in the spinal cord are rather constantly affected. However, in the porcine disease the lesions in the cerebral cortex and cerebellum are much more extensive and indiscriminately located than in polio-myelitis. No immunologic relationship of the viruses of the two diseases has been demonstrated.

Pathogenesis.—Following oral infection, the virus first invades and replicates in lymphatic tissue and epithelium of the colon without leading to observable lesions in these tissues. Viremia follows, which allows spread of the virus to the central nervous system through the blood stream. In the brain and cord the virus invades and replicates in neurons, glia, and capillary endothelial cells.

Signs.—Following an incubation period of ten to twenty days, the onset is usually accompanied by fever (104° to 105° F.), anorexia, lassitude, depression and sometimes slight incoordination, particularly of the rear limbs. These symptoms are followed within a few hours or, at most, one to three days, by a stage of irritability and by stiffness of the extremities, and in severe cases by tremors, nystagmus, violent clonic convulsions, prostration and coma. Convul-sions accompanied by loud squealing can be set off by a stimulus, such as a sudden noise. Stiffness and opisthotonus are the most persistent symptoms in some cases. Sudden drop in temperature followed by paralysis and death three or four days after onset is the usual course, although some animals die within twenty-four hours. Others survive but are left with a flaccid posterior paralysis. Usually, if held up on their feet, these swine will eat ravenously and can, in fact, be kept alive for long periods.

Swine of all ages are affected during epizootics, but once the disease is endemic, clinical disease is limited to newborn pigs and newly introduced pigs.

Lesions.—No gross lesions specific for Teschen disease have been demonstrated in animals succumbing to this infection. Microscopic lesions are limited to the central nervous system. The virus attacks neurons of brain and cord, producing changes referable to the destruction of these nerve cells. The lesions have a spe-cific distribution, a point which can be utilized to some extent in differential diagnosis. The spinal cord is constantly affected, the changes being principally limited to the ventral columns of the gray matter. The cerebellum also suffers rather intensely, the Purkinje, molecular and granular layers being involved in that order of decreasing severity. In some cases, the leptomeninges over the cerebellum are heavily infiltrated with lymphocytes. The thalamus also sustains considerable damage, and lesions of decreasing intensity occur in the basal nuclei, the base of the brain generally, olfactory bulbs, hippocampal gyrus, and the pons and medulla. The motor cortex, although more vulnerable than the rest of the cerebral cortex, is not a site of predilection.

In affected sites, multipolar nerve cells show degeneration of varying degree up to and including necrosis, accompanied by neuronophagia, inflammatory or glial nodules, occasional hemorrhage and rather diffuse infiltration of leukocytes, predominantly lymphocytes. Rarely are neutrophils a part of the exudate in this disease. Accumulations of lymphocytes in the perivascular (Robin-Virchow) spaces are often seen. They are usually adjacent to lesions in the gray matter and may extend into the white matter; otherwise the white matter is not involved.

Koestner (1966) has demonstrated that the earliest lesion in neurons was detachment of ribosomes from endoplasmic reticulum and disappearance of ribo-somal clusters followed by dilation of endoplasmic reticulum, and vesiculation.

Diagnosis.—The demonstration of typical microscopic lesions in the brain and

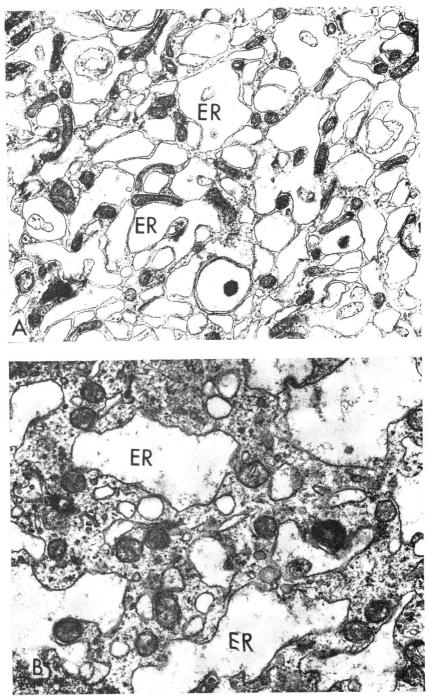

Fig. 10–5. Teschen Disease of swine (Porcine polioencephalomyelitis). *A*, Extensive vesiculation of neuronal endoplasmic reticulum cisternae (ER). ($\times$ 23,700). *B*, Higher magnification of the dilated endoplasmic reticulum cisternae (ER). Mitochondria are compressed ($\times$ 35,000). (Courtesy Dr. A. Koestner and American Journal of Pathology.)

Poliomyelitis of Mice

BODIAN, D., and HOWE, H. A.: The Significance of Lesions in Peripheral Ganglia in Chimpanzee and in Human Poliomyelitis. J. Exper. Med. *85*:231–241, 1947.

BODIAN, D.: Histopathological Basis of Clinic Findings in Poliomyelitis. Am. J. Med. *6*:563–578, 1949.

DANIELS, J. B., PAPPENHEIMER, A. M., and RICHARDSON, S.: Observations on Encephalomyelitis of Mice, DA Strain. J. Exper. Med. *96*:517–530, 1952.

OLITSKY, P. K.: Further Studies of the Agent in Intestines of Normal Mice Which Induces Encephalomyelitis. Proc. Soc. Exper. Biol. & Med. *43*:296–300, 1940.

——————: A Transmissible Agent (Theiler's Virus) in the Intestines of Normal Mice. J. Exper. Med. *72*:113–127, 1940.

OLITSKY, P. K., and SCHLESINGER, R. W.: Histopathology of CNS of Mice Infected with Virus of Theiler's Disease (Spontaneous Encephalomyelitis). Proc. Soc. Exper. Biol. & Med. *47*:79–83, 1941.

THEILER, M.: Spontaneous Encephalomyelitis of Mice—A New Virus Disease. Science *80*:122, 1934.

——————: Spontaneous Encephalomyelitis of Mice. J. Exper. Med. *65*:705–719, 1937.

THEILER, M., and GARD, S.: Encephalomyelitis of Mice. J. Exper. Med. *72*:49–67, 1940.

——————: Epidemiology of Mouse Encephalomyelitis. J. Exper. Med. *72*:79–90, 1940.

Pseudorabies

(Infectious Bulbar Paralysis, Aujeszky's Disease, Mad Itch)

Pseudorabies, a disease to which many species are susceptible, is caused by a virus of the herpes group termed *Herpesvirus suis*. The disease was first described by Aujeszky (1902) in Hungary, but is now kno wn to occur in many parts of the world, including the United States. Natural ¹nfection occurs in swine, cattle, dogs, cats, sheep, rats and mink, but is of greatest importance in cattle in which the disease is nearly always fatal. The infection is similar with respect to epizootiology, clinical signs and pathological changes to certain other herpesvirus infections such as *Herpesvirus B* (p. 380), and *Herpesvirus simplex* (p. 383).

Epizoötiology and Signs.—Swine and probably rats serve as the natural and reservoir hosts for *H. suis*. Swine are very susceptible to infection but adult animals rarely exhibit symptoms or die from the disease. In adult swine a mild febrile, nonfatal disease may occur but recovery is the rule. In piglets the infection is more severe, occurring as an acute illness which may lead to death in twenty-four to forty-eight hours without specific clinical signs. Piglets over four weeks of age may show signs of involvement of the central nervous system, usually as incoordination of the hind quarters, tremors, convulsions and eventual paralysis. Although not usual, older pigs may develop encephalitis and die of the infection. Intrauterine infection can occur leading to abortion and stillbirth.

Young and adult swine may excrete the virus in the absence of clinical disease, a situation analogous to *Herpesvirus simplex* in man. This may represent activation of a latent infection. Swine with a subclinical infection, by nuzzling with their snout, may transmit the disease to cattle. Sheep are susceptible to experimental exposure to the virus by scarification of the skin, subcutaneous injection and installation into nasal passages, oral cavity or conjunctival sac. The disease also occurs naturally among sheep which are housed with pigs, and it is transmitted by the nuzzling pigs in much the same manner that they convey the virus to cattle. Intense itching develops in the skin of the bovine at the point of contact after about fifty hours. Frenzied scratching of this area by the animal causes ulceration of the skin and secondary infection ensues. Paralysis may develop, and

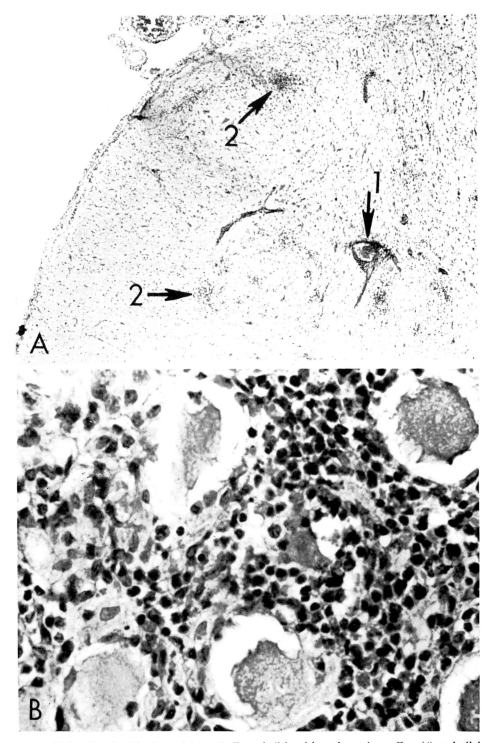

Fig. 10-7.—Pseudorabies in a piglet. *A*, Encephalitis with perivascular cuffing (*1*) and glial nodules (*2*). *B*, Semilunar ganglioneuritis with ganglion cell necrosis, capsule cell proliferation and a pleomorphic cellular infiltrate. (Courtesy Dr. H. J. Olander.)

cattle may die rather suddenly with indications of bulbar involvement. Rabbits are particularly susceptible to artificial exposure to this disease; guinea pigs are somewhat less so. Monkeys are also readily infected by experimental means. The virus may be transmitted through the abraded skin simply by rubbing the nose of an infected rabbit against it.

Lesions.—Following natural or experimental inoculation, *Herpesvirus suis* reaches the central nervous system by traveling up nerve fibers. Lesions occur in the nerve fibers, ganglia, and central nervous system in all species; their extent and distribution depending on the site of inoculation and duration of the illness. In general, central lesions are most extensive in the spinal ganglia, temporal cerebral cortex, and basal ganglia of the brain.

Local irritation and necrosis occur at the site of subcutaneous inoculation of **rabbits** and involve both fascia and musculature. The virus reaches the spinal ganglia, first affecting those on the side of the body where the inoculation was given. The lesions in the ganglia, which are believed to be the cause of the intense pruritus, consist of degeneration of neurons and proliferation of capsule cells and other glial cells. Intracranial inoculation of the rabbit is followed by lymphocytic proliferation in the meninges, proliferation of the subpial glia and necrosis of superficially placed nerve cells. Intranuclear inclusions are observed in cells of all embryonic layers: nerve cells, glia, capillary endothelium, sarcolemmal cells and Schwann cells. These inclusions, when stained by phloxine—methylene blue, reveal aggregations of coarse, pale pink granules or irregular, deeper pink granules. In the rabbit, death usually occurs as soon as the virus reaches the medulla and before microscopic lesions are visible at this site. Respiratory failure resulting from involvement of the medulla oblongata appears to be the cause of death. This may be true in other species as well.

In the **guinea pig,** the lesions are quite similar to those in the rabbit, although the guinea pig is somewhat more resistant to experimental infection. In the **monkey,** after intracerebral inoculation, degeneration and necrosis of cortical nerve cells are widespread, with intranuclear inclusions occurring in nerve and glial cells but not in mesodermal cells. No lesions are found in viscera.

In the **bovine** and **ovine,** the spontaneous disease resembles the experimental disease in the monkey. Moderate perivascular infiltration of lymphocytes and some foci of microglial proliferation are seen in the central nervous system, but most nerve cells are normal or exhibit only mild chromatolysis. A few inclusions are found.

In **swine,** the lesions in the central nervous system may be very mild or unrecognizable. There are vascular, perivascular and interstitial lesions with very slight nerve cell degeneration. Inclusion bodies are present but may be few in number. In addition to invasion of the nervous system, lesions are often present in other organs and tissues. Focal necrosis of pharyngeal mucosa, tonsils, lymph nodes, lungs, liver and adrenal cortex associated with intranuclear inclusion bodies in both epithelial and mesenchymal cells are frequently encountered. Invasion of tissues outside the nervous system is unusual in other species, although adrenal cortical necrosis with inclusion bodies has been reported in experimental pseudorabies in sheep.

Diagnosis.—Pseudorabies may be suspected in disease outbreaks in which animals die shortly after showing very severe pruritus limited to a segment of the skin. Cattle or sheep in which the disease appears are almost always closely

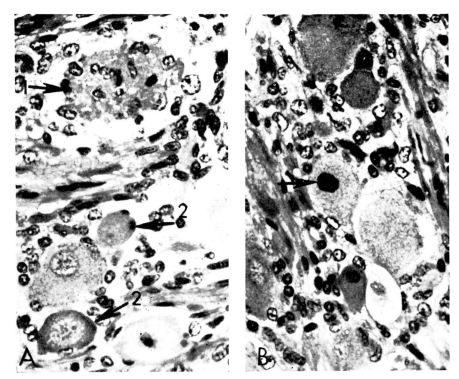

Fig. 10-8.—Pseudorabies in a lamb. *A*, Dorsal root ganglioneuritis with a neuronophagic nodule (*1*) and neuron necrosis (*2*). *B*, A neuron containing an intranuclear inclusion body. (Tissue courtesy Dr. R. M. McCraken and Dr. C. Dow.)

associated with swine or with wild rats. The microscopic lesions in the skin and the spinal ganglia are of some presumptive significance, but the final diagnosis of pseudorabies is dependent upon reproduction of the disease in experimental animals. This is most readily accomplished by the subcutaneous injection of rabbits with suspensions of nervous tissue from diseased animals. These rabbits will show intense, frenzied itching, with characteristic local inflammation of the skin; death is due to respiratory failure, and the chief pathological manifestations are necrotic changes in ganglion cells.

Pseudorabies

Aujeszky, A.: Über eine Neue Infektionskrankheit bei Haustiere. Zentralbl. f. Bakt., pt. 1, (Orig.), *32*:353–357, 1902.

Bergmann, B., and Becker, C.-H.: Studies on the Pathomorphology and Pathogenesis of Aujeszky's Disease. I. Histopathology of the Spinal Ganglia, Spinal Nerve Roots and Spinal Cord of Guinea Pigs After Experimental Infection. Path. Vet. *4*:97–119, 1967.

Boyse, E. A., *et al.*: The Spread of a Neurotropic Strain of Herpes Virus Into the Cerebrospinal Axis of Rabbits. Brit. J. Exp. Path. *37*:333–342, 1956.

Cernovsky, J.: Histopathology of the Central Nervous System in Aujeszky's Disease. Veterinářství *15*:176–178, 1965.

Corner, A. H.: Pathology of Experimental Aujeszky's Disease in Piglets. Res. Vet. Sci. *6*:337–343, 1965.

Csontos, L., and Szeky, A.: Gross and Microscopic Lesions in the Nasopharynx of Pigs with Aujeszky's Disease. Acta Vet. Hung. *16*:175–186, 1966.

Dow, C. and McFerran, J. B.: Experimental Aujeszky's Disease in Sheep. Am. J. Vet. Res. *25*:461–468, 1964.

————————: The Neuropathology of Aujeszky's Disease in the Pig. Res. in Vet. Sci. *3*:436–442, 1962. VB 504–63.

————————: The Pathology of Aujeszky's Disease in Cattle. J. Comp. Path. *72*:337–347, 1962. VB 827–63.

————————: Aujeszky's Disease in the Dog and Cat. Vet. Rec. *75*:1099–1101 and 1102, 1963. VB 1288–64.

————————: Experimental Studies on Aujeszky's Disease in Cattle. J. Comp. Path. *76*: 379–385, 1966.

————————: Experimental Studies on Aujeszky's Disease in Sheep. Brit. Vet J. *122*: 464–470, 1966.

FRASER, G., and RAMACHANDRAN, S. P.: Studies on the Virus of Aujeszky's Disease. I. Pathogenicity for Rats and Mice. J. Comp. Path. *79*:435–444, 1969.

GOTO, H., GORHAM, J. R., and HAGEN, K. W.: Clinical Observation of Experimental Pseudorabies in Mink and Ferrets. Jap. J. Vet. Sci. *30*:257–264, 1968.

HANSON, R. P.: The History of Pseudorabies in the United States. J. Am. Vet. Med. Assn. *124*:259–261, 1954.

HOWARTH, J. A., and DePAOLI, A.: An Enzootic of Pseudorabies in Swine in California. J. Am. Vet. Med. Assn. *152*:1114–1118, 1968.

HUCK, R. A., et al.: The Isolation of Aujeszky's Disease Virus From Dogs. Vet. Rec. *84*: 232, 1969.

HURST, E. W.: Studies on Pseudorabies. I. Histology of the Disease, with a Note on the Symptomatology. J. Exper. Med. *58*:415–433, 1933.

————————: Studies on Pseudorabies (Infectious Bulbar Paralysis—Mad Itch). II. Routes of Infection in the Rabbit, with Remarks on the Relation of the Virus to other Viruses Affecting the Nervous System. J. Exper. Med. *59*:729–749, 1934.

KAPLAN, A. S.: Herpes Simplex and Pseudorabies Viruses. Virology Monographs *5*:1–115, 1969.

KNOSEL, H.: Zur Kistopathologie der Aujeszky's Chen Krankheit bei Hund und Katze. Zenbtl. Vet. Med. *15B*:592–598, 1968.

————————: Histopathology of Aujeszky's Disease in Pigs. Deutsch tierarztl. Wschr. *72*: 279–282, 1965.

KOJNOK, J.: The Role of Carrier Sows in the Spreading of Aujeszky's Virus Carriership Among Fattening Pigs. Acta Vet. Hung. *15*:282–295, 1965.

————————: The Role of Pigs in the Spreading of Aujeszky's Disease among Sheep and Cattle. Acad. Sci. Hung. *12*:53–58, 1962.

LUCAS, A., METIANU, T., and ATANASIU, P.: Maladie D'Aujeszky Chez Le Chien en France. Annls. Inst. Pasteur, Paris *110*:130–135, 1966.

OLANDER, H. J., et al.: Pathologic Findings in Swine Affected With a Virulent Strain of Aujeszky's Virus. Pathologia Vet. *3*:64–82, 1966.

SHAHAN, M. S., KNUDSON, R. L., SEIBOLD, H. R., and DALE, C. N.: Aujeszky's Disease (Pseudorabies); A Review with Notes on Two Strains of the Virus. North Am. Vet. *28*: 440–449, 511–521, 1947.

SHOPE, R. E.: Experiments on the Epidemiology of Pseudorabies. I. Mode of Transmission of the Disease in Swine and Their Possible Role in its Spread to Cattle. J. Exper. Med. *62*: 85–99, 1935.

————————: Experiments on the Epidemiology of Pseudorabies. II. Prevalence of the Disease among Middle Western Swine and the Possible Role of Rats in Herd-to-Herd Infections. J. Exper. Med. *62*:101–117, 1935.

"Scrapie" of Sheep

"Scrapie" is the colloquial name of a disease of sheep and rarely goats, derived from the principal clinical manifestation which is almost continuous "scraping" of the skin against any reasonably stationary object as a result of the intense pruritus the animal suffers. The disease has been known in Scotland for at least two centuries, but has spread to Canada and the United States only in recent years. Present evidence indicates that the etiologic agent is a filtrable virus that can be experimentally transmitted by intracerebral passage of suspensions of medulla and spinal cord of affected animals. The virus which has not been seen with the electron microscope is unique in that it is resistant to heat, treatment with ether, acetone, formaldehyde, ribonuclease and deoxyribonuclease, and exposure to ionizing and ultraviolet radiation. These unusual properties suggest that the virus does not contain nucleic acid and is not dependent on a nucleic acid for its ability to replicate. These features clearly set the scrapie virus aside from other known infectious agents. It has been suggested that the transmissible agent is a small specific molecule (linkage substance) which combines with an incomplete DNA/polysaccharide subvirus or incomplete replicating factor which is always present in the susceptible recipient.

The disease appears to have a very prolonged incubation period, as much as one-and-one-half to five years in nature and from four to six months following intracerebral inoculation. The course of the disease is from two to twelve months. However, both the incubation period and course vary with the genotype of the sheep. Although certain individuals are resistant, the nature of the resistance is unknown. Mice, which are susceptible to experimental infection, are a useful laboratory animal. Many points remain obscure and further study of this interesting disease is needed. The disease "rida" in Iceland is probably the same as scrapie.

Signs.—The signs which appear in adult sheep are usually characterized at the outset by restlessness and a startled look, the eyes having a fixed and wild expression and the pupils being dilated. The sheep may hold its head down and wag it as if hunting a fly. Its movements are aimless and stiffness of the forelegs results in a trotting gait, a characteristic that gives the disease its German name, *Trabberkrankheit*. The animal usually grinds its teeth. Twitching, at first confined to the lips, soon involves the muscles of the shoulders and thighs as well. The voice may be altered. If startled, the animal may fall in an epileptiform seizure of rather brief duration. The skin irritation apparently starts in the lumbar region, then may involve the rest of the body surface. The intense pruritus causes the sheep to rub against objects rather continuously until the wool coat is almost completely lost. Scratching the back of an affected animal will cause it to grind its teeth and show a characteristic rapid twitching of the lips. Incoördination may be followed by paralysis and inability to stand, and finally the animal dies.

Lesions.—No characteristic gross lesion is found in this disease, the specific tissue alterations being limited to microscopic changes in the medulla oblongata, pons, midbrain and spinal cord. The most striking and diagnostic lesion is the presence of large vacuoles in the cytoplasm of neurons associated with rather diffuse astrogliosis and occasional accumulation of lymphocytes in the Virchow-Robin spaces. These lesions are most numerous in nuclei of the medulla and are not found in the cerebral cortex or cerebellum. Sections taken just anterior to the calamus scriptorius are most likely to contain affected cells, therefore should be selected for microscopic examination aimed at establishing the diagnosis. The nuclear masses in the medulla most frequently involved are the reticular formation, medial vestibular and lateral cuneate nuclei. Vacuolated neurons are found less frequently in the hypoglossal nuclei, the inferior olive, and the gray columns of the spinal cord. The possibility that vacuolization of nerve cells might be an artefact has been considered, and some controversy exists on this point. It does appear, however, that the altered neurons containing vacuoles represent one quite constant microscopic alteration recognizable in this disease. In some cases PAS-positive plaques are found in the molecular and granular layers of the cerebellum. Neutral fat can sometimes be demonstrated in the white matter, but otherwise demyelination is not obvious. The exact distribution of the tissue changes and the correlation between them and the symptoms are yet to be established. In the experimental disease in sheep, goats and mice, in addition to the changes described there is widespread status spongiosus. Lesions in muscles have been reported in some studies but the possibility exists that these changes are the result of a concurrent disease. More evidence is needed on many such facets of this disease.

Diagnosis.—The diagnosis is based upon the clinical symptoms and is confirmed by histologic examination of the brain and spinal cord with particular emphasis on the medulla oblongata, pons and midbrain. Especial study should be given sections from that area of medulla immediately cranial to the calamus scriptorius.

Scrapie

ADAMS, D. H., and FIELD, E. J.: The Infective Process in Scrapie. Lancet *1*:714–716, 1968.
BERTRAND, I., CARRÉ, H., and LUCAM, F.: La tremblante du mouton. Rec. Méd. Vet. *113*:586–603, 1937.
————: La tremblante du mouton. Rec. Méd. Vet. *113*:540–561, 1937.
BROWNLEE, A.: Histopathological Studies of Scrapie, an Obscure Disease of Sheep. Brit. Vet. J. *96*:254–259, 1940.
CHANDLER, R. L.: Encephalopathy in Mice Produced by Inoculation With Scrapie Brain Material. Lancet *1*:1378, 1961.
DICKINSON, A. G., *et al.*: Some Factors Controlling the Incidence of Scrapie in Cheviot Sheep Injected with a Cheviot-Passaged Scrapie Agent. J. Comp. Path. *78*:313–321, 1968.
GAJDUSEK, D. C., GIBBS, C. J., and ALPERS, M. (Eds.): Slow, Latent, and Temperate Virus Infections. Nat. Inst. Neurological Diseases and Blindness Monographs, No. 2, 1965.
GAJDUSEK, D. C.: Slow-Virus Infections of the Nervous System. New Eng. J. Med. *276*: 392–400, 1967.
GIBBONS, R. A., and HUNTER, G. D.: Nature of the Scrapie Agent. Nature (London) *215*: 1041–1043, 1967.
GRIFFITH, J. S.: Self-Replication of Scrapie. Nature *215*:1043–1044, 1967.
HADLOW, W. J.: Scrapie and Kuru. Lancet, September 5, 1959, pp. 289–290.
————: The Pathology of Experimental Scrapie in the Dairy Goat. Res. Vet. Sci. *2*:289–314, 1961. VB 549–562.
HOLMAN, H. H., and PATTISON, I. H.: Further Evidence on the Significance of Vacuolated Nerve Cells in the Medulla Oblongata of Sheep Affected with Scrapie. J. Comp. Path. & Therap. *53*:231–236, 1940–1943.
MORRIS, J. A., and GAJDUSEK, D. C.: Encephalopathy in Mice Following Inoculation of Scrapie Sheep Brain. Nature (London) *197*:1084–1086, 1963.
MOULD, D. L. and SMITH, W.: The Causal Agent of Scrapie. I. Extraction of the Agent from Infected Sheep Tissue. II. From Infected Goat Tissue. J. Comp. Path. *72*:97–105 and 106–112, 1962.
PALMER, A. C.: Studies in scrapie. Vet. Rec. *69*:1318–1328, 1957.
PATTISON, I. H., and JONES, K. M.: The Possible Nature of the Transmissible Agent of Scrapie. Vet. Rec. *80*:2–9, 1967.
PATTISON, I. H., GORDON, W. S., and MILLSON, G. C.: Experimental Production of Scrapie in Goats. J. Comp. Path. *69*:300–312, 1959.
PERRY, H. B.,: SCRAPIE: A transmissible hereditary disease of sheep. Nature (Lond) *185*: 441–443, 1960.
STOCKMAN, S.: Contribution to the Study of the Disease Known as Scrapie. J. Comp. Path. & Therap. *39*:42–59, 1926.
WILSON, D. R., ANDERSON, R. D., and SMITH, W.: Studies in Scrapie. J. Comp. Path. & Therap. *60*:267–282, 1950.
WRIGHT, P. A. L.: The histopathology of the spinal cord in scrapie disease of sheep. J. Comp. Path. *70*:70–83, 1960.
ZLOTNICK, I.: The histopathology of the brain stem of sheep affected with experimental scrapie. J. Comp. Path. *68*:428–438, 1958.
————: The Histopathology of the Brain of Goats Affected with Scrapie. J. Comp. Path. *71*:440–448, 1961.

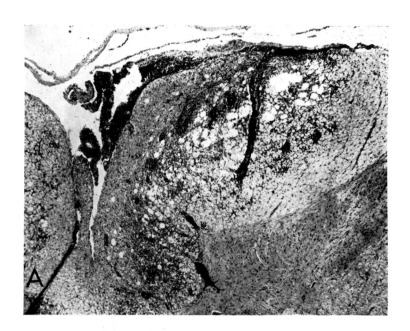

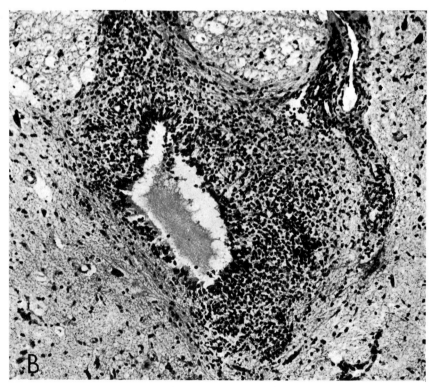

FIG. 10–9.—Visna. *A*, Leptomeningeal infiltrate, perivascular cuffing and microcavitation of lumbar spinal cord. *B*, Cellular infiltration surrounding central canal of cervical spinal cord. (Courtesy Dr. Páll A. Pálsson.)

VISNA

Visna is a chronic viral encephalomyelitis of sheep which was first reported in Iceland in 1935 by Sigurdsson, Thormar, and Palsson. The disease was eradicated in 1951 and has since been maintained as a laboratory infection of interest due to certain pathological similarities to multiple sclerosis of man. The causative virus is similar, or possibly identical to the agent of Maedi (p. 1116) a slow pulmonary infection of Icelandic sheep. The incubation period may be as long as two to three years.

Lesions.—A marked pleocytosis (increased number of cells in cerebrospinal fluid) appears prior to any detectable clinical signs; a distinguishing feature from scrapie in which pleocytosis does not occur. The first outward sign of the disease is paresis of the hind limbs which slowly progresses to total paraplegia and death over a course of several weeks to months. No characteristic gross change is present and microscopic lesions are limited to the central nervous system where the principal change is demyelination and destruction of paraventricular white matter of the cerebrum and cerebellum and focal demyelination of the spinal cord. There is an associated gliosis and sub-ependymal and perivascular lymphocytic infiltration. Mononuclear meningitis is usually present over both the brain and spinal cord.

Ressang *et al.* (1966) have reported a leucoencephalomyelitis in two sheep in the Netherlands which is pathologically similar to Visna. Both sheep were in the final stages of Zwoegerziekte (p. 1116) a pulmonary disease closely resembling Maedi.

Visna

RESSANG, A. A., STAM, F. C., and DeBOER, G. F.: A Meningo-leucoencephalomyelitis Resembling Visna in Dutch Zwoeger Sheep. Pathologia Vet. *3*:401–411, 1966.
SIGURDSSON, B., and PALSSON, P. A.: Visna of Sheep. A Slow Demyelinating Infection. Brit. J. Exp. Path. *39*:519–528, 1958.
SIGURDSSON, B., THORMAR, H., and PALSSON, P. A.: Cultivation of Visna Virus in Tissue Culture. Arch. ges. Virusforsch. *10*:368–381, 1960.
SIGURDSSON, B.: Observations on Three Slow Infections of Sheep, With General Remarks on Infections Which Develop Slowly and Some of Their Special Characteristics. Brit. Vet. J. *110*:341–354, 1954.
SIGURDSSON, B., PALSSON, P. A., and GRIMSSON, H.: Visna, A Demyelinating Transmissible Disease of Sheep. J. Neuropath. Exp. Neurol. *16*:389–403, 1957.
SIGURDSSON, B., PALSSON, P. A., and VAN BOGAERT, L.: Pathology of Visna (Transmissible Demyelinating Disease of Sheep in Iceland). Acta Neuropath. *1*:343–362, 1962.
THORMAR, H.: Physical, Chemical, and Biological Properties of Visna Virus and Its Relationship to Other Animal Viruses. Natl. Inst. of Neurological Diseases and Blindness Monograph No. *2*:335–340, 1965.

Mink Encephalopathy

Mink encephalopathy is a transmissible disease of mink which has been described in Wisconsin and Idaho. Although the transmissible agent has not been isolated, it is filterable and unusually resistant to heat, ether and formaldehyde, similar to the scrapie virus. The incubation period in the experimentally transmitted disease in mink is five to ten months. Ferrets and non-human primates can be experimentally infected.

The clinical signs are characterized by slowly progressive locomotor incoordination, excitability, late somnolence, and occasionally convulsions. Death follows a course of three to eight weeks. Lesions are restricted to the central nervous system where widespread neuronal degeneration and marked astrogliosis are found in the cerebrum, cerebellum, and brainstem. The gray matter may have a spongy appearance. Neurons, especially in the cerebellar peduncles, may contain cytoplasmic vacuoles similar to those seen in scrapie.

Mink Encephalopathy

BURGER, D., and HARTSOUGH, G. R.: Encephalopathy of Mink. II. Experimental and Natural Transmission. J. Infect. Dis. *115*:393–399, 1965.
————: Transmissible Encephalopathy of Mink. Nat. Inst. Neurol. Dis. and Blindness Monograph No. 2, 297–305, 1965.
ECKROADE, R. J., and ZU RHEIN, G. M.: Transmissible Mink Encephalopathy: Experimental Transmission to the Squirrel Monkey. Science *169*:1088–1090, 1970.
HARTSOUGH, G. R., and BURGER, D.: Encephalopathy of Mink. I. Epizoologic and Clinical Observations. J. Infect. Dis. *115*:387–392, 1965.
MARSH, R. F., *et al.*: A Preliminary Report on the Experimental Host Range of the Transmissible Mink Encephalopathic Agent. J. Infect. Dis. *120*:713–719, 1969.

Viral Encephalomyocarditis

A disease characterized chiefly by myocarditis was first described by Helwig and Schmidt (1945) in certain non-human primates, namely, the gibbon and chimpanzee, from which a viral agent has been transferred to mice and other animals with the production of encephalomyelitis and myocarditis. Since the initial reports, the virus has been isolated from several animal species and associated with either

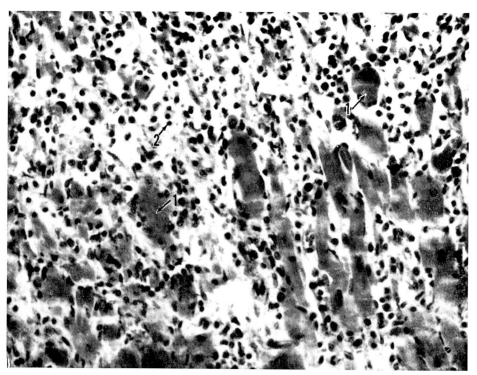

FIG. 10–10.—Encephalomyocarditis, myocardium (× 350) of a gibbon. Fragmented myocardial fibers (*1*) are separated by intense infiltration of lymphocytes (*2*) and plasma cells. (Courtesy of Armed Forces Institute of Pathology.) Contributor: Lt. Col. F. C. Helwig.

encephalomyelitis, myocarditis, or both. As a spontaneous disease in animals, the disease is of greatest importance in non-human primates and swine where the virus produces a fatal myocarditis without encephalitis. The demonstration of neutralizing antibodies in human sera indicates that this agent might well be infectious for man. Wild rats probably serve as a reservoir for the virus.

The principal lesion of this disease is interstitial myocarditis. The heart usually is dilated and there is some slightly blood-tinged pericardial effusion. Occasionally bilateral hydrothorax and pulmonary edema are observed. The interstitial myocarditis seen microscopically is characterized by necrosis of myocardial fibers and rather intense infiltration with polymorphonuclear and mononuclear cells. The experimentally induced disease in mice usually results in encephalomyelitis as well as myocarditis. Hamsters and rats have been reported susceptible, with the resultant disease similar to that seen in mice. The virus is reported to induce myelitis in horses, and myocarditis in cattle. Rabbits and guinea pigs are somewhat refractory to experimental infection. Although microscopic calcification of muscle bundles has been described in guinea pigs in which attempts have been made to induce the infection, this change may not be due to the virus of encephalomyocarditis.

Craighead (1966, 1968) has obtained two variant strains of encephalomyocarditis virus through serial passage in either brain tissue (E-strain) or heart tissue (M-strain). In mice the E strain is predominantly neurotropic, whereas the M strain principally affects the heart. In addition, the E strain produces necrosis of the acinar pancreas, parotid salivary gland and lacrimal gland. In contrast, the M strain, which also affects the lacrimal gland, produces necrosis of the islets of Langerhans and transient diabetes mellitus.

Viral Encephalomyocarditis

CRAIGHEAD, J. E.: Pathogenicity of the M and E Variants of the Encephalomyocarditis (EMC) Virus. II. Lesions of the Pancreas, Parotid and Lacrimal Glands. Am. J. Path. 48:375–386, 1966.
————: Pathogenicity of the M and E Variants of the Encephalomyocarditis (EMC) Virus. I. Myocardiotropic and Neurotropic Properties. Am. J. Path. 48:333–345, 1966.
CRAIGHEAD, J. E., and MCLANE, M. F.: Diabetes Mellitus: Induction in Mice by Encephalomyocarditis Virus. Science 162:913–914, 1968.
GAINER, J. H.: Encephalomyocarditis Virus Infections in Florida, 1960–1966. J. Am. Vet. Med. Assoc. 151:421–425, 1967.
GAINER, J. H., SANDEFUR, J. R., and BIGLER, W. J.: High Mortality in a Florida Swine Herd Infected with the Encephalomyocarditis Virus. An Accompanying Epizootiologic Survey. Cornell Vet. 58:31–47, 1968.
HELWIG, F. C., and SCHMIDT, E. C. H.: A Filter Passing Agent Producing Interstitial Myocarditis in Anthropoid Apes and Small Animals. Science 102:31–33, 1945.
ROCA-GARCIA, M., and SANMARTIN-BARBERI, C.: The Isolation of Encephalomyocarditis Virus from *Aotus* Monkeys. Am. J. Trop. Med. 6:840–852, 1957.
SCHMIDT, E. C. H.: Virus Myocarditis. Pathologic and Experimental Studies. Am. J. Path. 24:97–117, 1948.

Japanese B Encephalitis

A viral encephalitis, primarily of man but to which cattle, swine and horses are susceptible, has been described from the Far East. The natural infection is most prevalent in Japan but is known on Guam, Formosa, Okinawa and the Chinese mainland. The disease is insect-borne, transmitted by mosquitoes of the genus *Culex*. The demonstration of neutralizing and complement-fixing antibodies in cattle, swine and horses with no history of frank disease has been used to establish the presence of inapparent infection. In swine the virus is an important cause of abortion, stillbirth, and neonatal death. The sows are generally symptomless.

Lesions.—In fatal infections in man, neuronophagic nodules are observed in all parts of the gray matter, the thalamus, substantia nigra, nucleus basalis and anterior horns of the spinal cord being most severely involved. In the spinal cord, the lesions tend to become confluent, whereas, in the cerebral cortex and cerebellum, the lesions are generally discrete. The neuronophagic nodules indicate involvement of neurons as discussed under equine encephalomyelitis (p. 356).

In animals, including aborted and stillborn pigs, similar lesions are seen, particularly in the gray matter of the cerebral cortex and basal ganglia.

Diagnosis.—Although the presence of typical lesions may suggest Japanese B encephalitis, they cannot with certainty be differentiated from those of louping ill, Teschen disease or even equine encephalomyelitis. In order to make a definitive diagnosis, it is necessary to isolate the causative virus or demonstrate specific neutralizing antibody production following infection.

Japanese B Encephalitis

BURNS, K. F.: Congenital Japanese B Encephalitis of Swine. Proc. Soc. Exp. Biol., N.Y. 75:621–625, 1950.

BURNS, K. F., and MATUMOTO, M.: Japanese Equine Encephalomyelitis. J. Am. Vet. Med. Assn. 115:112–115, 167–170, 1949.

BURNS, K. F., and MATUMOTO, M.: Survey of Animals for Inapparent Infection with the Virus of Japanese B Encephalitis. Am. J. Vet. Research 10:146–149, 1949.

HAYMAKER, W., and SABIN, A. B.: Topographic Distribution of Lesions in the Central Nervous System in Japanese B Encephalitis. Arch. Neurol. & Psychiat. 57:673–692, 1947.

WEBSTER, L. T.: Japanese B Encephalitis Virus; Its Differentiation from St. Louis Encephalitis Virus and Relationship to Louping-ill Virus. J. Exper. Med. 67:609–618, 1938.

ZIMMERMAN, H. M.: Pathology of Japanese B Encephalitis. Am. J. Path. 22:965–991, 1946.

Herpesvirus B Infection of Monkeys
(Herpes-B, Herpesvirus simiae, B-virus)

The increasingly frequent use of monkeys of various species in medical research has stimulated interest in studies of the spontaneous diseases of these animals as a necessary corollary. In 1934, Sabin and Wright isolated a virus from the brain of a human patient who died following the bite of an apparently normal rhesus monkey (*Macaca mulatta*). The virus was shown subsequently to be carried by Old World monkeys of the genus *Macaca* in which little or no disease is usually evident. Based on the presence of clinical disease, virus isolation and/or serum neutralizing antibodies the following species have been incriminated as natural reservoir hosts for the virus: *M. mulatta* (rhesus); *M. fascicularis* (cynomolgus, crab-eating macaque); *M. fuscata* (Japanese macaque) and *M. arctoides* (stump-tail macaque).

The Disease in Monkeys.—The bulk of our knowledge of *Herpesvirus B* comes from studies with rhesus monkeys. Following infection, clinical disease characterized by vesicles and ulcers, particularly on the dorsal surface of the tongue and on the mucocutaneous junction of the lip, may develop, but it is not known if lesions invariably follow infection. In addition to the oral mucous membranes, vesicles and ulcers may also occur on the skin and the virus may cause conjunctivitis. These lesions heal uneventfully in seven to fourteen days. *Microscopically*, the lesions are characterized by ballooning degeneration and necrosis of epithelial cells and the presence of intranuclear inclusion bodies. Multinucleated epithelial cells containing intranuclear inclusion bodies are also usually present. Inclusion bodies may also be found in macrophages and in endothelial cells. During the course of clinical disease in the rhesus and cynamolgus monkey, visceral lesions may also develop. When present, these are characterized by foci of necrosis in the liver, associated with intranuclear inclusion bodies. In the central nervous system neuronal necrosis and gliosis associated with minimal perivascular cuffing with lymphocytes may be found. Intranuclear inclusion bodies occur in glial cells and neurons. The lesions are most frequent in the nucleus and tract of the descending branches of the trigeminal nerve, between the roots of origin of the facial and auditory nerves; and at the roots of the trigeminal and facial nerves.

These natural lesions have been shown to be intensified by the administration of cortisone and the intraspinal, intrathalamic and intramuscular inoculation of inactivated poliomyelitis vaccine. These are procedures used in the testing of the safety of this vaccine. In monkeys in which the disease has been thus activated, a diffuse encephalomyelitis may occur and the architecture of the spinal cord may be destroyed at the site of the inoculation. Lymphocytic infiltration of the meninges and nerve roots as well as neutrophils and focal demyelinization may be found in the lumbar region. Edema and necrosis occur as well as diffuse glial infiltration in the medulla and pons, particularly at the midline, and perivascular lymphocytic infiltration is extensive. Diffuse necrosis may be seen in the floor of the fourth ventricle and the inflammation may cause loss of ependymal cells and extend into the ventricle. Glial infiltrations are common in vestibular nuclei, medial longitudinal fasciculi, and nuclei of the spinal tracts of the fifth cranial nerve. Small glial foci may occur around the cerebral aqueduct, in the thalamus, putamen, caudate nucleus and in the parietal and temporal cortex. The hippocampus, occipital cortex, amygdaloid and hypothalamus are reportedly free of lesions in this accentuated form of the natural disease.

The infection spreads within a colony of monkeys *via* direct contact, fomites and probably aerosols until nearly 100 per cent of the colony has become infected as determined by the presence of serum neutralizing antibodies. Oral lesions are not encountered in every animal which is explained in part by failure to observe them.

Once a monkey is infected with *Herpesvirus B*, it should probably be considered infected for life. Although recurrence of lesions, as in *Herpesvirus simplex* infection in man, has not been recognized, periodic excretion of the virus in the absence of visible lesions may occur.

Herpesvirus B has not been demonstrated to produce spontaneous fatal disease in rhesus monkeys, but in the cynamolgus monkey the disease may be severe enough to lead to death.

The Disease in Man.—The principal importance of *Herpesvirus B* is not its hazards to the reservoir hosts but rather that the virus produces a fatal disease in man. Although the morbidity rate is low, of 18 cases reported, all but two have proved fatal. Most infections have followed a monkey bite. The disease is characterized clinically and pathologically by encephalomyelitis. Focal necrosis may occur in the liver, spleen, lymph nodes, and adrenals. Intranuclear inclusion bodies may be found in any affected tissue but have not been demonstrated in all cases.

Diagnosis.—A presumptive diagnosis can be made from the characteristic lesions. Due to the number of simian herpesviruses, definitive diagnosis requires isolation and identification of the virus. A rise in titre of serum neutralizing antibodies may support the diagnosis.

Herpesvirus B

DAVIDSON, W. L.: B Virus Infection in Man. Ann. N.Y. Acad. Sci. *85*:970–979, 1960.

ENDO, M., KAMINURA, T., AOYAMA, Y., HAYASHIDA, T., KINJO, T., KOLERA, YONO A., SUZUKI, K., TAIJIMA, Y., and ANDO, K.: Etude de Virus au Japan. Jap. J. Exp. Med. *30*: 227–233, 385–392, 1960.

GRALLA, E. J., CIECURA, S. J., and DELAHUNT, C. S.: Extended B-virus Anti-body Determinations in a Closed Monkey Colony. Lab. Anim. Care *16*:510–514, 1966.

HARTLEY, E. G.: Naturally-occurring "B" Virus Infection in Cynamolgus Monkeys. Vet. Rec. *76*:555–557, 1964.

HULL, R. N.: *The Simian Viruses, Virology Monographs 2*, Springer-Verlag, New York, 1968.

HUNT, R. D., and MELENDEZ, L. V.: Herpes Virus Infections of Non-Human Primates: A Review. Lab. Anim. Care *19*:221–234, 1969.

KEEBLE, S. A.: B Virus Infection in Monkeys. Ann. N.Y. Acad. Sci. *85* 960–969, 1960.

KEEBLE, S. A., CHRISTOFINIS, G. J., and WOOD, W.: Natural B-virus infection in rhesus monkeys. J. Path & Bact. *76*:189–199, 1958.

KIRSCHSTEIN, R. L., VAN HOOSIER, C. L., and LI, C. P.: Virus B-infection of the central nervous system of monkeys used for the poliomyelitis vaccine safety test. Am. J. Path. *38*: 119–125, 1961.

SABIN, A. B. and WRIGHT, A. M.: Acute ascending myelitis following a monkey bite, with isolation of a virus capable of reproducing the disease. J. Exper. Med. *59*:115–136, 1934.

SABIN, A. B.: Studies on the B Virus. I. The Immunological Identity of a Virus Isolated from a Human Case of Ascending Myelitis Associated with Visceral Necrosis. Brit. J. Exp. Path. *15*:248–269, 1934.

SHAH, K. V., and SOUTHWICK, C. H.: Prevalence of Antibodies to Certain Viruses in Sera of Free-Living Rhesus and of Captive Monkeys. Indian J. Med. Res. *53*:488–500, 1965.

Herpesvirus T Infection of Monkeys
(Herpesvirus M, Herpesvirus platarrhinae I)

Herpesvirus T infection has many similarities to *Herpesvirus B* infection discussed above; however, the virus is distinct and the susceptible hosts are New World monkeys. *Herpesvirus T* is carried as a latent viral infection by the squirrel monkey (*Saimiri sciureus*). Based on evidence derived from circulating serum neutralizing antibodies, cinnamon ringtail monkeys (*Cebus albifrons*) and spider monkeys (*Ateles spp.*) are also likely natural reservoir hosts. Although the morbidity is high, clinical disease is rarely seen in the reservoir host, and has only been documented in the squirrel monkey where the lesions consist of vesicles and ulcers of the oral mucous membranes. The microscopic features are identical to *Herpesvirus B* infection in the rhesus. Visceral lesions or changes in the central nervous systems are not known to occur. The disease in the reservoir hosts is not known to be fatal. Exacerbation of oral lesions is also not known to occur but as with *Herpesvirus B* infection, the virus can be excreted in the absence of visible lesions. All available evidence suggests that latent infection remains for life.

Marmosets (*Saguinus spp.*) and owl monkeys (*Aotus trivirgatus*) have a less fortunate relationship with *Herpesvirus T*. In these hosts *Herpesvirus T* produces an epizootic disease of high morbidity and mortality. The clinical features which develop following a seven- to ten-day incubation period are characterized by anorexia, lassitude, oral and labial vesicles and ulcers, ulcerative dermatitis (especially of the face), and occasionally conjunctivitis. Hyperesthesia, as evidenced by intense scratching, may be the most obvious sign. After a course of two to three days, most animals become moribund and die. **Gross** lesions consist of vesicles and/or ulcers of the skin, lips, oral cavity, esophagus, small intestine, cecum and colon. Hemorrhage is present in most lymph nodes, the adrenal cortices and occasionally in the lung. **Microscopically** variable sized foci of necrosis and intranuclear inclusion bodies are found in most organs and tissues of the body. Lesions are most frequent in the oral cavity, small and large intestine, liver, spleen, lymph nodes, adrenal cortex and various ganglia. Multinucleated giant cells are present in lesions of the oral cavity and skin. Encephalitis is not common and when present, it is not extensive.

Diagnosis.—In either the reservoir hosts or the fatally affected hosts the characteristic lesions allow for a presumptive diagnosis. However, due to the occurrence of other herpesviruses in New World monkeys, the virus should be isolated and identified. In owl monkeys the lesions of *Herpesvirus T* infection cannot be differentiated from those of *Herpesvirus simplex* infection.

Herpesvirus T

DANIEL, M. D., KARPAS, A., MELENDEZ, L. V., KING, N. W., and HUNT, R. D.: Isolation of Herpes-T Virus From a Spontaneous Disease in Squirrel Monkeys (*Saimiri sciureus*). Arch. Ges. Virusforsch *22*:324–331, 1967.
HOLMES, A. W., CALDWELL, R. G., DEDMON, R. E., and DEINHARDT, F.: Isolation and Characterization of a New Herpes Virus. J. Immunol. *92*:602–610, 1964.
HOLMES, A. W., DEVINE, J. A., NOWAKOWSKI, E., and DEINHARDT, F.: The Epidemiology of a Herpes Virus Infection of New World Monkeys. J. Immunol. *90*:668–671, 1966.
HUNT, R. D., and MELENDEZ, L. V.: Herpes Virus Infections of Non-Human Primates: A Review. Lab. Anim. Care *19*:221–234.
HUNT, R. D., and MELENDEZ, L. V.: Spontaneous Herpes-T Infection in the Owl Monkey (*Aotus trivirgatus*). Path. Vet. *3*:1–26, 1966.
KING, N. W., HUNT, R. D., DANIEL, M. D., and MELENDEZ, L. V.: Overt Herpes-T Infection in Squirrel Monkeys (*Saimiri sciureus*). Lab. Anim. Care *17*:413–423, 1967.
MELENDEZ, L. V., HUNT, R. D., GARCIA, F. G., and TRUM, B. F.: A Latent Herpes-T Infection in *Saimiri sciureus* (squirrel monkey). In *Some Recent Developments in Comparative Medicine*, R. N. T-W-Fiennes, Ed. pp. 393–397. London, Academic Press, 1966.

Herpesvirus Simplex Infection in Primates
(Herpesvirus hominus)

Herpesvirus simplex infection is one of the oldest viral diseases known to man. The use of the word herpes in medicine can be traced as far back as Hippocrates, and descriptions clearly related to the disease as we understand it in man today were published in the seventeenth century. There are also many early reports describing experimental transmission of *Herpesvirus simplex* to laboratory animals such as rabbits, guinea pigs, mice, rats and hamsters. Recently *H. simplex* has been shown to be an important spontaneous disease of owl monkeys (*Aotus trivirgatus*) a New World species, and gibbons (*Hylobates lar*) an anthropoid ape.

The Disease in Man.—Man is the natural and reservoir host for *H. simplex* assuming a role similar to the rhesus monkey with *Herpesvirus B* (p. 380), the squirrel monkey with *Herpesvirus T* (p. 382), and swine with *Herpesvirus suis* (p. 369). Primary infection occurs principally in young children taking the form of an acute gingivostomatitis which heals with no serious side effects. By adolescence or early adulthood, 90 to 95 per cent of all individuals have become infected

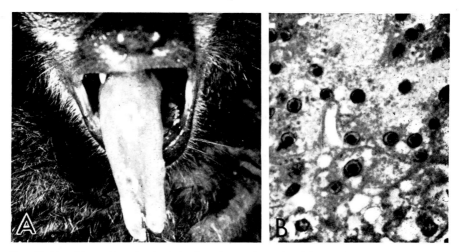

Fig. 10–11.—*Herpesvirus simplex* infection of an owl monkey (*Aotus trivirgatus*). *A*, Ulcerative glossitis. *B*, Intranuclear inclusion bodies in hepatocytes. (Courtesy New England Regional Primate Research Center, Harvard Medical School.)

as evidenced by the presence of serum neutralizing antibodies. Many people, despite the presence of serum neutralizing antibodies, suffer from periodic recurrence of secondary *H. simplex* infection for much of their lives, often with several episodes occurring each year. Recurrent lesions are believed to be the result of an activation of a latent infection which persists in all infected individuals for life. A variety of stimuli have been associated with activation, including fever ("fever blister"), colds ("cold sore"), fatigue, menstruation, emotional distress and certain foods. Recurrent lesions are characterized by small clusters of vesicles which rupture, leaving erosions or ulcers which heal in five to ten days. Hyperesthesia and neuralgia often precede the lesions and may persist for variable periods of time after healing. The mucocutaneous junction of the lip is the most frequent site, but the external nares, oral mucosa, conjunctiva, skin, esophagus, external genitalia, vagina and cervix are not uncommon locations. **Microscopic features** are ballooning degeneration, necrosis, intercellular edema, multinucleated giant cells and intranuclear inclusion bodies. Virus is readily isolated during the course and up to three weeks after recovery. Interestingly, virus can be recovered from a proportion of the population (7 to 20 per cent) in the absence of visible lesions.

H. simplex infection in man is not always a benign disease. In neonates and young children, primary infection may lead to a fatal generalized disease affecting most organs and tissues, and in adults fatal meningoencephalitis can develop. The lesions in both of these forms are characterized by focal necrosis and intranuclear inclusion bodies in the affected tissues. At present there is no satisfactory explanation for the occurrence of serious disease in the natural host for *H. simplex*. The finding is, however, not dissimilar from the effect of *H. suis* in its natural host, swine (p. 369), or for *H. canis* in its probable natural host, the dog (p. 389).

The Disease in Monkeys.—In owl monkeys *H. simplex* produces an epizootic disease with high morbidity and mortality. Following an incubation period of about seven days, there is a short clinical illness characterized by oral and labial ulceration, ulcerative dermatitis, conjunctivitis, anorexia, hyperesthesia, weak-

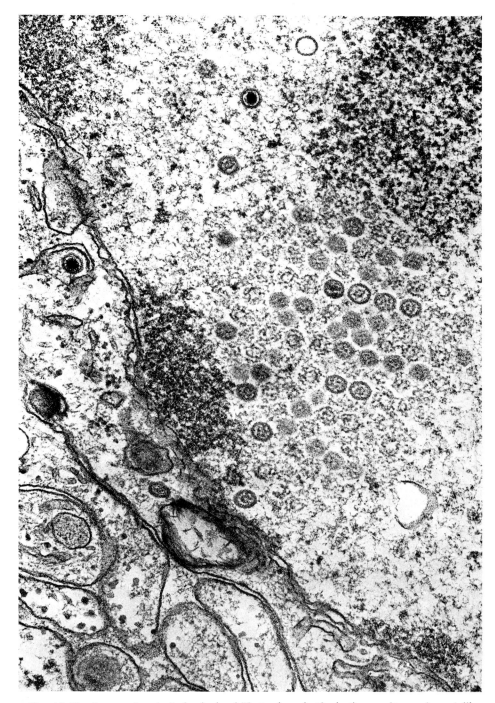

Fig. 10–12.—Intranuclear inclusion body of *Herpesvirus simplex* in tissue culture. A crystalline array of viral particles lies within the nucleus (× 50,000). (Courtesy Dr. J. E. Leestma and Laboratory Investigation.)

ness and incoordination. Death is the usual outcome in two to three days. Lesions are widespread and identical both in the gross and microscopic to those produced in this species by *Herpesvirus T*, with the exception that encephalitis is frequent in *H. simplex* infection. The encephalitis is similar to *H. simplex* infection in man; the lesions are most extensive in the temporal lobes of the cerebral

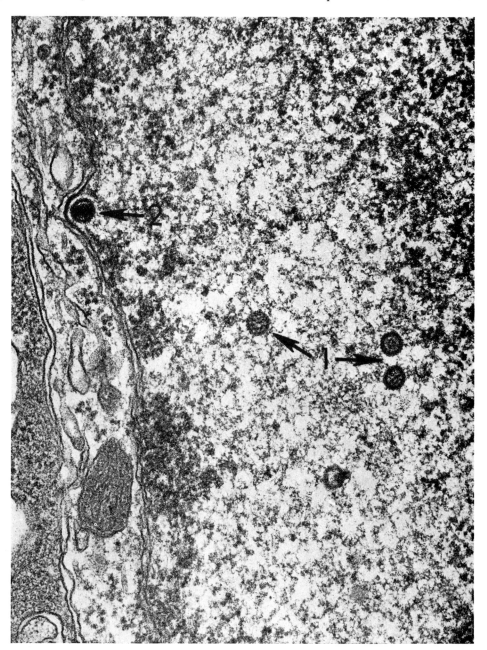

FIG. 10–13.—*Herpesvirus simplex* infection in tissue culture of nervous tissue. Note un-enveloped viral particles in the nucleus (*1*). A single virion (*2*) is approaching the bulging nuclear membrane, a stage preparatory to envelopment (× 40,000). (Courtesy Dr. J. E. Leestma and Laboratory Investigation.)

cortex with extension in the frontal, parietal and occipital lobes. Lesions may also occur in the thalamus and basal nuclei. The changes are principally characterized by widespread necrosis of neurons with many neurons containing intranuclear inclusion bodies. Gliosis and perivascular cuffing may or may not be prominent.

Diagnosis.—A presumptive diagnosis of *H. simplex* infection in owl monkeys can be made on the basis of history and pathological changes. However, generally the lesions cannot be distinguished from *Herpesvirus T* infection in this species, therefore definitive diagnosis requires viral isolation and identification. In addition to the owl monkey spontaneous *H. simplex* encephalitis has been reported in the gibbon, an anthropoid ape (*Hylobates lar*), and marmosets (*Saguinus spp.*) have been shown to be experimentally susceptible to the virus.

Herpesvirus simplex

BUDDINGH, G. J., SCHRUM, D. I., LANIER, J. C., and GUIDRY, D. J.: Studies of the Natural History of Herpes Simplex Infections. Pediatrics *11*:595–610, 1953.

CONSTANTINE, V. S., FRANCIS, R. D., and MONTES, L. F.: Association of Recurrent Herpes Simplex with Neuralgia. J. Am. Med. Assoc. *205*:131–133, 1968.

DEINHARDT, F., HOLMES, A. W., DEVINE, J., and DEINHARDT, J.: Marmosets as Laboratory Animals. IV. The Microbiology of Laboratory Kept Marmosets. Lab. Anim. Care *17*:48–70, 1967.

HUNT, R. D., and MELENDEZ, L. V.: Herpes Virus Infections of Non-Human Primates: A Review. Lab. Anim. Care *19*:221–234, 1969.

KAPLAN, A. S.: Herpes Simplex and Pseudorabies Viruses. Virology Monographs 1969. New York, Springer-Verlag, pp. 1–115.

KATZIN, D. S., CONNOR, J. D., WILSON, L. A., and SEXTON, R. S.: Experimental Herpes Simplex Infection in the Owl Monkey. Proc. Soc. Exp. Biol. Med. *125*:391–398, 1967.

LEESTMA, J. E., BORNSTEIN, M. B., SHEPPARD, R. D., and FELDMAN, L. A.: Ultrastructural Aspects of Herpes Simplex Virus Infection in Organized Cultures of Mammalian Nervous Tissue. Lab. Invest. *20*:70–78, 1969.

LEIDER, W., MAGOFFIN, R. L., LENNETTE, E. H., and LEONARDS, L. N. R.: Herpes Simplex Virus Encephalitis. Its Possible Association with Reactivated Latent Infection. New Eng. J. Med. *273*:341–347, 1965.

MELENDEZ, L. V., ESPAÑA, C., HUNT, R. D., DANIEL, M. D., and GARCIA, F. G.: Natural Herpes Simplex Infection in Owl Monkey (*Aotus trivirgatus*). Lab. Anim. Care *19*:38–45, 1969.

MILLER, J. K., HESSER, F., and TOMPKINS, V. N.: Herpes Simplex Encephalitis. Ann. Int. Med. *64*:92–103, 1966.

OLSON, L. C., BUESCHER, E. L., ARTENSTEIN, M. S., and PARKMAN, P. D.: Herpesvirus Infections of the Human Central Nervous System. New Eng. J. Med. *277*:1271–1277, 1967.

RHODES, A. J., and VANROOYEN, C. E.: *Textbook of Virology*. Baltimore, The Williams & Wilkins Co., 1962, pp. 136–146.

SMITH, P. C., YUILL, T. M., BUCHANAN, R. D., STANTON, J. S., and CHAICUMPA, V.: The Gibbon (*Hylobates lar*) A New Primate Host for *Herpesvirus hominis*. I. A Natural Epizootic in a Laboratory Colony. J. Infect. Dis. *120*:292–297, 1969.

SMITH, P. C., YUILL, T. M., and BUCHANAN, R. D.: Natural and Experimental Infection of Gibbons with Herpesvirus hominis. Ann. Prog. Report SEATO Med. Res. Lab. and SEATO Clinical Res. Cen., Bangkok, Thailand, pp. 258–261, 1958.

SZOGI, S., and BERGE, TH.: Generalized Herpes Simplex in Newborns. Acta Path. et microbiol. scandinav. *66*:401–408, 1966.

Additional Simian Herpesviruses

In addition to *Herpesvirus B*, *Herpesvirus T*, and *Herpesvirus simplex*, several other herpesviruses of non-human primates deserve brief mention. However, our knowledge of these agents is less complete.

A fatal systemic infection has been described in African green or vervet monkeys (*Cercopithecus aethiops*), an Old World species. The agent, tentatively called

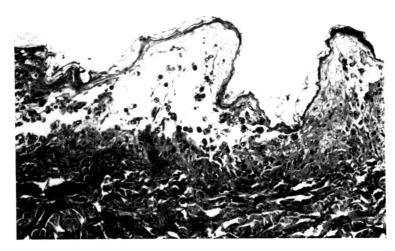

FIG. 10–14.—Liverpool vervet monkey virus infection. Vesicular dermatitis of a vervet monkey
(*Cercopithecus aethiops*). (Tissue courtesy Dr. E. Thorpe.)

the **Liverpool vervet monkey virus** was first isolated in England. The disease is
characterized by the development of a generalized vesicular rash which is followed by death in twenty-four to forty-eight hours. In addition to epidermal
vesicles, focal necrosis occurs in the lung, liver, and spleen. Intranuclear inclusion
bodies are found in all affected tissues. Lesions have not been described in the
oral cavity or central nervous system. The natural or reservoir host(s) for the
virus is not known. A similar disease entity has been described in patas monkeys
(*Erythrocebus patas*). The causative agent is a herpesvirus and resembles the
Liverpool vervet monkey virus but has not been completely classified.

An agent termed the **spider monkey herpesvirus** was isolated from a young
spider monkey which died of a generalized infection with oral and labial erosions
and ulcers. Further examples of spontaneous disease have not been reported.

Other herpesviruses have been reported for which no known natural disease
has been described. SA8 is a herpesvirus which is probably latent in vervet monkeys, SA15 is a herpesvirus which is probably latent in baboons, and *H. saimiri*
is a latent herpesvirus infection in squirrel monkeys (*Saimiri sciureus*). SA8 may
be capable of causing myelitis in vervet monkeys and *H. saimiri* is experimentally
oncogenic in marmosets and owl monkeys inducing malignant lymphoma with
leukemia.

Additional Simian Herpesviruses

CLARKSON, M. J., THORPE, E., and McCARTHY, K.: A Virus Disease of Captive Vervet
Monkeys (*Cercopithecus aethiops*) Caused by a New Herpesvirus. Arch. Ges Virusforsch. *22*:
219–234, 1967.
HULL, R. N.: *The Simian Viruses, Virology Monographs* 2, New York, Springer-Verlag,
1968.
HUNT, R. D., and MELENDEZ, L. V.: Herpes Virus Infections of Non-Human Primates: A
Review. Lab. Anim. Care *19*:221–234, 1969.
LENNETTE, E. H.: Workshop on Viral Diseases Which Impede Colonization of Nonhuman
Primates. Nat'l. Center for Primate Biology, Univ. of Calif. at Davis, May 22–24, 1968.

MALHERBE, H., and HARWIN, R.: Neurotropic Virus in African Monkeys. Lancet 2:530, 1958.

MALHERBE, H., HARWIN, R., and ULRICH, M.: The Cytopathic Effects of Vervet Monkey Viruses. S. A. Med. J. 37:407–411, 1963.

MALHERBE, H., and STRICKLAND-CHOLMLEY, M.: Virus from Baboons. Lancet 2:1300, 1969.

McCARTHY, K., THORPE, E., LAURSEN, A. C., HEYMANN, C. S., and BEALE, A. J.: Exanthematous Disease in Patas Monkeys Caused by a Herpes Virus. Lancet 2:856–857, 1968.

Herpesvirus Canis Infection of Dogs

Herpesvirus canis was first isolated, characterized and identified as the cause of a fatal systemic infection of neonatal puppies in 1965. From available evidence it appears that dogs are the natural and reservoir hosts for this herpesvirus, in a manner analogous to *Herpesvirus simplex* in man, *Herpesvirus B* in monkeys, and *Herpesvirus suis* in swine. A high percentage of dogs become infected with the virus without history of associated illness and the virus can be isolated from puppies and adult dogs in the absence of recognizable disease. Although adult dogs carry the virus as a latent infection, it has been shown to cause a mild tracheobronchitis. The occurrence of fatal infections in neonatal puppies appears to be analogous to the parallel condition of fatal *Herpesvirus simplex* in infants or fatal *Herpesvirus suis* in piglets. These are each an example of fatal disease in the same host which usually carries the virus as a latent infection.

Puppies are infected *in utero* or during birth by exposure to the virus in the vagina. The infection results in either stillbirth, or an acute fatal disease in the first three weeks of life. After three to five weeks of age, infection is usually inapparent.

Lesions.—The most striking **gross** pathological change is hemorrhage, especially of the renal cortices and lungs but the stomach, intestine, and adrenals may also contain hemorrhages. Serosanguinous fluid is usually present in the thoracic and abdominal cavities and there is splenomegaly and enlargement of lymph nodes. Variably sized grey foci are often present in the lungs, kidneys and liver. **Microscopically** the lesions in all tissues are characterized by focal necrosis and the presence of intranuclear inclusion bodies. These necrotizing lesions may be found in the lung, kidneys, liver, spleen, lymph nodes, adrenal, intestines and brain. Usually the lesions are most extensive in the kidneys and lungs. The lesions in the central nervous system are those of a disseminated, nonsuppurative encephalomyelitis with focal malacia of the cerebral cortex, cerebellar cortex, basal ganglia and grey columns of the spinal cord. Secondary lesions follow in the white matter. Infection in adult dogs is usually not associated with histopathological changes, but the virus may produce a catarrhal tracheobronchitis with intranuclear inclusions in the lining epithelium. Inclusion bodies in both neonates and adults may be difficult to demonstrate unless an acid fixative such as Zenker's fluid has been employed.

Diagnosis.—The characteristic necrotizing lesions and intranuclear inclusion bodies in neonatal or stillborn puppies allows for a presumptive diagnosis. Definitive diagnosis requires virus isolation and characterization. Dogs are natural hosts for this virus and subject to latent infection, therefore virus isolation in the absence of characteristic histopathological lesions must be approached with caution.

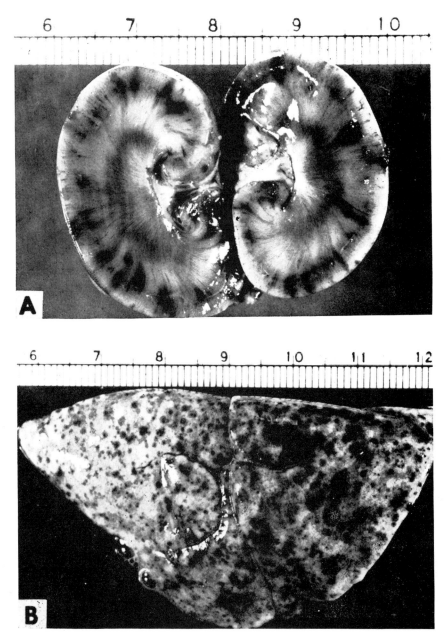

FIG. 10–15.—*Herpesvirus canis* infection in a puppy. *A*, Hemorrhage and necrosis in renal cortex. *B*, Numerous petechiae, ecchymoses and suffusion in the lung. (Courtesy Dr. T. J. Kakuk and Laboratory Animal Care.)

Herpesvirus canis

CARMICHAEL, L. E., STRANDBERG, J. D., and BARNES, F. D.:   Identification of a Cytopathogenic Agent Infectious for Puppies as a Canine Herpesvirus.   Proc. Soc. Exp. Biol. & Med. *120*:644–650, 1966.
CARMICHAEL, L. E., SQUIRE, R. A., and KROOK, L.:   Clinical and Pathologic Features of a Fatal Viral Disease of Newborn Pups.   Am. J. Vet. Res. *26*:803–814, 1965.
CORNWELL, H. J. C., WRIGHT, N. G., CAMPBELL, R. S. F., and ROBERTS, R. J.:   Neonatal Disease in the Dog Associated with a Herpes-Like Virus.   Vet. Rec. *79*:661–662, 1966.

Mims, C. A.: Effect on the Fetus of Maternal Infection with Lymphocytic Choriomeningitis (LCM) Virus. J. Infect. Dis. *120*:582–597, 1969.
————: Immunofluorescence Study of the Carrier State and Mechanism of Vertical Transmission in Lymphocytic Choriomeningitis Infection in Mice. J. Path. Bact. *91*:395–402, 1966.
Smadel, J. E., and Wall, M. J.: Identification of the Virus Lymphocytic Choriomeningitis. J. Bact. *41*:421–430, 1941.
Traub, E.: An Epidemic in a Mouse Colony Due to Lymphocytic Choriomeningitis. J. Exper. Med. *63*:533–546, 1936.

EPITHELIOTROPIC VIRAL DISEASES

Aphthous Fever

(Foot and Mouth Disease, Epizoötic Aphtha)

Aphthous fever is an important and widespread disease caused by a virus with strong epitheliotropic features. The disease occurs naturally in cloven-hoofed animals, the most important of which are cattle, sheep, goats and swine. It may also affect wild ruminants such as deer, goats and antelope, and under some conditions they act as reservoirs for the infection. Guinea pigs, suckling mice, birds and carnivores are susceptible to experimental inoculation with the virus. Natural infection may occur in man, in whom the disease is usually mild and limited to acute fever associated with the appearance of vesicles on the hands, feet and oral mucosæ.

Although aphthous fever is prevalent in all of Europe, Africa, much of Asia, and in some countries of South America, the disease has been prevented from re-entering the United States since 1929, when a severe outbreak occurred in California. This and previous outbreaks were stamped out by stringent quarantine of infected areas and slaughter of exposed and infected animals. In recent years important outbreaks have occurred in Mexico and Canada, but at the present writing appear to be under control.

The virus occurs in seven principal antigenic types. These, in the international nomenclature, are designated as "A," "O" (Vallée and Carré) and "C" (Waldmann), SAT-1, SAT-2, SAT-3 (Galloway, Brooksby and Henderson) (SA = South Africa) and Asia −1. Although the symptoms and lesions produced by each virus type are essentially similar, infection with one virus does not immunize against the others. In recent years numerous subtypes have been identified which are also antigenically distinct. These are designated by a subnumber, *i.e.*, A_5.

Pathogenesis.—Features of particular significance in this disease are the extreme infectiousness of the virus and the ease with which it can be carried, not only by infected animals and their products, but mechanically by man and other animals. It may be transported on the shoes or clothing of human beings, in or on the bodies of migratory birds or animals, as well as in such products as raw hides, milk, bedding and forage. Infection is presumed to occur *per os*, with primary aphthæ developing on the lips or oral mucosae. The virus soon gains access to the blood stream and is widely disseminated through the body, producing secondary lesions in epithelial tissues. Only the greater severity and wider dissemination of the secondary lesions distinguish them from primary lesions. The virus can be isolated from the blood during the febrile stage and becomes concentrated in the fluid of epithelial vesicles when the temperature falls.

Signs.—The signs are directly related to the lesions of the disease. Those in the oral mucosa produce excess salivation and make eating painful, thus causing the infected animal to refuse food and water. Smacking of the lips and tongue is characteristic. The epithelium of the dorsum of the tongue usually becomes eroded. Lesions of the feet may produce lameness. Aphthæ may be detected around other parts of the body which are lightly haired, such as the skin of the udder, the vulva and the conjunctiva.

In young animals (lambs and calves), acute gastro-enteritis and myocarditis are common and the mortality is very high. In animal populations which have experienced exposure to the disease, the mortality is low, rarely more than 5 per cent in adult animals, although certain virus strains can cause a mortality as high as 60 per cent.

Lesions.—On cattle, the distribution of the vesicular lesions is characteristic. The oral mucosa over the lips, dorsum of the tongue and palate is most severely involved. Lesions occur in the skin near the coronary band adjacent to the inter-digital space and are also frequent in other areas in which the hair is sparse, such as the vulva, teat and udder. The conjunctiva may be affected, as may be that part of the forestomach which is lined with squamous epithelium (rumen, reticulum and omasum). Small epidermal vesicles may also occur in grossly normal skin of the brisket, abdomen, hock, carpus, and perineum. In addition to these specific vesicular lesions, punctate hemorrhages or diffuse edema of the mucosa may be observed in the abomasum and small intestine. The mucosa of the large intestine may be hyperemic, blue-red, and some animals may bear subpleural, subepithelial or subepicardial hemorrhages. These, however, are not considered primary lesions.

The specific lesions in their early stages are microscopic and are limited to the epithelium at the sites of predilection. The lesion starts with localized "balloon" degeneration of cells in the middle of the stratum spinosum of the epithelium. Here the intercellular prickles are lost; the epithelial cells become round and detached from one another; their cytoplasm takes an intensely eosinophilic stain, and their nuclei are pyknotic. Edema fluid containing bits of fibrin accumulates between and separates the cells. Neutrophils infiltrate the epithelium at this stage. Liquefaction necrosis and accumulation of serum and leukocytes produce vesicles roofed over by the compressed stratum corneum, lucidum and granulosum and extending down to the basal layer, which usually remains in place over the heavily congested dermis. These small vesicles (aphthae) coalesce to form bullae which cause large areas of epithelium to be detached and easily shed or rubbed off. Loss of epithelium is most common on the dorsal surface of the anterior two-thirds of the bovine tongue which is separated by a transverse notch from a dorsal eminence occupying the posterior third of the tongue. The entire epithelium over the anterior area may be lost, leaving a raw, red surface which oozes blood. The pain from this denuded area explains the severe anorexia which is often a symptom. In addition to the virus, the vesicles contain necrotic epithelial cells, leukocytes, occasional erythrocytes and, in the late stages, bacteria. Small pleomorphic bodies have been described in lymphocytes and epithelial cells, but these have not been established as virus particles or specific "inclusions."

Lesions in the myocardium are most common in the fatal disease in very young calves or lambs but also occur in pigs and young goats. The lesions observed in the wall and septum of the left ventricle, seldom in the atria, appear as small, grayish foci of irregular size, which may give the myocardium a somewhat striped appearance (so-called tiger heart). Microscopically, hyaline degeneration and

Table 10–2—Susceptibility of Various Species

| Disease | Cattle | Swine | Horses | Sheep | Guinea Pig | Mouse | | Chick Em-bryo | Man |
						Adult	Unweaned		
Aphthous fever (Foot and mouth disease) . .	+	+	—	+	+	—	+	+	+
Vesicular stoma-titis	±*	+	+	+	+	+	+	+	+
Vesicular exan-thema . . .	—	+	±	—	—	—	—	?	—

* *Note:* Cattle are susceptible to vesicular stomatitis virus when injected by the lingual route but not when injected intramuscularly.

necrosis of myocardial fibers are accompanied by an intense lymphocytic, occasionally neutrophilic, infiltration. The myocardial lesion is not strictly specific for infections with the virus of foot and mouth disease, but it is believed to be the one that most commonly causes death of newborn animals.

In the skeletal muscle, lesions similar to those in the myocardium may be observed. Sharply delimited areas of necrosis are seen grossly as gray foci of various sizes and microscopically as necrosis of muscle bundles associated with rather intense leukocytic infiltration. A similar, but much more severe, acute myositis occurs in suckling mice experimentally inoculated with the virus. The susceptibility of the musculature of young mice is being utilized with increasing frequency in experimental study of the virus.

Diagnosis.—In the differential diagnosis of aphthous fever (foot and mouth disease), it is necessary to consider all other so-called "vesicular diseases" such as vesicular exanthema and vesicular stomatitis. These cannot be differentiated with absolute certainty by their symptoms and lesions. It is necessary, therefore, to isolate and identify the virus or to demonstrate complement-fixing or virus-neutralizing antibodies in recovered cases. The susceptibility of several animals to the viruses of these vesicular diseases varies, a point which may be used to some extent in differential diagnosis.

Table 10–2 indicates the differences in susceptibility of several species to experimental inoculation.

Aphthous Fever

DAUBNEY, R.: Foot and Mouth Diseases; the Fixed Virus Types. J. Comp. Path. & Therap. 47:259–281, 1934.

DOMANSKI, E., and FITKO, R.: Disturbances of the Pituitary and other Hormonal Glands after Foot and Mouth Disease. Proc. 16th Intern. Vet. Cong., Madrid. 2:421–423, 1959.

FRENKEL, H. S.: Histologic Changes in Explanted Bovine Epithelial Tongue Tissue Infected with the Virus of Foot and Mouth Disease. Am. J. Vet. Research 10:142–145, 1949.

GAILIUNAS, P.: Microscopic Skin Lesions in Cattle with Foot-and-Mouth Disease. Arch. Ges. Virusforsch. 25:188–200, 1968.

GAILIUNAS, P., COTTRAL, G. E., and SEIBOLD, H. R.: Teat Lesions in Heifers Experimentally Infected with Foot-and-Mouth Disease Virus. Am. J. Vet. Res. 25:1062–1069, 1964.

GALLOWAY, I. A., HENDERSON, W. M., and BROOKSBY, J. B.: Strains of the Virus of Foot and Mouth Disease Recovered from Outbreaks in Mexico. Proc. Soc. Exper. Biol. & Med. 69:57–63, 1948.

GILLESPIE, J. H.: Propagation of Type C Foot-and-Mouth-Disease Virus in Eggs and Effects of The Egg-Cultivated Virus on Cattle. Cornell Vet. 45:170–179, 1955.

PLATT, H.: Observations on the Pathology of Experimental Foot and Mouth Disease in Adult Guinea Pigs. J. Path. & Bact. 76:119–131, 1958.

PLATT, H.: Phagocytic Acitity in Squamous Epithelium and its Role in Cellular Susceptibility to Foot-and-Mouth Disease. Nature, Lond. 190:1075–1076, 1961. (VB 104–62.)

SEIBOLD, H. R.: The Histopathology of Foot and Mouth Disease in Pregnant and Lactating Mice. Am. J. Vet. Res. 21:870–877, 1960.

SKINNER, H. H.: Propagation of Strains of Foot and Mouth Disease Virus in Unweaned White Mice. Proc. Royal Soc. Med. 44:1041–1044, 1951.

VESICULAR STOMATITIS

The virus of vesicular stomatitis may naturally affect swine, cattle, horses and man, producing a disease which has close similarities to aphthous fever (foot and mouth disease), and vesicular exanthema. Vesicular stomatitis is present only in the warm months of the year, appearing in the late spring and disappearing with the coming of freezing weather. It is most common in cattle and horses, but severe outbreaks have been reported in swine in serum-producing biological plants. Insect vectors are believed to represent the principal means of transmission.

The lesions of vesicular stomatitis are usually described as vesicular, but Seibold and Sharp (1960) disagree with this concept as a consequence of their study of experimentally infected bovine tongues. These investigators found the basic histologic alterations to be (1) intercellular edema in the middle of the malpighian layer, resulting in a filigree appearance but not usually vesiculation; (2) necrosis of epithelial cells in the middle of the malpighian layer and usually sparing the basal layer; and (3) inflammatory cellular infiltration by heterophils and monocytes into the necrotic zones of epithelium. In some lesions, the intraepithelial edema becomes abundant enough to result in a vesicle but this occurs in less than 30 per cent of the experimental lesions. This observation is in agreement with several field experiences in which vesiculation was rarely observed clinically.

Non-vesiculated lesions terminate by dehydration of the superficial layers of epithelium-edema fluid apparently escaping through vertical cracks in the *stratum corneum*. Lesions with large vesicles or bullae usually lost the overlying epithelial layers leaving a thin layer of basal cells over the congested dermis. These eroded lesions would therefore have the characteristic red, raw appearance. Healing proceeds by regrowth of the epithelium from the remaining basal cells.

The susceptibility of various species to vesicular stomatitis in comparison to aphthous fever and vesicular exanthema is indicated in Table 10–2.

Lesions.—The lesions of vesicular stomatitis are essentially similar in distribution, location and microscopic appearance to those of aphthous fever and vesicular exanthema. The lesions of these three diseases cannot be definitively distinguished on morphologic grounds in spite of the less conspicuous vesiculation evident in vesicular stomatitis. Vesicular stomatitis, unlike aphthous fever, rarely causes myocarditis and is almost never fatal.

Vesicular Stomatitis

BROOKSBY, J. B.: Vesicular Stomatitis and Foot-and-mouth Disease Differentiation by Complement-fixation. Proc. Soc. Exper. Biol. & Med. 67:254–258, 1948.

CHOW, T. L., HANSEN, R. R., and McNUTT, S. H.: Pathology of Vesicular Stomatitis in Cattle. Proc. Am. Vet. Med. Assn., 1951, pp. 119–124.

CHOW, T. L., and McNUTT, S. H.: Pathological Changes of Experimental Vesicular Stomatitis of Swine. Am. J. Vet. Research, 14:420–424, 1953.

FIELDS, B. N., and HAWKINS, K.: Human Infection With the Virus of Vesicular Stomatitis During an Epizootic. New Eng. J. Med. 277:989–994, 1967.

FRANK, A. H., APPLEBY, A., and SEIBOLD, H. R.: Experimental Intracerebral Infection of Horses, Cattle and Sheep with the Virus of Vesicular Stomatitis. Am. J. Vet. Research, 6:28–38, 1945.

RIBELIN, W. E.: The Cytopathogenesis of Vesicular Stomatitis Virus Infection in Cattle. Am. J. Vet. Res. 19:66–73, 1958.

SEIBOLD, H. R. and SHARP, J. B., JR.: A Revised Concept of the Pathologic Changes of the Tongue in Cattle with Vesicular Stomatitis. Am. J. Vet. Res. 21:35–51, 1960.

SHAHAN, M. S., FRANK, A. H., and MOTT, L. O.: Studies on Vesicular Stomatitis with Special Reference to a Virus of Swine Origin. J. Am. Vet. Med. Assn. 108:5–19, 1946.

SRIHONGSE, S.: Vesicular Stomatitis Virus Infection in Panamanian Primates and Other Vertebrates. Amer. J. Epidem. 90:69–76, 1969.

SUDIA, W. D., FIELDS, B. N., and CALISHER, C. H.: The Isolation of Vesicular Stomatitis Virus (Indian Strain) and other Viruses From Mosquitoes in New Mexico, 1965. Amer. J. Epidem. 86:598–602, 1967.

TESH, R. B., PERALTA, P. H., and JOHNSON, K. M.: Ecologic Studies of Vesicular Stomatitis Virus. I. Prevalence of Infection Among Animals and Humans Living in an Area of Endemic VSB Activity. Amer. J. Epidem. 90:255–261, 1969.

Vesicular Exanthema

Vesicular exanthema is a viral disease of swine characterized by fever and vesicle formation in the epithelium of the snout, lips, nostrils, tongue, feet and mammary glands. It was first described in 1935, by Traum, whose observations were made on garbage-fed swine in California. The occurrence of this disease in a geographic area from which aphthous fever had been eliminated only with great economic loss, and the similarity of the symptoms and lesions of the two diseases, magnified its importance; actually, vesicular exanthema runs a mild, rapid course of about ten days and is almost never fatal. So that proper measures for control can be adopted, it is essential that it be differentiated from aphthous fever and vesicular stomatitis, which produce similar manifestations. Through slaughter and other control measures, vesicular exanthema is now believed to have been eradicated in the United States.

Lesions.—The lesions of vesicular exanthema appear sixteen to twenty-eight hours after experimental inoculation of vesicle fluid as slightly reddened areas at sites of inoculation. Abrupt rise in temperature to as high as 107° F. is accompanied or followed shortly by the appearance of small vesicles filled with clear or straw-colored fluid. The vesicles occur in the epithelium of the snout, nose, lips, gums, tongue, between digits, around the coronary band, on the ball of the foot, or even in the dew-claws. They may develop on the udder and teats of nursing sows. Vesicles sometimes coalesce. Spontaneous rupture of all vesicles occurs after a few days and is soon followed by healing. The covering of eroded areas becomes brown and dry and gradually sloughs off. After seven to ten days only slightly scarred areas are left at the sites of vesiculation. Ulceration and presumably secondary bacterial infections of lesions on the feet may cause a few of the heavier animals to remain lame for some time. The cutaneous lesions are believed to be morphologically indistinguishable from the intra-epithelial lesions of foot and mouth disease, but systemic lesions are not seen in vesicular exanthema.

Diagnosis.—The diagnosis of vesicular exanthema depends upon complement-fixation tests, animal inoculations or virus isolation and identification, which are necessary to distinguish it from foot and mouth disease (p. 395) or vesicular stomatitis (p. 398).

Vesicular Exanthema

BANKOWSKI, R. A., KEITH, H. B., STUART, E. E., and KUMMER, M.: Recovery of the Fourth Immunological Type of Vesicular Exanthema Virus in California. J. Am. Vet. Med. Assn. 125:383–384, 1954.

CRAWFORD, A. B.: Experimental Vesicular Exanthema of Swine. J. Am. Vet. Med. Assn. 90:380–395, 1937.
MADIN, S. H., and TRAUM, J.: Experimental Studies with Vesicular Exanthema of Swine. Vet. Med. 48:395–400, 1953.
TRAUM, J.: Vesicular Exanthema of Swine. J. Am. Vet. Med. Assn. 88:316–334, 1936.

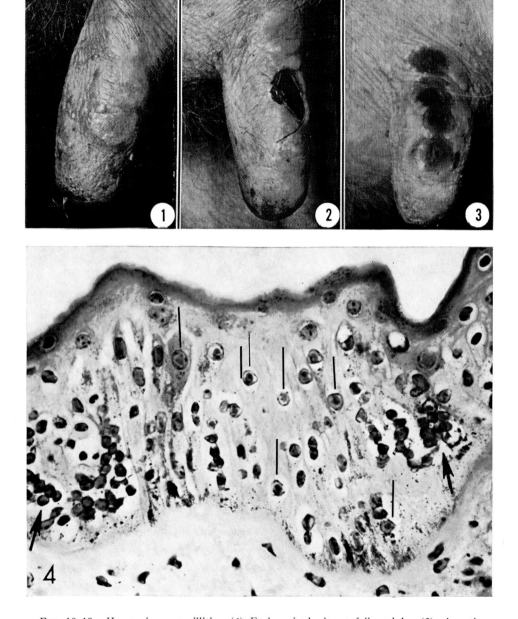

FIG. 10–18.—Herpesvirus mamillitis. (1) Early raised plaque followed by (2) ulceration, and (3) scab formation. (4) Epithelial cells of teat epithelium containing intranuclear inclusion bodies (bars). Multinucleated cells are also evident (arrows). (Courtesy Dr. W. B. Martin, Dr. I. M. Lauder and American Journal of Veterinary Research.)

BOVINE ULCERATIVE MAMILLITIS
(Bovine Herpesvirus Mamillitis)

Although recognized earlier, a specific ulcerative disease of the bovine teat caused by a herpesvirus was first reported by Martin, Martin, and Lauder (1964). The virus which is a distinct member of the herpesvirus group, is not distinguishable from the Allerton virus, a herpesvirus which was once thought to be associated with lumpy skin disease (now recognized as a poxvirus infection of cattle, p. 408).

The lesions of ulcerative mamillitis are usually confined to the teats, although lesions may spread to the skin of the udder. Beginning as local areas of erythema and edema, the lesions progress to vesicles which rupture, leaving scab-covered ulcers. Healing without visible scars generally occurs in ten to eighteen days, though lesions may persist up to three months. **Microscopically** the features resemble other localized herpesvirus induced lesions (see *Herpesvirus simplex*, *B*, and *T*, p. 380). In the epidermis there is ballooning degeneration, intercellular edema and necrosis leading to vesiculation. Multinucleated giant cells form within the epidermis. Intranuclear inclusion bodies are numerous in epithelial cells and giant cells. A cellular inflammatory response develops in the dermis.

Diagnosis.—The disease must be differentiated from cowpox (p. 403) and pseudocowpox (p. 404). Histologically the presence of giant cells and intranuclear inclusion bodies differentiates herpesvirus infections from poxvirus infections which are characterized by cytoplasmic inclusions. Viral isolation and identification allows for a definitive diagnosis.

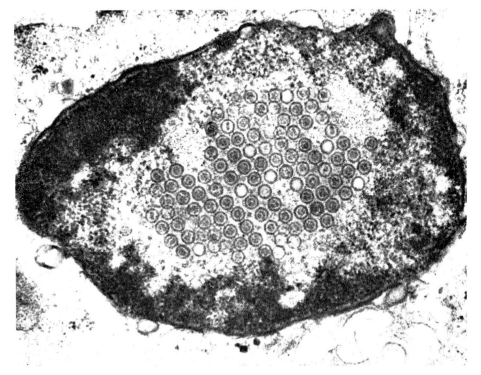

Fig. 10–19.—Herpesvirus mamillitis. Numerous viral particles form an inclusion body in an epidermal cell (× 42,000). (Courtesy Dr. W. B. Martin, Dr. I. M. Lauder and American Journal of Veterinary Research.)

Bovine Ulcerative Mamillitis

MARTIN, W. B., *et al.*: Pathogenesis of Bovine Mamillitis Virus Infection in Cattle. Am. J. Vet. Res. *30*:2151–2166, 1969.

——————: Bovine Ulcerative Mammillitis Caused by a Herpesvirus. Vet. Rec. *78*: 494–497, 1966.

——————: Characteristics of Bovine Mamillitis Virus. J. Gen. Microbiol. *45*:325–332, 1966.

MARTIN, W. B., MARTIN, B., and LAUDER, I. M.: Ulceration of Cows' Teats Caused by a Virus. Vet. Rec. *76*:15–16, 1964.

RWEYEMAMU, M. M., JOHNSON, R. H., and McCREA, M. R.: Bovine Herpes Mammillitis Virus. III. Observations on Experimental Infection. Brit. Vet. J. *124*:317–323, 1968.

RWEYEMAMU, M. M., JOHNSON, R. H., and TUTT, J. B.: Some Observations on Herpes Virus Mammillitis of Bovine Animals. Vet. Rec. *79*:810–811, 1966.

RWEYEMAMU, M. M., OSBORNE, A. D., and JOHNSON, R. H.: Observations on the Histopathology of Bovine Herpes Mammillitis. Res. Vet. Sci. *10*:203–207, 1969.

Pox in Animals

Animals and man are affected by related viral agents which cause the development of circumscribed cutaneous lesions (pocks) with or without other systemic symptoms. Generally speaking, each animal species is affected by a specific agent, but cross-infection and cross-immunization may occur. An historical example is found in the work of Jenner, who demonstrated that dairymen who had contracted a pox-like disease on their hands from contact with the teats and udders of cows affected with cowpox were immune to human smallpox (variola). Jenner applied the dried contents of cowpox lesions to scarified human skin to produce small innocuous lesions, and thus introduced the first successful method of artificial immunization (vaccination). The relationship of the numerous animal poxviruses to one another is not always clear, but the similarity of the viruses and the lesions they produce justifies their consideration as a group. Included in this section are smallpox, vaccinia, cowpox, pseudocowpox, horsepox, swinepox, sheeppox, goatpox, bovine papular stomatitis, contagious ovine ecthyma, fowlpox, rabbitpox, mousepox, monkeypox, Yaba virus infection, molluscum contagiosum, lumpy-skin disease and myxomatosis. The Shope fibroma and squirrel fibroma which are also caused by poxviruses are discussed on page 516.

Smallpox (*variola*).—This human disease is a highly contagious viral infection with a febrile onset, followed in a few days by characteristic cutaneous eruptions. Beginning as macules, these soon become papules, then vesicles and, finally, within about ten days, pustules, which undergo typical umbilication. The disease is observed in three clinical types: discrete, confluent and hemorrhagic, in order of mounting mortality. A mild form of the disease, *varioloid*, is seen in persons who have been partially immunized by vaccination. A milder form of the disease known as *alastrim* or *variola minor* is caused by an immunologically indistinguishable but less virulent strain of virus.

The cutaneous **lesion** in smallpox begins as a circumscribed zone of congestion and lymphocytic infiltration in the dermal papillæ underlying the affected epidermis. Epidermal cells swell, are isolated by extrusion of fluid between them and eventually become necrotic. Before necrosis occurs the epithelial cells contain eosinophilic cytoplasmic inclusions, **Guarnieri bodies,** composed of myriads of minute spherical granules, **Borrel** or **Paschen bodies,** believed to be the elementary visible form of the virus. As necrosis occurs in the affected epithelium, a clear vesicle forms and soon fills with neutrophils. This pustular lesion, which is from 2 to 4 mm. in diameter, appears grossly to be both elevated above the surface and embedded in the skin. The contents of the pustule become desiccated, producing an umbilicated lesion; healing follows and a deep, pitted scar is left. Hemorrhagic pneumonia, cutaneous and renal hemorrhages have been observed in fatal cases.

Vaccinia.—Vaccinia is the virus used for immunization of man against smallpox. The origin of the virus is obscure. It is classical to consider it to have been derived from cowpox, but continuous passage over many years through man, laboratory animals and tissue culture, have resulted in the "creation" of a laboratory virus which although infectious to a wide spectrum of animals, does not exist as a natural disease. Two major types of vaccinia occur, a dermatotropic strain and a neurotropic strain, properties developed by the method of propagating the virus in laboratory rabbits. The vaccinia virus, or very closely related viruses, have been isolated from spontaneous diseases in several animal species and certain of the pox diseases discussed in this section may not be distinct entities, but rather vaccinia infections. Vaccinia is known to be infectious for rabbits, mice, cattle, sheep, swine, monkeys, and man. The lesions produced in each of these species is similar to those described for smallpox.

Smallpox and Vaccinia

ARITA, I., and HENDERSON, D. A.: Smallpox and Monkeypox in Primates. Primates in Med. *3*:122–123, 1969.

DOWNIE, A. W., and DUMBELL, K. R.: Pox Viruses. Ann. Rev. Microbiol. *10*:237–252, 1956.

FENNER, F., and BURNET, F. M.: A Short Description of the Pox-Virus Group (Vaccinia and Related Viruses). Virology *4*:305–314, 1957.

FENNER, F.: The Biological Characters of Several Strains of Vaccinia, Cowpox, and Rabbitpox Viruses. Virology *5*:502–529, 1958.

GOODPASTURE, E. W., WOODRUFF, A. M., and BUDDINGH, G. J.: Vaccinal Infection of the Chorio-allantoic Membrane of the Chick Embryo. Am. J. Path. *8*:271–282, 1932.

LILLIE, R. D.: Smallpox and Vaccinia. Arch. Path. *10*:241–291, 1930.

JOKLIK, W. K.: The Poxviruses. Bacteriol. Rev. *30*:33–66, 1966.

LUM, G. S., SORIANO, F., TREJOS, A., and LLERENA, J.: Vaccinia Epizootic in El Salvador. Am. J. Trop. Med. Hyg. *16*:332–338, 1967.

NOBLE, J. JR., and RICH, J. A.: Transmission of Smallpox by Contact and by Aerosol Routes in *Macaca irus*. Bull. of World Health Org. *40*:279–286, 1969.

RHODES, A. J., and VANROOYEN, C. E.: *Textbook of Virology*. 5th Edition. Baltimore, The Williams & Wilkins Co., 1968.

WOLMAN, M.: Pathologic Findings in Hemorrhagic Smallpox (Purpura Variolosa): Report of Case with Special Reference to Feulgen's Reaction in Tissues. Am. J. Clin. Path. *21*: 1127–1138, 1951.

WOODROOFE, G. M., and FENNER, F.: Serological Relationships Within the Poxvirus Group: An Antigen Common to All Members of the Group. Virology *16*:334–341, 1962.

Cowpox.—This disease in cattle is caused by a virus closely related but distinguishable from vaccinia. The disease which is not common is mild, self-limiting, and its lesions are found only on the teats and udder. Microscopically the lesions resemble smallpox with vesiculation and cytoplasmic inclusions. The disease is spread by milking. Human infection may occur with lesions usually limited to the hands. Experimental infection can be induced in rabbits, guinea pigs, mice and monkeys. Cattle are also susceptible to vaccinia; infection usually resulting from exposure to a person recently vaccinated.

Cowpox

DOWNIE, A. W., and HADDOCK, D. W.: A Variant of Cowpox Virus. Lancet May 24, 1049–1050, 1952.
DOWNIE, A. W.: A Study of the Lesions Produced Experimentally by Cowpox Virus. J. Path. Bact. *48*:361–378, 1939.
————: The Immunological Relationship of the Virus of Spontaneous Cowpox to Vaccinia Virus. Brit. J. Exp. Path. *20*:158–176, 1939.
HESTER, H. R., BOLEY, L. E., and GRAHAM, R.: Studies on Cowpox. I. An Outbreak of Natural Cowpox and its Relation to Vaccinia. Cornell Vet. *31*:360–378, 1941.
MALTSEVA, N. N., AKATOVA-SHELUKHINA, E. M., YUMASHEVA, M. A., and MARENNIKOVA, S. S.: The Aetiology of Epizootics of Certain Smallpox Like Infections in Cattle and Methods of Differentiating Vaccinia, Cowpox and Swine Pox Viruses. J. Hyg. Epidem. Microbiol. Immunol. *10*:202–209, 1966.

Pseudocowpox.—The virus of pseudocowpox is called *paravaccinia* and is not related to vaccinia or cowpox. Paravaccinia virus is closely related to the viruses of contagious ovine ecthyma and bovine papular stomatitis. The lesions are limited to the teats and udders, appearing as red papules and vesicles. Microscopically there is proliferation of the subepithelial capillary network, vesicular degeneration of the epithelium and eosinophilic cytoplasmic inclusion bodies. Infection does not confer immunity. The disease is transmissible to man as "milkers' nodules" and oral lesions may develop in suckling calves.

Pseudocowpox

CHEVILLE, N. F., and SHEY, D. J.: Pseudocowpox in Dairy Cattle. J. Amer. Vet. Med. Assoc. *150*:855–861, 1967.
DUNCAN, A. G.: Milkers' Nodules. Canad. Med. Ass. J. *77*:339–342, 1957.
FRIEDMAN-KEEN, A. E., ROWE, S. P., and BANFIELD, W. G.: Milker's Nodules. Isolation of a Poxvirus from a Human Case. Science *140*:1335–1336, 1963.
HUCK, R. A.: A Paravaccinia Virus Isolated from Cows' Teats. Vet. Rec. *78*:503–504, 1966.
LAURENCE, B.: Cowpox in Man and Its Relationship With Milker's Nodules. Lancet *268*: 764–766, 1955.
LIEBERMANN, H.: Relationships Between Milker's Nodules, Udder Pox, Papular Stomatitis and Contagious Ecthyma. Z. arztl. Fortbildung. *61*:447–448, 1967.
NAGINGTON, J., LAUDER, T. M., and SMITH, J. S.: Bovine Papular Stomatitis, Pseudo-Cowpox and Milker's Nodules. Vet. Rec. *81*:306–313, 1967.
NAGINGTON, J., TEE, G. H., and SMITH, J. S.: Milker's Nodule Virus Infection in Dorset and Their Similarity to Orf. Nature *208*:505–507, 1965.
NEAL, E. J. E., and CALVERT, H. T.: Milkers' Nodules. Some Observations on True and False Cowpox Apropos An Outbreak in a Closed Community. Brit. J. Derm. *79*:318–324, 1967.

Horsepox.—Apparently an ancient disease of horses, horsepox is known in Europe but not in the United States. It is believed to be caused by an immunologically distinct virus, but the relationship of the horsepox virus to other poxviruses is not known. Lesions may occur on the lips, nose, oral mucosa, and genitalia. "Grease-heel" and papular dermatitis of the horse may represent other forms of horsepox.

Horsepox

ANDREWS, C., and PEREIRA, H. G.: *Viruses of Vertebrates*, 2nd Ed. Bailliere, Tindall and Cassell, London, 1967.
EBY, C. H.: A Note in the History of Horse Pox. J. Am. Vet. Med. Assn. *132*:420–422, 1958.
McINTYRE, R. W.: Virus Papular Dermatitis of the Horse. Am. J. Vet Res. *10*:229–232, 1949.

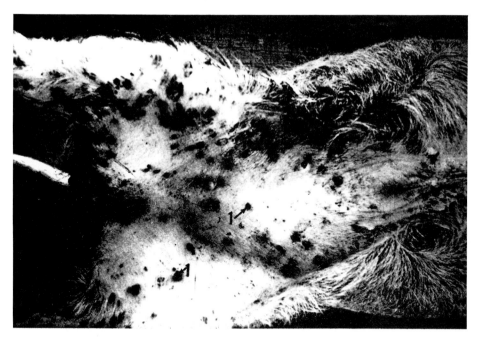

FIG. 10–20.—Swine pox, abdomen of a pig. Note hemorrhagic appearance of pox lesions (*1*).

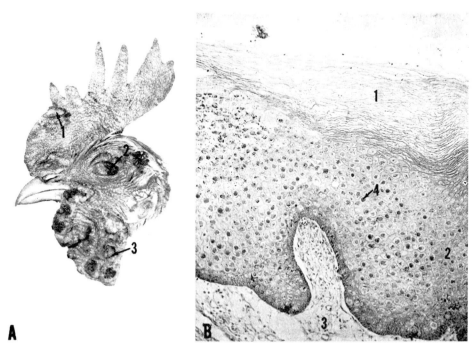

A

B

FIG. 10–21.—*A*, Fowl pox. Lesions on comb (*1*), eyelid (*2*), and wattle (*3*) of a chicken. Contributor: Dr. C. L. Davis. *B*, Canary pox. Lesions (× 100), skin of the foot of a canary. Wide layer of keratin (*1*), hyperplastic epidermis (*2*), edema in dermis (*3*), and Bollinger bodies (*4*). (Courtesy of Armed Forces Institute of Pathology.) Contributor: Dr. J. Andrade dos Santos.

Swinepox.—A common disease in the corn belt of the United States principally affects young swine. The virus of swinepox is not related to that of vaccinia and is believed to be transmitted by the swine louse, *Haematopinus suis*, though a vector is not necessary for transmission. The incubation period is five to seven days, following which erythematous areas, then papules, 4 to 5 mm. in diameter, appear. These lesions usually are limited to the underside of the body but may involve the skin generally. In the vesicular and pustular stages, the lesions often escape observation and are detected only when they have become umbilicated. Eosinophilic cytoplasmic inclusion bodies develop in epithelial cells. Swine are reported to be susceptible to vaccinia virus and this is the most common and severe form of pox in swine in Europe. True swinepox also occurs in Europe.

Swinepox

BLAKEMORE, F., and ABDUSSALAM, M.: Morphology of the Elementary Bodies and Cell Inclusions in Swine Pox. J. Comp. Path. *66*:373–377, 1956.
CHEVILLE, N. F.: The Cytopathology of Swine Pox in the Skin of Swine. Amer. J. Path. *49*:339–352, 1966.
DATT, N. S., and ORLANS, E. S.: The Immunological Relationship of the Vaccinia and Pigpox Viruses Demonstrated by Gel Diffusion. Immunology *1*:81–86, 1958.
DATT, N. S.: Comparative Studies of Pigpox and Vaccinia Viruses. II. Serological Relationship. J. Comp. Path. *74*:70–80, 1964.
KASZA, L., and GRIESEMER, R. A.: Experimental Swine Pox. Amer. J. Vet. Res. *23*:443–451, 1962.
McNUTT, S. H., MURRAY, C., and PURWIN, P.: Swine Pox. J. Am. Vet. Med. Assn. *74*:752–761, 1929.
MURRAY, C.: Swine Pox. J. Am. Vet. Med. Assn. *90*:326–330, 1937.
NAKAMATSU, M., GOGO, M., and MORITA, M.: Electron Microscopy of the Inclusion Bodies in Pigpox. Jap. J. Vet. Sci. *30*:289–297, 1968.

Sheeppox.—Only sheep are susceptible to the virus of sheeppox, however the virus is related to the viruses of goatpox and lumpy-skin disease. Sheeppox does not occur in the United States but is prevalent in North Africa, Asia, and Southern Europe. Sheeppox is a serious generalized disease, although cutaneous lesions occur in areas devoid of wool, such as the cheeks, lips and nostrils. Hemorrhages are often an aftermath of vesicle formation and later, pustules develop. Gelatinous edema of the subcutis may be observed. The disease has a tendency to become generalized, thus resembling smallpox, and mortality rates of 5 to 50 per cent have been reported.

Goatpox.—Goatpox exists in North Africa, the Middle East, and parts of Europe. The virus has a slightly longer incubation period and the disease is less severe than in sheeppox. The skin lesions are smaller than those of sheeppox and seldom are associated with hemorrhage. A viral dermatitis has been reported in India which may be related to goatpox.

Sheeppox and Goatpox

BENNETT, S. C. J., HORGAN, E. S., and MENSUR, A. H.: The Pox Disease of Sheep and Goats. J. Comp. Path. *54*:131–159, 1944.
KRISHNAN, E.: Pathogenesis of Sheeppox. Indian Vet. J. *45*:297–302, 1968.
LIKHACHEV, N. V., *et al.*: Some Studies on the Pathogenesis of Sheep Pox. Trudy Nauchno-Kontrol Inst. Vet. Preparatov. *12*:9–12, 1964. Vet. Bull. *35*:1736, 1965.
PALGOV, A. A.: Immunogenic Properties of Various Sheep Pox Virus Strains. Trudy Nauchno-Kontrol Inst. Vet. Preparatov. *12*:32–15, 1964. Vet. Bull. *35*:1735, 1965.

PLOWRIGHT, W., MacLEOD, W. G., and FERRIS, R. D.: The Pathogenesis of Sheep Pox in the Skin of Sheep. J. Comp. Path. *69*:400–413, 1959.
SEN, D. C.: Immunobiological Relationships of Goat Pox and Sheep Pox Viruses. Indian J. Med. Res. *56*:1153–1156, 1968.
SEN, K. C., and DATT, N. S.: Studies on Goat Pox Virus. 1. Host Range Pathogenicity. II. Serological Reactions. Indian J. Vet. Sci. *38*:388–393, and 394–398, 1968.
SHARMA, S. N.: Studies on Sheep and Goat Pox Viruses. Summary of Thesis, Agra Univ., 1966. Vet. Bull. *37*:4682, 1967.
VIGARIO, J. D., and FERRAZ, F. P.: Study of Sheeppox Virus Synthesis by Fluorescent Antibody Technique. Am. J. Vet. Res. *28*:809–813, 1967.

Fowl Pox (*avian pox, contagious epithelioma*).—There appear to be at least four pox viruses which affect different species of birds; those of fowl pox, canary pox, pigeon pox, and turkey pox. Although most infective for their homologous hosts, the viruses may also infect heterologous species. A great deal of experimental work has been accomplished with these agents, hence they are among the better known viruses. It was with the agent of fowl pox that Woodruff and Goodpasture (1930) demonstrated that a single elementary (Borrel) body separated from the inclusion (Bollinger) body was capable of inducing typical infection. The spontaneous lesions in chickens occur in the skin of the head, particularly the comb and wattles, or in the mucosa of the mouth or nasal passages, where a diphtheritic membrane forms. Lesions on the feet, legs and body are less common. A complete review of avian pox may be found in Biester and Schwarte (1965).

Fowl Pox
BIESTER, H. E., and SCHWARTE, L. H.: *Diseases of Poultry*, 4th Ed., Ames, Iowa, Iowa State University Press, 1965.
DANKS, W. B. C.: A Histochemical Study by Microincineration of the Inclusion Body of Fowl Pox. Amer. J. Path. *8*:711–716, 1932.
GOODPASTURE, E. W., WOODRUFF, A. M., and BUDDINGH, G. J.: Vaccinal Infection of the Chorio-allantoic Membrane of the Chick Embryo. Amer. J. Path. *8*:271–282, 1932.
WOODRUFF, C. E., and GOODPASTURE, E. W.: The Infectivity of Isolated Inclusion Bodies in Fowl Pox. Amer. J. Path. *5*:1–9, 1929.
————: Relation of Virus of Fowl Pox to Specific Cellular Inclusions in the Disease. Amer. J. Path. *6*:713–720, 1930.
WOODRUFF, C. E.: Comparison of the Lesions of Fowl Pox and Vaccinia in the Chick, with Especial Reference to the Virus Bodies. Amer. J. Path. *6*:169–173, 1930.

Mouse Pox (infectious ectromelia).—A viral disease of laboratory mice, mouse pox occurs in Europe and has, at times, been recognized in the United States. The causative agent is immunologically related to vaccinia and the disease may result in cutaneous or disseminated lesions. The clinical disease has been described as occurring in two forms, a rapidly fatal form with few or no cutaneous lesions, and a chronic form characterized by ulceration of the skin, particularly the feet, tail and snout. These are not dissimilar forms of the disease but rather represent different stages in the pathogenesis of the infection. The infection begins with a primary lesion of the skin characterized by edema, ulceration and ultimate scarring, which releases virus to the lymphatics and the blood stream enabling it to localize and multiply in the liver and spleen. Virus is released from these organs, localizes in other viscera (salivary gland, lung, pancreas, lymph nodes, Peyer's patches, small intestine, lung, kidney, urinary bladder) and in the skin. The localization in the epidermis results in secondary skin lesions characterized by a generalized papular rash which may progress to ulceration of the skin and gangrene of the extremities. If multiplication in the liver and spleen is exceptionally rapid, death may occur at this stage without premonitory clinical signs or a skin rash except for the primary lesion, which may be small, absent or overlooked. The lesions in this fulminating form of the disease are principally confined to the liver and spleen. In the liver focal areas of necrosis are randomly distributed without any lobular pattern. The splenic lesions are also characterized by focal necrosis, which affects both the lymphoid follicles and the intervening reticuloendothelial tissue. Other visceral lesions may include focal necrosis of lymph nodes, Peyer's patches, mucosa of the small intestine, lung, kidney, urinary bladder, pancreas and salivary gland. Eosinophilic, intracytoplasmic inclusion bodies may occur in all of these viscera. The primary and secondary skin lesions are characterized by spongiosis and ballooning degeneration of the epidermis, followed by necrosis and ulceration with a lymphocytic infiltration of the dermis. Eosinophilic intracytoplasmic inclusion bodies occur in the ballooned epithelial cells. During the stage of the secondary skin rash conjunctivitis and blepharitis are frequent, and ulcers may occur on the tongue and buccal mucous membranes. Mortality ranges from 50 to 100 per cent. If death does not occur in the stage of virus multiplication in the spleen and liver, recovery usually follows unless the secondary cutaneous lesions are exceptionally severe or if gangrene occurs. In recovered mice, hairless scars may be present in the skin and dense scars are usually present in the spleen.

The definitive diagnosis is based upon the demonstration of antihemagglutinins to vaccinia in the sera of convalescent mice or of cross-immunization of mice with the agents of vaccinia and mouse pox, or viral isolation and identification.

Mouse Pox

BRIODY, B. A.: The Natural History of Mousepox. *Viruses of Laboratory Rodents.* Nat. Cancer Inst. Monogr. 20:105–116, 1966.

DINGLE, J. H.: Infectious Diseases of Mice, in SNELL, G. D.: *Biology of the Laboratory Mouse*, Philadelphia, Blakiston, 1941, chap. 12, pp. 380–474.

FENNER, F.: Mousepox (Infectious Ectromelia of Mice): A Review. J. Immunol. 63: 341–373, 1949.

————: The Clinical Features and Pathogenesis of Mouse Pox (Infectious Ectromelia of Mice). J. Path. & Bact. 60:529–552, 1948.

SCHELL, K.: On the Isolation of Ectromelia Virus From the Brains of Mice From a "Normal" Mouse Colony. Lab. Anim. Care 14:506–513, 1964.

TRENTIN, J. J.: An Outbreak of Mouse Pox (Infectious Ectromelia) in the United States. I. Presumptive Diagnosis. Science 117:226–227, 1953.

TRENTIN, J. J., and BRIODY, B. A.: An Outbreak of Mouse Pox (Infectious Ectromelia) in the United States. II. Definitive Diagnosis. Science 117:227–228, 1953.

Lumpy-Skin Disease.—Lumpy-skin disease is a disease of cattle, restricted to Africa, caused by a poxvirus related to the viruses of sheeppox and goatpox. It is thought to be transmitted by insect vectors. The disease is characterized by a generalized cutaneous eruption of round, firm nodules, varying from 0.5 to 5 cm. in diameter. Nodules may also appear on oral, nasal and genital mucous membranes, and there is enlargement of the superficial lymph nodes. Mortality is generally low but may approach 10 per cent. Microscopically the nodule is characterized by the inflammatory reaction in the dermis composed of edema, perivascular collections of lymphocytes, macrophages, plasma cells and neutrophils and proliferation of fibroblasts. There is necrosis and vesicle formation in the overlying epidermis. Eosinophilic cytoplasmic inclusion bodies form in epithelial cells and macrophages. Necrosis of the entire nodule precedes healing which requires three to five weeks. Rabbits are experimentally susceptible to the virus.

Lumpy-Skin Disease

AYRE-SMITH, R. A.: The Symptoms and Clinical Diagnosis of Lumpy-Skin Disease. Vet. Rec. *72*:469–472, 1960.

MUNZ, E. K., and OWEN, N. C.: Electron Microscopic Studies on Lumpy-Skin Disease Virus Type "Neethling." Ondersterpoort. J. Vet. Res. *33*:3–8, 1966.

WEISS, K. E.: Lumpy Skin Disease. Virology Monographs *3*:109–131, 1968.

Monkey Pox. — Various species of non-human primates are naturally susceptible to three poxvirus infections; a vaccinia-related virus; Yaba virus; and a virus

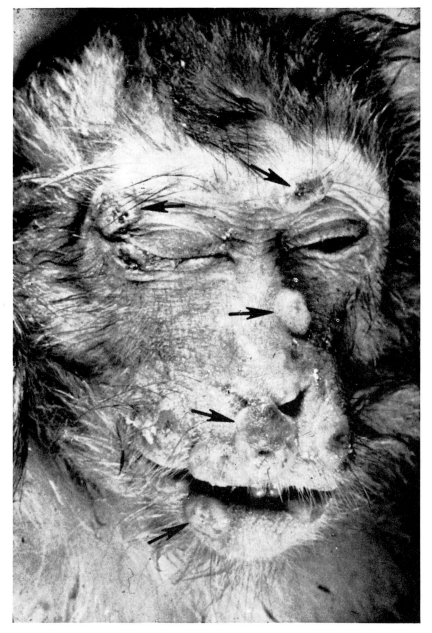

FIG. 10–22.—Monkey pox. Numerous elevated pocks on the skin of the face of a macaque infected with "Oregon" monkey pox. (Courtesy Dr. W. P. McNulty.)

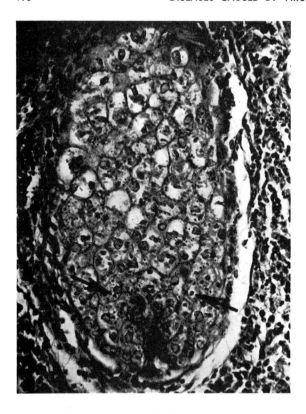

FIG. 10–23.—Oregon monkey pox. Cytoplasmic inclusion bodies (*arrows*) in epithelial cells of a hair bulb. (Courtesy Dr. W. P. Mc-Nulty.)

presently termed Yaba-like virus or Oregon virus. The vaccinia-related virus produces a pox disease resembling smallpox in its clinical and pathological manifestations in New-World monkeys, Old-World monkeys, and anthropoid apes. Lesions may occur on the skin, oral mucous membranes and be disseminated in various viscera.

The Oregon virus, which is distinct from vaccinia, produces a non-vesiculating pock with epidermal necrosis and marked hyperplasia similar to contagious ovine ecthyma. The disease has been termed benign epidermal monkey pox. Eosinophilic cytoplasmic inclusions are present in epidermal cells. The virus which is immunologically related to Yaba virus has been isolated from diseased Old-World monkeys of the genus *Macaca*. Natural infection has also been reported in humans in contact with diseased monkeys. An epidemic viral infection of man termed *tanapox* (named for the Tana River in Kenya) appears to be caused by the same virus (Downie *et al.*, 1971). The virus isolated from infected human beings has been named tanapox. Monkeys are the presumed source of infection.

Monkey Pox

CASEY, H. W., WOODRUFF, J. M., and BUTCHER, W. I.: Electron Microscopy of a Benign Epidermal Pox Disease of Rhesus Monkeys. Am. J. Path. *51*:431–446, 1967.

CHEVILLE, N., *et al.*: Cytopathic Changes in Lesions of a Pox Disease in Monkeys. Iowa State Univ. Vet. *30*:77–81, 1968. Vet. Bull. *39*:3328, 1969.

CRANDELL, R. A., CASEY, H. W., and BRUNLOW, W. B.: Studies of a Newly Recognized Poxvirus of Monkeys. J. of Infect. Dis. *119*:80–88, 1969.

DOWNIE, A. W., *et al.*: Tanapox: A New Disease Caused by a Pox Virus. Br. Med. J. *1*: 363–368, 1971.

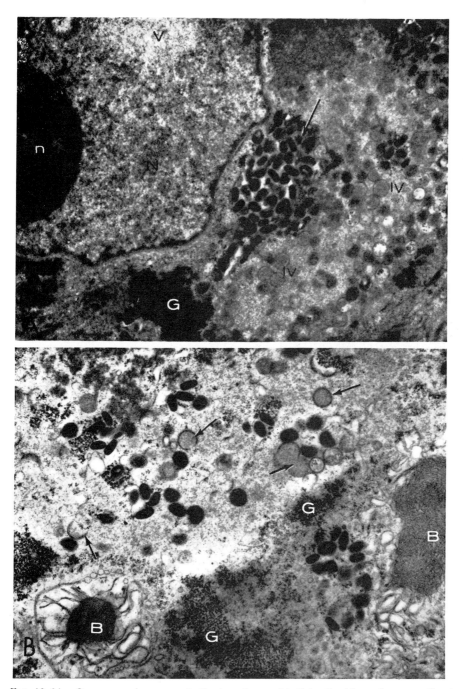

FIG. 10–24.—Oregon monkey pox. *A*, Portion of an epithelial cell with nuclear vacuolization (*V*); abundant mature viral particles (*arrow*) surrounded by immature particles (*IV*). G = glycogen, N = nucleus, n = nucleolus (× 17,000). *B*, Immature viral particles (*arrows*) and dense crystalloid bodies (*B*). G = glycogen (× 26,000). (Courtesy Dr. W. P. McNulty.)

GISPEN, R., VERLINDE, J. D., and ZWART, P.: Histopathological and Virological Studies on Monkeypox. Arch Ges. Virusforsch. *21*:205–216, 1967.

HALL, A. S., and McNULTY, W. P., JR.: A Contagious Pox Disease in Monkeys. J. Am. Vet. Med. Ass. *151*:833–838, 1967.

McCONNELL, S., et al.: Monkeypox: Experimental Infection in Chimpanzee (*Pan satyrus*) and Immunization with Vaccinia Virus. Am. J. of Vet. Res. *29*:1675–1680, 1968.

————— –: Protection of Rhesus Monkeys Against Monkeypox by Vaccinia Virus Immunization. Am. J. Vet. Res. *25*:192–195, 1964.

McNULTY, W. P., et al.: A Pox Disease in Monkeys Transmitted to Man. Arch. Derm. *97*: 286–293, 1968.

PETERS, J. C.: An Epizootic of Monkey Pox at Rotterdam Zoo. Int. Zoo Yearbook *6*: 274–275, 1966.

PRIER, J. E., et al.: Studies on a Pox Disease of Monkeys. II. Isolation of the Etiological Agent. Am. J. Vet. Res. *21*:381–384, 1960.

SAUER, R. M., et al.: Studies on a Pox Disease of Monkeys. I. Pathology. Am. J. Vet. Res. *21*:377–380, 1960.

ROUHANDEH, H., et al.: Properties of Monkey Pox Virus. Arch. Ges. Virusforsch. *20*: 363–373, 1967.

VON MAGNUS, P., ANDERSON, E. K., PETERSON, K. B.: A Pox-Like Disease in Cynomlgus Monkeys. Acta Path. Microbiol. Scand. *46*:156–176, 1959.

WENNER, H. A., et al.: Studies on Pathogenesis of Monkey Pox. III. Histopathological Lesions and Sites of Immunofluorescence. Arch. Ges. Virusforsch. *27*:179–197, 1969.

WENNER, H. A., MACASAET, F. D., and KAMITSUKA, P. S.: Monkey Pox. I. Clinical, Virologic and Immunologic Studies. Am. J. Epidem. *87*:551–566, 1968.

WENNER, H. A., et al.: Studies on Pathogenesis of Monkey Pox. II. Dose-response and Virus Dispersion. Arch. Ges. Virusforsch. *27*:166–178, 1969.

Yaba Virus Infection.

Yaba Virus Infection.—Yaba virus infection was first reported in Yaba, Nigeria. The virus which is distinct from vaccinia, produces self-limiting cutaneous "histiocytomas" composed of solid sheets of large foamy mononuclear cells which may contain eosinophilic cytoplasmic inclusion bodies. Various species of Old-World monkeys and man are susceptible to the virus.

Yaba Virus

AMBRUS, J. L., STRANDSTROM, H. V., KAWINSKI, W.: 'Spontaneous' Occurrence of Yaba Tumor in a Monkey Colony. Experimentia *25*:64–65, 1969.

AMBRUS, J. L., and STRANDSTROM, H. V.: Susceptibility of Old World Monkeys to Yaba Virus. Nature (London):*211*:876, 1966.

BEHBEHANI, A. M., et al.: Yaba Tumor Virus. I. Studies on Pathogenesis and Immunity. Proc. Soc. Exp. Biol. Med. *129*:556–561, 1968.

GRACE, J. T., and MIRAND, E. A.: Human Susceptibility to a Simian Tumor Virus. Ann. New York Acad. Sci. *108*:1123–1128, 1963.

GRACE, J. T., JR., and MIRAND, E. A.: Yaba Virus Infection in Humans. Exp. Med. Surg. *23*:213–216, 1965.

NIVAN, J. S. C., et al.: Subcutaneous Growths in Monkeys Produced by Poxvirus. J. Path. and Bact. *81*:1–14, 1961.

WOLFE, L. G., GRIESEMER, R. A., and FARRELL, R. L.: Experimental Aerosol Transmission of Yaba Virus in Monkeys. J. Nat. Cancer Inst. *41*:1175–1195, 1968.

Molluscum Contagiosum.

Molluscum Contagiosum.—Molluscum contagiosum is a disease of man caused by a distinct poxvirus. The lesions are characterized by epithelial hyperplasia and extremely large eosinophilic inclusion bodies which enlarge to eventually occupy a whole cell. A disease histologically similar has been described in chimpanzees.

Molluscum Contagiosum

DOUGLAS, J. D., et al.: Molluscum Contagiosum in Chimpanzees. J. Am. Vet. Med. Ass. *151*:901–904, 1967.

GOODPASTURE, W. E., and WOODRUFF, C. E.: Molluscum Contagiosum. Am. J. Path. *7*: 1–9, 1931.

Rabbitpox.—Outbreaks of pox have been described in rabbits caused by a virus indistinguishable from vaccinia. The disease may become generalized with necrotizing lesions in the oral mucous membranes, lungs, liver, adrenal, testicle, and lymph nodes, in addition to cutaneous pocks. The skin lesions lack the vesicular character seen in most other poxvirus infections. Inclusion bodies have not been reported.

Rabbitpox

CHRISTENSEN, L. R., BOND, E., and MATANIC, B.: "Pock-less" Rabbit Pox. Lab. Anim. Care *17*:281–296, 1967.
GREEN, H. S. N.: Rabbit Pox. I. Clinical Manifestations and Cause of the Disease. II. Pathology of the Epidemic Disease. J. Exp. Med. *60*:427–440, 441–456, 1934.

Contagious Ovine Ecthyma (Contagious Pustular Dermatitis, Infectious Labial Dermatitis, "Scabby Mouth," "Sore Mouth," "Orf").—Contagious ecthyma is an infectious poxvirus disease of sheep and goats in which vesicular or pustular lesions develop on the lips, oral mucous membranes, udder and rarely, feet. It is also transmissible to man. The virus is immunologically related to the viruses of bovine papular stomatitis and pseudocowpox. The virus also appears to be related to the virus of ulcerative dermatosis of sheep. Mild transitory pustular lesions, particularly on the forearm, characterize the human disease which has occurred after contact with infected sheep. Infection has been reproduced in sheep with material taken from such human lesions. The disease is known in the United States, Europe and Australia. Screwworm (*Cochliomyia macellaria* and *Callitroga americana*) infestation of lesions is a serious complication of this disease in southern parts of the United States. (See p. 809.)

The gross **lesions** appear as papules, vesicles, and then pustules, with necrosis and eventual sloughing of the affected areas. **Microscopically,** the lesions are sharply delimited, with the affected epidermis overlying a densely cellular dermis, richly vascular and infiltrated with leukocytes and edema. The basal epidermal layer proliferates and appears to grow downward into the dermis. The superficial layers of the epidermis undergo degenerative changes consisting of vacuolation, balloon degeneration, vesiculation and pustule formation. In lambs, the disease may be more fulminant and staphylococci are often present in the vesicles. Eosinophilic cytoplasmic inclusion bodies have been reported but they are transitory and their specificity is not established.

The **diagnosis** of contagious ecthyma is based on the characteristic lesions and isolation and identification of the virus. The disease must be differentiated from sheeppox and ulcerative dermatosis. The virus is immunologically distinct from sheeppox virus and although related, separable from the virus of ulcerative dermatosis. The absence of inclusions in ecthyma is a point of histologic differentiation, as is also the downgrowth of the basal layer of epidermis into the dermis which does not occur in sheeppox or ulcerative dermatosis. The widespread cutaneous distribution of the lesions of sheeppox and the preputial lesions of ulcerative dermatosis also aid in differential diagnosis.

Contagious Ovine Ecthyma

ABDUSSALAM, M.: Contagious Pustular Dermatitis. 2. Pathological Histology. J. Comp. Path. *67*:217–222, 1957.

——————: Contagious Pustular Dermatitis. 3. Experimental Infection (Rabbits). J. Comp. Path. 67:305–319, 1957.

——————: Contagious Pustular Dermatitis. 4. Immunological Reactions. J. Comp. Path. 68:23–35, 1958.

ABDUSSALAM, M., and COSSLETT, V. E.: Contagious Pustular Dermatitis Virus. 1. Studies on Morphology. J. Comp. Path. 67:145–156, 1957.

BOUGHTON, I. B., and HARDY, W. T.: Contagious Ecthyma (Sore Mouth) of Sheep and Goats. J. Am. Vet. Med. Assn. 85:150–178, 1934.

PARK, V. M., MACKERRAS, I. M., SUTHERLAND, A. K., and SIMMONS, G. C.: Transmission of Contagious Ecthyma from Sheep to Man. M. J. Australia 2:628–632, 1951.

THEILER, A.: Ecthyma Contagiosum of Sheep and Goats. Thirteenth and 14th Ann. Reports, Director, Vet. Ed. and Res., Union of South Africa, 1928, pp. 7–14.

WHEELER, C. E., and CAWLEY, E. P.: The Microscopic Picture of Ecthyma Contagiosum (orf) in Sheep, Rabbits, and Men. Amer. J. Path. 32:535–545, 1956.

Ulcerative Dermatosis

Ulcerative Dermatosis (Infectious Balanoposthitis, Ulcerative Vulvitis, Lip and Leg Ulceration).—Ulcerative dermatosis is a disease of sheep and goats characterized by an ulcerative dermatitis of the lips, legs, feet, prepuce and vulva. The virus is a member of the poxvirus group and is immunologically related to the virus of contagious ovine ecthyma. The lesions are poorly studied but reportedly non-specific in microscopic appearance and lack the hyperplasia of epidermis seen in contagious ecthyma.

Ulcerative Dermatitis

FLOOK, W. H.: An Outbreak of Venereal Disease Among Sheep (Ulcerative Dermatosis). J. Comp. Path. 16:374–375, 1903.

M'FADYEAN, J. A.: A Contagious Disease of the Generative Organ of Sheep. J. Comp. Path. 16:375–376, 1903.

ROBERTS, R. S., and BOLTON, J. F. A.: A Venereal Disease of Sheep. Vet. Rec. 57:686–687, 1945.

TRUEBLOOD, M. S.: Relationship of Ovine Contagious Ecthyma and Ulcerative Dermatosis. Cornell Vet. 56:521–526, 1966.

TUNNICLIFF, E. A.: Ulcerative Dermatosis of Sheep. Am. J. Vet. Res. 10:240–249, 1949.

Bovine Papular Stomatitis.—A mild disease which causes lesions in and around the mouth of young cattle has been recognized from time to time in Europe and the United States. It does not cause serious illness but in some respects simulates some features of certain important bovine diseases (aphthous fever, p. 395; vesicular stomatitis, p. 398; mucosal disease, p. 493; and viral diarrhea, p. 492). Several different names have been used to describe what may eventually prove to be a single disease entity: "pseudoaphthous stomatitis," *stomatitis papulosa bovis specifica*, "infectious ulcerative stomatitis," "proliferative stomatitis" and "esophagitis."

One viral agent has been isolated by Griesemer and Cole (1960), and the disease reproduced experimentally. This agent multiplies in tissue cultures of bovine kidney cells but does not produce any cytopathogenic effect in these cultures. Guinea pigs, weanling mice and chick embryos are apparently not susceptible. This virus may be the same as the infectious agent described by Olson and Palionis (1953) and Pritchard et al. (1958), because the diseases are similar but exact comparisons have not yet been made. The virus has recently been shown to be closely related to paravaccinia (pseudo-cowpox virus) and to share antigenic properties with the virus of contagious ecthyma. The virus is infectious for man producing erythematous papules on the hands and arms.

The disease affects young calves for the most part; clinical signs are mild and

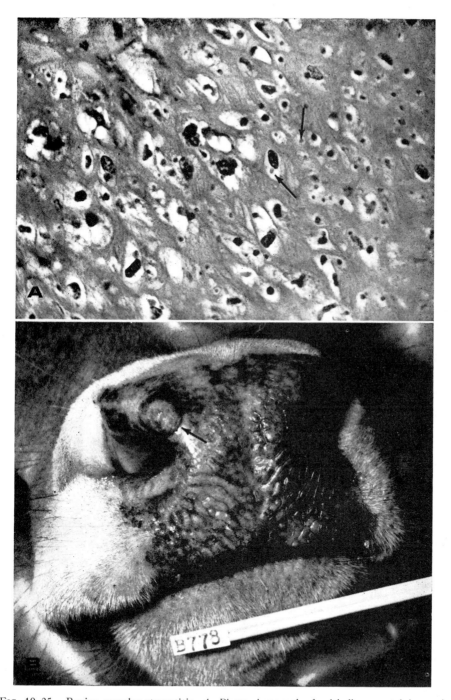

FIG. 10–25.—Bovine papular stomatitis. *A*, Photomicrograph of epithelium containing eosinophilic inclusion bodies (arrows). *B*, Muzzle of a calf with an experimentally induced papular lesion on nostril (arrow). (Courtesy of Dr. Richard A. Griesemer, Ohio State University.)

fever is not usually manifest although viremia evidently occurs. The course of the disease is prolonged—usually several weeks.

The **lesions** are found on the lips, muzzle, nostrils, gingivae, tongue and oral mucosa generally and, in sacrificed animals, in the esophagus, rumen, reticulum and omasum. The earliest lesions are recognized grossly as small hyperemic foci 2 to 4 mm. in diameter, often on the lower margin of the nostrils, occasionally on the palate or inner surface of the lips. In about a day the center of these foci become elevated from the surface to form a low convex whitish papule. At this time, the epithelium, seen microscopically, is focally hyperplastic and contains focal areas of hydropic degeneration (p. 43). These changes in the epithelium, up to 300 microns in diameter, are located for the most part in the superficial part of the *stratum spinosum*. Nuclei in these zones are often pyknotic and occasionally undergo karyorrhexis. As the disease progresses, the hydropic lesions move toward the surface and the affected epithelial cells often contain spherical cytoplasmic inclusion bodies which are up to 10 microns or more in diameter, homogenous, eosinophilic and usually only one in a cell. Congestion of the adjacent lamina propria usually gives the papular lesion a reddish or pink hue at this time. As the lesions reach the surface, they become grossly roughened and may become infiltrated by neutrophils. The thickened epithelium may become eroded, leaving an elevated ulcer. Superficial erosion of the epithelium may in some instances appear rather than ulcers. These may become filled with pyogenic granulation tissue. Confluence of lesions often occurs. Healing is usually uneventful but prolonged.

The **diagnosis** is usually based upon the mild clinical course, the gross and histologic appearance of the lesions and the isolation and identification of the virus.

Bovine Papular Stomatitis

BUTTNER, D., *et al.*: The Fine Structure of the Virions of Contagious Pustular Dermatitis and Bovine Papular Stomatitis. Arch. Ges. Virusforsch *14*:657–673, 1964.
CARSON, C. A., KERR, K. M., and GRUMBLES, L. C.: Bovine Papular Stomatitis: Experimental Transmission from Man. Am. J. Vet. Res. *29*:1783–1790, 1968.
CARSON, C. A., and KERR, K. M.: Bovine Papular Stomatitis with Apparent Transmission to Man. J. Am. Vet. Med. Assn. *151*:183–187, 1967.
GRIESEMER, R. A. and COLE, C. R.: Bovine Papular Stomatitis. I. Recognition in the United States. J. Am. Vet. M. A. *137*:404–410, 1960.
————: Bovine Papular Stomatitis. II. The Experimentally-produced Disease. Am. J. Vet. Res. *22*:473–481, 1961.
————: Bovine Papillary Stomatitis. III. Histopathology. Am. J. Vet. Res. *22*: 482–486, 1961.
MATTHIAS, D. and JAKOB, W.: Zur pathologischen Anatomie der Stomatitis papulosa infectiosa bovis. Mh. Vet. Med. *17*:265–271, 1962. (VB 4156–4162.)
OLSON, C., JR. and PALIONIS, T.: The Transmission of Proliferative Stomatitis of Cattle. J. Am. Vet. M. A. *123*:419–426, 1953.
PLOWRIGHT, W., and FERRIS, R. D.: Papular Stomatitis of Cattle in Kenya and Nigeria. Vet. Rec. *71*:718–722, 1959.
————: Papular Stomatitis of Cattle. II. Reproduction of the Disease With Culture-Passaged Virus. Vet. Rec. *71*:828–832, 1959.
PRITCHARD, W. R., CLAFLIN, R. M., GUSTAFSON, D. P., and RISTIC, M.: An Infectious Ulcerative Stomatitis of Cattle. J. Am. Vet. M. A. *132*:273–278, 1958.

Infectious Myxomatosis of Rabbits.—Infectious myxomatosis occurring spontaneously in South American rabbits was first described by Sanarelli in 1898. During the intervening years the malady has been observed in many other parts

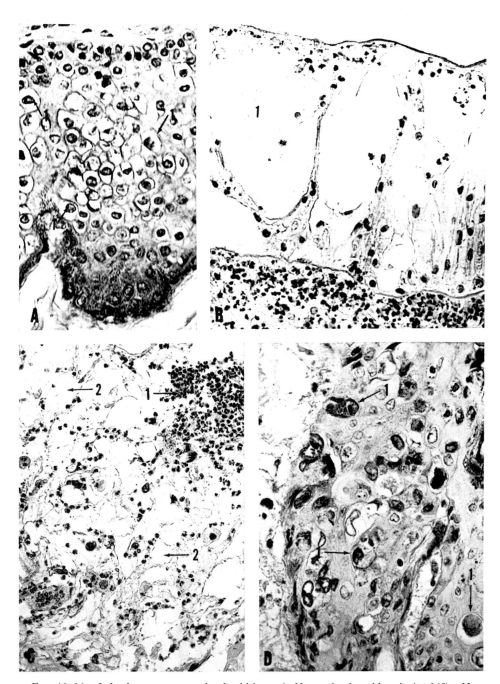

FIG. 10–26.—Infectious myxomatosis of rabbits. *A*, Hyperplastic epidermis (× 365). Note large cells with vacuoles surrounding nuclei (*1*). *B*, Large vesicle (*1*) in epidermis in a later stage (× 395). *C*, Microabscess (*1*) and edematous spaces (*2*) in dermis (× 235). *D*, Giant, distorted nuclei (*1*) in the epidermis (× 395). (Courtesy of Armed Forces Institute of Pathology.) Contributor: Dr. J. Andrade dos Santos.

of the world, where it has decimated the wild rabbits and threatened the domesticated rabbit population. In *Oryctolagus sp.* the disease is characterized by the appearance of firm, elevated nodules in the skin, particularly in the vicinity of the eyes, mouth, nose, ears and genitalia. Purulent conjunctivitis is a rather constant feature. The disease runs a rapid, highly fatal course, with death occurring a week or two after onset of symptoms.

The etiologic agent is a poxvirus which can be readily transmitted to susceptible rabbits but not to other animals. Its relation to the virus of the Shope fibroma (p. 516) is indicated by the immunity of rabbits against myxomatosis after infection with the fibroma virus. The virus exists in a natural state in wild rabbits in South America (*Sylvilagus braziliani*) and California (*Sylvilagus bachmani*) occurring as an enzootic disease characterized by local cutaneous swelling without systemic lesions or mortality. The disease is exceptionally rare in hares (*Lepus sp.*) which are naturally resistant to the virus. In the European, or common laboratory rabbit (*Oryctolagus cuniculus*), both wild and domestic, the virus produces a systemic disease with a mortality greater than 99 per cent. In Australia and probably Europe, following the deliberate introduction of the virus into wild populations of *Oryctolagus cuniculus*, attenuated strains of myxoma virus have evolved which are less virulent and result in a disease of lower mortality. Also the extreme lethality of myxomatosis has resulted in the evolution of a population of rabbits in these geographic areas with genetic resistance to the disease. Mosquitoes and fleas serve as mechanical vectors for natural transmission of the virus.

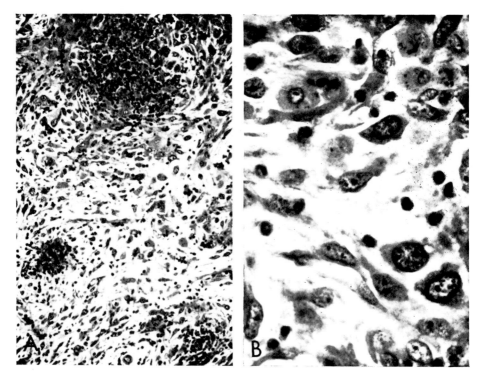

Fig. 10–27.—Infectious myxomatosis, rabbit. *A*, Replacement of a lymph node by large "myxoma" cells. *B*, Higher magnification of "myxoma" cells in a lymph node. (Tissue courtesy Dr. F. Fenner.)

The **lesions** in the skin are described by Rivers as numerous elevated, round or ovoid masses which sometimes cause the skin to appear purplish. Most of these nodules are firm and solid, but those near the genitalia may be edematous. Vesiculation of the epidermis over the lesions is grossly evident and the vesicles are replaced by crusts, if the animal survives long enough. On cut section, the consistency of the cutaneous nodules is firm and tough, the epidermis is thickened or vesiculated, and the corium and subcutis contain gelatinous material interspersed with numerous blood vessels. The nodules are sometimes attached to the underlying musculature. The lymph nodes become enlarged, solid and uniform in consistency.

Microscopically, the earliest change is increase in size and number of cells in the Malpighian layer, accompanied by the appearance of acidophilic granules which increase in number and evenutally fill the cytoplasm. Blue, rod-shaped bodies are sometimes seen among the acidophilic granules. The nuclei become swollen or vacuolated and their chromatin is fragmented. The cells undergo dissolution to form vesicles in the epidermis which subsequently coalesce into rather large bullæ. In the underlying corium, large, stellate or polygonal cells appear along with much amorphous material, many neutrophils and multinucleated cells. The nuclei of the stellate cells are swollen and contain some mitoses, and granules assumed to be ingested material are seen in the cytoplnsm. These cells are often concentrated around blood vessels, and the endothelial cells of some vessels increase in number and size.

In the lymph nodes, hyperplasia of lymphoid cells occurs; the reticulum cells in the follicles are increased in number and mixed with a few neutrophils and eosinophils. The medulla is edematous, especially around vessels, and contains collections of neutrophils, eosinophils, mononuclear cells and fibroblasts. Edema appears around small vessels, in the pulp and fibrin thrombi may be seen in the sinuses. Later many lymphocytes are lost and overgrowth of reticulo-endothelial cells interspersed with islands of neutrophils replaces most of the node. Later the reticulum may undergo cystic degeneration.

Diagnosis is based on the clinical features, along with the gross and microscopic lesions, which are characteristic of the disease. Confirmation can be obtained by transmission of the disease to susceptible rabbits or virus isolation.

Infectious Myxomatosis

FENNER, F., and RATCLIFFE, F. N.: *Myxomatosis.* Cambridge, Cambridge Univ. Press, 1965.
FENNER, F.: Myxomatosis. Brit. Med. Bull. *15*:240–245, 1959.
HURST, E. W.: Myxoma and the Shope Fibroma. I. Histology of Myxoma. Brit. J. Exp. Path. *18*:1–15, 1937.
RIVERS, T. M.: Observations on the Pathological Changes Induced by Virus Myxomatosum (Sanarelli). J. Exper. Med. *51*:965–976, 1930.
SANARELLI, G.: Das myxomatogene virus; Beitrag zum Studium der Krankheitserreger ausserhalb des Sichtbaren. Zentralbl. f. Bakt. *23*:865–873, 1898.
STEWART, F. W.: The Fundamental Pathology of Infectious Myxomatosis. Am. J. Cancer *15*:2013–2028, 1931.

Cytomegalic Inclusion Diseases

Cytomegalic inclusion diseases, which affect a variety of animal species including man, are caused by relatively host specific viruses termed cytomegaloviruses classified within the herpesvirus group. The viruses characteristically induce the formation of extremely large cells up to 40 microns in diameter which bear large intranuclear inclusion bodies. Most of the cytomegaloviruses have a particular affinity for salivary glands. The infection is most often latent or subclinical but under proper circumstances overwhelming, generalized and frequently fatal infection, can develop. Specific cytomegaloviruses have been isolated from man, guinea pigs, mice, rats, African green monkeys (*Cercopithecus aethiops*), swine (inclusion body rhinitis), ground squirrels and horses. Although viruses have not been isolated, lesions compatible with cytomegalovirus infection have been seen in the rhesus monkey (*Macaca mulatta*), cebus monkey, hamster, chimpanzee, gorilla, sheep, sand rat, and tarsier. As indicated, in most species the infection is of little concern, the principal importance lying in recognition and differential diagnosis. Therefore we will only elaborate on three cytomegalic inclusion diseases to illustrate the host virus relationships which may exist.

Cytomegalic Inclusion Disease in Man.—Based on the presence of complement fixing antibodies, cytomegalovirus infection is extremely common in man. Pathologically the infection can be divided into two forms. In the **localized** form of the disease, inclusion bearing megalocytes without associated tissue damage or inflammatory reaction are confined to the salivary gland. This is the most frequent expression of the disease in man and in various animal cytomegalovirus infection. **Generalized** cytomegalic inclusion disease, although less frequent, represents a serious and often fatal disorder. This form is most frequent in newborn children which are believed to have become infected *in utero*. Less frequently it is seen in children beyond the neonatal period. Characteristic megalo-

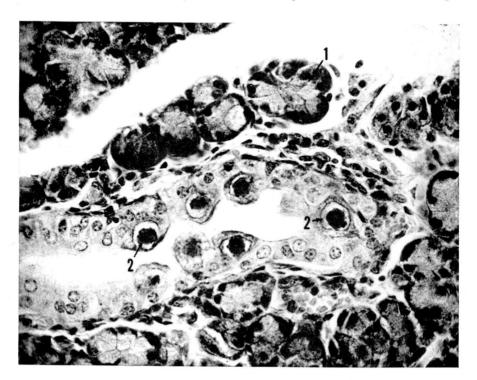

FIG. 10–28.—Salivary gland virus disease in guinea pig (× 395). Salivary acinar epithelium (*1*), intranuclear inclusions in epithelium of a duct (*2*). (Courtesy of Armed Forces Institute of Pathology.) Contributor: Major C. N. Barron.

cytes and inclusion bodies may be found in the salivary glands, kidneys, liver, lungs, adrenals, thyroids, pancreas, thymus, and brain, often associated with necrosis and cellular infiltration. Often the child is subnormal in size. Surviving children may develop hydrocephalus, microcephaly, microphthalmia and mental retardation. Generalized cytomegalic inclusion disease also occurs in adults, generally in association with neoplastic disease or immunosuppressive therapy.

Cytomegalic Inclusion Disease in Guinea Pigs.—This spontaneous viral disease of guinea pigs has been the subject of considerable investigation. The disease, although not uncommon, is usually occult and it is most frequently recognized by the finding of large eosinophilic or basophilic inclusion bodies in the nuclei of ducts of salivary glands. Experimental serial passage of the agent through young guinea pigs enhances its virulence until it can produce symptoms and even death. The infection is of interest in comparison with a cytomegalic inclusion disease of infants in which the inclusion bodies are similar. The causative agents of the human and animal disease, however, are distinct.

The intranuclear inclusions in the guinea pig disease are usually not accompanied by any specific necrosis or inflammatory changes. A salivary gland duct that otherwise appears normal may contain several enlarged epithelial nuclei with margination of chromatin and a large central mass, which is either eosino-

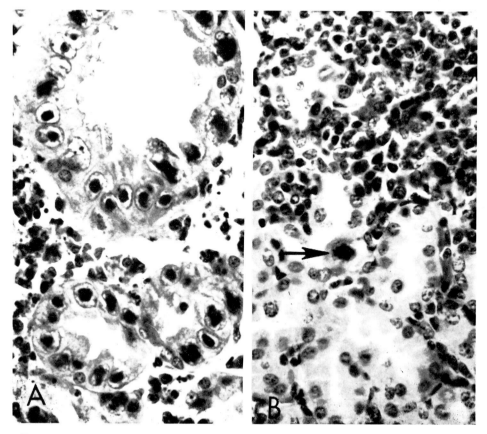

Fig. 10–29.—Inclusion body rhinitis of swine. *A*, Numerous intranuclear inclusion bodies in nasal glands. (Tissue courtesy Dr. J. R. Duncan.) *B*, Intranuclear inclusion body (*arrow*) in renal tubular epithelial cell and lymphocytic nephritis. (Courtesy Dr. D. F. Kelly.)

philic or slightly basophilic.   The inclusion body has some resemblance to that of canine hepatitis (p. 449).

The virus may disseminate through the body of the guinea pig, particularly when its virulence is enhanced by serial passage, but apparently it localizes in the submaxillary salivary gland even when introduced into the subcutis.   While the infection seldom causes much loss in colonies of laboratory animals, its presence makes the guinea pig unsuitable for research on other viruses whose lesions might be confused with those of the salivary gland virus.

Inclusion Body Rhinitis of Swine.—Inclusion body rhinitis of swine is a cytomegalovirus disease first described in Great Britain in 1955.   The disease, known to occur in Europe and the United States, principally affects two- to three-week-old piglets producing a mild catarrhal to purulent rhinitis.   Morbidity is high but the disease is of low mortality unless complicated by more serious secondary pathogens.   **Microscopically** the picture is dominated by inclusion bearing megalocytes in the glandular epithelium of the nasal cavity.   Recovery is usually uneventful.   In the experimentally induced disease, inclusion bodies are first seen ten days after infection and are usually absent by twenty-seven days.   Inclusion bearing megalocytes have also been described in the kidney and salivary gland.

Cytomegalic Inclusion Diseases

BLACK, P. H., HARTLEY, J. W., and ROWE, W. P.:   Isolation of a Cytomegalovirus from African Green Monkeys.   Proc. Soc. Exptl. Biol. & Med. *112*:601–605, 1963.

COLE, R., and KUTTNER, A. G.:   A Filterable Virus Present in the Submaxillary Glands of Guinea Pigs.   J. Exper. Med. *44*:855–873, 1926.

COWDRY, E. V., and SCOTT, G. N.:   Nuclear Inclusions Suggestive of Virus Action in the Salivary Glands of the Monkey, *Cebus fatuellus.*   Am. J. Path. *11*:647–658, 1935.

————:   Nuclear Inclusions in the Kidneys of Macacus Rhesus Monkeys.   Am. J. Path. *11*:659–668, 1935.

CRAIGHEAD, J. E., HANSHAW, J. B., and CARPENTER, C. B.:   Cytomegalovirus Infection After Renal Allotransplantation.   J. Am. Med. Assn. *201*:725–728, 1967.

DIOSI, P., BABUSCEAC, L., and DAVID, C.:   Recovery of Cytomegalovirus from the Submaxillary Glands of Ground Squirrels.   Arch. Ges. Virusforsch. *20*:383–386, 1967.

DIOSI, P., *et al.*:   Incidence of Cytomegalic Infection in Man.   Pathologia et Microbiologia *30*:453–468, 1967.

DONE, T. C.:   An "Inclusion-Body" Rhinitis of Pigs (Preliminary Report).   Vet. Rec. *67*:525–527, 1955.

DUNCAN, J. R., RAMSEY, F. K., and SWITZER, W. P.:   Electron Microscopy of Cytomegalic Inclusion Disease of Swine (Inclusion Body Rhinitis).   Am. J. Vet. Res. *26*:939–947, 1965.

DUVALL, C. P., *et al.*:   Recovery of Cytomegalovirus from Adults with Neoplastic Disease.   Ann. Int. Med. *64*:531–541, 1966.

FETTERMAN, G. H., *et al.*:   Generalized Cytomegalic Inclusion Disease of the Newborn.   Arch. Path. *86*:86–94, 1968.

GOODWIN, R. F. W., and WHITTLESTON, P.:   Inclusion-Body Rhinitis of Pigs: An Experimental Study of Some Factors That Affect the Incidence of Inclusion Bodies in the Nasal Mucosa.   Res. Vet. Sci. *8*:346–352, 1967.

HANSHAW, J. B.:   Cytomegalovirus Complement-Fixing Antibody in Microcephaly.   New Eng. J. Med. *275*:476–479, 1966.

HANSHAW, H. B.:   Cytomegaloviruses.   Virology Monographs *3*:1–23, New York, Springer-Verlag, 1968.

HARDING, J. D. J.:   Inclusion Body Rhinitis of Swine in Maryland.   Am. J. Vet. Res. *19*:907–912, 1958.

HSIUNG, G. D., *et al.*:   Characterization of a Cytomegalo-Like Virus Isolated From Spontaneously Degenerated Equine Kidney Cell Culture.   Proc. Soc. Exp. Biol. Med. *130*:80–84, 1969.

HUNT, R. D., MELENDEZ, L. V., and KING, N. W., JR.:   Cytomegalic Inclusion Disease in Sand Rats (Psammomys obesus): Histopathologic Evidence.   Am. J. Vet. Res. *28*:1190–1193, 1967.

JOHNSON, K. P.: Mouse Cytomegalovirus: Placental Infection. J. Infect. Dis. *120*:445–450, 1969.

KELLY, D. F.: Pathology of Extranasal Lesions in Experimental Inclusion Body Rhinitis of Pigs. Res. Vet. Sci. *8*:472–478, 1967.

KENDALL, O., *et al.*: Cytomegaloviruses as Common Adventitious Contaminants in Primary African Green Monkey Kidney Cell Cultures. J. Nat. Cancer Inst. *42*:489–496, 1969.

KUTTNER, A. G.: Further Studies Concerning the Filterable Virus Present in the Submaxillary Glands of Guinea Pigs. J. Exper. Med. *46*:935–956, 1927.

NAEYE, R. L.: Cytomegalic Inclusion Disease, The Fetal Disorder. Am. J. Clin. Path. *47*:738–744, 1967.

RABSON, A. S., *et al.*: Isolation and Growth of Rat Cytomegalovirus *In Vitro*. Proc. Soc. Exp. Biol. & Med. *131*:923–927, 1969.

RIFKIND, D.: Cytomegalovirus Infection after Renal Transplantation. Arch. Intern. Med. *116*:553–558, 1965.

RINKER, C. T., and McGRAW, J. P.: Cytomegalic Inclusion Disease in Childhood Leukemia. Cancer *20*:36–39, 1967.

SMITH, A. A., and McNULTY, W. P., JR.: Salivary Gland Inclusion Disease in the Tarsier. Lab. Anim. Care *19*:479–481, 1969.

VOGEL, F. S., and PINKERTON, H.: Spontaneous Salivary Gland Virus Disease in Chimpanzees. Arch. of Path. *60*:281–285, 1955.

TSUCHIYA, Y., ISSHIKI, O., and YAMADA, H.: Generalized Cytomegalovirus Infection in Gorilla. Jap. J. Med. Sci. Biol. *23*:71–73, 1970.

PNEUMOTROPIC VIRAL DISEASES

Equine Influenza

The term influenza has been in use for centuries to describe respiratory diseases of man and animals, often being used as a catch-all diagnosis for diseases of uncertain cause. Influenza should be restricted to those specific diseases caused by agents classified within the myxovirus group, as influenza viruses. Specific disease associated influenza viruses have been isolated from man, swine (p. 424), equines, and birds. Equine influenza virus was first isolated and identified in 1958 in Czechoslovakia (A/Equi 1 serotype). A second serotype (A/Equi 2) was isolated in 1963 in Miami. Both serotypes are of worldwide distribution, and cause similar syndromes which are highly infectious, spreading rapidly. Clinical signs include nasal discharge, cough, dyspnea, fever, depression and reluctance to move. The illness lasts two to seven days. The disease is rarely if ever fatal in adult horses, but death is reported in young foals. Secondary bacterial infection may complicate the disease in both adult and young animals. The pathologic effects of equine influenza virus have not been studied, however they probably mimic those of swine and human influenza viruses where the basic lesion is necrosis of respiratory epithelium.

Diagnosis.—Positive diagnosis depends on demonstrating serum neutralizing antibodies or isolation and identification of the virus. The clinical disease must be differentiated from other respiratory diseases. Equine rhinopneumonitis (p. 429) may resemble influenza but as a respiratory disease it is principally an infection of young horses. Differentiating features of equine viral arteritis (p. 498) include edema of the limbs, colic, diarrhea, conjunctivitis, and photophobia. Viral arteritis is also associated with abortion during the course or in early convalescence. Rhinovirus and parainfluenza virus infections of horses produce respiratory illnesses which are indistinguishable from influenza.

Equine Influenza

HOYLE, L.: The Influenza Viruses. Virology Monographs *4*:1–375, New York, Springer-Verlag, 1968.

McQueen, J. L., Steele, J. H., and Robinson, R. Q.: Influenza in Animals. Advances Vet. Sci. *12*:285–336, 1968.

Sinvinova, O., *et al.*: Isolation of a Virus Causing Respiratory Disease in Horses. Acta Virol. *2*:52–61, 1958.

Waddell, G. H., Teigland, M. B., and Sigel, M. M.: A New Influenza Virus Associated with Equine Respiratory Disease. J. Am. Vet. Med. Assn. *143*:587–590, 1963.

Swine Influenza

Swine influenza is an infectious respiratory disease of swine caused by a virus acting in synergy with a gram-negative bacterial organism, *Hemophilus influenzae suis*. The swine influenza virus is closely related to the viruses of human influenza; in fact, its transmission to laboratory animals (mice, ferrets) by Shope was the opening step to extensive work with similar viruses to which man is susceptible. In addition, Shope demonstrated that the swine lungworm (p. 765) can act as intermediate host and reservoir for the swine influenza virus during interenzoötic periods. The virus is introduced into susceptible pigs by lungworm larvae; infection is provoked by the presence of *H. influenzae suis*; then the disease can spread to other pigs in the herd by direct contact. Swine, ferrets and mice are susceptible to the experimental disease. There is some experimental evidence to indicate that 2 to 3 week old swine undergo severe pneumonia when inoculated with swine influenza virus during the migration of *Ascaris suum* larvae through the lungs.

Signs.—The disease principally affects young pigs; after an incubation period of twenty-four to forty-eight hours, they exhibit fever, rhinitis, cough and inappetence. These symptoms usually abate after three to five days, but in some cases transitory fever may recur within three weeks. Dyspnea associated with severe pulmonary involvement is observed in some cases, and death occurs following severe pneumonia. The mortality is usually not high (around 1 per cent) but in some outbreaks may assume serious proportions. The morbidity may approach 100 per cent.

Lesions.—The specific lesions of swine influenza are restricted to the trachea, bronchi, bronchioles, alveolar ducts and alveoli. The gross evidence of pathologic changes in these structures consists in part of mucopurulent exudate which lies over the tracheal and bronchial mucosæ and fills smaller branches of the bronchi. Plugging of these bronchi and bronchioles results in sharply demarcated prune-colored areas of atelectasis. Consolidation of lung parenchyma occurs around the bronchi, starting adjacent to their finer branches. Experimental intranasal exposure of swine to the virus alone results in atelectasis restricted to the pendant portions of the lung, especially in the cardiac, apical and intermediate lobes. The addition of *H. influenzae suis* to the inoculum produces more extensive pulmonary involvement: atelectasis extends to include the pendant portions of the diaphragmatic lobes, and peribronchial consolidation of the upper portions of all lobes occurs. Mucopurulent exudate in the bronchial system is also more extensive. Frank pneumonic consolidation and fibrinous pleuritis develop in affected animals exposed concurrently to unfavorable conditions (cold wet weather, shipping, etc.).

The microscopic changes that follow the intranasal instillation of swine influenza virus in mice, described by Dubin (1945), appear to parallel those that occur in swine. In mice, the virus produces necrosis of the lining cells of alveoli and bronchi and, to a smaller extent, those of the lower part of the trachea. Because

STENIUS, P. I.: Bovine Malignant Catarrh. A Statistical Histopathological and Experimental Study. Bull. Inst. Path. Vet. College, Helsinki, 1952.

Equine Viral Rhinopneumonitis

(Equine Virus Abortion)

A viral disease of the equine fetus, originally described in 1940 by Dimock *et al.*, under the term "equine virus abortion," has since become well established as a cause of intra-uterine death of near-term equine fetuses. It is a particular hazard in horse breeding establishments. In the same year, a filtrable virus was isolated by Jones and co-workers (1948) from young horses with a respiratory disease and was maintained for several years by serial passage through colts. This disease was responsible for a large number of deaths of horses in remount depots during World War II, usually from pneumonic complications. The disease was called equine influenza at the time, although no immunologic relationship could be demonstrated between this virus and that of swine or human influenza; furthermore, it had other characteristics quite different from those of the other influenza viruses. It is now recognized that the causative agent of rhinopneumonitis is a herpesvirus. Since the isolation of true influenza viruses from horses, with respiratory diseases, the use of the term influenza should be restricted to those diseases, and those diseases alone. The appropriate term for equine herpesvirus infection is now accepted as equine viral rhinopneumonitis.

In 1954, Doll and co-workers adapted to hamsters and chick embryos the viruses isolated by Dimock and Jones and demonstrated serologic and immunologic similarities between the two. They also showed that the virus causing the respiratory disease of young horses could produce intra-uterine death of near-term fetuses, in which the pathologic changes were characteristic of virus abortion. The lesions in fetuses dead of equine abortion and in animals with equine rhinopneumonitis also had distinct similarities, further evidence that the same etiologic agent was concerned. For this reason, equine viral abortion and equine rhinopneumonitis, although previously regarded as separate and distinct disease entities, can appropriately be considered together. The term equine viral rhinopneumonitis was first suggested by Doll for this disease complex which is now recognized to occur worldwide. Since further study on this subject is needed, future developments may cause revision of present concepts of the nature of these diseases. German workers have described a similar disease of viral etiology, but the agent has not yet been compared with those encountered in the United States. Another disease which can now be separated, on the basis of its etiology and pathology, from the clinical "influenza" group is equine viral arteritis, described by Doll *et al.* (p. 498).

Signs.—Infection of the fetus with the agent of virus abortion has some characteristic features from which a presumptive diagnosis can often be made. The disease almost exclusively affects the fetus during the eighth to the eleventh months of pregnancy, the majority of abortions being in the ninth and tenth months. The fetus is expelled from the uterus promptly after death or, in some cases, before the heart beat stops, usually with no more difficulty than is experienced in normal parturition. Complications such as retained placenta, delayed involution and postparturient metritis are seldom encountered following abortion due to this viral agent. The mare usually recovers promptly, showing little more

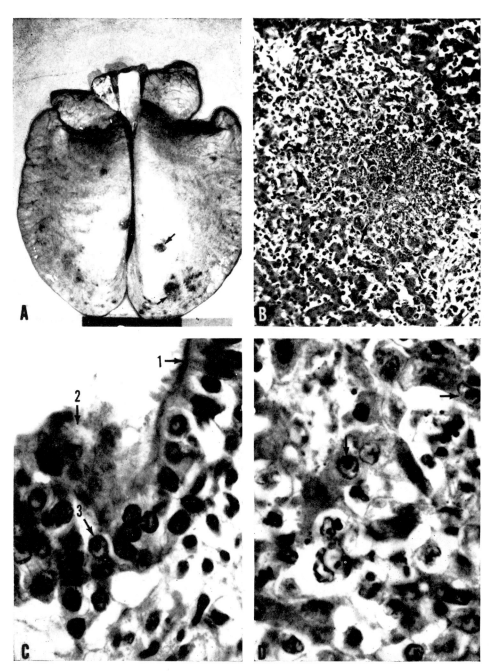

FIG. 10–30.—Equine rhinopneumonitis. *A*, Hemorrhages in pleura, lung of an aborted fetus. *B*, Focal necrosis (arrows) in liver (× 145). *C*, Erosion and proliferation of bronchiolar epithelium (× 825). Bronchiolar epithelium (*1*) which is desquamated and hyperplastic at (*2*) and contains intranuclear inclusions (*3*). *D*, Intranuclear inclusions (arrows) in liver cells (× 825). (Courtesy of Armed Forces Institute of Pathology.) Contributor: Dr. Rufus Humphrey.

than a slight transitory fever. A storm of abortions may occur, as many as 90 per cent of the pregnant mares in a band being affected, or the disease may be limited to only a small fraction of the susceptible mares.

In young horses from one to four years of age, the same virus produces a fever with abrupt onset about three days after intravenous or intranasal instillation of the virus. Slight congestion of nasal and conjunctival mucosæ occurs, the animal is somewhat depressed, and a dry, hacking cough may develop; the fever usually subsides in two to four days and the animal recovers promptly. In complicated cases observed in natural outbreaks in large groups of horses, however, severe respiratory symptoms may appear, particularly when beta hemolytic streptococci are also involved. Death may result from pneumonia or, in a few cases, from purpura hemorrhagica or streptococcal septicemia. One late sequel is damage to the left recurrent laryngeal nerve which produces paralysis of the vocal cords, causing characteristic sounds with each inspiration ("roaring").

Lesions.— In the aborted fetus, the lesions are typically found in the lungs, liver and lymph nodes, although some icteric discoloration, interlobular pulmonary edema and excess peritoneal fluid are significant gross findings. The changes in the liver, which usually is congested, may be seen grossly as tiny gray subcapsular foci, usually from 2 to 5 mm. in diameter, scattered throughout the lobules. Microscopically, these foci consist of sharply demarcated aggregations of necrotic liver cells. Liver cells surrounding the foci of necrosis very often contain small eosinophilic intranuclear inclusions (Fig. 10–30). Enlargement of the nucleus or margination of the chromatin is seldom associated with these inclusions, which usually are quite small although large enough to replace most of the internal structure of the nucleus. In the lung, interlobular edema and excessive pleural fluid are constant gross lesions. The microscopic changes in the lung consist of cellular debris in the lumen of the bronchi and bronchioles and partial or complete erosion of adjacent epithelium. In epithelial cells near the eroded areas, the nuclei contain eosinophilic inclusions like those in liver cells (Fig. 10–30). Similar intranuclear inclusions and foci of necrosis are found in the spleen and lymph nodes in many cases.

In the young adult animal, the lesions are often complicated by the effect of hemolytic streptococci and other bacteria which invade the respiratory system in association with the virus. Hemorrhagic or purulent bronchopneumonia is the most frequent finding in fatal cases but disseminated abscesses or purpura hemorrhagica (p. 1172) may also be found.

Diagnosis.— Diagnosis of this infection in an aborted equine fetus is confirmed by the demonstration of characteristic lesions with intranuclear inclusions in the lung, liver and other organs. Further confirmation may be accomplished by infection of suckling hamsters with suspensions of equine fetal tissues and demonstration of similar lesions in the liver of these animals; however, serial passage is usually necessary to adapt the virus to hamsters. Experimental intrauterine injection of mares in the ninth month of pregnancy almost invariably results in infection and abortion of the fetus, with characteristic lesions. Differential diagnosis of the respiratory form of rhinopneumonitis must include equine influenza (p. 423) and equine viral arteritis (p. 498).

Three equine herpesviruses (equine herpesvirus types 2, 3 and equine cytomegalovirus), distinct from equine rhinopneumonitis virus, have recently been reported. Their pathogenicity has not been studied, but it necessitates caution in identifying herpesvirus isolates from horses.   Recent reports have also associated a herpesvirus, believed to be distinct from equine rhinopneumonitis virus, with vulvitis and balanitis in horses.

Equine Rhinopneumonitis

DIMOCK, W. W.: The Diagnosis of Virus Abortion in Mares. J. Am. Vet. Med. Assn. *96*:665–666, 1940.

DOLL, E. R.: Intrauterine and Intrafetal Inoculations with Equine Abortion Virus in Pregnant Mares. Cornell Vet. *43*:112–121, 1953.

DOLL, E. R., RICHARDS, M. G., and WALLACE, M. E.: Adaptation of the Equine Abortion Virus to Suckling Syrian Hamsters. Cornell Vet. *43*:551–558, 1953.

————: Cultivation of the Equine Influenza Virus in Suckling Syrian Hamsters. Its Similarity to the Equine Abortion Virus. Cornell Vet. *44*:133–138, 1954.

DOLL, E. R., WALLACE, M. E., and RICHARDS, M. G.: Thermal, Hematological, and Serological Responses of Weanling Horses Following Inoculation with Equine Abortion Virus: Its Similarity to Equine Influenza. Cornell Vet. *44*:181–190, 1954.

DOLL, E. R., BRYANS, J. T., McCOLLUM, W. H., and CROWE, E. W.: Isolation of a Filterable Agent Causing Arteritis of Horses and Abortion by Mares. Its Differentiation from the Equine Abortion (Influenza) Virus. Cornell Vet. In press.

GIRARD, A., GREIG, A. S., and MITCHELL, D.: A Virus Associated With Vulvitis and Balanitis in the Horse: A Preliminary Report. Can. J. Comp. Med. *32*:603–604, 1968.

HATZIOLAS, B. C., and REAGAN, R. L.: Neurotropism of Equine Influenza-abortion Virus in Infant Experimental Animals. Am. J. Vet. Res. *21*:856–861, 1960.

JELEFF, W.: Beitrag zur fötalen Histopathologie des Virusaborts der Stute mit besonderer Berucksichtigung der Differentialdiagnose. Arch. Exp. Vet. Med. *11*:906–920, 1959.

JONES, T. C., and MAURER, F. D.: Neutralization Studies of the Viruses of Influenza A, Influenza B and Swine Influenza with Equine Influenza Convalescent Serums. Am. J. Vet. Research *3*:179–182, 1942.

JONES, T. C., and MAURER, F. D.: The Pathology of Equine Influenza. Am. J. Vet. Research *4*:15–31, 1943.

JONES, T. C. *et al.*: Transmission and Immunization Studies on Equine Influenza. Am. J. Vet. Research *9*:243–253, 1948.

JONES, T. C., DOLL, E. R., and BRYANS, J. T.: The Lesions of Equine Viral Arteritis. Cornell Vet. *47*: 52–68, 1957.

KARPAS, A.: Characterization of a New Herpes-Like Virus Isolated From Foal Kidney. Ann. Inst. Pasteur. Paris *110*:688–696, 1966.

MATUMOTO, M., ISHIZAKI, R., and SHIMIZU, T.: Serologic Survey of Equine Rhinopneumonitis Virus Infection Among Horses in Various Countries. Arch. Ges. Virusforsch. *15*:609–624, 1965.

McCOLLUM, W. H., DOLL, E. R., WILSON, J. C., and JOHNSON, C. B.: Isolation and Propagation of Equine Rhinopneumonitis Virus in Primary Monolayer Kidney Cell Cultures of Domestic Animals. Cornell Vet. *52*:164–173, 1962.

PASCOE, R. R., SPRADBROW, P. B., and BAGUST, T. J.: An Equine Genital Infection Resembling Coital Exanthema Associated with a Virus. Aust. Vet. *45*:166–170, 1969.

PLUMMER, G., BOWLING, C. P., and GOODHEART, C. R.: Comparison of Four Horse Herpesviruses. J. Virol. *4*:738–741, 1969.

SÁLYI, J.: Beitrag zur Pathohistologie des Virusabortus der Stuten. Arch. f. wissensch. u. prakt. Tierh. *77*:244–253, 1941–42.

STRAUB, M.: Histology of Catarrhal Influenzal Bronchitis and Collapse of Lung in Mice Infected with Influenza Virus. J. Path. & Bact. *50*:31–36, 1940.

WALDMAN, O., and KÖBE, K.: Der seuchenhafte infektiose Husten (infektiose Bronchitis) des Pferdes. Zentralbl. f. Bakt., pt. 1, (Orig.) *133*:49–59, 1934.

WESTERFIELD, C., and DIMOCK, W. W.: The Pathology of Equine Virus Abortion. J. Am. Vet. Med. Assn. *109*:101–111, 1946.

Chronic Murine Pneumonia

(Endemic Viral Pneumonia of the Rat, Chronic Bronchiectasis of Rats)

A chronic viral disease is a common cause of pulmonary disease in laboratory rats and frequently interferes with the use of these animals for experiments of certain types.   Mice are also susceptible but the disease is less frequent in mice. It is apparent from the work of Nelson (1946) that the etiologic agent is a filtrable virus transmitted from adult rats to suckling young, which, however may not exhibit symptoms or lesions until they reach old age. The disease can also be experimentally transmitted to young mice. The infection "smoulders" in a rat colony, rarely causing acute disease or death but eventually producing lesions which may cause symptoms or be misinterpreted as the result of some experimental procedure. This disease may occur together with "infectious catarrh" (p. 530) of rats, which is caused by *Mycoplasma pulmonis*, a "pleuropneumonia-like organism" (PPLO) and is characterized by upper respiratory and middle ear involvement, with middle ear infection (labyrinthitis) resulting in severe and characteristic clinical manifestations. Rats affected with murine pneumonia may exhibit few or no clinical signs, but in advanced cases "snuffles," roughness of the hair coat, torpor or dyspnea may be observed.

Lesions.—The lesions are limited to the lower respiratory tract. Grossly, they are discrete or disseminated, affecting one or many lobes. Discrete lesions are gray to red, indurated and somewhat depressed; lobes that are completely involved have a rubbery consistency and cobbled surface. Disseminated foci in several lobes appear as small circumscribed reddish brown masses of induration. The pleura is very rarely involved by adhesions or emphysema. The cut surface of the lung reveals cystic, dilated and thick-walled bronchi filled with mucoid material in the indurated zones. In old lesions, these bronchiectatic areas may be surrounded by a solid tissue and contain caseous exudate, thus superficially suggesting abscesses.

Microscopically, the dominant feature of full-blown lesions is the distended thick-walled bronchi which are surrounded by a heavy collar of lymphoid cells Eventually this change progresses to involve bronchioles as well. The adjacent alveolar parenchyma may be temporarily infiltrated with foamy macrophages, but in terminal stages it is collapsed (atelectatic) by the pressure of the enlarged bronchi and bronchioles. The bronchial tree is usually filled with mucus and cellular debris, but abscesses or frank pneumonic consolidation are not common. In advanced cases, lymphoid cells surround all branches of the bronchial tree; they may infiltrate the interstitial stroma diffusely, and form small collars around arterioles. Some peribronchial fibrosis may be evident around the dilated bronchi. Isolated or diffuse squamous metaplasia of the bronchial epithelium is observed in some cases.

Diagnosis.—Recognition of this disease usually depends upon discovery of the typical bronchiectasis at necropsy. The presence of the virus can be confirmed by passage of the agent to suckling mice in which it produces a frank, fatal pneumonia.

The virus of chronic murine pneumonia has not been characterized or grown in tissue culture. Viruses associated with pneumonia in rats and mice, which may or may not be related to the specific cause of chronic murine pneumonia, include grey lung virus (possibly a mycoplasma), enzootic bronchiectasis virus, mouse pneumonitis "virus" (a member of psittacosis group), pneumonia virus of mice (PVM), Sendai virus, and K virus. *Pasteurella pneumotropica* is often present in rats with chronic murine pneumonia and is considered by some to be of importance to the development of the disease.

Chronic Murine Pneumonia

BELL, D. P.: Chronic Respiratory Disease in a Caesarian-Derived and a Conventional Rat Colony. Lab. Anim. *1*:159–170, 1967.

BRENNAN, P. C., FRITZ, T. E., and FLYNN, R. J.: Murine Pneumonia: A Review of the Etiologic Agents. Lab. Anim. Care *19*:360–371, 1969.

EBBESEN, P.: Chronic Respiratory Disease in BAIB/c Mice. I. Pathology and Relation to Other Murine Lung Infections. II. Characteristics of the Disease. Am. J. Path. *53*:219–233 and 235–243, 1968.

INNES, J. R. M., McADAMS, A. J., and YEVICH, P.: Pulmonary Disease in Rats. A Survey with Comments on "Chronic Murine Pneumonia." Am. J. Path. *32*:141–159, 1956.

NELSON, J. B.: Studies in the Endemic Pneumonia of the Albino Rat. I. The Transmission of Communicable Disease to Mice from Naturally Infected Rats. II. The Nature of the Causal Agent in Experimentally Infected Mice. J. Exper. Med. *84*:7–23, 1946.

—————: Studies on Endemic Pneumonia of the Albino Rat. III. Carriage of the Virus like Agent by Young Rats and in Relation to Susceptibility. J. Exper. Med. *87*:11–19, 1948-

—————: Studies on Endemic Pneumonia of the Albino Rat. IV. Development of a Rat. Colony Free from Respiratory Infections. J. Exper. Med. *94*:377–386, 1951.

VENTURA, J., and DOMARADZKI, M.: Role of Mycoplasma Infection in the Development of Experimental Bronchiectasis in the Rat. J. Path. Bact. *93*:342–348, 1967.

Feline Viral Rhinotracheitis

Several viral agents have been isolated from cats during recent years, by the use of tissue culture techniques. Certain of these agents have been demonstrated to be etiologically related to a specific disease entity; on the other hand, some of them have not yet been clearly related to a disease entity. The viruses of panleukopenia (p. 475) and rabies (p. 351) fall in the category of agents which cause clearly recognizable disease in the cat. Among those which are not yet associated with a disease, is the agent isolated by Crandall and Madin (1960), and called "California feline isolate," even though it was recovered from cats with a non-fatal respiratory illness. The agent isolated by Fastier and called "kidney cell degenerating virus" does not appear at this writing to be related to any particular clinical disease. Several such agents have been isolated and others undoubtedly will be added to the list of such viruses if the present interest and work of virologists continue. As with other viral disease, the collaboration of virologists and pathologists in the study of such disease is often very productive.

The isolation and identification of a virus clearly related to an upper respiratory disease of cats, by Crandall and Maurer (1958), is of particular significance because the agent has been shown to be a widely disseminated disease of cats. Crandall and Maurer named this disease "feline viral rhinotracheitis," an apt designation which indicated its etiology as well as the species and anatomic structures affected. The virus has been characterized as a herpesvirus. The disease is manifest by sudden onset of sneezing and copious discharge of a mucous nasal exudate. This exudate may be seen clinging to the nostrils or on the forelegs as a result of the cat's efforts to clean its nose. Ulcerative glossitis frequently accompanies the respiratory signs. A transient fever occurs in the early stages. Young, recently weaned kittens are particularly susceptible, but the disease may affect cats of all ages. It is quite likely that this disease is responsible for much of the illness referred to as "coryza" which appears with such frequency in catteries and veterinary hospitals.

The **lesions** are confined to the nasal cavities, tongue, pharynx, larynx and trachea for the most part, only rarely involving the lungs. The virus attacks the respiratory and oral epithelium, resulting in necrosis of cells and, in early stages, the presence of intranuclear inclusions (Fig. 10–31). This change in the epithelium is followed by ulceration and attendant leukocytic infiltration. The intranuclear inclusions can also be demonstrated in tissue cultures of the virus

is expelled twenty-four to thirty-six hours after intrauterine death. Microscopically characteristic lesions in the fetus consist of focal necrosis in the liver, lymph nodes, spleen, and kidney. Intranuclear inclusion bodies may be found in each of these tissues, but they may be difficult to demonstrate owing to the extensive autolysis. Non-specific necrosis is seen in the placenta which is believed to develop subsequent to fetal death.

The pattern of IBR abortion and the fetal lesions are remarkably similar to equine rhinopneumonitis abortion in mares (p. 429). Both diseases are caused by herpes viruses.

Other Manifestations of IBR.—Experimentally IBR virus has been shown to cause mastitis characterized by focal necrosis and intranuclear inclusion bodies. The virus also causes conjunctivitis which may occur in conjunction with or independently of the respiratory disease. Encephalitis caused by IBR virus has been reported in calves in Australia and the United States. The lesions are characterized by neuronal necrosis and intranuclear inclusion bodies in neurons. Perivascular cuffing with lymphocytes and a mononuclear meningeal infiltration is also seen. In view of the neurotropism exhibited by most members of the herpesvirus group, this finding is not surprising.

Diagnosis.—A presumptive diagnosis of infectious bovine rhinotracheitis in any of its many forms can be based on characteristic clinical signs and the demonstration of necrotizing lesions containing intranuclear inclusion bodies. The diagnosis can be confirmed by isolation and characterization of the virus.

Infectious Bovine Rhinotracheitis

ABINANTI, F. R. and PLUMER, G. J.: The Isolation of Infectious Bovine Rhinotracheitis Virus from Cattle Affected with Conjunctivitis—Observations on the Experimental Infection. Am. J. Vet. Res. *22*:13–17, 1961.

BAKER, J. A., McENTEE, K., and GILLESPIE, J. H.: Effects of Infectious Bovine Rhinotracheitis-Infectious Pustular Vulvovaginitis (IBR-IPV) Virus on Newborn Calves. Cornell Vet. *50*:156–170, 1960.

BARENFUS, B., *et al.*: Isolation of Infectious Bovine Rhinotracheitis Virus from Calves with Meningoencephalitis. J. Am. Vet. Med. Assn. *143*:725–728, 1963.

CHEATHAM, W. J., CRANDELL, R. A.: Occurrence of intranuclear inclusions in tissue culture infected with virus of infectious bovine rhinotracheitis. Proc. Soc. Exptl. Biol. & Med., *96*: 536–538, 1957.

CHOW, T. L., DEEM, A. W., and JENSEN, R.: Infectious Rhinotracheitis in Cattle. II. Experimental Reproduction. Proc. U. S. Livestock San. Assn. (1955), pp. 151–167.

CHOW, T. L., PALOTAY, J. L., and DEEM, A. W.: Infectious Rhinotracheitis in Feedlot Cattle III. An Epizootiological Study in a Feedlot. J. Amer. Vet. Med. Assn. *128*:348–351, 1956.

CHOW, T. L. and DAVIS, R. W.: The Susceptibility of Mule Deer to Infectious Bovine Rhinotracheitis. Am. J. Vet. Res. *25*:518–519, 1964.

COLLIER, J. R., CHOW, T. L., BENJAMIN, M. M., and DEEM, A. W.: The Combined Effect of Infectious Bovine Rhinotracheitis Virus and *Pasteurella hemolytica* on Cattle. Am. J. Vet. Res. *21*:195–198, 1960.

CORNER, A. H., GREIG, A. S., and HILL, D. P.: A Histological Study of the Effects of the Herpesvirus of Infectious Bovine Rhinotracheitis in the Lactating Bovine Mammary Gland. Can. J. Comp. Med. Vet. Sci. *31*:320–330, 1967.

CRANDELL, R. A., CHEATHAM, W. J., and MAURER, F. D.: Infectious Bovine Rhinotracheitis —The Occurrence of Intranuclear Inclusion Bodies in Experimentally Infected Animals. Am. J. Vet. Res. *20*:505–509, 1959.

FRENCH, E. L.: A Specific Virus Encephalitis in Calves: Isolation and Characterization of the Causal Agent. Aust. Vet. J. *38*:216–221, 1962.

————: Relationship Between Infectious Bovine Rhinotracheitis (IBR) Virus and a Virus Isolated from Calves with Encephalitis. Aust. Vet. J. *38*:555–556, 1962.

GILLESPIE, J. H., McENTEE, K., KENDRICK, J. W., and WAGNER, W. C.: Comparison of Infectious Pustular Vulvovaginitis Agent with Infectious Bovine Rhinotracheitis Virus. Cornell Vet. *49*:288–297, 1959.

GILLESPIE, J. H., LEE, K. M., and BAKER, J. A.:   Infectious Bovine Rhinotracheitis. Am. J. Vet. Res. *18*:530–535, 1957.

GRIFFIN, T. P., HOWELLS, W. V., CRANDELL, R. A., and MAURER, F. D.:   Stability of the virus of infectious rhinoracheitis. Am. J. Vet. Res. *19*:990–992, 1958.

HALL, W. T. K., *et al.*:   The Pathogenesis of Encephalitis Caused by the Infectious Bovine Rhinotracheitis Virus. Aust. Vet. J. *42*:299–327, 1966.

JENSEN, R., GRINER, L. A., CHOW, T. L., and BROWN, W. W.:   Infectious rhinotracheitis in feedlot cattle. I. Pathology and symptoms. Proc. U. S. Livestock San. A. (1955):189–199.

KENDRICK, J. W., GILLESPIE, J. H., and McENTEE, K.:   Infectious Pustular Vulvovaginitis of Cattle. Cornell Vet. *48*:458–495, 1958.

KENDRICK, J. W., and STRAUB, O. C.:   Infectious Bovine Rhinotracheitis Infectious-Pustular Vulvovaginitis Virus Infection in Pregnant Cows. Am. J. Vet. Res. *28*:1269–1282, 1967.

KENNEDY, P. C., and RICHARDS, W. P. C.:   The Pathology of Abortion Caused by the Virus of Infectious Bovine Rhinotracheitis. Path. Vet. *1*:7–17, 1964.

MADIN, S. H., YORK, C. J., and McKERCHER, D. J.:   Isolation of the infectious bovine rhinotracheitis virus. Science. *124*:721–722, 1956.

McFEELY, R. A., MERRITT, A. M., and STEARLY, E. L.:   Abortion in a Dairy Herd Vaccinated for Infectious Bovine Rhinotracheitis. J. Am. Vet. Med. Assn. *153*:657–661, 1968.

McKERCHER, D. G.:   Infectious Bovine Rhinotracheitis. Adv. Vet. Sci. *5*:299–328, 1959.

McKERCHER, D. G., MOULTON, J. E., and JASPER, D. E.:   Virus and virus-like disease entities new to California. Proc. U. S. Livestock San. A. (1954).

McKERCHER, D. G., MOULTON, J. E., KENDRICK, J. W., and SAITO, J.:   Recent developments on upper respiratory disease of cattle. Proc. U. S. Livestock San. A. (1955): 151–167.

McKERCHER, D. G., MOULTON, J. E., MADIN, S. H., and KENDRICK, J. W.:   A Newly Recognized Virus Disease in Cattle. Am. J. Vet. Res. *18*:246–256, 1957.

McKERCHER, D. G., STRAUB, O. C., SAITO, J. K., and WODA, E. M.:   Comparative Studies of the Etiological Agents of Infectious Bovine Rhinotracheitis and Infectious Pustular Vulvovaginitis. Canad. J. Compar. Med. *23*: 320–328, 1959.

MILLER, N. J.:   Infectious Necrotic Rhinotracheitis of Cattle.   J. Am.Vet. Med. Assn. *126*: 463–467, 1955.

MITCHELL, D., and GREIG, A. S.:   The Incidence and Significance of Bovine Herpesvirus (Infectious Bovine Rhinotracheitis) Antibodies in the Sera of Aborting Cattle. Can. J. Comp . Med. Vet. Sci. *31*:234–238, 1967.

MOLELLO, J. A., *et al.*:   Placental Pathology. V. Placental Lesions of Cattle Experimentally Infected with Infectious Bovine Rhinotracheitis Virus. Am. J. Vet. Res. *27*:907–915, 1966.

OWEN, N. V., CHOW, T. L., and MOLELLO, J. A.:   Bovine Fetal Lesions Experimentally Produced by Infectious Bovine Rhinotracheitis Virus. Am. J. Vet. Res. *25*:1617–1626, 1964.

ROSNER, S. F.:   Infectious Bovine Rhinotracheitis: Clinical Review, Immunity and Control. J. Am. Vet. Med. Assn. *153*:1631–1638, 1968.

SATTAR, S. A., and BOHL, E. H.:   Some Studies of Infectious Bovine Rhinotracheitis (IBR) Virus Infection in Calves. Can. J. Comp. Med. *32*:587–592, 1968.

SAXEGAARD, F., and ONSTAD, O.:   Isolation and Identification of IBR IPV Virus from Cases of Vaginitis and Balanitis in Swine and from Healthy Swine. Nord. Vet. Med. *19*:54–57, 1967.

SNOWDON, W. A.:   The IBR-IPV Virus: Reaction to Infection and Intermittent Recovery of Virus from Experimentally Infected Cattle. Aust. Vet. J. *41*:135–142, 1965.

SCHWARZ, A. J. F., YORK, C. J., ZIRHEL, L. W., and ESTELA, L. A.:   Modification of Infectious Bovine Rhinotracheitis (IBR) Virus in Tissue Culture and Development of a Vaccine. Proc. Soc. Exptl. Biol. & Med. *96*:453–458, 1957.

VANKRUININGEN, H. A., and BARTHOLOMEW, R. C.:   Infectious Bovine Rhinotracheitis Diagnosed by Lesions in a Calf. J. Am. Vet. Med. Assn. *144*:1008–1012, 1964.

PANTROPIC VIRAL DISEASES

Canine Distemper

The common and serious disease of dogs known as canine distemper is caused by the filtrable virus originally described by Carré (1905) and later studied extensively by Laidlaw and Duncan (1926).   Bacterial organisms, particularly *Brucella bronchiseptica*, first isolated from fatal cases by Ferry (1911) and McGowan (1911), are now considered important secondary invaders, particularly in the presence of bronchopneumonia. The protean clinical manifestations of canine distemper have led to a great deal of confusion and difficulty, both in clinical diagnosis and experimental investigation of the disease. Many febrile diseases simulate certain of the features of canine distemper; in fact, only in recent years has clinical differentiation of such diseases as canine hepatitis and leptospirosis been possible. Not only are dogs susceptible to the virus, but also other members of the family *Canidae* (wolves, coyotes), *Mustelidae* (ferrets, mink), *Viverridae* (Binturong) and *Procyonidae* (raccoon).

Signs.—Exposure of susceptible dogs to the virus of Carré results in an acute fever which appears after seven or eight days of incubation. Within ninety-six hours the temperature usually drops rapidly to approximately normal levels where it remains until the eleventh or twelfth day, when it climbs to a second peak. This diphasic fever curve is a characteristic feature of the disease. Coryza, purulent conjunctivitis and bronchitis are manifest in varying degrees. Bronchopneumonia may occur. Very often, vesiculopustular lesions appear on the abdomen. In many cases, diarrhea leads to severe dehydration and emaciation. Nervous symptoms, characterized by chewing movements, excessive salivation, epileptiform seizures and occasionally neuromuscular tics, are prominent in some outbreaks, having been observed in 50 per cent of affected animals. Often neurological signs are not manifest until after the respiratory signs have abated. Blindness and paralysis are less frequent nervous manifestations. Hyperkeratosis of the digital pads develops in some cases. Although the disease may occur in a mild, nonfatal form, most animals with severe nervous and enteric symptoms succumb to the infection.

Considerable confusion concerning the nervous manifestations of this disease has existed and much is still to be learned, particularly about the pathogenesis of the lesions. Variants of the virus have been suggested as the causative agents in infection of the central nervous system. That such variants occur or that they are necessary to the production of the nervous symptoms, however, has never been established. Furthermore, evidence now available indicates that the virus of canine distemper can produce specific lesions of the central nervous system which develop in a high percentage of infected dogs even in the absence of clinically recognizable brain damage.

Lesions.—In the respiratory system, a purulent or catarrhal exudate may be found over the nasal and pharyngeal mucosæ. In microscopic sections, characteristic cytoplasmic and intranuclear inclusion bodies often are seen in cells associated with the exudate. These inclusions are eosinophilic when stained by hematoxylin and eosin and can be demonstrated distinctly by numerous other stains, particularly the Schorr S-3 stain. In the cytoplasm, they are round or ovoid and vary from 5 to 20 microns in diameter. They are usually homogeneous, sharply demarcated, and occasionally lie in vacuoles adjacent to the nucleus. The intranuclear inclusions, which are similar in appearance, cause only slight enlargement of the nucleus and little, if any, margination of the chromatin.

In the lung, the lesions may be manifested by a purulent bronchopneumonia in which bronchi and adjacent alveoli are filled with neutrophils, mucin and tissue debris. In early stages, the exudate may contain some blood, neutrophils and mononuclear cells. In other cases, collections of mononuclear cells lining alveolar walls or partially filling alveoli are the only evidence of infection. In some examples of this type multinucleated giant cells form in the bronchial lining, alveolar

15

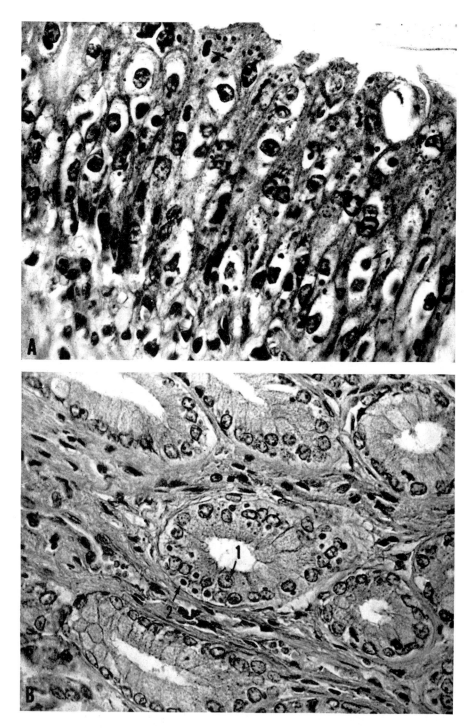

Fig. 10–33.—Canine distemper. *A*, Inclusion bodies (arrows) in cytoplasm of epithelium of urinary bladder (× 525). Contributor: Dr. C. L. Davis. *B*, Intranuclear (*1*) and cytoplasmic (*2*) inclusion bodies in gastric epithelium (× 470) (Courtesy of Armed Forces Institute of Pathology.) Contributor: Dr. E. E. Ruebush.

septa and free in alveoli. This form of giant cell pneumonia is similar to that associated with measles in man and monkeys (p. 454). Cytoplasmic and less frequent intranuclear inclusions are found in these giant cells, in other mononuclear cells and in cells of the bronchiolar and bronchial epithelium.

In the skin, particularly of the abdomen, a vesicular and pustular dermatitis may occur. The vesicles and pustules are confined to the Malpighian layer of the epidermis, but some congestion of the underlying dermis is usual and lymphocytic infiltration is occasional. Nuclear or cytoplasmic inclusion bodies may be present within epithelial cells, especially those of sebaceous glands. On the foot-pads, extensive proliferation of the keratin layer of the epidermis results in a clinically recognizable lesion which has given rise to the term "hard-pad disease." This lesion can develop in other diseases, for example, toxoplasmosis, and therefore is not descriptive of an entity.

The urinary epithelium, particularly of the renal pelvis and bladder, may show vascular congestion and microscopically demonstrable cytoplasmic or intranuclear inclusion bodies.

The stomach and intestines may contain large numbers of cytoplasmic and some intranuclear inclusions in the lining epithelium. Aside from these inclusions, few lesions are observed. In the large intestine, mucous exudate is often excessive; congestion and lymphocytic infiltration of the lamina propria may be demonstrable.

The spleen is often grossly enlarged and congested, and necrosis of lymphoid cells in the splenic follicles may be noted microscopically.

Of particular interest in the clinical diagnosis of distemper is the recent finding that cytoplasmic inclusions appear in some circulating neutrophils of affected dogs. The occurrence of these inclusions in leukocytes is good evidence that the virus is present but their absence is of little value in determining the absence of the virus. Less frequently similar inclusions are found in circulating lymphocytes. In some cases inclusion bodies can be demonstrated in conjunctival epithelium.

Distemper does not induce significant lesions in the liver, although inclusions may be present in biliary epithelium.

In the central nervous system, the canine distemper virus has an affinity for the myelinated portions of the brain and spinal cord; thus, in contrast to such infections as equine encephalomyelitis, Teschen disease, and poliomyelitis, the neurons are not primarily affected. The distribution and nature of the lesions in canine distemper, therefore, differ from those in most other viral encephalitides. The lesions of canine distemper in the nervous system were at one time thought to be due to some other agent and was often referred to as "McIntyre's Encephalitis." The lesions can be detected only by microscopic study. They vary in intensity and scope, usually in direct relation to the severity and duration of the clinical disease. The structures most constantly affected are the cerebellar peduncles (brachium pontis, brachium conjunctivum and restiform body), the anterior medullary velum, the myelinated tracts of the cerebellum, and the white columns of the spinal cord. The subcortical white matter of the cerebrum is usually spared. The lesions are characterized by rather sharply delimited areas of destruction, particularly in the myelinated tracts of the areas mentioned. Under the low power of the microscope, especially in tissue stained by Weil's method, sharply delimited holes of irregular size give the affected tracts a "spongy" appearance ("status spongiosa"). Associated with this appearance are increased numbers of microglia

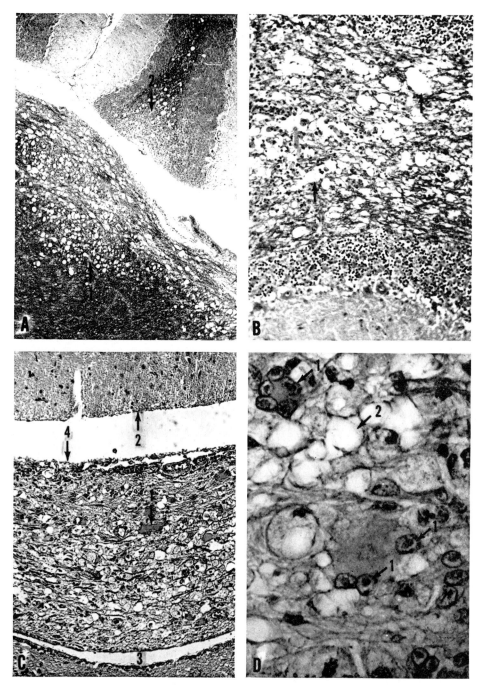

Fig. 10–34.—Canine distemper. Lesions in the central nervous system. *A*, Status spongiosus
in brachium pontis (*1*) and medullary part of folium (*2*) of cerebellum. Weil's stain (× 35).
(Courtesy of Armed Forces Institute of Pathology.) Contributor: Dr. J. R. M. Innes. *B*, Spongy
area in myelinated part of folium of cerebellum (× 150). H & E stain. Note large irregular
vacuoles (arrows) and increased numbers of cells. Contributor: Dr. C. H. Beckman. *C*, Lesion
in anterior medullary velum (× 100). H & E stain. "Gemistocytic" astrocytes (*1*) cerebellar
cortex (*2*), fourth ventricle (*3*) and artefactually detached pia mater (*4*). *D*, Higher magnification
(× 600) of *C*. Intranuclear inclusions (*1*) in gemistocytes with fused cytoplasm. Large droplets
of lipid (myelin) (*2*). (Courtesy of Armed Forces Institute of Pathology.) Contributor: Dr.
Elihu Bond.

and astrocytes and often collections of lymphocytes in the Virchow-Robin spaces around nearby vessels. Occasionally "gitter" cells are gathered around areas of necrosis in the white matter. Gemistocytic astrocytes or "gemistocytes" figure prominently in the exudate at many points. Intranuclear inclusions within "gemistocytes" and certain microglia are a characteristic feature of this lesion. In the cerebrum, the lesion is somewhat similar, but the most prominent microscopic feature is the apparent increase in the number of capillaries. This appearance may be due to proliferation of capillaries, or, more likely, to distention and congestion of blood vessels and loss of surrounding parenchyma causing the vasculature to appear more prominent. In many cases, lesions are limited to the cerebellar folia, the cerebellar peduncles, or the anterior medullary velum. In other cases, they are observed only in the anterior medullary velum, a very delicate tract lying over the roof of the fourth ventricle.

Although overshadowed by the changes in the myelinated tracts, degenerative changes also develop in neurons, apparently resulting from both primary viral invasion and retrograde lesions secondary to axon damage. There is pyknosis, chromatolysis, gliosis and neuronophagia. Rarely, cytoplasmic or nuclear inclusion bodies can be found in neurons. Neuronal necrosis may be present in the cerebral and cerebellar cortex, pontine and medullary nuclei and spinal cord. In most cases leptomeningitis, principally characterized by infiltrating lymphocytes, is present. Jubb, Saunders and Coates (1957) demonstrated that intraocular lesions occur in most cases of canine distemper. In the retina there is congestion, edema, perivascular cuffing with lymphocytes, degeneration of ganglion cells and gliosis. Neuritis of the optic nerve with demyelination and gliosis may also be present. Intranuclear inclusions are present in glia of the retina and optic nerve. The lesions lead to retinal atrophy of all layers. Swelling and proliferation of retinal pigment epithelium is also usually present.

According to one report (Crook and McNutt, 1959), inclusion bodies appeared in the bronchial epithelial cells as early as the fourth day after experimental intranasal infection of mink by means of aerosols. From the eighth to the thirty-second day inclusions were numerous and large. Inclusions appeared a little later in R.E. cells of spleen, epithelium of intrahepatic bile ducts, of bladder, renal pelvis, and intestine. Necrosis of lymphatic nodules of spleen, induced by pyknosis and karyolysis of individual cells appeared almost simultaneously. Lesions in ferrets were similar.

Diagnosis.—Post-mortem diagnosis can be based upon a history of the typical clinical disease and the demonstration of characteristic lesions and cytoplasmic and intranuclear viral inclusions. Isolation of the virus is difficult but possible when susceptible puppies or ferrets are used. Some strains do not grow well in tissue culture. If adaptable to tissue culture, the cytopathic effects include the formation of giant cells and inclusion bodies. Positive identification of the virus should be accomplished by neutralization or cross-immunization studies. The disease can be differentiated from canine hepatitis by the predilection of the virus of the latter disease for parenchymal cells of the liver and endothelium, where it produces typical margination of chromatin and large, rather basophilic intranuclear inclusions. The post-mortem diagnosis of canine distemper should not be made after examination of only one affected organ, but upon careful microscopic study of all organs, including the brain. During life, clinical diagnosis can be confirmed by finding typical inclusion bodies in smears of cells of the respiratory epithelium or peripheral blood. Unfortunately, these inclusions are not present in all cases, hence their absence does not preclude the diagnosis of distemper. A fluorescence antibody technique recently introduced offers an excellent method for the demonstration of the virus in tissue smears and sections. In dogs, toxoplasmosis often occurs in association with canine distemper. Lesions of both diseases should be sought if evidence of either infection is apparent.

Relationship Between Canine Distemper, Rinderpest and Measles.—Based on pathologic similarities, a relationship between canine distemper and measles was first suggested by Pinkerton, Smiley and Anderson (1945). Subsequently an immunologic relationship was demonstrated between the viruses of canine distemper and measles and the viruses of canine distemper and rinderpest. The viruses of these three diseases and the pathological processes are remarkably similar. As pointed out by Imagawa (1968), the main differences among measles, canine distemper and rinderpest viruses are indicated by their natural hosts: measles virus causing natural disease in man and monkeys; canine distemper virus causing natural disease in *Canidae* (dog, wolf, fox), *Mustelidae* (weasel, ferret, mink), and *Procyonidae* (raccoon), and rinderpest virus causing natural disease in species of the order *Artiodactyla* (cattle, water buffalo, camel, goats, sheep). The viruses which are morphologically and chemically similar are classified as paramyxoviruses. That they are immunologically related is clearly demonstrated with cross-immunity studies. Measles virus will protect dogs against distemper. Distemper virus provides limited protection against measles. Rinderpest virus protects dogs against distemper but distemper virus may or may not protect cattle against rinderpest. Measles virus can protect rabbits from rinderpest, however cattle are not protected against rinderpest by measles virus. Also hyperimmune sera from natural hosts to each agent neutralizes heterologous virus to some degree. Pathologically all three viruses produce multinucleated giant cells and both intranuclear and cytoplasmic eosinophilic inclusion bodies. A skin rash common to measles, may also develop in distemper and rinderpest and demyelinating encephalitis which is common in distemper, is occasionally seen in measles, and rarely in rinderpest. When adapted to experimental animals such as suckling mice, the pathological processes induced by the three viruses become indistinguishable.

Canine Distemper

APPEL, M. J. G.: Pathogenesis of Canine Distemper. Am. J. Vet. Res. *30*:1167–1182, 1969.
BROADHURST, J., MacLEAN, M. E., and SAURINO, V.: Nasal Inclusion Bodies in Dog Distemper. Cornell Vet. *28*:9–15, 1938.
BURKHART, R. L., POPPENSIEK, G. C., and ZINK, A.: A Study of Canine Encephalitis, with Special Reference to Clinical, Bacteriological and Postmortem Findings. Vet. Med. *45*:157–162, 1950.
BUSSELL, R. H., and KARSON, D. T.: I. Canine Distemper Virus in Ferret, Dog, and Bovine Kidney Cell Cultures. II. Canine Distemper Virus in Primary and Continuous Cell Lines of Human and Monkey Origin. Arch. Ges Virusforsch. *17*:163–182 and 183–202, 1965.
CABASSO, V. J.: Canine Distemper and Hardpad Disease. Vet. Med. *47*:417–423, 1952.
CABASSO, V. J., STEBBINS, M. R., and COX, H. R.: Experimental Canine Distemper Encephalitis and Immunization of Puppies Against It. Cornell Vet. *44*:153–167, 1954.
CARRÉ, H.: Sur la maladie des jeunes chiens. Compt. rend. Acad. d. sc. *140*:689–690, 1905.
CELLO, R. M., MOULTON, J. E., and McFARLAND, S.: The occurrence of inclusion bodies in the Circulating Neutrophils of Dogs with Canine Distemper. Cornell Vet. *49*:127–146, 1959.
COFFIN, D. L. and LIU, CHIEN: Studies on Canine Distemper Infection by Smears of Fluorescein-labeled Antibody. Virology *3*:132–145, 1947.

CORNWELL, H. J. C., *et al.*: Studies in Experimental Canine Distemper. II. Virology, Inclusion Body Studies and Haematology. J. Comp. Path. & Ther. *75*:19–34, 1965.

CORNWELL, H. J. C., *et al.*: Studies in Experimental Canine Distemper. I. Clinico-Pathological Findings. J. Comp. Path. Ther. *75*:3–17, 1965.

CROOK, E., and McNUTT, S. H.: Experimental Distemper in Mink and Ferrets. II. Appearance and Significance of Histopathological Changes. Am. J. Vet. Res. *20*:378–383, 1959.

DE MONBREUN, W. A.: Histopathology of Natural and Experimental Canine Distemper. Am. J. Path. *13*:187–212, 1937.

FERRY, N. S.: Etiology of Canine Distemper. J. Infect. Dis. *8*:399–420, 1911.

FISCHER, K.: Einschlusskörperchen bei Hunden mit Staupé Enzephalitis und Anderen Erkrankungen des Zentralnervensystems. Path. Vet. *2*:380–410, 1965.

GIBSON, J. P., GRIESEMER, R. A., and KOESTNER, A.: Experimental Distemper in the Gnotobiotic Dog. Path. Vet. *2*:1–19, 1965.

GILLESPIE, J. H.: Some Research Contributions on Canine Distemper. J. Am. Vet. Med. Assn. *132*:534–537, 1958.

GREENE, R. G., and EVANS, C. A.: A Comparative Study of Distemper Inclusions. Am. J. Hyg. *29*:73–87, 1939.

HURST, E. W., COOKE, B. T., and MELVIN, P.: Nervous Distemper in Dogs. A Pathological and Experimental Study with Some References to Demyelinating Diseases in General. Australian J. Exper. Biol. & M. Sc. *21*:115–126, 1943.

IMAGAWA, D. T.: Relationships Among Measles, Canine Distemper and Rinderpest Viruses. Prog. Med. Virol. *10*:160–193, 1968.

JUBB, K. B., SAUNDERS, L. Z., and COATES, H. V.: The Intraocular Lesions of Canine Distemper. J. Comp. Path. & Ther. *67*:21–29, 1957.

KING, L. S.: Disseminated Encephalomyelitis of the Dog. Arch. Path. *28*:151–162, 1939.

KOPROWSKI, H. *et al.*: A Study of Canine Encephalitis. Am. J. Hyg. *51*:63–75, 1950.

KRIESEL, H. R.: A Comparative Study of the Manifestations and Histopathology of Canine Distemper and Experimental Fox Encephalitis Infection in Dogs. Cornell Vet. *28*:324–330, 1938.

LAIDLAW, P. P., and DUNKIN, G. W.: Studies in Dog Distemper: III. The Nature of the Virus. J. Comp. Path. & Therap. *39*:222–230, 1926.

LENTZ, O.: Über spezifische Veränderungen an den Ganglienzellen wut—und staupekranker Tiere. Ein Beitrag zu unseren Kenntnissen über die Bedeutung und Entstehung der Negrischen Körperchen. Ztschr. f. Hyg. u. Infectionskr. *62*:63–94, 1908–1909.

MacINTYRE, A. B., TREVAN, D. J., and MONTGOMERIE, R. F.: Observations on Canine Encephalitis. Vet. Record *60*:635–648, 1948.

McGOWAN, J. P.: Some Observations on a Laboratory Epidemic Principally Among Dogs and Cats, in Which the Animals Affected Presented the Symptoms of the Disease Called Distemper." J. Path. & Bact. *15*:372–426, 1911.

PAGE, W. G., and GREEN, R. G.: An Improved Diagnostic Stain for Distemper Inclusions. Cornell Vet. *32*:265–268, 1942.

PERDRAU, J. R., and PUGH, L. P.: The Pathology of Disseminated Encephalomyelitis of the Dog (The "Nervous Form of Canine Distemper"). J. Path. & Bact. *33*:79–91, 1930.

PINKERTON, H., SMILEY, W. L., and ANDERSON, W. A. D.: Giant Cell Pneumonia with Inclusions. A Lesion Common to Hecht's Disease, Distemper and Measles. Am. J. Path. *21*:1–23, 1945.

RIBELIN, W. E.: The Incidence of Distemper in Canine Encephalitis Cases. Am. J. Vet. Research *14*:96–104, 1953.

WARREN, J.: The Relationships of the Viruses of Measles, Canine Distemper and Rinderpest. Adv. Virus Res. *7*:27–60, 1960.

WHITTEM, J. H., and BLOOD, D. C.: Canine Encephalitis, Pathological and Clinical Observations. Australian Vet. J. *26*:73–83, 1950.

WISNICKY, W., and WIPF, L.: Significance of Inclusion Bodies of Distemper. Am. J. Vet. Research *3*:285–288, 1942.

Infectious Canine Hepatitis

(Hepatitis Contagiosa Canis)

Although certain lesions of infectious canine hepatitis have been recognized for many years, its clinical features, its etiology and its actual existence as a separate disease were not established until the classic report of Rubarth appeared in 1947. The disease has since been recognized in many parts of the world and it is now possible to differentiate it from other diseases such as canine distemper. Rubarth pointed out that fox encephalitis virus, shown by Green to be infective for dogs, undoubtedly was identical to the virus of canine hepatitis. This has since been confirmed.

Signs.—Canine hepatitis principally affects young dogs. The infection is very common, but most often it goes unnoticed or is inapparent. When clinical disease is evident its course is rather variable but frequently peracute, with the first symptoms manifested only a few hours before death. More regularly, however, symptoms are apparent for several days before death or recovery occurs. The disease starts with apathy, followed by anorexia and, in many cases, intense thirst. Severe, disfiguring subcutaneous edema of the head, neck and ventral aspects of the trunk is a striking but rare manifestation. Vomiting and diarrhea, the latter with hemorrhage, are rather common symptoms, and abdominal pain is often expressed by moaning sounds. With onset the temperature is elevated, but it may fall abruptly to subnormal levels as death approaches. Symptoms referable to the central nervous system are uncommon and, when seen, take the form of clonic spasms of the extremities and neck, paralysis of the hind quarters, or, in a rare case, extreme agitation. The mucous membranes usually appear anemic, sometimes slightly icteric, but rarely deeply jaundiced. Petechiae may occur on the anemic membranes, particularly those of the gingiva. Generally the tonsils are reddened and swollen, with the result that tonsillitis is often the initial diagnosis. Copious lacrimation with hyperemic conjunctivae is rather common. In an occasional animal, diffuse, opaque cloudiness in the cornea of one eye is associated with a decrease in the visual acuity of that eye, its extent depending on the severity of the lesion. This corneal cloudiness disappears spontaneously if the animal recovers. In the urine, albumin may be present in significant amounts, but usually that is its only abnormality. Other clinicopathologic findings include: neutropenia and lymphopenia during the course with a lymphocytosis during recovery; prolonged bleeding and coagulation times; and elevation of SGOT and SGPT.

Lesions.—The virus of canine hepatitis has an obligate affinity for parenchymal and Kupffer cells of the liver and endothelial cells generally. Its lethal effect on cells of these types produces most of the lesions, both gross and microscopic, that can be attributed to the disease. Specific intranuclear inclusions, necrosis of cells and, in the case of endothelial cells, proliferation and increased vascular permeability with hemorrhage, are the pathologic evidence of this virus's affinity for these specific tissues. The only exceptions are seen in bone marrow and spleen where intranuclear inclusions may be observed in cells which, although difficult to identify, are probably reticulo-endothelial. In experimentally infected animals, it is possible to produce intranuclear inclusions in other tissues. For example, in animals injected via the cisterna magna with fox encephalitis virus, intranuclear inclusions develop in ependymal cells; in foxes inoculated by the testicular route, in interstitial cells; in dogs inoculated intraperitoneally, in the lining cells of the peritoneum. The gross appearance of the lesions is not diagnostic, for petechiæ in any location are the most common manifestation. The liver and spleen are usually congested and somewhat enlarged, and the gallbladder wall is edematous and thickened.

The liver is enlarged and usually contains an increased amount of blood, which can be detected both grossly and microscopically. In addition to congestion of myelin and occasional collections of glial cells are noted adjacent to affected vessels. These appear to be secondary to interference with circulation.

Carmichael (1964, 1965) has demonstrated that the ocular lesions which develop in dogs recovering from canine hepatitis are the result of an Arthus-type hypersensitivity reaction. Persistent virus within ocular tissues during the antibody response to the infection provides the proper prerequisites for an Arthus reaction. The principal lesion consists of iridocyclitis characterized by hyperemia, edema, and infiltration of plasma cells, neutrophils and lymphocytes. The cornea is edematous and infiltrated with neutrophils, lymphocytes and macrophages. Inclusion bodies are not present, although during the acute stages of the disease (prior to the hypersensitivity reaction) they may be numerous in the ciliary body and iris.

Ultrastructural studies have demonstrated that the inclusion bodies of infectious canine hepatitis contain viral particles, but that the bulk of the inclusion body is composed of finely granular electron-dense material. Degenerative changes develop in both the nucleus and cytoplasm of infected cells but no specific ultrastructural lesions, other than the presence of the virus, are present.

Diagnosis.—The diagnosis in the living animal is difficult because of the nonspecific nature of the symptoms. Microscopic demonstration of focal necrosis and intranuclear inclusions in surgically ablated tonsils or liver biopsy specimens is sufficient to confirm a presumptive clinical diagnosis. At necropsy, the diagnosis is not a problem. It is established by the demonstration of typical lesions associated with characteristic intranuclear inclusions. Fluorescent antibody techniques and viral isolation in tissue culture can be employed if necessary. This disease may occur in association with others, such as canine distemper or leptospirosis, hence may present a difficult but not insoluble diagnostic problem.

Infectious Canine Hepatitis

CARMICHAEL, L. E.: The Pathogenesis of Ocular Lesions of Infectious Canine Hepatitis. Path. Vet. *1*:73–95, 1964.
————: The Pathogenesis of Ocular Lesions of Infectious Canine Hepatitis. II. Experimental Ocular Hypersensitivity Produced by the Virus. Pathologia Vet. *2*:344–359, 1965.
COFFIN, D. L.: The Pathology of So-called Acute Tonsillitis of Dogs in Relation to Contagious Canine Hepatitis (Rubarth). J. Am. Vet. Med. Assn. *112*:355–362, 1948.
COFFIN, D. L., and CABASSO, V. J.: The Blood and Urine Findings in Infectious Canine Hepatitis. Am. J. Vet. Research *14*:254–259, 1953.
COFFIN, D. L., COONS, A. H., and CABASSO, V. J.: A Histological Study of Infectious Canine Hepatitis by Means of Fluorescent Antibody. J. Exper. Med. *98*:13–20, 1953.
CORREA, W. M.: Notas Preliminares sobré Hepatita a Virus dos Marrecos no Brasil. Rev. Fac. Med. Vet., Sao Paulo. *6*:43–52, 1957.
FUJIMOTO, Y.: Studies on Infectious Canine Hepatitis. I. Histopathological Studies on Spontaneous Cases. Jap. J. Vet. Res. *5*:51–70, 1957.
GIVAN, K. F., and JEZEQUEL, A.-M.: Infectious Canine Hepatitis: A Virologic and Ultrastructural Study. Lab. Invest. *20*:36–45, 1969.
GREEN, R. G., and DEWEY, E. T.: Fox Encephalitis and Canine Distemper. Proc. Soc. Exper. Biol. & Med. *27*:129–130, 1929.
GREEN, R. G., KATTER, M. S., SHILLINGER, J. E., and HANSON, K. B.: Epizoötic Fox Encephalitis. IV. The Intranuclear Inclusions. Am. J. Hyg. *18*:462–481, 1933.
GREEN, R. G., and SHILLINGER, J. E.: Epizoötic Fox Encephalitis. VI. A Description of the Experimental Infection in Dogs. Am. J. Hyg. *19*:362–391, 1934.
HUNT, R. D. *et al.*: A Histochemical Comparison of the Inclusion Bodies of Canine Distemper and Infectious Canine Hepatitis. Amer. J. Vet. Res. *24*:1248–1255, 1963. (VB 1343–64.)

INNES, J. R. M.: Hepatitis Contagiosa Canis (Rubarth) in Great Britain. Vet. Record 61:173–175, 1949.
LARIN, N. M.: Epidemiological Studies of Canine Virus Hepatitis (Rubarth's Disease). Vet. Res. 70:295–297, 1958.
MOULTON, J. E., and ZEE, Y. C.: Release of Infectious Canine Hepatitis Virus. Am. J. of Vet. Res. 30:2051–2065, 1969.
POPPENSIEK, G. C., and BAKER, J. A.: Persistence of Virus in Urine as Factor in Spread of Infectious Hepatitis in Dogs. Proc. Soc. Exper. Biol. & Med. 77:279–281, 1951.
RUBARTH, S.: An Acute Virus Disease with Liver Lesions in Dogs (Hepatitis Contagiosa Canis). A Pathologico-anatomical and Etiological Investigation. Acta. path. et microbiol. Scandinav. (Supp.) 69, 1947.
SAUNDERS, L. Z.: Jubb, K. V., and JONES, L. D.: The Intraocular Lesions of Hog Cholera. J. Comp. Path. 68:375–379, 1958.
SEIBOLD, H. R., and GREEN, J. E.: Virus-type Inclusions in the Epithelium of the Canine Renal Medulla. J. Am. Vet. Med. Assn. 125:385–386, 1954.
WRIGHT, N. G.: Experimental Infectious Canine Hepatitis. IV. Histological and Immuno-fluorescence Studies of the Kidney. J. Comp. Path. 77:153–158, 1967.

MEASLES

(Rubeola, Monkey Intranuclear Inclusion Agent—MINIA)

Measles is a highly infectious exanthematous viral disease of man, principally children. The virus and its pathologic effects are closely related to canine distemper and rinderpest. The relationships of these three agents are discussed on page 446. In addition to the characteristic exanthematous rash, measles infection in man may result in primary giant cell pneumonia and encephalomyelitis. Secondary bronchopneumonia is an important complication. Microscopically the rash is characterized by vesiculation and necrosis of epithelial cells with an associated inflammatory response in the dermis. Epithelial cells may contain intranuclear inclusion bodies and multinucleated giant cells are often present. The most characteristic pathologic feature is the Warthin-Finkeldly lymphoid giant cell which is found in lymph nodes, spleen, Peyer's patches, appendix, and tonsils. These cells contain up to 100 small, deeply basophilic nuclei which only rarely bear inclusions. Primary pneumonia is also characterized by giant cells, but here the cells have fewer/more leptochromatic nuclei, and both intranuclear and cytoplasmic eosinophilic inclusion bodies are often present. In measles encephalomyelitis there is congestion, hemorrhage, perivascular cuffing and demyelination.

Measles is also known to be infectious for several species of monkeys including rhesus (*Macaca mulatta*), cynomolgous (*M. fascicularis*), Taiwan macaque (*M. cyclopis*), baboons (*Papio spp.*), African green (*Cercopithecus aethiops*) and marmosets (*Saguinus sp.*). Although measles is rare in their native habitats, few rhesus monkeys escape infection once they are brought into captivity. Clinical disease is rarely recorded, either because it is mild or initial infection occurred enroute to the laboratory. However, monkeys may exhibit conjunctivitis and an exanthematous rash which lasts for three to four days. The disease is rarely if ever fatal. In newly imported animals dying of other causes, or killed in the course of experimentation, visceral lesions resulting from measles infection are encountered with some frequency, even in the absence of a rash. Most often these are characterized by giant cell pneumonia with intranuclear and cytoplasmic inclusion bodies within giant cells and respiratory epithelial cells. Lymphoid giant cells are less frequent than in human measles but may be present. Measles

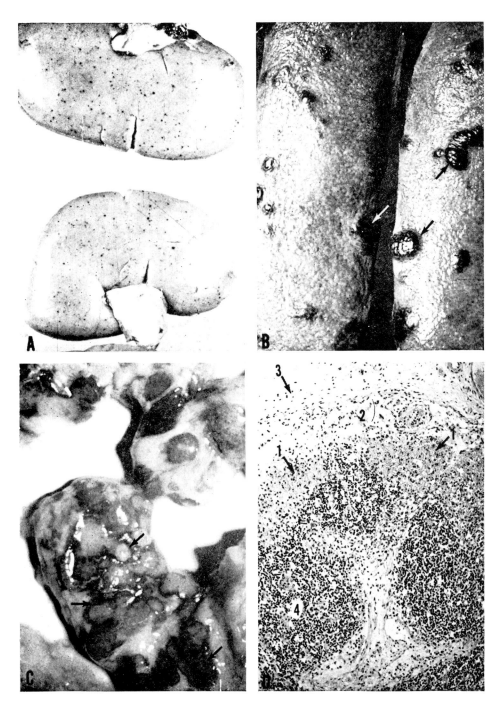

FIG. 10–40.—Hog cholera. *A*, Petechiae in the kidney. *B*, Infarcts (arrows) in the spleen. *C*, Hemorrhages (arrows) in lymph nodes. *D*, Hemorrhages (*1*) in cell-poor substance of lymph node (× 90). Note that the subcapsular sinusoids (*2*) and capsule (*3*) are not involved. Lymphoid follicle at (*4*). (Courtesy of Armed Forces Institute of Pathology.)

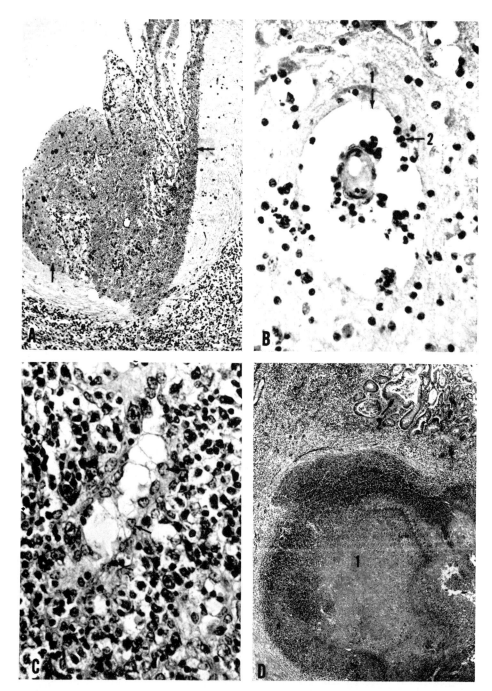

Fig. 10–41.—Hog cholera. *A*, Hemorrhage (arrows) in the pia mater (× 75). *B*, Edematous distention (*1*) of Virchow-Robin space and aggregation of a few leukocytes (*2*) in the cerebrum (× 220). *C*, Proliferation of endothelial nuclei (arrows) in a lymph node (× 410). Contributor: Lt. Col. F. D. Maurer. *D*, Sharply demarcated zone of necrosis (*1*) in the colon (× 35). Epithelium is indicated at (*2*). (Courtesy of Armed Forces Institute of Pathology.) Contributor: Lt. Col. F. D. Maurer.

eration. The large pyramidal cells are more likely to be damaged than are multi-polar cells of the cortex and gray nuclei. Some Purkinje cells may be affected. In the involved neurons, the nucleus is swollen and located peripherally; its chromatin is fragmented and the nucleolus is absent. There may be tigrolysis of the cytoplasm with vacuolation and loss of Nissl's granules. The cell membrane may be denticulated. Occasional neuronophagia and satellitosis are seen in the gray masses of the brain, cerebellum and cord. There is no demyelination. Inclusion bodies resembling those described by Joest and Degen (p. 367), in Borna disease and by Hurst (p. 358), in equine encephalomyelitis and poliomyelitis are found in a few cases but are not considered specific. These inclusions are intranuclear, round, homogeneous, acidophilic or occasionally basophilic, and several may be found in a single neuron.

In the spleen, infarction due to lesions in the arteries occurs in about 50 per cent of the cases. Grossly, the infarcts are sharply outlined, red in color, irregular in shape, and elevated (Fig. 10–40); some are definitely wedge-shaped. Microscopically, degenerative changes in the wall of follicular or trabecular arteries are characterized by proliferation of endothelium, hyalinization and necrosis in the media and adventitia with resultant thrombosis. Hemorrhagic infarction related to these vascular lesions is demonstrable as sharply demarcated areas of necrosis (Fig. 10–41).

Gross lesions are seen in one or more lymph nodes in more than 80 per cent of animals which die of hog cholera. Even in nodes of the same animal, they vary from swelling and hyperemia with bright red, subcapsular hemorrhages outlining the periphery of the node, to dense, dark-colored hemorrhages obscuring the entire nodal architecture. In the milder lesions, the fresh hemorrhage is confined to the cell-poor substance, which in porcine lymph nodes lies just beneath the cortical and adjacent to the trabecular sinuses.* The cortical sinuses, even in hemorrhagic nodes, seldom contain red blood cells. Pronounced changes are usually observed in the capillaries, arterioles and venules, particularly in the cell-poor substance. Swelling and proliferation of endothelial nuclei are striking and are accompanied by occlusion of the lumen and duplication of the vessels. Diffuse accumulation of erythrocytes may obscure most of the histologic features of nodes that are severely involved.

In the skin, erythematous areas resulting from cyanosis are the most common gross lesions. They usually appear as areas of purplish discoloration, 1 to 15 cm. in diameter, on the ventral surface of the abdomen and the thorax, the medial surface of the thigh and leg, on the ears, on the medial surface of the forearm, in the skin of the perineum and snout. Edema and necrosis with sloughing are very rare. The cyanotic changes usually can be readily detected in white-skinned swine, less easily in brown-skinned swine, and rarely in the black breeds. The typical changes in the vascular system also are responsible for these cutaneous lesions.

In the kidney, sharply demarcated petechiæ, from 1 to 5 mm. in diameter, are visible grossly just beneath the capsule and deep in the renal cortex. These petechiæ give the kidney a characteristic appearance which has been likened to that of a turkey egg (Fig. 10–40). Microscopically, hemorrhages are found in the interstitial stroma and in Bowman's spaces, and from the latter blood may flow

---

* The secondary follicles are located deep in the node near the trabeculae (Seifried & Cain, 1932). This is the reverse of the anatomic arrangement in most other species.

into the convoluted tubules. These hemorrhages are related to the typical lesions in the vasculature.

The digestive system is most obviously affected in animals dying after a more prolonged course. Diffuse catarrhal inflammation may be seen but is not specific for hog cholera. The characteristic lesion is a spherical ulcer in the mucosa, particularly of the colon. These ulcers are sharply circumscribed, single or multiple; they originate as small congested areas with adherent fecal material and develop into encrusted button-shaped foci ("button ulcers") a few millimeters in diameter. Cut section reveals a sharply demarcated zone of necrosis in the underlying mucosa and submucosa. This lesion develops following occlusion of a small artery by swelling and hydropic changes in its endothelium; thus the "button ulcer" is the result of infarction and evolves through the same sequence of events as do the infarcts in the spleen.

Diagnosis.—The diagnosis can usually be made on the basis of the clinical manifestations, gross and microscopic lesions. In the presence of fever without other symptoms, differentiation from acute systemic swine erysipelas may be a problem, but it can be solved by isolation of the organism of swine erysipelas from the blood stream. Acute arthritis, common in erysipelas, has specific diagnostic value because it does not occur in hog cholera. Teschen disease can be differentiated by the microscopic lesions found in the central nervous system. Confirmation of the diagnosis of hog cholera is accomplished by injection of blood or tissue filtrates from suspected swine into cholera-susceptible pigs, with controls receiving a large simultaneous dose of anticholera immune serum. The pigs receiving antiserum should remain well and the unprotected pigs sicken and die of hog cholera. This method obviously is suitable only for herd diagnosis. The virus can be isolated in tissue culture, but unfortunately most strains do not produce cytopathic effects. However, the presence of the virus can be demonstrated by the application of fluorescent antibody staining to infected cell cultures. This test has proven reliable and is replacing the older pig inoculation test. Fluorescent antibody staining can also be applied directly to tissue sections.

Hog Cholera

BEAMER, P. D. *et al.*: Sludged Blood in Three Young Pigs Experimentally Infected with Hog Cholera. Am. J. Vet. Research *10*:111–114, 1949.

CARBREY, E. A., *et al.*: Transmission of Hog Cholera by Pregnant Sows. J. Am. Vet. Med. Assn. *149*:23–30, 1966.

CHEVILLE, N. F., and MENGELING, W. L.: The Pathogenesis of Chronic Hog Cholera (Swine Fever), Histologic, Immunofluorescent, and Electron Microscopic Studies. Lab. Invest. *20*:261–274, 1969.

DE SCHWEINITZ, E. A., and DORSET, M.: A Form of Hog Cholera Not Caused by the Hog Cholera Bacillus. Circular 41, U.S.D.A., BAI, Washington, D.C., September 28, 1903.

DUNNE, H. W., and CLARK, C. D.: Embryonic Death, Fetal Mummification, Stillbirth, and Neonatal Death in Pigs of Gilts Vaccinated with Attenuated Live-Virus Hog Cholera Vaccine. Am. J. Vet. Res. *29*:787–796, 1968.

DUNNE, H. W. *et al*: A Study of an Encephalitic Strain of Hog Cholera Virus. Am. J. Vet. Research *13*:277–289, 1952.

DUNNE, H. W.: Hog Cholera. Chapt. 8 in Dunne, H. W., *Diseases of Swine*, 2nd Ed., Ames, Iowa, Iowa State Univ. Press, 1964.

DUNNE, H. W., SMITH, E. M., and RUNNELLS, R. A.: The Relation of Infarction to the Formation of Button Ulcers in Hog Cholera Infected Pigs. Proc. Am. Vet. Med. Assn., 1952, pp. 155–160.

DUNNE, H. W., REICH, C. V., HOKANSON, J. F., and LINDSTROM, E. S.: Variations in the Virus of Hog Cholera. A Study of Chronic Cases. Proc. Am. Vet. Med. Assn., 1955, pp. 148–153.

EMERSON, J. L., and DELEZ, A. L.: Cerebellar Hypoplasia, Hypomyelinogenesis, and Congenital Tremors of Pigs, Associated with Prenatal Hog Cholera Vaccination of Sows. J. Am. Vet. Med. Assn. *147*:47–54, 1965.

HELMBOLDT, C. F., and JUNGHERR, E. L.: Neuropathologic Diagnosis of Hog Cholera. Am. J. Vet. Research *11*:41–49, 1950.

————: Further Observations on the Neuropathological Diagnosis of Hog Cholera. Am. J. Vet Research *13*:309–317, 1952.

JONES, R. K., and DOYLE, L. P.: A Study of Encephalitis in Swine in Relation to Hog Cholera. Am. J. Vet. Research *14*:415–419, 1953.

KERNKAMP, H. C. H.: Lesions of Hog Cholera: Their Frequency of Occurrence. J. Am. Vet. Med. Assn. *95*:159–166, 1939.

————: The Blood Picture in Hog Cholera. J. Am. Vet. Med. Assn. *95*:525–529, 1939.

LEWIS, P. A., and SHOPE, R. E.: The Study of the Cells of the Blood as an Aid to the Diagnosis of Hog Cholera. J. Am. Vet. Med. Assn. *74*:145–152, 1929.

MENGELING, W. L., and PACKER, R. A.: Pathogenesis of Chronic Hog Cholera: Host Response. Am. J. Vet. Res. *30*:409–417, 1969.

MENGELING, W. L., and TORREY, J. P.: Evaluation of the Fluorescent Antibody-Cell Culture Test for Hog Cholera Diagnosis. Am. J. Vet. Res. *28*:1653–1659, 1967.

ROEHRER, H.: Histologische Untersuchungen bei Schweinepest. I. Lymphknotenveränderungen in akuten Fällen. Arch. f. Tierheilk. *62*:345–372, 1930–31.

————: Histologische Untersuchungen bei Schweinepest. II. Veränderungen im Zentralnervensystem in akuten Fällen. Arch. f. Tierheilk. *62*:439–462, 1930–31.

SEIFRIED, O.: Histological Studies on Hog Cholera. I. Lesions in the Central Nervous System. J. Exper. Med. *53*:277–289, 1931.

SEIFRIED, O., and CAIN, C. B.: Histological Studies on Hog Cholera. II. Lesions of the Vascular System. J. Exper. Med. *56*:345–349, 1932.

————: Histological Studies on Hog Cholera. III. Lesions in the Various Organs. J. Exper. Med. *56*:351–362, 1932.

SOLORZANO, R. R., *et al.*: The Diagnosis of Hog Cholera by a Fluorescent Antibody Test. J. Am. Vet. Med. Assn. *149*:31–34, 1966.

African Swine Fever

(Wart Hog Disease)

African swine fever, although immunologically distinct from hog cholera, has many features in common with that disease. Fortunately, African swine fever is principally restricted to Africa, where it causes devastating losses among domestic swine; however it has recently occurred in the Western hemisphere in Cuba. The disease is carried by wild swine (wart hogs) which apparently suffer little ill effect but transmit the virus with telling effect to domesticated swine. Mortality usually approaches 100 per cent in affected herds.

Clinical Manifestations.—A high fever characteristically precedes the appearance of other symptoms by several days. During this febrile period affected swine may appear well and have a hearty appetite, then in their final forty-eight hours, become depressed, weak, apathetic, cyanotic, develop cough and dyspnea, then die. With some strains of virus vomiting and diarrhea may be observed. Although unusual, a more protracted course, or recovery has been observed similar to "chronic" hog cholera (p. 456). Chronically infected swine carry and excrete the virus providing a potential source of infection.

Lesions.—Changes grossly evident in African swine fever are similar in many respects to those of hog cholera, but are generally more severe. Lymph nodes, especially adrenal, hepatic and gastric nodes, are usually diffusely hemorrhagic. Intralobular pulmonary edema is seen in about 40 per cent of the swine which succumb; petechiæ and ecchymoses are found in the pleura, pericardium and peritoneum in most cases. Edema and congestion are frequent in the gallbladder and in the adjacent liver. Very extensive perirenal, diffuse subcapsular and pelvic hemorrhages are encountered in a few cases. Hemorrhages into the renal cortex,

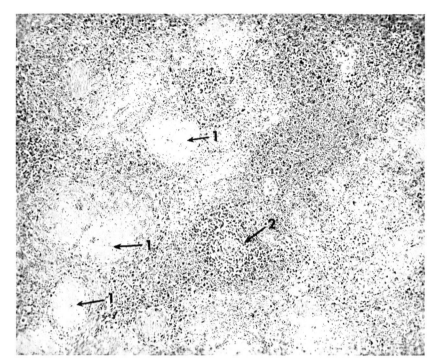

FIG. 10–42.—Spleen of a pig with African swine fever The splenic ellipsoids are enlarged and effaced by hyalin material (*1*). Lymphocytes (*2*) are for the most part necrotic or absent. (Courtesy of Colonel Fred D. Maurer and Armed Forces Institute of Pathology.)

if found at all, are very numerous. The spleen is engorged and swollen in about 10 per cent of the cases, while gastric ulceration is severe in about 20 per cent. Catarrhal enteritis is commonly manifest. The stomachs of about 80 per cent of the dead swine are full of feed, indicating the fulminant nature of the disease. Pneumonia is a rare complication.

The microscopic lesions in African swine fever have been studied critically and have been compared to those of hog cholera. The vascular lesions in African swine fever are similar to these of hog cholera but result in more severe circulatory disturbances (edema, hemorrhages, infarction). Severe karyolysis of lymphocytes occurs in African swine fever in contrast to hog cholera in which lymphopenia occurs but no severe destruction of lymphocytes is found in sections. A particularly striking lesion in the African disease is found in the ellipsoids of the spleen which become acellular and thus clearly demonstrated in tissue sections (Fig. 10–42).

"Chronic" infection is not associated with the acute lesions described. The most characteristic finding in such swine has been reported to be a pronounced chronic pericarditis.

Diagnosis.—The differentiation of hog cholera and African swine fever is not a problem at present because of the geographic separation of the two diseases. Should the African disease spread to the western hemisphere, however, the problem would become extremely critical. Although some differences in the clinical manifestations and gross lesions are apparent, they are insufficient for definitive diagnosis. Pigs immune to hog cholera can be killed with the virus of African swine fever, but in complete cross-immunity tests, it has proved to be very

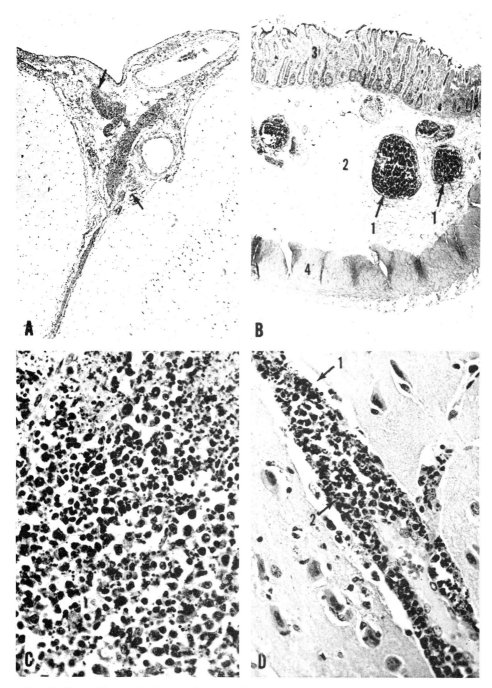

FIG. 10–43.—African swine fever. *A*, Hemorrhages (arrows) in the pia mater (× 50). *B*, Congested submucosal veins (*1*) edema in submucosa (*2*) hemorrhage in mucosa (*3*) of the colon (× 26). The muscularis is indicated at (*4*). *C*, Severe karyorrhexis involving lymphoid cells in a lymph node (× 395). *D*, A vein in the cerebral cortex (× 305). The Virchow-Robin space (*1*) is empty but the wall of the vein (*2*) is infiltrated by lymphoid cells. Courtesy of Lt. Col. F. D. Maurer.

difficult to immunize swine against the African disease. A significant finding which has aided the diagnosis of African swine fever is the growth of the virus in cultures of swine bone marrow and buffy coat in which the virus produces hemadsorption and cytopathic effect. Fluorescent antibody techniques have also shown promise.

African Swine Fever

DE KOCK, G., ROBBINSON, E. M., and KEPPEL, J. J. G.: Swine Fever in South Africa· Onderstepoort J. Vet. Sc. & Animal Ind., *14*:31–93, 1940.
DETRAY, D. E.: African Swine Fever. Adv. in Vet. Sci. *8*:299–333, 1963.
MALMQUIST, W. A., and HAY, D.: Hemadsorption and Cytopathic Effect Produced by African Swine Fever Virus in Swine Bone Marrow and Buffy Coat Cultures. Am. J. Vet. Res. *21*:104–108, 1960.
MAURER, F. D., GRIESEMER, R. A., and JONES, T. C.: The Pathology of African Swine Fever—A Comparison with Hog Cholera. Am. J. Vet. Res. *19*:517–539, 1958.
MONTGOMERY, R. E.: On a Form of Swine Fever Occurring in British East Africa (Kenya Colony). J. Comp. Path. & Therap. *34*:159–191, 243–262, 1921.
MOULTON, J., and COGGINS, L.: Comparison of Lesions in Acute and Chronic African Swine Fever. Cornell Vet. *58*:364–388, 1968.

Bluetongue of Sheep

(Catarrhal Fever of Sheep, "Soremuzzle")

This viral disease of sheep was first recognized in South Africa in 1902 and still remains a serious problem in that country. The first appearance of the disease outside South Africa was reported from Cyprus in 1949 (Gambles), but the virus was not identified in this or in a subsequent outbreak in Israel until 1952. Evidence that the disease had been introduced into the United States before 1951 is the report of Hardy and Price (1952), who observed a disease of sheep in Texas to which they applied the name "soremuzzle." They were unable to establish its cause and did not identify it with bluetongue. The following year McGowan (1953) reported a similar outbreak in California, and McKercher (1953) isolated the causative virus and demonstrated its identity with the agent of bluetongue, well known in South Africa.

The virus of bluetongue has been shown in South Africa and the United States to be transmitted by biting insects of the genus *Culicoides*.

Cattle, goats and deer are also susceptible to infection. In cattle the infection is usually not apparent although it may resemble the disease in sheep, only milder. Cattle may carry the virus for protracted periods of time with sporadic viremia adequate for insect transmission. In Africa the blesbok antelope is considered to represent a reservoir host for the virus. In deer the disease (and virus) is remarkably similar to *epizootic hemorrhagic disease* of deer.

Signs.—High fever is the first sign (105° F.), associated with reddening of the nasal and oral mucosae with excessive salivation. A watery discharge from the nostrils later becomes mucous and may dry to form crusts. Edematous swellings arise in the lips, tongue, ears, face and intermandibular space. Edema and cyanosis of the tongue are so striking that they have given the disease its name, even though they are not always present. Petechiæ soon appear on the oral and nasal mucosæ where the epithelium apparently becomes thickened and is shed, leaving excoriations and bleeding points. With subsidence of the fever, flushing of the skin and feet appears; the coronets become warm and tender, and

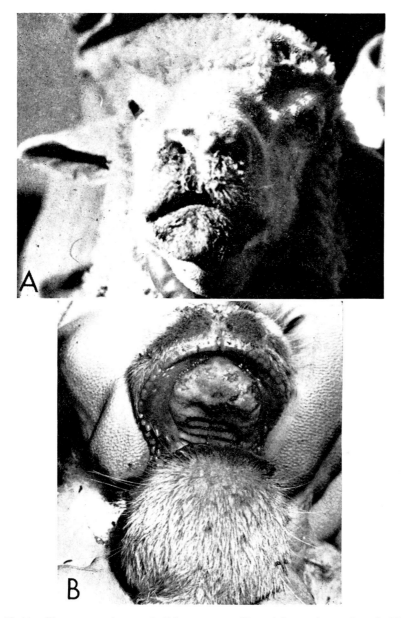

Fig 10-44 —Bluetongue, sheep. *A*, Edematous swelling of lips and nostrils. *B*, Ulcers of dental pad and swelling of lips and buccal mucosa. (Courtesy Dr. J. G. Bowne and Journal of the American Veterinary Medicine Association)

later the pink perioplic band turns red. Hemorrhage into the medullary canals of the growing horn at the junction of skin and hoof, according to Thomas and Neitz (1947), leaves a "streaky zone" parallel to the periople. This irregular zone, or line, persists but is moved away from the coronet with growth of the hoof, and its color gradually changes from bright red to brown because of the breakdown of hemoglobin in the exudate. The presence of this zone is of distinct value in identifying a previous attack of the disease. The changes in the hoof and adjacent

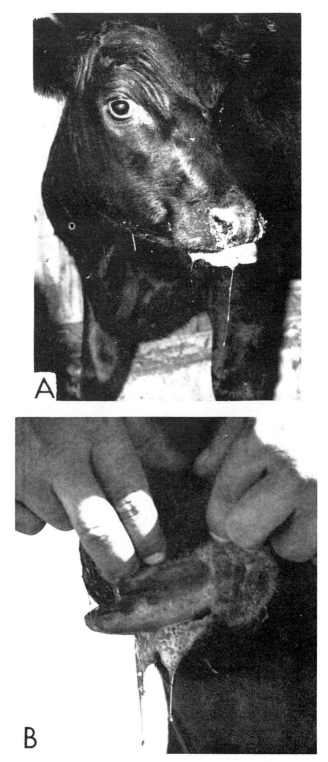

Fig. 10–45.—Bluetongue, shorthorn heifer. *A*, The muzzle is dry and cracked and a muco-purulent exudate surrounds the nares. *B*, Erosions on the lateral surface of the tongue. (Courtesy Dr. J. G. Bowne and Journal of the American Veterinary Medical Association.)

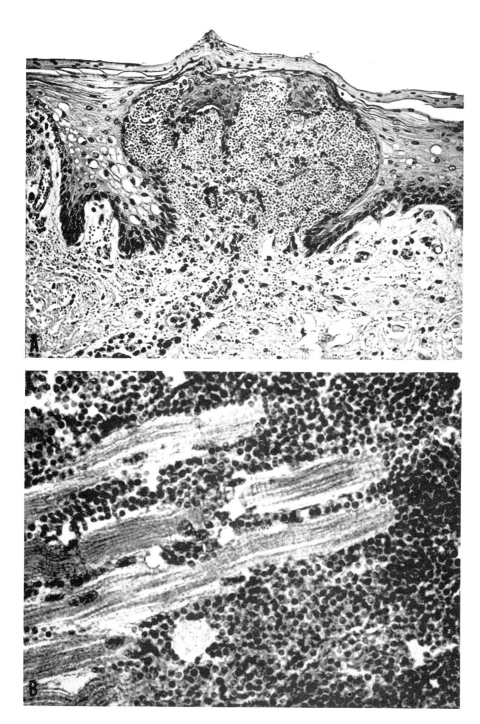

FIG. 10–46.—Bluetongue. Hemorrhages in the tongue of a year-old ewe. *A*, Hemorrhage into a lingual papilla (arrow) (× 190). *B*, Severe hemorrhage isolating muscle bundles in the tongue (× 560). (Courtesy of Armed Forces Institute of Pathology.) Contributor: Dr. W. S. Monlux.

skin are believed to be indications of an acute aseptic pododermatitis, as is laminitis in the equine.

The disease may terminate in severe emaciation, prostration, and muscular weakness (occasionally with torticollis) which may last three weeks or more, followed by pulmonary edema and death from pneumonia. In prolonged cases, a "break" in the growth of wool may cause the fleece to be shed.

The morbidity in mild outbreaks is usually about 50 per cent of a flock, with the mortality about 7 per cent. In severe outbreaks, however, losses from death may reach 50 per cent. Sheep of all ages are susceptible, but in the United States adults seem to be more often affected than lambs.

Lesions.—Although the gross manifestations of this disease apparently result from changes in the vascular system, the microscopic lesions of the vessels have not received adequate study. Severe engorgement is the most striking change in the vessels. Arteritis characterized by endothelial hyperplasia and an infiltration of neutrophils and lymphocytes in the adventitia has been reported in the oral mucosa, brain and placenta. Further study is needed, therefore, to establish the basic nature of the lesions in this disease. The changes around the mouth which characterize the disease clinically are most obvious at necropsy and consist of hyperemia, edema, cyanosis, and multiple hemorrhages in the tongue and cheeks, with erosion and even ulceration of the epithelium. The cyanosis and edema of the lips and tongue, however, are not constant findings. Similar lesions may be present on the dental pad, hard palate and gingivae.

The skin is hyperemic and the subcutis, particularly around the head and neck, is edematous. Microscopic examination of the hoof and adjacent skin reveals intense hyperemia of the vascular corium, most concentrated at the tips of the dermal papillæ, associated with edema and infiltration with neutrophils. The red "streak" or zone seen grossly in the wall of the hoof is the result of the accumulation of erythrocytes as well as neutrophils in the hollow medullary canals of the horny wall, which continue as channels from the dermal papillæ. At the periople, these channels may become dilated, although distal to the zone they are of capillary size.

The musculature usually contains foci of gross hemorrhage which are associated with microscopic evidence of necrotic changes in muscle bundles. These changes have been described as hyalinization and loss of striations in the muscle bundles and pyknosis of sarcolemmal nuclei, followed by coagulation, irregular swelling and fragmentation of sarcoplasm. Proliferation of sarcolemmal nuclei and occasional calcific stippling of sarcoplasm have been reported. The pathogenesis of these changes is not clear, but it is possible that they are brought about by disturbance of the blood flow to the muscles.

In the digestive system, extravasations of blood from the mucosa of the abomasum and duodenum may be seen. The liver may show microscopic evidence of slight fatty change at the periphery of the lobules. The endocardium may be the site of extravasation of blood and the pericardial sac may be distended with blood-tinged fluid. In the lungs edema may be succeeded by pneumonia which is not specific in character. In the spleen, slight congestion and enlargement are grossly apparent, and congestion, hemosiderosis and some neutrophilic infiltration of the red pulp, microscopically.

Bluetongue vaccine prepared from modified live virus and administered to pregnant ewes has been demonstrated to cause encephalopathic lesions in their progeny. The critical period for exposure appears to be between the fourth and eighth weeks of gestation. Lambs may be stillborn, spastic, or most often "dummies" which walk aimlessly, circle, bump into objects, are uncoordinated and do not nurse unless helped. The congenital anomalies in the nervous system range from hydrocephalus to subcortical cysts in the cerebrum and cerebellum with *ex vacuo* dilation of lateral ventricles. The studies of Young and Cordy (1964) have demonstrated that the lesions are the result of an acute necrotizing meningoencephalitis. Although the clinical and gross findings of swayback (enzootic ataxia, p. 1402) may be similar, the two processes may be differentiated in that swayback is a dysmyelinating disease in which inflammatory changes do not occur.

Diagnosis.—The clinical diagnosis may be made from the symptoms and gross lesions, but bluetongue must be differentiated from photosensitization, contagious ecthyma and sheep pox. At present isolation and identification of the virus are necessary to confirm the diagnosis.

Bluetongue

ANDERSON, C. K., and JENSEN, R.: Pathologic Changes in Placentas of Ewes Inoculated with Bluetongue Virus. Am. J. Vet. Res. *30*:987–999, 1969.
BOWNE, J. G., et al.: Bluetongue Disease in Cattle. J. Am. Vet. Med. Assn. *153*:662–668, 1968
DE KOCK, G., DUTOIT, R., and NEITZ, W. O.: Observations on Blue Tongue in Cattle and Sheep. Onderstepoort J. Vet. Sc. & Animal Ind. *8*:129–181, 1937.
DUTOIT, R. M.: The Transmission of Blue Tongue and Horsesickness by Culicoides. Onderstepoort J. Vet. Sc. & Animal Ind. *19*:7–16, 1944.
GAMBLES, R. M.: Blue Tongue of Sheep in Cyprus. J. Comp. Path. & Therap. *59*:176–190, 1949.
GRINER, L. A., et al.: Bluetongue Associated with Abnormalities in Newborn Lambs. J. Am. Vet. Med. Assn. *145*:1013–1019, 1964.
HARDY, W. T., and PRICE, D. A.: Soremuzzle of Sheep. J. Am. Vet. Med. Assn. *120*: 23–25, 1952.
HUTCHEON, D.: Malarial Catarrhal Fever of Sheep. Vet. Record. *14*:629–633, 1902.
LUEDKE, A. J., BOWNE, J. G., JOCHIM, M. M., and DOYLE, C.: Clinical and Pathological Features of Bluetongue in Sheep. Am. J. Vet. Res. *25*:963–970, 1964.
MCGOWAN, B.: An Epidemic Resembling Soremuzzle or Blue Tongue in California Sheep. Cornell Vet. *43*:213–216, 1953.
MCKERCHER, D. G., MCGOWAN, B., HOWARTH, J. A., and SAITO, J. K.: A Preliminary Report on the Isolation and Identification of the Blue Tongue Virus from Sheep in California. J. Am. Vet. Med. Assn. *122*:300–301, 1953.
MOULTON, J. E.: Pathology of Bluetongue of Sheep. J. Am. Vet. M. A. *138*:493–498, 1961.
RICHARDS, W. P. C., and CORDY, D. R.: Bluetongue Virus Infection: Pathologic Responses of Nervous Systems in Sheep and Mice. Science *156*:530–531, 1967.
SHULTZ, G., and DELAY, P. D.: Losses in Newborn Lambs Associated with Bluetongue Vaccination of Pregnant Ewes. J. Am. Vet. Med. Assn. *127*:224–226, 1955.
STAIR, E. L., ROBINSON, R. M., and JONES, P. L.: Spontaneous Bluetongue in Texas White-Tailed Deer. Pathologia Vet. *5*:164–173, 1968.
THOMAS, A. D., and NEIDTZ, W. O.: Further Observations on the Pathology of Blue Tongue in Sheep. Onderstepoort J. Vet. Sc. & Animal Ind. *22*:27–40, 1947.
YOUNG, S., and CORDY, D. R.: An Ovine Fetal Encephalopathy Caused by Bluetongue Vaccine Virus. J. Neuropath. Exp. Neurol. *23*:635–659, 1964.

Rift Valley Fever

Rift Valley fever is an acute viral disease which, in nature, principally affects sheep and cattle, causing heavy mortality in young lambs and calves and abortion in pregnant ewes and cows. Human beings may contract the infection during the course of an epizoötic among domestic animals or by handling the virus in the laboratory. Sometimes human cases of an influenzal type may provide the first indication of the existence of an epizootic of Rift Valley fever. Montgomery in 1912 was the first to report the disease as an acute and highly fatal infection of lambs, and Stordy published similar observations the year following. Both reports were from Kenya, British East Africa, where the disease occurred on farms in the Rift Valley, a geological depression that starts in Iran, continues through North and Central Africa and ends in eastern Transvaal. Like many other newly reported diseases of unknown etiology, this one was named for the location where it was first observed, and not until 1931 was it established as a distinct entity by Daubney, Hudson and Garnham (1931), who were the first to demonstrate that it could be transmitted to susceptible animals. Rift Valley fever has a wide distribution in Africa, but has not been recognized in domestic animals outside of that continent.

Although the virus may be transmitted to susceptible animals by inoculation of infected blood or serum, in nature it is usually transmitted by arthropod vectors. The culicine mosquitoes, particularly *Eretmapodites chrysogastor*, have been shown experimentally to be capable of transmitting the disease. Experimental transmission of the virus to goats, mice, rats, wild rodents and golden hamsters, as well as to its natural hosts, has been successful. The African buffalo, ferrets and monkeys, both New World and Old World, are susceptible, although some species of primates appear to have resistance. Cats merely exhibit transitory febrile symptoms, and dogs, guinea pigs, rabbits, mongooses, hedgehogs, tortoises, frogs and birds are refractory to artificial infection. Man is particularly susceptible and can easily become infected.

Signs.—After an extremely short incubation period, from twenty to seventy-two hours after infection, the course in young lambs is brief. They may be disinclined to move, refuse to eat, exhibit some form of abdominal pain, and shortly thereafter become recumbent and unable to rise. Death may occur within twenty-four hours. It is not unusual for lambs to die before symptoms are observed. In adult sheep also, the disease often is not recognized; the infected animal is found dead without having displayed any indication of illness. Vomiting may be observed as the only symptom, but pregnant ewes usually abort in the course of the illness or during convalescence. In cattle, the disease may appear as a storm of abortions, the symptoms also are frequently indefinite, being manifest by a brief febrile period with inappetence, profuse salivation, diarrhea, abdominal pain, roughened hair coat and cessation of lactation. Mortality in cattle is not high, but erosions of buccal mucosæ, necrosis of skin of udder or scrotum, laminitis and coronitis, may occur.

In man, the initial symptoms after an incubation period of from four to six days, are malaise, nausea, hyperthermia, epigastric pain and a sensation of fullness over the region of the liver. There is usually complete anorexia, followed by rigors, violent headache, characteristic flushing of the face, injection of the conjunctiva, photophobia, aching pains in the back and joints, vertigo, and sometimes epistaxis. The disease in man is rarely fatal and immunity follows recovery, but serious sequelæ such as thrombophlebitis, retinopathy and retinal detachment have been reported.

Lesions.—The disagreement in the literature concerning the characteristic gross and microscopic changes in Rift Valley fever indicate the need for further study. Varying manifestations in the susceptible species also create problems. According to Schultz (1951) and others, the most constant and characteristic lesions are found in the liver. In sheep, the organ is grossly enlarged, its surface is mottled gray to grayish red or purple and bears numerous gray to white, sub-capsular, opaque foci. Microscopically these foci are seen as areas of necrosis involving parenchymal cells near the central veins. The affected liver cells have swollen, eosinophilic, hyaline cytoplasm and pyknotic or fragmented nuclei, their appearance suggesting the Councilman bodies of yellow fever. Findlay (1933) has described intranuclear inclusions, but their specificity is in doubt. They have also been seen in experimental animals but inclusion bodies do not form in tissue culture. The studies of McGavran and Easterday (1963) suggest that the inclusion bodies represent a degenerative change, in that they were not formed of viral particles. The frequent "paracentral" location of the liver lesion is suggestive of the changes associated with anoxia. In lambs, the liver usually is gray to reddish brown, but sometimes ochre yellow, and the distribution of the gray necrotic lesions is likely to be more diffuse than in adult sheep.

The gallbladder wall may be thickened by edema and contain subserosal hemorrhages, particularly near its attachment to the liver.

The visible mucosæ are usually cyanotic and the vessels of the skin and subcutis are injected, particularly over the head and neck. The mammary gland may be

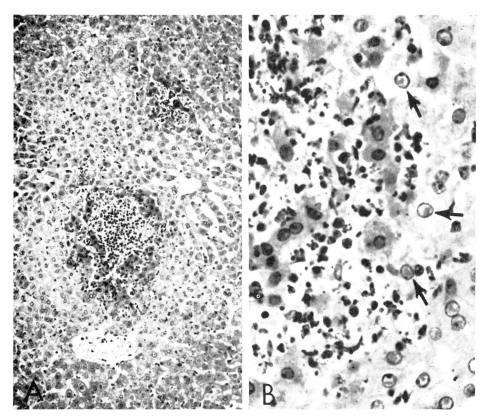

Fig. 10–47.—Rift Valley fever, experimental infection in a hamster. *A*, Focal hepatic necrosis accompanied by purulent inflammation. *B*, Higher magnification illustrating small eosinophilic intranuclear inclusion bodies (arrows) in hepatocytes.

grossly purple in color, but no mastitis is present. Hemorrhages may occur in the subcutis of the axillæ, medial and lower aspects of the limbs.

Hemorrhages may also be seen in the peritoneum of the gastro-intestinal tract and diaphragm as well as under the pleura, pericardium, endocardium and in the myocardium. Similar hemorrhages may occur in the submucosa and muscularis of the gastrointestinal tract, in the pancreas, kidney, adrenal, lung, thymus and lymph nodes (especially those of the mesentery). The lymph nodes are enlarged, moist appearing and reddened, and the mesenteric and periportal nodes may contain numerous hemorrhages. Necrotic foci among lymphoid cells, with infiltration of neutrophils, vascular congestion and edema, may be detected microscopically.

Ulceration of the intestinal mucosa may be seen in the terminal portion of the ileum, the cecum, and the initial part of the colon. Hemorrhagic lesions in some cases involve the entire gastro-intestinal tract but possibly are due to secondary factors.

The lungs are invariably hyperemic and edematous, often with subpleural and diffuse hemorrhages. Consolidation, particularly in the apical and cardiac lobes, may be fibrinous in character. In addition to bearing hemorrhages, the kidneys are usually slightly enlarged and show histologic evidence of nephrosis (swelling and loss of cell outline in tubular epithelium, albuminous casts in convoluted and collecting tubules, hemosiderin in tubular epithelium, congestion).

The spleen is usually enlarged and exhibits subcapsular petechiæ. The malpighian bodies are indistinct because of reduction of lymphocytes. In the red pulp hemorrhages with adjoining masses of pyknotic and fragmented nuclei may be seen, and sometimes collections of neutrophils.

Diagnosis.—Rift Valley fever should be suspected in outbreaks of highly fatal disease affecting both lambs and calves, especially if persons associated with the sick animals or who handle infective materials display mild febrile symptoms. In addition, the occurrence of abortion in adult animals and the presence of the gross and microscopic lesions, particularly those of the liver, are believed to permit a presumptive diagnosis. Neutralization of infective blood by immune serum, using mice as test animals, confirms the diagnosis. A serum neutralization test with mice may also be employed.

Rift Valley Fever

ALEXANDER, R. A.: Rift Valley Fever in the Union. J. South African Vet. Med. Assoc. 22:105–111, 1951.
DAUBNEY, R., HUDSON, J. R., and GARNHAM, P. C.: Enzoötic Hepatitis or Rift Valley Fever. An Undescribed Virus Disease of Sheep, Cattle and Man from East Africa. J. Path. & Bact. 34:545–579, 1931.
EASTERDAY, B. C.: Rift Valley Fever. Adv. Vet. Sci. 10:65–127, 1965.
EASTERDAY, B. C., McGAVRAN, M. H., ROONEY, J. R., and MURPHY, L. C.: The Pathogenesis of Rift Valley Fever in Lambs. Am. J. Vet. Res. 23:470–479, 1962.
FINDLAY, G. M.: Rift Valley Fever or Enzoötic Hepatitis. Tr. Roy. Soc. Trop. Med. & Hyg. 25:229–265, 1932.
————: Cytological Changes in the Liver in Rift Valley Fever with Special Reference to the Nuclear Inclusions. Brit. J. Exper. Path. 14:207–219, 1933.
FINDLAY, G. M., and HOWARD, E. M.: The Susceptibility of Rats to Rift Valley Fever in Relation to Age. Ann. Trop. Med. 46:33–37, 1952.
MACKENZIE, R. D., FINDLAY, G. M., and STERN, R. O.: Studies on Neurotropic Rift Valley Fever Virus: the Susceptibility of Rodents. Brit. J. Exper. Path. 17:352–361, 1936.
McGAVRAN, M. H., and EASTERDAY, B. C.: Rift Valley Fever Virus Hepatitis. Light and Microscope Studies in the Mouse. Am. J. Path. 42:587–607, 1963.

Sabin, A. B., and Blumberg, R. W.: Human Infection with Rift Valley Fever Virus and Immunity Twelve Years After Single Attack. Proc. Soc. Exper. Biol. & Med. *64*:385–389, 1947.

Schultz, K. C. A.: The Pathology of Rift Valley Fever or Enzoötic Hepatitis in South Africa. J. South African Vet. Med. Assn. *22*:113–120, 1951.

Schwentker, F. F., and Rivers, T. M.: Rift Valley Fever in Man. Report of a Fatal Laboratory Infection Complicated by Thrombophlebitis. J. Exper. Med. *59*:305-313, 1934.

Smithburn, K. C., Haddow, A. J., and Gillett, J. D.: Rift Valley Fever: Isolation of the Virus from Wild Mosquitoes. Brit. J. Exper. Path. *29*:107–121, 1948.

Feline Panleukopenia

(Feline Distemper, Feline Enteritis, Agranulocytosis)

Feline panleukopenia is a highly contagious and usually fatal febrile disease of domestic cats, other *Felidæ* and mink. It is caused by a virus and is characterized clinically by severe panleukopenia, fever and enteritis that results in extreme dehydration. Although the domestic house cat is the principal host, a variety of wild felines and raccoons, are susceptible. The disease runs a rapid course. Its onset is marked by lassitude and abrupt elevation of temperature to 104 to 105° F. The fever is diphasic; it falls after about twenty-four hours and rises approximately forty-eight hours later. Severe leukopenia involving all of the granulocytic series (agranulocytosis) and all other leukocytes is a constant feature. Vomiting and intractable diarrhea also may be observed. Death frequently occurs shortly after the second peak of temperature.

Lesions.—The gross lesions seen at necropsy usually consist of extreme dehydration and emaciation, with mucopurulent exudate on the nasal and lacrimal mucosæ. The mucosa of the terminal part of the ileum is often covered with hemorrhagic exudate. The lymph nodes of the mesentery are edematous and somewhat enlarged. The bone marrow of the long bones often appears greasy, yellowish or white, and semifluid. The lack of hematopoietic marrow is obvious.

The principal microscopic lesions are found in the gastro-intestinal tract and associated lymph nodes. The superficial layers of the mucosa in the small intestine are eroded and the remaining epithelium has undergone proliferation. The crypts are dilated with mucus and lined with irregular, hyperplastic epithelial cells. Here inflammatory infiltration of the lamina propria occurs, but little change is seen in the submucosa. In some cases granular, eosinophilic intranuclear inclusions have been described in the lining epithelium remaining at the sites of erosion. These inclusions, when present, are helpful in diagnosis.

The changes in the lymph nodes are reported to be characteristic. Early in the disease the mesenteric lymph nodes are edematous and hyperemic and there is proliferation of reticulo-endothelial cells. Erythrophagocytosis is seen in the center of the nodes, and intranuclear inclusions have been reported in a small percentage of monocytic cells.

As the disease progresses, the lymphoid cells become hyperplastic, and later, necrosis becomes evident. Marked hyperplasia of the secondary follicles may occur at some stages but appears to be transient, for it is not uniformly demonstrable post mortem. The changes in the spleen parallel those in the lymph nodes except that the large secondary nodules are not so prominent. The bone marrow is specifically inhibited; the normal hematopoietic marrow is usually replaced by fatty marrow.

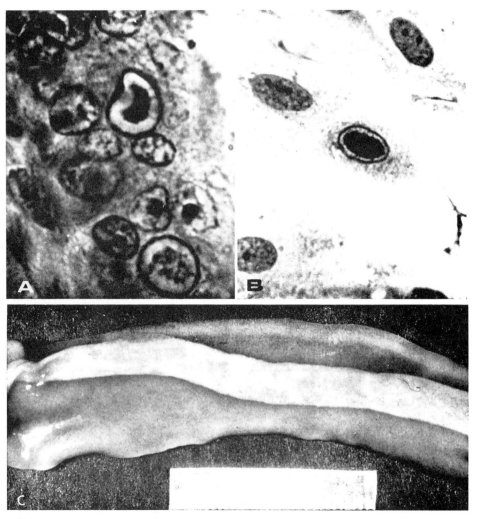

FIG 10–48 —*A*, Intranuclear inclusions of panleukopenia (infectious feline enteritis) virus. In intestinal epithelium of a cat five days following inoculation with the virus. *B*, Inclusion in culture of feline kidney cells five days after inoculation with virus. (Courtesy of Dr. John R. Gorham, Washington State University.) *C*, Fibrinous cast in the lumen of a seven-month-old male cat with panleukopenia. (Courtesy of Angell Memorial Animal Hospital.)

The studies by Rohovsky and Griesemer (1967) and Johnson, *et al.* (1967) on experimental panleukopenia in germfree cats are of particular interest. Enteric lesions were not observed in germfree cats, but consistently developed in specific pathogen-free cats. The most significant findings in germfree cats were lymphocytic destruction, reticulo-endothelial hyperplasia, severe thymic atrophy, and panleukopenia. These studies suggest that the intestinal lesions so characteristic of panleukopenia in conventional cats may not be a primary effect of the virus.

Diagnosis.—A presumptive diagnosis usually can be based upon the symptoms and the agranulocytosis. Demonstration of intranuclear inclusions in the epithelial cells of the small intestine is helpful in post-mortem diagnosis, but unfortunately they are not always present.

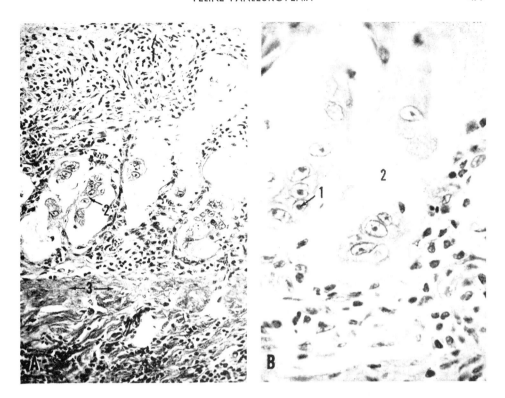

FIG. 10-49.—Feline panleukopenia. *A*, Wall of a small intestine (× 210) of a cat. Loss of epithelium at tips of villi (*1*), disorganization and proliferation of epithelial cells in crypts (*2*). Note collection of mucus. *B*, Higher magnification (× 590) to show intranuclear inclusions (*1*) and collections of mucus (*2*). (Courtesy of Armed Forces Institute of Pathology.) Contributor: Dr. J. T. Bryans.

Panleukopenia and Cerebellar Hypoplasia.—Kilham, Margolis and Colby (1967) have recently demonstrated that the virus of feline panleukopenia can produce cerebellar hypoplasia in kittens. The virus, when injected into the fetus or intravenously into a pregnant cat, invades cells of the external germinal layer of the fetal cerebellum producing intranuclear inclusion bodies and necrosis which leads to gross or microscopic "hypoplasia" of the cerebellum in the newborn kitten. Inclusion bodies may persist to the early neonatal period, but are usually not evident after birth. Virus, however, can be isolated from various tissues, especially the kidney, for several months. The virus has also been isolated from natural cases of cerebellar hypoplasia in kittens. Kilham (1966) had previously demonstrated that rat virus can induce cerebellar hypoplasia in kittens, rats, and hamsters. Although it appears that panleukopenia virus is an important cause of cerebellar hypoplasia in kittens, the relative importance of rat virus is undetermined. These studies are of great significance in that a viral etiology has been demonstrated for a disease accepted by many to represent a genetic abnormality.

Kilham's studies are also of interest in that they demonstrated that feline panleukopenia virus could also induce cerebellar hypoplasia in ferrets, a species not considered susceptible to classical panleukopenia.

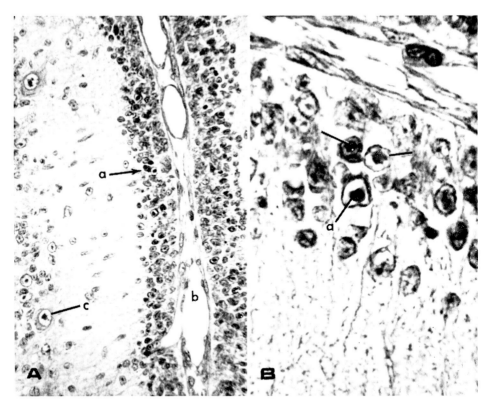

Fig. 10–50.—Cerebellum of a twenty-one-day old kitten which had received the panleukopenia virus at birth. *A*, Note intranuclear inclusions and necrotic cells in the cells of the germinal layer (*a*) adjacent to the vascular pia mater (*b*), Purkinje cells at (*c*). *B*, Higher magnification of *A*. Note intranuclear inclusions (*a*) and margination of chromatin in affected nuclei. (Courtesy of Dr. George Margolis, Dartmouth Medical School.)

Feline Panleukopenia

Bittle, J. L., York, C. J., Newberne, J. W., and Martin, M.: Serological Relationship of New Feline Cytopathogenic Viruses. Am. J. Vet. Res. *21*:547–550, 1960.

Bittle, J. L., Emery, J. B., York, C. J., and McMillen, J. K.: Comparative Study of Feline Cytopathogenic Viruses and Feline Panleukopenia Virus. Am. J. Vet. Res. *22*:374–378, 1961.

Cohen, D., Yohn, D. S., Pavia, R. A., and Hammon, W. McD.: The Relationship of a Feline Virus Isolated by Bolin to Feline Panleukopenia, Kidney Cell Degenerating Virus, and Two Feline Respiratory Viruses. Am. J. Vet. Res. *22*:637–643, 1961.

Hammon, W. D., and Enders, J. F.: A Virus Disease of Cats Principally Characterized by Aleucocytosis, Enteric Lesions and the Presence of Intranuclear Inclusion Bodies. J. Exper. Med. *69*:327–351, 1939.

Hersey, D. F. and Maurer, F. D.: Immunological Relationship of Selected Feline Viruses by Complement Fixation. Proc. Soc. Exp. Biol. *107*:645–646, 1961.

Johnson, G. R, Koestner, A., and Rohovsky, M. W.: Experimental Feline Infectious Enteritis in the Germfree Cat. An Electron Microscopic Study. Pathologia Vet. *4*:275–288, 1967.

Johnson, R. H., Margolis, G., and Kilham, L.: Identity of Feline Ataxia Virus with Feline Panleucopenia Virus. Nature, Lond. *214*:175–177, 1967.

Kilham, L., and Margolis, G.: Viral Etiology of Spontaneous Ataxis of Cats. Am. J. Path. *48*:991–1011, 1966.

Kilham, L., Margolis, G., and Colby, E. D.: Congenital Infections of Cats and Ferrets by Feline Panleukopenia Virus Manifested by Cerebellar Hypoplasia. Lab. Invest. *17*:465–480, 1967.

LAWRENCE, J. S., SYVERTON, J. T., SHAW, J. S., and SMITH, F. P.: Infectious Feline Agranulocytosis. Am. J. Path. *16*:333–354, 1940.

LAWRENCE, J. S. *et al.*: The Virus of Infectious Feline Agranulocytosis. II. Immunological Relation to Other Viruses. J. Exper. Med. *77*:57–64, 1943.

LUCAS, A. M., and RISER, W. H.: Intranuclear Inclusions in Panleukopenia of Cats. Am. J. Path. *21*:435–465, 1945.

RISER, W. H.: The Histopathology of Panleucopenia (Agranulocytosis) in the Domestic Cat. Am. J. Vet. Research *7*:455–465, 1946.

ROHOVSKY, M. W., and GRIESEMER, R. A.: Experimental Feline Infectious Enteritis in the Germfree Cat. Pathologia Vet. *4*:391–410, 1967.

SYVERTON, J. T. *et al.*: The Virus of Infectious Feline Agranulocytosis. I. Character of the Virus: Pathogenicity. J. Exper. Med. *77*:41–56, 1943.

FELINE INFECTIOUS PERITONITIS

Although the infectious agent has not been isolated, the studies of Zook, *et al.* (1968), clearly indicate that feline infectious peritonitis is caused by an agent less than 200 μ in smallest dimension. Also, viral particles 70 to 90 mμ in diameter have been seen within mesothelial cells of affected cats.

Signs.—The disease, which is most frequent in young cats, is characterized by persistent fever, anorexia, depression, weight loss and ascites leading to gradual abdominal enlargement. Other signs may include vomiting, diarrhea and dyspnea. The disease is invariably fatal following a course of two weeks to two months.

Lesions.—The abdominal cavity contains excessive fluid, often up to 1 liter. The fluid is yellow, viscid, and transparent, though it may contain flakes of fibrin. A grey-white granular exudate is present over all serosal surfaces being especially thick over the liver and spleen. A similar fibrinous exudate extends into the scrotum and may also be present in the thoracic cavity. Small, discrete white foci of necrosis are often present throughout the liver. In protracted cases organization of fibrinous exudate can result in severe distortion of abdominal viscera. Microscopically the peritonitis, or pleuritis, is a classical fibrinous inflammation (p. 156) consisting of layer of fibrin of varied thickness containing cellular debris overlying a zone of neutrophils, lymphocytes and macrophages. Fibroplasia and proliferation of capillaries may accompany the exudate in protracted cases. The inflammatory process may extend beneath the serosa into any of the affected tissues. The focal hepatic necrosis is accompanied by an inflammatory reaction. Similar necrotic foci may be found microscopically in the spleen, kidneys, pancreas, lymph nodes, and muscular layers of the gastrointestinal tract. While not usual, purulent and mononuclear meningitis may be seen.

Diagnosis.—The clinical signs are usually sufficient for diagnosis of the disease in the living animal. The gross and microscopic features are not duplicated by other forms of peritonitis.

Feline Infectious Peritonitis

WARD, J. M., *et al.*: An Observation of Feline Infectious Peritonitis. Vet. Rec. *83*:416–417, 1968.

WARD, B. C., and PEDERSON, N.: Infectious Peritonitis in Cats. J. Am. Vet. Med. Assn. *154*:26–35, 1969.

WOLFE, L. G., and GRIESEMER, R. A.: Feline Infectious Peritonitis. Path. Vet *.3*:255–270, 1966.

ZOOK, B. C., *et al.*: Ultrastructural Evidence for the Viral Etiology of Feline Infectious Peritonitis. Path. Vet. *5*:91–95, 1968.

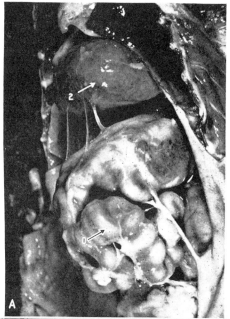

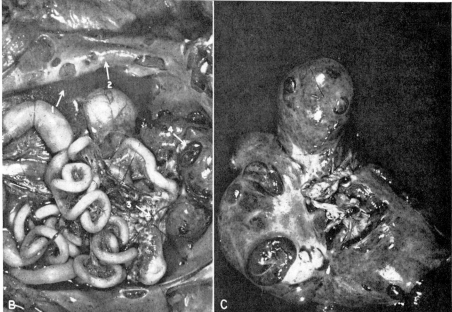

FIG. 10–51.—Infectious feline peritonitis. *A*, Organizing fibrinous peritonitis in a four-year-old female cat. The exudate binds the intestines together (*1*) and covers and compresses the liver (*2*). *B*, Chronic organizing peritonitis of unknown cause in a fifteen-year-old female cat. Cloudy fluid (*1*) distends the abdomen, the parietal peritoneum is thick and tough (*2*) the mesentery (*3*) is short and thick, and the liver (*4*) is compressed and distorted in shape by the exudate covering its capsule. *C*, Another view of the liver in *B*, with thick, tough fibrous exudate on the capsule, compressing and distorting the liver. (Courtesy of Angell Memorial Animal Hospital.)

effect is quantitative. The microscopic picture is one of hematopoietic marrow with myeloid and erythroid elements in approximately normal proportion. It is obvious from these findings that hematopoiesis is not depressed but rather stimulated, probably as the result of destruction of erythrocytes. Large numbers of reticulo-endothelial and lymphoid cells are interposed between the erythroid and myeloid elements.

Kidney.—*Acute Type.*—The kidneys are usually involved in the edema that affects the perirenal tissues, particularly in the region of the pelvis. Intense infiltration of immature lymphoid cells into the interstitital stroma of both cortex and medulla is especially prominent around blood vessels and occasionally around glomeruli. This lymphoid infiltration takes on a nodular distribution in some cases. There is generally an increased cellularity to the mesangium of the glomeruli. Immunoglobulins and complement have been demonstrated with immunofluorescent techniques.

Subacute and Chronic Types.—The lymphoid cells may be present in smaller numbers.

Other Organs.—*Acute Type.*—It is possible for all organs and tissues of the body to show evidence of the reticulo-endothelial hyperplasia described in spleen, lymph nodes, liver and kidney, but this change is not constant nor particularly distinctive. In the adrenal, lymphoid cell masses may separate parenchymal cells in much the same manner as in the liver. Endothelial cells of the adrenal have been reported to contain hemosiderin.

Subacute and Chronic Types.—No distinctive alterations are found in other organs.

Hematologic Changes.—The anemia is characteristically normocytic and normochromic. Reticulocytosis or other evidence of increased erythropoiesis are not evident. The anemia appears to result from a combination of hemolysis, erythrophagocytosis and a decreased production of erythrocytes. The response of the bone marrow has received little attention, although usually described as hyperplastic, there is little evidence of increased erythropoiesis. To the contrary, studies of Obara and Nakajima (1961) and McGuire, *et al.* (1969), indicate both a decrease in erythrocyte lifespan and production. Following an immediate lymphopenia, the disease is characterized by lymphocytosis and the appearance of iron-laden monocytes or siderocytes in the peripheral blood. Thrombocytopenia is a usual finding. Serum levels of gamma globulin are usually increased in the acute stages, and the Coomb's test is reportedly positive.

Diagnosis.—In the living animal, a presumptive diagnosis can be made from the symptoms and history, but unfortunately only the inoculation of a normal horse can prove the presence of the virus. Necropsy findings and the demonstration of characteristic microscopic lesions are of distinct value in establishing the diagnosis in an individual case.

The recent isolation of the virus and demonstration of cytopathic effects in horse leukocyte cultures by Kobayashi and Kono (1967) will hopefully lead to laboratory methods for accurate diagnosis which will not require horse inoculation. Also serologic methods have shown promise.

Equine Infectious Anemia

Brudnjak, Z. and Topolnik, E.: Diagnosis of Equine Infectious Anemia by the Use of Hydroxylamine-treated Rabbits. (Trans. title. CR. e. g.) Vet. Arkiv. *32*:117–120, 1962. VB 518–63.

Cohrs, P.: Verdauungsorgane, in Nieberle, K., and Cohrs, P.: *Lehrbuch der Speziellen Pathologischen Anatomie der Haustiere.* 3rd ed., Jena, Fischer, 1954, pp. 384–388.

De Kock, G.: A Contribution to the Study of the Virus, Haematology, and Pathology of Infectious Anaemia of Equines under South African Conditions. Ninth and 10th Reports of Veterinary Education and Research, Union of South Africa, 1923, pp. 253–313.

Dreguss, M. N., and Lombard, L. S.: *Experimental Studies in Equine Infectious Anemia*, Philadelphia, University of Pennsylvania Press, 1954.

Hasumi, K.: Recent Studies on Equine Infectious Anemia. Report IV. Pathogenicity of E.I.A. Virus. J. Cancer Virol. *2*:29–53, 1959.

Hjärre, A.: Die Leberveränderungen bei der Infektiösen Anämie des Pferdes. Münch. tierärztl. Wchnschr. *87*:26–31, 1936.

Ishi, S.: Equine Infectious Anemia or Swamp Fever. Adv. Vet. Sci. *8*:263–298, 1963.

Kobayashi, K., and Kono, Y.: Propagation and Titration of Equine Infectious Anemia Virus in Horse Leukocyte Culture. Nat. Inst. Anim. Health Quart. *7*:8–20, 1967.

Obara, J., and Nakajima, H.: Kinetics of Iron Metabolism in Equine Infectious Anemia. Jap. J. Vet. Sci. *23*:247–252, 1961.

————: Lifespan of ⁵¹Cr-Labeled Erythrocytes in Equine Infectious Anemia. Jap. J. Vet. Sci. *23*:207–209, 1961.

McGuire, T. C., Henson, J. B,. and Quist, S. E.: Viral-Induced Hemolysis in Equine Infectious Anemia. Am. J. Vet. Res. *30*:2091–2097, 1969.

————: Impaired Bone Marrow Response in Equine Infectious Anemia. Am. J. Vet. Res. *30*:2099–2113, 1969.

Rothenbacher, H. J., Ishida, K., and Barner, R. D.: Equine Infectious Anemia. II. The Sideroleukocyte Test as an Aid in the Clinical Diagnosis. Vet. Med. *57*:886–890, 1962. VB 1187–63.

Squire, R. A.: Equine Infectious Anemia: A Model of Immunoproliferative Disease. Blood *32*:157–169, 1968.

Stein, C. D.: The History and Distribution of Equine Infectious Anemia in the United States. Vet. Med. *36*:410–419, 1941.

Stein, C. D., Osteen, O. L., Mott, L. O., and Shahan, M. S.: Experimental Transmission of Equine Infectious Anemia by Contact and Body Secretions and Excretions. Vet. Med. *39*:46–52, 1944.

Rinderpest

(Cattle Plague)

Rinderpest has been a serious disease of cattle from antiquity and is today the foremost cause of death in cattle in Africa and Asia. Fortunately it is not present in the Western Hemisphere or in Europe. The mortality in cattle varies from 25 to 90 per cent, depending on the strains of virus involved and the resistance of the animals. The incubation period is from six to nine days after infection by contact, but only two or three days following experimental injection of the virus. In addition to cattle, sheep, swine, goats, deer, camels, and buffalo are susceptible to natural or artificial infection with rinderpest virus. The virus is immunologically and pathologically related to the viruses of canine distemper and measles. This interrelationship is discussed on page 446.

Signs.—The onset of illness is indicated by a sharp rise in temperature to 104 to 105° F. accompanied by restlessness, dryness of the muzzle, and constipation. Within a day or two, nasal and lacrimal discharges appear. Other manifestations are photophobia, depression, excessive thirst, starry coat, retarded rumination, anorexia, leukopenia and excessive salivation. A maculo-papular rash may develop on those parts of the body where the hair is fine. The fever usually reaches its peak on the third to the fifth day but drops abruptly with the onset of diarrhea, even though other symptoms are intensified. Lesions in the oral mucosa may appear by the second or third day of fever but usually do not become conspicuous until after the onset of diarrhea. As the diarrhea increases in severity, it is accompanied by abdominal pain, accelerated respiration, occasional cough, severe dehydration and emaciation, which are followed by prostration, subnormal temperature and death, usually after a course of six to twelve days.

Lesions.—The rinderpest virus has a particular affinity for lymphoid tissue and for epithelial tissues of the gastro-intestinal tract, in which it produces severe and characteristic effects.

In lymphoid tissue, the virus causes necrosis of lymphocytes, which is striking in microscopic sections of lymph nodes, spleen and Peyer's patches. The destruction of lymphocytes is first evidenced by a fragmentation of nuclei in the germinal centers, and in a short time most of the mature lymphocytes disappear. The lymph follicles are involved to various degrees, depending upon the severity and stage of the disease in which they are examined. Multinucleated giant cells containing eosinophilic cytoplasmic inclusion bodies are often present. Rarely intranuclear inclusions are seen in these cells. Edema and congestion of capillaries are also seen microscopically, but only the edema can be detected grossly. The destruction of lymphoid cells leaves a fibrillar, somewhat eosinophilic and acellular matrix in place of the lymphoid follicles. The matrix may be surrounded by lymphocytes, plasma cells, nuclear debris and macrophages. Although these changes in lymphoid tissue are essentially the same in lymph nodes and in the Peyer's patches, grossly they are seen to better advantage in the latter, which may be darkened with hemorrhage and slough out, leaving deep craters in the intestinal wall.

In the experimental disease in the rabbit, this affinity for lymphocytes is particularly well demonstrated in the Peyer's patches, in the sacculus rotundus and appendix, where rather characteristic lesions, grossly chalk-white, stand out individually in contrast to the adjacent flesh-colored tissues. When viewed from the serous surface, these collections of lymphoid follicles have the appearance of white hexagonal tile separated by dark cement.

In the digestive system of cattle, the rinderpest virus produces typical lesions in the epithelium, varying with the anatomical features of the parts of the digestive tract affected. Application of the virus to the oral mucosa does not readily produce infection, which suggests that the virus is carried to the oral mucosa by the blood stream. In the squamous epithelium of the oral cavity, the first evidence of the presence of the virus is necrosis of a few epithelial cells in the deep layers of the stratum malpighii. These affected cells have pyknotic and fragmented nuclei and irregular, eosinophilic cytoplasm; they appear shrunken and are separated from the adjoining epithelium by a clear space. As these necrotic areas increase in size and extend toward the surface, the cornified layer above them becomes elevated and causes them to appear grossly as tiny, grayish-white, slightly raised puncta. Multinucleated giant cells form in the stratum spinosum. Eosinophilic cytoplasmic inclusion bodies form in the mucosal epithelial cells and giant cells. Intranuclear inclusion bodies are reportedly rarely seen. Vesicles are not formed in this disease. The foci of necrosis in the epithelium usually remain discrete for a time, but later coalesce to form large areas of erosion. Since the basal layer of the squamous epithelium is rarely penetrated, ulcers seldom form. The erosions are shallow with a red, raw-appearing floor, bounded by essentially normal epithelium which provides a sharply demarcated margin. The lesions in the oral mucosa have a selective distribution: the inside of the lower lip, the adjacent gum, the cheeks near the commissures and the ventral surface of the

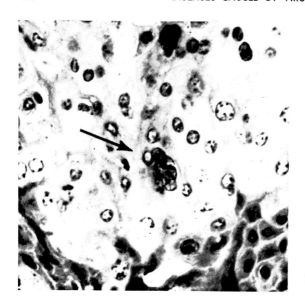

FIG. 10-53.—Rinderpest. A multi-nucleated giant cell in the lingual mucosa. A small intranuclear inclusion body is evident. (Courtesy Dr. W. Plowright.)

free portion of the tongue. In severe cases, they may extend from these sites to the hard palate and pharynx, and in fulminant cases to all the mucous surfaces of the tongue with the singular exception of the anterior seven-eighths of its dorsal surface. The esophageal lesions, particularly those of its upper third, are similar to those in the mouth and pharynx, but usually less severe. The rumen, reticulum and omasum rarely exhibit any lesions, although in a few instances small eroded foci are found in the omasal leaves.

The abomasum is one of the most common sites of the lesions of rinderpest. They are most severe and consistent in the pyloric region, where necrotic foci of microscopic size in the epithelium are accompanied by capillary congestion and hemorrhage in the underlying lamina propria. This results in the gross appearance of irregularly outlined, superficial streaks of color, ranging from bright red to dark brown. The lesions tend to follow the edges of the broad plicae as streaks extending into the fundus, but becoming more numerous and diffuse in the flattened portion of the pylorus. Edema may be extensive in the submucosa of plicae, involving an entire fold and causing it to appear grossly thickened and gelatinous on cross section. As necrosis of the epithelium progresses, the infected areas become slate colored and the epithelium sloughs away, leaving sharply outlined irregular erosions with a red, raw floor oozing blood. In cases of relatively longer standing, black clotted blood may partially or completely fill these pits in the mucosa. Often the most tenacious portion of the clot is at the periphery of the erosion and clings to the edges, leaving the center open. Deep ulceration occasionally occurs, with microscopic evidence of penetration of the muscularis mucosae. In fatal cases, the lumen of the abomasum is usually empty, except for blood-tinged mucous material.

In the small intestine severe lesions are less common than in the mouth, abomasum or large intestine, but streaks of hemorrhage and, less frequently, erosions along the crest of the folds of mucous membrane may be found, particularly in the initial part of the duodenum and terminal ileum. Peyer's patches

the course of the disease. Disturbances in distribution of body heat may be observed, with the ears, muzzle and extremities cold, and other parts of the body very warm to the touch. The nasal and oral mucosae are congested, varying from pink to red. The conjunctiva may be congested, but the eye is not otherwise involved. Dehydration and suspension of milk secretion and rumination occur in severe infections, and the animals so affected are weak and tend to be recumbent. Abortions are frequent following acute attacks, even in animals which appear to be recovering. Septic metritis following abortion may result in death. In the fetus, lesions similar to those of the adult may be seen in the oral cavity, esophagus and abomasum. Calves born alive may also exhibit signs and lesions of virus diarrhea. Congenital cerebellar hypoplasia has been noted in calves born to naturally and experimentally infected dams. Observation of infected herds has shown that from 33 to 100 per cent of the animals exhibit symptoms. The mortality is usually from 4 to 8 per cent.

Lesions.—At necropsy, except for general dehydration and emaciation of the carcass, the principal gross lesions are found in the gastro-intestinal tract. Sharply delimited, irregularly-shaped ulcers or erosions of the mucosa are found on the dental pad, palate, lateral surfaces of the tongue and inside of the cheeks. Ulcers may also occur on the muzzle and at the external nares, although usually the nasal mucosæ are merely reddened. On the mucous membrane of the pharynx, irregularly-shaped ulcers of varying size may be covered by a tenacious gray exudate. Necrotic lesions may be confined to the pharynx or may extend to the larynx. Some animals develop pneumonia.

In the esophagus, the entire mucous membrane may contain shallow erosions or ulcers with sharply delimited, irregular margins and a red base. At times these lesions coalesce to form elongated ulcers or erosions, with necrotic material adhering to some.

The abomasal mucosa may be diffusely reddened or may contain petechiæ and a few ulcers. Hemorrhages may be present in the leaves of the omasum. The mucosa of the small intestine is diffusely reddened, but prominent petechiæ and ulcers are found only in the cecum. Hemorrhages have been observed in the vaginal mucosa, subcutis generally and the epicardium.

Diagnosis.—The resemblance of the lesions of virus diarrhea to the gastro-intestinal lesions of rinderpest and the oral lesions of malignant catarrhal fever complicates the differential diagnosis. At present, cross-immunity and cross-serum neutralization tests can be used to distinguish rinderpest from virus diarrhea. Malignant catarrh can be differentiated by its slower spread and the characteristic ocular, nasal, and brain lesions which it produces. The recently described "mucosal disease" of cattle (below) also presents problems in differential diagnosis. At this writing it appears that an immunologically distinct viral agent is involved in mucosal disease, but further study is needed in order to distinguish clearly between virus diarrhea, mucosal disease, and malignant catarrh.

Mucosal Disease

A disease of cattle in the state of Iowa was reported, in 1953, by Ramsey and Chivers, who called it mucosal disease because its predominant effect appeared to be upon the mucosæ of the digestive tract. This disease, or disease complex, has some clinical or pathologic similarities to rinderpest (p. 486), malignant catarrh (p. 426), virus diarrhea (p. 492), and bovine hyperkeratosis (p. 938). Although present evidence indicates that mucosal disease is a separate entity, further research is needed to clarify its relationship to the other diseases of cattle with which it has features in common. Immunologic evidence now available indicates that the causative agent of this disease is different from that of rinderpest and probably from that of viral diarrhea. Obviously this is not the same disease as bovine hyperkeratosis, which is induced by ingestion of, or contact with, highly chlorinated naphthalenes.

Mucosal disease occurs chiefly in young bovines, six to fourteen months of age. The incidence of clinical cases is usually low, varying from 2 to 50 per cent, but the mortality in obviously affected animals is high, usually over 90 per cent. The principal symptoms are fever (106° F. at onset, soon returning to normal), inappetence, watery or bloody diarrhea, excessive salivation, dehydration, depression, and increased lacrimation. A foul smelling, mucopurulent exudate often hangs from the muzzle and nostrils. Erosions of the mucosa of the nostrils, muzzle, lips, tongue, gums and oral cavity are important lesions which can be observed in the living animal. Leukopenia may occur early in the course of the disease but leukocytosis is usually present when clinical signs become marked.

Lesions.—The most prominent changes found at necropsy are in the mucosae of the digestive tract. Erosions of epithelium are also observed in the oral mucosa over the tongue, gums, lips, cheeks and palate. Similar changes may occur in the pharynx, and severe erosions in the esophagus may cause most of its epithelium to be lost. Shallow erosions are often found in the leaves of the omasum and pillars of the rumen, where a few progress to hemorrhagic ulcers. Multiple, sharply circumscribed erosions, 1 to 1.5 mm. in diameter, with elevated margins, are seen in the folds of the fundus of the abomasum and are sometimes accentuated by a concentric red halo of petechiæ. Microscopically, these lesions result from atrophy and cystic changes in the gastric glands, but ulceration seldom occurs because the overlying epithelium remains relatively intact. Edema, congestion and occasional hemorrhage are common in the lamina propria and submucosa. In the small intestine, particularly over the Peyer's patches, focal areas of erosion are seen, some with thick, blood-flecked, tenacious mucus adhering to them. Necrosis and sloughing of lymphoid tissue and the mucosa over affected areas may be observed. The cecum, colon and rectum are usually affected, although in degrees varying from catarrhal inflammation, manifested by congestion and excess mucus, to hemorrhage, ulceration and necrosis of patches of mucosa. In the colon 10 to 20 cm. distal to the ileocecal valve, cysts 1 to 4 mm. in diameter may form in the mucosal wall. The lymph nodes of the intestinal tract are described as grossly normal or slightly edematous. The cervical or retropharyngeal lymph nodes have been observed to be grossly enlarged, but microscopic evidence of severe destruction of lymphocytes, as in rinderpest, has not been reported.

In some of the cases, large quantities of mucopurulent exudate with small underlying epithelial erosions may be found in the nares, but the rest of the respiratory system is not affected. The lesions in the remainder of the body are inconstant and not considered specific.

Diagnosis.—The diagnosis of mucosal disease presents many difficulties, stemming in part from the present incomplete state of knowledge of the disease. The disease can be suspected from its symptomatology and presumptively diagnosed from the gross and microscopic lesions, but definitive diagnosis must await immunologic differentiation of the causative agent. It is hoped that investigations now in progress will serve to define this entity more clearly and to provide the information needed for its specific recognition.

Virus Diarrhea—Mucosal Disease

BAKER, J. A., YORK, C. J., GILLESPIE, J. H., and MITCHELL, G. B.: Virus Diarrhea in Cattle. Am. J. Vet. Research *15*:525–531, 1954.

CARLSON, R. G., PRITCHARD, W. R., and DOYLE, L. P.: The Pathology of Virus Diarrhea of Cattle in Indiana. Am. J. Vet. Res. *18*:560–568, 1957.

GILLESPIE, J. H., and BAKER, J. A.: Studies on Virus Diarrhea. Cornell Vet. *49*:439–443, 1959.

GILLESPIE, J. H., BAKER, J. A., and McENTEE, K.: A Cytopathogenic Strain of Virus Diarrhea Virus. Cornell Vet. *50*:73–79, 1960.

GILLESPIE, J. H., *et al.*: The Isolation of Noncytopathic Virus Diarrhea Virus from Two Aborted Bovine Fetuses. Cornell Vet. *57*:564–571, 1967.

GILLESPIE, J. H.: Comments on Bovine Viral Diarrhea-Mucosal Disease. J. Am. Vet. Med. Assn. *152*:768–770, 1968.

LAMBERT, G., FERNELIUS, A. L., and CHEVILLE, N. F.: Experimental Bovine Viral Diarrhea in Neonatal Calves. J. Am. Vet. Med. Assn. *154*:181–189, 1969.

McCORMACK, P. E., ST.-GEORGE-GRAMBAUER, T. D., and PULSFORD, N. F.: Mucosa Type Disease of Cattle in South Australia. Austral. Vet. J. *35*:482–488, 1959.

MILLS, J. H. L., NIELSEN, S. W., and LUGINBUHL, R. E.: Current Status of Bovine Mucosal Disease. J. Am. Vet. Med. Assn. *146*:691–696, 1965.

OLAFSON, P., McCALLUM, A. D., and FOX, F. H.: An Apparently New Transmissible Disease of Cattle. Cornell Vet. *36*:205–213, 1946.

OLAFSON, P., and RICKARD, C. G.: Further Observations on the Virus Diarrhea (New Transmissible Disease) of Cattle. Cornell Vet. *37*:104–106, 1947.

PANDE, P. G. and KRISHNAMURTHY, D.: Incidence and Pathology of Some Recently Recognized Mucosal Disease-like Syndromes Amongst Cattle and Buffaloes in India. Bull. Off. Int. Epiz. *55*:706–714, 1961. (VB 127–62.)

PETER, C. P., *et al.*: Cytopathologic Changes of Lymphatic Tissues of Cattle with the Bovine Virus Diarrhea-Mucosal Disease Complex. Am. J. Vet. Res. *29*:939–948, 1968.

RAMSEY, F. K., and CHIVERS, W. H.: Mucosal Disease of Cattle. North Am. Vet. *34*: 629–633, 1953.

RAMSEY, F. K.: The Pathology of a Mucosal Disease of Cattle. Proc. Am. Vet. Med. Assn., 1954, pp. 162–167.

SALISBURY, R. M. *et al.*: A Mucosal Disease-like Syndrome of Cattle in New Zealand. Bull. Off. Int. Epiz. *56*:72–78, 1961. (VB 123–62.)

SCHULTZ, L. E.: Pathologisch-Anatomische Befunde bei der Sogenannten "Mucosal Disease" (Schleimhautkrankheit) des Rindes. Dtsche. Tierärzt. Wschr. *66*:582–586, 1959.

TAYLOR, D. O. N., GUSTAFSON, D. P., and CLAFLIN, R. M.: Properties of Some Viruses of the Mucosal Disease-Virus Diarrhea Complex. Am. J. Vet. Res. *24*:143–149, 1963.

TYLER, D. E., and RAMSEY, F. K.: Comparative Pathologic, Immunologic, and Clinical Responses Produced by Selected Agents of the Bovine Mucosal Disease-Virus Diarrhea Complex. Am. J. Vet. Res. *26*:903–913, 1965.

WALKER, R. V. L., and OLAFSON, P.: Failure of Virus Diarrhea of Cattle to Immunize Against Rinderpest. Cornell Vet. *37*:107–111, 1947.

WARD, G. M., *et al.*: A Study of Experimentally Induced Bovine Viral Diarrhea-Mucosal Disease in Pregnant Cows and Their Progeny. Cornell Vet. *59*:525–538, 1969.

WARD, G. M.: Bovine Cerebellar Hypoplasia Apparently Caused by BVD-MD Virus. A Case Report. Cornell Vet. *59*:570–576, 1969.

WHEAT, J. D., McKERCHER, D. G., and YORK, C. J.: Virus Diarrhea in California. California Vet. *8*:26–28, 35, 1954.

Epidemic Diarrheal Disease of Mice

(EDIM)

An enteric disease caused by a viral agent often presents a serious problem in colonies of laboratory mice, for it is hard to control and produces a very high mortality among suckling animals. Entire mouse colonies have been sacrificed in efforts to eliminate the disease.

Adult mice can become infected and eliminate the virus for varying periods of time in their feces, however clinical disease does not occur.

The disease appears in suckling mice ten to fifteen days of age but does not affect mice which have reached weaning age (twenty-two days). Although the nursing females are ostensibly normal, their affected young appear somewhat shrunken or dehydrated with dry whitish scales over the skin of the back and shoulder. Some mice have a cyanotic color, especially noticeable along the neck and between the shoulders. Diarrhea is evidenced by profuse soiling of the perineal region and tail with yellowish fecal material. Death often occurs soon after onset, but if mice survive more than two days, a tenacious somewhat darker material often stains the perianal region, and in such cases death may follow severe obstipation. In mild, uncomplicated cases, mice recover completely in two to five days, although the growth of some may be retarded.

The lesions in fatal cases have been described only to the extent that cytoplasmic inclusion bodies occur in the intestinal epithelium. These inclusions are probably, but not incontrovertibly, related to the disease and point toward its viral etiology. The inclusion bodies, described originally by Pappenheimer and Enders (1947), are spherical, sharply outlined, 1 to 4 microns in diameter, and sometimes surrounded by a narrow clear halo. Laidlaw's acid fuchsin-phosphomolybdic acid-orange G stain reveals these inclusions to be intensely fuchsinophilic. They are eosinophilic with hematoxylin and eosin stain and resemble the inclusion bodies of canine distemper (p. 440).

Epidemic Diarrheal Disease of Mice

CHEEVER, F. S., and MUELLER, J. H.: Epidemic Diarrheal Disease of Suckling Mice. I. Manifestations, Epidemiology and Attempts to Transmit the Disease. J. Exper. Med. 85:405-416, 1947.
————: Epidemic Diarrheal Disease of Suckling Mice. III. The Effect of Strain, Litter and Season on the Incidence of the Disease. J. Exper. Med. 88:309–316, 1948.
KRAFT, L. M.: Two Viruses Causing Diarrhea in Infant Mice in *The Problems of Laboratory Animal Disease.* Harris, R. J. C. (Ed.). New York, Academic Press, 1962, pp. 115–130.
PAPPENHEIMER, A. M., and ENDERS, J. F.: An Epidemic Diarrheal Disease of Suckling Mice. II. Inclusions in the Intestinal Epithelial Cells. J. Exper. Med. 85:417–422, 1947.
PAPPENHEIMER, A. M., and CHEEVER, F. S.: Epidemic Diarrheal Disease of Suckling Mice. IV. Cytoplasmic Inclusion Bodies in Intestinal Epithelium in Relation to the Disease. J. Exper. Med. 88:317–324, 1948.

LETHAL INTESTINAL DISEASE OF INFANT MICE
(LIVIM)

Lethal intestinal disease of infant mice is a viral infection of suckling mice characterized by diarrhea and high mortality. Although similar to EDIM infection (p. 495), the two diseases are caused by distinct viruses. LIVIM produces clinical disease in mice up to sixteen to twenty days of age. As in EDIM, adults can become infected and shed the virus in the feces without clinical signs. Suckling mice develop diarrhea, do not suckle, become severely dehydrated and almost completely inactive. The mortality is high. Few gross changes occur. The stomach is empty, the small intestine often distended with gas, and unformed feces are present in the colon. Microscopically multinucleated epithelial cells are present in the villi of the small intestine. These and other cells slough leaving

McCollum, W. H., Doll, E. R., Wilson, J. C., and Cheatham, J.: Isolation and Propagation of Equine Arteritis Virus in Monolayer Cell Cultures of Rabbit Kidney. Cornell Vet. 52:452–458, 1962.

Wilson, J. C., Doll, E. R., McCollum, W. H., and Cheatham, J.: Propagation of Equine Arteritis Virus Previously Adapted to Cell Cultures of Equine Kidney in Monolayer Cultures of Hamster Kidney. Cornell Vet. 52:200–205, 1962.

Aleutian Disease of Mink

A few years ago breeders of mink found that unusual colors in mink fur could bring a premium in the market place. This led to the selection of animals with any of several mutant genes which in the homozygous state could result in a coat color different from the wild type. One of the first of these unusual coats was a blue color, due to a single recessive gene, which came to be called "Aleutian." After animals with this color became reasonably numerous a serious disease appeared among them—hence the name "Aleutian Disease." It is now known that other types of mink are also susceptible but most natural cases occur in "Aleutian" or "Sapphire" mink (the latter are homozygous for the Aleutian gene [a] and for another mutant gene [p] as well. The disease is more rapidly progressive in mink homozygous for the Aleutian gene than in non-Aleutian type mink in which the disease is more protracted, lasting several months or years. The increased susceptibility of mink homozygous for the Aleutian gene is believed to be explained in part in that all such mink have an inherited anomaly of granule producing cells designated the Chediak-Higashi syndrome (p. 1171).

Hartsough is credited by Helmbolt and Jungherr (1958) with first recognizing the disease in 1946 and one of the first reports was by Hartsough and Gorham (1956). The disease is known in all parts of the world in which mink are raised.

The etiologic agent is a virus, approximately 50 mμ in size, which is partially resistant to formalin and heat. Natural transmission occurs both horizontally and vertically. Viremia is usually persistent throughout the course and virus is present in urine and saliva.

The disease is manifest in affected mink by lethargy, anorexia, cachexia, occasionally with fever which may reach 107° F. Blood often exudes from the mouth and sometimes from the anus. Young kits tend to die within a few days after signs of illness are seen but most adults live for several weeks. Some may survive for many months but among animals which show signs, 90 per cent or more can be expected to die.

There is a progressive thrombocytopenia and anemia. The anemia is believed to result from hemorrhage associated with defective hemostasis and depression of erythropoiesis secondary to uremia. The thrombocytopenia has been shown to result from episodic intravascular coagulation with removal of fibrinogen and platelets from the circulation. Intravascular coagulation with deposition of incompletely polymerized fibrin in glomeruli is believed to play an important role in the pathogenesis of glomerular lesions in Aleutian disease, although the glomerulonephritis may represent a form of immune-complex disease.

Of particular interest is the severe hypergammaglobulinemia, first reported by Henson et al. (1961) and subsequently confirmed by others. The changes in the serum proteins are the result of elevation in the gamma globulin fraction, due to increase in the 7 S components of euglobulin. In normal pastel or Aleutian mink, gamma globulin constitutes 15 to 20 per cent of the serum proteins. In mink affected with Aleutian Disease, the gamma globulin may constitute as much as 65 per cent of the serum proteins. The highest levels of gamma globulin are found in those cases with the most widespread accumulation of plasma cells in the tissues, a point to be described later.

The **lesions** of Aleutian Disease are characterized chiefly by disseminated focal accumulations of plasma cells in several organs; hyaline and inflammatory changes in the walls of small arteries; dilatation and proliferation of intrahepatic bile ducts; focal or diffuse interstitial fibrosis of the kidneys, glomerulonephritis, hemorrhages and focal encephalomalacia with non-suppurative leptomeningitis. The large number of plasma cells in the tissues is a consistent feature of the disease and is undoubtedly the source of the excessive gamma globulins found in the serum. Obel (1959) considered these plasma cells to be neoplastic but it must be realized that these cells appear quite well differentiated and do not usually compress, invade and displace normal tissue as decisively as frankly neoplastic cells can be seen to do. According to Helmbolt and Jungherr (1958), the lesions, consisting largely of plasma cells and lymphocytes, were found in a series of 40 cases in the following organs: liver (85 per cent), brain (80 per cent), kidney (60 per cent) and lung (48 per cent). Arteritis was noted in small arteries in about 28 per cent of their cases. These lesions were characterized by hyaline changes in the media, infiltration of media and adventitia by lymphoid cells and eventual occlusion of the lumen with hyalin. These changes are indistinguishable from those of periarteritis nodosa (p. 1159). In severely diseased mink, plasma cell infiltration and arteritis may be found in any organ or tissue. The kidneys not only contain arterial lesions and accumulations of lymphocytes and plasma cells, but focal or diffuse fibrosis of the interstitial tissues may be evident. Glomerular tufts may be thickened due to deposition of a hyalin PAS-positive material, and some convoluted tubules may be distended with protein. Leader (1963), and Henson and co-workers (1967, 1968) have described the pathogenesis and ultrastructural features of the renal lesions.

The gross lesions conform to those one would expect to result from the microscopic lesions in arteries. Small (3 mm.) ulcers are often found in the mouth, particularly on the gums and buccal mucosa and may be covered with a diphtheritic membrane. The kidneys are often three times normal size, pale orange to yellow color, frequently mottled with white punctate areas. Stellar hemorrhages may be seen in the renal capsule which is not usually adherent to the underlying cortex. The liver may be enlarged as much as twice normal size and have a mahogany color. The spleen is enlarged from twice to five times its normal size but otherwise not remarkable grossly. The lungs may contain patches of red color which are visible on the surface and extend deeply into the parenchyma. In a few cases, the colon may contain free blood and in others, the tissues may be obviously anemic.

Although the pathogenesis of Aleutian disease is still under intensive investigation, the presence of plasmacytosis, vascular lesions, and hypergammaglobulinemia suggest that it may represent an infectious autoimmune disease.

The **diagnosis** of Aleutian disease can be made with certainty from the histologic lesions which are distinguishable from infection with avian tubercle bacilli, page 626 (granulomas containing acid-fast bacilli); canine distemper, page 440 (cytoplasmic and intranuclear inclusion bodies); and steatitis, page 994 (inflammation and ceroid pigment in adipose tissues). The hypergammaglobulinemia is also useful to confirm presumptive diagnosis based upon clinical signs.

Aleutian Disease of Mink

BASRUR, P. K., GRAY, D. P., and KARSTAD, L.: Aleutian Disease (Plasmacytosis) of Mink. III. Propagation of the Virus in Mink Tissue Cultures. Canad. J. Comp. Med. & Vet. Sci. 27:301–306, 1963.

CHAPMAN, I. and JIMENEZ, F. A.: Aleutian-Mink Disease in Man. New Engl. J. Med. 269: 1171–1174, 1963.

EKLUND, C. M., et al.: Aleutian Disease of Mink: Properties of the Etiologic Agent and the Host Responses. J. Infect. Dis. 118:510–526, 1968.

GORHAM, J. R., LEADER, R. W., and HENSON, J. B.: Neutralizing Ability of Hypergammaglobulinemia Serum on the Aleutian Disease Virus of Mink. Fed. Proc. 47:265, 1963.

HARTSOUGH, G. R. and GORHAM, J. R.: Aleutian Disease in Mink. Nat. Fur News 28: 10–11, 38, 1956.

HELMBOLDT, C. F. and JUNGHERR, E. L.: The Pathology of Aleutian Disease in Mink. Am. J. Vet. Res. 19:212–222, 1958.

HENSON, J. B., et al.: The Sequential Development of Lesions in Spontaneous Aleutian Disease of Mink. Pathologia Vet. 3:289-314, 1966.

HENSON, J. B., et al.: The Sequential Development of Ultrastructural Lesions in the Glomeruli of Mink with Experimental Aleutian Disease. Lab. Invest. 19:153–162, 1968.

HENSON, J. B., GORHAM, J. R., and TANKA, Y.: Renal Glomerular Ultrastructure in Mink Affected by Aleutian Disease. Lab. Invest. 17:123–139, 1967.

HENSON, J. B., LEADER, R. W., and GORHAM, J. R.: Hypergammaglobulinemia in Mink. Proc. Soc. Exp. Soc. Biol. Med. 107:919–920, 1961.

HENSON, J. B., GORHAM, J. R., LEADER, R. W., and WAGNER, B. M.: Experimental Hypergammaglobulinemia in Mink. J. Exp. Med. 116:357–364, 1962.

KARSTAD, L.: Aleutian Disease. A Slowly Progressive Viral Infection of Mink. Current Topics in Microbiology and Immunology 40:9–21, 1967.

KARSTAD, L. and PRIDHAM, T. J.: Aleutian Disease of Mink. 1. Evidence of its Viral Etiology. Canad. J. Comp. Med. and Vet. Sci. 26:97–102, 1962.

KENYON, A. J., TRAUTWEIN, G., and HELMBOLDT, C. F.: Characterization of Blood Serum Proteins from Mink with Aleutian Disease. Am. J. Vet. Res. 24:168–173, 1963.

KENYON, A. J., HELMBOLDT, C. F., and NIELSEN, S. W.: Experimental Transmission of Aleutian Disease with Urine. Am. J. Vet. Res. 24:1066–1067, 1963.

KENYON, A. J. and HELMBOLDT, C. F.: Solubility and Electrophoretic Characterizations of Globulins from Mink with Aleutian Disease. Am. J. Vet. Res. 25:1535–1541, 1964.

LEADER, R. W., WAGNER, B. M., HENSON, J. B., and GORHAM, J. R.: Structural and Histochemical Observations of Liver and Kidney in Aleutian Disease of Mink. Am. J. Path. 43:33–53, 1963.

McKAY, D. G., et al.: Chronic Intravascular Coagulation in Aleutian Disease of Mink. Am. J. Path. 50:899–916, 1967.

OBEL, A-L.: Studies on a Disease in Mink with Systemic Proliferation of the Plasma Cells. Am. J. Vet. Res. 20:384–393, 1959.

PADGETT, G. A., GORHAM, J. R., and HENSON, J. B.: Epizootiologic Studies of Aleutian Disease. I. Transplacental Transmission of the Virus. J. Infect. Dis. 117:35–38, 1967.

TRAUTWEIN, G. W. and HELMBOLDT, C. F.: Aleutian Disease of Mink. 1. Experimental Transmission of the Disease. Am. J. Vet. Res. 23:1280–1288, 1962.

WAGNER, B. M.: Aleutian Disease of Mink. Arthritis and Rheumatism 6:386–391, 1963.

African Horse-Sickness

The apparently non-specific name, African Horse-Sickness, applies to a specific and important disease of *Equidæ*, caused by a virus which is transmitted by several species of *Culicoides*. The disease was apparently present in South Africa when the first European settlers brought their horses and mules into that country in the 18th Century and has in recent years crossed the boundaries of several other countries—namely, Egypt, Israel, West Pakistan, Afghanistan, Cyprus, Iraq, Syria, Lebanon, Turkey, India, Iran and Jordan. The entire problem has been adequately reviewed most recently by Maurer and McCully (1963).

The etiologic agent is a virus with many immunologically distinguishable strains. The globular virus particles (50 millimicrons in diameter) are filterable through Seitz E K filter pads, and are infective for mice by intracerebral inoculation. Specific strains which by passage via this route have become neurotropic for the mouse, are used extensively in the production of vaccine.

The **clinical features** of African Horse-sickness usually are described as conforming to one of four types. The first is the least serious and is more often observed in partially immune animals, particularly donkeys. Mild fever, anorexia, dyspnea and accelerated pulse rate may be all that is observed, followed by rapid recovery. The acute pulmonary form of the disease is recognized by an incubation period of three to five days, sudden onset of high fever (105–107° F.), severe dyspnea due to pulmonary edema—often with frothy exudates in the nostrils. Sweating and coughing may occur and death usually results within a few hours of onset of the pulmonary edema. This form has been described in dogs as well. A third clinical type of the disease is the subacute cardiac form in which the incubation period and course is usually longer than in the pulmonary form. It is distinguished by the occurrence of edema of the head and neck, lips, eyelids, cheek and tongue and most characteristically, edematous bulging of the supraorbital fossa. Petechiæ may appear on the ventral aspect of the tongue, abdominal pain and paralysis of the esophagus may be manifest and death usually is due to cardiac failure and hypoxia. In a fourth, mixed form, a combination of pulmonary and cardiac lesions are found at necropsy.

The **lesions** at necropsy usually can be correlated with the clinical form of the disease. The most striking changes are seen in the respiratory system. Hydrothorax usually accompanies the severe edema which involves the subpleural and interlobular stroma and fills alveoli in many lobules. Frothy fluid usually fills the bronchi, trachea and the rest of the upper respiratory tract. Fibrin and proteinaceous material are recognizable microscopically in the edematous tissues, and leukocytes may also be present. In some cases these leukocytes may be present in sufficient numbers to suggest bronchopneumonia. The cardiac lesions are also significant. Hydropericardium is usually present along with petechiae and inflammatory edema in the epicardium. Disseminated foci of myocardial necrosis are seen microscopically and are often accentuated by hemorrhages which may be recognized grossly. Sometimes edema may involve the adventitia of arterioles but otherwise, small blood vessels do not contain identifiable lesions. Depletion of lymphocytes is usually evident in the spleen and lymph nodes; reticulo-endothelial and plasma cells are usually increased in number although the spleen is not usually enlarged. Some lymph nodes may be grossly hemorrhagic. The gastrointestinal tract may be involved. Edema around the pharynx may account for the presumed paralysis of the esophagus which is noted in some descriptions of the clinical features. Hemorrhage is common in the gastric mucosa. The liver is usually only congested. Hemorrhage and edema may be found in the kidneys, particularly involving the peripelvic fat.

The **diagnosis** is usually made presumptively in enzootic regions from the clinical features and necropsy findings but should be confirmed by recovery and identification of the virus. The method presently most suitable involves the intracerebral inoculation of mice and subsequent neutralization tests to determine the antigenic type. Differentiation from equine viral arteritis (p. 498) should be considered because both diseases are characterized by edema and hemorrhage in the subcutis, heart and lungs. The specific lesions in the musculature of arterioles in arteritis would be useful but isolation and identification of the virus should also be undertaken.

African Horse-Sickness

BREESE, S. S., JR., OZAWA, Y., and DARDIRI, A. H.: Electron Microscopic Characterization of African Horse-sickness Virus. J. Am. Vet. Med. Assn. *155*:391–400, 1969.

HENNING, M. W.: *Animal Diseases of South Africa*, 3rd Ed., Pretoria, Central News Agency, Ltd., 1956.

LECATSAS, G., and ERASMUS, B. J.: Electron Microscopic Study of the Formation of African Horse-Sickness Virus. Arch. Ges. Virusforsch *22*:442–450, 1967.

MAURER, F. D. and McCULLY, R. M.: African Horsesickness—with Emphasis on Pathology. Amer. J. Vet. Res. *24*:235–266, 1963.

PIERCY, S. E.: Some Observations on African Horse-sickness Including an Account of an Outbreak Amongst Dogs. East African Agric. J. *17*:1–3, 1951.

REID, N. R.: African Horse-sickness. Brit. Vet. J. *118*:137–142, 1961.

MARBURG AGENT DISEASE

(Marburg Virus Disease; Vervet Monkey Disease)

First described in 1967 in Marburg and Frankfurt, Germany, and Belgrade, Yugoslavia, Marburg Agent disease is principally of importance as an infection of man contracted from vervet monkeys (African green monkey; *Cercopithecus aethiops*). Of 30 cases reported in 1967, 7 were fatal. The majority of cases occurred in laboratory workers in contact with monkey tissues; four occurred in hospital personnel caring for the patients. Following an incubation period of five to seven days, the clinical course was characterized by fever, headache, backache, prostration, vomiting, diarrhea and an exanthematous rash. The rash later become hemorrhagic, and bleeding developed in the lungs and gastrointestinal tract. Pathological findings were dominated by widespread focal necrosis especially of the liver, lymphatic tissues, kidney, pancreas, adrenals and skin. Non-suppurative encephalitis with glial nodules and hemorrhage was also present.

The agent, although apparently a virus, has not at present been fully characterized or classified. However, the isolate, as well as human patient tissues were highly virulent for vervet monkeys and also for rhesus monkeys (*Macaca mulatta*), squirrel monkeys (*Saimiri sciureus*), guinea pigs, and hamsters. The disease, which is uniformly fatal, mimics the picture seen in man. In guinea pigs and hamsters, intracytoplasmic granules considered to represent the infective agent, are found in hepatocytes and epithelial cells of the kidney and lung. Infected animals excrete infectious material and all tissues are infective. The disease has developed in uninoculated monkeys housed with experimentally infected animals.

Although the disease has not been recorded since, it provides a tragic example of the possible consequences which may result from intimate contact with poorly studied species.

Marburg Agent Disease

BECHTELSHEIMER, H., JACOB, H., and SOLCHER, H.: Zur Neuropathologie due Dursch Grune Meerkatzen (*Cercopithecus aethiops*) Ubertragenen Infektionskrankheiten in Marburg. Deutsch. Med. Wschr. *93*:602–604, 1968.

————: The Neuropathology of an Infectious Disease Transmitted by African Green Monkeys (*Cercopithecus aethiops*). Germ. Med. Mth. *14*:10–12, 1969.

BOWEN, E. T. W., *et al.*: Vervet Monkey Disease: Studies on Some Physical and Chemical Properties of the Causative Agent. Br. J. of Exp. Pathology *50*:400–407, 1969.

GEDIGK, P., BECHTELSHEIMER, H., and KORB, G.: Die Pathologische Anatomie der Marburg-Virus – "Krankheit(Sog. "Marburger Offenkrankeit"). Deutsch. Med. Wschr. *93*:590–601, 1968.

KALTER, S. S., RATNER, J. J., and HEVERLING, R. L.: Antibodies in Primates to the Marburg Virus. Proc. Soc. Exp. Biol. & Med. *130*:10–12, 1969.

17

Korb, G., Bechtelsheimer, H., and Gedigk, P.: Die Wichtigsten Histologischen Befunde Bei der Marburg Virus Krankheit. Jahrgang *19*:1089–1096, 1968.

Kissling, R. E., *et al.*: Agent of Disease Contracted from Green Monkeys. Science *160*: 888–890, 1968.

Martini, G. A.: Marburg Agent Disease: In Man. Royal Soc. of Trop. Med. Hyg. *63*: 295–302, 1969.

Saenz, A. C.: Disease in Laboratory Personnel Associated with Vervet Monkeys. I. A General Report on the Outbreak. Primates in Med. *3*:129–134, 1969.

Siegert, R., Shu, H. L., and Slenczka, W.: Isoberung und Identifizierung des "Marburg-Virus." Deutsch. Med. Wschr. *93*:616–619, 1968.

Simpson, D. I. H.: Vervet Monkey Disease: Transmission to the Hamster. Br. J. Exp. Path. *50*:389–392, 1969.

Simpson, D. I. H., Zlotnik, I., and Rutter, D. A.: Vervet Monkey Disease. Experimental Infection of Guinea Pigs and Monkeys with the Causative Agent. Br. J. Exp. Path. *49*:458–464, 1968.

Simpson, D. I. H.: Marburg Agent Disease: In Monkeys. Royal Soc. Trop. Med. Hyg. *63*:303–309, 1969.

Zlotnik, I., Simpson, D. I. H., and Howard, D. M. R.: Structure of the Vervet-Monkey Disease Agent. Lancet *2*:26–28, 1968.

Zlotnik, I.: Marburg Agent Disease: Pathology. Trans. Roy. Soc. Trop. Med. Hyg. *63*:310–327, 1969.

Zlotnik, I., and Simpson, D. I. H.: The Pathology of Experimental Vervet Monkey Disease in Hamsters. Brit. J. Exp. Path. *50*:393–399, 1969.

SIMIAN HEMORRHAGIC FEVER

Simian hemorrhagic fever is a highly infectious disease of monkeys caused by a virus tentatively considered a member of the Arbovirus group, although there is no evidence that arthropods play a role in transmission. The disease, which has only been reported in Old-World primates, of the genus *Macaca* (*M. mulatta*, *M. fascicularis*, *M. arctoides*) has occurred in primate colonies in Washington, D. C., California, England and Russia. Clinical signs include rapid onset, fever, facial edema, cyanosis, anorexia, dehydration, epistaxis, melena, and cutaneous, subcutaneous and retrobulbar hemorrhage. The course runs ten to fifteen days and the mortality rate is high. The gross and microscopic lesions are dominated by hemorrhage which may be found in most any organ or tissue, although almost constantly in the skin, nasal mucosa, lung, gastrointestinal tract, perirenal tissues, renal capsule, adrenal and periocular tissues. There is marked splenomegaly and necrosis of lymphocytic follicles of the spleen, lymph nodes, tonsils and Peyer's patches. Thrombi are frequent in small veins and capillaries. Degenerative changes may occur in the liver, kidney, brain, and bone marrow which are believed to be due to blood stasis and hypoxia.

The disease must be differentiated from **Kyasanur Forest Disease** which is an arbovirus infection of Old World monkeys (*M. radiata* and *Presbytis entellus*) and man, transmitted by a tick, *Haemophysalis spinigera*. Kyasanur Forest Disease has not been described outside India. The hemorrhagic tendencies are generally more severe in simian hemorrhagic fever and marked splenomegaly and lymphocytic necrosis are not features of Kyasanur Forest Disease. Non-suppurative encephalomyelitis may occur in Kayasanur Forest Disease. Mice are susceptible to Kyasanur Forest Disease but the virus of simian hemorrhagic fever does not kill mice, a point which can aid differentiation. Definitive diagnosis of either infection requires virus isolation and identification.

Simian Hemorrhagic Fever

Allen, A. M., *et al.*: Simian Hemorrhagic Fever. II. Studies in Pathology. Amer. J. Trop. Med. *17*:413–421, 1968.

IYER, C. G. S., *et al.*: Kyasanur Forest Disease. VII. Pathological Findings in Monkeys, *Presbytis entellus* and *Macaca radiata*, Found Dead in the Forest. Indian J. Med. Res. *48*: 276–286, 1960.

PALMER, A. E., *et al.*: Simian Hemorrhagic Fever. I. Clinical and Epizootiologic Aspects of an Outbreak Among Quarantined Monkeys. Amer. J. Trop. Med. *17*:404–412, 1968.

TAURASO, N. M., *et al.*: Simian Hemorrhagic Fever. III. Isolation and Characterization of a Viral Agent. Am. J. Trop. Med. & Hyg. *17*:422–431, 1968.

WEBB, H. E., and BURSTON, J.: Clinical and Pathological Observations With Special Reference to the Nervous System in *Macaca radiata* infected With Kyasanur Forest Disease Virus. Trans. Royal Soc. Trop. Med. & Hyg. *60*:325–331, 1966.

WEBB, H. E.: Kyasanur Forest Disease Virus Infection in Monkeys. Lab. Anim. Handb. *4*:131–134, 1969.

WEBB., H. E., and CHATTERJEA, J. B.: Clinico-Pathological Observations on Monkeys Infected with Kyasanur Forest Disease Virus, with Special Reference to the Haemopoietic System. Brit. J. Haemat. *VIII*:401–413, 1962.

TUMOR-FORMING VIRAL DISEASES

Since the momentous studies of Ellerman and Bang in 1908 and Rous in 1911, the role of viruses in carcinogenesis has steadily received more and more attention. Extensive studies have uncovered many more oncogenic viruses, have provided considerable insight on the interactions of oncogenic viruses and tumor cells, and have led to several intriguing hypotheses to explain spontaneous cancer in man and animals. However, despite the present effort and the sophistication of tumor virus research it is not known how a virus transforms a normal cell into a neoplastic cell.

Much of the current experimentation with oncogenic viruses is conducted with *in vitro* methods. Such an approach has allowed the use and study of human cells (or any other animal) and viruses in a relatively simple, controlled system. In tissue culture systems many oncogenic viruses produce characteristic changes of the cells which are transmitted hereditarily to their progeny. This phenomenon is called transformation. Whether transformed cells are in fact the same as neoplastic cells is unknown, but the discovery of transformation has greatly aided the study, and has led to much of our present understanding of oncogenic viruses. The criteria of transformation as stated by Habel (1968) are "(1) Increased growth rate, shorter doubling time; (2) Unlimited lifetime in culture, establish as permanent lines; (3) Lack of contact inhibition, produce multi-layered clones; (4) Chromosomal abnormalities, increased incidence and types; (5) Production of tumors on transplantation to immunologically compatible host."

Aside from their ability to induce neoplasia, oncogenic viruses do not fall into a unique category. Their physical and chemical characteristics are varied, as are those of viruses causing acute non-neoplastic infections. Oncogenic viruses may contain either DNA or RNA. DNA tumor viruses and RNA tumor viruses differ in their relationship to the infected transformed cell. DNA tumor viruses can either multiply, producing more virus which leads to the death of the cell (as in non-tumor virus infection) or transform the cell without production of more viral particles. In the transformed cell the DNA of the virus enters into a permanent association with the cell, becoming a true set of genes of the cell and its descendants. Virus cannot be demonstrated by usual techniques, however recent studies have provided means of demonstrating the masked viral DNA. The absence of recognizable viral particles in many tumors believed to be of viral origin may be explained by this unique relationship of viral and cellular DNA.

RNA tumor viruses behave in an entirely different manner from DNA tumor viruses. In the transformed cell, viral RNA is continuously produced, often (but not always) maturing to complete viral particles recognizable by standard virological techniques.

The presence of a tumor virus does not always lead to cellular transformation and neoplasia, no more so than infection with non-tumor viruses always lead to recognizable disease. What determines full expression of an oncogenic virus remains a mystery but clearly important are host genotype and various modifying environmental factors.

The following discussion of tumor forming viral diseases does not review the voluminous literature describing experimental studies with these agents designed to elucidate the mechanisms of viral induction of tumors but rather presents the clinical, gross and microscopic features of the diseases as they occur naturally.

Viral Oncogenesis

DULBECCO, R.: Viruses in Carcinogenesis. Ann. Int. Med. *70*:1019–1030, 1969.
————: Cell Transformation by Viruses: Two Minute Viruses are Powerful Tools for Analyzing the Mechanism of Cancer. Science *166*:962–968, 1969.
HABEL, K.: Tumor Viruses. Yale J. Biol. & Med. *37*:473–484, 1965.
————: The Biology of Viral Carcinogenesis. Cancer Res. *28*:1825–1831, 1968.
HUEBNER, R. J., and TODARO, G. T.: Oncogenes of RNA Tumor Viruses as Determinants of Cancer. Proc. Natl. Acad. of Sci. *64*:1087–1094, 1969.
RAPP, F.: The Role of the Viral Genome in Oncogenesis. Cancer Res. *28*:1832–1834, 1968.
SYLVERTON, J. T.: Present Status of Studies on Tumor-Producing Viruses. J. Nat. Cancer Inst. Monograph No. *4*:345–353, 1959.
WILNER, B. I.: *A Classification of the Major Groups of Human and Other Animal Viruses.* 4th Ed. Minneapolis, Burgess Pub. Co., pp. 1–250, 1964.

Papillomatosis in Animals

(Common Warts, Verrucæ Vulgaris)

The common wart that adorns the finger of the small boy has its counterpart in nearly every animal species. In some animals, these warts are precise lesions that fastidiously refuse to grow anywhere but in a selected type of epithelium— in the mouth, for example. In others, massively huge and roughly keratinized warts indiscriminately involve large areas of the skin. Most warts are known from observation to be infectious by contact, and many have been shown by experiment to be transmissible with bacteria-free suspensions of macerated wart tissue. In cutaneous papillomas of the rabbit and goat, transformation of simple hyperplastic squamous epithelium to frankly malignant squamous cell carcinoma has been demonstrated. Thus it appears that papillomatoses represent infectious diseases caused by viruses and characterized by benign hyperplasia of stroma and epithelium, which may, under certain circumstances, undergo malignant change. These viruses may therefore be considered among those which induce tumor formation. They are classified in the papovavirus group.

Bovine Cutaneous Papillomatosis.—In the bovine species, cutaneous papillomatosis is more frequent than in any other domestic animal. Its viral etiology seems to be well established. The disease is more common and severe in young animals; only partial immunity to reinfection develops, and neutralizing antibodies are not demonstrable in bovine serum. The disease is generally self-limiting and recovery without treatment is the usual course; but when lesions occur on the genitalia (see Fibropapillomas), they may interfere with reproduction.

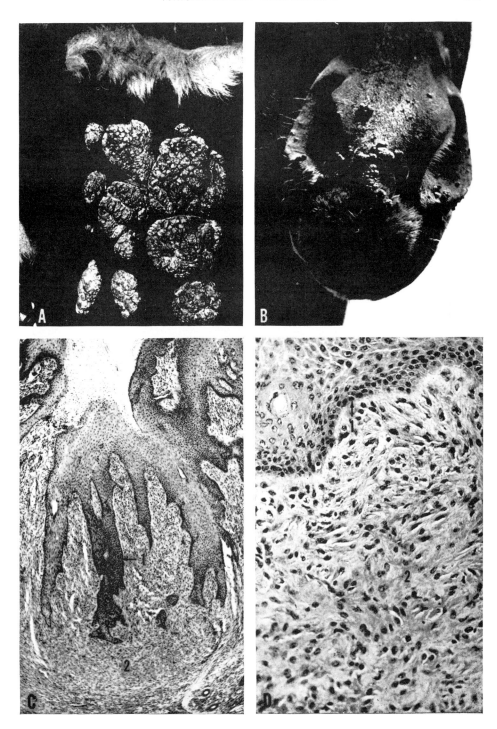

FIG. 10–56.—*A*, Bovine papillomatosis (warts) neck of a Hereford steer. *B*, Equine papillomatosis, nose of a horse. Photographs courtesy of Dr. Carl Olson, Jr. *C*, Experimentally transmitted bovie papillomatosis (× 35) 41 days after inoculation. Note elongated growth of epidermis (*1*) and cellular dermis (*2*). *D*, Higher magnification (× 210) with hyperplastic but sharply demarcated epidermis (*1*) and richly cellular dermis (*2*). (Courtesy of Armed Forces Institute of Pathology.) Contributor: Dr. Carl Olson, Jr.

An outbreak of papillomatosis described by Bagdonas and Olson (1953) involved 82 (74.5 per cent) of a herd of 110 Hereford cattle in the course of two and one-half years. The incubation period following intimate natural contact was three and one-half to four months and the duration of disease was one to five and one-half months, all animals recovering spontaneously. Papillomas were observed by these workers to be most frequent on the neck, chin, shoulder and dewlap; less common on the ears, eyelids, throat, lips and elsewhere. The site of the lesions depends to a great extent upon points of skin contact between affected and susceptible animals.

Lesions.—The typical bovine wart appears grossly as a rough, cauliflower-like mass of varying size and irregular shape, elevated above the skin surface and attached by either a narrow stalk or a broad base. The lesions are first seen as numerous, closely spaced elevations of the skin, which are round and smooth but soon become rough and horny (Fig. 10–56).

Microscopically, the lesions are made up of greatly thickened epidermis, which is both acanthotic and hyperkeratotic, supported in elongated fronds by a core of hyperplastic dermis. In some lesions, particularly those induced experimentally by intradermal injection of the virus, overgrowth of the connective tissue elements of the dermis is a dominant feature. Thus the virus can induce proliferative growth in both epidermis and dermis. Electron microscopic and immunofluorescent studies indicate that the virus is present in the epithelial portion and the fibromatous portion of the papilloma. Epithelial cells of the stratum spinosum occasionally contain intranuclear eosinophilic, homogenous structures which may represent viral inclusion bodies.

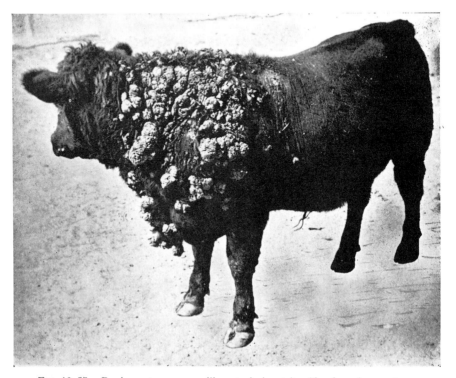

Fig. 10–57.—Bovine cutaneous papillomatosis (warts). Aberdeen-Angus steer.

Fibropapillomas of Bovine Genitalia.—Certain papillary lesions of the penis of young bulls and vagina of cows have been shown by numerous workers to be transmissible, and McEntee (1950) has demonstrated that they are caused by the virus of cutaneous bovine papillomatosis. These fibropapillomas differ from ordinary warts not only in their location, but also in their structure, which is characterized by intense proliferation of connective tissue elements with only slight overgrowth of the overlying epithelium (Fig. 10–58). Interlacing bundles of large, spindle-shaped cells suggest fibroma or fibrosarcoma. Loss of epithelium and secondary infection may result in leukocytic infiltration and edema which increase the cellularity of the lesion and add to the difficulties of interpretation by the uninitiated pathologist. This specific entity is readily recognized, however, by one familiar with its characteristics. The lesions in the genitalia often present surgical problems and may recur after excision, but they do not metastasize and are usually self-limiting.

Olson *et al.* (1959) have experimentally demonstrated that the bovine papilloma virus can induce fibromas and polyps of the bovine urinary bladder similar to the naturally occurring tumors associated with chronic enzootic hematuria (p. 1298). Olson and associates (1965) subsequently isolated a virus, resembling the bovine papilloma virus, from spontaneous urinary bladder tumors of cattle. Experimentally the bovine papilloma virus has also been shown to induce fibromatous meningeal tumors in calves and hamsters, and fibromatous tumors in the skin of horses, hamsters, and mice.

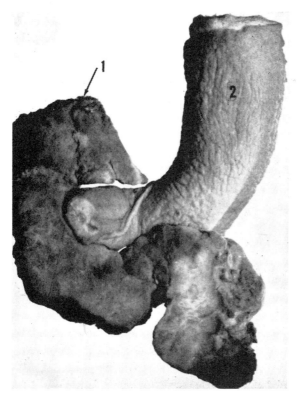

FIG. 10–58.—Bovine fibropapillomatosis. Large roughly irregular mass (*1*) on the glans penis (*2*) of a bull.

Equine Sarcoid.—The pathological characteristics of this growth are presented in the chapter on Neoplasms (p. 196). The entity was first recognized by Jackson (1936) in South Africa, who found evidence suggesting that it was transferable from one part of the horse's body to another. He also thought that the abnormal proliferation was primarily epidermal, the underlying dermis later becoming affected and assuming a preponderant role. In these two respects he perceived a resemblance to the common warts (papillomas), which are known to have a viral origin.

Olson (1948) has experimentally demonstrated what Jackson suspected, that the lesion can be transplanted from one cutaneous site to another in the same horse (autotransplantation). Later Olson and Cook (1951) were able to produce a lesion resembling equine sarcoid by inoculating the horse's skin with material from bovine papillomas (warts), a unique crossing of species boundaries. Ragland and Spencer (1969) have confirmed these findings in ponies.

Equine Cutaneous Papillomatosis.—Common warts are most frequent on the nose, muzzle and lips of horses during their first and second years of life. These lesions are experimentally transmissible to horses by exposure of scarified skin to triturated suspensions of warts, before or after filtration through bacteria-retaining filters; calves, lambs, dogs, rabbits and guinea pigs are not susceptible. Natural transmission between horses appears to occur through simple contact. The incubation period is two to three months; the duration of the lesions is about two months, spontaneous regression having occurred in all reported cases. Reinfection is rarely observed in animals which have recovered from the disease.

The papillomas of this equine disease are usually small, discrete, and attached by a narrow stalk, but in some cases they are very numerous and may be confluent. Small papillomas may appear as elongated, elevated nodules with a smooth surface, but larger ones have the rough surface characteristic of warts in other species.

Microscopically, hyperplastic, folded layers of squamous epithelium are supported by a thin core of connective tissue continuous with the dermis. Acanthosis and hyperkeratosis are prominent features in the affected epidermis. The outer layers of the acanthotic prickle cell layer exhibit so-called balloon degeneration, and aggregations of keratohyaline granules may be present in the cells. The lesions in general do not differ basically from those of papillomatosis in other species.

Canine Oral Papillomatosis.—Infectious papillomas have been known for many years (McFadyean and Hobday, 1898) to occur in the oral cavity of young dogs. These lesions are transmissible by contact or through injection of bacteria-free suspensions of wart material, but will grow only on the oral mucosa, skin and other epithelial surfaces being refractory to infection. Only dogs are susceptible; attempts to infect guinea pigs, rabbits, rats, mice, monkeys and kittens have been unsuccessful. Although cutaneous warts do occur in dogs, apparently they are not caused by the same virus that induces the oral lesions. The duration of oral papillomas is usually from three to five months.

The lesions may be single but more often are multiple, and in some dogs are so numerous as to interfere with mastication and deglutition. They occur anywhere on the oral mucosa, in the cheeks, tongue, palate or pharynx, but do not extend below the epiglottis or into the esophagus. The papillomas are sharply

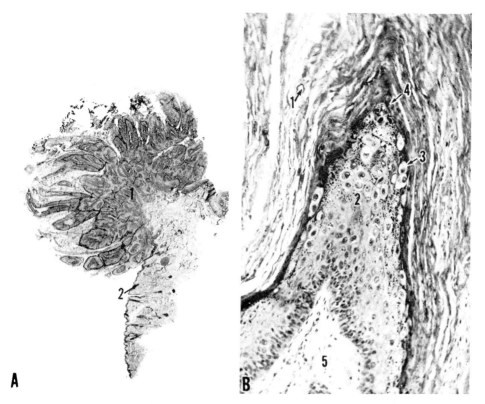

FIG. 10-59.—Canine oral papillomatosis. *A*, A verrucous mass (*1*) arising from the junction of oral mucosa and skin (*2*) (× 7). *B*, Higher magnification (× 160). Note extensive layer of keratin (*1*), long fronds of hyperplastic epidermis (*2*) containing some vacuoles (*3*) and eleidin granules (*4*). (Courtesy of Armed Forces Institute of Pathology.) Contributor: Dr. S. Pollock.

delimited, single or confluent cauliflower-shaped masses with a roughened surface, elevated from the oral mucosa.

Microscopically, the earliest lesion is seen as a sharply circumscribed segment of hyperplastic epithelium in which mitotic figures are frequent. The prickle cell layer becomes progressively thicker as the lesion grows; some cells lose their intercellular bridges and there is beginning papillary formation. Hyperkeratosis becomes a prominent feature, and although cells of the malpighian layer remain normal in size, the squamous cells become larger, their cytoplasm vacuolated or filled with albuminous material. The nuclei of the squamous cells either become greatly enlarged, or, in the outer layers, shrunken and distorted. The superficial cells apparently drop out, leaving a meshwork in the thick keratin layer. In old lesions, a few cytoplasmic inclusions, 1 to 5 microns in diameter, may be seen just under the keratin layer. These are interpreted as keratohyaline masses. In some sections basophilic inclusions fill nuclei of epithelial cells. Viral particles have been demonstrated in epithelial nuclei and correlated with the development of the basophilic inclusions. The underlying corium is relatively unchanged, but it sends out long vascular fronds to support the finger-like projections of hyperplastic epithelium. A few plasma cells and lymphocytes may be seen in the stroma underlying old lesions.

Cutaneous Papillomatosis of Rabbits.—An infectious papillomatosis of wild cottontail rabbits (*Sylvilagus*) was originally investigated by Shope (1933), hence is often referred to as the Shope papilloma. The warts in this disease are usually found in cases of natural infection involving the skin of the inner surface of the thighs, abdomen, or about the neck and shoulders. The lesions are black or gray, 0.5 to 1.0 cm. in diameter and 1.0 to 1.5 cm. in height, and are covered with a thick layer of keratin. They can be transmitted without difficulty from one cottontail rabbit to another by injecting or applying filtered or unfiltered wart suspensions to scarified skin. Recently, evidence has been obtained to indicate that certain arthropods may transmit the virus of this disease. Although domestic rabbits (*Oryctolagus*) can be infected, the disease cannot be perpetuated in series in such breeds. However, once established in a domestic rabbit, the papillomas can persist for long periods, undergo malignant transformation and kill the animal by metastasis. When these tumors become carcinomatous, they lose their pigment and differentiated characteristics, assume the features of squamous cell carcinoma, and can be transplanted to other domestic rabbits.

Oral Papillomatosis of Rabbits. — Spontaneous papillomatosis of the oral cavity of domestic rabbits (*Oryctolagus*) has been described by Parsons and Kidd (1943) and demonstrated to be the result of a virus infection. The viral agent is distinct from the Shope papilloma virus (p. 513) which affects the epithelium of the skin but not of the mouth. These spontaneous papillomas are small, discrete, gray-white nodules, either sessile or pedunculated. Usually multiple and sometimes numerous, they are almost always situated on the under surface of the tongue, occasionally on the gums, and rarely on the floor of the mouth. The lesions are predominantly small, with a smooth dome-shaped surface, but occasionally are larger, sometimes attaining a diameter of 5 mm., with a rugose, cauliflower-like surface.

Microscopically, the lesions appear as discrete nodules of thickened, folded, hyperplastic epithelium, supported by sharply demarcated stroma which may form delicate papillæ. In lesions of long standing, the prominent changes are seen in epithelial cells; those of the malpighian layer become large, coarsely vacuolated and irregularly polyhedral in shape. The nuclei of all layers, particularly of the prickle cells, become enlarged, vesicular and may contain eosinophilic or basophilic inclusion bodies. The inclusions have been demonstrated to contain viral particles. There is little tendency toward excessive keratinization of the affected epithelium; the outer layers merely appear denser and more eosinophilic in stained sections.

Caprine Papillomatosis. — Papillomatosis of goats may occur in either of two forms. Davis and Kemper (1936) described cutaneous warts on the head, face, shoulder, neck and upper part of the forelimb, but not on the teats and udder, in one herd of Saanen goats. Moulton (1954) reported papillomatosis limited to the teats and udder in another herd of goats of the same breed. The outbreak described by Moulton was initiated by the introduction of an infected goat into the herd, with the strange result that 50 to 150 black goats were affected, while not one of the 50 white goats exhibited lesions. The disease in this herd was of long duration, papillomas persisting more than five months with little sign of regression. Some of them looked like cutaneous horns, reaching a length of 3 cm., and usually having a rod-like or conical, rather than a papillary, shape. Massive discoid tumors develop in some instances, with frank squamous cell carcinomas arising by dissociation and downgrowth of epithelium. Although there was no

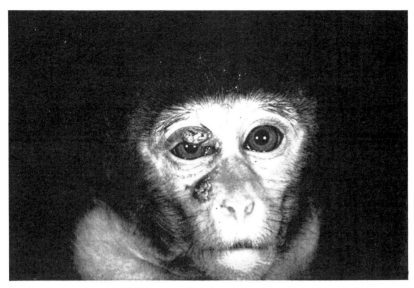

FIG. 10–60.   Cutaneous papillomatosis of the face of a rhesus monkey (*Macaca mulatta*).
(Courtesy New England Regional Primate Research Center, Harvard Medical School.)

generalized metastasis, one of these squamous cell carcinomas metastasized to the supramammary lymph node.   Of 7 advanced lesions examined microscopically, 4 showed evidence of malignant transformation.   Moulton was unable to cultivate the agent in chick embryos, and transmission to other goats was not attempted.

Papillomatosis of Monkeys.—A papillomatous lesion of the skin of a brown Cebus monkey, described by Lucké, Ratcliffe and Breedis (1950), was experimentally transmitted to another skin site on the same monkey and later to 11 of 13 other monkeys.   Both Old and New World monkeys were included in the susceptible group.   The incubation period was about two weeks; regression of the lesions occurred between the fourth and eighth months, and no evidence of malignancy was seen during a subsequent eight-month period of observation.   This record adds another to the species of animals in which papillomatosis has been observed.

Papillomatosis

BAGDONAS, V., and OLSON, C. JR.:   Observations on the Epizoötiology of Cutaneous Papillomatosis (Warts) of Cattle.   J. Am. Vet. Med. Assn. *122*:393–397, 1953.
————: Observations on Immunity in Cutaneous Bovine Papillomatosis.   Am. J. Vet. Research *15*:240–245, 1954.
BROBST, D. F., and DULAC, G. C.:   Meningeal Tumors Induced in Calves with the Bovine Cutaneous Papilloma Virus.   Pathologia Vet. *6*:135–145, 1969.
BROBST, D. F., and HINSMAN, E. J.:   Electron Microscopy of the Bovine Cutaneous Papilloma.   Pathologia Vet. *3*:196–207, 1966.
BROBST, D. F., and OLSON, C.:   Histopathology of Urinary Bladder Tumors Induced by Bovine Cutaneous Papilloma Agent.   Cancer Res. *25*:12–19, 1965.
CHEVILLE, N. F., and OLSON, C. L.:   Cytology of the Canine Oral Papilloma.   Am. J. Path. *45*:848–872, 1964.
COOK, R. H., and OLSON, C. JR.:   Experimental Transmission of Cutaneous Papilloma of the Horse.   Am. J. Path. *27*:1087–1097, 1951.
DALMAT, H. T.:   Arthropod Transmission of Rabbit Papillomatosis.   J. Exper. Med. *108*:9–20, 1958.
DAVIS, C. L., and KEMPER, H. E.:   Common Warts (Papillomata) in Goats.   J. Am. Vet. Med. Assn. *88*:175–179, 1936.

DeMonbreun, W. A., and Goodpasture, E. W.: Infectious Oral Papillomatosis of Dogs. Am. J. Path. 8:43–56, 1932.

Fujimoto, Y., and Olson, C.: The Fine Structure of the Bovine Wart. Path. Vet. 3:659–684, 1966.

Gordon, D. W., and Olson, C.: Meningiomas and Fibroblastic Neoplasia in Calves Induced with the Bovine Papilloma Virus. Cancer Res. 28:2423–2431, 1968.

Jackson, C.: The Incidence and Pathology of Tumours of Domesticated Animals in South Africa. Onderstepoort J. Vet. Sc. & Animal Ind. 6:1–460, 1936.

Lucké, B., Ratcliffe, H., and Breedis, C.: Transmissible Papilloma in Monkeys. Federation Proc. 9:337, 1950.

McEntee, K.: Transmissible Fibropapillomas of the External Genitalia of Cattle. Rep. New York State Veterinary College, Cornell Univ., Ithaca, N. Y., 1950–51, p. 28.

——————: Fibropapillomas on the External Genitalia of Cattle. Cornell Vet. 40:304–312, 1950.

McFadyean, J., and Hobday, F.: Note on the Experimental Transmission of Warts in the Dog. J. Comp. Path. & Therap. 11:341–344, 1898.

Moulton, J. E.: Cutaneous Papillomas on the Udders of Milk Goats. North Am. Vet. 35:29-33, 1954.

Olson, C. Jr.: Equine Sarcoid; A Cutaneous Neoplasm. Am J. Vet. Research 9:333–341, 1948.

Olson, C., and Cook, R. H.: Cutaneous Sarcoma-like Lesions of the Horse Caused by the Agent of Bovine Papilloma. Proc. Soc. Exper. Biol. & Med. 77:281–284, 1951.

Olson, C., et al.: A Urinary Bladder Tumor Induced by a Bovine Cutaneous Papilloma Agent. Cancer Res. 19:779–782, 1959.

Olson, C., Pamukcu, A. M., and Brobst, D. F.: Papilloma-Like Virus From Bovine Urinary Bladder Tumors. Cancer Res. 25:840–849, 1965.

Parsons, R. J., and Kidd, J. G.: Oral Papillomatosis of Rabbits: A Virus Disease. J. Exper. Med. 77:233–250, 1943.

Penberthy, J.: Contagious Warty Tumours in Dogs. J. Comp. Path. & Therap. 11:363–365, 1898.

Ragland, W. L., and Spencer, G. R.: Attempts to Relate Bovine Papilloma Virus to the Cause of Equine Sarcoid: Equidae Inoculated Intradermally With Bovine Papilloma Virus. Am. J. Vet. Res. 30:743–752, 1969.

——————: Attempts to Relate Bovine Papilloma Virus to the Cause of Equine Sarcoid: Immunity to Bovine Papilloma Virus. Am. J. Vet. Res. 29:1363–1366, 1968.

Rdzok, E. J., Shipkowitz, N. L., and Richter, W. R.: Rabbit Oral Papillomatosis: Ultrastructure of Experimental Infection. Cancer Res. 26:160–166, 1966.

Richter, W. R., Shipkowitz, N. L., and Rdzok, E. J.: Oral Papillomatosis of the Rabbit: An Electron Microscopic Study. Lab. Invest. 13:430–438, 1964.

Robl, M. G., and Olson, C.: Oncogenic Action of Bovine Papilloma Virus in Hamsters. Cancer Res. 28:1596–1604, 1968.

Rous, P., and Beard, J. W.: The Progression to Carcinoma of Virus-induced Rabbit Papillomas (Shope). J. Exper. Med. 62:523–548, 1935.

Segre, D., Olson, C. Jr., and Hoerlein, A. B.: Neutralization of Bovine Papilloma Virus with Serums from Cattle and Horses with Experimental Papillomas. Am. J. Vet. Research, 16:517–520, 1955.

Shope, R. E.: Infectious Papillomatosis of Rabbits. J. Exper. Med. 58:607–624, 1933.

Tajima, M., Gordon, D. E., and Olson, C.: Electron Microscopy of Bovine Papilloma and Deer Fibroma Viruses. Am. J. Vet. Res. 29:1185–1194, 1968.

Voss, J. L.: Transmission of Equine Sarcoid. Am. J. Vet. Res. 30:183–191, 1969.

Watrach, A. M.: The Ultrastructure of Canine Cutaneous Papilloma. Cancer Res. 29:2079–2084, 1969.

Shope Fibroma

Fibromas occurring naturally in the skin of wild cottontail rabbits (*Sylvilagus*) were described by Shope in 1932 and shown to be caused by a filtrable virus, classified as a poxvirus. These lesions are also transmitted experimentally to domestic rabbits (*Oryctolagus*) and the agent was demonstrated to be related to that of infectious myxomatosis (p. 416). The fibroma virus produces an effective immunity to subsequent infection by myxomatosis, although in other respects there is no resemblance between the two diseases.

The lesions in the Shope fibroma are often multiple and are described as elevations of the skin by a fibrous mass; the overlying epidermis is thickened and sends bulbous proliferating epithelium deep into the tumor. Large eosinophilic inclusions occur in the cytoplasm of the affected epidermal cells.

Viruses similar to the Shope fibroma virus have been reported to cause fibromas in brush rabbits (*Sylvilagus*) in California, fibromas in hares (*Lepus*) in Europe and fibromas in grey squirrels in North America.

Shope Fibroma

CILLI, V.: Aspetti Virologici del Fibroma di Shope e suoi Rapporti con il Mixoma di Sanarelli. G. Mal. Infet. Parassit. *10*:1017–1040, 1958.
SHOPE, R. E.: A Transmissible Tumor-like Condition in Rabbits. J. Exper. Med. *56*:793–802, 1932.
————: A Filterable Virus Causing a Tumor-like Condition in Rabbits and its Relationship to Virus Myxomatosum. J. Exper. Med. *56*:803–833, 1932.

Avian Leukosis Complex

The term avian leukosis has largely replaced "leukemia" as the designation for a group of avian diseases which are characterized by autonomous proliferation of leukocytes and their precursors. The subject is of such general interest to pathologists that it will be discussed briefly even though poultry pathology is outside the scope of this book. Ellerman and Bang in 1908, transmitted avian leukosis with bacteria-free and cell-free filtrates to establish it as the first neoplastic disease of proved viral etiology. The transmissibility of the disease has been amply confirmed by extensive research during the past fifty years, which also has revealed a pattern of pathologic manifestations so complicated that the exact etiologic interrelationships are not yet clear. Difficulties in detecting immunologic differences between agents and the mixture of pathologic patterns in nature as well as in the laboratory have added to the complexity of the problem. The classification of the various entities within this complex, which Jungherr (1952) has based on the pathologic manifestations, is of value in an understanding of avian leukosis. His classification of the avian leukosis complex is as follows:

Lymphomatosis   Erythroblastosis
  neural   Granuloblastosis
  ocular   Myelocytomatosis
  visceral
  osteopetrotic

As indicated, this represents a pathologic classification and not an etiologic classification. Based on etiologic factors, the following classification modified from that of Biggs (1961) is more appropriate:

Marek's Disease (Neurolymphomatosis; Ocular lymphomatosis)
Leukoses
  Lymphoid Leukosis
  Myeloid Leukosis
  Erythroblastosis

There are at least five viruses, or strains of virus, responsible for the pathologic entities. These are: (1) virus of visceral lymphomatosis or lymphoid leukosis virus, (2) avian erythroblastosis virus, (3) myeloblastosis virus, (4) osteopetrosis virus, and (5) neurolymphomatosis virus, or Marek's disease virus. The first three agents which are morphologically similar RNA viruses, generally induce the pathologic picture for which they are named, but the type of neoplasm produced may vary. Under proper circumstances these agents may induce renal carcinomas, fibrosarcomas, hemangioendotheliomas, as well as other tumors morphologically distinct from leukosis. At present the osteopetrosis virus is not believed to be closely related to the viruses of the leukosis complex, *i.e.*, lymphomatosis, erythroblastosis and myeloblastosis viruses. Neurolymphomatosis and ocular lymphomatosis are now believed to be caused by a herpesvirus, a DNA virus. To compound the confusion, Marek's disease virus can also induce "visceral lesions" which are essentially identical to those of visceral lymphomatosis.

Leukemia is not a feature of neurolymphomatosis (Marek's disease), visceral lymphomatosis (lymphoid leukosis), or myelocytomatosis, but invasion of peripheral blood is a constant feature of erythroblastosis and granuloblastosis (myeloid leukosis).

The following descriptions describe the pathological features of the various entities as classified by Jungherr (1952).

Neural Lymphomatosis (Marek's disease, fowl paralysis, range paralysis, polyneuritis, neurolymphomatosis gallinarum, neurogranulomatosis).—This disease occurs in poultry flocks throughout the world, primarily affecting birds between two and five months of age but sparing neither older nor younger ones. The principal manifestations are flaccid paralysis of one or both wings or legs, occasionally with involvement of other muscles. The lesions are found in the large peripheral nerve trunks (brachial plexus, femoral nerve, sciatic nerve, etc.), where dense infiltration of the nerve by lymphoid cells results in diffuse or localized enlargements, which are usually bilaterally asymmetrical. Microscopic examination discloses large numbers of lymphoid cells infiltrating all layers of the nerve, separating nerve bundles by long narrow columns of cells in some places, forming solid nodules in others. Sometimes definite microscopic lesions are demonstrable in nerves in which gross changes could not be detected. Microscopic examination thus constitutes the most precise method of diagnosis available at present.

Ocular Lymphomatosis (Iritis, uveitis, gray eye, epidemic blindness, etc.).—Ocular manifestations, usually in older birds, are encountered most frequently in flocks in which neural lymphomatosis is present. The iris in the affected chicken is thickened with annular or diffuse masses which decrease the size and distort the shape of the pupil. Pigment is lost in affected areas and the iris appears gray or white. The anterior chamber sometimes contains turbid exudate. The histologic features are characteristic. The iris, less often the entire anterior uveal tract, is distorted by massive infiltration with lymphoid cells. These include both large and small lymphocytes; heterophils are rare, and their presence in large numbers is indicative of some other disease. Granular coagulation is often observed in the anterior chamber, but leukocytes are less frequent. Grayish discoloration of the iris should arouse suspicion of the disease, but the diagnosis should be confirmed by microscopic examination.

Visceral Lymphomatosis (Lymphocytoma, big liver disease, lymphatic leukosis, visceral lymphomata, lymphocythaemia or myelolymphomatosis, hemocytoblastic myelosis, lymphoadenoma, lymphomyelosis, lymphosarcoma, lymphocytomatosis, etc.).—Visceral lymphomatosis may be considered the most common avian neoplastic disease. It occurs particularly in adult birds, often in association with ocular or neural lymphomatosis. The disease is characterized as its name implies, by proliferation of lymphoid cells in any or all of the visceral organs, often with displacement of much of the normal tissue. This results in indefinite outward manifestations which depend upon the severity and location of visceral involvement. Loss of flesh, diarrhea, enlargement of the abdomen, paleness of the mucosæ, and palpable enlargement of the liver may be observed in living birds. The gross lesions are extremely variable. The liver, spleen and kidney are most frequently affected, but any tissue of the body may be involved. The liver is usually greatly enlarged as the result of infiltration by lymphoid cells which appear as nodular or diffuse gray areas. The spleen usually contains similar gray nodules, the smaller ones diffusely spread through the parenchyma, the larger ones forming solid nodules which elevate the capsule. The kidneys, heart, lungs, mesentery and other tissues may also be involved by lymphoid tumors. The microscopic features of visceral lymphomatosis may be summarized as diffuse or nodular infiltration of organs by immature lymphoid cells which displace normal tissue. In some cases, proliferation of endothelial cells has been observed, apparently resulting from action of the lymphomatosis agent.

Osteopetrotic Lymphomatosis (Thick leg disease, marble bone, akropachia —ossea, osteopetrosis gallinarum, etc.).—A disease of the bones of poultry has been associated with the agent of lymphomatosis by Jungherr (1938). The lesions are quite different from those of other components of the avian leukosis complex, which suggests that this classification should be tentative until more can be learned. This rather rare disorder is characterized by thickening of the diaphysis of the long bones of the extremities, although in extreme cases it may involve all the bones. The changes are often bilaterally symmetrical and start with solid osseous thickening of the bone cortex, which eventually obliterates the marrow cavity and gives the bones a characteristic gross and radiographic appearance. Microscopically, the bone cortex and marrow are replaced by inward growth of sheets of new bone which eventually appears solid and heavily calcified. A prominent mosaic pattern results from the irregular lines of growth and calcification.

Erythroblastosis (Erythroleukosis, anemia, leukomyelose, oligoerythrocythemia, erythromyelosis, etc.).—Transmission experiments have disclosed an agent that produces intense intravascular proliferation of primitive erythroblastic cells which find their way in great numbers into the circulating blood. The disease is rarely recognized as a natural occurrence, for in most instances it is mixed with other entities of this complex. It causes diffuse enlargement of visceral organs with little tendency to form discrete tumors. Hemoglobin pigment may be deposited in the tissues in abnormally large amounts and anemia is often a prominent feature. Blood smears reveal many hemoglobin-free precursors of erythrocytes.

Granuloblastosis (Leukemic myeloid or myelotic leukosis, leukocythemia, leukomyelosis, leukemic myeloblastosis, etc.).—Neoplastic proliferation of primitive cells of the granulocytic series has been observed in association with similar overgrowth of cells of the erythrocytic type. Apparently it was this mixed form of erythroblastosis and granuloblastosis that was described by Ellerman and Bang and shown by them to be transmissible. What distinguishes the disease from erythroblastosis is the nature of the leukemic cells in the circulating blood, which are primitive cells of the granulocytic type. Thus, myeloblasts and promyelocytes may appear in abundance, although mature heterophils are not especially increased in number. This disease also may result in anemia.

Myelocytomatosis (Aleukemic myeloid leukosis, leukochloroma, myelocytoma, myelocytomatosis, myeloma, aleukemic myeloblastosis).—In this disease, multiple yellowish tumors form in the muscles and viscera or along the ribs or on other parts of the skeleton. The tumors are made up of solid masses of myelocytes which contain acidophilic granules of the mature heterophil or eosinophil. The blood picture is usually aleukemic, although in rare instances immature myelocytes appear in the circulation.

Avian Leukosis

BIESTER, H. D. and SCHWARTE, L. H.: *Diseases of Poultry*, 4th Ed., Ames, Iowa, Iowa State Univ. Press, 1965.
BIGGS, P. M.: A Discussion on the Classification of the Avian Leukosis Complex and Fowl Paralysis. Brit. Vet. J. *117*:326–334, 1961.
BURMESTER, B. R.: The Vertical and Horizontal Transmission of Avian Visceral Lymphomatosis. Sympos. Quart. Biol. *27*:471–477, 1962.
ELLERMANN, V., and BANG, O.: Experimentelle Leukämie bei Hühnern. Zentralbl. f. Bakt., pt. I, (Orig.) *46*:595–609, 1908.
FURTH, J.: Observations with a New Transmissible Strain of the Leucosis (Leucemia) of Fowls. J. Exper. Med. *53*:243–267, 1931.
————: Lymphomatosis, Myelomatosis and Endothelioma of Chickens Caused by a Filterable Agent. I. Transmission Experiments. J. Exper. Med. *58*:253–275, 1933.
————: Recent Experimental Studies on Leukemia. Physiol. Rev. *26*:47–76, 1946.
HELMBOLDT, G. F., and FREDRICKSON, T. N.: The Pathology of Avian Leukemia in *Experimental Leukemia*. Rich, M. A. (Ed.), New York, Appleton-Century-Crofts, 1968, pp. 233–259.
JOHNSON, E. P.: A Study of Lymphomatosis of Fowls. Va. Agri. Exper. Sta. Tech. Bull. 44, 1932.
JUNGHERR, E., and LANDAUER, W.: Studies in Fowl Paralysis. III. A Condition Resembling Osteopetrosis (Marble Bone) in Common Fowl. Storrs Agri. Exper. Sta. Bull. 222, Storrs, Connecticut, 1938.
JUNGHERR, E.: The Avian Leukosis Complex, in BIESTER, H. E., and SCHWARTE, L. H.: *Diseases of Poultry*. 3rd ed., Ames, Iowa State College Press, 1952, pp. 453–519.
OLSON, C. JR.: A Study of Transmissible Fowl Leukosis. J. Am. Vet. Med. Assn. *89*: 681–705, 1936.
PAPPENHEIMER, A. M., DUNN, L. C., and CONE, V.: A Study of Fowl Paralysis (Neurolymphomatosis Gallinarum). Storrs Agri. Exper. Sta. Bull. 143, Storrs, Connecticut, 1926.
————: Studies on Fowl Paralysis (Neuro-lymphomatosis Gallinarum). I. Clinical Features and Pathology. J. Exper. Med. *49*:63–86, 1929.
STEWART, H., SNELL, K., DUNHAM, L. J., and SCHLYEN, S.: *Transplantable and Transmissible Tumors of Animals*, Section 12, Fascicle 40, Atlas of Tumor Pathology, Washington, D.C., AFIP, 1957.

Infectious Avian Sarcomas

Of particular interest in the field of oncology are the malignant avian neoplasms which can be transmitted by bacteria-free and cell-free materials. The Rous sarcoma (chicken tumor I, Rous sarcoma No. 1), an example of such a tumor, was originally observed in 1910 by Rous as a fibrosarcoma occurring spontaneously in the right breast region of a barred Plymouth Rock hen. Rous transplanted this tumor to other locations in the same hen, then to other genetically related hens. Later he transmitted the tumor to hens by means of cell-free filtrates of the neoplasm. The sarcoma increased in virulence upon successive passage in the laboratory until 90 to 100 per cent of young chickens could be successfully infected. This tumor has been maintained in the laboratory over the years; much has been learned from it about neoplastic growth and it still is used in cancer research laboratories.

VIRAL INDUCED MALIGNANT LYMPHOMA

That malignant lymphomas are infectious diseases has been the subject of countless investigations and reports. Few of these studies have led to the isolation of oncogenic viruses but each has contributed to the overall effort in cancer research. The gross and microscopic features of this form of neoplasia have been

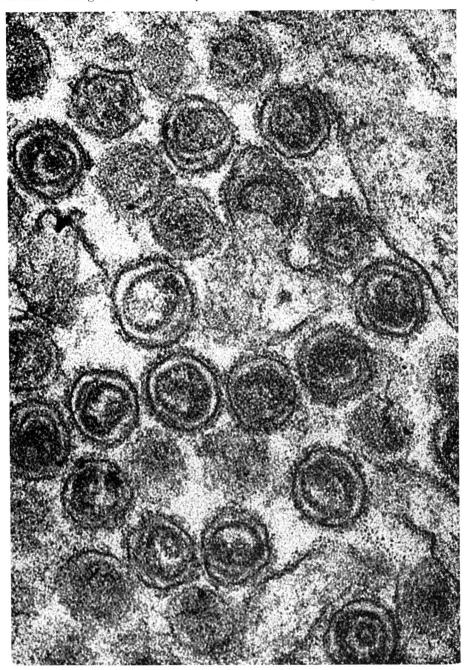

FIG. 10–61.—Feline malignant lymphoma virus. Intracellular mature C-type viral particles (approximately 150,000 ×). (Courtesy Dr. G. H. Theilen.)

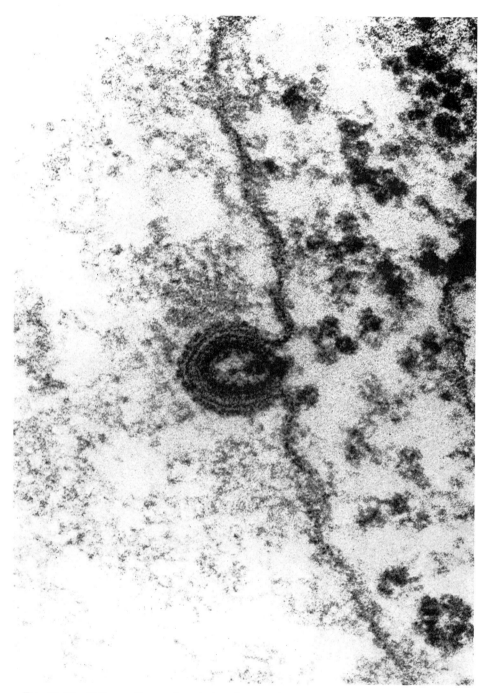

Fig. 10–62.—Feline malignant lymphoma virus. Advanced stage of the budding process of the C-type virus from the cytoplasmic membrane of a lymphocyte (approximately 200,000 ×). (Courtesy Dr. G. H. Theilen.)

discussed in Chapter 7. The basic morphology of malignant lymphoma varies little whether of proven viral etiology or not. The mouse was the first mammalian species in which malignant lymphoma was demonstrated to be caused by a virus. The virus, now known as Gross's virus, seems to be the causative agent of malignant lymphoma as commonly seen in many inbred strains of mice. Since the identification of this virus, several additional viruses have been isolated which induce malignant lymphoma in mice. All of these agents are RNA viruses. Only recently has evidence been gathered to suggest that malignant lymphomas in other mammals are caused by viruses. A specific RNA virus has been isolated and incriminated in malignant lymphoma in the cat. Cell-free transmission has been apparently demonstrated in the rat, guinea pig and dog, and considerable epizootiological evidence points toward a viral cause in cattle. In addition, viral particles have been observed in malignant lymphoma cells of cats, dogs, and cattle.

DNA viruses have also been demonstrated to induce malignant lymphoma. The herpesvirus of Marek's disease has already been mentioned (p. 518). *Herpesvirus saimiri* causes malignant lymphoma in several species of non-human primates. In man the Epstein-Barr virus is suspected as causally related to Burkitt's lymphoma as well as infectious mononucleosis, Hodgkin's disease and nasopharyngeal carcinoma.

Viral Induced Malignant Lymphoma

DUTCHER, R. M. (Ed.).: *Comparative Leukemia Research 1969*, Bibliotheca Haematologica, No. 36, 1970.
RICH, M. A. (Ed.).: *Experimental Leukemia*, New York, Appleton-Century-Crofts, 1968.

Mammary-tumor Milk Virus

It has been known for many years that the offspring of hybrid mice produced by pairs from two inbred strains have an increased incidence of certain mammary tumors if their mothers are descendants of strains in which the incidence of mammary tumors is high. Bittner demonstrated in 1936 that a factor in the milk of the mice from the affected strains is responsible for the production of these tumors, even though they do not appear until the offspring mature. The frequency of tumors could be sharply reduced in mice with the same genetic background by putting them to nurse on foster mothers that did not carry the factor. The mammary-tumor milk agent is known to be a virus. The virus, which is transmitted in milk, infects infant mice when nursing, whether or not the mother has mammary cancer, as infected mice may be "latently" infected and excrete virus in the absence of disease. Newly infected mice may similarly transmit the virus to their offspring without developing mammary tumors. Once infected, development of mammary tumors requires a genetic susceptibility and appropriate hormone influence which is usually provided by pregnancy.

Not all mammary tumors in mice are related to this virus, for several transplantable tumors have been recognized in mice which are free of the milk agent. The murine mammary tumor associated with the milk agent is of much interest in experimental oncology, as it provides a link in the chain of evidence pointing toward the viral etiology of neoplasia.

Mammary-tumor Milk Virus

GROSS, L.: Oncogenic Viruses. *International Series of Monographs on Pure and Applied Biology*, Vol. 11. New York, Pergamon Press, 1961.

S. E. Polyoma Virus

The virus first described by Sarah E. Stewart and Bernice E. Eddy of the National Institutes of Health serves to illustrate the complexities, contradictions and surprises encountered by investigators studying viruses in relation to neoplasms. The agent now called the S. E. (after Stewart and Eddy) Polyoma virus was first encountered by Stewart in the course of an experiment to repeat the success of Gross, in 1951, in transmitting spontaneous lymphocytic leukemia of the mouse with cell-free extracts. To her surprise, mice (of the C_3H/Hen strain) inoculated with cell-free extracts of lymphomatous mouse tissue, did not acquire leukemia but, after eight to ten months, developed multiple tumors of the parotid salivary glands. Hybrid mice (C_3H_f X AKR) inoculated with similar extracts, on the other hand, developed leukemia early in life. In further experiments with cell-free extracts of leukemic mouse tissues, pleomorphic tumors of salivary glands, kidneys, mammary gland, thymus and adrenal appeared following inoculation of this cell-free material. Subsequently it was shown that the material contained a virus which could be cultivated in cultures of monkey kidney cells and mouse embryo tissues. At this writing good evidence has been accumualted to establish this agent as a virus; much of this knowledge has been summarized by Eddy, 1960.

A few points are of interest concerning the pathologic effects of this virus. First, its presence results in intranuclear inclusion bodies in renal epithelium Second, several host species are susceptible; for example, mice, Syrian hamsters, Chinese hamsters, rabbits and rats. Third, a wide variety of neoplasms appear in these hosts following introduction of the polyoma virus. Some of these tumors are summarized by Stewart, 1960, as follows:

1. Pleomorphic tumors of salivary glands and mucous glands of head and neck.
2. Renal cortical tumors and renal sarcomas.
3. Epithelial thymomas.
4. Mammary adenocarcinomas and epidermoid carcinomas.
5. Bone tumors.
6. Mesotheliomas.
7. Subcutaneous sarcomas and hemangioendotheliomas.
8. Medullary adrenal carcinomas.
9. Other tumor types—thyroid adenocarcinoma and epidermoid carcinoma.

Eddy (1969) has recently published a comprehensive review on this agent.

Polyoma

EDDY, B. E.: The Polyoma Virus (B). Adv. Virus Res. 7:91–102, 1960.
————: Polyoma Virus. Virology Monographs 7:1–114, 1969.
STEWART, S. E.: The Polyoma Virus (A). Adv. Virus Res. 7:61–90, 1960.

THE LUCKÉ FROG KIDNEY CARCINOMA

Lucké described a carcinoma of the kidney, in 1934, as a frequent spontaneous tumor of the leopard frog (*Rana pipiens*) particularly in Northern New England States. He later suggested that the disease was caused by a transmissible virus. Present evidence supports that the neoplasm is caused by a virus of the herpesvirus group.   The tumors may occur in one or both kidneys as single or multiple white nodules.   Microscopically they appear as typical adenocarcinomas with the unique exception that eosinophilic intranuclear inclusion bodies are often present.

Lucké Carcinoma

GROSS, L.:   Oncogenic Viruses.   *International Series of Monographs on Pure and Applied Biology*, Vol. 11.   New York, Pergamon Press, 1961.
LUCKÉ, B.:   A Neoplastic Disease of the Kidney of the Frog, *Rana pipiens*.   Am. J. Cancer *20*:352–379, 1934.
————:   Carcinoma in the Leopard Frog.   Its Probable Causation by A Virus.   J. Exp. Med. *68*:457–468, 1938.

Canine Venereal Tumor

(Transmissible Lymphosarcoma, Venereal Granuloma, Infectious Sarcoma, Venereal Lymphosarcoma, Histiocytoma, Canine Condyloma)

The canine venereal tumor is of great historical interest as the first neoplasm to be successfully transplanted from one host to another.   A Russian veterinarian, M. A. Novinsky, was the first to demonstrate that this tumor could be transplanted to other dogs, a feat which earned him the title "Forefather of Experimental Oncology" in Russian literature.   This neoplasm is readily reproduced by the experimental transfer of viable cells from one dog to another, and in nature is spread by coitus or other contact.   In spite of this evidence of its infectious nature, no microbial agent has been demonstrated, nor has the tumor been transmitted by cell-free filtrate.   This neoplasm is described more fully on page 236.

Canine Venereal Tumor

KARLSON, A. G. and MANN, F. C.:   The Transmissible Venereal Tumor of Dogs: Observations on Forty Generations of Experimental Transfers.   Ann. New York Acad. Sc. *54*:1197–1213, 1952.
STEWART, H., SNELL, K., DUNHAM, L. J., and SCHLYEN, S.:   *Transplantable and Transmissible Tumors of Animals*, Section 12, Fascicle 40, Atlas of Tumor Pathology, Washington, D. C., AFIP, 1957.

References

General Virology

ANDREWES, C., PEREIRA, H. G.:   *Viruses of Vertebrates*.   2nd Ed., London, Baillière, Tindall and Cassell, 1967.
BIESTER, H. E. and SCHWARTE, L. H.:   *Diseases of Poultry*.   3rd ed., Ames, Iowa State College Press, 1952.
CABASSO, V. J.:   Emerging Classification of Animal Viruses—A Review.   Avian Diseases *9*: 471–489, 1965.
HAGAN, W. A. and BRUNER, D. W.:   *The Infectious Diseases of Domestic Animals*.   4th ed., Ithaca, N. Y., Comstock Publishing Co., 1961.
HENNING, M. W.:   *Animal Diseases of South Africa*.   3rd ed., S. Africa, Central News Agency, Ltd., 1956.
HUCK, R. A.:   The Classification of Viruses.   Vet. Bul. *34*:239–253, 1964.
KELSER, R. A. and SCHOENING, H. W.:   *Manual of Veterinary Bacteriology*.   5th ed., Baltimore, Williams & Wilkins Co., 1948.
LWOFF, A.:   The Concept of Virus.   J. Gen. Microbiol. *17*:239–253, 1957.
MELNICK, J. L.:   Summary of Classification of Animal Viruses, 1968.   Progr. Med. Virol. *10*:487–489, 1968.
MERCHANT, I. A. and PACKER, R. A.:   *Veterinary Bacteriology and Virology*, 5th ed., Ames, Iowa, Iowa State College Press, 1956.
RHODES, A. J. and VAN ROOYEN, C. E.:   *Textbook of Virology*.   2nd ed., Baltimore, The Williams & Wilkins Co., 1953.
RIVERS, T. M.:   *Viral and Rickettsial Infections of Man*.   Philadelphia, J. B. Lippincott Co., 1948.

11

Diseases Caused by Organisms of Uncertain Classification

INTRODUCTION

Diseases to be considered in this chapter are specific entities caused by identifiable infectious organisms. Although several important diseases of animals and man are included here, the relationship of the causative organisms to other infectious agents is not completely settled. Thus the appellation, "of uncertain classification." It seems useful to group these diseases together because the causative agents are not true viruses as defined in Chapter 10, and they are also distinguishable from simple bacteria (Chapter 12), higher bacteria (Chapter 13) and protozoa (Chapter 14). Although no unifying pathologic features appear in this chapter as a whole, the related causative agents usually result in similar pathologic manifestations. For this reason, a short description of the family of organisms precedes the section in which the disease is described. Further details may be found by consulting the references listed, particularly Merchant and Packer (1956) and Bergey (1957).

REFERENCES

BREED, R. S., MURRAY, E. G. D., and SMITH, N. R.: *Bergey's Manual of Determinative Bacteriology*, 7th ed., Baltimore, Williams & Wilkins Co., 1957.
FREUNDT, E. A.: *The Mycoplasmataceæ*, Monograph, State Serum Institute, Copenhagen, 1958.
MERCHANT, I. A. and PACKER, R. A.: *Veterinary Bacteriology and Virology*, 5th ed., Ames, Iowa, Iowa State College Press, 1956.

THE PLEUROPNEUMONIA GROUP

The organism isolated by Nocard in 1898 from cases of bovine pleuropneumonia is the prototype of a group of similar organisms. The inelegant expression "pleuropneumonia-like-organism" or "PPLO" abounds in the literature, but, hopefully, may eventually be replaced by better terms as more is learned about the organisms. Part of the difficulty stems from the variable nature of the organisms and the historical development of knowledge about them. Currently, these organisms are classified in the order *Mycoplasmatales* which includes one genus, *Mycoplasma*. Several organisms now classified in this genus have been isolated from animals with specific disease and from apparently healthy animals as well. The pathogenic properties of these organisms in many instances have not been easily established but several now are definitely accepted as pathogens.

The organisms in this group may be either saprophytic or parasitic and may be cultivated on solid or liquid media. Polymorphism is a strong feature of these organisms as elementary bodies, rings, globules, and filaments may occur. Many of these forms will pass through filters which retain ordinary bacteria, a feature which at one time led to their classification among the viruses. Most of them grow aerobically and the parasitic species usually require a medium with high protein content. On suitable solid media, tiny glistening, adherent colonies are formed which can be recognized with the dissection microscope. The organisms themselves are best stained with Giemsa's stain and are visible under ordinary oil-immersion microscopy.

Bovine pleuropneumonia is an infectious disease of cattle caused by a specific organism, currently called *Mycoplasma mycoides* (Novak, 1929). Some of the synonyms for this organism are: "pleuropneumonia organism," *Asterococcus mycoides* (Borrell, 1910), *Coccobacillus mycoides peripneumoniæ* (Martiznovski, 1911), *Micromyces peripneumoniæ bovis contagiosæ* (Frosch, 1923), *Mycoplasma peripneumoniæ* (Novak, 1929), *Astromyces peripneumoniæ bovis* (Wroblewski, 1931), and *Borrelomyces peripneumoniæ* (Turner, Campbell and Dick, 1935).

A similar pleuropneumonia in goats is caused by an organism now classified as *Mycoplasma mycoides* var *capri*.

The disease has been known as a specific entity for over two hundred years. In the nineteenth century it spread from Europe to many parts of the world, including the United States. It was eliminated from this country before 1892 by an intensive campaign involving slaughter and quarantine of infected and exposed animals and fortunately has not reappeared. About 1854, the disease was introduced from Holland into South Africa where it spread rapidly, causing the death of over 100,000 cattle in a two-year period. It has remained an extremely important disease in Africa, second only to rinderpest as an economic problem. At present the disease is distributed over much of the world with the exception of the western hemisphere. A feature that adds to the difficulty of controlling the spread of pleuropneumonia is that it may exist in a symptomless form in some animals which, nonetheless, are carriers.

The disease affects cattle primarily, although buffalo, goats and sheep apparently are susceptible to artificial infection. Mice, rabbits, guinea pigs, horses, camels and swine are not susceptible.

Signs.—In the typical case, after a prolonged and variable incubation period, the animal exhibits pneumonia which clinically is indistinguishable from that of nonspecific etiology. In the acute stage, a dry and painful cough, which later becomes moist, is followed by labored respiration with grunting, halting expiration. When the lungs are extensively involved, respiratory distress is exhibited by dyspnea so severe that the animal stands with its elbows turned out. In the later stages, there may be mucopurulent discharge from the nose and sometimes edematous infiltration of the lower thorax. Weakness and emaciation usually become apparent, and swelling of the joints (polyarthritis) is sometimes seen in young calves. The organism may invade the placenta and fetus resulting in abortion.

Lesions.—In the typical case of pleuropneumonia, the lesions of the lung are characteristic. They usually are limited to one lung, occasionally are bilateral, but never symmetrically involve contralateral lungs. The pleural cavity over the affected lung usually contains an excess of pleural fluid which may be blood-

Table 11–1.—Diseases Caused by Organisms of Uncertain Classification

THE PLEUROPNEUMONIA GROUP

Disease	*Organism*
Bovine pleuropneumonia	*Mycoplasma mycoides*
Murine arthritis	*Mycoplasma arthritidis*
Infectious catarrh of rats	*Mycoplasma pulmonis*
Ovine pneumonia and arthritis	*Mycoplasma spp.*
Polyserositis and arthritis in swine	*Mycoplasma hyorhinis*
Arthritis in swine	*Mycoplasma hyoarthrinosa, Mycoplasma granularum*
Bovine mastitis and metritis	*Mycoplasma agalactiae, v. bovis*
Caprine and swine mastitis	*Mycoplasma agalactiae*
Bovine vaginitis	*Mycoplasma bovigenitalium*
Pneumonia in swine	*Mycoplasma spp.*

THE RICKETTSIAL GROUP

Disease	*Organism*
Salmon disease of dogs and foxes	*Neorickettsia helmintheca*
Heartwater disease of cattle	*Cowdria ruminantium*
Q fever of man	*Coxiella burnettii*
Typhus fever of man	*Rickettsia prowazekii*
Murine typhus of man	*Rickettsia typhi*
Rocky Mountain spotted fever	*Rickettsia rickettsii*
Boutonneuse fever of man	*Rickettsia conorii*
Scrub typhus of man (Tsutsugamushi fever)	*Rickettsia tsutsugamushi*
Rickettsial pox of man	*Rickettsia akari*
Trench fever in man	*Rickettsia quintana*
Rickettsiosis of cattle	*Ehrlichia bovis*
Canine ehrlichiosis	*Ehrlichia canis*
Febrile disease of sheep	*Ehrlichia ovina*
Tick-borne fever of cattle	*Rickettsia phagocytophilia*
Equine ehrlichiosis	*Ehrlichia sp.*

THE BARTONELLA GROUP

Disease	*Organism*
Oroya fever, verruga peruana or Carrion's disease of man	*Bartonella bacilliformis*
Parasite of voles	*Grahamella talpae*
Eperythrozoonosis of swine	*Eperythrozoon suis*
Eperythrozoonosis of cattle	*Eperythrozoon wenyoni*
Eperythrozoonosis of voles	*Eperythrozoon dispar*
Eperythrozoonosis of deer mice	*Eperythrozoon varians*
Eperythrozoonosis of sheep	*Eperythrozoon ovis*
Eperythrozoonosis of mice	*Eperythrozoon coccoides*
Haemobartonellosis, rat and mouse	*Haemobartonella muris*
Haemobartonellosis, cat	*H. felis*
Haemobartonellosis, dog	*H. canis*
Haemobartonellosis, gray-backed deer mouse	*H. peromyscii, var. maniculate*
Haemobartonellosis, vole	*H. microtii*
Haemobartonellosis, guinea pig	*H. tyzzeri*
Haemobartonellosis, cattle	*H. bovis*
Haemobartonellosis, buffalo	*H. sturmani*
Haemobartonellosis, deer mouse	*H. peromyscii*
Haemobartonellosis, short-tailed shrew	*H. blarinae*
Haemobartonellosis, gray squirrel	*H. sciuri*

THE ANAPLASMA GROUP

Disease	*Organism*
Bovine anaplasmosis	*Anaplasma marginale, Anaplasma centrale*
Ovine and Caprine anaplasmosis	*Anaplasma ovis*

Table 11–1.—Diseases Caused by Organisms of Uncertain Classification (Cont.)

THE PSITTACOSIS-LYMPHOGRANULOMA-TRACHOMA GROUP

Psittacosis—man and animals (Ornithosis, Parrot Fever)	*Chlamydia psittaci* and *C. ornithosis*
Sporadic Bovine Encephalomyelitis	*C. pecoris*
Feline pneumonitis	*C. felis*
Polyarthritis in sheep	*Chlamydia sp.*
Polyarthritis in calves	*Chlamydia sp.*
Epizootic Bovine Abortion	*Chlamydia sp.*
Enzootic Abortion of Ewes	*Chlamydia sp.*
Enteritis in Cattle	*Chlamydia bovis*
Pneumonia in cattle and sheep	*Chlamydia sp.*
Pneumonitis in man	*C. pneumoniae, C. louisianae, C. illini*
Pneumonitis mice	*C. bronchopneumoniae*
Trachoma of man	*C. trachomatis*
Guinea pig inclusion conjunctivitis	*Chlamydia sp.*
Conjunctivitis and keratitis of sheep, cattle and goats	*Colesiota conjunctivae*
Conjunctivitis and keratitis in chickens	*Co. conjunctivae-galli*

LEPTOSPIROSIS

Leptospirosis in man (Weil's disease)	*Leptospira icterohemorrhagiae, L. canicola, L. pomona*
Leptospirosis in dogs	*L. canicola, L. icterohemorrhagiae, L. pomona*
Leptospirosis in cattle, swine, man, horses, dogs	*L. pomona* (also other serotypes)

stained and include strands of fibrin; as a rule the pleura is adherent to the thoracic wall at some points. The parenchyma does not collapse when the thorax is opened but remains firm and raised above the relatively normal adjacent lung tissue. The cut surface has a marbled appearance with red and grayish areas of parenchyma separated by thick yellowish interlobular septa. The presence of unequally distended lymph spaces often imparts a "beaded" appearance to these septa. In cases of long standing, zones of necrosis within groups of lobules tend to become sequestrated from the adjacent lung and surrounded by a dense layer of connective tissue. Within these sequestra, which often are large, the original configuration of lung parenchyma may be retained for a time. Eventually abscesses may form in the encapsulated tissue and their rupture may cause an acute exacerbation of the symptoms, or the entire sequestrum may be converted to scar tissue.

The outstanding histologic characteristic of the lung is the separation of the lobules into distinct compartments by the heavily thickened interlobular septa, in which there is not only edema but organization as well. The lobules contain areas in which the alveoli are patent, although they are completely consolidated in many others. A particularly intense infiltration of round cells, chiefly lymphocytes and plasma cells, is seen around blood vessels and bronchi. Similar focal collections of leukocytes are found within the interlobular septa.

The lesions in other organs are not specific for this disease, but in the liver there may be round cell infiltration in the hepatic triads and some necrosis of individual liver cells near central veins. These necrotic liver cells are acidophilic, have dark pyknotic nuclei and are believed by some to be the result of gradual anoxia. In the spleen, the germinal centers may be enlarged, mature lymphocytes decreased in number, plasma cells increased, and red blood cells and blood pigment present in excessive amounts.

Diagnosis.—The diagnosis may be established by the history, the clinical symptoms, the gross and microscopic lesions, and recovery of the organism. A complement fixation test can also be used to establish the nature of the infection in acute cases but is less significant in long-standing cases because the complement-fixing antibody gradually decreases in titer.

Pleuropneumonia

DAUBNEY, R.: Contagious Bovine Pleuropneumonia. Note on Experimental Reproduction and Infection by Contact. J. Comp. Path. & Therap. *48*:83–96, 1935.
JOHNSTON, L. A. Y., and SIMMONS, G. C.: Bovine Pneumonias in Queensland with Particular Reference to the Diagnosis of Contagious Bovine Pleuropneumonia. Aust. Vet. J. *39*:290–294, 1963. VB 823–64.
METTAM, R. W. M.: Contagious Pleuropneumonia of Goats in East Africa. Pan African Agri. & Vet. Conf., Bull. 8E, 1929.

Murine Arthritis

Arthritis is a reasonably frequent occurrence in laboratory rats and mice. In many instances this disease is associated with the presence of *Mycoplasma arthritidis*, a rather ubiquitous organism originally isolated by Klieneberger (1938) from the submaxillary gland of a rat. The organism has also been recovered from infected joints, heart blood, abscesses, a transmissible sarcoma and submaxillary glands of rats. It is also pathogenic for mice but most other laboratory animals are refractory to infection. The joints of the limbs are most frequently involved. Usually only a single joint is involved but occasionally two or more are affected. The joints are swollen, hot, tender and fixed as in acute arthritis (p. 1078) in any species. After a time, proliferation of synovia and accumulation of fluid in the joint is accompanied by the appearance of purulent and lymphocytic inflammation in the adjacent tissues. Other organisms may also cause arthritis in these species; among them are *Streptococci* and *Streptobacillis moniliformis*.

Murine Arthritis

FREUNDT, E. A.: Arthritis Caused by *Streptobacillus moniliformis* and Pleuropneumonia-like Organisms in Small Rodents. Lab. Invest. *8*:1358–1375, 1959.
SOKOLOFF, L.: Osteoarthritis in Laboratory Animals. Lab. Invest. *8*:1209–1217, 1959.

Infectious Catarrh of Rats and Mice

Respiratory disease in laboratory rats and mice often interferes with experiments using these species and may cause serious mortality. Although the evidence is not as complete as desirable, it is Nelson's (1962) opinion that a virus is the principal etiologic agent in chronic murine pneumonia (p. 432) which may be made more severe by the presence of *Mycoplasma*. In his opinion *Mycoplasma* are the sole etiologic agent in certain infections of the upper respiratory tract, middle and internal ear, collectively named "infectious catarrh." Other investigators believe that *Mycoplasma* are the primary cause of chronic murine pneumonia. No doubt these organisms can and do induce pulmonary lesions, but their role as the sole cause of chronic murine pneumonia remains to be established.

Several organisms of the pleuropneumonia group have been recovered from infected mice and rats but their relation to one another has not been established.

Mycoplasma pulmonis, isolated by Klieneberger and Steabben (1937) appears to be the most important one in infectious catarrh. *Mycoplasma neurolyticum* and *M. arthritidis* (p. 530) may also be recovered from the conjunctiva and nasal passages of rodents.

Purulent rhinitis is manifest in the rat and mouse by nasal discharge, coughing, sneezing and snuffling. Involvement of the inner ear results in twisting and rotary movements of the affected animal. A rat held up by the tail will exhibit characteristic rapid twisting or twirling motions. Postmortem examination is usually necessary to establish the diagnosis. Purulent exudate in the nasal cavities, middle and internal ear may be recognizable grossly but in some instances can be detected only by aspiration of material with a capillary pipette. This material is cultured for *Mycoplasma*, used for animal inoculation (usually mice) and smeared on a slide and stained to demonstrate the presence of leukocytes and pleomorphic organisms.

Murine Catarrh

GOGOLAK, F. M.: The Histopathology of Murine Pneumonitis Infection and the Growth of the Virus in the Mouse Lung. J. Infect. Dis. *92*:254–272, 1953.
KLIENEBERGER, E. and STEABBEN, D. B.: On a Pleuropneumonia-like Organism in Lung Lesions of Rats, with Notes on the Clinical and Pathological Features of the Underlying Condition. J. Hyg. (Cambr.) *37*:143–153, 1937.
KOHN, DENNIS F., and KIRK, B. E.: Pathogenicity of *Mycoplasma Pulmonis* in Laboratory Rats. Lab. Anim. Care *19*:321–329, 1969.
NELSON, J. B.: Chronic Respiratory Disease. In *The Problems of Laboratory Animal Disease*, pp. 157–168, ed. by R. J. C. Harris, New York, Academic Press, 1962.

Mycoplasma in Ovine Pneumonia and Arthritis

The situation is not clear at this writing, but it seems likely that organisms of the pleuropneumonia group may be important in pneumonia and arthritis in sheep and goats. *Mycoplasma* occur in affected lungs and joints of sheep, sometimes in association with a virus of the psittacosis-lymphogranuloma group (p. 556). The report of Boidin *et al.* (1958) indicate that *Mycoplasma* recovered from pneumonic lungs of sheep will produce septicemia and localize in joints of lambs injected with cultures of the organism. A rickettsial-type organism, isolated from the same pneumonic lungs, appears to cause the more severe natural disease in which lungs and joints may be involved. Further studies are needed to clarify these points gleaned from research done in widely separated parts of the world.

Cordy (1955) described a fatal disease of goats characterized by septicemia and arthritis caused by a *Mycoplasma*. In addition to fibrinopurulent arthritis, fibrinous pleuritis, pericarditis and peritonitis, and lymphadenitis were almost constant findings.

Mycoplasma agalactiae, which is pathogenic to goats and to a lesser extent sheep, localizes in the mammary gland causing mastitis, but it may also localize in the joints and produce arthritis.

Ovine Pneumonia and Arthritis

BOIDIN, A. G., CORDY, D. R., and ADLER, H. E.: A Pleuropneumonia-like Organism and a Virus in Ovine Pneumonia in California. Cornell Vet. *48*:410–430, 1958.
CORDY, D. R., ADLER, H. E., and YAMAMOTO, R.: A Pathogenic Pleuropneumonia like Organism from Goats. Cornell Vet. *45*:50–68, 1955.

COTTEW, G. S., and LLOYD, L. C.:   An Outbreak of Pleurisy and Pneumonia in Goats in Australia Attributed to a Mycoplasma Species. J. Comp. Path. *75*:368–374, 1965.

HAMDY, A. H., POUNDEN, W. D., and FERGUSON, L. C.: Microbial Agents Associated with Pneumonia in Slaughtered Lambs. Am. J. Vet. Res. *20*:87–90, 1959.

HAMDY, A. H., and SANGER, V. L.:   Characteristics of a Virus Associated with Lamb Pneumonia. Am. J. Vet. Res. *20*:84–86, 1959.

McGOWAN, B., MOULTON, J. E., and SHULTZ, G.:   Pneumonia in California Lambs. J. Am. Vet. Med. Assn. *131*:318–323, 1957.

Polyserositis and Arthritis in Swine

Inflammatory lesions in the pericardium, pleura, peritoneum and joints are often encountered in young swine. In many instances the etiologic factors are diverse or unknown but good evidence is now available indicating that *Mycoplasma hyorhinis* is one agent capable of causing such lesions. McNutt *et al.* (1945) appears to be the first to recognize that an infectious agent (distinguishable from *Erysipelothrix rhusiopathiæ*) could be recovered from synovia of young arthritic pigs by inoculation of chick embryos. Material from the infected chick embryos caused arthritis, pleuritis, peritonitis and pericarditis when injected by various routes into young pigs. Switzer, in 1953, demonstrated a similar agent from the nasal passages of swine with atrophic rhinitis and observed intracellular organisms in chick embryos. These organisms were subsequently characterized in the pleuropneumonia group (Carter and McKay, 1953) and named *Mycoplasma hyorhinis* by Switzer (1955).

Although *Mycoplasma* are generally thought to be species-specific, it is of interest that Cordy *et al.* (1958) demonstrated that an organism, originally isolated from infected goats, was also infective for young swine. Polyserositis and arthritis was produced experimentally in these animals.

Polyserositis and polyarthritis have been reproduced by experimental inoculation of young pigs with pure cultures of *Mycoplasma hyorhinis*. The lesions of the experimental disease are described in detail by Roberts *et al.* (1963). The pericarditis, pleuritis, and peritonitis (collectively sometimes spoken of as "polyserositis") is rather characteristic; each serous surface is affected in essentially the same way. Within six days following intraperitoneal instillation of organisms, fibrinopurulent exudate may be seen grossly on serous surfaces. This exudate becomes more extensive at ten days following inoculation but wanes by the thirtieth day. The peritoneum and pleura are severely involved, the pericardium much less so in the experimental disease. The full-blown lesion consists of fibrinopurulent exudate on the serous surface, with swelling and disorganization of the serosal lining cells. Underlying these cells are lymphocytes, macrophages and plasma cells. Hyperemia and vascularization are features during this stage. As the disease runs its course, after fifteen to thirty days, the fibrinous exudate may organize (p. 156) particularly over the pleura and peritoneal surfaces. This results in adhesions which may persist for a long time. In an occasional case severe exudation in the pericardial sac may lead to organizing epicarditis which eventually interferes with cardiac function. The lymphocytic exudate sometimes extends into the subpleural alveoli and Glisson's capsule of the liver but otherwise does not affect parenchymatous organs. The tunica vaginalis may be affected by extension from the peritoneum. In some cases, lymphocytic leptomeningitis may be demonstrable. Numerous joints may become involved in this infection with swelling, congestion and pain evident from lameness. In the least severely affected joints and early in the course of the disease, the joint capsule may be slightly hyperemic and the synovial fluid excessive in volume. In more severely affected joints, the synovial fluid becomes yellow or turbid and may contain strands of fibrin. Neutrophils are numerous in such synovial fluid. The synovial membranes may become edematous, and hyperemic and yellowish in color. The membranes are seen microscopically to contain large numbers of lymphocytes and macrophages. The villi are edematous, redundant and hyperemic. Nodules of lymphocytes sometimes form. In young swine, disorganization may be seen in the columns of cartilage in the epiphyseal plate. The cartilage columns lose their straight orderly arrangement and are distorted and irregular, with congested vascular spaces between them. Fibrous thickening of the joint capsule may result in partial or complete ankylosis of the affected joint.

Mycoplasma hyoarthrinosa and *Mycoplasma granularum* are two mycoplasmas distinct from *Mycoplasma hyorhinis* which have recently been reported to induce polyarthritis in swine. The disease differs from that induced by *Mycoplasma hyorhinis* in that it affects older swine and is not associated with polyserositis or meningitis. The synovial exudate in *Mycoplasma hyoarthrinosa* infection is reported to often be serosanguinous, a point which may be of value in differential diagnosis.

The **diagnosis** of Mycoplasma infections is based upon the gross and microscopic lesions and the demonstration of the organisms by cultural methods.

The "fibrinous-serosa-joint inflammation" of young pigs called "Glässer's Disease," is pathologically nearly identical to *M. hyorhinis* infection, but Hjärre and Wramby (1942) associated "Glässer's Disease" with swine influenza and infection with *Hemophilus influenzae suis*. Based on recent evidence it now seems reasonably certain that *H. influenzae suis* and *M. hyorhinis* are distinct causes of polyserositis and arthritis in swine. Hjärre reserves the eponym Glässer's disease for the disease caused by *H. influenzae suis* and distinguishes it from mycoplasmoses in that purulent meningitis is found in 80 per cent of spontaneous cases of Glässer's disease, whereas purulent meningitis is not a feature of mycoplasma infection. However, as noted above meningitis may develop in *M. hyorhinis* infection. For accurate differentiation attempts should be made to culture both organisms, but such efforts have often led to the isolation of both.

Polyserositis

CARTER, G. R. and McKAY, K. A.: A Pleuropneumonia-like Organism Associated with Infectious Atrophic Rhinitis of Swine. Canad. J. Comp. Med. *17*:413–416, 1953.

CORDY, D. R., ADLER, H. E., and YAMAMOTO, R.: A Pathogenic Pleuropneumonia-like Organism from Goats. Cornell Vet. *45*:50–68, 1955.

CORDY, D. R., ADLER, H. E., and BERG, J.: The Pathogenicity for Swine of a Pleuropneumonia-like Organism from Goats. Cornell Vet. *48*:25–30, 1958.

DUNCAN, J. R., and ROSS, R. F.: Fine Structure of the Synovial Membrane in *Mycoplasma hyorhinis* Arthritis of Swine. Amer. J. Path. *57*:171–186, 1969.

GLÄSSER, K., HUPKA, E., and WETZEL, R.: *Die Krankheiten des Schweines.* 5th ed., Hanover, Germany, M. and H. Schaper Verlag, 1950.

HJÄRRE, A.: Enzootic Virus Pneumonia and Glasser's Disease of Swine. Adv. Vet. Sci. *4*: 235–263, 1958.

HJÄRRE, A. and WRAMBY, G.: On Fibrinös Serosa-ledinflammation (Glässer) Hos Svin. Skand. vet.-tidskr, *32*:257–289, 1942.

KING, S. J.: Porcine Polyserositis and Arthritis—With Particular Reference to Mycoplasmosis and Glasser's Disease. **Aust. Vet. J. *44*:227–230, 1968.**

Leece, J. C.: Porcine Polyserositis with Arthritis Isolation of a Fastidious Pleuropneumonia-Like Organism and Hemophilus Influenzae Suis. Ann. New York Acad. Sci. 79:670–676, 1960.

McNutt, S. H., Leith, T. S., and Underbjerg, G. K.: An Active Agent Isolated from Hogs Affected with Arthritis. Am. J. Vet. Res. 6:247–251, 1945.

Moore, R. W., Redmond, H. E., and Livingston, C. W., Jr.: Pathologic and Serologic Characteristics of a Mycoplasma Causing Arthritis in Swine. Amer. J. Vet. Res. 27:1649–1656, 1966.

Neil, D. H., et al.: Glasser's Disease of Swine Produced by the Intratracheal Inoculation of Haemophilus suis. Can. J. Comp. Med. 33:187–193, 1969.

Roberts, E. D., Switzer, W. P., and Ramsey, F. K.: Pathology of the Visceral Organs of Swine Inoculated with Mycoplasma hyorhinis. Am. J. Vet. Res. 24:9–18, 1963.

—————: The Pathology of Mycoplasma hyorhinis Arthritis Produced Experimentally in Swine. Am. J. Vet. Res. 24:19–31, 1963.

Robinson, F. R., Moore, R. W., and Bridges, C. H.: Pathogenesis of Mycoplasma hyoarthrinosa Infection in Swine. Amer. J. Vet. Res. 28:483–496, 1967.

Switzer, W. P.: Mycoplasmosis. In Diseases of Swine. 2nd Ed., Dunne, H. W. (Ed.). Ames, Iowa State Univ. Press, 1964, pp. 498–507.

—————: Studies on Infectious Atrophic Rhinitis of Swine. I. Isolation of a Filterable Agent from the Nasal Cavity of Swine with Atrophic Rhinitis. J. Am. Vet. Med. Assn. 123:45–47, 1953.

—————: Studies on Infectious Atrophic Rhinitis. IV. Characterization of a Pleuropneumonia-like Organism Isolated from the Nasal Cavities of Swine. Am. J. Vet. Res. 16:540–544, 1955.

Mycoplasma in Bovine Mastitis and Metritis

An organism, tentatively named *Mycoplasma agalactiæ* var. *bovis* was isolated by Hale *et al.* (1962) from the mammary gland of one of several cows affected with severe mastitis. Instillation of pure cultures of this organism into mammæ of normal heifers resulted in a characteristic mastitis. The organism is therefore believed to be the etiologic agent. No *Streptococci* or other bacterial pathogen could be demonstrated.

The **lesions** are described to involve mammary acini, interlobular ducts and interstitial stroma. In early stages, purulent exudate fills acini—usually all acini in a lobule. The interlobular ducts may also be filled with neutrophils and the epithelium is hyperplastic. As the disease progresses, squamous metaplasia (p. 96) becomes evident in the ductal epithelium and some ducts and acini are filled with lipogranulomatous exudate (p. 166). The interstitial stroma is at first infiltrated by plasma, lymphocytes and plasma cells but eventually organization of the exudate leads to fibrosis. Eosinophils are reportedly a frequent component of the exudate in both natural and experimental *Mycoplasma* mastitis.

Mycoplasma were isolated from tne bovine genital tract by Edward *et al.* (1947), but the pathogenicity of the organism remained in doubt until Hartman *et al.* (1964), and Hirth and Nielsen (1966), produced endometritis, salpingitis and localized peritonitis in heifers by intrauterine injection of pure cultures of *Mycoplasma agalactiae* var. *bovis*. This organism may be responsible for some cases of sterility and low fertility in bovine animals.

The **lesions** in experimentally infected cows were not visible grossly and were limited to the uterus, oviduct and related peritoneum. The endometrium was at first edematous, then infiltrated with lymphocytes and plasma cells. Neutrophils soon were evident in the lumen. The lymphocytic inflammation often extended to the serosal surfaces of the uterus and oviducts. In long-standing lesions, collections of lymphocytes, and sometimes eosinophils, were noted in the stroma surrounding deep uterine glands. The **diagnosis** of this infection will depend upon isolation and identification of the causative organisms from infected mammary glands or genitalia in which lesions are present. The overall significance of this infection in bovine mastitis and metritis is yet to be determined.

Recently Afshar (1967) suggested that *Mycoplasma bovigenitalium* is the cause of bovine granular venereal disease (bovine granular vulvovaginitis). When the organism was applied to scarified vaginal mucosa a vaginitis closely mimicking the natural disease was produced. The lesions consist of granular elevations of the vulvo-vaginal epithelium and a mucopurulent discharge. Microscopically the lesions are characterized by nodular collections of lymphocytes, thinning and necrosis of the epithelium, hyperemia and an infiltration of eosinophils.

Mycoplasmas have also been suggested as causes of inflammatory diseases of the external and internal genital organs of bulls. They have been isolated with frequency from bulls (as well as from cows) but their exact significance and importance also remain to be determined in the bull.

Bovine Mastitis and Metritis

AFSHAR, A.: Genital Diseases of Cattle Associated with Mycoplasma. V. B. *37*:879–884, 1967.

EDWARD, D. C., HANCOCK, J. L., and HIGNETT, S. L.: Isolation of a Pleuropneumonia-like Organism from the Bovine Genital Tract. Vet. Rec. *59*:329–330, 1947.

HALE, H. H., HELMBOLDT, C. F., PLASTRIDGE, W. N., and STULA, E. F.: Bovine Mastitis Caused by a *Mycoplasma* species. Cornell Vet. *52*:582–591, 1962.

HARTMAN, H. A., TOURTELLOTTE, M. E., NIELSEN, S. W., and PLASTRIDGE, W. N.: Experimental Bovine Uterine Mycoplasmosis. Res. Vet. Sci. *5*:303–310, 1964.

HIRTH, R. S., and NIELSEN, S. W.: Experimental Pathology of Bovine Salpingitis Due to Mycoplasma Insemination. Lab. Invest. *15*:1132–1133, 1966.

KARBE, E., NIELSEN, S. W., and HELMBOLDT, C. F.: Pathology of Experimental Mycoplasma Mastitis in the Cow. Zentbl. Vet. Med. *14B*:7–31, 1967.

ROVOZZO, G. C., LUGINBUHL, R. E., and HELMBOLDT, C. F.: A *Mycoplasma* from a Bovine Causing Cytopathogenic Effects in Calf Kidney Tissue Culture. Cornell Vet. *53*:560–566, 1963.

Mycoplasma in Swine Pneumonia

A pneumonia of swine designated virus pig pneumonia or enzootic pneumonia of swine has been recognized for years, however, a specific causative virus has not been isolated. Recently evidence has been presented that the syndrome is caused by a *Mycoplasma* which has been termed *M. suipneumoniae* by Rosdiven *et al.* and *M. hyopneumoniae* by Maré and Switzer (1965, 1966). Additional research is required before Mycoplasma can be accepted as the sole cause; however, until a virus can be isolated and shown to reproduce the disease we will consider the syndrome in this section. Clinically the disease is chronic and characterized principally by poor weight gains and cough. In addition to lobular pneumonia, gross changes include enlargement of pulmonary lymph nodes and serofibrinous pleuritis, peritonitis and pericarditis. The latter changes are reminiscent of mycoplasma polyserositis and arthritis in swine (p. 532).

Microscopically the pneumonia is characterized by a slight to marked peribronchial, perivascular, and alveolar septal infiltration of lymphocytes and macrophages. Neutrophils may be present in alveoli but the pneumonia is not purulent. Occasionally a non-purulent encephalitis is encountered.

Mycoplasma in Swine Pneumonia

HJÄRRE, A.: Enzootic Virus Pneumonia and Glasser's Disease of Swine. Adv. Vet. Sci. 4:235–263, 1958.

HUHN, R. G.: Enzootic Pneumonia of Pigs: A Review of the Literature. V.B. 40:249–257, 1970.

GOODWIN, R. F. W., POMEROY, A. P., and WHITTLESTONE, P.: Production of Enzootic Pneumonia in Pigs with a Mycoplasma. Vet. Rec. 77:1247–1249, 1965.

MARÉ, C. J., and SWITZER, W. P.: Mycoplasma hyopneumoniae. A. Causative Agent of Virus Pig Pneumonia. Vet. Med. Small Anim. Clin. 60:841–846, 1965.

————: Virus Pneumonia of Pigs: Drug and Ether Sensitivity of a Causative Agent. Am. J. Vet. Res. 27:1671–1675, 1966.

————: Virus Pneumonia of Pigs: Filtration and Visualization of a Causative Agent. Am. J. Vet. Res. 27:1677–1685, 1966.

————: Virus Pneumonia of Pigs: Propagation and Characterization of a Causative Agent. Am. J. Vet. Res. 27:1687–1693, 1966.

TERPSTAR, J. E., AKKERMANS, J. P. W. M., and POMPER, W.: A Mycoplasma as a Cause of Enzootic Pneumonia of a Swine. Neth. J. Vet. Sci. 2:5–11, 1969.

URMAN, H. K., UNDERDAHL, N. R., and YOUNG, G. A.: Comparative Histopathology of Experimental Swine Influenza and Virus Pneumonia of Pigs in Disease-free Antibody Devoid Pigs. Am. J. Vet. Res. 19:913–917, 1958.

THE RICKETTSIAL GROUP

Microorganisms classified in the Family *Rickettsiaceæ* (order: Rickettsiales) includes several causative agents of disease in man and animals. The organisms are minute obligate parasites which are found in the cytoplasm of tissue cells but not in erythrocytes. The organisms are very frequently transmitted from one vertebrate species to another by arthropod vectors. Five pathogenic genera are presently included in this family: *Rickettsia, Coxiella, Cowdria, Ehrlichia,* and *Neorickettsia*. The genus *Rickettsia* contains seven species which are pathogenic for man, each organism having a specific intermediate host-vector. *R. prowazekii* is louse-borne and the cause of typhus fever; *R. typhi* is carried by fleas from natural infections of rats and mice to produce murine typhus in man; *R. rickettsii* is the cause of Rocky Mountain Spotted Fever and is transmitted to man from naturally infected squirrels, rabbits and mice by several species of ticks, particularly *Dermacentor andersoni* (wood tick), *D. variabilis* (dog tick) and *Haemaphysalis leporis-palustris* (rabbit tick). *Rickettsia conorii* is the cause of Boutonneuse fever of man; its vector is a dog tick *Rhipicephalus sanguineus*, although the dog does not apparently become infected. The guinea pig is susceptible to experimental infection but the rabbit, sheep, pig, and pigeon are resistant. *Rickettsia tsutsugamushi* is the causative agent in scrub typhus and tsutsugamushi fever in man, and is transmitted by trombiculid mites and is also pathogenic for rhesus monkeys, gibbons, guinea pigs, hamsters, voles, rats, gerbilles and mice. Rickettsial pox in man is caused by *R. akari* which is transmitted by the mite, *Allodermanyssus sanguineus*. Mice and guinea pigs are susceptible. *Rickettsia quintana* is the causative agent of trench fever in man and is transmitted by the body louse, *Pediculus humanus*.

The second genus of interest is *Coxiella*, which currently holds only one species, *Coxiella burnetti*, the etiologic agent in Q fever of man. One species in the third genus in this group, *Cowdria ruminantium*, is of interest as the causative organism in "heartwater" of cattle.

The genus *Ehrlichia* contains three species: *E. bovis* (*Rickettsia bovis;* mild disease in cattle); *E. ovina* (*Rickettsia ovis;* mild disease of sheep) and *E. canis*

(*Rickettsia canis*) the cause of canine ehrlichiosis which is discussed later.   A disease of horses has been described in California which is tentatively considered to be caused by an *Ehrlichia sp.*   Tick-borne fever, a mild illness in cattle and sheep, is caused by an organism tentatively termed *Rickettsia phagocytophilia.*

Neorickettsia helmintheca, the cause of salmon poisoning in dogs, is the only member of the fifth genus.

Salmon Disease of Dogs and Foxes

("Salmon Poisoning")

A febrile, often fatal, disease of dogs and foxes has been known for some time to be associated with a diet that includes salmon, trout, and other fish.   It has been recognized that the disease is related to infection by a small intestinal fluke, *Troglotrema (Nanophyetus) salmincola,* whose encysted metacercariae are carried in fish of the family Salmonidae, which thus serve as intermediate hosts.   More recent observations indicate that a rickettsial organism is the probable etiologic agent of the disease, the fluke acting only as a reservoir for the infection.   This complex biologic pattern in host-parasite relationship is of unusual interest.   The disease is not spread by contact, but can be produced by feeding the dog or fox fish which are infected with metacercariae of *Troglotrema salmincola.*   It can be transmitted by intraperitoneal injection of blood of an infected dog, suspensions of washed flukes from infected dogs, or metacercariae from fish.

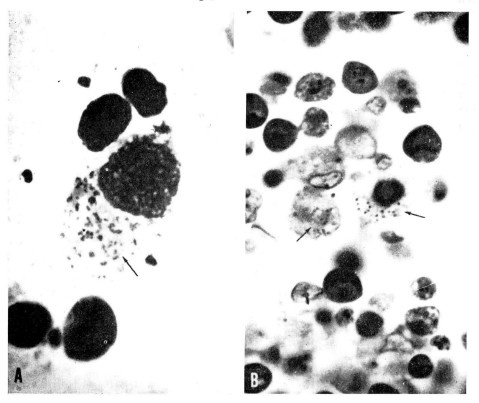

Fig. 11–1.—"Salmon Disease" in a dog. *A*, Smear from a mesenteric lymph node ($\times$ 1500). Giemsa stain.   *B*, Section from another lymph node ($\times$ 500).   Giemsa stain.   Arrows indicate organism, *Neorickettsia helmintheca.*   Photographs courtesy of Dr. Wm. J. Hadlow.

Signs.—The signs usually appear about five days after the ingestion of infected fish, starting as a fever which continues four to eight days. Anorexia is a characteristic feature, and is accompanied by depression, weakness, and weight loss. Vomiting and diarrhea, with scant, yellowish, watery, or occasionally bloody and mucoid feces, accompanied by tenesmus, are prominent manifestations. Occasionally a serous nasal discharge is observed, and a tenacious conjunctival exudate may collect at the inner canthus of the eye.

Lesions.—According to Cordy and Gorham (1950), lymphoid tissues suffer particularly in this disease; the visceral nodes of the abdomen may be enlarged to six times normal size (Fig. 24–8), with the somatic lymph nodes somewhat less severely affected. These enlarged nodes are usually yellowish with prominent white follicles in their cortex. Some edema may surround them, and occasionally an opaque grayish fluid can be expressed from a nodule. The tonsils, which are enlarged and yellowish with prominent follicles and occasional petechiæ, may be everted from the fossæ.The spleen is often enlarged. The splenic follicles are prominent in foxes but unrecognizable in dogs. The lymphoid tissue of the intestinal tract is especially hyperplastic (Fig. 24–8). The intestinal contents may include free blood, especially in animals in which flukes have damaged the intestinal mucosa. Petechiæ usually are seen in the intestinal mucosa, particularly over the enlarged lymphoid follicles. Bleeding from small ulcers may be noted in the pylorus. Intussusception of the small intestine is not uncommon. Although the liver often appears grossly normal, rupture is a possibility, with hemoperitoneum as the usual consequence. Hemorrhages have been observed in the gallbladder and the urinary bladder. The lungs usually are studded with many bright or dark red subpleural hemorrhagic puncta, 5 to 20 mm. in diameter.

The microscopic findings, prominent in the lymph nodes, are dominated by hyperplasia of reticulo-endothelial elements and depletion of small lymphocytes. Foci of necrosis are frequent and many include hemorrhages. Elementary bodies of *Neorickettsia* in reticulo-endothelial cells, both in sinuses and parenchyma, are demonstrated by Giemsa or Macchiavello's stain. The thymus in younger dogs is the site of prominent changes, including depletion of small lymphocytes, proliferation of reticulo-endothelial cells, increase in neutrophils, and the presence of small islands of necrosis throughout the gland. In the intestine, flukes may be demonstrated deep in the intestinal villi and occasionally in duodenal glands. There is surprisingly little tissue reaction to these flukes aside from a few foci of neutrophils and slight increase in lymphoid and plasma cells in the lamina propria. Small hemorrhages in the intestinal mucosa or submucosa may be seen, although not necessarily in relation to the flukes. According to Hadlow (1957), the brain contains microscopic lesions in 91 per cent of fatal cases. These changes consist of: "(a) slight to moderate accumulation of mononuclear cells in the leptomeninges, most intense over the cerebellum, (b) cellular exudative and proliferative changes in sheaths of small and medium-sized intracerebral blood vessels; and (c) focal collections of glial, mesenchymal cells, or both." The intracerebral lesions, less intense than those of the meninges, occur in the cerebral cortex, brain stem, and cerebellum. Similar lesions may occur in the neurohypophysis. Aside from the hemorrhages which are recognized grossly, microscopic changes in other viscera are minimal and believed to be nonspecific.

Diagnosis.—Of particular significance in the diagnosis of this disease are the small intracytoplasmic "elementary" bodies in reticulo-endothelial cells in lymphoid tissue and occasionally in large mononuclear cells of liver, lungs, and blood. These bodies are coccoid or coccobacillary in shape and uniformly about 0.3 micron in diameter. With Giemsa's stain, these bodies are purple; with Macchiavello's stain, red or blue; with Levaditi's method, black or dark brown; with hematoxylin and eosin, pale bluish violet. They are gram-negative. In some cells, they form nearly solid "plaques" filling the cytoplasm. In some smears, they are found free, apparently released from ruptured cells. They have not been observed in epithelium, endothelium, fibroblasts or muscle cells.

Salmon Disease

CORDY, D. R., and GORHAM, J. R.: The Pathology and Etiology of Salmon Disease in the Dog and Fox. Am. J. Path. 26:617–637, 1950.

HADLOW, W. J.: Neuropathology of Experimental Salmon Poisoning of Dogs. Am. J. Vet. Res. 18:898–908, 1957.

PHILIP, C. B., HADLOW, W. J., and HUGHES, L. E.: Neorickettsia helmintheca, a new Rickettsia-like Disease Agent of Dogs in Western United States Transmitted by a Helminth. Proc. 6th Internat. Cong. Microbiol. (Rome) 4:70–82, 1953.

CANINE EHRLICHIOSIS
(Canine Rickettsiosis)

Caused by *Ehrlichia canis*, canine ehrlichiosis is principally of importance in Africa and India although it exists in the United States, Southeast Asia and the Caribbean. The disease is transmitted by the tick, *Rhipicephalus sanguineus*. The organism multiplies in reticulo-endothelial cells, lymphocytes and monocytes and can be visualized in stained smears of peripheral blood or tissue impressions, although often with difficulty. The life cycle of the parasite is not as yet completely understood, but three intracellular forms can be recognized. Initial bodies are small (1 to 2 μ) spherical structures which are believed to develop into larger bodies described as mulberry bodies or morulae composed of multiple subunits. The morula is thought to dissociate to small granules called elementary bodies. The disease is usually mild except in young puppies or when complicated by another disease such as infection with *Babesia canis*. Ewing (1965, 1969) describes the clinical signs as recurrent fever, serous nasal discharge, photophobia, vomiting, splenomegaly and signs of central nervous system derangement.

Aside from marked splenomegaly there are no characteristic gross changes. Microscopically in the spleen there is a reduction in mature lymphocytes and pronounced hyperplasia of immature lymphocytes and reticulo-endothelial cells. Similar changes occur to a lesser degree in other lymphoid organs. Excessive numbers of lymphoreticular cells may be present in the kidney, liver, pancreas, myocardium and lamina propria and submucosa of the small intestine and colon. In the central nervous system perivascular and meningeal accumulations of mononuclear cells are evident. Focal hepatic necrosis and interstitial pneumonia are also reported as frequent findings. Diagnosis is dependent upon demonstration of the causative organism.

Cytoplasmic inclusions similar to those of *Ehrlichia canis* have been demonstrated in circulating and tissue monocytes in dogs with a transmissible hemorrhagic disease. Based on this finding Huxsoll *et al.* (1970) have suggested that *Ehrlichia canis* may be the cause of the disease. The disorder, which has been described as *tropical canine pancytopenia* in United States military dogs in

Southeast Asia, is characterized by epistaxis, dyspnea, anemia, leukopenia and prolonged bleeding time, with normal coagulation and prothrombin times. Pathologic findings are dominated by hemorrhage, especially on serosal and mucosal surfaces. Microscopically numerous plasma cells are present in the meninges, kidney and lymphoreticular tissues.

Canine Ehrlichiosis

EWING, S. A.: Canine Ehrlichiosis. Adv. in Vet. Sci. *13*:331–353, 1969.
EWING, S. A., and BUCKNER, R. G.: Manifestations of Babesiosis, Ehrlichiosis, and Combined Infections in the Dog. Am. J. Vet. Res. *26*:815–828, 1965.
HUXSOLL, D. L., *et al.*: *Ehrlichia canis*—The Causative Agent of a Haemorrhagic Disease of Dogs. Vet. Rec. *87*:587, 1970.
STANNARD, A. A., GRIBBLE, D. H., and SMITH, R. S.: Equine Ehrlichiosis: A Disease with Similarities to Tick-Borne Fever and Bovine Petechial Fever. Vet. Rec. *84*:149–150, 1969.
WALKER, J. S., *et al.*: Clinical and Clinicopathologic Findings in Tropical Canine Pancytopenia. J. Am. Vet. Med. Assn. *157*:43–55, 1970.

"Heartwater" of Cattle, Sheep and Goats

The name of this disease, which is rather important on the African Continent, is derived from its characteristic lesion: hydropericardium. The causative agent, *Cowdria* (formerly *Rickettsia*) *ruminantium* is an intracellular parasite which is transmitted by ticks (genus *Amblyomma*). It is currently differentiated from the *Rickettsia* which may be transmitted through the egg to succeeding generations of ticks. *C. ruminantium* may be carried through metamorphosis of larva to nymph or nymph to adult, but not through the egg. The organism is a tiny rod-shaped, often diplococcoid organism which can be demonstrated with Giemsa's stain in endothelial cells of the jugular vein, vena cava, renal glomerular capillaries and cerebral gray matter. It is gram-negative, cannot be cultivated on artificial media and is not demonstrable in the circulating blood.

The clinical manifestations are high fever and nervous manifestations, death resulting from systemic infection—often with distention of the pericardial sac by serous exudate.

"Heartwater"

HAIG, D. A.: Tickborne Rickettsioses in South Africa. Adv. Vet. Sci. *2*:307–325, 1955.
HENNING, M. W.: *Animal Diseases of South Africa*, 3rd ed., Pretoria, Central News Agency, Ltd., 1956.
PIENAAR, J. G., *et al.*: Studies on the Pathology of Heartwater (Cowdria Rickettsia) Ruminantium Cowdry, 1926. I. Neuropathological Changes. Onderstepoort J. Vet. Res. *33*:115–138, 1966.

Q Fever

A febrile disease of slaughterhouse workers was originally described in Australia by Derrick (1937), who named the disease "Q" fever (Q for Query, *i.e.*, of questionable or unknown etiology). The disease is known to occur in widely scattered parts of the world, including the United States and Europe. The infectious agent, now classified with the rickettsial organisms and called *Coxiella burnetti* (*Rickettsia burnetii*, *R. diaporica*), is harbored by cattle, sheep and probably other species and can be transmitted by ticks (*Dermacentor andersoni, D. occidentalis, Rhipicephalus sanguineus, Otobius megnini*, and others). Man may acquire the infection by contact with freshly slaughtered infected cattle or by consuming raw milk or butter in which the organisms are present. The organisms can be passed through filters which retain most bacteria, but they are demonstrable in tissues stained by Giemsa or Macchiavello methods, where they appear as minute pleomorphic organisms in the form of lanceolate rods, 0.05 micron in width and 0.5 micron long, as bipolar forms about 1.0 micron in length, or as diplobacillary forms which attain a length of 1.5 microns. Clusters of these organisms appear in the cytoplasm of tissue cells and occasionally are seen extracellularly. *Coxiella burnetii* are poorly stained by ordinary bacterial methods, thus conforming to the characteristics of other rickettsiæ.

Organisms have been recovered from cows which exhibited no signs of infection, and post-mortem examination of such animals has disclosed few, if any, specific lesions. It is necessary to study the tissues of experimentally infected guinea pigs for information concerning the lesions of Q fever. According to Lillie (1942), the lesions in guinea pigs are characterized by focal perivascular exudation of lymphoid cells, less often monocytes and fibroblasts, and "vascular endotheliosis," particularly in the myocardium, lungs, alveolar tissue generally, adrenals, renal cortex and medulla and epididymis. In the lungs small foci made up of collections of epithelioid cells are seen in alveoli and some lymphocytes and other mononuclear cells are located in the interalveolar stroma. In later stages of the disease, small nodules of epithelioid cells are found in the spleen, liver, and vertebral marrow; less often in the heart, mediastinal and mesenteric fat, pancreas, kidney, adrenal, bladder mucosa, testicle and brain. These small granulomas often contain large, multinucleated giant cells which may replace the entire nodule. Serous exudate is common in alveolar tissues of the renal pelvis and rare in the epididymis.

In mice inoculated intranasally or intraperitoneally, Perrin and Bengston (1942) have shown that nodular or patchy, granulomatous lesions develop in the spleen, liver, kidneys and adrenals. Nodular and patchy areas of aplasia and necrosis also occur in the bone marrow. Proliferative changes in the lung and exudation of mononuclear cells are also observed in mice inoculated intranasally.

Diagnosis.—Recognition of infection in cattle is dependent upon the isolation and identification of organisms, usually by inoculation of guinea pigs. Neutralization tests using convalescent serum to protect guinea pigs are of value in differential diagnosis. A complement-fixation test is also employed.

Q Fever

Davis, G. E., Cox, H. R., Parker, R. R., and Dyer, R. E.: A Filter-passing Infectious Agent Isolated from Ticks. I. Isolation from *Dermacentor andersoni*, Reactions in Animals and Filtration Experiments. II. Transmission by *Dermacentor andersoni*. III. Description of the Organism and Cultivation Experiments. IV. Human Infection. Pub. Health Rep. *53*:2259–2282, 1938.

Derrick, E. H.: "Q" Fever, a New Fever Entity: Clinical Features, Diagnosis and Laboratory Investigation. Med. J. Australia 2:281–299, 1937.

Lillie, R. D.: Pathologic Histology in Guinea Pigs Following Intraperitoneal Inoculation with the Virus of "Q" Fever. Pub. Health Rep. 57:296–306, 1942.

Parker, R. R., Bell, E. J., and Stoerner, H. G.: "Q" Fever—A Brief Survey of the Problem. J. Am. Vet. Med. Assn. *114*:55–60, 124–130, 1939.

Perrin, T. L., and Bengston, I. A.: The Histopathology of Experimental "Q" Fever in Mice. Pub. Health Rep. *57*:790–798, 1942.

THE BARTONELLA GROUP

In this category will be considered diseases which are caused by organisms presently classified in the Family *Bartonellaceæ*. These small, markedly pleomorphic organisms are found in erythrocytes of several species. The organisms take Giemsa's stain intensely but are only lightly stained with aniline dyes. They are gram-negative. They are distinguished from protozoa by the absence of recognizable cytoplasm around their nucleus.

Four genera currently make up this family: *Bartonella*, *Haemobartonella*, *Grahamella*, and *Eperythrozoon;* each of them contains parasitic species. *Bartonella bacilliformis*, the only species now recognized in this first genus, is the cause of a disease syndrome of man called Oroya fever, verruga peruana, or Carrion's Disease. This organism parasitizes the erythrocytes, reticulo-endothelial system and vascular endothelium, occurring in the form of tiny polymorphous cocci and rods. Human bartonellosis is of considerable importance in South America, particularly in Peru and Colombia, but also occurs in Central America. It is transmitted by several species of *Phlebotomus*.

The third genus in this Family, *Grahamella*, consists of rod to club-shaped organisms, 0.1 to 1.0 microns in size and occur in the erythrocytes of several hosts. Only one species, *Grahamella talpæ*, a parasite of voles, is currently recognized although the organisms seen in other hosts may be different enough to be eventually considered as separate species. These organisms stain light blue with Giemsa's stain; the club-shaped ends of the organism are usually a darker blue.

The fourth genus, *Eperythrozoon*, includes organisms which appear in the plasma and on the erythrocytes of affected animals. The organisms are 1 to 2 microns in length, appearing in short, coccoid rods or in ring shapes. They are gram-negative, but by Giemsa's method stain bluish or pinkish violet. Splenectomy of susceptible animals may activate latent infections. The species which

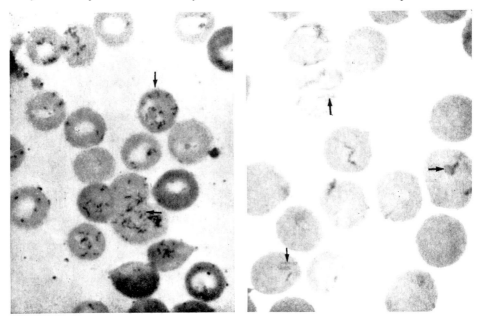

Fig. 11–2.—Left, Bartonella (arrows) in human blood (× 1650).
Right, *Haemobartonella muris* in rat blood (× 1970).

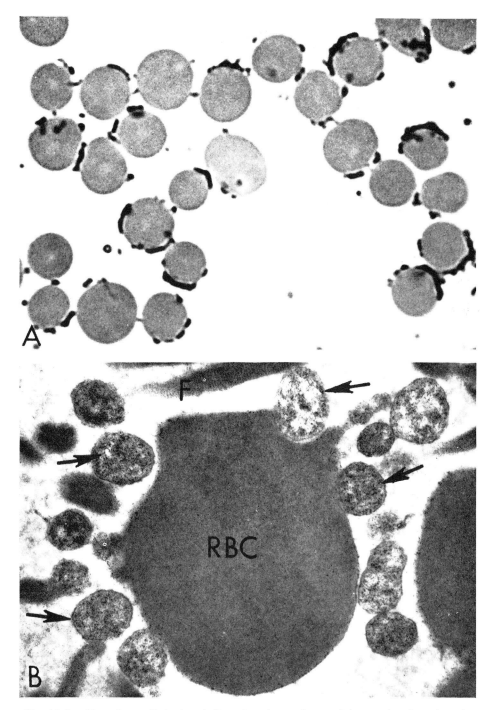

FIG. 11–3.—*Haemobartonella bovis*. *A*, Organisms (arrows) on periphery and surface of erythrocytes (RBC) from a splenectomized calf. *B*, Coccoid and rod shaped organisms (arrows) on an erythrocyte (× 40,000). F = fibrin. (Courtesy Dr. C. F. Simpson and American Journal of Veterinary Research.)

have been described and named include: *Eperythrozoon suis* and *E. parvum*, in swine; *E. wenyoni*, in cattle; *E. dispar*, in voles; *E. varians*, in gray-backed deer mice; *E. ovis*, in sheep; and *E. coccoides*, in mice. The disease caused by these organisms will be described later under **Eperythrozoonosis.**

In contrast to *Bartonella*, *Hæmobartonella* species are parasites of the red blood cells only with no demonstrable extra-erythrocytic forms. As many as 22 different species have been distinguished on the basis of their morphology and host range, but many of these species may not be valid. However, several species have been named from various hosts: *Hæmobartonella muris*, from the rat and mouse; *H. peromyscii* var *maniculati*, the gray-backed deer mouse; *H. microtii*, the vole; *H. tyzzeri*, the guinea pig; *H. bovis*, cattle; *H. sturmanii*, buffalo; *H. peromyscii*, the deer mouse; *H. blarinæ*, the short-tailed shrew; *H. sciuri*, the gray squirrel; *H. felis*, the cat; and *H. canis*, the dog. *Hæmobartonella muris* is of particular interest because of its widespread distribution in laboratory rodents. These organisms usually produce an infection which remains latent until splenectomy or some other deleterious incident causes the organisms to multiply rapidly and produce severe anemia. *Hæmobartonella* are predominantly rods less than 1 micron in length, but a variety of coccoid, filamentous, dumbbell or curved forms may be seen on the surface of erythrocytes or within their cytoplasm. Ultrastructural studies have demonstrated that the organisms lie in intimate contact with the erythrocytes, and that the parasites do not penetrate the erythrocytes. A distinct intervening space is present between the plasmalemma of the erythrocyte and the limiting membrane of the organism.

Rats are more severely affected by the disease, but mice are susceptible and infections have been encountered in guinea pigs, hamsters, dogs, cats and cattle. The lesions are those which should be expected in hemolytic anemia from any cause. The diagnosis is established with the aid of blood smears, stained with Giemsa's or Wright's stain. The organisms may be cultured with difficulty on semisolid blood or serum agar.

Feline Infectious Anemia.—The studies of Flint and co-workers (1959) have done much to clarify the clinical and etiologic aspects of this disease which is now being recognized with increasing frequency in the domestic cat. Most of the available evidence points toward the parasite of erythrocytes, *Hemobartonella felis*, as the etiologic agent. This organism is seen as coccoid, ring or rod-shaped bodies on the erythrocytes of affected cats. These are best seen in blood smears stained with Giemsa's or Wright's stain (Fig. 11–4). The natural mode of transmission is not known but the disease has been reproduced following the injection of 0.5 ml. of feline blood containing parasitized erythrocytes. In contrast to the situation in rodents and dogs in which splenectomy is necessary to cause overt disease, cats are naturally susceptible to this disease and fatal illness often results.

In its earliest stages, feline infectious anemia (hemobartonellosis) is manifest by fever, anorexia, depression and macrocytic, hemolytic anemia. The anemia is evidenced by pale, occasionally icteric, mucous membranes, weakness and a characteristic blood picture in which the hemoglobin and packed cell volumes are severely decreased. The hemoglobin levels usually decrease from a normal of 11 grams per 100 ml. of blood to as low as 1.5 grams in severe cases. Levels of 6.0 grams of hemoglobin per 100 ml. of blood or lower are usually considered typical of this disease. Macrocytosis and anisocytosis are usually prominent features and,

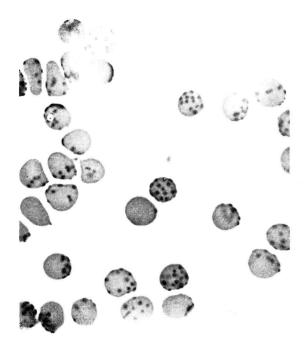

Fig. 11–4.—*Haemobartonella felis* on the erythrocytes of cat with feline infectious anemia. Giemsa (× 1200). (Photograph by Dr. Rue Jensen, contributed by Dr. Jean C. Flint, Colorado State University.)

in early stages, nucleated erythrocytes are present in large numbers. Reticulocytes are also increased in number and some of them may contain the organisms, *Hemobartonella felis*. These organisms are not readily demonstrable in all stages of the disease, a fact which complicates the diagnostic problem in many cases.

The leukocyte count in the acute stage is usually elevated, a point of diagnostic significance in eliminating panleukopenia (p. 475), but as the disease progresses, the leukocyte count gradually falls. After a prolonged illness, leukopenia may be severe and abnormal "reticulo-endothelial cells" may appear in the peripheral circulation.

Severely affected animals may die with evidences of a severe hemolytic anemia, others may recover, with or without treatment, and still others will undergo relapses and eventually die following a prolonged illness. The *lesions* in fatal cases have not been adequately documented and the cases of prolonged duration present some particularly challenging problems in the post-mortem recognition of fatal cases, and in understanding the pathogenesis of the disease. The post-mortem findings in cats which die following an acute episode are usually quite characteristic. Icterus is a feature in some acute cases and the spleen is enlarged many times and its cut surface is dark, firm and bulges when cut. Microscopically, this appearance is found to be due to congestion and extramedullary hematopoiesis. Hemoglobin may stain the urine in the bladder and hemorrhages may be present, particularly on serous surfaces. Fatty infiltration may be evident in pale yellowish color of the liver and central or paracentral necrosis may also be seen in microscopic sections of this organ. These changes are believed to be secondary to the anemia. The bone marrow is usually solidly red in the long bones and is seen microscopically to contain large numbers of hematopoietic cells in approximately normal proportions. The lymph nodes are usually grossly enlarged and moist in all parts of the body and microscopic sections reveal the enlargement to be due to reactive hyperplasia.

The lesions found at necropsy of animals which die after the prolonged illness, described previously, are often subtle and at this point are not clearly understood. The reactive hyperplasia of lymph nodes seen in the acutely fatal case, is also a feature of the illness of longer duration, and the spleen may be large but not as hyperplastic. Icterus is rarely evident and the bone marrow is hyperplastic. Ulceration of intestinal mucosae may be present, and sometimes hemorrhage may follow this ulceration. (See color plate II.)

Hemobartonella

BENJAMIN, M. M. and LUMB, W. V.: *Haemobartonella canis* Infection in a Dog. J. Am. Vet Med. Assn. *135*:388–390, 1959.

CARR, D. T., and ESSEX, H. E.: Bartonellosis: A Cause of Severe Anemia in Splenectomized Dogs. Proc. Soc. Exper. Biol. & Med. *57*:44–45, 1944.

FLINT, J. C., and MOSS, L. C.: Infectious Anemia in Cats. J. Am. Vet. Med. Assn. *122*:45–48, 1953.

FLINT, J. C., ROEPKE, M. H., and JENSEN, R.: Feline infectious anemia. I. Clinical aspects. Am. J. Vet. Res. *19*:165–168, 1958.

FLINT, J. C., ROEPKE, M. H., and JENSEN, R.: Feline infectious anemia. II. Experimental cases. Am. J. Vet. Res. *20*:33–40, 1959.

INGLE, R. T.: *Bartonella* Infection in a Dog. North Am. Vet. *27*:501–502, 1946.

LOTZE, J. C., and BOWMAN, G. W.: The Occurrence of *Bartonella* in Cases of Anaplasmosis and in Apparently Normal Cattle. Proc. Helminth. Soc., Washington, D.C. *9*:71–72, 1942.

MULHERN, C. R.: A Note on Two Blood Parasites of Cattle, (*Spirochaeta theileri* and *Bartonella bovis*), Recorded for the First Time in Australia. Australian Vet. *22*:118–119, 1946.

SIMPSON, C. F., and LOVE, J. N.: Fine Structure of Haemobartonella bovis in Blood and Liver of Splenectomized Calves. Am. J. Vet. Res. *31*:225–231, 1970.

SMALL, E., and RISTIC, M.: Morphologic Features of Haemobartonella felis. Am. J. Vet. Res. *28*:845–851, 1967.

TANAKA, H., *et al.*: Fine Structure of *Haemobartonella muris* as Compared with *Eperythrozoon coccoides* and *Mycoplasma pulmonis*. J. Bact. *90*:1735–1749, 1965.

TYZZER, E. E.: "Interference" in Mixed Infections of *Bartonella* and *Eperythrozoon* in Mice. Am. J. Path. *17*:141–153, 1941.

————: A Comparative Study of *Grahamellæ*, *Haemobartonellæ* and *Eperythrozoa* in Small Mammals. Proc. Am. Philos. Soc. *85*:359–398, 1942.

VENABLE, J. H., and EQUING, S. A.: Fine Structure of Hemobartonella canis (Rickettsiales: Bartonellacea) and Its Relation to the Host Erythrocyte. J. Parasit. *54*:259–268, 1968.

WEINMAN, D.: On the Cause of the Anemia in *Bartonella* Infection of Rats. J. Infect. Dis. *63*:1–9, 1938.

WEINMAN, D., and PINKERTON, H.: Carrion's Disease. III. Experimental Production in Animals. Proc. Soc. Exper. Biol. & Med. *37*:594–595, 1937.

Eperythrozoonosis

In recent years increasing numbers of parasites which attack red blood cells have been discovered in animals. Organisms grouped in the genus *Eperythrozoön* are among the latest of these to be recognized. This genus is considered to be related to *Bartonella*, *Hæmobartonella*, and *Grahamella*, because each group contains organisms of similar morphology, all parasitize erythrocytes and the diseases which result from their presence are all quite similar. Each organism can be clearly distinguished by its specific immunologic effects upon the host, hence it is of practical importance to identify clearly the causative agent in each of these infections of erythrocytes.

Eperythrozoön are seen in blood smears stained by Giemsa's method as tiny pleomorphic structures which are within the erythrocytes, lying on their surface or free in the plasma. The organisms are delicate pale purple to pinkish purple and are predominantly in ring-shapes 0.5 to 1.0 micron in diameter or occasionally slightly larger. Triangular, ovoid, rod, dumbbell and tennis-racket shapes may be seen. One to a dozen organisms may be present in a single red blood cell and large numbers uniformly distributed through the plasma. Organisms are much more numerous in blood smears taken at the height of infection.

The mode of transmission is not clearly established for all species of *Eperythrozoön*, but arthropods are generally suspected. *Eperythrozoön coccoides*, which infects mice, has been shown to be transmitted by a louse, *Polyplax serrata*. Biting flies have been tentatively incriminated as vectors in other hosts. Experimental infection is greatly facilitated by the use of splenectomized animals.

The **clinical manifestations** of eperythrozoönosis are best known and quite similar in sheep and swine. In both species, evidence of infection may appear spontaneously, particularly in young animals, exposed to other deleterious influences, such as helminthic parasitism, or may be brought forth by splenectomy of animals which are already harboring the infection. The natural disease in swine has been called "ictero-anemia" and has recognized similarities to anaplasmosis of herbivora. It is of course distinguished with difficulty from anaplasmosis when sheep are involved. The symptoms start with fever (104 to 107° F.) which appears six to ten days following exposure or splenectomy of animals with latent infection. This is accompanied by gradually increasing depression and weakness. The total red blood cell count drops precipitously to 1 to 2 million per cubic millimeter, hemoglobin is decreased to 2 to 4 grams per 100 ml., and the packed red cell volume goes down to 4 to 7 per cent. The icteric index is elevated to 18 to 25 and the sedimentation rate is greatly accelerated, reaching 75 mm. per minute in some cases. The white cell count is usually not changed, although leukocytosis occurs in a few cases. Death may occur in an acute episode, such as described, but animals more frequently recover but then are prone to have repeated recrudescences.

Lesions.—The gross lesions are compatible with the hemolytic anemia resulting from the effect of *Eperythrozoön* upon the red blood cells. Icterus is a prominent feature, the blood is thin and watery, the liver is yellowish brown and the gallbladder contains thick gelatinous bile. Hydropericardium and ascites are present in some cases and the heart is pale and flabby. Petechiæ may be seen in the mucosa of the urinary bladder. The bone marrow is predominantly red rather than fatty.

Microscopic changes are seen in the bone marrow, which is hyperplastic, and the liver, which is rich in hemosiderin, shows some fatty change and central or paracentral necrosis of liver lobules. The latter is presumed to be an effect of anoxia. The organisms are difficult to demonstrate in tissue sections.

Diagnosis.—Eperythrozoönosis must be differentiated from anaplasmosis, bartonellosis, babesiosis, and other hemolytic anemias. The differentiation is most readily made by the precise identification of the causative organisms in the erythrocytes.

Eperythrozoon

Adams, E. W., *et al.*: Eperythrozoonosis in a Herd of Purebred Landrace Pigs. J. Am. Vet. Med. Assn. *135*:226–228, 1959.

Neitz, W. O.: *Eperythrozoonosis* in Sheep. Onderstepoort J. Vet. Sc. & Ind. *9*:9–30, 1937.

SPLITTER, E. J.: *Eperythrozoon suis*, the Etiologic Agent of Ictero-anemia or Anaplasmosis-like Disease in Swine. Am. J. Vet. Research *11*:324–330, 1950.
SPLITTER, E. J., and WILLIAMSON, R. L.: Eperythrozoonosis in Swine. A Preliminary Report. J. Am. Vet. Med. Assn. *116*:360–364, 1950.

ANAPLASMOSIS

The classification of the anaplasma has not been established with any certainty. Once considered protozoa, they are now included in the Order *Rickettsiales*, Family *Anaplasmataceae*. Their structure, and the disease induced, closely resembles the structure and diseases associated with other families in this order (Rickettsiaciae, p. 536; Chlamydiaciae, p. 550; Bartonellaceae, p. 542). Three species are recognized within the single genus of this family: *Anaplasma marginale*, *Anaplasma centrale* and *Anaplasma ovis*.

Anaplasma marginale which parasitizes the red cells of cattle, causes an important disease of world-wide distribution. The disease is unusual in that infection results in overt disease only in adult animals; most young calves undergo an inapparent infection unless splenectomized prior to exposure. Fever of short duration is manifest in adult cattle but may be undetected or overshadowed by the later findings. Anemia is the essential effect produced by the organism and is manifest by weakness, pallor of mucosae, accelerated respiration, jaundice, decreased red cell count and hemoglobin, occasionally muscular trembling, depression, anorexia and excessive salivation. Anemia results from increased destruction of parasitized erythrocytes by the reticulo-endothelial system and not by

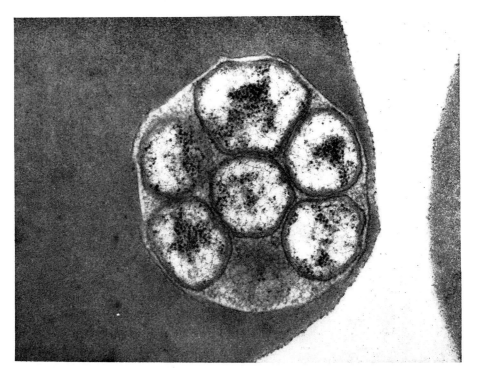

FIG. 11–5.—*Anaplasma marginale*. An anaplasma body (marginal body) containing six subunits (initial bodies) (× 60,000). (Courtesy Dr. C. T. Simpson and American Journal of Veterinary Research.)

hemolysis, therefore hemoglobinuria is not seen. Autoimmunity has been suggested as a cause of the erythrocyte destruction but this has not been confirmed. Death occurs in many cases but recovery is not infrequent, the recovered animals remaining carriers of the infection for some time.

The organism, *Anaplasma marginale*, is a tiny spherical body, 0.3 to 0.8 micron in diameter which is found within the cytoplasm of erythrocytes near the periphery of the cell. It is best demonstrated in blood smears with Giemsa stain. Recent studies by Ristic and Watrach (1963) with the electron microscope and with fluorescent antibody indicate that four developmental stages of Anaplasma are recognizable in infected erythrocytes. These stages are (*a*) early stage, consisting of "initial bodies"—the infective form, (*b*) mixed population stage with marginal and initial bodies, (*c*) stage of vigorous growth and transfer and (*d*) massive multiplication with a predominance of marginal bodies. According to these workers, after penetration of the erythrocytic cell membrane by "initial bodies," the organisms reproduce by binary fission and pass through the above described 4 stages of development, then are transferred to other mature erythrocytes by direct contact between cells. Simpson and co-workers (1967) described the initial body as spherical and surrounded by a double membrane. The marginal body contains up to six subunits (initial bodies) and is surrounded by a single membrane. Microfibrillar structures between erythrocytes appear to facilitate exchange of organisms. A fluorescence technic using acridine orange has been shown to be useful by Gainer (1961) in identifying *Anaplasma* as has the fluorescence antibody technic described by Ristic and Watrach (1963). The infection can be transmitted to a normal animal by carrying over a minute amount of blood. This can occur by the use of improperly sterilized bleeding needles, or by dehorning or castration without prior aseptic precautions, but usually in nature is spread by bites of ticks (*Boöphilus annulatus*, and others), biting flies (*Tabanus sp.*) and less often by mosquitoes (*Psorophora sp.*). Ticks are the most important vectors in that they can carry the organisms for long periods of time. The transfer *in utero* between bovine mother and fetus has also been reported. The presence of carriers has long posed a problem in the control of the disease. The detection of such carriers is rarely possible by examination of blood smears but a complement-fixation test can be used to detect carriers.

Lesions.—The gross post-mortem findings in fatal cases are those of severe anemia, with pallor of the tissues and occasionally icterus. The spleen is usually greatly enlarged, with reddish-brown pulp and enlarged splenic follicles. The liver is enlarged, has rounded edges, and is yellowish in cases with icterus. The gallbladder is usually distended with dark grumous bile. Petechiae in the pericardium may be encountered, and catarrhal inflammation may be evident in the gastro-intestinal tract. The microscopic findings indicate severe demands upon the hematopoietic system, with hyperplasia of the bone marrow and extra-medullary hematopoiesis in the spleen and other organs. *Anaplasma* can be demonstrated with difficulty in erythrocytes in tissue sections.

The number of organisms demonstrable in smears of peripheral blood is highly variable. Prior to the onset of anemia, the majority of erythrocytes may harbor organisms but with their sudden removal from the circulation their numbers decrease. Immature erythrocytes (reticulocytes) which enter the circulation in response to the anemia are, for reasons poorly understood, resistant to the parasites.

Whether *Anaplasma centrale* warrants consideration as a separate species is doubtful; it may be a variant of *A. marginale*. It produces a very mild infection in cattle, and has been employed to immunize cattle to *A. marginale*. *A. centrale* usually localizes near the center of the red blood cell.

Anaplasma ovis is infectious for sheep and goats. Cattle are not susceptible. The disease is mild, only rarely resulting in clinical signs of anemia.

Diagnosis.— The diagnosis is based upon the clinical signs and demonstration of *Anaplasma* in erythrocytes. The complement-fixation test can be used for the detection of clinically silent carriers.

Anaplasmosis

BROCK, W. E., *et al.*: Autoantibody Studies in Bovine Anaplasmosis. Am. J. Vet. Res. *26*: 250–253, 1965.

CHRISTENSEN, K. F., and HOWARTH, J. A.: Anaplasmosis Transmission by Dermacentor Occidentalis Taken from Cattle in Santa Barbara County, California. Am. J. Vet. Res. *27*: 1473–1475, 1966.

ESPANA, C., ESPANA, E. M., and GORGALEZ, D.: *Anaplasma marginale.* I. Studies with Phase Contrast and Electron Microscopy. Am. J. Vet. Res. *20*:795–805, 1959.

FRANKLIN, T. E., and REDMOND, H. E.: Observations on the Morphology of *Anaplasma marginale* with Reference to Projection or Tails. Am. J. Vet. Res. *19*:252–253, 1958.

GAINER, J. H.: Demonstration of *Anaplasma marginale* with the Fluorescent Dye, Acridine Orange, Comparisons with the Complement-Fixation Test and Wright's Stain. Am. J. Vet. Res. *22*:882–886, 1961.

GATES, D. W., and ROBY, T. O.: The Status of the Complement-Fixation Test for the Diagnosis of Anaplasmosis in 1955. Ann. New York Acad. Sci. *64*:31–39, 1956.

JONES, E. W., *et al.*: *Anaplasma marginale* Infection in Young and Aged Cattle. Am. J. Vet. Res. *29*:535–544, 1968.

JONES, E. W., *et al.*: *Anaplasma marginale* Infection in Splenectomized Calves. Am. J. Vet. Res. *29*:523–533, 1968.

KREIER, J. P., RISTIC, M., and SCHROEDER, W.: Anaplasmosis, XVI. The Pathogenesis of Anemia Produced by Infection with Anaplasma. Am. J. Vet. Res. *25*:343–352, 1964.

KUTTLER, K. L.: Clinical and Hematologic Comparison of *Anaplasma marginale* and *Anaplasma centrale* Infections in Cattle. Am. J. Vet. Res. *27*:941–946, 1966.

LOTZE, J. C., and YIENGST, M. J.: Mechanical Transmission of Bovine Anaplasmosis by the Horsefly, *Tabanus sulcifrons* (Macquart). Am. J. Vet. Res. *2*:323–326, 1941.

————: Studies on the Nature of Anaplasma. Am. J. Vet. Res. *3*:312–320, 1942.

PIERCY, P. L.: Transmission of Anaplasmosis. Ann. New York Acad. Sci. *64*:40–48, 1956.

RISTIC, M., and WATRACH, A. M.: Studies in Anaplasmosis. II. Electron Microscopy of *Anaplasma marginale* in Deer. Am. J. Vet. Res. *22*:109–116, 1961.

————: Anaplasmosis. VI. Studies and a Hypothesis Concerning the Cycle of Development of the Causative Agent. Am. J. Vet. Res. *24*:267–277, 1963.

RYFF, J. F., WEIBEL, J. L., and THOMAS, G. M.: Relationship of Ovine to Bovine Anaplasmosis. Cornell Vet. *54*:407–414, 1964.

SCHMIDT, H.: Manifestations and Diagnosis of Anaplasmosis. Ann. New York Acad. Sci. *64*:27–30, 1956.

SCHROEDER, W. R., and RISTIC, M.: Anaplasmosis. XVII. The Relation of Autoimmune Processes to Anemia. Am. J. Vet. Res. *26*:239–245, 1965.

SIMPSON, C. F., KLING, J. M., and LOVE, J. N.: Morphologic and Histochemical Nature of *Anaplasma marginale*. Am. J. Vet. Res. *28*:1055–1065, 1967.

THE PSITTACOSIS LYMPHOGRANULOMA-TRACHOMA GROUP

The fourth Family of organisms classified in the Order *Rickettsiales* is named *Chlamydiaceae* and includes several pathogens which affect human subjects and several which cause disease in other animals. These organisms are all minute, pleomorphic, usually coccoid bodies which have not been cultivated in the absence of living cells. Various classifications set forth include from one to five genera within this family. Although certain of these have become firmly entrenched in the literature there is little evidence to consider the members of this family as belonging to separate genera: some have not even been cultured. Rake (7th edition *Bergey's Manual*) presents five genera; *Chlamydia*, *Colesiota*, *Ricolesia*, *Miyagawanella* and *Colettsia*. In order to reduce confusion as well as to recognize that the similarities between the various "genera" outweigh their differences, several authors have proposed that the entire group be considered as a single genus. Brumpt (1938) proposed *Miyagawanella*, Jones, Rake and Stearns (1945) proposed *Chlamydia* and Meyer (1953) proposed *Bedsonia*. Page (1966) recently reviewed the taxonomy of the family and has provided convincing taxonomical and scientific evidence in support of the desirability of recognizing *Chlamydia* (Jones, Rake and Stearns, 1945) as the name of the genus under which all of the species of the psittacosis lymphogranuloma-trachoma group be included. In this section we will consider all members as belonging to the genus *Chlamydia* with the exception of certain organisms so poorly characterized that their taxonomic position cannot be established at present. When considered necessary, synonyms will be provided which will hopefully not perpetuate confusion.

The important members of the genus *Chlamydia* include: *C. trachomatis*, the cause of trachoma in man; *C. oculogenitale*, the cause of lower urinary infection and conjunctivitis in man; *C. psittaci*; the cause of psittacosis in man and psittacine birds; *C. ornithosis* a similar organism to *C. psittaci* but which is found in numerous non-psittacine birds and mammals; *C. felis*, the cause of feline pneumonitis; *C. ovis*, the cause of enzootic abortion in ewes; *C. lymphogranulomatosis*, the cause of human lymphogranuloma venereum; *C. bronchopneumoniae*, a presumed cause of pneumonitis in mice; *C. pneumonia*, *C. louisianae*, and *C. illini*, three species which produce "viral" pneumonia (pneumonitis) in man; *C. pecoris*, the cause of sporadic bovine encephalomyelitis; and *C. bovis*, suggested as a cause of bovine enteritis. Agents which presumably will also be classified as *Chlamydia* are recognized as causes of pneumonia in calves, lambs and goats, abortion in cattle, arthritis in calves, and guinea pig inclusion conjunctivitis.

Certain organisms have been so poorly characterized that it is not possible to ascertain whether they should be classified as *Chlamydia*. *Colesiota conjunctivae* (*Rickettsiae conjunctivae*, *Ricolesia bovis; R. conjunctivae bovis*) has been found in association with conjunctivitis of sheep, goats and cattle in South Africa. Apparently this organism is not the cause of keratoconjunctivitis in cattle in the United States (p. 1415). Conjunctivitis and keratitis in chickens in South Africa is caused by another organism, *Colesiota conjunctiva-galli* (*Ricolesia conjunctivae*). *Ricolesia lestoquardii* (*Rickettsia conjunctivae-suis*) causes conjunctivitis and keratitis in swine.

Psittacosis Group

BRUMPT, E.: *Rickettsia intracellulaire stomacale* (*Rickettsia culicis* N. Sp.) de *Culex fatigans*. Ann. de Parasitologie *16*:153–158, 1938.

JONES, H., RAKE, G., and STEARNS, B.: Studies on Lymphogranuloma venereum. III. The Action of the Sulfonamides on the Agent of Lymphogranuloma venereum. J. Infect. Dis. *76*: 55–69, 1945.

MEYER, K. F.: Psittacosis Group. Ann. New York Acad. Sci. *56*:545–556, 1953.

PAGE, L. A.: Revision of the Family *Chlamydiaceae* Rake (*Rickettsiales*): Unification of the Psittacosis-Lymphogranuloma Venereum-Trachoma Group of Organisms in the Genus Chlamydia Jones, Rake and Stearns, 1945. Int. J. Systemat. Bacteriol. *16*:223–252, 1966.

Psittacosis

(Ornithosis, Parrot Fever)

A febrile pulmonary disease of man, believed since the latter half of the nineteenth century to be contracted from sick parrots ("parrot fever"), is now known to be caused by an infectious agent harbored not only by parrots, but also by a wide variety of other birds. Psittacine birds (Family Psittacidæ), including parrots, parakeets, cockatoos, macaws, cockatiels and masked love birds, were the first in which the infection was demonstrated, both in an inapparent form and with obvious signs of illness. Several birds, including finches, canaries and rice birds, are known to acquire the infection by contact with parrots and to transport the disease to man. Pigeons, ducks, fulmars, sea gulls, chickens and, more recently, turkeys have been shown to be naturally infected and to serve as reservoirs for human infection. It is probable that the distribution of the agent of psittacosis will eventually be found to be much wider and to include many more hosts than presently recognized.

Etiology.—The causative agent of psittacosis consists of coccoid elementary bodies which are between the rickettsiæ and the filtrable viruses in size. Elementary particles of psittacosis, generally designated as LCL (Levinthal-Cole-Lillie) bodies, are similar to those of feline pneumonitis (p. 555) and undergo a developmental cycle in the cells of the host. The smallest elementary particles, perfectly spherical in shape, increase in size under favorable conditions and become embedded in a homogeneous ground substance, forming a plaque 3 to 12 microns in diameter. These large bodies divide repeatedly, becoming smaller and smaller until the elementary body stage is again reached. These particles (LCL bodies) measure 0.280 to 0.380 micron in diameter and may be found in all sizes of this range in smears from infected pericardial or peritoneal exudate or organs of infected birds. The tinctorial features of these bodies are helpful in their recognition: with Castañeda's stain for rickettsia the large bodies are usually blue and the smaller ones red; with the Giemsa's stain they are bluish, and with Macchiavello's method for rickettsia they are red.

The agent grows rapidly within the host cells, soon filling the cytoplasm and killing the cell. Rupture of the cytoplasmic membrane allows the infective particles to escape and become available to parasitize other tissue cells. The organism has been called *Microbacterium multiforme psittacosis*; it is classified in the seventh edition of Bergey's Manual of Determinative Bacteriology as *Miyagawanella psittaci*, and is generally referred to by virologists as the psittacosis "virus," a member of the psittacosis-lymphogranuloma group of infectious agents. The preferred name at present is *Chlamydia psittaci*.

Clinical Manifestations.—The disease in man is manifest by sudden onset of a febrile illness with upper respiratory involvement, usually accompanied by pneumonia or pneumonitis and severe debility. Although the disease is not usually fatal, deaths occur with alarming frequency in some outbreaks. Antibiotic therapy has reduced the death rate dramatically.

In birds, psittacosis may appear as a fulminant, highly fatal disease or as a smouldering inapparent infection demonstrable only by laboratory study or by appearance of the disease in human contacts. Infection in birds does not produce characteristic clinical manifestations; hence necropsy and laboratory examination are necessary for definitive diagnosis. Infected parrots or parakeets are sleepy, listless and refuse to eat. Their wings droop and their feathers can be pulled out easily. After two or three weeks of illness, greenish and occasionally blood-tinged feces stain the feathers around the cloaca. Mortality is likely to be higher in parrots than in parakeets, but losses, particularly among young birds, may be great in both species.

Lesions.—Psittacine birds that die of the disease or are sacrificed while they have definite symptoms are emaciated, and many maculæ, 2 to 4 mm. in diameter, are seen on the skin over the body and legs. The nares may be plugged with mucopurulent exudate. Fibrinous or fibrinopurulent exudates are found over the pericardial sac, peritoneum, pleura or air sacs. The liver is enlarged, its edges are rounded and it is yellowish, with mottling or patchy discoloration in shades of green or brown. In some cases it may be studded with petechiæ and small yellowish foci of necrosis. The spleen is rather constantly enlarged, dark blood red, and occasionally yellowish necrotic foci are seen on its surface. The kidneys may be swollen, pale and friable. The lungs are only rarely affected and the changes are limited to a few small areas of consolidation.

In parrots, parakeets, and other psittacine birds with latent infection, the spleen may be greatly enlarged, but no other gross lesions are apparent.

The microscopic changes in tissues in acute symptomatic psittacosis are associated with the presence of the organism in various tissue cells. The spleen is moderately to intensely infiltrated by mononuclear cells containing organisms and its hemosiderin content is often increased. Hyperplasia of the reticuloendothelial cells is commonly observed. The liver often contains focal lesions involving isolated islands of parenchymal cells which undergo necrosis and replacement by a mass of hyaline amorphous material. Fibrin and lymphocytes may be noted on the liver capsule and the portal areas are rich in lymphocytes and plasma cells. The tubular epithelium of the kidney may be packed with large numbers of LCL bodies. Destruction of this epithelium is followed by interstitial accumulation of epithelioid and lymphocytic cells. In the lungs, a few alveoli may contain serous exudate, but frank pneumonic consolidation is rare. The superficial mucosa of the intestine is usually eroded and the underlying lamina propria and submucosa are infiltrated with lymphocytes and plasma cells.

Diagnosis.—The clinical manifestations and gross features at necropsy are generally insufficient for definite diagnosis. Necropsies must be performed by aseptic methods with adequate protection for the prosector, and especial care must be taken to prevent desiccation and subsequent scattering of any infective material. Histologic study of smears or sections of peritoneal or pericardial lesions, liver or spleen stained by the Macchiavello, Castañeda or Giemsa method will disclose intracellular organisms in most acute cases. Intracranial or intraperitoneal injection of mice with tissue suspensions from birds suspected of having the infection in a symptomless form usually causes death in four or five days, and organisms are demonstrable in the mouse tissues. In some instances at least one blind passage is required to establish the agent in mice. The organism also grows well in embryonated eggs and tissue culture.

The complement-fixation test is also of value in the detection of antibodies in birds that have latent infections or are convalescent.

Psittacosis

BEASLEY, J. N., DAVIS, D. E., and GRUMBLES, L. C.: Preliminary Studies on the histopathology of Experimental Ornithosis in Turkeys. Am. J. Vet. Res. *20*:341–349, 1959.

BEASLEY, J. N., WATKINS, J. R., and BRIDGES, C. H.: Experimental Ornithosis in Calves. Am. J. Vet. Res. *23*:1192–1199, 1962.

BLAND, J. C. W., and CANTI, R. G.: The Growth and Development of Psittacosis Virus in Tissue Cultures. J. Path. & Bact. *40*:231–241, 1935.

LILLIE, R. D.: The Pathology of Psittacosis in Animals and the Distribution of Rickettsia Psittaci in the Tissues of Man and Animals. Nat. Inst. Health Bull. 161, pp. 47–66, 1933.

MEYER, K. F.: Ornithosis and Psittacosis, in Biester, H. E., and Schwarte, L. H.: *Diseases of Poultry*. 3rd ed, Ames. Iowa State College Press, 1952, pp. 569–618.

PIERCE, K. R., MOORE, R. W., CARROLL, L. H., and BRIDGES, C. H.: Experimental Ornithosis in Ewes. Am. J. Vet. Res. *24*:1176–1188, 1963.

TOMLINSON, T. H. JR.: An Outbreak of Psittacosis at the National Zoological Park, Washington, D.C. Pub. Health Rep. *56*:1073–1081, 1941.

Sporadic Bovine Encephalomyelitis

A disease of young calves and, less frequently, older cattle, described by McNutt in Iowa, has now been reported in several midwestern states, Idaho, South Dakota, California, Oklahoma and Texas, as well as Australia, Europe and Japan. It probably is more widespread than published reports indicate. The disease is caused by a visible infectious agent which appears to belong in the lymphogranuloma-psittacosis group and currently designated *Chlamydia pecoris*.

Signs.—The onset is sudden with fever (105° to 107° F.), anorexia, depression, decreased activity, excessive salivation with drooling and nasal discharge soon appearing. Dyspnea with a cough is observed in about half the cases, but diarrhea, either mild or severe, is more common. Within a few days calves have difficulty in walking, exhibiting stiffness and knuckling in the fetlock joints. They move aimlessly in circles, stagger and fall with the head extended in opisthotonos. In the final stages, the limbs appear weak or paralyzed; death occurs in five to seven days in most cases, rarely being delayed for as long as a month.

Although calves are most susceptible, the report of Menges *et al.* (1953) indicates that adult cattle are also subject to the infection. These authors reported 21 herds totalling 1,774 cattle of all ages, of which 269 (15 per cent) exhibited symptoms and 75 (28 per cent of those affected) died from the disease. Among 892 calves in these herds, however, 224 (25 per cent) contracted the disease and 64 (29 per cent of those affected) died. Outbreaks of sporadic bovine encephalomyelitis usually follow introduction of new animals into a herd and must be differentiated clinically from "shipping fever," rabies, malignant catarrhal fever, and listeriosis.

Lesions.—The most constant gross lesion in fatal cases is serofibrinous peritonitis. Excessive amounts of clear yellow peritoneal fluid are present in early cases; in more prolonged cases adhesive strands of fibrin form an exudate over the omentum, liver and spleen. The spleen is sometimes enlarged. A similar fibrinous exudate lies over the pleura and pericardium in about half the fatal cases. A patchy lobular pneumonia may be seen in a few instances. The brain and spinal cord usually appear edematous and their vasculature is congested.

The microscopic lesions consist of fibrinous peritonitis, pleuritis, pericarditis and perisplenitis, with the addition of severe diffuse meningo-encephalomyelitis. The entire brain and spinal cord are involved in an intense inflammatory reaction, the meninges at the base of the brain being particularly affected. Proliferation of vascular endothelium and infiltration of the vessel walls with mononuclear and occasionally polymorphonuclear cells may be observed. Severe damage to neurons, both in brain and cord, has been described and is believed by some to be secondary to the severe vascular lesions. Minute elementary bodies are demonstrable in mononuclear cells in the serosal exudates and in the brain or spinal cord. These bodies occur singly or in small clusters in the cytoplasm of these cells. They vary in size but usually are less than a micron in diameter. They stain a pink-red color with Macchiavello's stain.

In guinea pigs, a fatal disease may be experimentally induced with this agent, the organisms being demonstrable in the guinea pig tissues. Chick embryos are also susceptible; the embryos are killed in five to seven days, after adaptation of the agent.

Diagnosis.—The gross and microscopic lesions are characteristic although not diagnostic of sporadic bovine encephalomyelitis. Demonstration of the typical elementary bodies is very helpful. Transmission of this disease to the guinea pig with subsequent demonstration of the elementary bodies is confirmatory. All clinical and pathologic data must be carefully evaluated to eliminate rabies, "shipping fever," listeriosis, and malignant catarrhal fever.

Sporadic Bovine Encephalomyelitis

LITTLEJOHNS, I. R., HARRIS, A. N. A., and HARDING, W. B.: Sporadic Bovine Encephalomyelitis. Austr. Vet. J. *37*:53, 1961. (VB 3956-61.)

McNUTT, S. H.: A Preliminary Report of an Infectious Encephalomyelitis of Cattle. Vet. Med. *35*:228–231, 1940.

McNUTT, S. H., and WALLER, E. F.: Sporadic Bovine Encephalomyelitis (Buss Disease). Cornell Vet. *30*:437–448, 1940.

MENGES, R. W., HARSHFIELD, G. S., and WENNER, H. A.: Sporadic Bovine Encephalomyelitis. Studies on Pathogenesis and Etiology of the Disease. J. Am. Vet. Med. Assn. *122*: 294–299, 1953.

OMORI, T., ISHII, S., and MATUMOTO, M.: Miyagawanellosis of Cattle in Japan. Am. J. Vet. Res. *21*:564–573, 1960.

PRICE, D. A. and HARDY, W. T.: Sporadic Bovine Encephalomyelitis—Isolation and Antibiotic Susceptibility of a Texas Strain. J. Am. Vet. Med. Assn. *128*:308–310, 1956.

TUSTIN, R. C., MARÉ, J., and VAN HEERDEN, A.: A Disease of Calves Resembling Sporadic Bovine Encephalomyelitis. J. S. Afr. Vet. Med. Assn. *32*:117–123, 1961. (VB 129–62.)

WENNER, H. A., HARSHFIELD, G. S., CHANG, T. W., and MENGES, R. W.: Sporadic Bovine Encephalomyelitis. II. Studies on the Etiology of the Disease. Isolation of Nine Strains of an Infectious Agent from Naturally Infected Cattle. Am. J. Hyg. *57*:15–29, 1953.

WENNER, H. A., MENGES, R. W., and CARTER, J.: Sporadic Bovine Encephalomyelitis. A Serologic Survey of Cattle in the Midwestern United States. Cornell Vet. *45*:68–77, 1955.

Feline Pneumonitis

Feline pneumonitis, a chlamydial infection of domesticated cats, is a problem in catteries and in experimental laboratories where cats are congregated. The disease starts as an acute upper respiratory infection, with sneezing and catarrh; later symptoms are nasal and conjunctival mucous discharges, transitory fever and some inappetence. The disease runs a course of about two weeks and terminates fatally in a small percentage of cases. It may be adapted to mice by serial passage of infected material inoculated intranasally. A feature of value in the recognition of the disease is the presence of elementary bodies of the organism which can be demonstrated most readily in the lung tissues of experimentally infected mice and occasionally in feline tissues.

Lesions.—Aside from catarrhal inflammatory changes in the upper respiratory passages, the principal lesions are usually found in the lungs. Sharply demarcated patches of what appears to be consolidation may be seen in the various lobes.

These patches are usually light reddish brown to gray or even prune colored, contrasting sharply with the light pink lung tissue.

Microscopic examination reveals that these affected areas are distributed around terminal bronchioles and consist principally of alveolar collapse rather than consolidation, although in some areas inflammatory cells, lymphoid and polymorphonuclear, fill the alveoli. Of diagnostic significance is the presence of elementary bodies, which usually appear in loose aggregates in the cytoplasm of epithelial and mononuclear cells. These bodies are tiny spherical structures, approximatelyone-half micron in diameter. In smears, they stain selectively with Macchiavello's stain, appearing brightly eosinophilic in color and usually coccoid in shape. In some instances the elementary bodies coalesce into a plaque, forming a solid eosinophilic body which distends the cytoplasm of epithelial and occasionally of leukocytic cells. These organisms are currently called *Chlamydia felis* (*Miyagawanella felis*).

Schachter, Ostler and Meyer (1969) have described a case of acute keratoconjunctivitis in man caused by the feline pneumonitis agent.

Feline Pneumonitis

BAKER, J. A.: A Virus Causing Pneumonia in Cats and Producing Elementary Bodies. J. Exper. Med. *79*:159–172, 1944.

SCHACHTER, J., OSTLER, H. B., and MEYER, K. R.: Human Infection with the Agent of Feline Pneumonitis. Lancet. May 31:1063–1065, 1969.

Polyarthritis of Sheep

One form of so-called "stiff-lamb-disease" is not the result of lesions in the muscles (p. 1049) but in the joints. Various organisms have been incriminated from time to time, including *Erysepelothrix rhusiopathiæ* (*insidiosa*) (p. 585) and organisms in the pleuropneumonia group (p. 531). A specific and rather widespread cause of arthritis appears to be an agent of the psittacosis-lymphogranuloma group of agents. This agent (*Chlamydia spp.* or *Miyagawanella spp.*) may be isolated from joints, feces, cerebrospinal fluid, urine, blood and viscera. Affected lambs are detected by a characteristic lameness involving one or more joints. Some lambs are depressed, with a high fever (106° F.), others lose weight and are slow to recover. Some animals appear to recover completely but others remain permanently lame.

The **lesions** in early stages consist for the most part of serofibrinous or fibrinous synovitis, occasionally with edema around the affected joint and greenish-gray masses of material in the articular spaces. Microscopically, affected synovial membranes are edematous, lining cells are swollen, often disorganized, detached and covered with fibropurulent debris. The subsynovial connective tissue contains granulomatous accumulations of mononuclear cells. In most examples, large numbers of elementary bodies can be demonstrated in smears or sections of synovia or joint fluid stained with Giemsa's or Macchiavello's stain; however, arthritis may persist in the absence of demonstrable organisms.

The **diagnosis** can be made by isolation of the infective agent in chick embryos, tissue culture or guinea pigs and demonstration of elementary bodies in association with characteristic lesions.

Polyarthritis of Sheep

MENDELOWSKI, B. and SEGRE, D.: Polyarthritis in Sheep. I. Description of the Disease and Experimental Transmission. Am. J. Vet. Res. *21*:68–73, 1960.

MENDLOWSKI, B., KRAYBILL, W. H., and SEGRE, D.: Polyarthritis in Sheep. II. Characteristics of the Causative Virus. Am. J. Vet. Res. *21*:74–80, 1960.

NORTON, W. L., and STORZ, J.: Observations on Sheep with Polyarthritis Produced by an Agent of the Psittacosis-Lymphogranuloma Venereum Trachoma Group. Arthr. & Rheum. *10*:1–12, 1967.

SHUPE, J. L. and STORZ, J.: Pathologic Study of Psittacosis-Lymphogranuloma Polyarthritis of Lambs. Am. J. Vet. Res. *25*:943–951, 1964.

STORZ, J., *et al.*: Polyarthritis of Lambs Induced Experimentally by a Psittacosis Agent. J. Infect. Dis. *115*:9–18, 1965.

STORZ, J., SHUPE, J. L., JAMES, L. F., and SMART, R. A.: Polyarthritis of Sheep in the Intermountain Region Caused by a Psittacosis-Lymphogranuloma Agent. Am. J. Vet. Res. *24*:1201–1206, 1963.

Polyarthritis of Calves

In essentially analogous circumstances as described under polyarthritis of sheep (p. 556) a variety of infectious organisms are capable of inducing polyarthritis in calves. *Mycoplasma mycoides* (p. 527) infection and vaccination can cause polyarthritis and unidentified *Mycoplasma sp.* have been isolated from polyarthritis by Moulton (1953) and Simmons and Johnson (1963). *Erysipelas insidiosa* and a variety of other bacteria (Salmonella, Pasteurella, Diplococci, Streptococci, Staphylococci, etc.), often following umbilical infection, are also known to cause polyarthritis. Recently studies by Storz and colleagues (1966) indicate that polyarthritis in calves can result from infection by a psittacosis-lymphogranuloma agent. The organism has been isolated from field cases of polyarthritis and shown to induce arthritis following experimental inoculation. The agent is antigenetically related to the agent of polyarthritis of sheep and guinea pig inclusion conjunctivitis. The infection as described by Storz *et al.* principally affected calves one to three weeks of age and was characterized by involvement of practically all joints of the limbs as well as vertebral and mandibular articulations. The joints were swollen and the synovial tissues edematous and thickened. The synovial fluid of the joints and tendon sheaths was increased in volume, was turbid, yellow-grey and contained numerous flakes of fibrin. Large plaques of fibrin often adhered to the synovial tissue and filled the pouches of the joint cavities. Cellular elements of the synovial fluid were increased in number and elementary bodies could be demonstrated in monocytic cells and synovial cells in smears stained with Giemsa.

Polyarthritis of Calves

HUGHES, K. L., *et al.*: Polyarthritis in Calves Caused by Mycoplasma sp. Vet. Rec. *78*: 276–281, 1966.

MOULTON, J. E., RHODE, E. R., and WHEAT, J. D.: Erysipelatous Arthritis in Calves. J. Am. Vet. Med. Assn. *123*:335–340, 1953.

SIMMONS, G. C., and JOHNSTON, L. A. Y.: Arthritis in Calves Caused by *Mycoplasma sp.* Aust. Vet. J. *39*:11–14, 1963.

STORZ, J., *et al.*: Polyarthritis of Calves: Isolation of Psittacosis Agents from Affected Joints. Am. J. Vet. Res. *27*:633–641, 1966.

STORZ, J., *et al.*: Polyarthritis of Calves: Experimental Induction by a Psittacosis Agent. Am. J. Vet. Res. *27*:987–995, 1966.

EPIZOOTIC BOVINE ABORTION

First described in California in 1956 by Howarth, epizootic bovine abortion (EBA) represents an important cause of abortion in cattle in the United States and Europe. It is caused by a *Chlamydia sp.*, however, the natural mode of transmission is unknown. The disease has many similarities to enzootic abortion

of ewes (EAE) (p. 558).   Pregnant cattle are susceptible to experimental infection
with the EAE agent and pregnant sheep are susceptible to experimental infection
with the EBA agent, however, the exact relationship of the two agents and diseases requires further study.

Epizootic bovine abortion is principally a disease of the fetus causing abortion,
stillbirth or birth of weak calves which die within a few days.   No clinical evidence
of disease is seen in the cow either before or after abortion.   Abortions usually
occur between the seventh and ninth months of gestation but earlier abortion
may occur.   The abortion rate may exceed 75 per cent of the pregnant animals
in a herd.   The pathological features have been described in detail by Kennedy
et al. (1960) and Kwapien et al. (1970).   Gross findings in the fetus include subcutaneous edema, pleural and peritoneal effusion, generalized enlargement of lymph
nodes, splenomegaly, petechiae on the oral mucous membrnaes, larynx, trachea
and conjunctivae, small grey foci in the myocardium and kidneys, and most
characteristically a swollen, friable, coarsely nodular liver.   Microscopically the
basic histologic change is described as a granulomatous inflammatory process that
may involve any or all body organs, but in particular the liver, meninges, brain,
kidney, heart, and skin.   Individual lesions consist of focal necrosis and collections
of macrophages, epithelioid cells, lymphocytes and neutrophils.   Lesions in lymph
nodes may contain Langhans type giant cells.   Marked reticuloendothelial
hyperplasia accounts for the gross lymphadenopathy and splenomegaly.   The
placenta in natural abortion has been described as edematous but of little diagnostic value.   In the experimental disease necroses of cotyledons, edema, accumulation of fibrinopurulent exudate and a leathery tough consistency have been
described.   The clinical, gross and microscopic findings should allow presumptive
diagnosis which can be supported by demonstrating cytoplasmic elementary
bodies in impression smears of placenta or fetal organs stained by Macchiavello,
Giemsa or Gimenez techniques.   Definitive diagnosis requires isolation of the
infectious agent.

Epizootic Bovine Abortion

Kennedy, P. C., Olander, H. J., and Howarth, J. A.:   Pathology of Epizootic Bovine
Abortion.   Cornell Vet. *50*:417–429, 1960.
Kwapien, R. P., *et al.*:   Pathologic Changes of Placentas from Heifers with Experimentally
Induced Epizootic Bovine Abortion.   Am. J. Vet. Res. *31*:999–1015, 1970.
Howarth, J. A., Moulton, J. E., and Brazier, L. M.:   Epizootic Bovine Abortion Charac-
terized by Fetal Hepatopathy.   J. Am. Vet. Med. Assn. *128*:441–449, 1956.
McKercher, D. G., *et al.*:   Epizootiologic and Immunologic Studies of Epizootic Bovine
Abortion.   Cornell Vet. *56*:433–450, 1966.
McKercher, D. G.:   Cause and Prevention of Epizootic Bovine Abortion.   J. Am. Vet.
Med. Assn. *154*:1192–1196, 1969.
Storz, J.:   Comparative Studies on EBA and EAE, Abortion Diseases of Cattle and Sheep
Resulting from Infection with Psittacosis Agents *in Abortion Diseases of Livestock*.   Faulkner,
L. C. (Ed.).   Springfield, Charles C Thomas, 1968.
Storz, J., *et al.*:   Epizootic Bovine Abortion in the Intermountain Region.   Some Recent
Clinical, Epidemiologic, and Pathologic Findings.   Cornell Vet. *57*:21–37, 1967.
Storz, J., *et al.*:   The Isolation of a Viral Agent from Epizootic Bovine Abortion.   J. Am.
Vet. Med. Assn. *137*:509–514, 1960.

ENZOOTIC ABORTION OF EWES

First reported in 1950 by Stamp in Scotland, enzootic abortion of ewes has
since been recognized in Europe and the United States.   The disease is caused by
Chlamydia ovis; closely related to the causative agent of epizootic bovine abortion

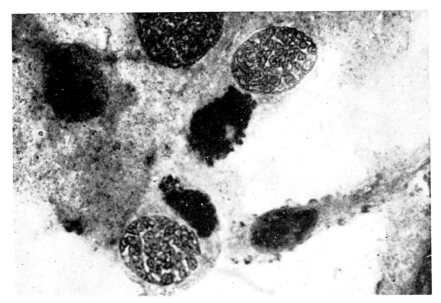

Fig. 11–6.—Chlamydial inclusions sixty hours after infection *in vitro* with the agent of ovine abortion. (Courtesy Dr. J. Storz.)

(p. 557). Abortion is usually in the last month of gestation, but earlier abortion, stillbirth and birth of weak lambs may occur. Fetal membranes are often retained which results in clinical disease in the ewe, otherwise specific signs of infection are not seen in the ewe. Placentitis is the major lesion. Cotyledons are grey to dark red and the periplacentome is thickened, opaque yellow-pink and covered with a flaky clay colored exudate. The uterine surface of the chorion is of tough, granular consistency, pink-yellow and covered with a flaky yellowish exudate. Microscopically there is focal necrosis, edema, vasculitis and a mononuclear cell infiltration. Cytoplasmic elementary bodies can be demonstrated in tissue sections or smears stained by the Giemsa, Macchiavello or Gimenez techniques. Lesions in the lamb are not striking, but resemble those of epizootic bovine abortion (p. 557) but of lesser degree. Diagnosis is based on clinical and pathological findings supported by demonstration of elementary bodies or isolation of the infectious agent.

Enzootic Abortion of Ewes

PARKER, H. D., HAWKINS, W. W., JR., and BRENNER, E.: Epizootiologic Studies of Ovine Virus Abortion. Am. J. Vet. Res. *27*:869–877, 1966.

PARKER, H. D.: A Virus of Ovine Abortion—Isolation from Sheep in the United States and Characterization of the Agent. Am. J. Vet. Res. *21*:243–250, 1960.

PAVLOV, N., and VESSELIVOVA, A.: Morphology of the Natural Infection in Lambs with the Virus of Lamb Abortion. Zentbl. Vet. Med. *12B*:517–526, 1965.

STAMP, J. T., *et al.*: Enzootic Abortion in Ewes. I. Transmission of the Disease. Vet. Rec. *62*:251–254, 1950.

STORZ, J.: Comparative Studies on EBA and EAE, Abortion Diseases of Cattle and Sheep Resulting from Infection with Psittacosis Agent *in Abortion Diseases of Livestock*. Faulkner, L. C. (Ed.). Springfield, Charles C Thomas, 1968.

STUDDERT, M. J.: Bedsonia Abortion of Sheep. II. Pathology and Pathogenesis with Observations on the Normal Ovine Placenta. Res. Vet. Sci. *9*:57–61, 1968.

STUDDERT, M. J., and McKERCHER, D. G.: Bedsonia Abortion of Sheep. I. Aetiological Studies. Res. Vet. Sci. *9*:48–56, 1968.

STUDDERT, M. J., and KENNEDY, P. C.: Enzootic Abortion of Ewes. Nature, London, *203*:1088–1089, 1964.

TUNNICLIFF, E. A.: Ovine Virus Abortion. J. Am. Vet. Med. Assn. *136*:132–134, 1960.

CHLAMYDIAL AGENTS IN PNEUMONIA OF CATTLE AND SHEEP

Organisms of the psittacosis lymphogranuloma-trachoma group have been demonstrated to cause pneumonia in cattle, sheep and goats which are usually referred to as **enzootic pneumonia.** The relationship of the agents incriminated as primary causes of pneumonia to those causing abortion, arthritis and encephalitis is not entirely clear at present. Cattle have been shown to be experimentally susceptible to ovine pneumonia isolates and sheep to the bovine isolates. The disease which is principally, but not exclusively, of importance in young animals is clinically non-specific, characterized by fever, nasal discharge, cough, dyspnea and depression. Lesions, which are comparable in cattle and sheep, are most often restricted to the anterior lobes of the lung. Microscopically the lesions are dominated by an extensive infiltration of lymphocytes, macrophages, and plasma cells particularly in the bronchiolar mucosa and surrounding bronchioles and blood vessels, but also within alveolar septae. The exudate often has a follicular arrangement and compresses bronchioles and alveoli. Bronchioles and alveoli contain macrophages and variable numbers of neutrophils but marked purulent exudate is lacking unless secondary bacterial invaders initiate a more characteristic picture of bronchopneumonia as is often the case. There is proliferation and epithelialization of alveolar lining cells which contributes to alveolar consolidation. As in other infections caused by *Chlamydia sp.* elementary bodies are more easily demonstrated in tissue impressions than tissue sections. Positive diagnosis requires isolation of the causative organism.

Chlamydial Pneumonia of Cattle and Sheep

CARTER, G. R., and ROWSELL, H. C.: Studies on Pneumonia of Cattle. II. An Enzootic Pneumonia of Calves in Canada. J. Am. Vet. Med. Assn. *132*:187–190, 1958.

DUNGWORTH, D. L., and CORDY, D. R.: The Pathogenesis of Ovine Pneumonia. II. Isolation of Virus from Faeces: Comparison of Pneumonia Caused by Faecal, Enzootic Abortion and Pneumonitis Viruses. J. Comp. Path. & Therap. *72*:71–79, 1962.

———: The Pathogenesis of Ovine Pneumonia. I. Isolation of a Virus of the PL Group. J. Comp. Path. & Therap. *72*:49–70, 1962.

MATUMOTO, M., *et al.*: Studies on the Disease of Cattle Caused by a Psittacosis-Lymphogranuloma Group Virus (Miyagawanella). VI. Bovine Pneumonia Caused by This Virus. Jap J. Exptl. Med. *25*:23–34, 1955.

McKERCHER, D. G.: A Virus Possibly Related to the Psittacosis-Lymphogranuloma-Pneumonitis Group Causing a Pneumonia in Sheep. Science *115*:543–544, 1952.

OMAR, A. R.: The Aetiology and Pathology of Pneumonia in Calves. V.B. *36*:260–273, 1966.

PALOTAY, J. L., and CHRISTENSEN, M. S.: Bovine Respiratory Infections. I. Psittacosis-Lymphogranuloma Venereum Group of Viruses as Etiological Agents. J. Am. Vet. Med. Assn. *134*:222–230, 1959.

PHILLIP, J. I. H., *et al.*: Pathogenesis and Pathology in Calves of Infection by Bedsonia Alone and by Bedsonia and Reovirus Together. J. Comp. Path. *78*:89–99, 1968.

STORZ, J.: Psittacosis-Lymphogranuloma Agents in Bovine Pneumonia. J. Am. Vet. Med. Assn. *152*:814–819, 1968.

LEPTOSPIROSIS

Spirochetal organisms of the genus *Leptospira* are responsible for a wide variety of infectious processes in man and animals. Animals often act as the reservoir

The microscopic appearance of these lesions is characteristic. Convoluted tubules undergoing degenerative changes are surrounded or replaced by large dense masses of cells, including lymphocytes, plasma cells, macrophages, occasional neutrophils and sometimes small nests of erythrocytes. Although convoluted tubules are severely affected, glomeruli are often spared or involved only secondarily. Except in cases treated with antibiotics, silver preparations demonstrate leptospirae in the lumen of tubules or in the cytoplasm of the tubular epithelium. The organisms occur singly or in tangled nests (Fig. 11–9).

Lesions resulting from uremia are found elsewhere in the body. They include severe gastric hemorrhages with microscopic depositis of calcium in the gastric mucosa and calcareous deposits in the walls of the aorta and large arteries (Fig. 22–12).

Bovine Leptospirosis.—Leptospiral organisms have been recovered from, or demonstrated in, tissues of cattle which were manifesting a wide gamut of clinical symptoms. Organisms have been demonstrated in tissue from bovine animals exhibiting symptoms of mastitis; fever, icterus, emaciation and hemoglobinuria; abortion; occasional anemia, transient leukopenia and death, particularly involving young animals. The variety of clinical signs that may occur in bovine leptospirosis not only indicates the need for laboratory tests to establish the diagnosis, but also emphasizes the importance of maintaining a critical attitude regarding all evidence pointing toward the infection. It now appears, however, that leptospiræ are well established as an agent of disease in the bovine species. The principal serotype found in cattle in the United States is *Leptospira pomona*.

Lesions.—The disease in cattle in many respects parallels its counterpart in dogs. It may occur in an acute septicemic form or as a chronic nephritic type of disease. The latter is rarely fatal. The lesions in these two bovine types are similar to those observed in dogs. In the *acute* case, icterus, a swollen yellowish liver and petechiae are the principal gross findings, as in the dog. Hemolytic anemia, which is not a feature of the canine disease, accounts for hemoglobinuria and partially contributes to the icterus and hepatic lesions. Microscopic changes include portal hepatic lymphocytic infiltration, with splenic hemosiderosis in some outbreaks and severe centrilobular necrosis of the liver in others. In certain outbreaks in Israel, leptospirosis, with organisms of the *L. grippotyphosa* serotype, took a protracted clinical course. The microscopic lesions included hepatic cell dissociation, cholangitis and congestion and hemosiderosis of the spleen. In the kidneys, swelling and disorganization of convoluted tubular epithelium were associated with bile pigment and hemoglobin in the lumen.

Animals that survive the systemic disease are found to have grayish to white focal lesions in the kidney parenchyma. These foci are usually discrete and scattered through the cortex, not concentrated at the corticomedullary junction as is often the case in dogs. Microscopically, the principal lesions are based upon changes in the tubular epithelium. The epithelial cells and affected tubules have granular, swollen or vacuolated cytoplasm, sometimes associated with fragmentation of the cytoplasm and detachment of the cells. These affected tubules are surrounded by dense masses of leukocytes, chiefly lymphocytes and plasma cells. In some cases, syncytial giant cells of the Langhans' type have been described. Leptospirae are usually, but not constantly, demonstrable in sections impregnated with silver, located within affected tubular epithelium or in the lumen of the tubule.

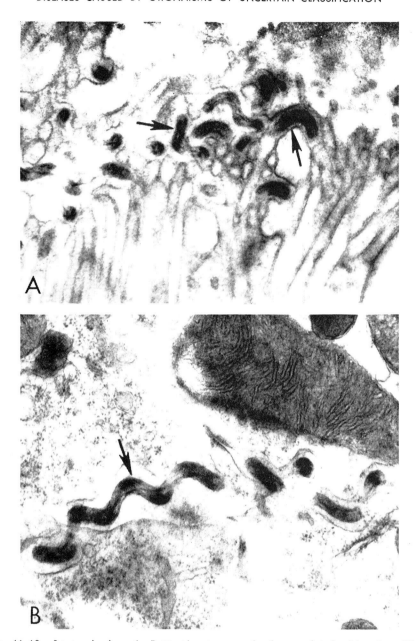

FIG. 11–10.—Leptospirosis.   *A*, *Leptospira pomona* closely associated with microvilli of a proximal convoluted tubule cell in the kidney of a hamster.   *B*, *Leptospira pomona* within a proximal tubule cell in the kidney of a hamster.   (Courtesy Dr. N. G. Miller and American Journal of Veterinary Research.)

Leptospiral abortion, which usually occurs in the latter half of pregnancy, is not associated with specific lesions in the placenta or fetus.

Porcine Leptospirosis.—Swine are susceptible to several serotypes of leptospirae.   In the United States *L. pomona* appears to be the most important organism.   The disease has not been studied as extensively in swine as it has in dogs and cattle but it is recognized that infection with leptospirae may occur as a subclinical infection or be associated with acute hepatitis and icterus, subacute or chronic nephritis and reproductive disorders characterized by abortion, stillbirths and the birth of weak litters which may die.

The gross and microscopic manifestations of leptospirosis in swine have not been adequately studied. Renal lesions have been described which mimic those in cattle. There is tubular degeneration and an intense focal lymphocytic infiltration. Leptospirae are demonstrable in the lumens and epithelium of the tubules and in the nodules of lymphocytic infiltration. In the pig, like most other susceptible species, leptospirae localize in the kidneys and are shed in the urine for protracted periods of time.

Stillborn pigs and aborted fetuses, which are mainly expelled in the last third of gestation, are often macerated, precluding accurate examination. The most characteristic lesion in abortuses and stillborns is focal necrosis of the liver, without significant cellular infiltration. Organisms can generally be isolated but may be difficult to demonstrate in tissues.

Leptospirosis in Other Species.—Leptospirosis is known to occur in a variety of other animal species, but data are insufficient to assess the relative importance of the infection as a disease. However, brief mention of the disease in horses is warranted. Serologic evidence indicates that leptospirosis is a relatively common infection in horses. Bryans (1955) demonstrated agglutinins for *L. icterohemorrhagiae*, *L. pomona* or *L. canicala* in 30 per cent of 512 mature horses. In horses inoculated with *L. pomona* he observed a mild transient disease characterized by fever, hemolytic anemia and icterus. In contrast to other species leptospirae were not present in the urine of the experimentally infected horses. The relationship of leptospirosis to periodic ophthalmia in horses is discussed on page 1421.

Both old and new world non-human primates are experimentally susceptible to leptospirosis, but the natural disease has not been described in new world species and appears to be infrequent in old world species. Cats are susceptible to several serotypes of leptospira but infection has not been associated with clinical or pathological changes. Disease resembling acute leptospirosis in cattle has been reported in sheep naturally infected with *Leptospira sp.*

Leptospirosis

AREAN, V. M.: The Pathologic Anatomy and Pathogenesis of Fatal Human Leptospirosis (Weil's Disease). Am. J. Path. *40*:393–423, 1962.

BAKER, J. A. and LITTLE, R. B.: Leptospirosis in Cattle. J. Exper. Med. *88*:295–307, 1948.

BOHL, E. H., POWERS, T. E., and FERGUSON, L. C.: Abortion In Swine Associated with Leptospirosis. J. Am. Vet. Med. Assn. *124*:262–264, 1954.

BRYANS, J. T.: Studies on Equine Leptospirosis. Cornell Vet. *45*:16–50, 1955.

BURDIN, M. L.: Renal Histopathology of Leptospirosis Grippotyphosa in Farm Animals in Kenya. Res. Vet. Sci. *4*:423–430, 1963. VB 3849–63.

BLOOM, F.: Histopathology of Canine Leptospirosis. Cornell Vet. *31*:266–268, 1941.

BREESE, S. S., JR., GOCHENOUR, W. S., JR., and YAGER, R. H.: Electron Microscopy of Leptospiral Strains. Proc. Soc. Exper. Biol. & Med. *80*:185–188, 1952.

CHAUDHARY, R. K., FISH, N. A., and BARNUM, D. A.: Experimental Infection with L. pomona in Normal and Immune Piglets. Can. Vet. J. *7*:106–112, 1966.

COFFIN, D. L. and MAESTRONE, G.: Detection of Leptospires by Fluorescent Antibody. Am. J. Vet. Res. *23*:159–164, 1962.

CORDY, D. R., and JASPER, D. E.: The Pathology of an Acute Hemolytic Anemia of Cattle in California Associated with Leptospira. J. Am. Vet. Med. Assn. *120*:175–178, 1952.

DE FREITAS, D. C. *et al.*: Notas sobre Leptospirose Equina (in Brazil). Arq. Inst. Biol. S. Paulo *27*:93–96, 1960. VB 1788–62.

FEAR, F. A., *et al.*: A Leptospirosis Outbreak in a Baboon (*Papio sp.*) colony. Lab. Anim. Care *18*:22–28, 1968.

FENNESTAD, K. L., and BORG-PETERSEN, C.: Experimental Leptospirosis in Pregnant Sows. J. Infect. Dis. *116*:57–66, 1966.

GOCHENOUR, W. S., JR., JOHNSTON, R. V., YAGER, R. H., and GOCHENOUR, W. S.: Porcine Leptospirosis. Am. J. Vet. Research *13*:158–160, 1952.

GOCHENOUR, W. S., JR., GLEISER, C. A. and WARD, M. K.: Laboratory diagnosis of leptospirosis. Ann. New York Acad. Sci. *70*:421–426, 1958.

GSELL, O.: Leptospirosis Pomona, die Schweinehüterkrankheit. Schweiz. med. Wchnschr. *76*:237–241, 1946.

HADLOW, W. J., and STOENNER, H. G.: Histopathologic Findings in Cows Naturally Infected with *Leptospira pomona*. Am. J. Vet. Research *16*:45–56, 1955.

HARTLEY, W. J.: Ovine Leptospirosis. Aust. Vet. J. *28*:169–170, 1952.

HEUSSER, H.: Die periodische augenentzündung, eine Leptospirose? Schweiz. Arch. f. Tierheilk. *90*:287–312, 1948.

IMBABI, S. E., *et al.*: Experimental Leptospirosis: Leptospira Canicola Infection in Calves. Am. J. Vet. Res. *28*:413–419, 1967.

JACUSIEL, F.: Problem of Leptospirosis in Israel. Refuah Vet. *6*:121–124, 1949.

JONES, T. C., ROBY, T. O., DAVIS, C. L., and MAURER, F. D.: Control of Leptospirosis in War Dogs. Am. J. Vet. Research *6*:120–128, 1945.

LANGHAM, R. F., MORSE, E. V., and MORTER, R. L.: Experimental leptospirosis V. *Leptospira pomona* infection in swine. Am. J. Vet. Res. *19*:395–400, 1958.

LANGHAM, R. F., MORSE, E. V., MORTER, R. L.: Pathology of experimental ovine leptospirosis. *Leptospira pomona* infections. J. Infect. Dis. *103*:285–290, 1958.

LUCKE, V. M., and CROWTHER, S. T.: The Incidence of Leptospiral Agglutination Titres in the Domestic Cat. Vet. Rec. *77*:647–648, 1965.

MEYER, K. F., STEWART-ANDERSON, B., and EDDIE, B.: Canine Leptospirosis in the United States. J. Am. Vet. Med. Assn. *95*:710–729, 1939.

MICHNA, S. W., and CAMPBELL, R. S. F.: Leptospirosis in Pigs: Epidemiology, Microbiology and Pathology. Vet. Rec. *84*:135–138, 1969.

MILLER, N. F., and WILSON, R. B.: Electron Microscopic Study of the Relationship of Leptospira Pomona to the Renal Tubules of the Hamster During Acute and Chronic Leptospirosis. Am. J. Vet. Res. *28*:225–235, 1967.

MINETTE, H. P.: Leptospirosis in Primates Other than Man. Am. J. Trop. Med. & Hyg. *15*:190–198, 1966.

MINETTE, H. P., and SHAFFER, M. F.: Experimental Leptospirosis in Monkeys. Am. J. Trop. Med. & Hyg. *17*:202–212, 1968.

MONLUX, W. S.: III. Clinical Pathology of Canine Leptospirosis. Cornell Vet. *38*:109–121, 1948.

————: Pathology of Canine Leptospirosis. Cornell Vet. *38*:199–208, 1948.

MORTON, H. E., and ANDERSON, T. F.: Morphology of *Leptospira icterohemorrhagiæ* and *L. canicola* as Revealed by the Electron Microscope. J. Bact. *45*:143–146, 1943.

MOULTON, J. E., and HOWARTH, J. A.: The demonstration of *Leptospira canicola* in hamster kidneys by means of fluorescent antibody. Cornell Vet. *57*:524–532, 1957.

MURPHY, J. C., and JENSEN, R.: Experimental Pathogenesis of Leptospiral Abortion in Cattle. Am. J. Vet. Res. *30*:703–713, 1969.

REINHARD, K. R., TIERNEY, W. F., and ROBERTS, S. J.: A Study of Two Enzoötic Occurrences of Bovine Leptospirosis. Cornell Vet., *40*:148–164, 1950.

REINHARD, K. E.: A Clinical Pathologic Study of Experimental Leptospirosis of Calves. Am. J. Vet. Research *12*:282–291, 1951.

REINHARD, K. R., and HADLOW, W. J.: Experimental Bovine Leptospirosis—Pathological, Hematological, Bacteriological and Serological Studies. Proc. Am. Vet. Med. Assn. *1954*: pp. 203–216.

ROBERTS, S. J.: Sequelae of leptospirosis in horses on a small farm. J. Am. Vet. Med. Assn. *133*:189–194, 1958.

ROTH, E. E.: Leptospirosis in Wildlife in the United States. Proc. Am. Vet. Med. Assn. *1964*: pp. 211–218.

SHIVE, R. J., *et al.*: Leptospirosis in Barbary Apes (*Macaca sylvana*). J. Am. Vet. Med. Assn., *155*:1176–1178, 1969.

SLEIGHT, S. D., LANGHAM, R. F., and MORTER, R. L.: Experimental Leptospirosis: the Early Pathogenesis of *Leptospira pomona* Infection in Young Swine. J. Infect. Dis. *106*: 262–269, 1960.

SMITH, R. E., REYNOLDS, I. M., and SAKAI, T.: Experimental leptospirosis in pregnant ewes. III. Pathologic features. Cornell Vet. *50*:115–122, 1960.

YAGER, R. H., GOCHENOUR, W. S., JR., and WETMORE, P. W.: Recurrent Iridocyclitis (Periodic Ophthalmia) of Horses. I. Agglutination and Lysis of Leptospiras by Serums Deriving from Horses Affected with Recurrent Iridocyclitis. J. Am. Vet. Med. Assn. *117*: 207–209, 1950.

12

Diseases Due to Simple Bacteria

The micro-organisms which the bacteriologist classifies as the simple bacteria (order Eubacteriales) are ubiquitous in nature, and include many pathogenic species. It is convenient to consider the diseases caused by such pathogens together, even though they compose a group that is undeniably heterogeneous. Among them are some of the diseases first shown to be caused by specific bacteria and consequently used for studies that established basic principles of etiology and immunology. While data concerning the causative organisms of many of the diseases are plentiful, very little has been recorded in regard to the pathogenesis and the nature of the specific lesions. While these earlier investigations had their place in the development of bacteriology as an important science, it is no longer enough to isolate an organism and, using it, to reproduce a disease in another animal. The disease itself must be precisely identified and the relation of the suspected etiologic agent to the specific disease must be clearly established. The need for thoroughness is emphasized by the doubts that now exist concerning the actual role of some of these organisms that for years have been considered the sole cause of specific diseases. The challenge to the pathologist is clear. It is for him to investigate the conditions under which these diseases occur and the precise effects of the pathogen on the host. Even some of the first of these diseases to be recognized, anthrax, for example, could be restudied with profit in the light of present day knowledge and with modern techniques.

In this chapter the student will note that infections caused by simple bacteria commonly are fulminant and overwhelming, although more prolonged or even smoldering infections may occur. The tissue reactions are often serous, fibrinous or hemorrhagic in severe infections of short duration, with purulent and granulomatous changes appearing in those of increasingly longer duration. In many fulminant diseases the recognizable morphologic changes are subtle and easily overlooked, necessitating careful observation and good pathologic technique.

REFERENCES

Cohrs, P.: *Lehrbuch der Speziellen pathologischen Anatomie der Haustiere.* 4th ed., Jena, Fischer, 1954.

Hagan, W. A., and Bruner, D. W.: *The Infectious Diseases of Domestic Animals.* 4th ed., Ithaca, Comstock Publishing Co., 1961.

Kelser, R. A., and Shoening, H. W.: *Manual of Veterinary Bacteriology.* 5th ed, Baltimore, Williams & Wilkins Co., 1948.

Merchant, I. A. and Packer, R. A.: *Veterinary Bacteriology and Virology.* 5th ed, Ames, Iowa, Iowa State College Press, 1958.

Smith, Louis D. S.: A key for tentative recognition of bacteria commonly encountered in clinical bacteriology. Am. J. Vet. Res. *13*:430–432, 1952.

19

ANTHRAX

Anthrax is not only of current significance as an infection of animals and man, but also of historical interest for it was investigated intensively by the founders of bacteriology. Robert Koch, in 1876, was the first to isolate the causative organism in pure culture and to reproduce the disease with the culture. Pasteur, Rous and Chamberland, in 1881, demonstrated active immunization with attenuated anthrax cultures in the famous experiment at Pouilly-le-Fort. Their dramatic demonstration of the immunizing properties of attenuated cultures of anthrax bacilli, before a special French Commission, has been hailed for years as a significant milestone in the history of bacteriology.

Anthrax is principally a disease of herbivorous animals, but it may affect a wide variety of species, including man. Sheep and cattle are most susceptible; horses and mules are slightly more resistant to natural infection. Swine are even more resistant, as are dogs, cats, and other species, although anthrax does occur in these animals. In the more susceptible species (sheep, cattle, horses), the disease is usually seen as a fulminant septicemia. In the more resistant animals (swine), the disease may be localized and confined to the regional lymph nodes, particularly those of the cervical region. Man usually acquires anthrax from contact with infected animals or animal products (hides, wool, shaving brushes made from infected hog bristles), the disease being manifest as a localized, persistent cutaneous pustule, malignant carbuncle, or as a systemic often fatal disease, "woolsorters' disease."

The causative organism, *Bacillus anthracis*, is a relatively large, encapsulated, rod-shaped bacillus, which produces spores and grows well under aerobic conditions and is gram-positive. In smears from the tissues, it often appears as chains of square-ended rods but spores are not formed until there has been exposure to air. Giemsa's stain should reveal red capsules on a minority of the organisms. It is the only pathogenic member of a large group of closely related aerobic bacilli. The organism grows in soil and organic material, hence a region in which infection

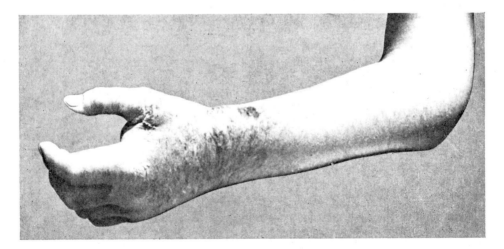

FIG. 12–1.—Cutaneous anthrax in man. This man and his wife skinned a cow recently dead of anthrax. The carcass was fed to hogs which soon exhibited "quinsey." *Bacillus anthracis* was isolated in pure culture from the lesion illustrated, from the swine, and the cow. The wife escaped infection. (Courtesy of Dr. Hubert Schmidt.)

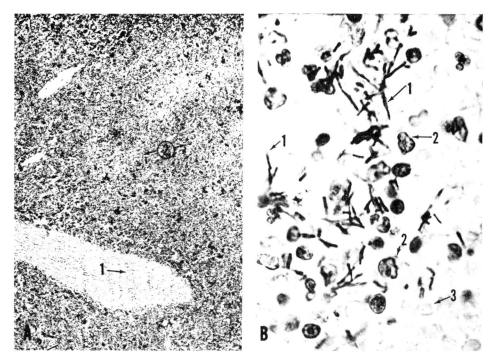

Fig. 12–2.—A, Anthrax. Spleen (× 62) in a fatal bovine case. H & E stain. Lymphoid elements are obscured and trabeculae (1) are widely separated by the massive hemorrhage (2). B, Spleen of a guinea pig which was experimentally infected with anthrax from a bovine (× 1500). Gram's stain of a tissue section. Note gram-positive bacilli (1), lymphoid cells (2), and erythrocytes (3). (Courtesy of Armed Forces Institute of Pathology.) Contributor: Dr. C. L. Davis.

has flourished may be rendered potentially hazardous for many years after the disease has apparently been eliminated. On the other hand, infected animal products are the chief source of virulent organisms. Aside from carcasses of animals dead of the disease, animal wastes and such products as wool, bristles, and hides from abattoirs have been implicated in many infections. Inadequately sterilized fertilizer and bone meal may harbor virulent anthrax bacilli. Infection can apparently follow ingestion or inhalation of spores or vegetative forms of the organism. It has also been produced by experimental inoculation through various routes.

The **signs** of anthrax are variable and may be overlooked in cases of short duration, death being the first indication of the presence of disease. In those instances in which symptoms have been observed, anthrax is recognized as a febrile disease with manifestations of depression, weakness, bloody discharges from body orifices, cyanosis, dyspnea and occasional edematous subcutaneous swellings. Most animals so affected die within a few hours or a day. Swine which have fed upon the carcasses of diseased sheep or cattle may exhibit nothing more than local infection of the pharynx, with enlargement of the cervical lymph nodes. The cutaneous form, malignant carbuncle of man, ordinarily is not recognized in animals.

Lesions.—The gross lesions in fatal cases of the disseminated form of anthrax include edematous and hemorrhagic changes in any part of the body, particularly in serous membranes. The spleen is greatly enlarged and engorged with dark, unclotted blood. Lymph nodes are usually swollen, edematous, and occasionally hemorrhagic. Lesions in other organs are inconstant, although hemorrhages and swelling may occur in the intestinal tract, liver and kidneys. In localized infections in swine, edema and hemorrhages are seen in the pharynx and cervical lymph nodes. In cases of longer standing, the lymph nodes become enlarged and solid, with yellowish foci surrounded by fibrous connective tissue.

The microscopic findings in generalized cases are dominated by the presence of large numbers of anthrax bacilli in the blood and most other tissues. These large rod-shaped organisms can be demonstrated in smears or tissue sections, but they cannot be distinguished from saprophytic bacilli without culturing them and determining their pathogenicity in laboratory animals. In the spleen, the architecture is obscured by the presence of large numbers of erythrocytes. The lymphoid follicles are not discernible; only the trabeculæ remain as tiny islands in a sea of red cells and nuclear débris which floods the splenic sinuses and the cords of Bilroth. Bacilli are readily demonstrated in sections of the spleen with Gram's stain (Fig. 12–2). The precise means by which the organisms produce their lethal effects upon the tissues is not known. It is postulated that a toxin is produced by growth of the bacilli *in vivo*, but no such toxin has been demonstrated from organisms grown *in vitro*.

Localized infection in lymph nodes of swine result in foci of necrosis surrounded by a layer of granulation tissue. Giant cells usually are not present.

Diagnosis.—Presumptive diagnoses are made largely upon the basis of the history (few premonitory symptoms, with sudden death of several animals in a herd) and the characteristic gross lesions found at necropsy. The diagnosis is confirmed by demonstration of *Bacillus anthracis* in large numbers in blood and tissues of animals dead of the disease. It is important that the organisms be identified and differentiated from saprophytes upon the basis of pathogenicity as well as morphologic and cultural characteristics. Inoculation of organisms, usually intraperitonelly, kills a mouse in twelve to twenty-four hours, a guinea pig in twenty-four to thirty-six hours. Organisms are readily seen in and cultured from the tissues of such inoculated animals.

Anthrax

FRIED, B. M.: The Infection of Rabbits with the Anthrax Bacillus by Way of the Trachea. Arch. Path. *10*:213–223, 1930.

GLEISER, C. A.: Pathology of Anthrax Infection in Animal Hosts. Fed. Proc. *26*:1518–1521, 1967.

STILES, G. W.: Isolation of the *Bacillus anthracis* from Spinose Ear Ticks *Ornithodorus Megnini*. Am. J. Vet. Research *5*:318–319, 1944.

CLOSTRIDIAL INFECTIONS

Bacterial organisms of the genus *Clostridium* are sporulating, anaerobic bacteria of rather large size, usually about 0.8 micron in width and 3 to 8 microns in length. Most members of the genus are non-pathogenic and are commonly found in soil and intestinal tracts of man and animals. Several members of the group are responsible for a number of important diseases of man and animals. Some of these will be described briefly. Pathogenic members of the genus are listed in Table 12–1.

Blackleg.—The causative agent of blackleg, *Clostridium chauvoei* (*C. feseri, Bacillus chauvoei*, bacillus of symptomatic anthrax), produces an acute, highly

Table 12–1.—Pathogenic Clostridiae

Species	Disease
Cl. chauvoei	Blackleg
Cl. septicum	Malignant edema, Braxy
Cl. hemolyticum	Bovine bacillary hemoglobinaria
Cl. novyi	Black disease
Cl. perfringens	
Type A	Gas gangrene
B	Lamb dysentery
C	Struck
D	Enterotoxemia
E	Enterotoremia
F	Hemorrhagic enteritis (enteritis necroticans) in man
Cl. sordelli	Wound infections
Cl. carnis	Wound infections
Cl. histolyticum	Wound infections
Cl. botulinum	Botulism (See Table 12–2)
Cl. tetani	Tetanus

fatal disease of cattle and occasionally of other species, such as sheep, goats and swine. The infection appears sporadically in certain areas where the organisms live in the soil. It runs an acute, usually fatal course, and affected animals are often found dead though signs of illness have not been observed.

The **lesions** consist of crepitant swellings in the musculature, particularly of the extremities, which produce a stiff characteristic extension of the limbs a short time after death. Affected muscles incised at necropsy are dark brown or dark red, streaked with black. Some areas appear moist and upon pressure yield dark, gas-filled exudate. Other groups of muscles are dry and sponge-like, with numerous gas bubbles. A peculiar sweetish odor may be noticed. The subcutaneous tissues overlying affected muscles are usually yellowish, gelatinous, blood-tinged and contain gas bubbles. Similar lesions are rather frequently demonstrated in the heart, rarely in tongue (could be confused here with "woody tongue") or even as diffuse hemorrhagic lesions in the lung.

Microscopically, the essential lesions are found in the skeletal musculature. Gas bubbles in the fixed tissues are indicated by spherical spaces separating muscle bundles and fascia. There are irregular areas of necrosis and collections of neutrophils and lymphocytes along the muscle septa. Edema is infrequent. Gram-positive organisms are demonstrable in the sections, appearing singly or in small irregular clumps.

The pathogenesis of the disease is not understood. It does not appear to result from wound infection. The disease is most frequent in young animals (six months to two years of age) on a good plane of nutrition.

The **diagnosis** may be confirmed by the characteristic gross lesions, and by demonstration of fairly numerous single or possibly paired bacilli with rounded ends and occasional spores near but not at the end of the cell. As is typical of the Clostridia, the spore is of somewhat greater diameter than the bacillus in which it forms. The organism grows only under strict anaerobic conditions.

Bovine Bacillary Hemoglobinuria.—A disease apparently first described in California in 1916 by K. F. Meyer, it occurs principally in sharply delimited geographic areas in the Western United States and has been reported in New Zealand. It is characterized by sudden onset of hemoglobinuria, high fever, collapse and death within a day or two. Affected cattle are found at necropsy to have large areas of infarction in their livers as the most constant lesion although hemorrhages and hematuria are also prominent. Vawter and Records (1926) isolated *Clostridium hemolyticum (Clostridium hemolyticus bovis)* from early cases and were able to produce fatalities but not characteristic lesions in cattle. In more recent years the disease has been observed to spread with certain cattle imported into Montana and its occurrence has been more frequent in regions in which *Fasciola hepatica* (liver fluke, p. 796) is prevalent.

Many aspects of the pathogenesis of this disease remain to be explained but available evidence suggests that following ingestion of *Cl. hemolyticum*, the bacteria localize in the liver and remain latent until an anaerobic environment is created by hepatic injury. Migration of liver flukes is believed to represent an important mode of initiating hepatic damage with resultant activation of the organism. Exotoxins produced by *Cl. hemolyticum* contribute to further hepatic damage with the production of the characteristic "infarct." Venous thrombi, which are usually present in the liver, enhance the development of the lesion, but are not believed to initiate the process. Olander, *et al.* (1966) described activation of the disease by liver biopsy and have reproduced the disease in rabbits.

Diagnosis is based on the pathologic findings (hepatic infarct, hemoglobinuria) and isolation of *Cl. hemolyticum*. The disease must be differentiated from many other situations which in the bovine are accompanied by hemoglobinuria. According to Van Ness and Erickson (1964), *Cl. hemolyticum* finds favorable growth conditions in marshy land in which the water supply is alkaline (pH 8.0 or higher) and is rich in organic matter.

Malignant Edema.—Originally isolated by Pasteur, who called it *"Vibrion septique," Clostridium septicum* is another ubiquitous organism that grows in soil but may produce infection in animals. Malignant edema is seen as a sequel of wounds, such as those incurred in shearing or docking, or in parturition attended by unskilled persons who ignore aseptic precautions. It is most frequent in horses, sheep and cattle, and is rare in dogs and cats.

The disease is characterized by a febrile course of short duration with hot, painful swelling at sites of infection. These swollen areas later become even more edematous, but less painful and cooler. At necropsy, the involved tissues are edematous, frequently hemorrhagic, and contain some gas bubbles. Septicemia often occurs, with hemorrhages distributed throughout the body. The lungs are congested and edematous. Serous, blood-tinged effusion from the peritoneum may also be observed. *Clostridium septicum* is readily demonstrable in the affected tissues.

Braxy.—Braxy (bradsot) is an acute infection of sheep caused by *Clostridium septicum* characterized by hemorrhagic abomasitis. The disease is principally of importance in Scotland and Scandinavia. The infection mainly affects young sheep and usually occurs during the winter months. Death is sudden with few or no clinical signs. The wall of the abomasum is thickened, edematous, and contains hemorrhages. Similar lesions may be encountered in the small intestine. The large causative bacilli can be seen in tissue section and readily isolated from the lesions.

Black Disease.—Also known as infectious necrotic hepatitis, black disease is an acute fatal infection of sheep and rarely cattle, caused by *Clostridium novyi*. The organism is widely distributed in soil as three strains (A, B, C), and is a frequent inhabitant of the intestinal tract of sheep. The type B organism is the most frequent strain in black disease. In a high percentage of animals in enzootic areas *Cl. novyi* pass through the intestinal wall and lodge in the liver where they remain as a latent infection. An anaerobic environment produced by the migration of liver flukes (*Fasciola hepatica* [p. 796], *Dicrocoelium dendriticum* [p. 799]), activates the bacteria which release exotoxins, further contributing to hepatic necrosis and producing fatal toxemia. Death may result without premonitory signs. Pathological changes include characteristic multiple foci of necrosis in the liver, petechiae on the epicardium and endocardium, and hydropericardium. Marked subcutaneous venous congestion causes a dark discoloration of the pelt which resulted in the name black disease.

Diagnosis is based on pathological findings and isolation of *Cl. novyi.*

Gas gangrene, the human counterpart of malignant edema, is a wound infection caused by *Clostridium spp.* Improved treatment of wounds, particularly war wounds, has greatly reduced the incidence of this infection. In addition to malignant edema discussed above, clostridial wound infections in animals include *Cl. perfringens, Cl. novyi, Cl. sordelli, Cl. feseri, Cl. histolyticum,* and *Cl. carnis.*

Tetanus.—Tetanus or "lockjaw" occurs in man and animals. It has become far less frequent than in the past because of more effective treatment of wounds, and widespread use of tetanus toxoid. The causative organism, *Clostridium tetani,* is a normal inhabitant of the intestinal tract of herbivorous animals and grows

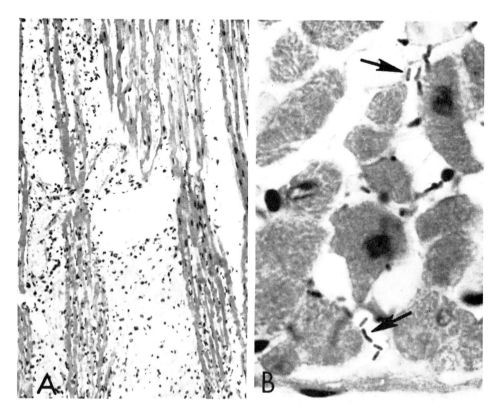

FIG. 12–3.—Blackleg, bovine muscle. *A,* Fragmented myofibers are separated by edema, cellular infiltration and gas bubbles. *B,* The large causative bacilli demonstrated with Giemsa stain. (Courtesy Dr. C. L. Davis.)

well in humus-rich soil. It is a Gram-positive, sporulating rod-shaped bacillus which is anaerobic. Tetanus is usually a sequel of wounds, often insignificant ones such as nail-pricks, or those produced by castration, docking or shearing, or even during parturition. The anaerobic environment of certain wounds allows germination of the spores, multiplication of the organism and release of exotoxin. The exotoxin is not histolytic and probably does not contribute to local tissue destruction. The toxin is a neurotoxin which becomes fixed to the gray matter of the central nervous system where it diminishes or abolishes synaptic inhibition.

The disease is characterized by prolonged spasmodic contractions of muscles, with extension of limbs, stiffness and immobilization. The muscles of mastication are often affected, immobilizing the jaws. The entire musculature is eventually involved and death follows. Diagnosis is based on clinical signs and history of trauma, however a wound is often not demonstrable and if present the bacilli are difficult to demonstrate. Specific lesions have not been described.

Enterotoxemia.—Clostridial infections associated with enteric disease in lambs and other species are discussed in Chapter 24, p. 1211.

Botulism.—*Clostridium botulinum*, another member of this group of anaerobic sporulating pathogens, is responsible for an extremely serious food intoxication, botulism. This disease is most important in man, resulting from consumption of inadequately sterilized canned food in which the organisms have produced their powerful neurotoxin. Wild ducks which feed upon the muddy contaminated bottoms of shallow ponds or lakes may contract the disease, and losses in some

Table 12–2.—Botulism in Animals and Man

Type	Principal Victims	Commonest Vehicles	Greatest Frequency	Reference
A	Man, chicken	Canned vegetables and fruits, meat and fish	Western United States	Leuchs, 1910 Burke, 1919
B	Man, horse	Meat, usually pork; silage and forage	Eastern United States, Europe	Leuchs, 1910 Burke, 1919
Ca	Wild birds	Fly larvae, rotting vegetation	North and South America, South Africa, Australia	Bengston, 1922 Pfenninger, 1924
Cb	Cattle, sheep, horse, mink	Silage, carrion	Australia, Europe, North America	Seddon, 1922 Pfenninger, 1924
D	Cattle	Carrion	South Africa	Theiler and Robinson, 1927 Meyer and Gunnison, 1928
E	Man, mink	Fish and marine animal foods	United States, Canada, Japan, Northern Europe	Gunnison, Cummings and Meyer, 1936.
F	Man	Liver paste	Denmark	Dolman, 1961

instances have been great.   Botulism also occurs in chickens fed spoiled canned foods (beans, etc.), and in that species it causes a peculiar torticollis, aptly named "limber neck."   Nutritionally deficient cattle which have fed upon animal carcasses have acquired botulism from the bits of decaying meat clinging to the bones.   No specific lesions are known.   (See also pp. 954 and 1009.)

Clostridium botulinum produces several antigenically distinguishable toxins, each requiring a specific antitoxin.   These toxins have different host ranges and are usually found in specific food products or environments.   Table 12–2, adapted from Scholtens and Coohon (1964), summarizes some of these relationships:

Although immunologically distinct, the pharmacologic effects of the toxins are identical.   They do not act on the central nervous system, but rather on the peripheral nervous system at the myoneural junction.   Their paralytic effect is apparently mediated through the prevention of the release of acetylcholine.   How the release of acetylcholine is inhibited is not known.

Clostridial Infections

BALDWIN, E. M., JR., FREDERICK, L. D., and RAY, J. D.: The Control of Ovine Enterotoxemia by the use of *Clostridium perfringens* Type D. Bacteria. Am. J. Vet. Research *9*: 296–303, 1948.

BRITTON, J. W., and CAMERON, H. S.: So-called Enterotoxemia of Lambs in California. Cornell Vet. *34*:19–30, 1944.

————: Experimental Reproduction of So-called Enterotoxemia. Cornell Vet. *35*:1–8, 1945.

DURAND, M., LOQUERIE, R., and HASCHICK, S.: (An Outbreak of Blackleg Caused by *Clostridium welchii*.) Arch. Inst. Pasteur, Tunis *39*:73–81, 1962.   VB 116–63.

GITTEO, M.: Botulism in mink: an outbreak caused by type-C toxin. Vet. Rec. *71*: 868–871, 1959.

HARSHFIELD, G. S., CROSS, F., and HOERLEIN, A. B.: Further Studies on Overeating (Enterotoxemia) of Feedlot Lambs. Am. J. Vet. Research *3*:86–91, 1942.

HELMY, N.: Experimental clostridial infection in dogs. Tijdschr Diergeneesh *83*: 1089–1096, 1958.

JASMIN, A. M.: Enzyme activity in *Clostridium hemolyticum* toxin. Am. J. Vet. Res. *8*:289–293, 1947.

KALMBACH, E. R.: Western Duck Sickness: a Form of Botulism. U.S.D.A. Tech. Bull. 411, 1934.

MACRAE, D. R., MURRAY, E. G., and GRANT, J. G.: Entero-Toxaemia in Young Suckled Calves. Vet. Record *55*:203–204, 1943.

MARSH, H., and TUNNICLIFF, E. A.: Enterotoxemia in Feedlot Lambs in Connection with an Outbreak of Coccidiosis. J. Am. Vet. Med. Assn. *104*:13–14, 1944.

MARSHALL, S. C.: The isolation of *Clostridium hemolyticum* from cattle in New Zealand. N. Z. Vet. J. *7*:115–119, 1959.

MEYER, K. F.: Studies to diagnose a fatal disease of cattle in the mountainous regions of California. J. Am. Vet. Med. Assn. *48*:552–565, 1916.

MUTH, O. H.: Control of Pulpy Kidney Disease (Entero-Toxemia) of Lambs. J. Am. Vet. Med. Assn. *104*:144–147, 1944.

MUTH, O. H., and MORRILL, D. R.: Control of Enterotoxemia (Pulpy Kidney Disease) in Lambs by the Use of Alum Precipitated Toxoid. Am. J. Vet. Research *7*:355–357, 1946.

OLANDER, H. J., HUGHES, J. P., and BIBERSTEIN, E. L.: Bacillary Haemoglobinuria: Induction by Liver Biopsy in Naturally and Experimentally Injected Animals. Pathologia Vet. *3*:421–450, 1966.

PAMUKCU, A. M.: Hemorrhagic encephalomyelitis due to botulism in cattle in Turkey. Zentralblatt für Veterinärmed *1*:707–722, 1954.

QUINLIVAN, T. D. and WEDDERBURN, J. F.: Bacillary haemoglobinuria in cattle in New Zealand. N. Z. Vet. J. *7*:113–115, 1959.

QUORTRUP, E. R., and SUDHEIMER, R. L.: Detection of Botulinus Toxin in the Blood Stream of Wild Ducks. J. Am. Vet. Med. Assn. *102*:264–266, 1943.

RECORDS, E. and VAWTER, L. R.: Bacillary hemoglobinuria of cattle and sheep. Bull. No. 173, Univ. of Nevada, June, 1945.

SAFFORD, J. W. and SMITH, L. deS.: A study of the epizootiology of bacillary hemoglobinuria. Proc. 91st Ann. Meet. Am. Vet. Med. Assn., 1954, pp. 159–161.

SCHOLTENS, R. G. and COOHON, D. R.:   Botulism in Animals and Man, with Special Reference to Type E, *Clostridium botulinum*. Sci. Proc. AVMA. 224–230, 1964.

SMITH, L. D.:   The control of bacillary hemoglobinuria. Proc. 60th Ann. Meet. U. S. Livestock San. Assoc., Chicago, 1956, pp. 135–138 (VB 1716–1958).

SINCLAIR, K. B.:   Black Disease—A Review. Brit. Vet. J.*112*:196–200, 1956.

SMITH, L. D. S.:   Clostridial Diseases of Animals. Adv. Vet. Sci. *3*:463–524, 1957.

VAN KAMPEN, K. R., and KENNEDY, P. C.:   Experimental Bacillary Hemoglobinuria. II. Pathogenesis of the Hepatic Lesion in the Rabbit. Pathologia Vet. *6*:59–75, 1969.

————: Experimental Bacillary Hemoglobinuria: Intrahepatic Detection of Spores of Clostridium Haemolyticum by Immunofluorescence in the Rabbit. Am. J. Vet. Res. *29*: 2173–2177, 1968.

WRIGHT, G. P.:   The Neurotoxins of *Clostridium botulinum* and *Clostridium tetani*. Pharmacol. Rev. *7*:413–465, 1955.

VAN NESS, G. B. and ERICKSON, K.:   Ecology of Bacillary Hemoglobinuria. J. Am. Vet. Med. Assn. *144*:492–496, 1964.

VAWTER, L. R. and RECORDS, E.:   Recent studies on ictero-hemoglobinuria of cattle. J. Am. Vet. Med. Assn. *68*:494–513, 1926.

STREPTOCOCCAL INFECTIONS

Certain of the gram-positive spherical organisms which occur in chains and are classified in the genus *Streptococcus* are pathogenic for man and animals. The incidence of these infections has decreased greatly during the last few years because of the widespread use of antibiotics. Some are still seen from time to time and will be discussed briefly. Some of the more important pathogenic streptococci are listed in Table 12–3, subdivided according to Lancefield's serologic groups and their associated diseases.

Strangles (Adenitis Equorum).—Strangles is an infectious respiratory disease of young horses characterized by sudden onset of fever and upper respiratory catarrh, followed by acute swelling and later by abscess formation in the submaxillary, parapharyngeal and other lymph nodes. A beta-hemolytic streptococcus, *Streptococcus equi*, is constantly present in pure culture in the abscesses and is generally conceded to be the cause of the disease. Strangles may occur in connection with, and be accentuated by, outbreaks of equine rhinopneumonitis (p. 429), but the work of Bazeley (1943) indicates that *Streptococcus equi* alone can

Table 12–3.—*Streptococcal Infections*

Lancefield Group	Species	Disease
A	*S. pyogenes*	Scarlet fever in man. Various pyogenic infections. Occasionally a cause of bovine mastitis.
B	*S. agalactiae*	Bovine mastitis.
C	*S. equi* *S. zooepidemicus* *S. dysgalactiae* *S. equisimilis* *S. genitalium*	Strangles. Various pyogenic infections. Bovine mastitis. Respiratory infection in man. Equine genital infection and abortion.
D	*S. faecalis*	Usually not pathogenic.
E	*S. uberis* *Streptococcus spp.*	Bovine mastitis. Cervical lymphadenitis in swine.
F thru O	*Streptococcus spp.*	Various species in these groups have been isolated from infections of the respiratory and genital mucous membranes of man and animals, and bovine mastitis.

produce the disease. Experimentally, new, rapidly growing cultures of these streptococci have been shown to produce the disease, while older cultures are avirulent.

The symptoms are characteristic, although they vary strikingly in severity. The edematous swelling of the pharyngeal regions may produce inspiratory dyspnea, which gives the impression that the animal is strangling. The submaxillary lymph nodes become enlarged, hot, and soon form abscesses which yield large quantities of creamy yellowish pus when they rupture spontaneously or are incised. In uncomplicated cases, recovery usually follows drainage of the abscess, but in some the infection spreads to other lymph nodes or reaches the general circulation. In such cases, abscesses may form in any organ but are more frequent in the lungs, kidneys, liver, spleen and less common in the brain. Fatal outcome may be expected in overwhelming infections or in those instances in which abscesses form in a critical organ.

Lesions.—Organisms that penetrate the respiratory mucosa cause acute inflammation in the adjoining structures, particularly the lymph nodes, where abscesses form. In some cases, abscesses of microscopic size have been demonstrated in parapharyngeal lymph nodes by one of us (Jones) within twenty-four hours of the first evidence of fever. Such abscesses may become encapsulated or, more commonly, rupture into the oral or pharyngeal cavities or through the skin of the intermandibular region. Catarrhal or purulent rhinitis in addition to

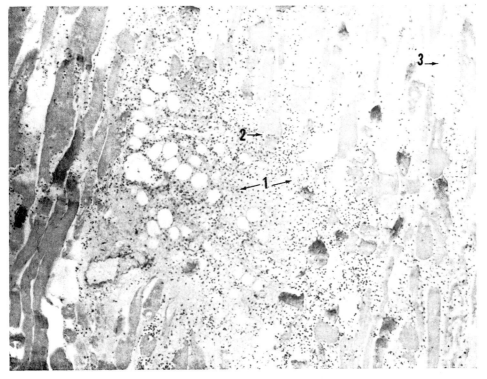

FIG. 12–4.—Inflammatory edema in panniculus muscle of a horse with purpura hemorrhagica following respiratory infection with *Streptococcus pyogenes* (× 100). Septic emboli were found in adjacent tissues. Note cellular and albuminous exudate (*1*), and fragmented muscle bundles (*2*). (Courtesy of Armed Forces Institute of Pathology.) Contributor: Army Veterinary Research Laboratory.

lymphadenitis is an unvariable feature in fatal cases. Metastatic abscesses occur in the lung (sometimes with cavitation), liver, kidney, spleen, and occasionally the brain. Septicemia is sometimes observed with abscesses few or absent.

Purpura hemorrhagica may be a complication of strangles, and in such cases large subcutaneous areas of edema and hemorrhage are associated with septic emboli in blood vessels of the tissues involved (see p. 1172).

Diagnosis.—The clinical history, the presence of characteristic gross lesions, and the demonstration of *Streptococcus equi* in abscesses are sufficient to establish the diagnosis at necropsy. Demonstration of the organisms in submaxillary or other abscesses will confirm the clinical diagnosis in living animals.

Streptococcal Mastitis.—Bovine mastitis is widespread, particularly in dairy herds, and constitutes an important economic problem. Gram-positive coccoid organisms, occurring in short or long chains (streptococci), are commonly associated with inflammation of the bovine mammary gland and are generally regarded as important in the etiology. Other factors, such as trauma and exposure to cold, may be influential in the production of the lesions, but *Streptococcus agalactia* is an obligate parasite of the mammary gland, and the mastitis produced by *Streptococcus agalactiae* represents a specific contagious disease of cattle. Other streptococci which do not require the mammary gland for survival are also of importance as causes of mastitis but the associated diseases are not solely dependent upon the presence of the bacterium as is the case with *Streptococcus agalactiae*. These include *Streptococcus uberis, Streptococcus dysgalactiae, Streptococcus fecalis, Streptococcus zooepidemicus*, and members of Lancefield groups G and L. In a few instances, streptococci of human origin (*Streptococcus pyogenes*) may be involved in outbreaks of bovine mastitis and contribute to concomitant epidemics of "septic sore throat" in persons who drink the milk. Bovine mastitis is described more fully in Chapter 26 (p.1327).

Genital Infections.—*Streptococcus genitalium* is encountered in the cervix and uterus of mares, where it is believed to contribute to inflammation which may result in sterility. The organisms in the genital tract are usually accompanied by catarrhal inflammation, which sometimes is followed by purulent exudation. When conception does occur in infected mares, the fetus is usually aborted during the early months of pregnancy. The lesions in aborted fetuses are not distinctive even though *Streptococcus genitalium* may be present throughout their tissues.

Cervical Lymphadenitis of Swine.—Abscesses (jowl abscess) are not infrequent in the cervical lymph nodes of swine. Streptococci of Lancefield group E are the most commonly isolated organisms, however, other bacterial species have also been isolated with frequency. The latter include group C streptococci, *Corynebacterium pyogenes, Pasteurella multocida*, and *Staphylococcus aureus*. Streptococcal cervical lymphadenitis is one of the most common diseases of guinea pigs.

Neonatal Streptococcal Infections.—Streptococcal infections are a particular hazard of the neonatal period in man and most domestic animals, particularly foals, calves, lambs and pigs. Infection is usually thought to gain entrance by way of the umbilicus but there is little evidence to substantiate this portal of entry. The infection most often results in suppurative polyarthritis ("joint-ill") and meningitis, but localization in the valvular endocardium, kidneys, and choroid of the eye are not infrequent, especially in lambs. Despite the virulence of streptococci in neonates, the strains usually isolated from neonates are not pathogenic for adult animals.

Wound Infections.—Local purulent inflammation may follow infection of wounds by streptococci and this may spread to distant organs. The tissue reaction is basically purulent, although encapsulation of abscesses may occur, giving the lesion a more granulomatous appearance as healing takes place.

Streptococcal Infections

ARMSTRONG, C. H., and PAYNE, J. B.: Bacteria Recovered From Swine Affected With Cervical Lymphadenitis (Jowl Abscess). Am. J. Vet. Res. *30*:1607–1612, 1969.
ARMSTRONG, C. H., BOEHM, P. N., and ELLIS, R. P.: Experimental Transmission of Streptococcic Lymphadenitis (Jowl Abscess) of Swine. Am. J. Vet. Res. *31*:823–829, 1970.
BAZELEY, P. L.: Studies with Equine Streptococci. 5. Some Relations between Virulence of *Streptococcus equi* and Immune Response in the Host. Australian Vet. J. *19*:62–85, 1943.
BLAKEMORE, E., ELLIOTT, S. D., and HART-MERCER, J.: Studies on Suppurative Polyarthritis (Joint-Ill) in Lambs. J. Path. & Bact. *52*:57–82, 1941.
ELLIOTT, S. D., ALEXANDER, T. J. L., and THOMAS, J. H.: Streptococcal Infection in Young Pigs. II. Epidemiology and Experimental Production of the Disease. J. Hyg. Camb. *64*: 213–220, 1966.
GIBBONS, W. J.: The Histopathology of Mastitis. Cornell Vet. *28*:240–249, 1938.
FIELD, H. I., BUTAIN, D., and DONE, J. T.: Studies on Piglet Mortality. I. Streptococcal Meningitis and Arthritis. Vet. Rec. *66*:453–455, 1954.
GUNNING, O. V.: Joint-Ill in Foals (Pyosepticemia). Vet. J. *103*:47–67, 104–111, 129–148, 1947.
JONES, F. S.: The Streptococci of Equines. J. Exper. Med. *30*:159–178, 1919.
MILLER, W. T., and JOHNSON, H. W.: Differential Staining of Sections of Unpreserved Bovine Udder Tissue Affected with Mastitis. U.S.D.A., Washington, D. C., Circular No. 514, 1939.
MITCHELL, C. A., and PLUMMER, P. J. G.: Septic Arthritis Caused by *Streptococcus equi*. Canad. J. Comp. M. *6*:24–25, 1942.
MORRILL, C. C.: A Histopathological Study of the Bovine Udder. Cornell Vet. *28*:196–210, 1938.
MURPHY, J. M.: The Relationship of Teat Mucous Membrane Topography to Age, Breed, and Incidence of Udder Infection in Cows. Cornell Vet. *35*:41–47, 1945.

STAPHYLOCOCCAL INFECTIONS

Coccoid bacterial organisms, which are gram-positive and occur in packets, are classified in the genus *Staphylococcus*. Occasionally they are pathogenic for man and animals. These organisms are widespread in nature and are frequent inhabitants of the normal skin. It is not surprising, therefore, that staphylococci commonly infect wounds and are present in cutaneous abscesses, boils and furuncles. Staphylococci are frequent inhabitants in both veterinary and human hospitals and represent a serious threat to surgical, debilitated, and diseased patients. Many strains (particularly hospital strains) are resistant to a variety of antibiotics and present formidable therapeutic problems. Some strains produce toxins which cause gastro-enteritis ("food poisoning") in man following consumption of contaminated food in which the bacteria have been allowed to grow.

Granulomatous Staphylococcal Mastitis.—Occurring with moderate rarity, and reported from Europe, the United States and Australia, this bovine disease has gone under the etiologically incorrect name of "actinomycotic mastitis." The pathological and etiological characteristics are also those of the granulomatous disease which has been known as "botryomycosis." Since the older writers mention botryomycosis as occurring in the udders of mares, we presume it is correct to say that mares are subject to this form of mastitis, although there appear to be no reports of it in recent times. Lesions identical to those described below in the mammary gland (botryomycosis) may be encountered in other animal species and in a variety of tissues including the skin, skeletal muscle and uterus.

One or more quarters of the udder are hard and moderately enlarged but neither hot nor painful, the onset being insidious and unperceived. The flow of milk is negligible or non-existent, but the general health of the animals has generally been unimpaired.

Microscopic study reveals that each interlobular septum, normally so thin as to be almost imperceptible, has proliferated until it forms a distinct fibrous capsule. The average diameter of these roughly spherical lobules is about a centimeter, and the whole affected area, which may be the entire quarter, is composed of these circular compartments packed together. Inside each fibrous capsule is a zone of reticulo-endothelial granulation tissue entirely comparable to that of actinomycosis (p. 616) and actinobacillosis (p. 619). Within the granulation tissue there are one or, as a rule, several minute abscesses, or masses of polymorphonuclear neutrophils. Within each focus of purulent exudate (p. 158), there are brilliant, red-staining (hematoxylin and eosin) "rosettes" which also closely simulate the rosettes of actinomycosis and actinobacillosis, showing however, less tendency to form "clubs" at the periphery. The Gram stain shows these rosettes to be packed with cocci, although the organisms often have died out in the center, the oldest part of the colony (Fig. 12–5, p. 582).

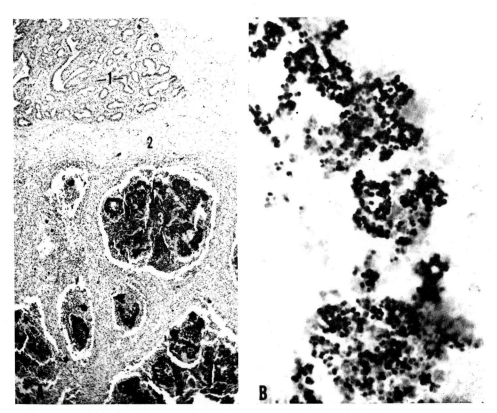

Fig. 12–5.—Granulomatous staphylococcal mastitis, udder of a cow. *A*, Mammary lobules (*1*) are separated by dense bands of connective tissue (*2*) from the colonies of staphylococci (*3*) which are surrounded by a narrow zone of pus (× 48). *B*, Part of a bacterial colony stained by Gram's method (× 1000). Note spherical staphylococci. Courtesy of Dr. E. A. Benbrook.

Grossly, the outlines of the lobular capsules are readily seen on the cut surface and a droplet of pus may ooze from each barely visible abscess. The rosettes are seldom sufficiently firm that they can be felt with the fingers, as they usually can be in actinomycosis.

Cultural studies of the causative cocci have shown that they differ in no significant manner from *Staphylococcus aureus*. Various theories have been proposed as to why this staphylococcus should produce a chronic granulomatous reaction so different from the acute sero-fibrino-purulent form which is the rule. It is believed that a delicately close balance between pathogenicity of the invader and the resistance of the host may well be the reason. **Diagnosis** should be practically certain from the gross examination of the tissue, but histopathological examination with demonstration of the organism leaves no room for doubt. Cultural or direct microscopic examination of the milk reveals only *Staphylococcus aureus* with no evidence of its granulomatous propensities.

Staphylococcal Infections

ALBISTON, H. E.: Actinomycosis of the Mammary Gland of Cows in Victoria. Australian Vet. J. *6*:2–22, 1930.
DENNIS, S. M.: Perinatal Staphylococcal Infections of Sheep. Vet. Rec. *79*:38–40, 1966.
DERBYSHIRE, J. B.: The Pathology of Experimental Staphylococcal Mastitis in the Goat. J. Comp. Path. & Therap. *68*:449–454, 1958.
MORRILL, C. C.: A Histopathological Study of the Bovine Udder. Cornell Vet. *28*:196–210, 1938.
PATTISON, I. H.: Histological Examination of the Teats of Goats Affected With Streptococcal Mastitis. J. Comp. Path. & Therap. *62*:1–5, 1952.
SMITH, H.: Two Cases of Actinomycotic Mastitis. J. Am. Vet. Med. Assn. *84*:635–644, 1934.
SPENCER, G. R. and McNUTT, S. H.: Pathogenesis of Bovine Mastitis. Am. J. Vet. Research *11*:188–198, 1950.

VIBRIOSIS

A disease of the genital system of several species, especially ruminants, is caused by one of the true bacteria, *Vibrio fetus*. This organism is one of about twenty related species in the genus *Vibrio* which includes *V. comma*, the cause of Asiatic cholera in man; *V. metchnikovii*, the cause of acute enteritis in chickens; *V. jejuni*, the etiologic agent in an acute enteritis of calves and mature cattle (p. 1210), and *Vibrio coli*, a cause of dysentery in swine (p. 1210).

Vibrio fetus (Spirillum fetus) is a rather pleomorphic organism, most commonly seen in comma- and S-shaped forms measuring 0.2 to 0.5 microns in width and 1.5 to 5.0 microns in length. Electron micrographs disclose polar flagellæ on the comma-shaped organisms and bipolar flagellæ on the S-forms. The organisms may form spirals and usually contain granules at one end of the cell. They are motile, Gram-negative and stain very well with alkaline methylene blue, crystal violet or carbol fuchsin. Enriched media and microaerophilic conditions are required for maximum growth, particularly for primary recovery from tissues or exudates.

The ewe and cow are most susceptible but the pregnant guinea pig and hamster may be infected and aborted by experimental exposure. The organism kills chick embryos but is reported not to affect rabbits, swine, rats or mice. In one case a pregnant woman reportedly aborted following exposure to a cow which had recently aborted due to infection with *Vibrio fetus*.

In cattle the transmission is entirely venereal either by coitus or in the course of artificial insemination. The infection in cattle is principally characterized by temporary infertility and prolonged estrus cycles. The cow is infected during breeding, and although fertilization and implantation are normal, *Vibrio fetus* soon kills the embryo and incites endometritis. Neither the death of the embryo nor the endometritis are manifest by clinical signs. Endometritis may prevent conception at succeeding estrus periods but most cattle will conceive prior to resolution of the disease. Recovered cows are usually resistant to reinfection. Rarely, *V. fetus* will cause late abortion. The infection in the bull does not induce lesions or affect sterility. Bulls usually recover spontaneously but certain bulls and cows can carry the organism for protracted periods of time.

In contrast to cattle, vibriosis in sheep is not a venereal disease. The oral route is believed to be the principal means of transmission. The infection is characterized by late abortion, stillbirth, or birth of weak lambs, which usually die soon after birth. Following abortion certain ewes may carry the organism. Birds (magpies and crows) have also been demonstrated to carry *V. fetus*.

The **lesions** of vibriosis in cattle are subtle. In experimentally induced disease, Estes and coworkers (1966) described the lesions as a subacute diffuse muco-purulent endometritis. The uterine glands contain neutrophils, lymphocytes, eosinophils and sloughed epithelium. The uterine mucosa is infiltrated with lymphocytes, plasma cells, neutrophils and eosinophils, especially beneath the surface epithelium, and around uterine glands and blood vessels.

In sheep the placenta is intensely invaded, becomes necrotic, detached, and the fetus is aborted. Autolytic changes in natural cases usually preclude adequate pathologic study of the fetus and placentae. Studies of experimentally induced vibriosis in sheep by Jensen, Miller and Molello (1961) have provided the following concepts of the pathogenesis of the disease: Maternal bacteremia with *V. fetus* is followed by localization of the organisms in the hilar zone of the placentomes; arteriolitis results in the vessels in the septums and capillary walls become necrotic, some thrombosed; *Vibrio fetus* penetrate from the maternal blood through capillaries or arterioles to gain access to the hematomas formed between the chorion and the septums; the bacteria proliferate in the hematoma and stimulate accumulation of leukocytes in the hematoma and septums. At this point the organisms gain access to the epithelial cells of the chorion by active penetration or by phagocytosis. These cells become engorged with organisms. From these infected chorionic epithelial cells (or from the hematoma) organisms gain access to the adjacent chorionic capillaries; these cells become engorged with bacteria and some lumens are occluded. From this point the organisms have free access to the fetal circulation. Edema of the chorionic villi is conspicuous at this time and desquamation between septum and villus results in separation. The fetus dies, presumably as the result of bacteremia and possibly toxemia but also possibly influenced by hypoxia resulting from separation of maternal and fetal placenta. The fetus and placentæ decompose rapidly, sometimes become macerated, and are expelled to contaminate the environment. Vulvitis and vaginitis very often follow. As indicated, lesions of diagnostic significance are generally absent in the fetus, but in about 10 per cent of the aborted fetuses lesions are present in the liver which are of aid to diagnosis. These consist of a focal necrotizing hepatitis, which is observable grossly as varying-sized tan to gray foci 1 mm. to 2 cm. in **diameter.**

Osborne and Smibert (1964) have suggested that vibrionic abortion may be the result of a hypersensitivity to *Vibrio fetus* toxin, rather than an infectious process. Their experimental studies clearly demonstrated allergic phenomena, but whether this explains natural vibrionic abortion will require further investigation.

The **diagnosis** in sheep is usually based upon clinical signs and gross lesions, usually confined to the uterus, its contents, vagina and vulva. The uterine wall is edematous, the placentomes swollen, soft, and pale. Purulent exudate and blood may accumulate between the chorion and endometrium in interplacentomal areas of the uterus. Smears of the placenta usually reveal typical organisms in large numbers. Confirmation by culture and identification of the organisms is advisable.

In cattle the clinical signs should cause suspicion of vibriosis but confirmation is necessary to differentiate trichomoniasis (p. 707). If the abortus is viable, the organism can be cultured. However, this is not usual, hence culture of cervico-vaginal mucus should be attempted. The agglutination test employed on cervical mucus is also of value. Culture can also be employed on preputial scrapings for diagnosis of infection in the bull. Infected bulls can also be identified by test-mating to disease-free heifers.

Vibriosis

DOZSA, LESLIE: The Effect of Vibrio Bubulus on the Bovine Endometrium. J. Am. Vet. Med. Assn. *147*:620–625, 1965.
DOZSA, L., MITCHELL, R. G., and OLSON, N. O.: Histologic Changes of the Uterine Mucosa Following the Duration of *Vibrio* Infection and the Subsequent Development of Immunity Am. J. Vet. Res. *23*:769–776, 1962.
ESTES, P. C., BRYNER, J. H., and O'BERRY, P. A.: Histopathology of Bovine Vibriosis and the Effects of Vibrio Fetus Extracts on the Female Genital Tract. Cornell Vet. *56*:610–622, 1966.
FAULKNER, L. C.: *Abortion Diseases of Livestock*. Springfield, Charles C Thomas, 1968.
JENSEN, R., MILLER, V. A., and MOLELLO, J. A.: Placental Pathology of Sheep with Vibriosis. Am. J. Vet. Res. *22*:169–185, 1961.
MEINERSHAGEN, W. A., *et al.*: Magpies As a Reservoir of Infection for Ovine Vibriosis. J. Am. Vet. Med. Assn. *147*:843–845, 1965.
OSBORNE, J. C., and SMIBERT, R. M.: Vibrio Fetus Toxin. I. Hypersensitivity and Aborti-Facient Action. Cornell Vet. *54*:561–572, 1964.
OSBORNE, J. C.: Pathologic Responses in Animals After Vibrio Fetus Toxin Shock. Am. J. Vet. Res. *26*:1056–1067, 1965.
REDMAN, D. R., TRAPP, A. L., HAMDY, A. H., and BELL, D. S.: Ovine Vibriosis in Ohio. J. Am. Vet. Med. Assn. *143*:1094–1095, 1963.
SAMUELSON, J. D., and WINTER, A. J.: Bovine Vibriosis: The Nature of the Carrier State in the Bull. J. Infect. Dis. *116*:518–592, 1966.

SWINE ERYSIPELAS

Swine erysipelas is a very important disease in many parts of the world. Not only does the causative organism produce infections in swine but also in a wide variety of other species, including birds (turkeys, chickens, geese, ducks, pigeons, parrots, and quail and many other wild species), sheep, fish, and porpoises. It is responsible for "erysipeloid" of man, particularly of persons who work in slaughter-houses and fish markets. The cutaneous lesions of "erysipeloid" are usually local but may explode into a fulminant disease with widespread exanthematous or bullous lesions on the hands, face or over the body.

The causative organism, *Erysipelothrix rhusiopathiae* (*E. insidiosa*), is small, pleomorphic, and rod-shaped, either straight or curved. It is Gram-positive and may have a beaded appearance. The organism forms tiny colonies on ordinary agar media. It survives for long periods in decaying flesh and in water, and is resistant to such preservative processes as salting, smoking and pickling. A rapid and economical method for isolating and identifying *E. rhusiopathiae*, using triple sugar iron agar has been described (Vickers and Bierer, 1958).

In swine, the disease presents diverse manifestations that often make its clinical recognition difficult. It may appear as an acute febrile disease with high mortality, death occurring before any specific lesions can be detected. In less severe infections, appearance of rhomboid-shaped areas of intense erythema in the skin are characteristic and have suggested the common name, "diamond skin disease," frequently applied to this entity. These erythematous lesions may progress to necrosis, with large patches of epidermis sloughing as healing occurs. Another frequent clinical manifestation results from localization of organisms in the joints. Arthritis in one or more joints is manifested by sudden onset of painful hot swelling, particularly of the carpal or tarsal articulations. Vegetative endocarditis is a common sequel and may result in sudden death. Hypersensitivity appears to play an important role in this disease but evidence is still accumulating on this point. Attempts to induce arthritis or other chronic lesions with killed or avirulent organisms have not substantiated these thoughts.

Lesions.—In acute septicemic cases of swine erysipelas, nonspecific lesions such as hemorrhages may be seen in serous surfaces and elsewhere. Specific lesions of diagnostic significance develop as the disease progresses. The distinguishing lesions of the less florid disease are found in the skin, synovial membranes and endocardium. The cutaneous lesions, which are most common on the abdomen but may occur anywhere on the skin, vary in size but are almost always of diamond, rhomboid or rectangular shape, sharply demarcated from the adjacent normal skin. At first they are bright red, but later they become purplish and eventually a dark bluish color. Necrosis in older lesions accounts for darkening of the skin; the overlying epidermis dries and eventually peels off. Forcible removal of scabs from an incompletely healed lesion uncovers a raw, bleeding surface. The reason for the shape of the skin lesions is not thoroughly understood, although the lesions themselves are believed to result from bacterial thrombosis of small cutaneous vessels. More thorough studies of the morphologic changes in the skin are definitely needed.

In affected joints, lesions of more chronic nature may be recognized grossly. The joint capsule is obviously enlarged, thickened, distended with excessive fluid, and the articular surfaces are roughened. Rugose thickening of the joint capsule is particularly evident at the margins of the articular surfaces. Microscopically, the joint capsule is seen to be infiltrated with lymphoid cells, occasional nests of neutrophils are present and the synovial lining is prominent and often thrown up into folds. Cell detritus and leukocytes may be found free in the lumen of the joint capsule.

Lesions in the heart are usually the consequence of subacute bacterial endocarditis. Most prominent are the large, irregularly coarse masses on the leaves of the mitral (bicuspid) valve or, less often, on the pulmonary valves. These nodular masses project into the lumen of the left ventricle and at times almost occlude it. The material adheres rather tenaciously to the valve leaflets, but it

some serotypes (various beta hemolytic Group O) of *Escherichia coli* are primary enteric pathogens and are capable of producing a severe, contagious gastro-enteritis in young animals known as colibacillosis (calves, foals, pigs, sheep, dogs).

In addition to gastro-enteritis, the infection sometimes progresses to septicemia, meningitis and arthritis. In all species profuse diarrhea is the principal sign of infection, though infants with septicemia or meningitis may die in the absence of signs referable to the gastrointestinal tract. *Escherichia coli* appears to be one of the principal pathogens of **"calf scours."** Lesions vary from minimal hyper-emia to catarrhal enteritis to hemorrhagic enteritis. In *Escherichia coli* septi-cemia, the principal findings are multiple petechiae and ecchymoses on serous surfaces, epicardium, endocardium, meninges, etc. The pathogenesis of the dis-ease is most often dependent on the production of an enterotoxin by the bacilli, comparable to cholera in man (*Vibrio comma*), but some strains of *Escherichia coli* cause disease by penetrating intestinal epithelial cells as in shigellosis (p. 607). *Escherichia coli*, also of Group O, are responsible for edema disease of swine which is discussed in Chapter 24 (p. 1213).

Klebsiella pneumoniae (Friedlander's bacillus) may cause upper respiratory infection and pneumonia in man and animals. In animals infection with this bacillus is most important in non-human primates where in addition to pneumonia it often is associated with septicemia.

Coliform Bacilli

BOTES, H. J. W.: Fatal Enterobacterial Septicaemia in Lambs. J. S. Afr. Vet. Med. Assn. *37*:17–25, 1966.

DuPONT, H. L., *et al.*: Pathogenesis of *Escherichia coli* Diarrhea. New Engl. J. Med. *285*: 1–9, 1971.

Fox, M. W., and HAYNES, E.: Neonatal Colibacillosis in the Dog. J. Small Anim. Pract. 7 599–603, 1966.

GAY, C. C.: *Escherichia coli* and Neonatal Disease of Calves. Bact. Rev. *29*:75–101, 1965.

GLANTZ, P. J., and ROTHENBACHER, H.: Isolation of *Escherichia coli* Serotype 055:K59(B5): H19 from Calves with Meningitis and Septicemia. Am. J. Vet. Res. *26*:258–261, 1965.

GYLES, C. L., and BARNUM, D. A.: A Heatlabile Enterotoxin from Strains of *Escherichia coli* Enteropathogenic for Pigs. J. Infect. Dis. *120*:419–426, 1969.

MONTEVERDE, J. J., and GARBERS, G. V.: Enterobacterial Infections in Horses. I. *Escherichia coli* 023 H16 in Fatal Septicaemia and Polyarthritis. Revta Med. Vet. B. Aires *45*: 263–270, and 273–279, 1964.

MOON, H. W., NIELSEN, N. O., and KRAMER, T. T.: Experimental Enteric Colibacillosis of the Newborn Pig: Histopathology of the Small Intestine and Changes in Plasma Electrolytes. Am. J. Vet. Res. *31*:103–112, 1970.

NIELSON, N. O., MOON, H. W., and ROE, W. E.: Enteric Colibacillosis in Swine. J. Am. Vet. Med. Assn. *153*:1590–1606, 1968.

STALEY, T. E., JONES, E. W., and CORLEY, L. D.: Attachment and Penetration of *Escherichia coli* into Intestinal Epithelium of the Ileum in Newborn Pigs. Amer. J. Path. *56*:371–392, 1969.

INFECTIONS DUE TO CORYNEBACTERIUM

Bacterial organisms classified in the genus *Corynebacterium* are involved in a wide variety of lesions in many domestic and wild animals, as well as in man. The best known organism in this genus is *Corynebacterium diphtheriæ*, the causative agent of human diphtheria. Other members of this group are often referred to collectively as "diphtheroid bacteria." The lesions produced by various species of *Corynebacterium* show much variety; the tissue reaction to some is essentially suppurative as it is to many of the simpler bacteria; the reactions to others is granulomatous. Because of these variations in pathologic characteristics, it is rather difficult to place these infections in a single group, but since the bacteriologic classification in current use includes this genus within the order Eubacteriales all infections with *Corynebacterium* will be discussed together.

The bacteria making up this genus are Gram-positive, nonacid-fast, occasionally "beaded" in stained sections, and grow slowly on ordinary media, some species producing hemolysis on blood agar. Artificial inoculation of laboratory animals usually gives rise to purulent reactive lesions.

Corynebacterium pyogenes is a common and important organism in pyogenic processes in cattle, swine, sheep and goats. In cattle, the organisms are found in abscesses, many of which are heavily encapsulated, and in necrotic and suppurative pneumonias they have also been isolated from the suppurative arthritis and umbilical infections in calves, and from those of purulent metritis and mastitis in cows. In swine, the "diphtheroid" organisms produce diseases resembling those of cattle; infection often follows farrowing and arthritis is a common manifestation. In sheep and goats, purulent pneumonias and abscesses in the upper respiratory tract have been described.

Corynebacterium renale is commonly associated with "bacillary" pyelonephritis of cattle, in which chronic purulent cystitis and urethritis accompany the inflammatory changes in the ureters and renal pelvis. Horses and sheep may become infected, but dogs rarely. *Corynebacterium suis* has been associated with a similar cystitis and pyelonephritis in swine.

Corynebacterium pseudotuberculosis (*C. ovis*, Preiz-Nocard bacillus) is the cause of ulcerative lymphangitis of horses and caseous lymphadenitis or pseudotuberculosis of sheep and goats. The lesions in the latter have some distinctive features, hence will be described in more detail.

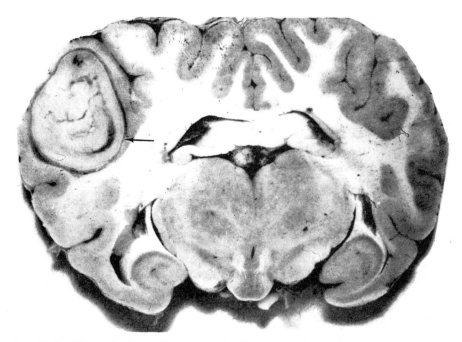

Fig. 12–8.—Abscess in the cerebral cortex of a three-year-old male deer. *Corynebacterium pseudotuberculosis* was recovered in pure culture from the abscess.

Corynebacterium kutscheri (C. pseudotuberculosis murium) is the cause of pseudo-tuberculosis in mice and rats. The lesions consist of disseminated caseopurulent foci particularly in the lungs, lymph nodes, liver, and kidneys (see also *Pasteurella pseudotuberculosis*, p. 609).

Corynebacterium equi is involved in a specific pneumonia of foals and has been isolated from arthritic joints in lambs and from granulomatous lesions in swine. In foals, the infection may be limited to the lungs, with lobular distribution of lesions, or it may be systemic, with abscess formation in many viscera. The microscopic lesion is often characterized by the large numbers of macrophages in the exudate. These cells usually contain demonstrable bacteria in large numbers.

OVINE CASEOUS LYMPHADENITIS

(Pseudotuberculosis of Sheep and Goats)

Caseous lymphadenitis often occurs as an inapparent infection in sheep and goats, but occasionally causes overt disease and sometimes death. Symptoms are rarely recorded, although superficial lymph nodes may become abscessed and lesions in the lungs may produce respiratory symptoms. The entity is most likely to be encountered as an incidental finding in slaughtered animals. The causative organism is *Corynebacterium pseudotuberculosis (Corynebacterium ovis)*, a gram-positive diphtheroid bacillus, but the mode of infection is unknown.

Lesions.—The lesions are found in the lungs and lymph nodes, particularly the prescapular, prefemoral and mediastinal nodes, and less often in the kidney and other viscera. Microscopic evidence indicates that the lesion starts as a

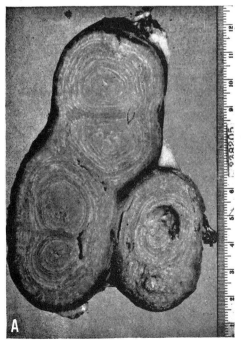
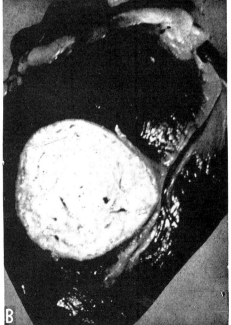

FIG. 12–9.—Caseous lymphadenitis. *A*, Thoracic lymph nodes of a sheep. Note concentric laminations. (Courtesy of Armed Forces Institute of Pathology.) Contributor: Dr. C. L. Davis. *B*, A lesion in the myocardium of a sheep. Photograph courtesy of Dr. C. L. Davis.

small nidus of epithelioid cells but is soon overtaken by caseation necrosis, which becomes the predominant feature. The central caseous mass is soon surrounded by a thin layer of epithelioid cells admixed with lymphocytes, to which an external reinforcing layer of fibrous connective tissue is added. As the lesion grows, the epithelioid and fibrous reactive layers undergo necrosis, the epithelioid layer dying earlier. While the fibrous layer still remains visible, new reactive layers form outside it and successively become necrotic. The result is a spherical, onion-like, concentrically laminated mass which may reach a diameter of several centimeters. Calcification may occur, but giant cells are not seen.

The gross appearance of lymph nodes is characteristic, the entire node being greatly enlarged and almost replaced by a single globoid lesion. In cross section it is seen to be concentrically laminated, layers of fibrous capsule alternating with caseous, friable material that may be greenish and occasionally gritty. In the lungs, the lesions may resemble an abscess with a central, semifluid mass of yellowish or greenish pus.

Diagnosis.—The gross and microscopic features, if typical, are practically diagnostic. Identification of the causative organism depends upon demonstrating its diphtheroid morphology and accepted cultural characteristics. Pathogenicity tests are commonly unfruitful.

Corynebacterium Infections

FELDMAN, W. H., MOSES, H. E., and KARLSON, A. G.: *Corynebacterium equi* as a Possible Cause of Tuberculous-like Lesions of Swine. Cornell Vet. *30*:465–481, 1940.

FOSS, J. O.: Identification of *Corynebacterium renalis* from the Kidney and Bladder of a Horse. J. Am. Vet. Med. Assn. *104*:27, 1944.

GIDDENS, W. E., JR., et al.: Pneumonia in Rats Due to Infection with Corynebacterium Kutscheri. Pathologia Vet. *5*:227–237, 1968.

HUGHES, J. P., BIBERSTEIN, E. L., and RICHARDS, W. P. C.: Two Cases of Generalized *Corynebacterium pseudotuberculosis* Infection in Mares. Cornell Vet. *52*:51–62, 1962.

HULL, F. E., and TAYLOR, E. L.: Abscess Affecting the Central Nervous System of Sheep. Am. J. Vet. Research *2*:356–357, 1941.

MARSH, H.: *Corynebacterium ovis* Associated with Arthritis in Lambs. Am. J. Vet. Res. *8*:294–298, 1947.

PERCY, D. H., RUHNKE, H. L., and SOLTYS, M. A.: A Case of Infectious Cystitis and Pyelonephritis of Swine Caused by Corynebacterium suis. Canad. Vet. J. *7*:291–292, 1966.

SCHECKMEISTER, I. L.: Pseudotuberculosis in Experimental Animals. Science. *123*:463–464, 1956.

SOLTYS, M. A.: Corynebacterium suis Associated with a Specific Cystitis and Pyelonephritis in Pigs. J. Path. Bact. *81*:441–446, 1961.

BRUCELLOSIS

The discovery and identification of three species of bacteria now grouped in the genus *Brucella*, were important steps in the development of knowledge concerning the complex disease of man and animals now known as brucellosis. *Brucella melitensis*, the first to be recognized, was isolated in 1887 from the spleen of patients dead of "Mediterranean" or "gastric fever" (later "Malta fever") by David Bruce, whose name is identified with the organism and the disease. It was several years later (1905) before the infection was traced to the milk goat, which even today is the most common source of the organism, although it also has been isolated from the milk of infected cattle and from aborted fetuses of sheep.

A second step, in 1897, was the isolation and identification of *Brucella abortus* from aborted bovine fetuses and fetal membranes by the Danish veterinarian,

Frederick Bang. The infection of cattle caused by that organism has since been known as "Bang's disease" or "Bang's abortion disease." Eventually it was proved that the causative organism was ubiquitous, natural infections occurring not only in cattle, but in man, horses, fowl, sheep, dogs, deer and bison. One important source of infection for man is cow's milk, although contact with aborted bovine fetuses or slaughtered cattle has also produced the disease. The characteristic undulating or recurrent fever often observed in the human disease has given rise to the name "undulant fever."

The third organism to be included in the genus *Brucella* was originally identified by Traum in 1914 in aborted swine fetuses. This organism, *Brucella suis*, also infects man and, in addition, has been isolated from naturally infected horses, cattle, fowl, and dogs. The disease in man, usually acquired from contact with swine, differs little from brucellosis caused by *Brucella abortus*, except that it tends to be more severe and persistent.

The three species of the genus Brucella (*melitensis, abortus* and *suis*) are similar in morphologic and other characteristics but can be differentiated by bacteriologic methods. Some bacteriologists, however, contend that each of these is but a strain of the same species. For our purposes, members of the genus *Brucella* may be described as small, Gram-negative bacillary organisms varying from 0.4 to 3.0 microns in length and 0.4 to 0.8 micron in width, with coccoid forms outnumbering rod forms under some cultural conditions. *Brucella abortus* differs from *Br. suis* and *Br. melitensis* in one particular cultural characteristic: it requires reduced oxygen tension for initial cultivation on artificial media, although after several passages it will grow under ordinary atmospheric conditions. Of importance to the laboratory study of these organisms is the high susceptibility of the guinea pig to artificial infection. In that rodent it produces a septicemic disease with multiple lesions grossly resembling those of tuberculosis.

Recently two new species have been included in the genus *Brucella*: *Brucella ovis* which causes chronic epididymitis in rams and *Brucella canis* which causes abortion in dogs. Neither of these organisms represents a public health problem, although exposure of laboratory workers to large numbers of *Brucella canis* has resulted in human infection.

Clinical Signs.—Each of the five species of brucella has an affinity for the male and female reproductive organs and the clinical signs are referable to these systems, most often presenting as abortion or epididymitis and orchitis. However, the organisms may localize in other organs and tissues such as mammary gland, lymph nodes, joints, bone, and cartilage resulting in diverse clinical signs. *Bovine brucellosis*, which is usually spread by contact with infective uterine discharges, is principally characterized by abortion between the seventh and eighth months of gestation. Although once a major cause of abortion, bovine brucellosis is no longer a significant cause of bovine abortion in the United States, owing to the use of strain 19 vaccine and testing programs. In bulls the principal clinical sign is tserility. Swelling of the scrotum may be observed but clinical signs of orchitis are usually not obvious. Strain 19 vaccine is pathogenic for bulls producing identical lesions to natural infection.

Brucellosis in *swine*, which is usually transmitted by coitus, causes abortion between the second and third months of gestation. Orchitis occurs in infected boars. Skeletal localization appears to be more frequent in swine than in other species. *Brucella melitensis* infection in sheep and goats is associated with late abortion. It is not an important infection in the United States. *Brucella ovis* is principally associated with epididymitis in rams, though reportedly invasion of the pregnant uterus occurs which can result in abortion. *Brucella canis* infection in dogs causes abortion between forty-five and fifty-five days of gestation, and epididymitis and orchitis.

Lesions.—The lesions of brucellosis in animals are as protean as are the clinical manifestations. The tendency of the organisms to circulate throughout the body in the blood stream at one stage and to localize in certain organs at a later stage is typical but differs between species. It is difficult to generalize about the anatomic manifestations of brucellosis, but since the basic tissue response appears to be the same in all lesions, it will be described before the gross manifestations are discussed.

When living *Brucella* organisms localize in tissues, they attract phagocytic cells. After they are engulfed, they grow and multiply in the cytoplasm of these cells, hence the predominant manifestation is the accumulation of epithelioid cells. Thus an early lesion in a nonsensitized animal will appear microscopically as a tiny nodule of epithelioid cells surrounded by a narrow zone of lymphocytes. As the disease progresses and the host becomes sensitized to the organisms, caseous necrosis occurs in the center of larger lesions and fibrous tissue is laid down at the periphery. Necrosis of cells attracts neutrophils and lymphocytes which may become important elements of the tissue reaction. Frank abscesses are rarely formed, for the tissue reaction is not purulent. In some instances inflammation is diffuse; epithelioid cells, lymphocytes and neutrophils make up the exudate and nodules or frank granulomas seldom form.

The **gross** lesions are often subtle and rarely diagnostic. They have been most clearly described in organs which exhibit manifestations recognizable clinically. The bovine placenta, for example, is believed to show specific changes when infected with *Brucella abortus*. (See p. 1318.) In early placental lesions, the fetal cotyledons are dull and granular in appearance and the intercotyledonary chorion is edematous. Microscopically, many organisms may be demonstrated in chorionic epithelial cells. More advanced lesions appear as yellowish granular necrotic areas on the surface of the fetal cotyledons, the rest of the chorion is opaque and thickened, with a leathery consistency. A sticky, brownish, odorless exudate, which resembles soft caramel candy, may adhere to the chorion. The aborted fetus is edematous with serosanguinous fluid in the body cavities. Fetal bronchopneumonia is nearly always present; characterized principally by a mononuclear cell infiltrate with lesser numbers of neutrophils.

The bovine mammary gland and the supramammary lymph nodes are common sites of localization of *Brucella abortus*, and induration may be the result. Microscopically, diffuse inflammation has been demonstrated, with lymphocytes and neutrophils predominating and collections of epithelioid cells and occasional Langhans' giant cells present in some areas (p. 1318). The epididymis and testicle of the bull occasionally exhibit lesions due to localization of *Br. abortus*. The scrotum becomes enlarged and indurated, features which can be detected in the living animal. The thickened tunica vaginalis usually surrounds large areas of thick fibrous connective tissue which may compress or replace the testicle or epididymis. In rare instances, necrosis of the contents of the sac formed by the tunica may result in suppuration, rupture and discharge of the contents. *Br. abortus* can usually be recovered in pure culture from the affected scrotal contents.

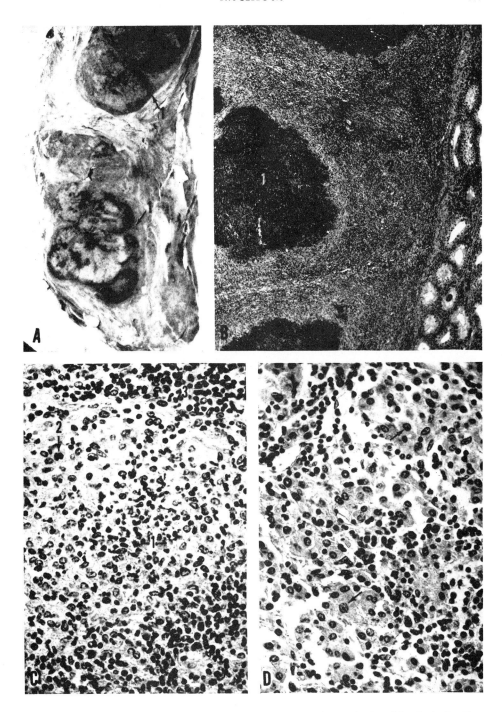

FIG. 12–10.—Brucellosis. *A*, Granulomatous lesions (*1*) in the seminal vesicle of a bull. Contributor: Bureau of Animal Industry, U. S. Department of Agriculture. *B*, Necrotic foci (*1*) surrounded by epithelioid granulation tissue (*2*), displacing seminiferous tubules (*3*) of swine testicle. Contributor: Dr. H. C. H. Kernkamp. *C*, Experimental brucellosis, lung of a guinea pig (× 300). Necrotic center (*1*) surrounded by epithelioid cells (*2*) and lymphocytes (*3*). *D*, Another field of *C* (× 300). Epithelioid cells (arrows) mixed with lymphocytes. (Courtesy of Armed Forces Institute of Pathology.) Contributor: Dr. J. Victor.

In swine, *Brucella suis* most frequently produces lesions in the uterus, but may also localize in other organs. The infected uterine mucosa usually bears tiny white to yellowish nodules which may reach a diameter of 5 mm. These nodules are firm and sometimes contain a central caseous mass. Similar lesions may occur in the spleen, liver, kidney, lymph nodes and bone. Large abscesses, also attributed to this organism, have been described in the spleen, subcutis, thorax and tendon sheaths of swine. Similar inflammatory processes have been noted in the epididymis, testicle and seminal vesicles of the boar. Generalized infections have also been reported to produce granulomatous lesions diffusely distributed throughout the viscera.

In rams, *Brucella ovis* infection characteristically involves the tail of the epididymis. The lesions begin as perivascular edema and lymphocytic infiltration with subsequent hyperplasia and degeneration of the tubular epithelium and intertubular fibrosis. Escape of spermatozoa from damaged tubules incites a granulomatous response which accounts for the major alteration of the epididymis. Primary lesions do not occur in the testicle, however stasis results in secondary testicular degeneration. Fetal lambs experimentally infected with *Brucella ovis* develop inflammatory changes in the lung, liver, lymph nodes, spleen, and kidneys. The nature of the lesions vary from reticulo-endothelial hyperplasia to well-formed nodules of reticulo-endothelial cells, lymphocytes and plasma cells. Necrosis and a cellular infiltration occur in the placenta.

Brucella canis infection in the bitch is accompanied by uterine and placental lesions analogous to bovine brucellosis. Bronchopneumonia is seen in aborted pups. The organism causes epididymitis and orchitis in infected males.

In horses, *Brucella bovis* has been isolated from the persistent necrotizing and purulent lesions involving the ligamentum nuchæ. These lesions may occur near the occipital attachment of the ligamentum nuchæ; at this site the age-old name "poll evil" indicates some of its clinical characteristics. In the region of the thoracic attachment of the ligamentum nuchæ, similar necrotizing and purulent lesions have led to its being called "fistulous withers." Other organisms, such as *Spheropherus necrophorus*, have also been recovered from such lesions, but Brucella appear to be the important pathogens.

Brucella abortus infection is occasionally reported in dogs. The lesions which have been attributed to infection include arthritis, orchitis, epididymitis, and abortion.

Diagnosis.—The precise diagnosis of brucellosis is often difficult, either in man or animals. The agglutination test and skin sensitivity (brucellin) tests are used but neither is infallible. Isolation of the organism in cases with suggestive symptoms and lesions is generally necessary for definitive diagnosis.

Brucellosis

ANDERSON, W. A. and DAVIS, C. L.: Nodular Splenitis in Swine Associated with Brucellosis. J. Am. Vet. Med. Assn. *131*:141–145, 1957.
BIBERSTEIN, E. L., *et al.*: Epididymitis in Rams. Study on Pathogenesis. Cornell Vet. *54*: 27–41, 1964.
BROWN, I. W., FORBUS, W. D., and KERBY, G. P.: The Reaction of the Reticulo-endothelial System in Experimental and Naturally Acquired Brucellosis of Swine. Am. J. Path. *21*: 205–232, 1945.
CARMICHAEL, L. E.: Canine Abortion Caused by *Brucella Canis*. J. Am. Vet. Assn. *152*: 605–616, 1968.

CLEGG, F. G., and RORRISON, J. M.: Brucella Abortus Infection in the Dog: A Case of Polyarthritis. Res. Vet. Sci. 9:183–185, 1968.

DEYOE, B. L.: Histopathologic Changes in Male Swine with Experimental Brucellosis. Am. J. Vet. Res. 29:1215–1220. 1968.

DELEZ, A. L., HUTCHINGS, L. M., and DONHAM, C. R.: Studies in Brucellosis in Swine. VI. Clinical and Histological Features of Intracutaneous Reactions to Fractions of Brucella suis. Am. J. Vet. Res. 8:225–234, 1947.

FELDMAN, W. H., and OLSON, C.: Spondylitis of Swine Associated with Bacteria of the Brucella Group. Arch. Path. 16:195–210, 1933.

HAMILTON, P. K.: The Bone Marrow in Brucellosis. Am. J. Clin. Path. 24:580–587, 1954.

HILL, W. A., VAN HOOSIER, G. L., JR., and McCORMICK, N.: Enzootic Abortion in a Canine Production Colony. I. Epizootiology, Clinical Features, and Control Procedures. Lab. Anim. Care 20:205–208, 1970.

HOFSTAD, M. S.: The Changes Produced by Brucella abortus in the Milk and Udder of Cows Infected with Bang's Disease. Cornell Vet. 32:289–294, 1942.

HUDDLESON, F. I.: Brucellosis in Man and Animals, New York, The Commonwealth Fund, 1939.

JACOB, KL.: Das bruzellöse Granulom. Path. Vet. 1:41–63, 1964.

JONES, L. M., et al.: Taxonomic Position in the Genus Brucella of the Causative Agent of Canine Abortion. J. Bact. 95:625–630, 1968.

KENNEDY, P. C., FRAZIER, L. M., and McGOWAN, B.: Epididymitis in Rams: Pathology and Bacteriology. Cornell Vet. 53:303–319, 1963.

KERNKAMP, H. C. H., ROEPKE, M. H., and JASPER, D. E.: Orchitis in Swine Due to Brucella suis. J. Am. Vet. Med. Assn. 108:215–221, 1946.

LANGENEGGER, J. and SZEDHY, A. M.: (Brucellosis of Domestic Equidæ: Isolation of Brucella abortus from Bursitis of the Withers in Brazil.) Arq. Inst. Biol. Anim. Rio de J. 4:49–63, 1963. VB 1193–64.

McCORMICK, N., et al.: Enzootic Abortion in a Canine Production Colony. II. Characteristics of the Associated Organisms, Evidence For Its Classification as Brucella canis, and Antibody Studies on Exposed Humans. Lab. Anim. Care 20:209–214, 1970.

McERLEAN, B. A.: Undulating Fever, Posterior Paresis and Arthritis in a Dog Apparently Due to Brucellosis. Vet. Rec. 79:567–569, 1966.

OSBURN, B. I.: The Relation of Fetal Age to the Character of Lesions in Fetal Lambs Infected with Brucella ovis. Path. Vet. 5:395–406, 1968.

OSBURN, B. I., and KENNEDY, P. C.: Pathologic and Immunologic Responses of the Fetal Lamb to Brucella ovis. Path. Vet. 3:110–136, 1966.

PEERY, T. M. and BELTER, L. F.: Brucellosis and Heart Disease. II. Fatal Brucellosis. A Review of the Literature and Report of New Cases. Am. J. Path. 36:673–697, 1960. VB 3516–60.

TULAREMIA

The history of tularemia begins in 1910 with the isolation of a bacterial organism from lesions of a "plague-like disease" of ground squirrels by McCoy. He named the organism *Bacterium tularense* after Tulare County, California, in which the first infected ground squirrels had been found. The organism was subsequently designated *Pasteurella tularensis* and more recently *Francisella tularensis* has been proposed. Accidental infection of laboratory workers with this organism was soon to follow and eventually the natural occurrence of the human disease was established. A human disease in Utah, for several years popularly known as "deer-fly fever," was later identified as tularemia. Localized cutaneous ulceration and lymphadenitis followed the bite of a blood-sucking fly, *Chrysops discalis*, which is probably responsible for spread of the disease among wild animals. A more important source of human infection was established by Francis (1925) who demonstrated tularemia organisms in the livers of wild rabbits collected from a market in Washington, D.C. "Rabbit-fever," well known among men in the rabbit market, also proved to be tularemia, a form of the disease that still is the most common.

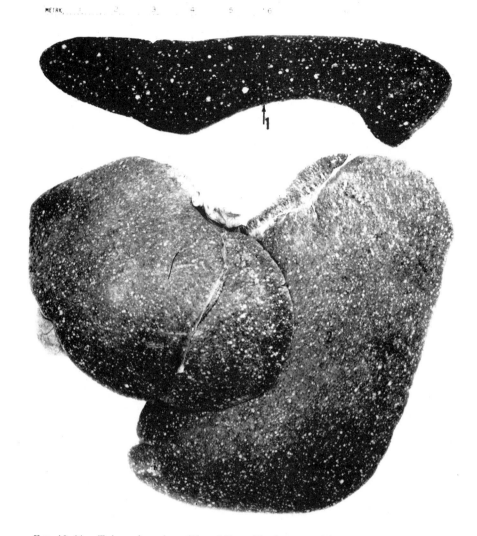

Fig. 12–11.—Tularemia, spleen (*1*) and liver (*2*) of a ground hog (*Marmota flaviventer*). Note uniform distribution of tiny white foci. (Courtesy of Armed Forces Institute of Pathology.) Contributor: Dr. E. Francis.

"Conjunctivitis tularensis" in persons who have dressed wild jack rabbits is also recognized as a form of tularemia. The disease in all its forms is limited to laboratory workers or to persons who handle wild rabbits or wild rodents, and is now known to be distributed over practically the entire United States. Although wild rabbits and rodents are the common reservoir of infection, tularemia has been recognized in dogs. Most mammals are undoubtedly susceptible, and in the laboratory the guinea pig is very readily infected.

In man, the first sign of tularemia usually is a small cutaneous indurated swelling at the site of an insect bite or on the fingers or hands following the dressing of wild rabbits. Hot, painful swelling, occasionally with suppuration, soon extends to the regional lymph nodes; the cutaneous lesion may ulcerate; other

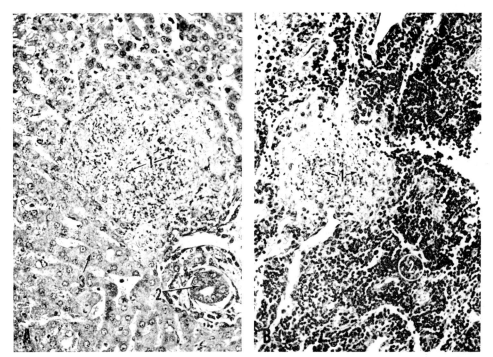

Fig. 12–12.—Tularemia. *A*, Liver of a rabbit (× 120). Note necrotic focus (*1*) near portal area containing bile duct (*2*). Intact liver columns (*3*). *B*, Lymph node (× 210) of a rabbit. Necrotic lesions (*1*) displacing lymphoid cells (*2*). (Courtesy of Armed Forces Institute of Pathology.) Contributor: Dr. W. J. Hadlow.

lymph nodes and the abdominal viscera may become involved. Widespread involvement of lymph nodes and viscera generally results in death.

In rabbits and ground squirrels, the disease is usually recognized by the discovery of multiple chalky focal lesions scattered through the liver, spleen and lymph nodes. These vary from pin-point size to large irregularly shaped foci several millimeters in diameter.

Microscopically, a central mass of caseous necrosis is surrounded by a zone of lymphocytes, mixed with a few neutrophils and macrophages. Early lesions may have a purulent core, but it is soon replaced by necrotic tissue debris. Thrombosis of small blood vessels is frequent and areas of necrosis may coalesce. The causative organisms, being Gram-negative, are difficult to demonstrate in tissue sections but are present in large numbers, particularly in phagocytes at the margin of lesions.

The **diagnosis** can be made upon the basis of the gross and microscopic lesions and the isolation of the causative organisms. Increased agglutination-antibody titer is of value in nonfatal human cases. Tularemia must be differentiated from other diseases which produce similar lesions in the liver. These include, Tyzzer's disease (p. 612), salmonellosis (p. 604), listeriosis (p. 610), toxoplasmosis (p. 684), and mouse pox (p. 407).

Tularemia

Coffee, W. M., and Miller, J.: Acute Canine Tularemia. J. Am. Vet. Med. Assn. *102*: 210–212, 1943.
Francis, E.: Tularemia. J. Am. Med. Assn. *84*:1243–1250, 1925.

20

GOODPASTURE, E. W., and HOUSE, S. J.: The Pathologic Anatomy of Tularemia in Man. Am. J. Path. *4*:213–226, 1928.
GRATZL, E.: Spontane Tularamie bei Hunden. Wein. tierarztl. Mschr. *47*:489–499, 1960. (VB 1379–61.)
JOHNSON, H. N.: Natural Occurrence of Tularemia in Dogs Used as a Source of Canine Distemper Virus. J. Lab. & Clin. Med. *29*:906–915, 1944.
QUIN, A. H., JR.: Tularemia, a Disease Transmissible from Animal to Man. North. Am. Vet. *6*:36–38, 1925.

GLANDERS

An age-old respiratory disease of equines and man, glanders is now very rare in the United States but still common in some parts of Asia. The respiratory mucosae and lungs are most frequently affected, but disseminated lesions may occur. Nasal involvement is indicated by a copious and persistent nasal discharge which is first catarrhal, later purulent. Ulceration often occurs in the nasal mucosa and chronic cough may indicate pulmonary infection. Cutaneous involvement ("farcy") produces indolent ulcers in the skin with thickening of the superficial lymphatics, sometimes leading to abscesses in superficial lymph nodes.

The causative organism, *Malleomyces mallei* (*Loefferella mallei*, *Pfeiferella mallei*, *Bacillus mallei*, *Actinobacillus mallei*), is a short rod-shaped organism with rounded ends. It is gram-negative, non-sporulating, aerobic, and an obligate parasite. Infection is passed from one animal to another through inhalation of nasal exudates or possibly by ingestion of contaminated food or water. Man

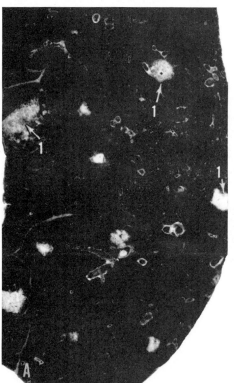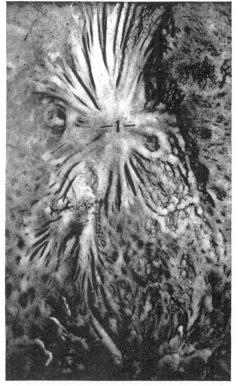

FIG. 12–13.—Glanders. *A*, Sharply demarcated consolidated lesions (*1*) in the lung of a horse. (Courtesy of Armed Forces Institute of Pathology.) Contributor: Capt. R. A. Kelser. *B*, Scar (*1*) in the nasal mucous membrane of a horse. Museum specimen courtesy School of Veterinary Medicine, Texas A&M University.

appears to have rather good resistance, but when infection does take place, the outcome is usually fatal. Guinea pigs, dogs, rabbits and cats are susceptible to the disease, and guinea pigs are most adaptable to laboratory investigation. Intraperitoneal injection of infected material into male guinea pigs (Strauss Test) will result in acute purulent orchitis in three or four days and the organisms can be isolated in pure culture from the testicular lesions.

Lesions.—The nasal lesions of glanders appear as erosive, deep ulcerations of the mucosa, particularly over the septum. After a prolonged course, the ulcers heal, leaving star-shaped scars. The pulmonary lesions are usually discrete granulomatous nodules resembling tubercles but occasionally they coalesce. In a few cases, the disease is manifested as acute purulent bronchopneumonia. The granulomas usually have a caseous necrotic center surrounded by epithelioid cells, a few giant cells and some lymphocytes. Granulomas occasionally occur in the liver, spleen, or other viscera.

The skin lesions, most frequent on the legs, appear as persistent ulcers connected by tortuous, indurated, thick-walled lymphatics. Superficial lymph nodes often become involved, suppurating and discharging thick tenacious pus. Healing occurs slowly with scarring, and the healed areas may break down, leaving persistent indolent ulcers.

Diagnosis.—Clinical diagnosis is usually confirmed by means of the intradermal mallein test which has been an effective means for detecting asymptomatic infections and making control of the disease possible. Diagnosis at necropsy is based upon the presence of typical lesions and the demonstration of *Malleomyces mallei* by cultural methods or guinea pig inoculation.

MELIOIDOSIS

An organism which is in some ways similar to the causative agent of glanders is *Malleomyces pseudomallei* (*Pseudomonas pseudomallei, Loefferella mallei, Flavobacterium pseudomallei, Bacilli whitmori, Loefferella whitmori, Pfeiferella whitmori*). However the causative agents of glanders and melioidosis can be distinguished from one another by their morphology and biochemical characteristics. Although infection may be latent melioidosis is frequently a fatal disease of man, non-human primates, rabbits, guinea pigs, goats, swine, horses and cattle and is most important in Laos, Thailand and Ceylon.

According to Omar (1963), the lesions are characterized by the formation of granulomatous nodules with a caseous center which in some cases become purulent. The solid, granulomatous nature of the nodules distinguishes them from frank abscesses. The organisms are found in colonies in the nodules' caseous center, surrounded by layers of granulation tissue which give the gross appearance a laminated character. Giant cells are seldom seen but purulent reaction, particularly in confluent nodules, is not infrequent.

In young swine, the lungs are most frequently affected by bronchopneumonia and the intrathoracic lymph nodes are edematous or contain granulomas. In adult swine, nodules are more apt to be seen involving lungs, thoracic lymph nodes, liver, spleen and less often other lymph nodes. Affected goats usually are found to be emaciated, have a head tilt and terminally are comatose. The lesions are usually more widely distributed than in swine and the nodules smaller. Ulcers may be found in the mucosa of the nasal septum and trachea; nodules and consolidated areas occur in the lungs, and multiple nodules are evident in the respiratory lymph nodes, spleen and liver. A few nodules may be found in the heart, wall of the cecum, bladder wall and mesentery. Nodules are also described in the lung of the affected horse, 2 to 3 mm. in diameter, with a yellowish caseous center. The lungs may be edematous and consolidated, peritoneal effusion evident and occasionally purulent pyelitis may be associated with the presence of the organism.

The **diagnosis** is dependent upon demonstration of the causative organism, *Malleomyces pseudomallei* in characteristic lesions and their isolation and identification.

Glanders and Melioidosis

FOURNIER, J.: La Mélioidose et le B. De Whitmore Controverses Épidémiologiques et Taxonomiques. Bull. Soc. Path. Exot. *58*:753–765, 1965.

MENDELSON, R. W.: Glanders. U. S. Armed Forces Med. J. *1*:781–784, 1950.

NGUYEN-BA-LUONG: La Melioidose Porcine au Viet-Nam. Bull. Off. Int. Epiz. *56*:964–976, 1964.

OMAR, A. R., CHEAH KOK KHEONG, and MAHENDRANATHAN, T.: Observations on Porcine Melioidosis in Malaya. Brit. Vet. J. *118*:421–429, 1962. VB 416–63.

OMAR, A. R.: Pathology of Melioidosis in Pigs, Goats and a Horse. J. Comp. Path. *73*:359–372, 1963.

RETNASABAPATHY, A., and JOSEPH, P. G.: A Case of Melioidosis in a Macaque Monkey. Vet. Rec. *79*:72–73, 1966.

STRAUSS, J. M., et al.: Melioidosis With Spontaneous Remission of Osteomyelitis in a Macaque (*Macaca nemestrina*). J. Am. Vet. Med. Assn. *155*:1169–1175, 1969.

THONN, S. et al.: Note sur une Epizootie de Mélioidose Porcine au Cambodge. (Outbreak of Melioidosis in Pigs in Cambodia.) Rev. Elevage. *13*:175–179, 1960. VB 1004–61.

SALMONELLOSIS

The genus *Salmonella* is made up of many species of antigenically related bacterial organisms which are Gram-negative, rod-shaped, 0.4 to 0.6 micron wide and 1 to 3 microns long. They do not form spores, are usually motile, and in culture regularly ferment glucose but not lactose. All the known species are pathogenic for man, animals, or both. A complex system of antigenic analysis is used to identify and classify the types of organisms making up this genus. A wide variety of diseases are associated with Salmonella, including fowl typhoid (*Salmonella gallinarum*) an enteric and septicemic disease of adult poultry; pullorum disease (*S. pullorum*) a similar infection of young chicks; equine abortion (*S. abortus-equi*); mouse typhoid (*S. typhimurium*); enteritis and septicemia in pigs (*S. choleraesuis*), horses (*S. typhimurium*), monkeys (*S. anatum, S. typhimurium*), and cattle (*S. dublin, S. typhimurium*); ovine abortion (*S. abortus-ovis*); typhoid fever in man (*S. typhosa*); and paratyphoid fever in man (*S. paratyphi*). This represents only a partial list of the numerous known serotypes of salmonellac Certain of these cause specific diseases and are host specific, such as *S. abortus-equi* in equine abortion, and *S. typhosa* in human typhoid fever. Other serotypes are not host specific, producing disease, usually gastroenteritis or septicemia, in a variety of hosts. For example *S. typhimurium* produces gastroenteritis, occasionally leading to septicemia, in cattle, horses, rodents, and man. These organisms are often secondary invaders in virus diseases, such as hog cholera, but are believed to contribute greatly to losses from death. Overcrowding, transport and exposure to cold also increase susceptibility to salmonellae. The infections are most frequent and of greatest concern in young animals. Recovered animals may become carriers and shed salmonellae in their feces, representing a serious obstacle to control of the infection.

Salmonella, often originating in birds or mammals, are responsible for a specific "food poisoning" in man. These organisms produce a toxin which causes severe gastro-enteritis with nausea, vomiting, cramps and diarrhea, which characteristically appears eighteen to twenty-four hours following ingestion of contaminated food. Fatalities are uncommon, but explosive outbreaks can be very alarming and involve large numbers of people.

Lesions.—The lesions of salmonellosis or "paratyphoid fever" in animals are those of enterocolitis and septicemia. The stomach and proximal small intestine are usually spared with enteritis commencing in the ileum and extending through the colon. The mucosa is hyperemic to frankly hemorrhagic, thickened, often covered with a red, yellow or grey exudate and may contain distinct ulcers. Microscopically in the mucosa there is hemorrhage, edema, necrosis and a marked leukocytic infiltration principally composed of macrophages. Lesions in other organs are less consistent. Although not pathognomonic, more specific lesions are found in the liver. These include small foci of necrosis and the so-called "paratyphoid nodules" ("typhoid" nodules in typhoid fever of man). The latter consist of small aggregations of reticulo-endothelial cells (histiocytes, macrophages) which may occur in association with or independent of hepatic necrosis. The Kupffer cells become prominent and the sinusoids may contain numerous leukocytes.

Reticulo-endothelial hyperplasia is present in lymph nodes and the spleen, which may cause enlargement of these tissues. Hemorrhage and necrosis is common in mesenteric lymph nodes. In septicemic cases there are, invariably, petechiae or ecchymoses on the pleura, peritoneum, endocardium, kidney and meninges.

Of especial interest is the recent study by Innes, Wilson and Ross (1956) of an epizootic disease associated with *Salmonella enteritidis* infection in hamsters. This highly fatal disease was reproduced experimentally in other hamsters with *Salmonella* which had been recovered from spontaneous cases; the organisms were then demonstrated in the induced disease. The lesions included erosion of intestinal epithelium and necrosis of intestinal lymphoid nodules with characteristic focal necrosis in liver and spleen. Of particular interest, however, was the occurrence of phlebothrombosis in the pulmonary veins, with few or no pneumonic changes but occasionally accompanied by septic emboli in the renal glomeruli.

Abortion in mares caused by *S. abortus-equi* is no longer a common disease in the United States. Characteristically, most abortions caused by this agent occur between the sixth and ninth months of gestation. The placenta is edematous and contains focal hemorrhage and necrosis. There is usually edema and hemorrhage of the fetus but specific lesions are lacking. Infected foals born at term are weak and die within a few days often with suppurative polyarthritis.

Diagnosis.—Salmonellosis can be suspected on the basis of gross and histopathologic findings, however the lesions are not specific and isolation of the causative agent in association with lesions is necessary for confirmation.

Salmonellosis

ARMSTRONG, W. H.: Occurrence of *Salmonella typhimurium* Infection in Muskrats. Cornell Vet. *32*:87–89, 1942.
ARSOV, R., and DHAWEDKAR, R. G.: Clinico-Microbiological and Immunological Studies on Experimental Oral Infection in Pregnant Sheep with Salmonella Abortus Ovis. Indian Vet. J. *46*:1–5, 1969.

BRUNER, D. W., and MORGAN, A. B.: Salmonella Infection of Domestic Animals. Cornell Vet. 39:53–63, 1949.

COBURN, D. R., ARMSTRONG, W. H., and WETMORE, P. W.: Observations on Bacterin Treatment of *Salmonella Typhimurium* Infections in Chinchillas. Am. J. Vet. Res. 3:96–99, 1942.

CORDY, D. R., and DAVIS, R. W.: An Outbreak of Salmonellosis in Horses and Mules. J. Am. Vet. Med. Assn. 108:20–24, 1946.

GOOD, R. C., MAY, B. D., and KAWATOMARI, T.: Enteric Pathogens in Monkeys. J. Bact. 97:1048–1055, 1969.

GORHAM, J. R., CORDY, D. R., and QUORTRUP, E. R.: Salmonella Infections in Mink and Ferrets. Am. J. Vet. Research 10:183–192, 1949.

INNES, J. R. M., WILSON, C., and ROSS, M. A.: Epizoötic *Salmonella enteritidis* Infection Causing Septic Pulmonary Phlebothrombosis in Hamsters. J. Infect. Dis. 98:133–141, 1956.

KENT, T. H., FORMAL, S. B., LABREC, E. H.: Salmonella Gastroenteritis in Rhesus Monkeys. Arch. Path. 82:272–279, 1966.

PETERSON, K. J., and COON, R. E.: Salmonella Typhimurium Infection in Dairy Cows. J. Am. Vet. Med. Assn. 151:344–350, 1967.

SEGHETTI, L.: Observations Regarding *Salmonella choleraesuis* (var. *kunzendorf*) Septicemia in Swine. J. Am. Vet. Med. Assn. 109:134–137, 1946.

SMITH, H. W., and JONES, J. E. T.: Observation On Experimental Oral Infection With Salmonella Dublin in Calves and Salmonella Choleraesuis in Pigs. J. Path. Bact. 93:141–156, 1967.

STEVENS, A. J., GIBSON, E. A., and HUGHES, L. E.: Salmonellosis: The Present Position in Man and Animals. III. Recent Observations on Field Aspects. Vet. Rec. 80:154–161, 161–167, 177, 1967.

TAKEUCHI, A., and SPRINZ, H.: Electronmicroscope Studies of Experimental Salmonella Infection in the Preconditioned Guinea Pig. II. Response of the Intestinal Mucosa to the Invasion by Salmonella Typhimurium. Amer. J. Path. 51:137–161, 1967.

SHIGELLA INFECTION OF FOALS

A specific infection of equines appearing during the neonatal period is caused by *Actinobacillus equuli*, formerly *Shigella equuli* (*Shigella equirulis*, *Shigella viscosa*). The organism, a tiny rod-shaped bacterium which is Gram-negative and non-sporulating, may be distinguished by its cultural and antigenic characteristics. It has been recovered in numerous instances from newborn foals, the disease being contracted *in utero*, at parturition, or during the first few days after birth. Most infected foals die within the first three days of life, sometimes within eighteen hours, but others may survive for a month or longer. Occasionally adult horses are affected. The organisms have been isolated from involved joints, fetal membranes, viscera (especially kidneys), umbilical cord or heart blood, and occasionally from infected verminous lesions in mesenteric arteries (p. 753). *Actinobacillus equuli* is the most common cause of *pyosepticemia neonatorum*, "joint-ill," "navel ill," or "septicemia of foals."

The disease must be suspected in newborn foals which are weak, unable to stand or nurse, have swollen, hot and painful joints, fever, and depression, or which die suddenly with a few days of birth.

Lesions.—Lesions may be difficult to discern in foals which die shortly after birth with a fulminant, septicemic infection, but if the foal survives a few days, gross lesions may become recognizable. Infected joints are enlarged and contain excessive amounts of synovial fluid admixed with sanguineous or purulent exudate. The most characteristic gross changes are observed in the kidney (Fig. 5–4B), in which tiny gray foci, all approximately equal in size, are uniformly distributed throughout the cortex. The renal medulla may contain hemorrhages but it is remarkably free from the gray foci which are demonstrable microscopically as tiny abscesses. These abscesses result from a shower of bacterial emboli which lodge in the capillaries, particularly in the glomerular tufts. Similar abscesses may occur in other organs but much less frequently than in the kidney.

Diagnosis can be confirmed by isolation of the organisms or by demonstration of typical gross and microscopic lesions in which the bacteria are present.

Shigellosis (foals)

DIMOCK, W. W., EDWARDS, P. R., and BULLARD, J. F.: *Bacterium viscosum equi:* a Factor in Joint-ill and Septicemia in Young Foals. J. Am. Vet. Med. Assn. *73*:163–172, 1928.
EDWARDS, P. R.: Studies on *Shigella equirulis.* Kentucky Agr. Exper. Sta. Bull. No. 320, 1931.

BACILLARY DYSENTERY
(Shigellosis)

Primates are the only hosts which are naturally susceptible to infection with dysentery bacilli. The disease is well known in man and has been described in a variety of non-human primate species. It represents a disease of particular importance and frequency in Old-World monkeys. *Shigella flexneri* is the most prevalent pathogen, but *Sh. sonnei,* and *Sh. dysenteriae* also occur with frequency. The strains of these shigellae species are infectious to man but they are not the strains which produce severe dysentery in man, and, fortunately, transmission from monkey to man is rare. The infection is readily transmissible between monkeys and often occurs as an epizootic. Control is hampered by infectious carriers which shed the bacilli in the absence of clinical disease.

Clinically the dysentery varies from mild diarrhea to severe watery or mucoid diarrhea mixed with blood. Animals become dehydrated, and rapidly lose condition. The pathologic changes are varied, nonspecific, and usually confined to the colon. The colonic mucosa is swollen, and granular, with patchy or diffuse hemorrhage. Ulceration may or may not be present. The intestinal lumen contains varied quantities of mucus and blood. Other findings may include serosal petechiae, hyperemia of the mesentery and enlarged and hemorrhagic mesenteric lymph nodes.

Microscopically the colitis is characterized by hyperemia, edema, hemorrhage, necrosis and desquamation of the mucosal epithelium. Large numbers of neutrophils and macrophages infiltrate the mucosa. The submucosa is usually edematous and hyperemic, but only rarely is there necrosis or cellular exudation.

Diagnosis requires isolation and identification of the causative organism.

Bacillary Dysentery

FORMAL, S. B., *et al.*: Fluorescent-Antibody and Histological Study of Vaccinated and Control Monkeys Challenged with *Shigella flexneri.* J. Bact. *91*:2368–2376, 1966.
MANNHEIMER, H. S., and RUBIN, L. D.: An Epizootic of Shigellosis in a Monkey Colony. J. Am. Vet. Med. Assn. *155*:1181–1185, 1969.
TAKEUCHI, A., FORMAL, S. B., and SPRINZ, H.: Experimental Acute Colitis in the Rhesus Monkey Following Peroral Infection with *Shigella flexneri:* An Electron Microscopic Study. Amer. J. Path. *52*:503–529, 1968.
TAKEUCHI, A., *et al.*: Experimental Bacillary Dysentery—An Electron Microscopic Study of the Response of the Intestinal Mucosa to Bacterial Invasion. Amer. J. Path. *47*:1011–1044, 1965.
LAPIN, B. A., and YAKOOVLEVA, L. A.: *Comparative Pathology in Monkeys.* Springfield, Charles C Thomas, 1963.

PASTEURELLOSIS

"Pasteurellosis" is the designation for all animal diseases associated with organisms of the genus *Pasteurella*, named for Louis Pasteur who was the first to describe a member of this genus, the agent of fowl cholera (*Pasteurella multocida*). Recently *Yersinia* has been recommended to replace *Pasteurella* as the official designation for this genus. In view of the seesawing that generic names are often subjected to, we will continue to employ *Pasteurella* and wait the test of time. Five pathogenic species are included in the genus. *Pasteurella tularensis*, the cause of tularemia, has been considered earlier in this chapter (p. 599). *Pasteurella Yers* *pestis*, the cause of plague, is principally of importance as a pathogen to man and wild rodents. *Pasteurella pseudotuberculosis*, the cause of pseudotuberculosis, is discussed separately (p. 609).

Included in this section, designated pasteurellosis, are diseases of mammalian species associated with *Pasteurella multocida* and *Pasteurella hemolytica*. These two species have been isolated from a variety of animals, but the associated diseases are most readily grouped bacteriologically, for the clinical and pathologic manifestations are varied, often obscure, and poorly understood. Because septicemia with widespread hemorrhages is often the principal or only gross lesion, the term "hemorrhagic septicemia" has been applied to this group of diseases. A pneumonic form generally referred to as "shipping fever," is another frequent expression of pasteurellosis. Continuing research is needed to establish the exact causal role of these bacteria, the possible influence of as yet unknown viruses, and the effect of other deleterious factors. It cannot be stated unequivocally that *Pasteurella* is the sole cause of hemorrhagic septicemia, even though organisms of this generic type are commonly or constantly recovered from fatal cases.

Clinical names which have been applied to the pasteurelloses occurring in various species include: hemorrhagic septicemia and shipping fever of cattle; fowl cholera; swine plague; "snuffles," pneumonia and septicemia in rabbits; and pneumonia and hemorrhagic septicemia in sheep. *Pasteurella multocida* and *Pasteurella hemolytica* have also been associated with meningitis and arthritis in calves, bovine mastitis and ovine mastitis.

Lesions.—The gross lesions in fatal cases of pasteurellosis are diverse and hardly specific. In cattle, losses following shipping ("shipping fever," "shipping pneumonia") are usually the result of pneumonia, consolidation of the lung being most frequent in the apical portions, less often extending to the diaphragmatic lobes. Interlobular edema may be present but is seldom prominent, nor are hemorrhages outstanding in the bovine disease. Pneumonic pasteurellosis is usually associated with *Pasteurella hemolytica*. Organisms are reportedly numerous in the pneumonic areas of the lung. Widespread petechiae are the principal findings in "hemorrhagic septicemia" of cattle which is believed to be caused by *Pasteurella multocida*. In rabbits, upper respiratory symptoms ("snuffles") may be followed by pleuritis and pneumonia or by acutely fatal septicemia in which the blood teems with *Pasteurella*. Petechiae on the pericardium and serous surfaces are often the only lesions evident grossly. Fowl cholera most commonly affects chickens, but ducks, swans, turkeys, geese and other birds are susceptible. The disease is usually an overwhelming, fulminant bacteremia in these species. Pathologic changes observed at necropsy may be limited to a few petechiae on the heart and pericardium, swelling of the spleen and slight congestion of the upper part of the digestive tract. Swine may be infected with *Pasteurella* as a complication or sequel of hog cholera or swine influenza. Pneumonic lesions are commonly found at necropsy of swine.

Biberstein and Kennedy (1959) have described a septicemic disease of lambs associated with the presence of *Pasteurella hemolytica*. This is apparently similar to the disease described by Stamp (1955) in Scotland. The important gross lesions in fatal cases were hemorrhages on serosal surfaces, with congestion and edema in lungs and lymph nodes. Bacterial colonies, rarely associated with much inflamation, were demonstrated microscopically in the lungs, liver, spleen and adrenal cortex. These colonies were often in capillaries and were considered to be characteristic of the disease.

In man *Pasteurella multocida* is one of the more common organisms found in infected wounds resulting from animal (dog and cat) bites.

Pasteurellosis

BIBERSTEIN, E. L., KENNEDY, P. C.: Systemic pasteurellosis in lambs. Am. J. Vet. Res. *20*: 94–101, 1959.

CARTER, G. R.: Pasteurellosis: *Pasteurella multocida* and *Pasteurella hemolytica*. Advances Vet. Sci. *11*:321–379, 1967.

ERICSON, C. and JUHLIN, I.: A case of *Pasteurella multocida* infection after a cat bite. Acta. Path. Microbiol. Scand. *46*:47–50, 1951.

HAGEN, K. W.: Enzootic pasteurellosis in domestic rabbits, I Pathology and Bacteriology. J. Am. Vet. Med. Assn. *133*:77–80, 1958.

ROGERS, R. J., and ELDER, J. K.: Purulent Leptomeningitis in a Dog Associated With An Aerogenic *Pasteurella multocida*. Aust. Vet. J. *43*:81–82, 1967.

STAMP, J. T., WATT, J. A. A., and TOMLINSON, J. R.: *Pasteurella hemolytica* septicemia in lambs. J. Comp. Path. *65*:183–196, 1955.

THOMSON, R. G., BENSON, M. L., and SAVAN, M.: Pneumonic Pasteurellosis of Cattle: Microbiology and Immunology. Can. J. Comp. Med. *33*:194–206, 1969.

PSEUDOTUBERCULOSIS

Pseudotuberculosis is principally a disease of guinea pigs, other rodents and birds caused by *Pasteurella pseudotuberculosis*. However, natural infections have been recorded in numerous animal species, including man, rabbits, mice, deer, cats, swine, monkeys, sheep, goats, chinchilla, mink, horses, and a variety of birds and exotic mammals. The infection can occur as a rapidly fatal acute septicemia in which a few specific lesions are encountered, or more usually as a subacute or chronic infection characterized by discrete, white or gray nodules in the liver, spleen, lungs and lymph nodes. **Microscopically,** the nodules consist of a necrotic core containing pus and bacteria, surrounded by a zone of macrophages. In lesions of longer duration, epithelioid cells may be present and peripheral fibrous encapsulation commences. Giant cells are absent. **Diagnosis** usually requires isolation and identification of *Pasteurella pseudotuberculosis*. The disease must be differentiated from *Corynebacterium kutscheri* infection (p. 593).

Yersinia enterocolitica infection, which is also known as pseudotuberculosis, produces essentially identical lesions in man and animals. Most frequently this infection involves the intestines and mesenteric lymph nodes. The causative agent is closely related to *P. pseudotuberculosis* and no doubt the two have been confused.

Pseudotuberculosis

FELDMAN, W. H., and KARLSON, A. G.: Pseudotuberculosis *in Diseases Transmitted from Animals to Man.* Hull, T. G. (Ed.), 5th Ed., Springfield, Charles C Thomas, 1963, pp. 605–623.

Leader, R. W., and Baker, G. A.:   A Report of Two Cases of *Pasteurella pseudotuberculosis* Infection in the Chinchilla.   Cornell Vet. *44*:262–267, 1954.

Langford, E. V.:   *Pasteurella pseudotuberculosis* Associated with Abortion and Pneumonia in the Bovine.   Can. Vet. J. *10*:208–211, 1969.

Mair, N. S., *et al.*: *Pasteurella pseudotuberculosis* Infection in the Cat: Two Cases. Vet. Rec. *81*:461–462, 1967.

Mair, N. S., *et al.*:   *Yersinia enterocolitica* Infection in the Bushbaby (Galago) Vet. Rec. *86*: 69–71, 1970.

Nilehn, B.:   Studies on *Yersinia enterocolitica*, with Special Reference to Bacterial Diagnosis and Occurrence in Human Enteric Disease.   Acta Path. Microbiol. Scand. Suppl. 206:1–48, 1969.

LISTERIOSIS

A small, rod-shaped, gram-positive bacterial organism, *Listeria* (formerly *Listerella*) *monocytogenes*, has been found in association with a number of diseases of man and animals and is undoubtedly the principal cause of some of them. Pure cultures of the organism have been obtained from human patients with meningitis, chickens with lesions of myocardial necrosis, rabbits with mononucleosis, and certain rodents (Gerbille) with liver lesions. The most important infection of lower animals occurs in cattle, sheep and goats in the form of encephalomyelitis (Listerella or Listeria encephalitis or "circling disease"). The organism has been recovered in cases of abortion in man, cattle, sheep and goats, as well as from the central nervous system of young swine which died with nervous manifestations. A systemic or septicemic form of listeriosis has been described in man, calves, lambs, swine, dogs, cats, rodents, and birds. *Listeria* has also been found incidentally in bovine mesenteric lymph nodes.

It is obvious that the clinical manifestations of listeriosis are diverse, since they include abortion in man, cattle, sheep and goats, and meningeal or encephalitic infection in man, cattle, sheep, goats and swine, and systemic (septicemic) infec-

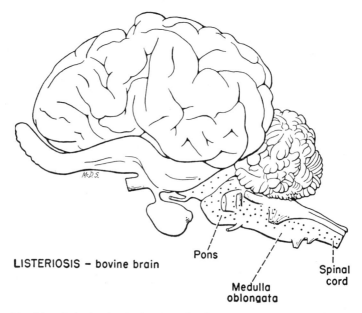

LISTERIOSIS – bovine brain

Pons

Medulla oblongata

Spinal cord

Fig. 12–14.—Listeriosis, bovine brain. Localization of lesions indicated by dots in pons, medulla and spinal cord. Compare with Fig. 10–17.

tion in man, cattle, sheep, swine, dogs, cats and rodents. Involvement of the central nervous system, considered most characteristic of the disease in ruminants, is manifested by abnormal posturing of the animal's head and neck and its walking aimlessly in a circle ("circling"). The conditions under which infection is likely to occur are poorly understood, although evidence points to certain feeding practices as predisposing to the disease.

Lesions.—The lesions are best approached by considering listeriosis in these forms: (1) encephalitis, (2) septicemia and (3) abortion.

Encephalitis.—The lesions in the central nervous system can be recognized only by microscopic examination and are confined to the brain stem, particularly the medulla oblongata and spinal cord. The primary lesion is a circumscribed collection of mononuclear cells, with or without neutrophils, in close proximity to blood vessels. Diffuse cellular infiltration and frank micro-abscesses may occur, but there is relatively little tissue necrosis. Nerve cells can be destroyed, but the lesions are not restricted to gray matter. In some cases, the gasserian ganglia are involved. The organisms, being gram-positive, can be demonstrated in tissue sections without difficulty with appropriate stains. They are found in the center of the lesions in the medulla oblongata or spinal cord. Intense meningeal infiltration of lymphoid cells is a characteristic accompaniment.

Visceral lesions similar to those described below in septicemic listeriosis may be encountered in both cattle and sheep with listeric encephalitis.

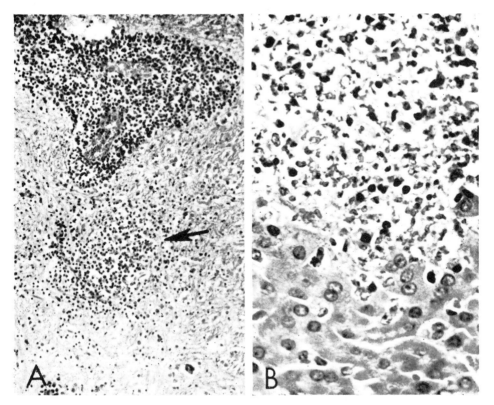

Fig. 12–15.—Listeriosis. *A*, Brain of a cow. Note perivascular cuffing and a "microabscess" (arrow). Courtesy Dr. C. L. Davis. *B*, Liver of a rat. There is focal necrosis with a moderate infiltration of neutrophils. (Courtesy Animal Research Center, Harvard Medical School.)

Septicemia.—Generalized listeriosis is most frequent in newborn and infants. The most characteristic lesion in this form is focal necrosis of the liver and less frequently of the spleen, lymph nodes, lungs, adrenals, myocardium, gastrointestinal tract and brain. Microscopically the lesions consist of focal areas of necrosis infiltrated with mononuclear cells and some neutrophils. The organisms are easily demonstrated with appropriately stained tissue sections.

Abortion.—Listeric abortion in animals is principally of importance in cattle and sheep. Abortion usually occurs in the last quarter of gestation without signs of infection in the dam. The fetus dies *in utero* and may be severely autolyzed when finally expelled. If not obscured, focal hepatic necrosis containing stainable organisms in the fetal liver is the principal lesion of diagnostic value.

Diagnosis.—The diagnosis of listeric encephalitis can be confirmed in suspicious cases by demonstration of the typical microscopic lesions which as indicated above include the combination of (1) micro-abscesses, diffuse purulent inflammation or glial nodules, (2) perivascular accumulation of lymphocytes, (3) lymphocytic leptomeningitis, and the gram-positive organisms associated with these lesions. Although the lesions in listeric septicemia and abortion are less specific than in listeric encephalitis, demonstration of the organisms within the necrotic lesions allows presumptive diagnosis. Confirmation can be made by isolation of the organisms in appropriate culture media inoculated with suspensions of tissue.

Listeriosis

ATTLEBERGER, M. H., and SEIBOLD, H. R.: Listeria Infection of Bovine Mesenteric Lymph Nodes. J. Am. Vet. Med. Assn. *128*:202–204, 1956.

BIESTER, H. E., and SCHWARTE. L. H.: Listerella Infection in Swine. J. Am. Vet. Med. Assn. *96*:339–342, 1940.

BORMAN, G., OLSON, C., SEGRE, D.: The trigeminal and facial nerves as pathways for infection of sheep with *Listeria monocytogenes*. Am. J. Vet. Res. *21*:993–1000, 1960.

CORDY, D. R. and OSEBOLD, J. W.: The neuropathogenesis of Listeria encephalemyelitis in sheep and mice. J. Infect. Dis. *104*:164–173, 1959.

GRAY, M. L., and KILLINGER, A. H.: Listeria Monocytogenes and Listeric Infections. Bact. Rev. *30*:309–382, 1966.

HARCOURT, R. A.: Listeria Monocytogenes in a Piglet. Vet. Rec. *78*:735, 1966.

JAKOB, W.: Further Experiments on the Pathogenesis of Cerebral Listeriosis in Sheep. I. Pathological Changes Caused by Freshly-Isolated Strains. Arch. Exp. Veterinaermed. *20*: 367–381, 1966.

KIDD, A. R. M., and TERLECKI, S.: Visceral and Cerebral Listeriosis in a Lamb. Vet. Rec. *78*:453–454, 1966.

KING, L. S.: Primary Encephalomyelitis in Goats Associated with Listerella Infection. Amer. J. Path. *16*:467–478, 1940.

OLAFSON, P.: Listerella Encephalitis (Circling Disease) of Sheep, Cattle, and Goats. Cornell Vet. *30*:141–150, 1940.

PULST, H.: Listeriosis in a Foal. Mh. Veterinaermed. *19*:742–744, 1964.

RITTENBACH, P., and MARTIN, J.: Experimental Listeriosis in Domestic and Experimental Animals. VIII. Experimental Listerial Abortion in Ewes. Arch. Exp. Veterinaermed. *19*: 681–730 1965.

SMITH, R. E., REYNOLDS, I. M., and BENNETT, R. A.: *Listeria Monocytogenes* and Abortion in a Cow. J. Am. Vet. Med. Assn. *126*:106–110, 1955.

SMITH, R. E., REYNOLDS, I. M., and CLARK, G. W.: Experimental Ovine Listeriosis. I. Inoculation of Pregnant Ewes. Cornell Vet. *58*:169–179, 1968.

YOUNG, S.: Listeriosis in Cattle and Sheep. pp. 95–107, *in Abortion Diseases of Livestock*. Faulkner, L. C. (Ed.). Springfield, Charles C Thomas, 1968.

TYZZER'S DISEASE

Tyzzer's disease is principally an infection of mice caused by *Bacillus piliformis*, a gram-negative, curved rod 10 to 40 μ long and 0.5 μ or less wide. The organism is an obligate intracellular parasite which has only been cultivated in tissue culture. *B. piliformis* appears to live as a saprophyte in many mouse colonies, producing disease under adverse environmental conditions and other forms of stress. The gross lesions consist of circular gray-white foci 1 to 2 mm. in diameter on the capsular and cut surfaces of the liver. Microscopically, these foci consist

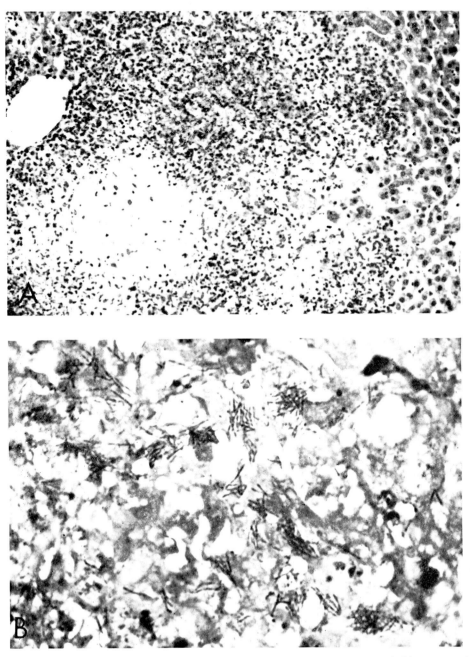

FIG. 12–16.—Tyzzer's disease in a mouse. *A*, Focal hepatic necrosis surrounded by a zone of inflammatory cells. *B*, Filamentous *Bacillus piliformis* in the cytoplasm of hepatocytes (Gomori's methenamine silver stain). (Tissue courtesy Dr. C. L. Davis.)

of focal areas of hepatic necrosis surrounded by a zone of neutrophils and a lesser number of lymphocytes and macrophages. Numerous organisms are present around the necrotic foci in the inflammatory zone and in intact hepatocytes. They usually cannot be seen in hematoxylin and eosin stained tissue sections, but are clearly evident in sections stained by the Giemsa, Gomori's methenamine silver and methylene blue techniques. Organisms are also found in intestinal epithelial cells, occasionally resulting in necrotizing enteritis. The mesenteric lymph nodes may contain small abscesses. Though usually of lesser importance as a spontaneous infection, Tyzzer's disease has been observed in rabbits, monkeys, rats, and gerbils. Necrotizing myocarditis has been reported in rabbits.

Tyzzer's Disease

ALLEN, A. M., *et al.*: Tyzzer's Disease Syndrome in Laboratory Rabbits. Amer. J. Path. *46*:859–882, 1965.

CARTER, G. R., WHITENACK, D. L., and JULIUS, L. A.: Natural Tyzzer's Disease in Mongolian Gerbils (*Meriones unguiculatus*). Lab. Anim. Care *19*:648–651, 1969.

FUJIWARA, K., *et al.*: Tyzzer's Disease in Mice: Pathologic Studies on Experimentally Infected Animals. Jap. J. Exp. Med. *33*:181–194, 1963.

PORT, C. D., RICHTER, W. R., and MOISE, S. M.: Tyzzer's Disease in the Gerbil (*Meriones unguiculatus*). Lab. Anim. Care *20*:109–111, 1970.

SAUNDERS, L. Z.: Tyzzer's Disease. J. Nat. Cancer Inst. *20*:893–897, 1958.

TYZZER, E. E.: A Fatal Disease of the Japanese Waltzing Mouse Caused by Spore-Bearing Bacillus (*Bacillus piliformis*, N. Sp.). J. Med. Res. *38*:307–338, 1917.

Chapter

13

Diseases Caused by Higher Bacteria and Fungi

The diseases to be described in this chapter have been grouped together not only for the reason that their causative agents are related, but also because the reactions these agents provoke in their hosts have certain striking similarities. Many of these diseases are characterized by the formation of epithelioid granulation tissue and thus may be conveniently classified as the "infectious granulomas." Included in this group are:

Actinomycosis	Pseudotuberculosis	Cryptococcosis
Actinobacillosis	Aspergillosis	Histoplasmosis
Nocardiosis	Epizoötic lymphangitis	Mucormycosis
Dermatophilus infection	Blastomycosis	Nasal granuloma of cattle
Tuberculosis	Coccidioidomycosis	Sporotrichosis
Paratuberculosis	Rhinosporidiosis	Protothecosis
Leprosy	Maduromycosis	Geotrichosis

The superficial mycoses also have a different reaction pattern, influenced more perhaps by the cutaneous habitat of the organism than by its intrinsic properties. Although possibly redundant, it is nonetheless pertinent to point out that the more closely organisms are related biologically, the more nearly identical will be the tissue reactions of their parasitized hosts. The infectious granulomas are of particular importance to the pathologist, because his techniques are especially valuable in arriving at their precise diagnosis.

General

BAKER, R. D. *et al.* (ed).: International Symposium on Opportunistic Fungus Infections. Lab. Invest. *11*:1017–1241, 1962.

CONANT, N. F. *et al.*: *Manual of Clinical Mycology.* 2nd ed., Philadelphia, W. B. Saunders Co., 1954.

CONNOLE, M. D., and JOHNSTON, L. A. Y.: A Review of Animal Mycoses in Australia. Vet. Bull. 37:145–153, 1967.

EMMONS, C. W., BINFORD, C. H., and UTZ, J. P.: *Medical Mycology.* 2nd ed. Philadelphia, Lea & Febiger, 1970.

METZGER, J. F., KASE, A., and SMITH, C. W.: Identification of Pathogenic Fungi in Surgical and Autopsy Specimens by Immunofluorescence. Mycopathologia. *17*:335–344, 1962. VB 467–63.

KAPLAN, W. and KAUFMAN, L.: The Fluorescent Antibody Technique and Fungal Diseases. Proc. 66th Ann. Meet. U. S. Livestock Sanit. Assn. Washington, 1962. pp. 417–425. 1963. VB 3875–63.

SAUNDERS, L. Z.: Fungous Diseases, in HULL, T. G.: *Diseases Transmitted from Animals to Man*, 4th ed., Springfield, Charles C Thomas, 1955, Chap. 23.

————: Systemic Fungous Infections in Animals. Cornell Vet. *38*:213–238, 1948.

ACTINOMYCOSIS

Actinomycosis is a disease of cattle, man and some other species, caused by a specific organism, *Actinomyces bovis* (*Actinomyces israeli* in man). The name of this disease has often been applied erroneously to somewhat similar infections, such as actinobacillosis and nocardiosis, which are caused by different etiologic agents. The most frequent and obvious manifestation of actinomycosis in cattle is the hard, irregular enlargement that results from infection of the mandible or, less often, the maxilla, and gives the disease its common name, "lumpy jaw." Similar infection of the mandible has been observed in wild ruminants such as elk. In dogs, actinomycosis usually affects soft tissues and may become generalized. In man, the cheek, mouth, skin of the chest, appendix and intestine are the usual sites of involvement. Actinomycotic infection of the porcine mammary glands is not uncommon, and the organisms also have been identified in association with *Brucella abortus* in equine "fistulous withers."

Lesions. — The organisms grow in tenacious colonies of microscopic size, located in tiny purulent centers surrounded by dense granulation tissue which displaces the nearby normal tissues. When the organisms penetrate bone, it becomes enlarged and honeycombed as a result of destructive rarefaction and regenerative proliferation. The cut surface of the lesion usually is white and glistening from the dense connective tissue in which the small abscesses are embedded. Occasional sinus tracts may be demonstrated, with drainage through the skin or into the oral cavity. Expression of the yellowish pus from the abscesses yields tiny, hard masses called "sulfur granules" because of their gross consistency and yellowish color. Microscopically, these masses may appear as rosettes, and although early investigators considered them the "ray fungus," they are now known to be merely separate colonies of actinomyces organisms growing in characteristic fashion. In sections stained with hematoxylin and eosin, a colony appears as an eosinophilic, irregularly-shaped mass, 20 or more microns in diameter, surrounded by a zone of radially arranged projections with rounded ends, their shape suggesting Indian clubs or baseball bats. These radiating clubs are usually coarse, 3 to 10 microns in diameter and 10 to 30 microns in length, and brightly eosinophilic in color. Although their exact nature is not understood, it appears likely that they are a product of the cells of the host, rather than of the infecting organism.

The central part of the colony can be demonstrated by Gram's stain to be made up of a tangled mass of gram-positive, rod-shaped or long filamentous organisms, which are often beaded and occasionally branched. Beyond the radiating clubs there is usually a zone of neutrophils, surrounded by an outer area of large mononuclear (epithelioid) cells with abundant, often foamy, cytoplasm. Giant cells of the Langhans' type and lymphocytes are occasionally found in this region. The dense, moderately vascular connective tissue that separates the many abscesses from one another usually encapsulates the entire lesion.

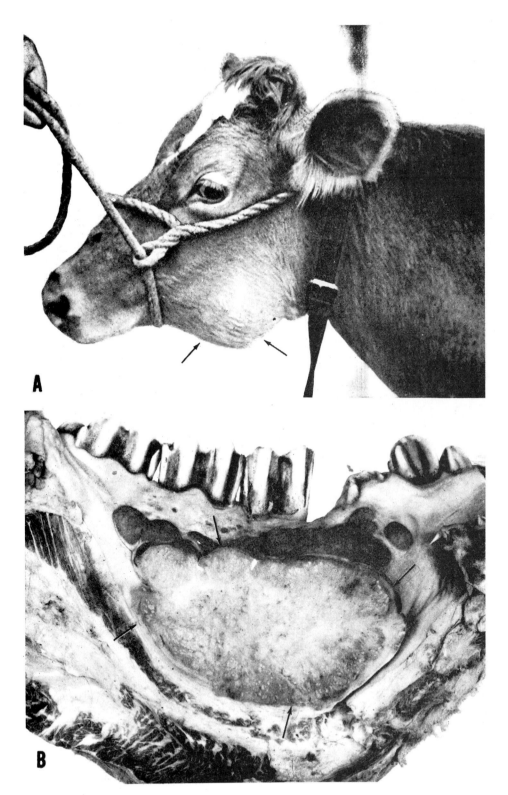

Fig. 13–1.—Actinomycosis. *A*, Lesions in mandible of a Guernsey cow. Case from clinic of College of Veterinary Medicine, Iowa State College. *B*, Gross specimen from mandible of a similar case. (Courtesy of Armed Forces Institute of Pathology.) Contributor: Major Lytle, V.C.

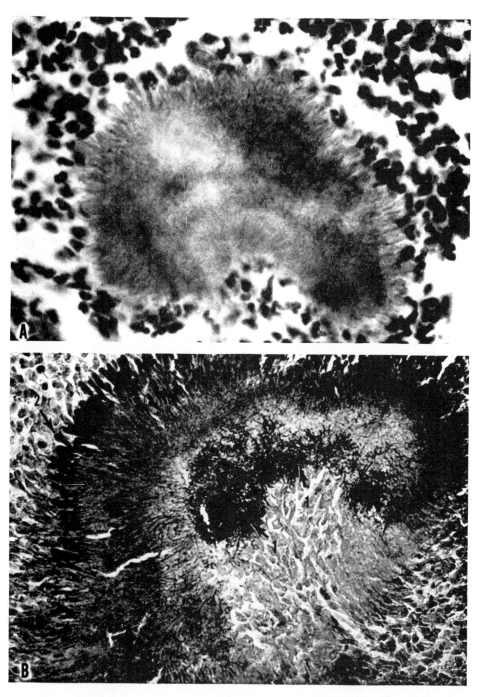

Fig. 13–2.—Actinomycosis. *A*, Colony of *Actinomyces bovis* ($\times$ 500), in a tissue section stained with hematoxylin and eosin. Contributor: Major Lytle, V.C. *B*, A similar colony of *Actinomyces bovis* ($\times$ 500) in a tissue section stained by Gram's method. Note tangled, branching, Gram-positive organisms in the center (*1*) surrounded by zones of radiating club-shaped structures (*2*). (Courtesy of Armed Forces Institute of Pathology.) Contributor: Dr. H. R. Seibold.

The colonies of actinomyces may become calcified in cases of long standing, in which event they assume a gritty texture as blue-staining granules of calcium salts replace the organisms.

Diagnosis.—The characteristic lesions can be identified positively by using Gram's stain on sections of fixed tissue to differentiate the gram-positive organisms at the center of the colonies. Organisms can also be demonstrated in smears of fresh, unfixed material stained by Gram's method. Successful cultures must be maintained under reduced oxygen tension, but they are seldom essential for diagnosis. The rosettes with the shiny, refractile, radiating clubs can be demonstrated in wet preparations of fresh pus compressed under a coverglass and examined with reduced illumination.

Differential diagnosis must include other granulomatous infections, but in particular actinobacillosis, nocardiosis and staphylococcosis (botryomycosis). The morphology of the bacterial colonies, and individual organisms and their staining reactions, which differ in each of these infections, allow ready differentiation.

ACTINOBACILLOSIS

Infection with *Actinobacillus lignieresi* (from the Latin *lignum* meaning wood) produces signs and gross lesions that resemble those of actinomycosis but differ in several respects. This organism may infect the jaw of cattle; but with far greater frequency it invades the tongue ("woody tongue"), lymph nodes of the

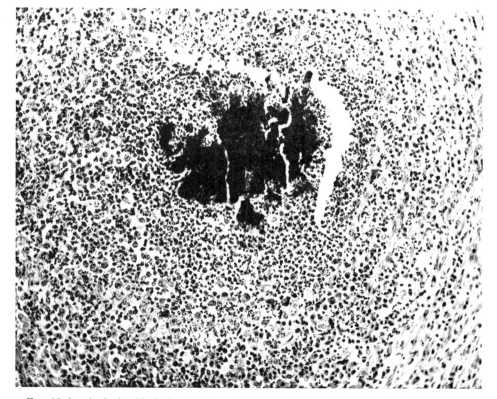

FIG. 13–3.—Actinobacillosis, lung of a cow (× 160). Colony of *Actinobacillus lignieresi* in the center of a tiny abscess. (Courtesy of Armed Forces Institute of Pathology.) Contributor: Dr. C. L. Davis.

head, neck and thorax, less often the lung, and rarely other organs. This infection in cattle is therefore much more frequent in soft tissues than in bones—a point of differentiation from actinomycosis. In the rare instances in which actinobacillosis occurs in sheep, it affects the soft tissues and lymph nodes related to the mouth and pharynx. Generalized infections have been described in man and experimentally inoculated guinea pigs. Localized soft tissue infection has been reported in dogs.

Lesions.—Microscopically, the lesions closely resemble actinomycosis, with discrete colonies of organisms surrounded by radiating clubs, suspended in pus, and encapsulated with rather dense connective tissue. The colonies tend to be much smaller, the radiating clubs longer and more slender, and the purulent exudate more abundant than in actinomycosis. Gram's stain of smears or sections reveals gram-negative, rod-shaped organisms in the center of the colonies, but they may be difficult to detect because of the acidophilic staining of the background.

In the tongue, where the abscesses are usually small, diffuse proliferation of connective tissue sometimes causes such great enlargement that the stiff, partially immobile tongue protrudes from the mouth. This is the so-called "woody tongue" of cattle. In lymph nodes, the usual change consists of the formation of an abscess, one to several centimeters in diameter, filled with thick, smooth, shiny pus which has marked cohesive, but slight adhesive properties. In the lungs and other tissues, the abscesses are usually much smaller.

Diagnosis.—In tissue sections, gram-negative material in the center of the colonies suffices to distinguish actinobacillosis from actinomycosis, nocardiosis and staphylococcus infections ("botryomycosis"). Demonstration of rosettes and the absence of gram-positive organisms in fresh preparations also establish the diagnosis in bovine material. Culture and identification of the organisms may be used to confirm the diagnosis further.

Actinobacillosis and Actinomycosis

AWAD, F. I.: Nocardiosis of the Bovine Udder and Testes. Vet. Rec. *72*:341–342, 1960.

CARB, A. V., and LIN, S-K.: *Actinobacillus ligniersii* Infection in a Dog. J. Am. Vet. Med. Assn. *154*:1062–1067, 1969.

COLEMAN, M., and GEORG, L. K.: Comparative Pathogenicity of *Actinomyces naeslundii* and *Actinomyces israelii*. Appl. Microbiol. *18*:427–432, 1969.

GINSBERG, A., and LITTLE, A. C. W.: Actinomycosis in Dogs. J. Path. & Bact. *60*:563–572, 1948.

MARTIN, H. M.: Actinomycosis of the Dog and Cat. University of Pennsylvania Bulletin, Veterinary Extension Quarterly, No. 87:15–19, June 16, 1942.

MENGES, R. W., LARSH, H. W., and HABERMANN, R. T.: Canine Actinomycosis. J. Am. Vet. Med. Assn. *122*:73–78, 1953.

PINE, L. and OVERMAN, J. R.: Determination of the Structure and Composition of the "Sulphur Granules" of Actinomyces Bovis. J. Gen. Microbiol. *32*:209–223, 1963. VB 4260–63.

ROBBOY, S. J., and VICKERY, A. L.: Tinctorial and Morphologic Properties Distinguishing Actinomycosis and Nocardiosis. New Eng. J. Med. *282*:593–596, 1970.

RYFF, J. F.: Encephalitis in a Deer due to *Actinomyces bovis*. J. Am. Vet. Med. Assn. *122*: 78–80, 1953.

SAUTTER, J. H., ROWSELL, H. C., and HOHN, R. B.: Actinomycosis and Actinobacillosis in Dogs. North Am. Vet. *34*:341–346, 1953.

SHAHAN, M. S., and DAVIS, C. L.: The Diagnosis of Actinomycosis and Actinobacillosis. Am. J. Vet. Research *3*:321–328, 1942.

SWERCZEK, T. W., SCHIEFER, B., and NIELSEN, S. W.: Canine Actinomycosis. Zentbl. Vet. Med. *15B*:955–970, 1968.

TILL, D. H., and PALMER, F. P.: A Review of Actinobacillosis With a Study of the Causal Organism. Vet. Rec. *72*:527–533, 1960.

NOCARDIOSIS

Infections with aerobic, gram-positive, filamentous organisms, which under some conditions have "acid-fast" staining properties, occur in man and animals, particularly dogs. The organisms have been known under several names (*Actinomyces asteroides, Cladothrix asteroides, Actinomyces gypsoides*) but at present are grouped in the genus *Nocardia* (*Nocardia asteroides*) from which comes the name nocardiosis. The lesions and organisms are sufficiently unlike those of actinomycosis to permit their differentiation.

In dogs, infection of the lungs and pleura or skin is most common, although systemic infection can occur and the organisms may localize in peritoneal and pleural cavities, in the brain, or in any visceral organ. The **lesions** are seen microscopically as tangled, indistinct colonies of organisms surrounded by necrotic cellular debris, purulent exudate and granulation tissue. The colonies are not surrounded by radiating clubs. The organisms can usually be demonstrated in the tissues as gram-positive, branching filaments, which are acid-fast when appropriately stained. Cultural identification of the organism is necessary to establish the diagnosis, although presumptive diagnoses can be made from tissue sections.

Nocardiosis is less frequent in other species but is a sporadic cause of bovine mastitis and pneumonia in monkeys. The lesions in these or other species are similar to those described in the dog.

Nocardia farcinica (which may be identical to *Nocardia asteroides*) is reportedly the cause of a disease of cattle known as bovine farcy. The infection is not known in the United States but has been described in the Sudan, the Far East and Latin America. The disease occurs as a chronic suppurative granulomatous inflammation of the skin, lymphatics and draining lymph nodes, usually confined to the limbs. In fatal infections there is metastasis to the lungs, liver, spleen and internal lymph nodes.

Nocardiosis

AWAD, F. I. and KARIB, A. A.: Studies on Bovine Farcy (Nocardiosis) among cattle in the Sudan. Zbl. Vet. Med. 5:265–272, 1958.

BOHL, E. H., JONES, D. O., FARRELL, R. L., CHAMBERLAIN, D. M., COLE, C. R., and FERGUSON, L. C.: Nocardiosis in the Dog. J. Am. Vet. Med. Assn. 122:81–85, 1953.

BROWN, A. R. and OSBORNE, A. D.: A Case of Canine Nocardiosis. Vet. Rec. 74:371–373, 1962. VB 2568–62.

CUTTINO, J. T., and McCABE, A. M.: Pure Granulomatous Nocardiosis: A New Fungus Disease Distinguished by Intracellular Parasitism. Am. J. Path. 25:1–47, 1949.

GINSBERG, A., and LITTLE, A. C. W.: Actinomycosis in Dogs. J. Path. & Bact. 60:563–572, 1948.

JONAS, A. M., and WYAND, D. S.: Pulmonary Nocardiosis in the Rhesus Monkey. Importance of Differentiation from Tuberculosis. Path. Vet. 3:588–600, 1966.

KINCH, D. A.: A Rapidly Fatal Infection Caused by Nocardia caviae in a Dog. J. Path. Bact. 95:540–546, 1968.

MOSTAFA, I. E.: Bovine Nocardiosis (Cattle Farcy). A Review. Vet. Bull. 36:189–193, 1966.

PIER, A. C.: Nocardiosis in Animals. Proc. 66th Ann. Meet. U. S. Livestock Sanit. Assn. Washington, 1962, pp. 409–415, 1963. VB 3872–63.

PIER, A. C., GRAY, D. M., and FORSATTI, M. J.: *Nocardia asteroides*—A Newly Recognized Pathogen of the Mastitis Complex. Am. J. Vet. Res. 19:319–331, 1958.

RODRIGUEZ, I. G.: Aportacion al Estudio de las Nocardiosis del Caballo. Una Enzootia de Nocardiosis Equina. Bol. Inf. Cons. Col. Vet. Esp. 8:747–757, 1961. VB 1416–62.

SWERCZEK, T. W., TRUTWEIN, G., and NIELSEN, S. W.: Canine Nocardiosis. Zentbl. Vet. Med. 15B:971–978, 1968.

THORDAL-CHRISTENSEN, A., and CLIFFORD, D. H.: Actinomycosis (Nocardiosis) in a Dog. Am. J. Vet. Research 14:298–306 1953.

DERMATOPHILUS INFECTION
(Cutaneous Streptothricosis)

Infection by the actinomycete *Dermatophilus congolensis* has been termed mycotic dermatitis, cutaneous streptothricosis, lumpy wool, strawberry foot rot,

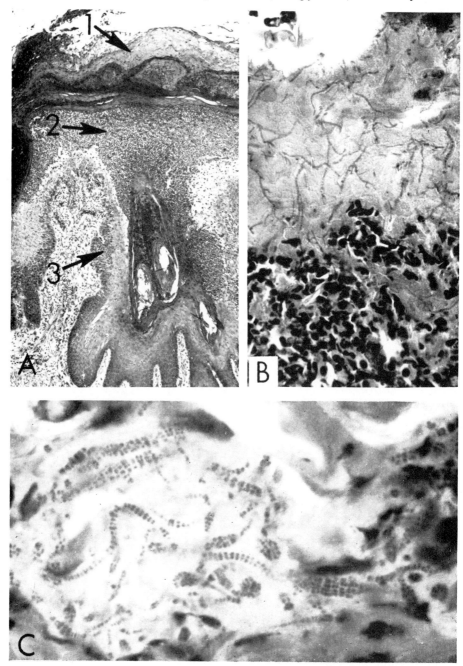

Fig. 13–4.—Dermatophilus infection, skin, owl monkey (*Aotus trivirgatus*). *A*, Characteristic lamination of cornified epithelium (*1*), purulent exudate (*2*) and regenerating epithelium (*3*). *B*, Mycelia in cornified epithelium. *C*, Characteristic multidimensional division of *Dermatophilus congolensis*. (Courtesy Dr. N. W. King, Jr.)

cutaneous actinomycosis and other terms which contain erroneous implications regarding the nature of the causal agent. Dermatophilus infection (the preferred designation) has been described in cattle, sheep, goats, deer, horses, dogs, monkeys and man. Rabbits, mice and guinea pigs have been experimentally infected. In each of these species with the exception of man, the gross and histopathologic changes are similar. The infection is limited to the skin producing raised, alopecic, and sometimes papillomatous lesions covered by thick keratinaceous incrustations. The lesions may be well circumscribed or confluent and may affect any portion of the body. The microscopic features are unique and best understood by explaining the pathogenesis of the infection. The organism invades and multiplies within the epidermis as branching filaments which divide in a characteristic multidimensional fashion, giving rise to multiple rows of coccoid organisms. They do not invade the dermis, but induce an extensive purulent exudate beneath the epidermis, separating it from the dermis. The invaded epidermis cornifies and a new epidermis forms under the exudate which in turn is invaded by hyphae at the periphery of the lesion. A second inflammatory exudate separates the new epidermis from the dermis and a third epithelium is generated. The process is repeated resulting in a thick scab composed of alternate strata of cornified epidermis and exudate. The organism can usually be seen in hematoxylin and eosin stained tissue sections and are clearly seen as gram-positive filaments or chains of cocci in sections stained with the Gram's technique.

The disease is transmitted by the coccoid forms which result from the multidimensional division of the hyphae. This stage, known as a zoospore, is motile and released when the scabs are exposed to moisture. Transmission can be direct or indirect through contaminated water or grasses. Insect transmission which has been demonstrated with flies and ticks, is believed to be a principal means of spreading zoospores.

Diagnosis can usually be made from the morphology of the exudate and demonstration of the organisms. If necessary, the organism can be cultured.

Dermatophilus Infection

BENTINCK-SMITH, J., FOX, F. H., and BAKER, D. W.: Equine Dermatitis (Cutaneous Streptothricosis) Infection with Dermatophilus in the U.S. Cornell Vet. *51*:334–349, 1961.
BRIDGES, C. H., and ROMANE, W. M.: Cutaneous Streptothricosis in Cattle. J. Am. Vet. Med. Assn. *138*:153–157, 1961.
GORDON, M. A.: The Genus Dermatophilus. J. Bact. *88*:509–522, 1964.
LERICHE, P. D.: The Transmission of Dermatophilosis (Mycotic Dermatitis) in Sheep. Aust. Vet. J. *44*:64–67, 1968.
RICHARD, J. L., and PIER, A. C.: Transmission of Dermatophilus congolensis by Stomoxys Calcitrans and Musca Domestica. Am. J. Vet. Res. *27*:419–423, 1966.
ROBERTS, D. S.: Dermatophilus Infection. Vet. Bull. *37*:513–521, 1967.
————: The Histopathology of Epidermal Infection with the Actinomycete, *Dermatophilus congolensis*. J. Path. Bact. *90*:213–216, 1965.
SEARCY, G. P., and HULLAND, T. J.: Dermatophilus dermatitis (streptothricosis) in Ontario. I. Clinical Observations. II. Laboratory Findings. Can. Vet. J. *9*:7–15 & 16–21, 1968.

NECROBACILLOSIS

Several necrotizing disease processes involving herbivorous animals have been associated with the presence of a certain anaerobic, non-sporulating, gram-negative, filamentous organism, currently named *Spherophorus necrophorus* (*Fusiformis necrophorus*). There is little doubt that this organism can be recov-

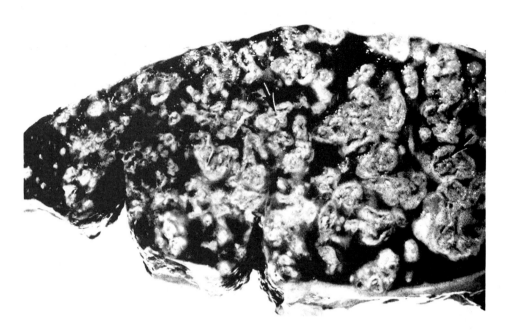

FIG. 13–5.—Necrobacillosis. Irregularly shaped necrotic and encapsulated lesions (arrows) in a bovine spleen. Photograph courtesy of Dr. Wm. J. Hadlow.

ered from animal lesions, but there is serious question that it is the sole, or even the primary cause of disease. Since these lesions are encountered with some frequency, it appears advisable to describe them briefly and express the hope that future research will contribute to a better understanding.

In horses, a severe necrotizing disease of the feet appears in animals which are forced to remain for long periods in deep, manure- and urine-soaked mud. This "gangrenous dermatitis" usually starts at the heel or in the deep structures of the frog and results in irregular areas of sharply demarcated necrosis involving large amounts of tissue. It often produces serious disability.

In cattle, necrophorus organisms are found in the elevated, tenacious, necrotic plaques of the larynx, pharynx and trachea, commonly referred to as "calf diphtheria." They also have been demonstrated in bovine cases which terminated fatally in pneumonia. Large, sharply delimited foci of necrosis also occur in the liver and spleen of adult cattle, particularly those which are heavily fed. The hepatic lesions are associated with ulcerations of the rumen and are discussed further in Chapter 24, page 1231. In the Sudan, the disease in cattle has been reported to involve the subcutis, lymph vessels and nodes with occasional spread to internal organs or in some cases the internal organs are infected without apparent lesions in the subcutis. (See "bovine farcy" p. 621.) Foot rot of cattle (infectious pododermatitis) is invariably associated with *Spheropherus necrophorus.*

Ulcerative, necrotizing stomatitis and enteritis (p. 1206) in swine have been questionably attributed to *Spherophorus necrophorus* as has a disfiguring type of rhinitis ("bullnose"). The similarity of the external appearance of the nose of affected swine is some evidence that this latter entity might have been confused in the past with atrophic rhinitis (Chapter 21, p. 1094).

In sheep the necrophorus organism is associated with an obligate parasite, *Fusiformis nodosus,* and possibly a third organism, *Spirochaeta penortha,* in ovine "foot rot." Foot abscess and "lip and leg ulceration" have also been ascribed to necrophorus infection. However, it is quite doubtful that this organism is the cause of these disease conditions in sheep.

Necrobacillosis

Britton, J. W.: An unusual infection in a foal. Cornell Vet. *37*:391–393, 1947.

Egerton, J. R., Roberts, D. S., and Parsonson, I. M.: The Aetiology and Pathogenesis of Ovine Foot-Rot. I. A Histological Study of the Bacterial Invasion. J. Comp. Path. *79*: 207–215, 1969.

Jensen, R., Flint, J. C., and Griner, L. A.: Experimental hepatic necrobacillosis in beef cattle. Am. J. Vet. Res. *15*:5–14, 1954.

Mackey, D. R.: Calf Diphtheria. J. Am. Vet. Med. Assn. *152*:822–823, 1968.

Marsh, H.: Necrobacillosis of the rumen in young lambs. J. Am. Vet. Med. Assn. *104*:23–25 1944.

Roberts, D. S., and Egerton, J. R.: The Aetiology and Pathogenesis of Ovine Foot-Rot. II. The Pathogenic Association of *Fusiformis nodosus* and *F. necrophorus.* J. Comp. Path. *79*:217–227, 1969.

Simon, P. C., and Stovell, P. L.: Diseases of Animals Associated with Sphaerophorus necrophorus: Characteristics of the Organism. Vet. Bull. *39*:311–315, 1969.

TUBERCULOSIS

Tuberculosis remains one of the most prevalent and devastating diseases of man and animals in spite of great strides made in its control and treatment. It occurs in all species of domestic animals and birds and in most wild animals, but presents a particularly serious problem in cattle, swine, domestic birds and captive subhuman primates. Throughout most of the world, the bovine disease is widespread, but in the United States, Denmark and some other countries its incidence has been greatly reduced by tuberculin testing and elimination of infected animals. In these countries, the control of bovine tuberculosis has dramatically reduced the prevalence of infection of the bovine type in man and animals.

The causative agents are acid-fast bacilli classified in the genus *Mycobacterium.* Three principal species cause tuberculosis, *i.e.,* human, bovine, and avian organisms presently classified as *M. tuberculosis, M. bovis,* and *M. avium* respectively (Wayne *et al.* 1969). These organisms produce similar lesions, closely resemble one another morphologically, being small acid-fast bacillary forms, but vary in cultural characteristics, antigenic composition, and pathogenicity to various species. Tubercle bacilli of human type are found most frequently in man but may infect other animals, both under natural and experimental conditions. Cattle usually are infected with the bovine type but are susceptible to the human type and may contract the disease from human sources. Birds most frequently harbor tubercle bacilli of the avian type. Swine are susceptible to all three types; they may be exposed to the bovine type by ingestion of excrement from infected cattle, to the avian, by eating infected chickens, and to the human, by consumption of infected garbage or contact with human wastes. In man, the bovine organisms may also be responsible for lesions, especially those in non-pulmonary sites—intestinal tract, lymph nodes, bones and joints. Such lesions are most common in children who drink milk from tuberculous cows. In rare instances, tubercle bacilli of the avian type are known to have caused human infection. In dogs, infection of the human type usually results from close association with man, and infections of the bovine type also may occur. Horses are susceptible to organisms of both human and bovine types, and in rare instances, have been reported to be infected with the avian type. Cats have found to be susceptible to and most often infected with the bovine type, but in a recent instance a Siamese cat had severe lesions in lymph nodes and lung from which an avian type tubercle bacillus was recovered. Captive nonhuman primates, espe-

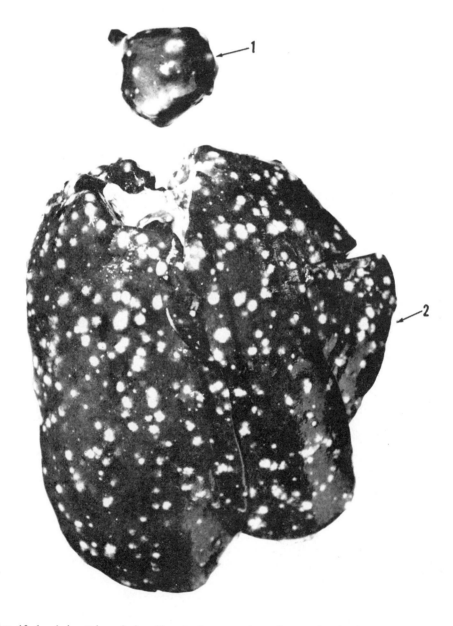

FIG. 13–6.—Avian tuberculosis. Sharply demarcated, confluent tubercles in spleen (1) and liver (2) of a chicken. Photograph courtesy of Dr. Wm. J. Hadlow.

cially Old-World monkeys and anthropoid apes, are very susceptible to organisms of the human type, and consequently the disease is an important problem in zoos and laboratories. New-World species are also susceptible, but reports in these species have been fewer.

Most mammals have considerable natural resistance to the avian type bacilli

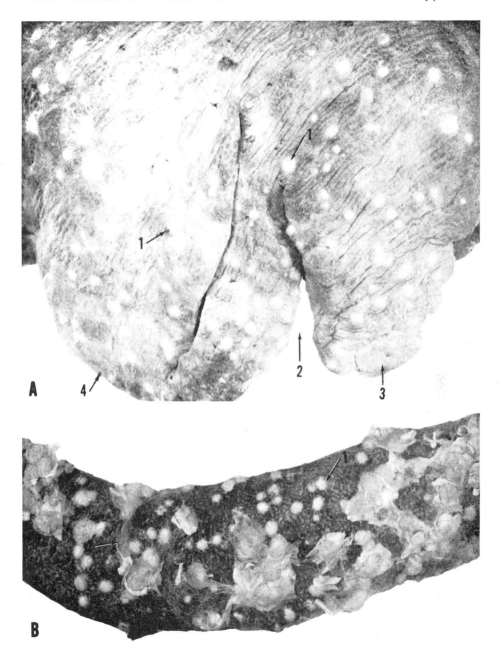

Fig. 13-7.—Tuberculosis in swine. *A*, Lung. Sharply demarcated nodules (*1*) elevating the pleura. Cardiac notch (*2*), apical lobe (*3*) and inferior border (*4*) of the lung. *B*, Nodules in the spleen (*1*), adhesions of mesentery (*2*). (Courtesy of Armed Forces Institute of Pathology.) Contributor: Dr. B. A. Walter.

but it has been reported in cats, cattle, swine, man, horses, sheep, goats, dogs and monkeys. Usually the infection is limited to lymph nodes, and tubercles are often not detectable grossly.

Atypical mycobacteria, culturally distinct from the three classical tubercle bacilli, have become increasingly important as causes of tuberculosis in man.

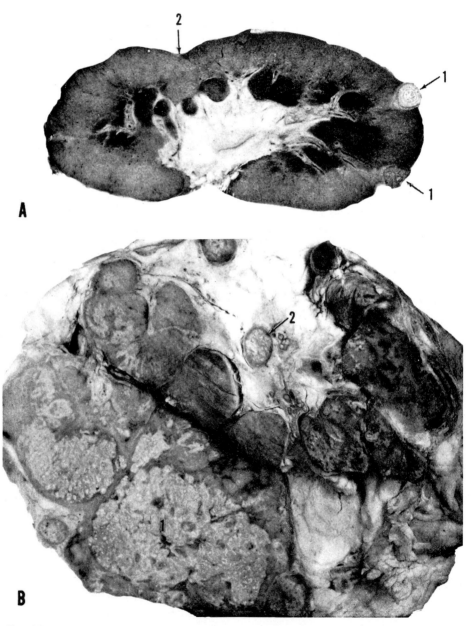

FIG. 13–8.—Tuberculosis in swine. *A*, Spherical subcapsular lesions in kidney (*1*). Note depressed zone in cortex (*2*) indicating an old infarct. *B*, Large (*1*) and small (*2*) confluent tubercles in mesenteric lymph nodes. (Courtesy of Armed Forces Institute of Pathology.) Contributor: Dr. B. A. Walter.

Classified on cultural characteristics as *scotochromagens, photochromagens, non-photochromagens* and *rapid growers* these organisms present unique therapeutic problems in that they are often resistant to the usual chemotherapeutic compounds employed against tuberculosis. Their role in animal tuberculosis has not been established.

Lesions.—The characteristic microscopic lesion is the tubercle, starting as a cluster of neutrophils surrounding the invading bacilli but replaced in a few hours by a whorl of epithelioid (endothelioid, reticulo-endothelial) cells, which usually represents the earliest stage encountered. The epithelioid cells encircle and engulf the bacteria but do not inhibit the growth of the lesion. As the tubercle bacilli multiply and produce toxic substances, the adjacent cells undergo caseous necrosis and more epithelioid granulation tissue is laid down around the caseous center. The cells making up the granulation tissue have abundant, foamy, pale, acidophilic cytoplasm and round, often eccentrically placed, nuclei. These cells may coalesce to form Langhans' giant cells, which are syncytial cells as much as 50 microns in diameter, with huge irregular masses of pale acidophilic cytoplasm and a number of round nuclei arranged in the form of a wreath or crescent at the periphery. The cell wall may be so indistinct that the cytoplasm appears to blend with adjacent tissues.

Langhans' giant cells may contain droplets of lipid and tubercle bacilli, the latter being demonstrable with acid-fast stains. Tubercle bacilli in varying numbers can also be demonstrated in the cytoplasm of epithelioid cells and in the caseous necrotic debris. The granulation tissue is usually surrounded by a zone of lymphocytes, arranged diffusely, in clumps, or near blood vessels. As the lesion ages, it becomes encapsulated by connective tissue of varying thickness. Calcification may occur in the caseous center of the tubercle except in avian tuberculosis where it is practically unknown.

A simple tubercle is usually between 1 mm. and 2 cm. in diameter, but larger conglomerate tubercles may be formed by the growth and coalescence of one or more adjacent single tubercles. Although they may attain almost any shape and size, the structural relations still persist. If the bacteria in the lesion are eventually overcome, the tubercle will be reduced to a small mass of fibrous or hyaline scar tissue. This is recognized as a healed tubercle. If healing does not take place, secondary infection with other organisms may occur, to be followed by suppuration or by liquefaction necrosis that produces cavitation.

Infection with tubercle bacilli does not always result in the formation of typical tubercles. This is particularly true of meningeal tuberculosis, a rapidly fatal infection, in which the pathologic changes consist of a scanty fibrinous or fibrino-purulent exudate on the surface of the pia mater and only a scattering of epithelioid cells in the meninges. Tissue reaction of a similar diffuse type may occur in overwhelming infections in sensitized animals.

The gross appearance of a tubercle, whether deep in soft tissue like liver and lungs, or bulging from a mucous or serous surface, is usually that of a firm or hard, white, gray or yellow nodule. On cut section its yellowish, caseous, necrotic center is dry and solid in contrast to the pus in an abscess. Calcification is common in many animals, and in sectioning a tubercle a gritty sensation and grating sound indicate the presence of calcareous material.

Occasionally a tubercle breaks into a blood vessel or by other means the blood is seeded with large numbers of tubercle bacilli which lodge in capillaries of the

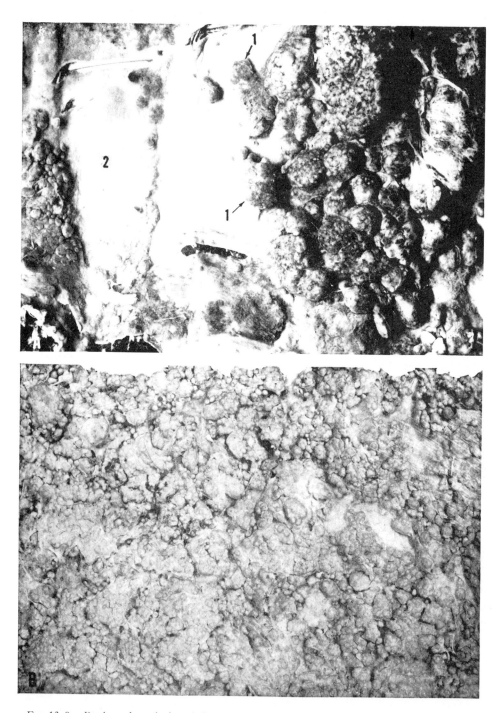

Fig. 13–9.—Bovine tuberculosis. *A*, Involvement of pleura by coarse nodules (*1*). Inner surface of rib (*2*). Contributor: Major Lytle, V.C., U.S. Army. *B*, Tuberculous involvement of the omentum of a cow. (Courtesy of Armed Forces Institute of Pathology.) Contributor: Station Veterinarian, U.S. Army, Fort Bayard, N.M.

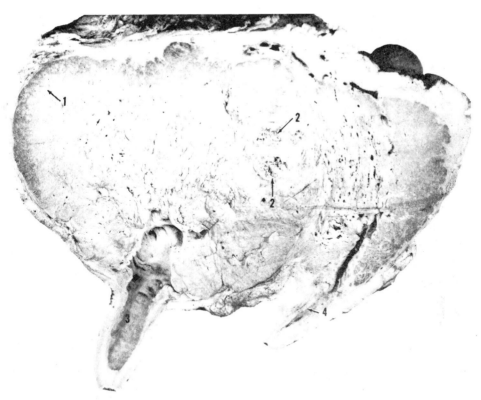

Fig. 13–10.—Tuberculous mastitis, udder of a cow. Tiny discrete tubercles are seen at (*1*), confluent lesions with central necrosis at (*2*). (Courtesy of Armed Forces Institute of Pathology.) Contributor: Major Lytle, V.C., U.S. Army.

parenchyma of visceral organs, where they give rise to myriad tubercles, 2 to 3 mm. in diameter, all of the same age and size. Because this lesion suggested a sprinkling of millet seeds to early observers, they gave the name **miliary tuberculosis** to infection of this rapidly fatal type.

Lesions in Different Species.—Although the general features of tuberculosis are evident in lesions from most species, certain differences in tissue reaction are more or less specific. In the **bovine,** calcification is often prominent, particularly in lymph nodes. Disseminated tubercles over the pleural and peritoneal surfaces are also fairly common. The appearance of these individual tubercles, usually from 0.5 to 1.0 cm. in diameter, gives this manifestation a common descriptive name—"pearl disease." Of particular interest are certain bovine skin lesions which, though histologically indistinguishable from those of typical tuberculosis, are not caused by infection with tubercle bacilli. Acid-fast bacilli, which apparently do not cause systemic disease, produce these tuberculoid lesions. The organisms involved can be shown by bacteriologic methods to differ from the usual tubercle bacilli, but they do produce sensitivity to bovine tuberculin, a point of considerable practical importance.

In the **horse,** the lesions of tuberculosis are usually of chronic, proliferative character and rarely exhibit caseation or calcification. In **birds** also, calcification is seldom observed. The lesions of tuberculosis of the avian type in swine appear as multiple encapsulated foci, a few millimeters in diameter, scattered throughout

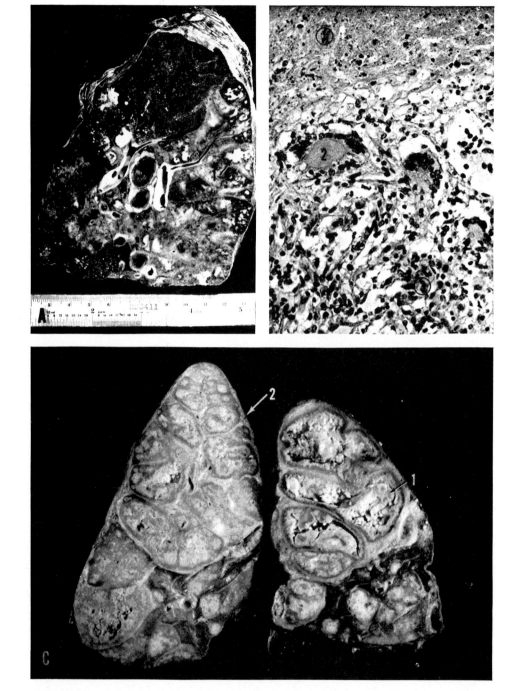

FIG. 13–11.—*A*, Lobular pneumonia of tuberculosis, lung of a tapir. The white foci (*1*) represent pus in consolidated lobules, contrasting with less consolidated lung (*2*). Contributor: National Zoological Park. *B*, Margin of a tubercle in a bovine lung (× 260). Caseous necrosis (*1*) Langhans' giant cell (*2*) and epithelioid cells (*3*). *C*, Consolidated apical lobes of a bovine lung. Same as Case *B*. Note caseous areas (*1*) and thickening of pleura (*2*) and interlobular septa. (Courtesy of Armed Forces Institute of Pathology.) Contributor: Dr. Wm. H. Feldman.

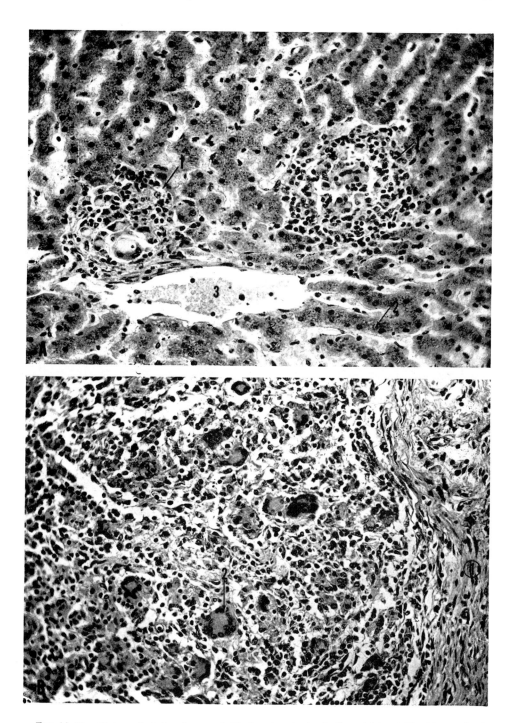

FIG. 13–12.—Tuberculosis in a horse. *A*, Early tubercles in the liver (*1*) (× 260). Liver cell columns (*2*), central vein (*3*). *B*, Margin of a well-developed tubercle in the liver (× 260). The lesion is encapsulated (*1*) and contains many Langhans' giant cells (*2*) and epithelioid cells (*3*). (Courtesy of Armed Forces Institute of Pathology.) Contributor: Dr. J. R. M. Innes.

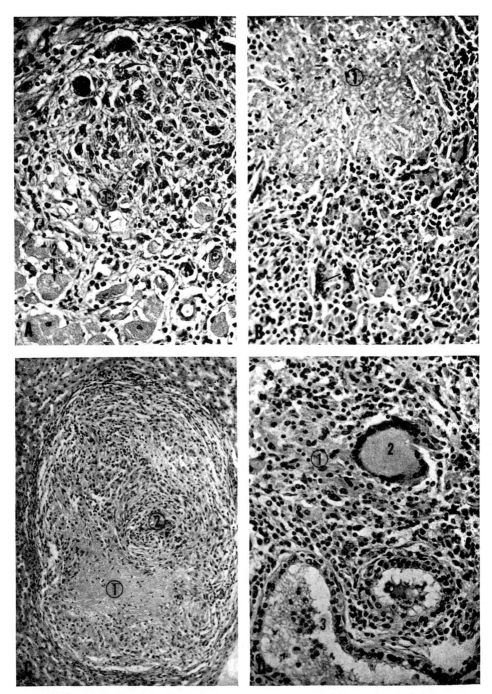

Fig. 13–13.—Tuberculous lesions in different species. *A*, Tuberculous myocarditis in a pig (× 260). Note epithelioid cells (*1*) displacing myocardial fibers (*2*). Contributor: Dr. C. L. Davis. *B*, Tubercle in the spleen of a pig (× 260). Caseous necrosis (*1*), epithelioid cells (*2*) and giant cells (*3*). Contributor: Dr. C. L. Davis. *C*, Confluent tubercles in the liver of a dog (× 100). Note caseous necrosis (*1*) and epithelioid cells (*2*). Giant cells are absent. Contributor: Dr. R. B. Oppenheimer. *D*, Tuberculous mastitis in a cow (× 260). Note epithelioid cells (*1*), Langhans' giant cell (*2*) and mammary acinus (*3*). (Courtesy of Armed Forces Institute of Pathology.) Contributor: Dr. Wm. H. Feldman.

the lymph nodes particularly of the head and cervical region. In **dogs,** pulmonary lesions rarely calcify, nor is caseation a prominent feature; diffuse infiltration of epithelioid cells usually predominates, but Langhans' giant cells are rare. In **nonhuman primates,** the disease is usually pulmonary and may run a fulminating course; miliary lesions are frequent, caseation is often prominent, and calcification is rare. Langhans' giant cells may be numerous or absent. A Siamese cat infected with the avian type organism was found to have granulomatous, calcified lesions in lymph nodes and diffuse consolidation of the lungs with epithelioid cells in which no giant cells, caseous necrosis nor calcification were present.

Pathogenesis. — Inhalation of tubercle bacilli commonly precedes the formation of a primary lesion in the lung, usually in one of the diaphragmatic lobes. If the infection is overcome, this lesion may heal, leaving only a dense hyaline scar. This process, however, sensitizes the animal to products of tubercle bacilli, causing the tissues to respond much more violently to subsequent exposures. If the primary lesion does not heal, the infection may travel via the lymphatic channels along the respiratory tree toward the tracheal and bronchial lymph nodes. Secondary tubercles developing along the course of these lymphatics, which lie adjacent to the bronchial epithelium, may protrude into the bronchi, rupture, and discharge virulent bacilli into the lumen, thus permitting infection of terminal alveoli and resulting in tuberculous pneumonia. It is also possible for bacilli that are discharged into the respiratory passages to be coughed up and then swallowed, thus infecting the digestive system secondarily. Organisms may also gain access to the blood by rupture of veins or through lymphatics, and thus be carried to any part of the body. Infection of the digestive tract in children in all probability results from ingestion of infected milk, meat or other food. In any species, circumscribed lesions develop in the mucosa or submucosa and the organisms may spread by way of the lymphatics to lymph nodes and thence to other tissues. Spread to bone, spleen, kidneys, genitalia and mammary glands from intestinal lesions is not uncommon. Skin lesions may develop as a consequence of systemic dissemination or by direct contact when tubercle bacilli presumably gain access through abraded skin.

Hypersensitivity in Tuberculosis. — Cellular hypersensitivity (delayed hypersensitivity) and cellular immunity play an important role in the pathogenesis of tuberculosis and account for the (1) striking difference between the reaction of an animal previously exposed to tuberculosis versus an animal which has never been infected and (2) effectiveness of tuberculin testing.

In previously exposed or vaccinated animals the cellular reaction around tubercle bacilli develops within a few days whereas in an unexposed individual, tubercle bacilli may remain at the site of inoculation and proliferate without inciting a response for as long as a week. Exposure to mycobacterial proteins results in hypersensitivity which is expressed in the response of macrophages and lymphocytes which, when re-exposed, or continuously exposed, are stimulated to proliferate and emigrate from the blood stream and accumulate at the site of tubercle bacilli or their extracts. Cellular hypersensitivity requires about ten to fourteen days to develop following natural infection. An increased capacity of macrophages to destroy tubercle bacilli is associated with the development of hypersensitivity. The latter cellular immunity which is closely linked with hypersensitivity but which is probably dependent on mycobacterial lipids and polysaccharides, is mainly nonimmunological in nature because it shows little specificity to tubercle bacilli; the "immune" macrophages having increased ability to destroy a variety of infectious agents. In contrast, cellular hypersensitivity is relatively specific to tuberculin. The net effect of calling forth "immune" macrophages is beneficial in overcoming infection and preventing its spread. However, if the mycobacterial products responsible for hypersensitivity are present in high concentrations, they cause necrosis of "sensitized" macrophages which contributes to caseous necrosis of the reactive nodule of macrophages and lymphocytes. Obviously circulatory phenomena and toxic products derived from the dying cells also contribute to necrosis. Delayed hypersensitivity is also held responsible, at least in part, for the liquefaction of the caseous foci, which provides an ideal locale for proliferation of tubercle bacilli separated from the host's defense reaction.

Thus hypersensitivity provides (1) a means of diagnosis (tuberculin), (2) the principal mechanism of combatting and resolving tuberculosis and (3) a detrimental effect by killing macrophages (epithelioid cells).

Diagnosis.—The diagnosis of tuberculosis in the living animal may be based upon x-ray findings, the tuberculin test, and demonstration of the organisms in exudates or excretions. In tissues obtained surgically or at necropsy, demonstration of acid-fast organisms within typical tubercles is sufficient to establish the diagnosis, although bacteriologic isolation of the organism is necessary to establish its type.

Tuberculosis

BOUGHTON, E.: Tuberculosis Caused by *Mycobacterium avium*. Vet. Bull. *39*:457–465, 1969.
BUILBRIDE, P. D. L., ROLLINSON, D. H. H. L., *et al.*: Tuberculosis in the Free-Living African (Cape) Buffalo (*Syncerus caffer caffer*, Sparrman). J. Comp. Path. *73*:337–348, 1963. VB 811–64.
CASSIDY, D. R., MOREHOUSE, L. G., and McDANIEL, H. A.: *Mycobacterium avium* infection in cattle: A Case Series. Am. J. Vet. Res. *29*:405–410, 1968.
CERNV, L.: (Tuberculosis in Mink.) Veterinarstvi *13*:152–154, 1963. VB 4208–63.
DANNENBERG, A. M.: Cellular Hypersensitivity and Cellular Immunity in the Pathogenesis of Tuberculosis: Specificity, Systemic and Local Nature, and Associated Macrophage Enzymes. Bact. Rev. *32*:85–102, 1968.
ENGLERT, H. K. and NASSAL, J.: Untersuchungen über das pathologisch-histologische Bild der durch die 3 Typen des Tuberkulose-erregers hervogerufenen Veränderungen beim Rind. Rindertuberk. u. Brucellose. *10*:21–27, 1961. VB 2048–61.
FELDMAN, W. H.: Histology of Experimental Tuberculosis in Different Species. Arch. Path. *11*:896–913, 1931.
————: Spontaneous Tuberculous Infections in Dogs. J. Am. Vet. Med. Assn. *85*: 653–663, 1934.
FELDMAN, W. H., and FITCH, C. P.: Histologic Features of the Intradermic Reactions to Tuberculin in Cattle. Arch. Path. *22*:495–509, 1936.
FELDMAN, W. H.: *Avian Tuberculosis Infections*, Baltimore, Williams & Wilkins Co., 1938.
HIX, J. A., JONES, T. C., KARLSON, A. G.: Avian Tubercle Bacillus Infection in a Cat. J. Am. Vet. Med. Assn. *138*:641–647, 1961.
INNES, J. R. M.: The Pathology and Pathogenesis of Tuberculosis in Domesticated Animals Compared with Man. Brit. Vet. J. *96*:42–50, 96–105, 391–407, 1940.
————: Tuberculosis in the Horse. Brit. Vet. J. *105*:373–383, 1949.
LESSLIE, I. W. and DAVIES, D. R. T.: Tuberculosis in a horse caused by the Avian type tubercle bacillus. Vet. Rec. *70*:82–84, 1958.
LINDSEY, J. R., and MELBY, E. C., JR.: Naturally Occurring Primary Cutaneous Tuberculosis in the Rhesus Monkey. Lab. Anim. Care *16*:369–385, 1966.
MARTIN, H. M.: Tuberculosis in the Dog. University of Pennsylvania Bulletin, Veterinary Extension Quarterly, No. 101, pp. 19–22.
MILLER, C. E., and KINARD, R.: A Case of Generalized Bone Tuberculosis in a Rhesus Monkey. Lab. Anim. Care *14*:264–267, 1964.

MORELAND, A. F.: Tuberculosis in New World Primates. Lab. Anim. Care 20:262–264, 1970.

NIELSEN, S. W., and SPRATLING, F. R.: Tuberculous Spondylitis in a Horse. Br. Vet. J. 124:503–508, 1968.

STAMP, J. T.: Tuberculosis of the Bovine Udder. J. Comp. Path. & Therap. 53:220–230, 1943.

WAYNE, L. G., RUNYON, E. H., and KUBICA, G. P.: Mycobacteria: A Guide to Nomenclatural Usage. Amer. Rev. Resp. Dis. 100:732–734, 1969.

PARATUBERCULOSIS

(Johne's Disease)

Paratuberculosis is a specific infection with an acid-fast organism, *Mycobacterium paratuberculosis*, which is known to affect cattle, sheep and goats, and is suspected of causing disease in swine, horses, and monkeys. It is a wasting illness with a prolonged course, during which intractable diarrhea results in dehydration, emaciation, and eventually in death. The disease is of worldwide distribution and constitutes an important economic problem in cattle but is less frequently encountered in other species. Many laboratory animals are resistant, however infection has been established in rabbits, mice, rats, hamsters, guinea pigs and moles. Successful transmission in both laboratory animals and ruminants usually requires exposure at an early age.

Infection in cattle and sheep does not always lead to clinical disease, however even in the absence of recognizable infection the organism is shed in the feces providing a source of infection for young animals. Although lesions are usually restricted to the intestinal tract and lymph nodes, the organism can infect the uterus which may lead to congenital infection and abortion.

Lesions.—The terminal part of the ileum is the most common site of the specific lesions which also occur in the remainder of the small and large intestines and the mesenteric lymph nodes. Microscopic sections reveal the lamina propria of

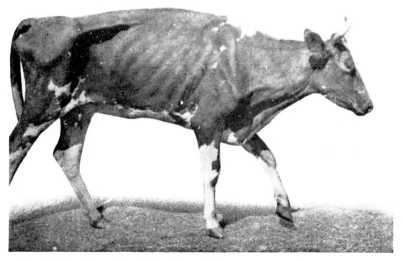

FIG. 13–14.—Paratuberculosis. Emaciation and dehydration are significant features in this affected cow.

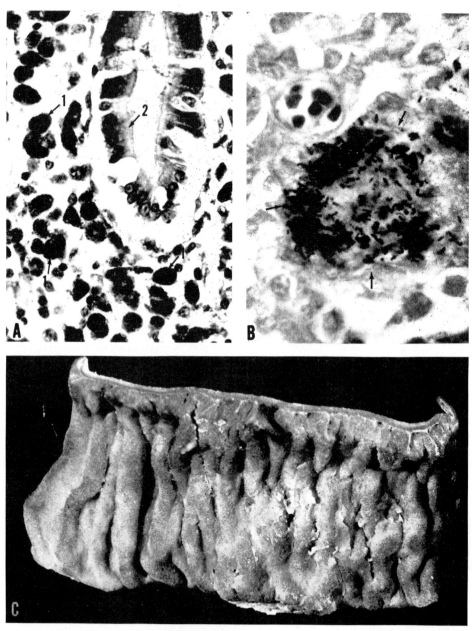

FIG. 13–15.—Paratuberculosis (Johne's Disease). *A*, Large macrophages laden with bacilli (*1*) in the lamina propria of the small intestine (× 440). Intestinal crypts (*2*) are separated from each other by the cellular exudate. Contributor: USAF School of Aviation Medicine. *B*, Higher magnification (× 1000) of a single macrophage (arrows) filled with bacilli. Acid-fast stain. Contributor: Dr. C. L. Davis. *C*, Small intestine of a cow. Note thick, rugose mucosa. (Courtesy of Armed Forces Institute of Pathology.) Contributor: Dr. Edward Records.

the mucosa to be closely packed with large, discrete epithelioid cells that have abundant foamy cytoplasm and are frequently multinucleated. These cells also infiltrate and thicken the submucosa but leave the muscularis mucosæ and muscularis intact. Nests of these same epithelioid cells may be found in mesenteric lymph nodes, but seldom elsewhere. In impression smears or sections through these lesions, Ziehl-Neelsen's stain demonstrates quantities of acid-fast, rod-shaped organisms crowding the cytoplasm of the epithelioid cells. Secondary changes in the intestinal mucosa in paratuberculosis include edema which results from local interference with circulation, nests of neutrophils, and increased numbers of eosinophils, the latter perhaps explainable on the basis of helminthic parasitism. Of importance is the absence of caseous necrosis, nodule formation, calcification and increased vascularization. In contrast to cattle, nodule formation with necrosis and calcification has been described in sheep and goats.

The gross appearance is directly related to the microscopic changes. The affected intestinal wall is thickened, sometimes edematous, and its mucosal surface bears many broad, closely placed, transverse folds, or rugæ. These rugæ result from thickening of villi and give the surface a corrugated appearance, which does not disappear when the intestinal wall is stretched.

Although lesions are usually confined to the intestines and lymph nodes, generalized infection has been described in both naturally and experimentally infected cattle, sheep and goats with lesions in the liver, spleen, lungs, kidneys, uterus, placenta and non-mesenteric lymph nodes.

Diagnosis.—The gross lesions in the intestine are highly suggestive, but confirmation of the diagnosis depends on the demonstration of epithelioid cells containing acid-fast bacilli in huge numbers in smears or sections of mucosa or submucosa. In about 60 per cent of affected cattle, the lesions and organisms extend into the colon and rectum, which makes it possible to diagnose the disease in the living animal by microscopic examination of mucosal scrapings collected per rectum.

The diffuse nature of the lesions, their confinement to the intestinal mucosa and mesenteric lymph nodes, and the presence of myriads of acid-fast bacilli serve to differentiate paratuberculosis from tuberculosis, in which nodule formation, fibrosis, abscess formation, necrosis, calcification, and but few acid-fast bacilli are characteristic. In sheep and goats, lesions with caseation and calcification require greater caution in differentiating tuberculosis, however the diffuse distribution of the lesions of paratuberculosis usually allows this distinction.

The intradermal johnin test and the complement-fixation test are aids to clinical diagnosis, but neither is completely satisfactory.

Paratuberculosis

DOYLE, T. M.: Foetal Infection in Johne's Disease. Vet. Rec. 70:238, 1958.
GILMOUR, N. J. L.: Recent Research on Johne's Disease. Vet. Rec. 77:1322–1326, 1965.
HALLMAN, E. T., and WITTER, J. F.: Some Observations on the Pathology of Johne's Disease. J. Am. Vet. Med. Assn. 83:159–187, 1933.
HARDING, H. P.: Experimental Infection with *Mycobacterium johnei*. 2. Histopathology of Infection in Experimental Goats. J. Comp. Path. 67:37–52, 1957.
————: The Histopathology of *Mycobacterium johnei* Infection in Small Laboratory Animals. J. Path. Bact. 78:157–169, 1959.
HATAKEYAMA, H. *et al.*: An Outbreak of Johne's Disease among Sheep in Japan. Nat. Int. Anim. Hlth. Quart. Tokyo 3:21–31, 1963. (In Engl.)
HOLE, N. H.: Johne's Disease. Adv. Vet. Sci. 4:341–387, 1958.

HOWARTH, J. A.: Paratuberculous Enteritis in Sheep. Cornell Vet. 27:223–234, 1937.

KOPECKY, K. E., LARSEN, A. B., and MERKAL, R. S.: Uterine Infection in Bovine Paratuberculosis. Am. J. Vet. Res. 28:1043–1045, 1967.

KLUGE, J. P., et al.: Experimental Paratuberculosis in Sheep After Oral, Intratracheal, or Intravenous Inoculation: Lesions and Demonstration of Etiologic Agent. Am. J. Vet. Res. 29:953–962, 1968.

LARSEN, A. B., and KOPECKY, K. E.: Mycobacterium Paratuberculosis in Reproductive Organs and Semen of Bulls. Am. J. Vet. Res. 31:255–258, 1970.

————: Studies on the Intravenous Administration of Johnin to Diagnose Johne's Disease. Am. J. Vet. Res. 26:673–675, 1965.

LARSEN, A. B., VARDAMAN, T. H., and MERKAL, R. S.: An Extended Study of a Herd of Cattle Naturally Infected with Johne's Disease. I. The Significance of the Intradermal Johnin Test. Am. J. Vet. Res. 24:91–93, 1963.

LOMINSKI, I., CAMERON, J., and ROBERTS, G. B. S.: Experimental Johne's Disease in Mice. J. Path. Bact. 71:211–221, 1956.

MERKAL, R. S., et al.: Experimental Paratuberculosis in Sheep After Oral, Intratracheal, or Intravenous Inoculation: Serologic and Intradermal Tests. Am. J. Vet. Res. 29:963–969, 1968.

MERKAL, R. S., et al.: Immunologic Mechanisms in Bovine Paratuberculosis. Am. J. Vet. Res. 31:475–486, 1970.

M'FADYEAN, J.: Histology of the Lesions of Johne's Disease. J. Comp. Path. & Therap. 31:73–87, 1918.

MINETT, F. C.: The diagnosis of Johne's disease by cultural methods. J. Path. & Bact. 54: 209–219, 1942.

NAKAMATSU, M., FUJIMOTO, Y., and SATOH, H.: The Pathological Study of Paratuberculosis in Goats, Centered Around the Formation of Remote Lesions. Jap. J. Vet. Res. 16: 103–120, 1969.

OMAR, A. R., LIM, S. Y., and RETNASABAPATHY, A.: Placentitis and Abortion in a Cow Probably Caused by Mycobacterium johnei. Kajian Vet. Singapore 1:39–43, 1967.

RAJYA, B. S. and SINGH, C. M.: Studies on the Pathology of Johne's Disease in Sheep. III. Pathologic Changes on Sheep with Naturally Occurring Infections. Am. J. Vet. Res. 22:189–203, 1961.

RANKIN, J. D.: The Experimental Production of Johne's Disease in Laboratory Rabbits. J. Path. Bact. 75:363–366, 1958.

————: The Present Knowledge of Johne's Disease. Vet. Rec. 70:693–697, 1958.

SIMON, J. and BREWER, R. L.: Investigation of Johne's Disease in Three Cattle Herds. J. Am. Vet. M. A. 143:263–266, 1963.

TAYLOR, A. W.: Experimental Johne's Disease in Cattle. J. Comp. Path. 63:355–367, 1953

LEPROSY OF BUFFALOES

(Lepra Bubalorum)

A disease of water buffaloes (carabao) characterized by persistent cutaneous and subcutaneous nodules on the legs and lower parts of the abdomen and thorax occurs in Java and other East Indian countries. It is of particular interest because of the similarity of its histologic features to those of human leprosy. Apparently the disease is uncommon and ordinarily does not result in death or serious disability. The causative organism, although demonstrable in tissue, has not been cultured successfully. A similar but even less frequent disease (Lepra bovinum) has been described in cattle in the East Indies.

Lesions.—The cutaneous nodules result from accumulation of large numbers of epithelioid cells in the dermis. Microscopically, these individually discrete cells are seen to have greatly distended, foamy, often vacuolated cytoplasm in which numerous acid-fast bacilli are demonstrable. The large vacuoles are believed to be the result of lipid production by the bacilli and are identical to those in the large "lepra cells" of human leprosy. Giant cells of Langhans' type may be seen, but caseation necrosis and calcification do not occur. The gross appearance of the lesion is not distinctive. A solid, uniform nodule, with a diameter as

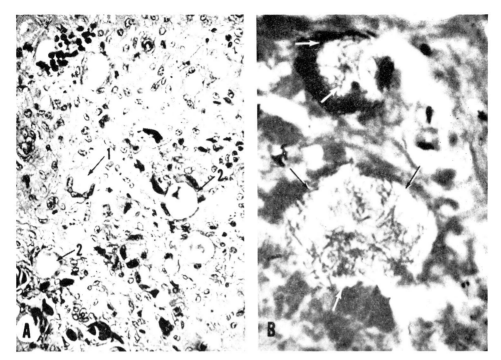

Fig. 13–16.—Leprosy of buffaloes. *A*, A section of a dermal nodule (× 300). Giant cells (*1*) and large macrophages, many containing large "globules" (*2*). *B*, Higher magnification (× 1250) of a section stained for acid-fast bacilli. The "globules" (arrows) are filled with acid-fast organisms. (Courtesy of Armed Forces Institute of Pathology.) Contributor: Dr. K. W. Wade.

great as 4 to 5 cm., may be firmly attached to the dermis and elevate the epidermis.

Diagnosis.—In countries where the disease occurs, the diagnosis can be made on the basis of the collections of "lepra cells" in the dermis, these cells being laden with acid-fast bacilli.

MURINE LEPROSY

Murine leprosy, a spontaneous disease of rats and mice which closely resembles human leprosy, was first described in 1902, by Stefansky. This disease has been studied extensively during the intervening years in attempts to gain information applicable to its human counterpart. The murine infection has been propagated by transfer of tissue suspensions containing the acid-fast bacilli, but the organisms have not been successfully cultivated outside the body of living animals. Progressive disease has been established in mice and rats and nonprogressive infection has been produced in rabbits and monkeys, but not in guinea pigs.

The lesions in murine leprosy are the result of aggregations of cells packed with bacilli, diffusely infiltrating the dermis, subcutis and all viscera except the kidney, or forming nodules in these tissues. These enlarged cells with foamy cytoplasm laden with acid-fast bacilli are called "lepra cells." They usually are derived from the reticulo-endothelial system but occasionally from epithelial cells of the epidermis, testicular tubules or epididymis. Some "lepra" cells contain such excessive numbers of bacilli and such quantities of lipid that they form vacuolated "globi," identical with those that occur in human or bovine leprosy (Fig. 13–16).

While murine leprosy occurs as a spontaneous disease in laboratory rodents, it is of particular importance as a symbiont which can be studied to gain information applicable to human leprosy.

Granulomas resembling the nodular lesions of leprosy have been described in frogs, but their significance and relationship to leprosy have not been established.

Leprosy

KRAKOWER, C., and GONZALES, L. M.: Mouse Leprosy. Arch. Path. *30*:308–329, 1940.
LOBEL, L. W. M.: Lepra Bubalorum. Internat. J. Leprosy *4*:79–96, 1936.
MACHICAO, N., and LA PLACA, E.: Lepra-like Granulomas in Frogs. Lab. Investigation *3*:219–227, 1954.
PINKERTON, H., and SELLARDS, A. W.: Histological and Cytological Studies of Murine Leprosy. Am. J. Path. *14*:435–442, 1938.
SELLARDS, A. W., and PINKERTON, H.: The Behavior of Murine and Human Leprosy in Foreign Hosts. Amer. J. Path. *14*:421–434, 1938.
STEFANSKY, W. K.: Eine lepraähnliche Erkrankung der Haut und der Lymphdrüsen bei Wanderratten. Zentralbl. f. Bakt., Orig. (pt. 1), *33*:481–487, 1903.

ASPERGILLOSIS

Infection with mycotic organisms of the genus *Aspergillus*, particularly *A. fumigatus*, is most prevalent in birds but may occur in mammals. The organisms are extremely common in nature, occurring on foodstuffs and plants as a white, fluffy mold. Young chickens and turkey poults are believed to become infected from contaminated bedding, usually while they are in the brooder stage of growth, hence the term "brooder pneumonia." Captive penguins, especially the King or

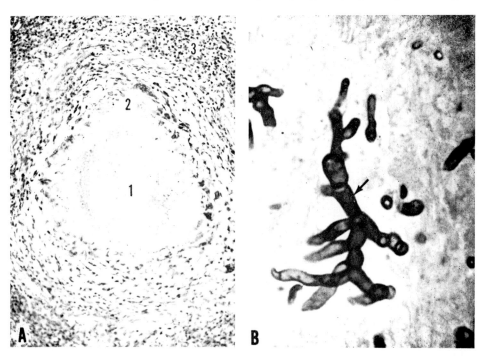

FIG. 13–17.—Aspergillosis. *A*, Granuloma in lung of a chick (× 185). Necrotic center (*1*) of the granuloma is surrounded by giant cells (*2*) and lymphocytes (*3*) in connective tissue. *B*, Gridley fungus stain of a section (× 840) to demonstrate the septate, branching fungus. (Courtesy of Armed Forces Institute of Pathology.) Contributor: Dr. C. L. Davis.

Emperor varieties in zoölogical gardens, are particularly susceptible to aspergillosis. Horses, cats, and rarely sheep and cattle have been reported to be infected. In man, the body openings, especially the external ear, are more frequently involved than the lungs. *Aspergillus fumigatus* is the most important cause of mycotic abortion (p. 671) in cattle. Debilitating conditions and prolonged antibiotic therapy predispose to infection in both man and animals.

Lesions.—The disease in birds may take several forms: (1) a diffuse pneumonic form, (2) a nodular pulmonary form, or (3) a diffuse infection of the air sacs. Aspergillosis in the first two forms may also occur in mammals. Gross examination of the lungs may disclose areas of consolidation, either diffuse or nodular, and thickening of the walls of air sacs (in birds) with a white moldy growth on the surface. The infection may become generalized or may be limited to one organ. Spherical nodules suggesting tuberculosis may be seen in the lungs and occasionally in other viscera.

Microscopically, the nodular lesions consist of a central core of caseation necrosis in which the organisms are found, surrounded by a wide zone of epithelioid granulation tissue. Giant cells of the foreign body type may be present, as well as lymphocytes and fibroblasts. The organisms in these granulomas appear as short, slender, septate, branching filaments, 3 or 4 microns wide and about 8 microns long. The organisms are poorly stained with hematoxylin and eosin, but stains for glycogen (PAS, Bauer's, Gridley's fungus) differentiate the mycelia by

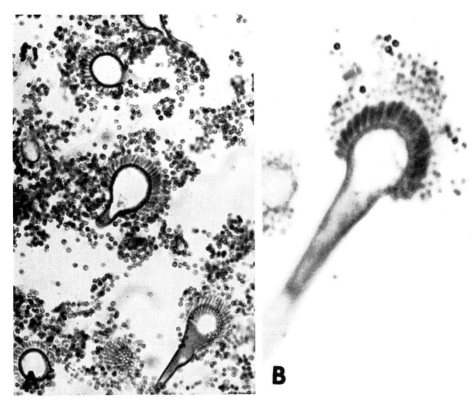

FIG. 13–18.—Aspergillosis, lung of a chicken. *A*, Conidiophores of *Aspergillus fumigatus*. These sporulating structures only form in the presence of a high oxygen tension. *B*, Higher magnification of a conidiophore.

coloring the cell wall intensely.   Short mycelia may appear to be almost spherical, but true spores are not found.   On surfaces exposed to air, such as those of air sacs and the lining of external orifices and trachea, the organisms may produce long aerial mycelia bearing conidiophores which project into the lumen.   The mycelial growth in these sites is like that in cultures on artificial media.   In cattle, club formation surrounding the fungi is sometimes seen similar to that in actino-mycosis and certain other mycotic infections.

Diagnosis.—The diagnosis can be confirmed by demonstrating the character-istic organisms with their slender, dichotomously branching septate hyphae, in tissue sections, or recovering them in cultures from typical lesions.

Aspergillosis

AINSWORTH, G. C., and REWELL, R. E.: The Incidence of Aspergillosis in Captive Wild Birds. J. Comp. Path. & Therap. *59*:213–224, 1949.

AUSTWICK, P. K. C.: The Presence of *Aspergillus fumigatus* in the Lungs of Dairy Cattle. Lab. Invest. *11*:1065–1072, 1962.

DAVIS, C. L., and SCHAEFER, W. B.: Cutaneous Aspergillosis in a Cow. J. Am. Vet. Med. Assn. *141*:1339–1343, 1962. VB 1497–63.

EGGERT, M. J., and ROMBERG, P. F.: Pulmonary Aspergillosis in a Calf. J. Am. Vet. Med. Assn. *137*:595–596, 1960.

GRIFFIN, R. M.: Pulmonary Aspergillosis in the Calf. Vet. Rec. *84*:109–111, 1969.

MOHLER, J. R., and BUCKLEY, J. S.: Pulmonary Mycosis of Birds—with Report of a Case in a Flamingo. U.S.D.A. Circular 58, Washington, D. C., 1904.

TAN KHENG KHOO, KENJI SUGAI, and TAN KIM LEONG: Disseminated Aspergillosis. Case Report and Review of the World Literature. Amer. J. Clin. Path. *45*:697–703, 1966.

BLASTOMYCOSIS

(North American Blastomycosis—Gilchrist's Disease)

Blastomycosis is an infectious disease of man and animals caused by a fungus, *Blastomyces dermatitidis* (*Zymonema dermatitidis, Gilchristia dermati-tidis*).   In man, the disease occurs as a cutaneous mycosis or as a pulmonary infection which may precede fatal dissemination.   In animals, principally dogs, the pulmonary form leading to dissemination is observed more commonly. Blastomycotic mastitis in a mare has been reported by Benbrook, Bryant and Saunders (1948).   Sheldon (1966) has described pulmonary blastomycosis in a cat and Easton (1961) described a case of cutaneous blastomycosis in a cat which are apparently the only reported examples of feline blastomycosis in North America.   Although the frequency and distribution of the disease in animals are not accurately known, it appears to be most frequent in the Missouri Valley of the United States.

South American Blastomycosis is of interest to contrast with North American Blastomycosis which is to be considered in greater detail.   The South American disease is caused by *Paracoccidioides braziliensis*, an organism which also affects man and animals but which can be differentiated in tissues by its manner of bud-ding.   This organism reproduces in tissues by multiple budding in contrast to the single bud which grows out from the cell wall of each spherule of *Blastomyces dermatitidis* (Fig. 13–19).

Lesions.—In the human skin, intra-epithelial abscesses with epithelioid reaction in the dermis and subcutis, ulceration and slow healing of the epidermis are described.   In the lungs of dogs, circumscribed gray nodules of solidification may

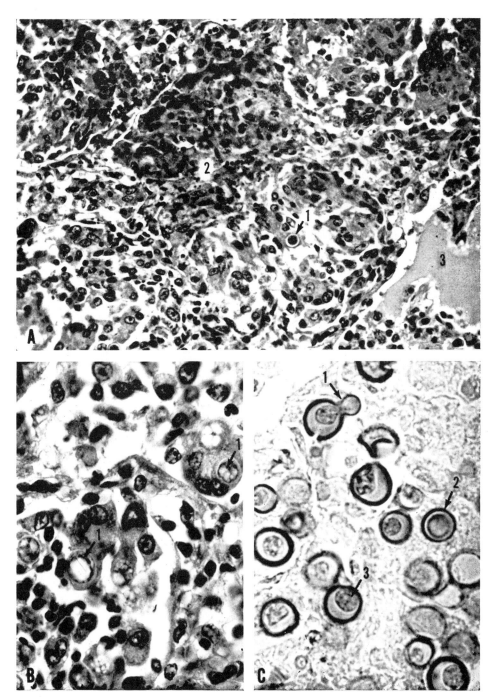

Fig. 13–19.—Blastomycosis in canine lung. *A, Blastomyces dermatitidis* (*1*) surrounded by large masses of epithelioid cells (*2*), alveolus (*3*) (× 210). Contributor: Dr. W. H. Riser. *B,* Numerous organisms (*1*) in macrophages in alveoli in a fulminant case (× 660). Contributor: Dr. J. R. Rooney II. *C,* Higher magnification (× 1050) of a section stained with Gridley's fungus stain. Note budding (*1*), thick walls (*2*), and the internal structure of the organisms (*3*). (Courtesy of Armed Forces Institute of Pathology.) Contributor: Dr. C. G. Loosli.

be seen in some cases, and diffuse consolidation of the lung, with the cut surfaces yielding purulent exudate, in others. Microscopically, the pulmonary lesion is characterized by intensive infiltration by reticulo-endothelial cells in which foci of neutrophils and diffusely distributed lymphocytes may be found. Caseation necrosis may occur, and although some fibroblasts are recognizable, there is little tendency toward encapsulation of the lesions. Multinucleated giant cells of the foreign body type may be seen, but Langhans' giant cells are rare. Calcification is infrequent.

The causative organisms are found in the lesions, free or in macrophages, as spherical, yeast-like cells, 8 to 20 microns in diameter, with double-contoured walls. In hematoxylin and eosin-stained sections, the organisms usually are seen as a central granular mass surrounded by a refractile, double-contoured unstained zone which is bounded by a thin outer wall. An occasional cell may be seen extruding a daughter cell (budding). Stains for bound glycogen (PAS, Bauer's, Gridley's fungus) will stain the outer wall of the organism selectively, differentiating it more clearly from the surrounding tissue.

The lesions may be limited to the lungs, but dissemination with abscess formation has been described in the subcutis, spleen, kidneys, lymph nodes, liver, brain, adrenals, eye and intestines.

Diagnosis.—Microscopic examination of affected tissues is necessary to establish the diagnosis. The organisms can be demonstrated readily in typical lesions and can be stained differentially with glycogen stains (PAS, Bauer's, Gridley's fungus). They are larger than *Histoplasma capsulatum* (p. 660), smaller than *Coccidioides immitis* (below) a fungus which contains endospores and does not reproduce by budding, and they do not have the wide, mucicarmine-staining capsule of *Cryptococcus neoformans* (p. 657). The tissue reactions in histoplasmosis and crytpococcosis are also unlike that of blastomycosis. Cultural identification of the organisms is of value, but it is more important that any fungus recovered in culture also be demonstrated in characteristic lesions.

Blastomycosis

BENBROOK, E. A., BRYANT, J. B., and SAUNDERS, L. Z.: Blastomycosis in the Horse. J. Am. Vet. Med. Assn. *112*:475–478, 1948.
EASTON, K. L.: Cutaneous North American Blastomycosis in a Siamese Cat. Can. Vet. J. *2*:350–351, 1961.
KURTZ, H. J., and SHARPNACK, S.: Blastomyces dermatitidis Meningoencephalitis in a Dog. Path. Vet. *6*:375–377, 1969.
LACROIX, L. J., RISER, W. H., and KARLSON, A. G.: Blastomycosis in the Dog. North Am. Vet. *28*:603–606, 1947.
SAUNDERS, L. Z.: Cutaneous Blastomycosis in the Dog. North Am. Vet. *29*:650–652, 1948.
SEIBOLD, H. R.: Systemic Blastomycosis in Dogs. North Am. Vet. *27*:162–168, 1946.
SHELDON, W. G.: Pulmonary Blastomycosis in a Cat. Lab. Anim. Care *16*:280–285, 1966.
TREVINO, G. S.: Canine Blastomycosis with Ocular Involvement. Path. Vet. *3*:652–658, 1966.
WILLIAMSON, W. M., LOMBARD, L. S., and GETTY, R. E.: North American Blastomycosis in a Northern Sea Lion. J. Am. Vet. Med. Assn. *135*:513–514, 1959.

COCCIDIOIDOMYCOSIS
(Coccidioidal Granuloma)

Coccidioidomycosis has been recognized as a human disease since 1892, when the first case was reported by Posada from Argentina. It is most prevalent in the arid regions of southwestern United States, but its distribution is generally

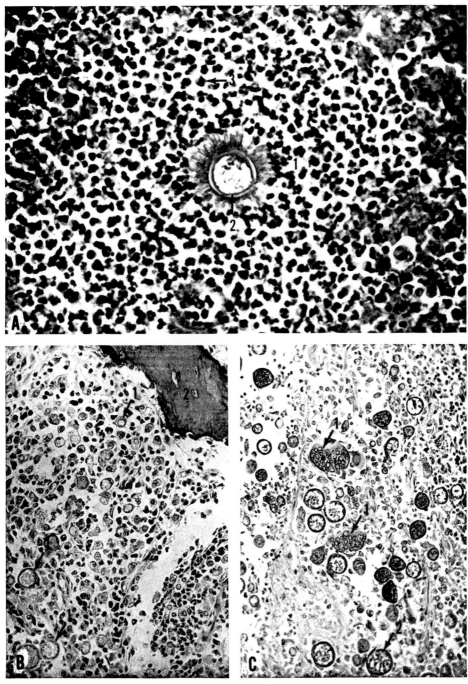

FIG. 13–20.—Coccidioidomycosis. *A*, Lesions in a mediastinal lymph node of a cow (× 100). Note radiating club-shaped structures (*1*) around the thick-walled organism (*2*) which lies in a pool of neutrophils (*3*). Contributor: Dr. H. R. Seibold. *B*, Lesion in bone marrow of a dog (× 185). Organisms (*1*) of various sizes in macrophages which replace the normal marrow. Bone trabecula (*2*). *C*, Another section of *B* stained with Gridley's fungus stain (× 235). Large organisms (*1*) filled with endospores which are just starting to develop in smaller organisms (*2*). (Courtesy of Armed Forces Institute of Pathology.) Contributor: Dr. H. A. Smith.

world-wide. Coccidioidomycosis was first recognized as a spontaneous infection of animals by Giltner, who reported a bovine case in 1918. It is now known to occur in a wide variety of wild and domesticated animals, including wild deer, mice, pocket mice, grasshopper mice, Kangaroo rats, pack rats, ground squirrels, gorillas, monkeys, dogs, sheep and cattle. The disease has also been reported in a horse (Zontine, 1958). In man, the disease may occur as an acute, febrile, upper respiratory infection with a short, favorable course (so-called "Valley Fever") or as a progressive intractable disease with disseminated lesions and fatal outcome. In animals, the disease usually assumes the chronic progressive form, although an inapparent pulmonary infection has been recognized in cattle.

The causative organism, *Coccidioides immitis* (*Oidium coccidioides*), may live in the soil, and inhalation of spores from this source will initiate the disease in either man or animals. Direct transmission from one animal host to another apparently does not occur, although certain rodents have been suspected of being reservoirs of infection. The organisms grow well in cultures, producing aerial mycelia which form a small, fluffy-white, spherical colony. In tissues, however, mycelial structures are not observed, the fungus taking the form of spherules 5 to 50 microns in diameter with double-contoured walls. Reproduction in tissues is by endosporulation, hence endospores may be found in some of the larger spherules.

Signs are absent in many cases, particularly in cattle, and the first indications of infection are lesions of pulmonary lymph nodes found in apparently healthy animals at the time of slaughter. Generalized infections run a slow course; the signs are nonspecific and may include emaciation, inappetence, low grade fever and occasional cough.

Lesions.—The gross lesions of coccidioidomycosis resemble those of tuberculosis in many respects. They may appear as discrete or confluent granulomas, with or without suppuration or calcification. In cattle, the lesions often are limited to small nodules in the lungs and, more frequently, to nodules or diffuse enlargements of bronchial or mediastinal lymph nodes. Large or small purulent foci may be surrounded by a wide band of granulation tissue and a fibrous capsule. Incision of an affected lymph node may permit the expression of thick yellowish pus. In the disseminated form of the disease, as in the dog, grayish nodules of various sizes may be found in the lungs, lymph nodes, liver, spleen, meninges, bone marrow, and other organs. The nodules are usually irregular in size and shape and may or may not exude material when put under pressure. At times a close relation to the larger blood vessels may be demonstrated.

The microscopic appearance is characteristic but varies to some extent in relation to the developmental stage of the fungus which predominates in the lesion. The largest spherules, often filled with endospores, are usually surrounded by a wide zone of epithelioid cells, admixed with a few neutrophils and some lymphocytes. In cattle, these large spherules may be surrounded by a corona of radiating club-shaped structures (Fig. 13–20), somewhat resembling the "rosette" around a colony of *Actinomyces bovis* (p. 616). When the wall of a large spherule ruptures, releasing its endospores, the tissue reaction becomes rich in neutrophils and lymphocytes, with fewer epithelioid cells. As these endospores mature, leukocytes and epithelioid cells tend to predominate in the inflammatory exudate. As organisms in all stages may occur in a single lesion, mixed tissue reactions are common. The organisms within the cytoplasm of Langhans' giant cells are clearly seen in sections stained with hematoxylin and eosin, but stains for bound glycogen (PAS,

Gridley's fungus Bauer's) will demonstrate the double-contoured wall selectively. In the liver, spleen and lung, the lesions are usually spherical and sharply circumscribed and obviously are expanding to displace normal tissues; in lymph nodes and bone marrow, the feature of circumscription is usually lost. In the meninges, spherical nodules of microscopic size, containing one or two organisms in a mantle of epithelioid cells, may appear in the pia-arachnoid.

Diagnosis.—Microscopic demonstration of the organisms in characteristic lesions usually establishes the diagnosis. When organisms are few, special stains (PAS, Gridley's fungus, Bauer's) are helpful in revealing them. The size of the largest spherules (up to 50 microns), the presence of endospores and absence of budding serve to distinguish *Coccidioides immitis* from *Blastomyces dermatitidis* (p. 644) or *Cryptococcus neoformans* (p. 657). The spherules of *Haplosporangium parvum* (p. 649) may be very similar in appearance and even larger in size, but they do not contain endospores.

Coccidioidomycosis

ASHBURN, L. L., and EMMONS, C. W.: Spontaneous Coccidioidal Granuloma in the Lungs of Wild Rodents. Arch. Path. *34*:791–800, 1942.
CRANE, C. S.: Equine Coccidioidomycosis. Vet. Med. *57*:1073–1074, 1962. VB 1503–63.
DAVIS, C. L., STILES, G. W., and McGREGOR, A. N., JR.: Pulmonary Coccidioidal Granuloma; a New Site of Infection in Cattle. J. Am. Vet. Med. Assn. *91*:209–215, 1937.
EMMONS, C. W.: Coccidioidomycosis. Mycologia *34*:452–463, 1942.
FARNESS, O. J.: Coccidioidal Infection in a Dog. J. Am. Vet. Med. Assn. *97*:263–264, 1940.
FORBUS, W. D., and BESTEBREURTJE, A. M.: Coccidioidomycosis: A Study of 95 Cases of the Disseminated Type with Special Reference to the Pathogenesis of the Disease. Mil. Surgeon *99*:653–719, 1946.
GILTNER, L. T.: Occurrence of Coccidioidal Granuloma (Oidiomycosis) in Cattle. J. Agric. Research *14*:533–542, 1918.
HUGENHOLTZ, P. G. *et al.*: Experimental coccidioidomycosis in dogs. Am. J. Vet. Res. *19*:433–439, 1958.
MADDY, K. T.: Disseminated coccidioidomycosis of the dog. J. Am. Vet. Med. Assn. *132*:483–489, 1958.
McKENNEY, F. D., TRAUM, J., and BONESTELL, A. E.: Acute Coccidiomycosis in a Mountain Gorilla (*Gorilla beringeri*). J. Am. Vet. Med. Assn. *104*:136–140, 1944.
REED, R. E., HOGE, R. S., and TRAUTMAN, R. J.: Coccidioidomycosis in Two Cats. J. Am. Vet. M. A. *143*:953–956, 1963.
REHKEMPER, J. A.: Coccidioidomycosis in the horse. A pathologic study. Cornell Vet. *49*:198–211, 1959.
SMITH, H. A.: Coccidioidomycosis in Animals. Am. J. Path. *24*:223–233, 1948.
STILES, G. W., and DAVIS, C. L.: Coccidioidal Granuloma (Coccidioidomycosis). Its Incidence in Man and Animals and its Diagnosis in Animals. J. Am. Med. Assn. *119*:765–769, 1942.
ZONTINE, W. J.: Coccoidomycosis in the horse, a case report. J. Am. Vet. Med. Assn. *132*:490–492, 1958.

HAPLOMYCOSIS (ADIASPIROMYCOSIS)

A mycotic organism with wide geographic distribution, originally called *Haplosporangium parvum*, and most recently named *Emmonsia parva*, has been reported to produce infection in many wild animals such as ground squirrels, pocket mice, white-footed mice, Kangaroo rats, pine squirrels, muskrats, beavers, rock and cottontail rabbits, mink, martins, skunks, weasels, wood rats and raccoons. Both of us (Jones and Hunt) have observed organisms with the morphology of *H. parvum* in sections of lungs of nine-banded armadillos. The name for the disease produced by this organism was proposed by Emmons (1948).

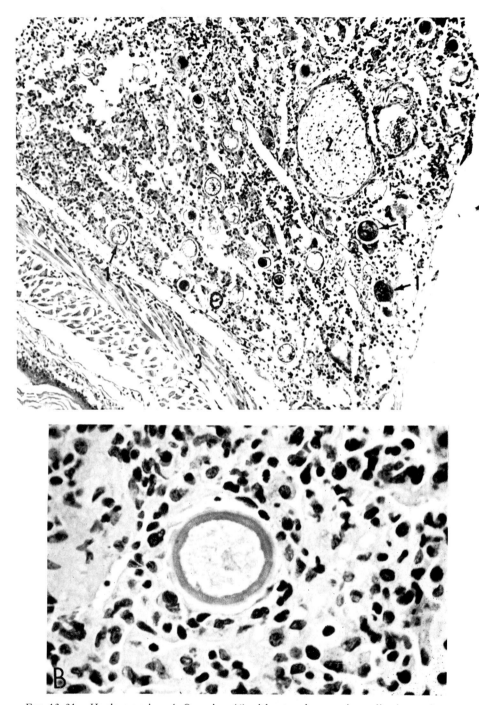

FIG. 13–21.—Haplomycosis.   A, Organism (1) without endospores in mediastinum of a mouse. Nerve (2), esophagus (3). Preparation courtesy Dr. R. T. Haberman.   B, A single spherule in the lung of an armadillo. Note thick wall and absence of endospores. Courtesy Animal Research Center, Harvard Medical School.

Although skin sensitivity of cattle to products of growth of *Haplosporangium* (haplosporangin) has been demonstrated and gross contamination of barnyard soils is known, natural infection of domesticated animals has not been recognized. However, it is altogether possible that domestic animals may become infected if conditions are suitable.

Emmons and Jellison (1960) have pointed out that the organism described above was improperly classified and have accepted its classification by Ciferri and Montemartini (1959) in a new genus as *Emmonsia parva*. Emmons and Jellison also suggest that a parasitic form of this genus be called *Emmonsia crescens* (n.sp.). The large spherule formed in tissues by *E. crescens*, which grows in size but does not form endospores, is called an *adiaspore* by these authors. Further, they suggest that the disease be called *adiaspiromycosis*, indicating a mycosis in which no multiplication or dissemination of the organism occurs beyond its original site of implantation.

Although *Haplosporangium parvum* may occur naturally in the same animals that harbor *Coccidioides immitis* (p. 646), these two organisms apparently are only distantly related and can be differentiated both in tissues and in culture. *Haplosporangium* is uninucleate, does not produce progressive disease in rodents, reproduces in culture by means of sporangioles rather than arthrospores, and does not produce endospores in tissues. The lesions observed in spontaneous infections with this organism are usually limited to the lungs, which suggests inhalation of the organisms. In the tissues of the host, the organisms grow from rather minute forms to large (up to 270 microns) spherical structures with thick, double-contoured walls. Endospores are not formed in tissues, in fact, no reproduction of organisms takes place in tissues, hence the disease is not progressive and the extent of involvement is related to the number of organisms inhaled. In spite of the very large size of some of the spherules of *Haplosporangium*, only a mild tissue reaction is evoked in the host. Epithelioid cells and occasional giant cells are seen engulfing the organisms (Fig. 13–21). Mild lymphocytic infiltration may be present, but neutrophils are few and usually are adjacent to smaller spherules which appear to be increasing in size.

Haplomycosis

ASHBURN, L. L., and EMMONS, C. W.: Experimental Haplosporangium Infection. Arch. Path. *39*:3–8, 1945.
EMMONS, C. W.: Coccidioidomycosis and Haplomycosis. Proc. Fourth Internat. Cong. Trop. Med. & Malaria *2*:1278–1286, Washington, D. C., 1948.
EMMONS, C. W., and ASHBURN, L. L.: The Isolation of *Haplosporangium parvum* (n. sp.) and *Coccidioides immitis* from Wild Rodents. Their Relationship to Coccidioidomycosis. Pub. Health Rep. *57*:1715–1727, 1942.
EMMONS, C. W. and JELLISON, W. L.: *Emmonsia crescens sp. n.* and Adiaspiromycosis (Haplomycosis) in Mammals. Ann. New York Acad. Sci. *89*:91–101, 1960.
MENGES, R. W., and HABERMANN, R. T.: Isolation of *Haplosporangium parvum* from Soil and Results of Experimental Inoculations. Am. J. Hyg. *60*:106–116, 1954.

RHINOSPORIDIOSIS

Infection of the nasal mucosæ with a fungus, *Rhinosporidium seeberi*, is known in man, horses, cattle and dogs. It is common in man in India and is rarely reported in North and South America. In animals, as in man, the organism invades the subepithelial stroma of the nasal mucosa where it induces chronic inflamma-

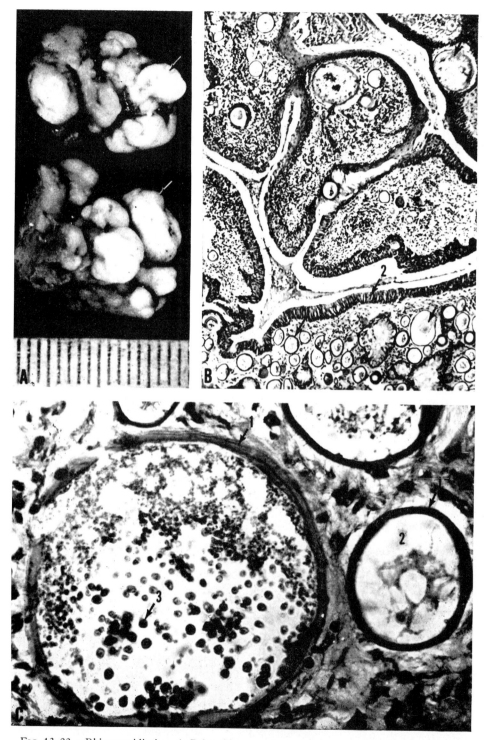

FIG. 13–22.—Rhinosporidiosis. *A*, Polypoid masses from nasal mucosa of a horse. *B*, Section (× 100) of one of the polyps. *Rhinosporidium seeberi* containing endospore (*1*) or as empty cysts, elevating the mucous membrane (*2*). *C*, The organism (× 600); note thick wall (*1*), empty organisms (*2*), and others containing small and large (*3*) endospores. (Courtesy of Armed Forces Institute of Pathology.) Contributor: Col. M. W. Hale.

tion and often results in polyp formation. The polyps are single or multiple, irregular in size and shape, and may become large enough to occlude the nasal passages. In the horse in the Americas, the nasal polypi are reportedly limited in extent, amenable to surgery, and probably self-limited in duration.

Microscopic examinations of the polyps discloses a stroma filled with spherical organisms (Fig. 13–22) with a thick double-contoured wall. These spherules vary in size, depending upon their stage of development, the largest (sporangium) measuring nearly 300 microns and the smallest (spore) about 2.0 microns in diameter. The round daughter cells, or endospores, formed within the sporangium are released by rupture of the cell wall at the so-called pore, where it is thinnest. In the spore form, the organisms gain access to the tissues where they continue their life cycle, developing into sporangia containing innumerable endospores. The fragmented cell walls from mature organisms appear to excite the most intense tissue reaction, which in places may encapsulate the organism with dense connective tissue. The growing, living organisms attract inflammatory infiltration consisting principally of lymphocytes with few epithelioid cells.

Rhinosporidiosis

AINSWORTH, G. C. and AUSTWICK, P. K. C.: Fungal Diseases of Animals. Rhinosporidiosis. Review Series No. 6, Commonwealth Bureau of Animal Health. Common. Agric. Bureaux, Farnham Royal, Bucks, England 44–45, 1959.
MYERS, D. D., SIMON, J., and CASE, M. T.: Rhinosporidiosis in a Horse. J. Am. Vet. Med. Assn. *145*:345–347, 1964.
SMITH, H. A. and FRANKSON, M. C.: Rhinosporidiosis in a Texas Horse. Southwest Vet. *15*:22–24, 1961.
WELLER, C. V., and RIKER, A. D.: *Rhinosporidium seeberi:* Pathological Histology and Report of the Third Case from the United States. Am. J. Path. *6*:721–732, 1930.
ZSCHOKKE, E.: Ein rhinosporidiom beim Pferd. Schweitz. Arch. f. Tierheilk. *55*:641–650, 1913.

NASAL GRANULOMA OF CATTLE

Polypoid or sessile masses in the nasal cavity of cattle have occasionally been reported from some parts of the country. This so-called nasal granuloma appears to be a definite clinical entity. Although its etiology is not clearly established, there is evidence that fungi may be involved, and it is possible that more than one causative agent may be concerned. There is little to suggest a relation between nasal granuloma in cattle in the United States and rhinosporidiosis (above), although such a possibility must be admitted. Spherical organisms, undoubtedly fungal, were described in histologic sections of nasal granulomas, and cultures of *Helminthosporum* recovered from these lesions by Davis and Shorten (1936) but the disease was not reproduced experimentally. Comparisons of the infection with haplomycosis and coccidioidomycosis (p. 646) have been made, but no conclusions reached.

The lesions are confined to the external nares and appear as nodules which project from any part of the nasal mucosa into the nasal cavity (Fig. 13–23). The resulting partial obstruction may be accentuated by accumulation over the nodules of mucous and purulent exudates which also stream from the external nostrils. The nodules have a glistening surface and are grayish yellow to red on cut section. Microscopically, the lesions underlying the elevated and often ulcerated nasal epithelium consist of granulation tissue in which epithelioid and foreign body

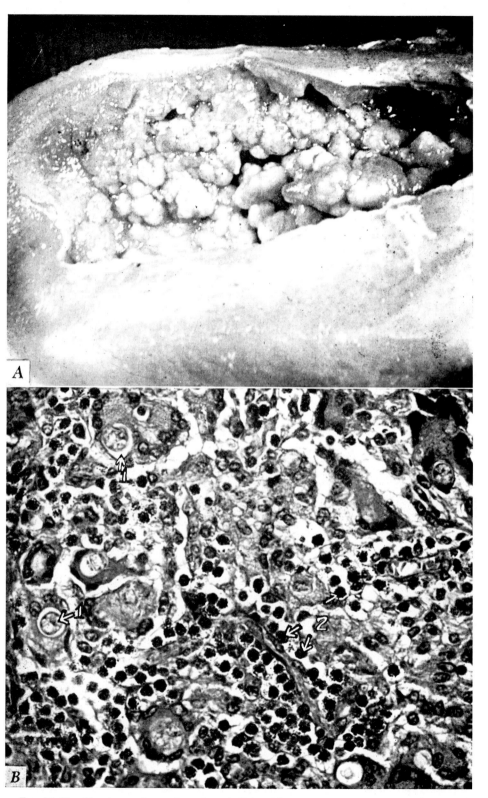

FIG. 13–23.—Nasal granuloma of cattle. *A*, Polypoid masses on nasal septum. Photograph courtesy of Dr. C. L. Davis. *B*, Section of a nasal granuloma. H & E, × 400. Note fungal organisms (*1*) and eosinophils (*2*).

giant cells predominate. Lymphocytes and eosinophils may make up a large part of some lesions. Spherical bodies, with thick walls and indistinct contents suggesting a fungus, are often seen within epithelioid and giant cells. In some reported cases, these organisms have not been found, although the possibility remains that they were present in parts of the lesion not examined microscopically.

Bridges (1960) has reviewed the problem of bovine nasal granuloma, has studied material from previously reported cases and published three new cases from central Texas. He was able to demonstrate both pigmented and non-pigmented hyphae and chlamydospores in the lesions and by comparing their morphologic features, determined that these organisms were a species of *Helminthosporum*. This organism has been isolated from cases of maduromycosis suggesting that nasal granuloma is merely a form of this latter disease. It is apparent that the Texas lesion is somewhat different from that of rhinosporidiosis as it is known in South America, and also differs from the bovine nasal granuloma of cattle in India, in which a fluke, *Schistosoma nasalis*, is demonstrable.

Nasal Granuloma

BRIDGES, C. H.: Maduromycosis of Bovine Nasal Mucosa (Nasal Granuloma of Cattle) Cornell Vet. *50*:469–484, 1960.

CREECH, G. T., and MILLER, F. W.: Nasal Granuloma in Cattle. Vet. Med. *28*:279–284, 1933.

DAVIS, C. L., and SHORTEN, H. L.: Nasal Swelling in a Bovine. J. Am. Vet. Med. Assn. *89*:91–96, 1936.

DIKMANS, G.: Nasal Granuloma in Cattle in Louisiana. North Am. Vet. *15*:20–24, 1934.

ROBINSON, V. B.: Nasal Granuloma. Am. J. Vet. Research *12*:85–89, 1951.

MADUROMYCOSIS

(Maduromycotic Mycetoma, Madura Foot)

An age-old disease of barefooted people ("Madura foot") was originally named after an area in which the disease was first described (Madura, India). Many different organisms have been recovered from such cases and may well have etiologic significance. One of these, *Nocardia madurae*, does not yet appear to be important in animals and does not result in the pathologic lesions which are usually classified as maduromycosis. The causative organisms currently grouped under this term, in tissues, form definite colonies or "grains" which are composed of cohesive masses of large segmented mycelial filaments with well-defined walls, chlamydospores or other spores and, in most cases, pigment (Fig. 13–24). Fungi which do not produce pigment are involved in "white-grained maduromycosis"; those colonies which contain pigment are visible to the unaided eye as "black grains," suggesting tiny bits of coal.

Among the fungal organisms which have been identified from lesions characteristic of maduromycosis are the following: *Allescheria boydii*, *Curvularia geniculata* and *Brachycladium spiciferum*. Only the latter two named have been recovered and identified in cultures.

Lesions.—The lesions of maduromycosis are distinguished by the presence of discrete black or brown colonies of fungi which appear grossly as tiny black or brown flecks ("grains") 1 to 3 mm. wide, embedded in a large mass of granulation tissue. These colonies are tenaciously discrete and can be expressed by pressure from the narrow zone of pus which surrounds them. The lesions in animals are

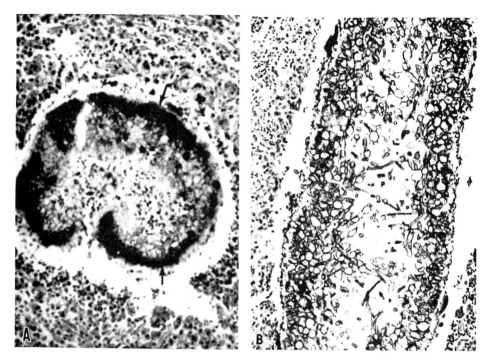

FIG. 13–24.—Maduromycosis. *A*, Nasal granuloma in a horse (× 224). Note pigment in tenaceous colony. (Courtesy of Armed Forces Institute of Pathology.) Contributor: Dr. Leon Z. Saunders. *B*, Granuloma of one year's duration in the foot of a dog (× 130). *Curvularia geniculata* was isolated from this lesion. Note colony of organisms without pigment.

most frequent on the extremities but may involve the nasal mucosa, peritoneum or skin at any site. The coiled glands of the foot pad of dogs appear to be sites of predilection. These mycotic granulomas may become quite large and are generally very resistant to any treatment short of surgical excision.

The microscopic appearance is quite distinctive. Colonies of the fungi are seen as brown, irregularly spherical bodies embedded within a pocket of neutrophils. These purulent centers are separated by abundant amounts of granulation tissue richly infiltrated with macrophages, plasma cells and lymphocytes. The organisms in the fungal colony cling together tenaciously and form an outer coronal zone made up of coarse, irregular, often swollen hyphæ and thick-walled chlamydospores. The center of the colony is usually less dense and contains many branching, septate hyphæ. The hyphæ are of irregular length but rarely more than 10 microns in width. The chlamydospores have thicker walls, are usually spherical and may attain a diameter of 25 microns or more. The periodic-acid Schiff (PAS), Bauer's and Gridley's fungus stains are particularly useful in demonstrating the morphology of the fungi in tissue sections (Fig. 13–24).

Diagnosis.—The diagnosis may be confirmed by demonstration of typical fungal colonies in characteristic granulomas. Organisms can be cultured without difficulty with appropriate techniques.

Maduromycosis

BRIDGES, C. H.: Maduromycotic Mycetomas in Animals. *Curvularia geniculata* as an Etiological Agent. Am. J. Path. *33*:411–427, 1957.

Bridges, C. H., and Beasley, J. N.: Maduromycotic Mycetomas in Animals—*Brachycladium spiciferum*, Bainier as an Etiologic Agent. J. Am. Vet. Med. Assn. *137*:192–201, 1960.
Brodey, R. S., *et al.*: Mycetoma in a Dog. J. Am. Vet. Med. Assn. *151*:442–451, 1967.
Seibold, H. R.: Mycetoma in a Dog. J. Am. Vet. Med. Assn. *127*:444–445, 1955.

CRYPTOCOCCOSIS

(Torulosis, European Blastomycosis)

Cryptococcosis is being recognized with increasing frequency in many animal species and is well known in man. The causative organism, *Cryptococcus neoformans* (*Cryptococcus hominis*, or *Torula histolytica*), is a yeast-like fungus which may live in a nonparasitic state in nature. The organisms are found in soil, manure and dust, from which sources both animals and man may be infected. Direct transmission of the disease between animals or from animals to man has not been demonstrated. In man, and in some animals as well, the organism has an affinity for the cerebrospinal meninges, but it may attack the respiratory system, the mammary gland, or several systems of the body.

Cryptococcosis has been reported in cattle, swine, horses, cats, dogs, marmoset (*Saguinus sp.*), rhesus (*Macaca mulatta*) and Taiwan monkeys (*M. cyclopis*), and the cheetah. The manifestations of cryptococcosis depend upon the organs or systems involved, therefore no constant clinical syndrome can be described. In cats, nasal obstructions resembling neoplasms have been associated with pulmonary infection and subsequently the meninges have been involved. Outbreaks of intractable mastitis have been reported in dairy cattle, but though the supramammary lymph nodes were involved, dissemination throughout the

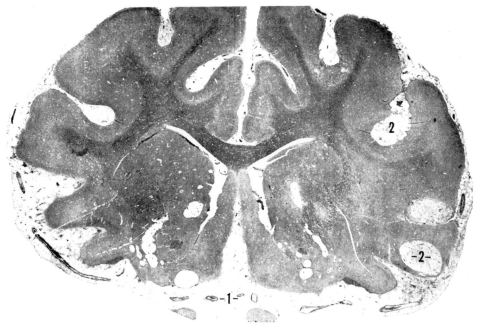

Fig. 13–25.—Cryptococcosis, brain of a cat. Large masses of organisms in leptomeninges (*1*) give them an edematous appearance and result in distention of depths of sulci (*2*). (Courtesy of Armed Forces Institute of Pathology.) Contributor: Dr. John Mills.

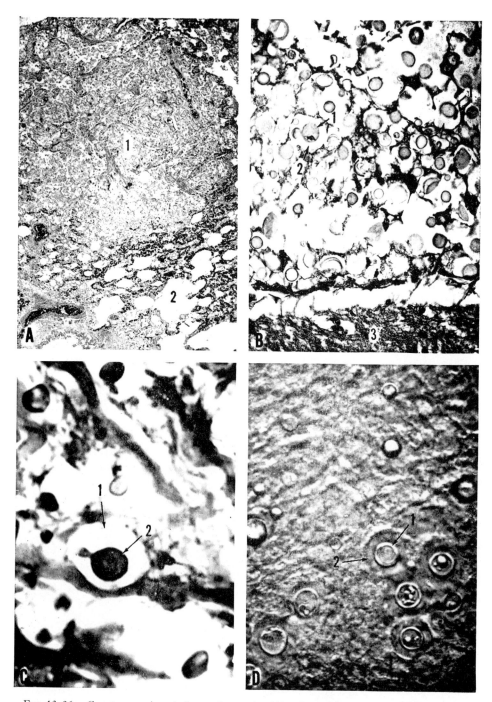

FIG. 13–26.—Cryptococcosis. *A*, Lung of a cat ($\times$ 48). Consolidated area (*1*) filling and compressing alveoli (*2*). *B*, Organisms in pia mater of a cat ($\times$ 300). Note spherical organisms (*1*) surrounded by a wide, clear capsule (*2*). Cerebral cortex (*3*). Contributor: Dr. John Mills. *C*, Organisms in cat lung ($\times$ 1045), same case as *A*. Note wide unstained capsule (*1*) surrounding a budding organism (*2*). (Courtesy of Armed Forces Institute of Pathology.) Contributor: Dr. Jean Holzworth. *D*, Unstained smear preparation viewed with phase contrast. Cell body (*1*) and capsule (*2*) ($\times$ 925).

body was the exception. Not infrequently, in many species, the presenting symptom is enlargement of lymph nodes.

Lesions.—The gross lesions are not diagnostic. In the lungs, peritoneum, nasal mucosæ and similar structures, they appear as granulomatous nodules sometimes with ulceration of the contiguous mucous membranes. Affected lymph nodes are enlarged, apparently from edema, and the cut surfaces have a definitely mucinous quality. The involved meninges are thickened with translucent material grossly resembling edema. In the mammary gland, diffuse or patchy induration may be observed. While the gross changes are inconclusive, the microscopic findings are diagnostic. The organisms occur in tissues as ovoid or spherical, thick-walled, yeast-like bodies which occasionally show single budding and are surrounded by a wide gelatinous capsule (Fig. 13–26). The cell inside the capsule is usually 5 to 20 microns in diameter; the capsule increases the over-all diameter to a maximum of 30 microns. In sections stained with hematoxylin and eosin, the cell wall and sometimes its contents are visible, but the capsule remains unstained. This capsule stains selectively by the mucicarmine technique and the periodic acid-Schiff (PAS) method for glycogen. In most situations, the organisms grow and multiply rapidly, forming a cystic space occupied by myriads of organisms whose mucoid capsules account for the glistening appearance and slimy consistency encountered grossly. This is a prominent feature in the brain, the organisms growing in the pia mater over the surface and deep into the cerebral convolutions where they form cystic areas and displace the brain parenchyma. Cystic lesions may occur in lungs, adrenal glands, lymph nodes and mammary glands. In such sites, the tissue reaction of the host is difficult to detect, although occasional macrophages with engulfed organisms may be found. In some sites, the organisms are less numerous and the tissue reaction much more profound. In lesions of this type, which may be adjacent to a cystic lesion, numerous endothelial cells with an admixture of lymphocytes are partially or completely surrounded by connective tissue. This granulomatous reaction is particularly prominent in some cases of cryptococcal mastitis but has also been observed in lesions in the brain, lung and other organs.

Diagnosis.—The diagnosis is readily made from characteristic microscopic lesions in which the organisms can be demonstrated and identified culturally or morphologically. The wide mucoid capsule which selectively absorbs the mucicarmine stain differentiates *Cryptococcus neoformans* in tissue from *Blastomyces dermatitidis* (p. 644). The budding of *Cryptococcus neoformans*, as well as its smaller size and capsule, serves to distinguish it from *Coccidioides immitis* (p. 646) which produces endospores and is not encapsulated.

Cryptococcosis

BALLARINI, G. and BREGA, A.: (Abomasal Erosions Associated with Cryptococcus Neoformans in a Cow.) Ital. Nuova Vet. *38*:237–245, 1962. VB 1133–63.
BARRON, C. N.: Cryptococcosis in Animals. J. Am. Vet. Med. Assn. *127*:125–132, 1955.
BERGMAN, F.: Pathology of Experimental Crytococcosis . . . in Mice. Acta Path. Microbiol. Scand. Supp. No. 147, pp. 160. (In English.) VB 385–62.
ERWIN, C. F. P. and RAC. R.: Cryptococcosis infection in a horse. Austral. Vet. J. *33*:97–98, 1957. (Vet. Bull. 390, 1958.)
GARNER, F. M., FORD, D. F., and ROSS, M. A.: Systemic Cryptococcosis in 2 Monkeys. J. Amer. Vet. Med. Assn. *155*:1163–1168, 1969.
HERIN, V. and DORMAL, R.: (Cerebral *Cryptococcus Neoformans* Infection in a Horse in the Congo.) Ann. Soc. belge Med. trop. *42*:865–970, 1962. VB 3099–63.

HOLZWORTH, J.: Cryptococcosis in a Cat. Cornell Vet. *42*:12–15, 1952.

HOLZWORTH, J., and COFFIN, D. L.: Cryptococcosis in the Cat. Cornell Vet. *43*:546–550, 1953.

HOWELL, J. McC., and ALLAN, D.: A Case of Cryptococcosis in the Cat. J. Comp. Path. *74*:415–418, 1964.

INNES, J. R. M., SEIBOLD, H. R., and ARENTZEN, W. P.: The Pathology of Bovine Mastitis Caused by *Cryptococcus neoformans*. Am. J. Vet. Research *13*:469–475, 1952.

JOHNSTON, L. A. Y. and LAVERS, D. W.: Cryptococcal Meningitis in a Cat in North Queensland. Aust. vet. J. *39*:306–307, 1963. VB 828–64.

KAVIT, A. Y.: Cryptococcic Arthritis in a Cocker Spaniel. J. Am. Vet. Med. Assn. *133*:386–389, 1958.

LITTMAN, M. L. and ZIMMERMAN, L. E.: *Cryptococcosis (Torulosis, or European Blastomycosis)*. New York, Grune & Stratton, 1956.

OLANDER, H. J., REED, H., and PIER, A. C.: Feline Cryptococcosis. J. Am. Vet. Med. Assn. *142*:138–143, 1963.

ROBERTS, E. D. *et al.*: Feline Cryptococcosis. Iowa State Univ. Vet. *26*:30–33, 1963–64.

RUBIN, L. F., and CRAIG, P. H.: Intraocular Cryptococcosis in a Dog. J. Amer. Vet. Med. Assn. *147*:27–32, 1965.

SEIBOLD, H. R., ROBERTS, C. S., and JORDAN, E. M.: Cryptococcosis in a Dog. J. Am. Vet. Med. Assn. *122*:213–215, 1953.

SIMON, J., NICHOLS, R. E., and MORSE, E. V.: An Outbreak of Bovine Cryptococcosis. J. Am. Vet. Med. Assn. *122*:31–35, 1953.

SMITH, D. L. T., FISHER, J. B., and BARNUM, D. A.: Generalized *Cryptococcus neoformans* Infection in a Dog. Canad. M.A.J. *72*:18–20, 1955.

SUTMÖLLER, P., and POELMA, F. G.: *Cryptococcus neoformans* infection (torulosis) of goats in the Leeward Islands Region. W. Ind. Med. J. *6*:225–228, 1957.

TAKOS, M. J., and ELTON, N. W.: Spontaneous Cryptococcosis of Marmoset Monkeys in Panama. A.M.A. Arch. Path. *55*:403–407, 1953.

TRAUTWEIN, B. and NIELSEN, S. W.: Cryptococcosis in 2 Cats, a Dog and a Mink. J. Am. Vet. Med. Assn. *140*:437–442, 1962.

WAGNER, J. L., PICK, J. R., and KIRGMAN, M. R.: *Cryptococcus neoformans* Infection in a Dog. J. Amer. Vet. Med. Assn. *153*:945–949, 1968.

WEIDMAN, F. D., and RATCLIFFE, H. J.: Cryptococcosis in a Cheetah at the Philadelphia Zoo. Arch. Path. *18*:362–369, 1934.

HISTOPLASMOSIS

Histoplasmosis is an infectious, but not contagious, mycotic disease of man and lower animals. The causative organism, *Histoplasma capsulatum*, grows readily in culture media and soil as a white to brown mold which bears spores of two types: spherical, minutely spiny *microconidia*, 3 to 4 microns in diameter, and spherical, or rarely clavate, *macroconidia*, 8 to 12 microns in diameter, with evenly spaced, finger-like projections over the surface. The parasitic phase in the mammalian host develops from either of these conidia into a yeast-like form.

Although for many years the disease in man was believed to occur only as a rare, consistently fatal, disseminated infection, it is now known that an acute nonfatal form is much more prevalent both in man and lower animals. The disease is not spread by direct contact between hosts, but it may appear in animals and man sharing the same environment. So-called "epidemics" of histoplasmosis are thus related to an environmental source of infection rather than to spread of contagion from host to host. Both the benign inapparent and the fatal disseminated forms of the disease occur in a wide variety of animals, including dogs, cats, cattle, horses, guinea pigs, bats, rats, mice, woodchucks, skunks, opossums, foxes and raccoons. It has been reported from many parts of the United States, South and Central America, and less frequently other parts of the world, but apparently is most common in certain regions of the United States, specifically those bordering the Missouri, Ohio and Mississippi Rivers. This impression may be misleading and merely reflect the more thorough studies that have been conducted in these areas. It is highly probable that most cases of histoplasmosis, both animal and human, are neither recognized nor reported.

The benign form of the disease in animals is seldom recognized unless pulmonary lesions are present or organisms are recovered at necropsy, although in some instances x-ray examination has revealed lesions in subjects with histoplasmin sensitivity. Benign histoplasmosis in man may become apparent as an acute febrile pneumonitis with weight loss and adenopathy, or by roentgenologic evidence of dense, sometimes calcified "coin lesions" in the lungs, usually associated with histoplasmin sensitivity. The fatal disseminated form in animals, observed most frequently in dogs, usually runs a prolonged course with progressive loss of weight, lymphadenopathy, diarrhea, weakness, anemia, hepatomegaly, and ascites. Although histoplasmosis is difficult to recognize in the living animal, it has been diagnosed from the symptoms and course and confirmed by demonstration of organisms in the circulating blood.

Lesions.—The dominant feature of the tissue changes in histoplasmosis is the extensive proliferation of reticulo-endothelial cells (macrophages, endothelioid, epithelioid cells), many of which contain yeast forms of the causative organism, either a few, or so many that the cytoplasm is distended and tremendously enlarged. It is the proliferation of reticulo-endothelial cells that causes displacement of normal tissues, interference with function and gross enlargement of organs.

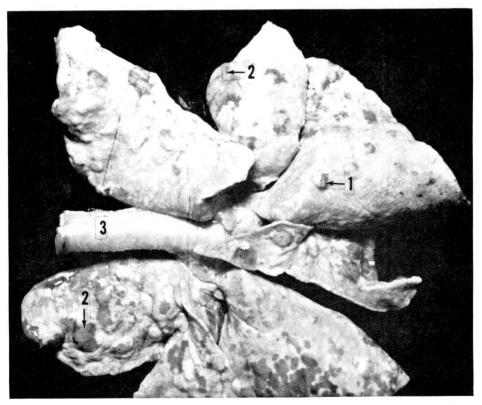

Fig. 13–27.—Histoplasmosis. Nodules (*1*) in the lung of a dog. Consolidated lobules (*2*). Trachea (*3*). (Courtesy of Armed Forces Institute of Pathology.) Contributor: Dr. Karl S. Harmon.

The disease has been more adequately studied in the dog, hence the following remarks on the lesions will apply especially to the dog.

The lungs in the benign form may show only a few discrete, well-encapsulated nodules or islands of epithelioid cells, some of which may contain demonstrable organisms. With recovery these lesions regress to fibrocalcareous nodules which remain in the lung for years. In the disseminated form, the alveoli and interstitial stroma may be flooded with lymphocytes, plasma cells and epithelioid cells, many containing organisms. The yeast-like bodies, which are always located in the cytoplasm, are irregularly egg-shaped and measure from 2 by 3 to 3 by 4 microns. In sections stained with hematoxylin and eosin, a central, spherical, usually basophilic body is surrounded by an unstained zone, which, in turn, is encircled by a thin cell wall. This may give the effect of a capsule around the central body, but the organism has no true capsule; the clear halo is actually within the cell wall. By the periodic acid-Schiff (PAS), Bauer's or Gridley's fungus method, the wall is stained selectively, leaving its contents unstained, thus the organism appears as an empty red ring. These stains are particularly useful in visualizing organisms when only a few are present and in differentiating them from other phagocytized particles, especially tissue debris.

The lymph nodes in the disseminated disease are tremendously enlarged by the proliferation of cells of the reticulo-endothelium. Grossly, the nodes are firm and uniform in appearance, not unlike those of malignant lymphoma. The reticulo-endothelial proliferation in severely affected nodes may obliterate the normal nodal architecture. Necrosis, purulent inflammation and calcification are seldom observed, nor are multinucleated giant cells common. The predominant cell is mononuclear with tremendously expanded cytoplasm, often packed with organisms. Lymphocytes and plasma cells may be present in smaller numbers.

The spleen is enlarged to several times its normal size, light gray and firm as the result of the reticulo-endothelioid proliferation which masks much of the splenic architecture.

The liver is also enlarged, firm, and light gray because of the diffuse interlobular and intralobular proliferation of reticulo-endothelial cells. These cells displace liver parenchyma and thus obviously interfere with liver function. As elsewhere, there is little tendency for encapsulation of the lesions in the disseminated form. Lymphocytes and plasma cells may be present in varying numbers.

The intestine, when involved, has a thickened rugose or nodular mucosal surface and its wall is thickened by reticulo-endothelial proliferation in the lamina propria and submucosa. Ulceration is unusual. The lymph nodules and adjacent lymph nodes are greatly enlarged, their architecture distorted by the characteristic large macrophages laden with organisms. The ileocecal junction and the adjacent lymph nodes are often severely affected.

The adrenal glands may be largely replaced by macrophages filled with organisms. This is particularly striking in fatal cases, but less so in affected animals sacrificed before the terminal stages of the disease.

Other organs, including skin, pancreas, heart, genitalia, and kidneys, are usually less severely affected but may be involved by the characteristic reticulo-endothelial proliferation.

Diagnosis.—In the living animal the diagnosis can be established by demonstration of typical reticulo-endothelial proliferation and organisms in tissues at

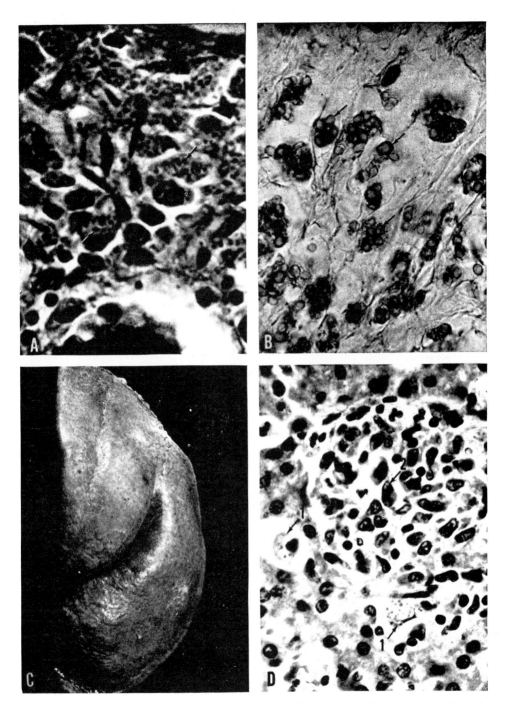

FIG. 13–28.—Histoplasmosis. *A*, Macrophages (arrows) laden with *Histoplasma capsulatum* in submucosa of the ileum (× 1000) of a dog. Contributor: Dr. R. F. Birge. *B*, Organisms (arrows) stained by Gridley's fungus stain. The cell wall is stained red, causing the organisms to look larger than in *A*, although the magnification is the same (× 1000). *C*, Enlarged gray liver of a dog. Same as Case *B*. Contributor: Dr. Karl S. Harmon. *D*, Lesion in the liver (× 630) of a dog. Note macrophages laden with organisms (*1*) and reticuloendothelial cells (*2*). (Courtesy of Armed Forces Institute of Pathology). Contributor: Dr. H. R. Seibold.

biopsy (tonsils, lymph node, liver). In some cases macrophages containing *H. capsulatum* can be demonstrated in smears of the circulating blood. Microscopic examination of tissue sections usually permits definitive diagnosis, but in some cases identification of the organisms in cultures is advisable. The organism of epizoötic lymphangitis (p. 664) cannot be differentiated in tissue sections, hence cultures are necessary to distinguish these two infections. However, the different geographical distribution and the anatomical location of the two diseases usually eliminate difficulty. Some malignant neoplasms (malignant lymphoma, reticulum cell sarcoma), in which tissue necrosis and phagocytosis of cell debris have occurred, may have gross and microscopic features erroneously suggesting histoplasmosis but can be distinguished by the absence of unequivocal organisms. Stains for bound glycogen (PAS, Bauer's, Gridley's fungus) are helpful in differential staining of the organisms. Differentiation of other mycotic organisms is not difficult in tissue sections because *Blastomyces dermatitidis* (p. 644) is larger and exhibits budding; *Coccidioides immitis* (p. 646) is much larger and forms endospores; and *Cryptococcus neoformans* (p. 657) is larger, has a wide mucoid capsule, and displays prominent budding.

Histoplasmosis

BIRGE, R. F., and RISER, W. H.: Canine Histoplasmosis. North Am. Vet. *26*:281–287, 1915.
CORDY, D. R.: Histoplasmosis in a Dog. Cornell Vet. *39*:339–343, 1949.
CORREA, W. M., and PACHECO, A. C.: Naturally Occurring Histoplasmosis in Guinea Pigs. Can. J. Comp. Med. Vet. Sci. *31*:203–206, 1967.
DEL FAVERO, J. E., and FARRELL, R. L.: Experimental Histoplasmosis in Gnotobiotic Dogs. Am. J. Vet. Res. *27*:60–66, 1966.
DE MONBREUN, W. A.: The Dog as a Natural Host for *Histoplasma capsulatum*. Am. J. Trop. Med. *19*:565–588, 1939.
EMMONS, C. W.: Histoplasmosis. Bull. New York Acad. Med. *31*:627–638, 1955.
EMMONS, C. W., and ASHBURN, L. L.: Histoplasmosis in Wild Rats. Pub. Health Rep. *63*:1416–1422, 1948.
FARRELL, R. L., and COLE, C. R.: Experimental Canine Histoplasmosis with Acute Fatal and Chronic Recovered Courses. Amer. J. Path. *53*:425–445, 1968.
HARMON, K. S.: Histoplasmosis in Dogs. J. Am. Vet. Med. Assn. *108*:60–62, 1948.
LAMAS DA SILVA, J. M., BARBOSA, M., and HIPOLITO, O.: (*Histoplasma capsulatum* Infection in a Dog in Brazil.) Arq. Esc. Vet. Minas Gerais. *13*:101–106, 1962.
MENGES, R. W., HABERMANN, R. T., SELBY, L. A., and BEHLOW, R. F.: *Histoplasma capsulatum* Isolated from a Calf and a Pig. Vet. Med. *57*:1067–1070, 1962. VB 1909-63.
MENGES, R. W., et al.: Ecologic Studies of Histoplasmosis. Amer. J. Epidem. *85*:108–119, 1967.
PANCIERA, R. J.: Histoplasmic (Histoplasma capsulatum) Infection in a Horse. Cornell Vet. *59*:306–312, 1969.
ROWLEY, D. A., HABERMANN, R. A., and EMMONS, C. W.: Histoplasmosis: Pathologic Study of Fifty Cats and Fifty Dogs from Loudon County, Virginia. J. Infect. Dis. *95*:98–108, 1954.
SEIBOLD, H. R.: Histoplasmosis in a Dog. J. Am. Vet. Med. Assn. *109*:209–211, 1946.
SELBY, L. A., MENGES, R. W., and HABERMANN, R. T.: Survey for Blastomycosis and Histoplasmosis Among Stray Dogs in Arkansas. Am. J. Vet. Res. *28*:345–349, 1967.
TOMLINSON, W. J., and GROCOTT, R. G.: Canine Histoplasmosis. A Pathologic Study of the Three Reported Cases and the First Case Found in the Canal Zone. Am. J. Clin. Path. *15*:501–507, 1945.

EPIZOÖTIC LYMPHANGITIS

Epizoötic lymphangitis is a disease of the skin and superficial lymphatics of horses, caused by a mycotic organism currently known as *Histoplasma farciminosum (Cryptococcus farciminosus, Blastomyces farciminosus, Saccharomyces farciminosus, Endomyces farciminosa, Saccharomyces equi* or *Zyomonema farcimi-*

nosum). This organism is yeast-shaped in tissue but forms mycelia in cultures, in many respects resembling *Histoplasma capsulatum* (p. 660). The disease probably no longer occurs in the United States, but still is common in some other countries, notably China. The clinical features are those of chronic indurative ulceration of the skin, especially of the limbs, with thickening of the superficial lymphatics, enlargement of regional lymph nodes, formation of abscesses and discharge of purulent material, followed by the development of new indolent ulcers. Less frequently infection may occur as conjunctivitis, and rarely becomes generalized involving internal viscera.

The mode of transmission is not established. Direct contact does not appear important unless infective material is conveyed to previously injured skin. Experimentally, flies (*Musca* and *Stomoxys*) have been shown capable of transmitting the infection.

With the exception of rabbits, most laboratory animals are refractory to infection.

Lesions.—Sections of the cutaneous lesions reveal granulomatous tissue reactions with a predominance of large macrophages, their cytoplasm distended with oval organisms, each about 2.0 × 3.0 microns and enveloped by a thin capsule. The central mass of the fungus is demonstrable in sections stained with hematoxylin and eosin; the peripheral capsule remains unstained. Stains for bound glycogen (PAS, Bauer's and Gridley's fungus stain) identify the capsule selectively, staining it red and leaving the central body unstained. The organisms are very similar to *Histoplasma capsulatum* in tissues; in fact, their appearance suggests that the two organisms should be carefully compared. Mycelial forms of *H. farciminosum* have been described in tissues but are usually absent.

The **diagnosis** of epizoötic lymphangitis can be confirmed by the demonstration of typical organisms in characteristic lesions, in tissue sections, cultures or stained smears of exudate.

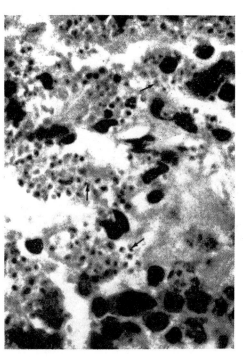

Fig. 13–29.—Epizoötic lymphangitis, skin of a mule (× 1200). Large numbers of *Histoplasma farciminosum* (arrows) are seen in macrophages. (Courtesy of Armed Forces Institute of Pathology). Contributor: Ninth Medical Service Detachment Laboratory, U.S. Army.

Epizoötic Lymphangitis

SINGH, T.: Studies on Epizootic Lymphangitis. I. Modes of Infection and Transmission of Equine Histoplasmosis (*Epizootic lymphangitis*). Indian J. Vet. Sci. *35*:102–110, 1965.
SINGH, T., and VARMANI, B. M. L.: Studies on Epizootic Lymphangitis: A Note on Pathogenicity of *Histoplasma farciminosum* (Rivolta) for Laboratory Animals. Indian J. Vet. Sci. *36*:164–167, 1966.
————: Some Observations on Experimental Infection with *Histoplasma farciminosum* (Rivolta) and the Morphology of the Organism. Indian J. Vet. Sci. *37*:47–57, 1967.

MUCORMYCOSIS

(Phycomycosis)

One of the less frequent infectious granulomas of animals is caused by fungi which grow in tissue as coarse, nonseptate, branching, filamentous organisms. One of the more frequently isolated fungi has been known by various names (*Mucor corymbifer, Lichtheimia corymbifer*), but the name currently preferred by mycologists is *Absidia corymbifera*. Infections with species of the genera *Mucor, Rhizopus, Hyphomyces, Entomophthora*, as well as other members of the class *Phycomycetes* are also occasional causes of mucormycosis in animals. Even though the identity of the causative organisms is somewhat unsettled, and several organisms may be involved, mucormycosis is an acceptable designation for the disease. It has been described in a wide variety of animals including man, generally affecting lymph nodes of one or more systems but occasionally producing disseminated lesions. In man, the lungs or ears appear to be sites of predilection, but infection may occur in the eye, brain, meninges and gastric mucosa. Earlier reports of isolation of *Mucor sp.* from bovine placenta with necrotic hemorrhagic lesions and from bovine fetal tissues must be accepted with caution, because the organisms recovered could easily have been contaminants. Recent reports by Gleiser (1953) of the disease in 2 dogs and 1 bovine, and by Davis (1955) relative

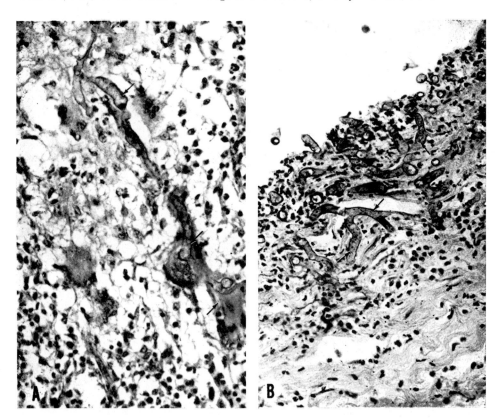

FIG. 13–30.—Mucormycosis. *A*, Bovine mesenteric lymph node (× 310). Note long mycelium (arrows) in a large giant cell. Preparation courtesy of Dr. C. L. Davis. *B*, Organisms (arrows) in the depths of an ulcer in the stomach of a dog (× 130). (Courtesy of Armed Forces Institute of Pathology.) Contributor: Dr. M. A. Troy.

to 11 cases in cattle and 1 in a pig, present convincing evidence that this organism can produce a lesion within which the fungus can be demonstrated. Of interest is a report by Gitter and Austwick (1959) in which *Rhizopus microsporus* and *Candida albicans* were both reported to be isolated from gastric lesions in suckling pigs. Bridges and Emmons (1961) have described cutaneous mycotic granulomas in 8 horses from which *Hyphomyces destruens* was isolated. Lesions of mucormycosis are usually found in the course of postmortem examination of animals slaughtered for food or which have died from some other cause. The organisms, however, will cause a fatal generalized infection in mice or rabbits when injected intravenously.

Lesions.—The gross lesions of mucormycosis are rather nonspecific. Ulcers with raised edges may occur in the stomach; affected lymph nodes in cattle may be enlarged and replaced by yellowish granulomas with caseous or calcareous foci within them. Similar caseous lesions may be seen in any affected organ.

Microscopically, epithelioid granulation tissue with varying degrees of necrosis and calcification replaces normal tissues. Lymphocytic infiltration may be intense and giant cells are often present. In cattle, particularly in the mesenteric lymph nodes, eosinophils are often conspicuous. The organisms appear in giant cells or necrotic zones as irregular, coarse hyphæ, which are often branched but rarely septate. The organisms are readily demonstrable with hematoxylin and eosin stains but are more distinctly outlined by the periodic acid-Schiff (PAS) reaction. There can be little doubt that this organism grows in tissue and that host cells react specifically to its presence.

Diagnosis.—Specific diagnosis should be based upon demonstration of characteristic organisms in typical granulomatous lesions. Isolation of organisms from the lesions is necessary for their further identification and study, but histologic demonstration of the fungus within tissues which are obviously reacting to its presence is critical in establishing the causal relationship in an individual lesion. Identification of the organism recovered from cultures is not decisive, because this fungus grows free in nature and can easily contaminate cultures taken under many circumstances.

Mucormycosis

Bridges, C. H., and EMMONS, C. W.: A Phycomycosis of Horses Caused by *Hyphomyces destruens*. J. Am. Vet. Med. Assn. *138*:579–589, 1961.
DAVIS, C. L., ANDERSON, W. A., and McCRORY, B. R.: Mucormycosis in Food-producing Animals. J. Am. Vet. Med. Assn. *126*:261–267, 1955.
GISLER, D. B., and PITCOCK, J. A.: Intestinal Mucormycosis in the Monkey (*Macaca mulatta*). Am. J. Vet. Res. *23*:365–366, 1962.
GITTER, M. and AUSTWICK, P. K. C.: Mucormycosis and moniliasis in a litter of suckling pigs. Vet. Rec. *71*:6–11, 1959.
GLEISER, C. A.: Mucormycosis in Animals. J. Am. Vet. Med. Assn. *123*:441–445, 1953.
GREGORY, J. E., GOLDEN, A., and HAYMAKER, W.: Mucormycosis of the Central Nervous System. Bull. Johns Hopkins Hosp. *73*:405–419, 1953.
HALL, J. E.: Multiple Maduromycotic Mycetomas in a Colt Caused by Helminthosporium. Southwest Vet. *18*:233–234, 1965.
HESSLER, J. R., *et al.*: Mucormycosis in a Rhesus Monkey. J. Am. Vet. Med. Assn. *151*: 909–913, 1967.
MARTIN, J. E., *et al.*: Rhino-Orbital Phycomycosis in a Rhesus Monkey. J. Am. Vet. Med. Assn. *155*:1253–1257, 1969.
SHIRLEY, A. G. H.: Two Cases of Phycomycotic Ulceration in Sheep. Vet. Rec. *77*: 675–677, 1965.
SYMEONIDIS, A., and EMMONS, C. W.: Granulomatous Growth Induced in Mice by *Absidia corymbifera*. A.M.A. Arch. Path. *60*:251–258, 1955.

SPOROTRICHOSIS

Sporotrichosis is a fungous disease which occurs both in man and animals, the horse being the most frequently affected lower animal.   The causative organism, *Sporotrichum schenkii*, grows as a mold with aerial mycelia in culture but is restricted to irregular club or cigar-shaped forms in tissues.   Chronic peritonitis and orchitis can be produced experimentally in male rats, mice and hamsters by the intraperitoneal injection of material containing *S. schenkii*.   In experimentally induced lesions, the organisms are much more numerous and more easily seen and identified.   The disease runs a slow, obstinate course and does not become generalized.

The **lesions** of sporotrichosis occur in the skin and cutaneous lymphatics, particularly over the legs, thorax and abdomen.   Spherical nodules, from 1 to 4 cm. in diameter, are formed in the dermis and subcutis along the course of cutaneous lymphatics, which are thickened and pursue a tortuous course between the nodules.   Occasionally the nodules ulcerate, yield small amounts of thick, creamy pus, and then heal very slowly.   Microscopic sections of the nodules reveal a purulent center surrounded by a wide band of epithelioid granulation tissue containing giant cells and lymphocytes. The lesion is usually surrounded by a very dense connective-tissue capsule. The organisms in the lesion are not demonstrable with ordinary hematoxylin and eosin stains, but are stained by the periodic acid-Schiff (PAS) method or by modifications of this technique, such as the Gridley's fungus stain. The bound glycogen in the capsule of the organism makes it possible to visualize it in tissue sections. Demonstration of the organisms in sections, cultures or laboratory animals is necessary to distinguish sporotrichosis from the cutaneous form of glanders ("farcy") (p. 602), which is clinically similar.

Sporotrichosis

DAVIS, H. H., and WORTHINGTON, E. W.:   Equine Sporotrichosis.   J. Am. Vet. Med. Assn. *145*:692–693, 1964.
JONES, T. C. and MAURER, F. D.:   Sporotrichosis in Horses.   Bul. U. S. Army Med. Dept. No. *74*:63–73, 1944.
KAPLAN, W. and OCHOA, A. G.:   Application of the Fluorescent Antibody Technique to the Rapid Diagnosis of Sporotrichosis. J. Lab. Clin Med. *62*:835–841, 1963. VB 1251–64.

CANDIDIASIS

(Moniliasis, Thrush)

Candidiasis, caused by species of the fungus *Candida* (most usually *Candida albicans*) is principally a superficial mycosis of mucous membranes.   It is encountered most frequently in avian species affecting the mouth, esophagus, crop and proventriculus.   Superficial infection of oral mucous membranes is also the most common form of candidiasis in mammals, where it has been seen in man, cats, cattle, swine and non-human primates.   Systemic candidiasis, though rare, has been described in man, mice and calves.   Infection may also involve the skin of man and animals and in man, *Candida sp.* may cause bronchitis, pneumonia and vulvovaginitis.   It has been reported as a cause of bovine mastitis and abortion. Candidiasis is most common in young animals, debilitated patients and as a complication of protracted antibiotic therapy.   The gross *lesions* in the superficial form of candidiasis are characterized by a white pseudomembrane overlying the skin or mucous membranes. Microscopically the membrane is composed of masses of entangled pseudohyphae and budding yeast-like organisms 3 to 4 microns in diameter, which invade the epithelium, but rarely beyond the basal layer. The organism can be difficult to discern in hematoxylin and eosin stained tissue sections but are clearly demonstrated with the periodic acid-Schiff, Gridley and Gomori methenamine silver techniques. A leukocytic infiltration predominantly composed of neutrophils and lymphocytes accumulates beneath the epidermis. Lesions in systemic candidiasis, which may involve various internal organs but in particular the kidneys, are characterized by necrosis and suppuration. Rarely is a granulomatous reaction encountered.

Diagnosis is dependent upon demonstration of the organisms in characteristic lesions.

Candidiasis

GOETZ, M. E., and TAYLOR, D. O. N.: A Naturally Occurring Outbreak of Candida tropicallis Infection in a Laboratory Mouse Colony. Amer. J. Path. *50*:361–369, 1967.
GOLDSTEIN, E., *et al.*: Studies on the Pathogenesis of Experimental Candida guilliermondii Infection in Mice. J. Infect. Dis. *115*:293–302, 1965.
KAUFMANN, A. F., and QUIST, K. D.: Thrush in a Rhesus Monkey: Report of a Case. Lab. Anim. Care *19*:526–527, 1969.
KRAL, F., and USCAVAGE, J. P.: Cutaneous Candidiasis in a Dog. J. Am. Vet. Med. Assn. *136*:612–615, 1960.
MILLS, J. H. L., and HIRTH, R. S.: Systemic Candidiasis in Calves on Prolonged Antibiotic Therapy. J. Am. Vet. Med. Assn. *150*:862–870, 1967.
REYNOLDS, I. M., MINER, P. W., and SMITH, R. E.: Cutaneous Candidiasis in Swine. J. Am. Vet. Med. Assn. *152*:182–186, 1968.

PROTOTHECOSIS

Colorless algae of the genus *Prototheca*, though usually saprophytic, have been reported to cause disease in man and animals. Although the infection appears to

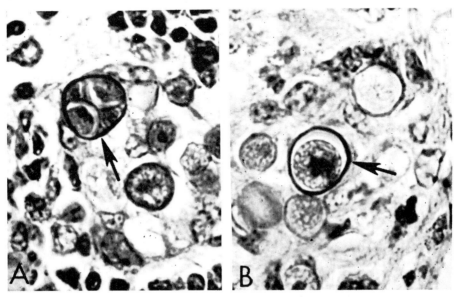

FIG. 13–31.—Protothecosis, bovine lymph node. *A*, Several organisms, one composed of four daugher cells within a single cell wall (arrow), Mayer's mucicarmine stain. *B*, Single organisms have distinct cell walls (arrow) and one or more nuclei, Mayer's mucicarmine stain. (Courtesy Dr. G. Migaki and Pathologia Veterinaria.)

be rare, *Prototheca spp.* have been associated with cutaneous granulomas in man, dogs and deer, generalized infection in dogs, mastitis in cattle and granulomatous lymphadenitis in man, deer and cattle. In tissue section, *Prototheca spp.* appear as round to oval organisms 3 to 20 microns in greatest diameter, with a refractile wall, granular cytoplasm and a single nucleus. Reproduction occurs by endosporulation which gives rise to single organisms containing several daughter cells (endospores). The cell wall stains poorly in hematoxylin and eosin stained tissue sections but is strongly positive to stains for carbohydrate (PAS, Gridley's, Baurer's, G.M.S.). Tissue reaction may be minimal or the organism may incite granulomatous inflammation characterized by central necrosis surrounded by macrophages, epithelioid cells, lymphocytes and foreign body and Langhans' type giant cells.

Diagnosis requires demonstration of the organism in tissue section. Positive identification of the organism requires isolation on artificial medium, but isolation in the absence of demonstrating tissue invasion should be viewed with caution.

Protothecosis

FRANK, N., *et al.*: Prototheca, A Cause of Bovine Mastitis. Am. J. Vet. Res. *30*:1785–1794, 1969.

MIGAKI, G., GARNER, F. M., and IMES, G. D., JR.: Bovine Protothecosis. A Report of Three Cases. Path. Vet. *6*:444–453, 1969.

POVEY, R. C., *et al.*: A Case of Prothothecosis in a Dog. Path. Vet. *6*:396–402, 1969.

VAN KRUININGEN, H. J.: Prototheccal Enterocolitis in a Dog. J. Am. Vet. Med. Assn. *157*: 56–63, 1970.

VAN KRUININGEN, H. J., GARNER, F. N., and SCHIEFER, B.: Protothecosis in a Dog. Path. Vet. *6*:348–354, 1969.

GEOTRICHOSIS

Geotrichosis is a rare mycosis of man and animals caused by *Geotrichum candidum*, a fungus common on fruits, vegetables and dairy products. It has been described as causing mastitis and abortion in cattle, lymphadenitis in swine and a systemic infection in a dog. In man, geotrichosis has been described as a chronic bronchitis, stomatitis, enteritis, conjunctivitis, dermatitis, and disseminated mycosis. The **lesions** described by Lincoln and Adcock (1968) in a dog consisted of necrotizing pneumonia, lymphadenitis, nephritis, adrenalitis and mycocarditis; well-defined granulomas in the liver, spleen, bone marrow and brain; and a mononuclear chorioiditis of the eye. Organisms were associated with each of these lesions, occurring as intra- and extracellular round to ovoid yeast-like cells 3 to 7 microns in diameter. Branching, septate hyphae and chains of round yeast-like cells resembling pseudohyphae of *Candida albicans* (p. 668) were also present. **Diagnosis** requires demonstration of the organism in tissue section and differentiation from *Candida albicans* (p. 668). Isolation of the organism is necessary for positive identification but cannot be relied upon as the sole means of diagnosis owing to the near ubiquitous presence of *Geotrichum spp.* in nature.

Geotrichosis

LINCOLN, S. D., and ADCOCK, J. L.: Disseminated Geotrichosis in a Dog. Path. Vet. *5*: 282–289, 1968.

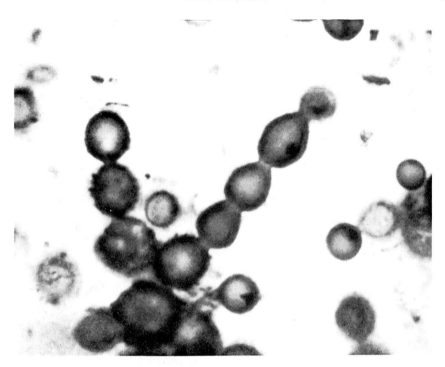

Fig. 13–32. Lobo's disease, Atlantic bottlenose dolphin. A branching chain of the fungus *Loboa loboi*. Courtesy Dr. G. Migaki.

LOBO'S DISEASE

Lobo's disease, or keloidal blastomycosis, is a chronic granulomatous infection of the skin caused by a fungus *Loboa loboi*. Aside from a single description of the disease in an Atlantic bottlenose dolphin (*Tursiops truncatus*) by Migaki and associates (1971) the infection has been reported only in man, where the occurrence is restricted to Brazil, Surinam and Costa Rica; the dolphin was from Florida waters. The lesions, which are localized in the skin without visceral involvement, are characterized by dense collections of histiocytes and multinucleated giant cells with little proliferation of fibrous connective tissue. Small collections of neutrophils are usually present. The causative organisms are principally located within histiocytes and giant cells appearing as round to oval yeast-like bodies 5–10 μ in diameter containing a faintly basophilic central body 1 to 2 u in diameter. They are often arranged in branching chains connected by short, thick tubes. They are best demonstrated with stains for carbohydrates (PAS, Gridley). Diagnosis is dependent on demonstrating the characteristic organisms in tissue sections; the fungus has not been successfully cultured.

Lobo's Disease

Migaki, G., Valerio, M. G., Irvine, B., and Garner, F. M.: Lobo's Disease in an Atlantic Bottlenose Dolphin. J. Amer. Vet. Med. Assn. 15 Sep 1971.

Bovine Mycotic Abortion.—Premature expulsion of the bovine fetus upon occasion has been demonstrated to be associated with an infection of the placenta by one of several species of moulds. The demonstration of granulomatous lesions in relation to the presence of fungi in the placenta may be accepted as good evidence that these organisms cause infection which may result in abortion. Perhaps a better name would be "mycotic placentitis," because the placenta is principally involved even though the fetus may also be infected.

Twenty-four species of fungi have been isolated from cases of "mycotic abortion" but it appears that *Aspergillus fumigatus* is the most frequent pathogen— it has been recovered in 60 per cent of the reported cases. *Absidia ramosa*, *Absidia corymbifera* and *Rhizopus* and *Mucor spp.* (see p. 666) have also been recovered with some frequency. Other species are rarely reported and some doubt may remain as to the pathogenic significance of some of them. Infection is generally believed to result from dissemination of organisms via the circulation rather than by direct infection of the genital tract. One of the facts that support this belief is that the disease has been reproduced experimentally by the intravenous injection of fungal spores.

The **lesions** of mycotic abortion are found in the placenta of the aborted bovine fetus but the affected dam rarely exhibits any signs or lesions which could characterize the disease. Affected placentae are described as having enlarged, thickened cotyledons which retain much of the maternal placenta, are thickened at the margins and necrotic in the center. The intracaruncular zones may have a thickened, leathery appearance. Hemorrhage and hyperemia are reported to be prominent in histologic sections of early lesions and are accompanied by neutrophilic and eosinophilic leukocytes. Necrosis tends to separate the maternal and fetal layers of the placenta and the organisms are demonstrable in this zone by appropriate staining techniques (Gridley's, Baurer's, PAS). The organisms are also recoverable from these lesions with suitable culture media. Although thick, encrusted, corrugated lesions have been seen in bovine fetuses from which fungi (*Aspergillus fumigatus*, particularly) were isolated, the histologic nature of the cutaneous lesions have not been determined. The organisms may be recovered from the stomach of aborted bovine fetuses but no lesions have been described in the stomach.

Equine Mycotic Abortion.—It is of interest to record that lesions have been found by Mahaffey and Adam (1964) in the placentae of Thoroughbred mares, indicating that fungi may also be a cause of abortion in the equine species. These workers have demonstrated fungal organisms histologically in lesions in equine placentæ and have isolated organisms identified as *Aspergillus* and *Mucor species*. Further studies will be required to determine the significance of these infections in *Equidæ*.

Cysewski and Pier (1968) have experimentally induced mycotic abortion in ewes with intravenous inoculation of spores of *Aspergillus fumigatus*. The role of fungi in spontaneous abortion of ewes has not been established.

Mycotic Abortion

AINSWORTH, G. C. and AUSTWICK, P. K. C.: *Fungal Diseases of Animals*, Rev. Series 6, 1959. Commonwealth Agric. Bureaux, Farnham Royal, Bucks, England.
BRIDGES, C. H.: Mycotic Diseases in Mammalian Reproduction in *Comparative Aspects of Reproductive Failure*. K. Benirschke, Ed. New York, Springer-Verlag, 1967.
CYSEWSKI, S. J., and PIER, A. C.: Mycotic Abortion in Ewes Produced by *Aspergillus fumigatus*: Pathologic Changes. Am. J. Vet. Res. *29*:1135–1151, 1968.
MAHAFFEY, L. W. and ADAM, N. M.: Abortions Associated with Mycotic Lesions of the Placenta in Mares. J. Am. Vet. Med. Assn. *144*:24–32, 1964.

DERMATOMYCOSES
(Trichophytosis, Ringworm, Favus, Tinea, Superficial Mycoses)

Dermatomycoses are those infections of the skin and its adnexae caused by the dermatophytic fungi (dermatophytes). These fungi comprise many species which inhabit the skin of man or animals and produce lesions under certain conditions. Not only may animals serve as reservoirs for human infection, but man may transmit his infection to animals. The dermatomycoses are characterized by growth of organisms upon or within the hairs, in the stratum corneum of the epidermis, in the hair follicles or the nails. The infection does not disseminate to deeper structures of the body.

The generally accepted mycologic classification of the dermatophytes proposed by Emmons (1934) on the basis of their morphologic characteristics in cultures separates these fungi into three genera (*Trichophyton*, *Microsporum* and *Epidermophyton*) which include all species pathogenic for man and animals. Practically all of the human pathogens in this group also produce lesions in animals. Unfortunately the fungi that cause particular lesions in animals have not always been adequately identified, and several fungi can cause lesions that are clinically indistinguishable. Therefore, precise association of specific agents with characteristic lesions is not always possible. The plethora of synonyms and duplication of names are also confusing to the student. Table 13–1 condenses essential information concerning some identified fungi of this group with their current names and the lesions with which they may be associated. The student is referred to the papers of Georg and associates (1954, 1957, 1959) relative to the clinical and mycological differentiation of the dermatomycoses.

In man, superficial mycoses are often classified by the anatomic site of the lesions as well as their clinical appearance. Several different fungi may be in-

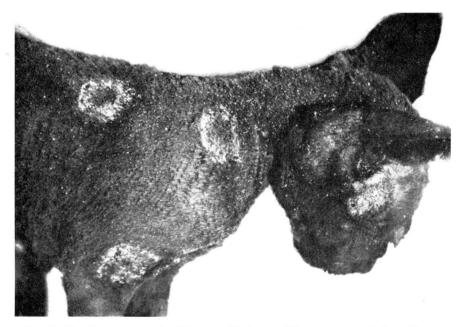

Fig. 13–33.—Dermatomycosis ("ringworm") due to *Microsporum canis*, in a kitten. (Courtesy of Angell Memorial Animal Hospital.)

Table 13–1.—Dermatomycoses

Dermatophyte	Disease	Hosts Commonly Affected
Genus *Trichophyton* (Malmsten, 1845)		
T. mentagrophytes . . .	Ringworm, tinea barbae	Mice, rats, muskrats, chinchillas, cattle, man, horses, sheep, dogs, cats, swine, goats, rabbits, and guinea pigs
T. rubrum	Ringworm, tinea barbae	Dogs, foxes, primates, mice, squirrels, muskrats, etc.
T. tonsurans	Tinea capitis	Man
T. schoenleini	Tinea favosa	Man, cats, mice, rats, and rabbits
T. concentricum . . .	Tinea imbricata, tropical ringworm	Man
T. violaceum	Tinea imbricata	Man
T. verrucosum	Tinea favosa, ringworm	Cattle, man, horses, dogs, and sheep
T. megnini	Tinea favosa	Man
T. gallinae	Favus, tinea	Chickens and turkeys, man
T. equinum	Ringworm, tinia barbae	Children, horses
T. quinkeanum	Ringworm	Children and adults, horses
Genus *Microsporum* (Gruby, 1843)		
M. canis	Sporadic ringworm	Dogs, cats, man, sheep, monkeys
M. audouini	Epidemic ringworm of scalp	Children, dogs, monkeys
M. gypseum	Sporadic ringworm of scalp, favus	Children and adults, dogs, cats, horses
M. nanum	Ringworm	Swine
M. distortum	Ringworm	Monkeys, dogs
Genus *Epidermophyton* (Sabouraud, 1910)		
E. floccusum	Tinea pedis ("athlete's foot")	Man

volved in one clinical entity. Animals are often the source of these organisms, hence some reference to these human entities is of interest. **Tinea pedis,** "athlete's foot" or ringworm of the feet, is associated with *Epidermophyton floccosum,* various species of *Trichophyton* and rarely species of *Microsporum* or *Candida albicans.* **Tinea unguium,** ringworm of the nails, is caused by *Trichophyton rubrum* and occasionally *Candida albicans.* **Tinea cruris,** ringworm of the groin or "jockey itch" results from infection with *Epidermophyton floccosum* and species of *Trichophyton.* **Tinea corporis,** ringworm of the body, is caused by various species of *Trichophyton* and *Microsporum,* involves the glabrous (smooth and hairless) skin and results in either simple scaling or deep granulomas. **Tinea imbricata,** scaly ringworm, is a disease of the tropics and is apparently caused by a single fungus, *Trichophyton concentricum.* **Tinea barbae,** "barber's itch," or ringworms of the beard, is caused by various species of *Trichophyton* and *Microsporum.* The lesions may be superficial or deep and infection is often contracted from animals, particularly cattle. **Tinea capitis,** ringworm of the scalp and hair, is most common in children but may affect adults. The causative organisms, various species of *Trichophyton* and *Microsporum,* may be acquired by contact with infected animals or children. *Microsporum audouini* is most commonly involved but *M. canis* and *M. gypseum* produce deeper, more severe lesions. *T. tonsurans* also is known to produce widespread fungous infections of the scalp. Tinea favosa, favus or

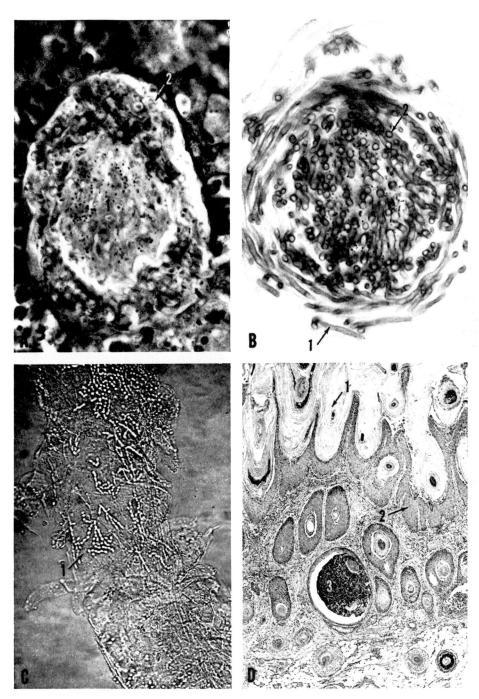

FIG. 13-34.—Dermatomycosis. *A*, Hair follicle (× 730) in the skin of a monkey. Hematoxylin and eosin stain. Organisms are indistinctly seen in hair (*1*) and surrounding it (*2*). *B*, Replicate section of *A*, (× 730) stained with Gridley's fungus stain. Note hyphae of fungi in longitudinal (*1*) and cross section (*2*). *C*, A fresh preparation of hair, showing fungi on surface (*1*) of the hair. *D*, Skin of monkey (× 35). Same case as *A* and *B*. Note severe hyperkeratosis (1), acanthosis (2), and abscess in one hair follicle (*3*). (Courtesy of Armed Forces Institute of Pathology.) Contributor: Dr. Mervin G. Rhoades.

honeycomb ringworm, is also a chronic dermatophytosis caused by *Trichophyton schoenleini*, *T. violaceum* or *Microsporum gypseum*. It is usually limited to the scalp and is characterized by yellowish, cup-shaped crusts (scutula) which have a peculiar "mousey" odor. The disease may produce scarring or permanent alopecia and may spread to the glabrous skin and nails.

The clinical recognition of some of the superficial mycoses is facilitated by the use of filtered ultraviolet light (Wood's light) to examine the lesions in a darkened room. Some species, particularly of *Microsporum*, exhibit fluorescence under the ultraviolet light, making it possible to recognize mild infections. In dogs and cats, *Microsporum canis* is the commonest cause of ringworm but *Trichophyton mentagrophytes* and *Microsporum gypseum* are recovered occasionally by suitable cultural methods. Cattle and horses are more apt to be infected with *Trycophyton mentagrophytes*.

Lesions.—The lesions of dermatomycosis are limited to the hairs, nails, epidermis and dermis. The fungi grow within or upon the surface of the stratum corneum or the hairs. Growth of the fungi often binds hairs together or causes them to shed, depending upon the fungus and host. Dry, scaly or powdery crusts may form, or the hair may be bound together in a *scutulum* which leaves a red, sometimes raw and bleeding surface when it is removed. The lesions are often circumscribed and may involve any part of the skin surface. The name "ringworm" is suggested by the circinate lesions that sometimes result from the outward growth of the organisms from the healing areas in the center.

The microscopic appearance of the lesions is subtle and easily overlooked in routine sections. Thickening of the stratum corneum may be all that can be seen in sections stained with hematoxylin and eosin, but special methods, such as Bauer's stain, the periodic acid-Schiff (PAS) reaction and the Gridley's fungus stain, often make it possible to recognize the fungi in tissue sections. Hypertrophy of the epidermis occurs in severe cases, accompanied by congestion and lymphocytic infiltration of the underlying dermis. In deeper infections in which the hair follicles are involved, severe destruction of the follicle with much resulting inflammation in the dermis may be seen. Organisms also can be identified in hairs and skin scrapings, cleared with a concentrated aqueous solution of sodium or potassium hydroxide and examined under the microscope, using decreased illumination.

Dermatomycosis

BANKS, K. L., and CLARKSON, T. B.: Naturally Occurring Dermatomycosis in the Rabbit. J. Am. Vet. Med. Assn. *151*:926–929, 1967.

CONNOLE, M. D.: A Review of Dermatomycoses of Animals in Australia. Aust. Vet. J. *39*:130–134, 1963. VB 3871–63.

EMMONS, C. W.: Dermatophytes. Natural Grouping Based upon the Form of the Spores and Accessory Organs. Arch. Dermat. & Syph. *30*: 337–362, 1934.

ERRINGTON, P. L.: Observations on a Fungus Skin Disease of Iowa Muskrats. Am. J. Vet. Research *3*:195–201, 1942.

FOWLE, L. P., and GEORG, L. K.: Suppurative Ringworm Contracted from Cattle. Arch. Derm. & Syph. *56*:780–793, 1947.

FUENTES, C. A., BOSCH, Z. E., and BOUDET, C. C.: Occurrence of *Trichophyton mentagrophytes* and *Microsporum gypseum* on Hairs of Healthy Cats. J. Invest. Dermat. *23*:311–313, 1954.

FUENTES, C. A., and ABOULAFIA, R.: *Trichophyton mentagrophytes* from Apparently Healthy Guinea Pigs. Arch. Dermat. & Syph. *71*:478–480, 1955.

GEORG, L. K.: The Diagnosis of Ringworm in Animals, Vet. Med. *49*:157–166, 1954.

GEORG, L. K., KAPLAN, W. and Canap, L. B.: Equine ringworm with special reference to *Trichophyton equinum*. Am. J. Vet. Res. *18*:798–810, 1957.

GEORG, L. K.: Animal Ringworm and Public Health. Diagnosis and Nature. Booklet, U. S. Dept. of Health, Education and Welfare, Public Health Service, Communicable Disease Center, 1959.

GINTHER, O. J.: Clinical Aspects of *Microsporum nanum* Infection in Swine. J. Am. Vet. Med. Assn. *146*:945–953, 1965.

HOERLEIN, A. B.: Studies on Animal Dermatomycoses. I. Clinical Studies. Cornell Vet. *35*:287–298, 1945.

————: Studies on Animal Dermatomycoses. II. Cultural Studies. Cornell Vet. *35*: 299–307, 1945.

KAPLAN, W., HOPPING, J. L., and GEORG, L. K.: Ringworm in Horses Caused by the Dermatophyte, *Microsporum gypseum*. J. Am. Vet. Med. Assn. *131*:329–332, 1957.

MENGES, R. W., and GEORG, L. K.: An Epizoötic of Ringworm among Guinea Pigs Caused by *Trichophyton mentagrophytes*. J. Am. Vet. Med. Assn. *128*:395–398, 1956.

PARRISH, H. J., and CRADDOCK, S.: A Ringworm Epizoötic in Mice. Brit. J. Exper. Path. *12*:209–212, 1931.

14

Diseases Due to Protozoa

In man's scheme of classification of the animal kingdom, unicellular animals are grouped in one phylum: Protozoa. In a current classification (Kudo, 1966), Protozoa are divided into two subphyla: Plasmodroma and Ciliophora. Subphylum Plasmodroma is arranged in four classes:

Class 1. Mastigophora—protozoa with one or more flagella; three types of nutrition (**holophytic**—synthesizing simple carbohydrates from carbon dioxide and water by chlorophyll contained in chloroplasts, **holozoic**—involving capture, ingestion, digestion and assimilation of organic materials and excretion of waste products, **saprozoic**—utilizing simple dissolved organic or inorganic compounds requiring no enzymes or special organelles); free-living and parasitic; parasitic genera include: *Trypanosoma, Leishmania, Giardia, Trichomonas, Histomonas* and *Hexamita.*

Class 2. Sarcodina—protozoa with thin pellicle; form pseudopodia; free-living and parasitic; parasitic genera in the order Amoebida include: *Hartmanella, Acanthamoeba, Endamoeba, Entamoeba, Endolimax* and *Iodamoeba.*

Class 3. Sporozoa—without locomotor organs; produce spores at end of life cycle; all parasitic; include following genera: *Eimeria, Isospora, Klossiella, Hepatozoon, Plasmodium, Haemoproteus, Leukocytozoon, Babesia* and *Theileria.* Three genera of uncertain position may be considered in this class: *Sarcocystis, Besnoitia* and *Toxoplasma.*

Class 4. Cnidosporidia—formerly grouped with the Sporozoa; have unique spores with one to six polar filaments; one or more sporoplasms; parasites of bees, silkworms and fishes; two genera of interest: *Nosema* and *Encephalitozoon.*

The Subphylum Ciliophora contains protozoa with cilia, cirri or other compound ciliary structures for locomotion; two kinds of nuclei—a macronucleus and micronucleus; holozoic and saprozoic nutrition; majority are free living—few are parasitic. Of two classes, Suctoria and Ciliata, only the latter contains a parasitic genus of interest in this text: *Balantidium.*

In this chapter, the effect of protozoa upon various animal hosts will be described and the life cycle of some of the parasitic protozoa will be outlined, with emphasis on those features that influence pathogenesis. In some instances, the effects upon the host have been rather clearly demonstrated and the tissue changes are well known; in others, practically nothing is known. The poorly understood protozoan diseases of animals, therefore, present many challenges to the research-minded veterinary pathologist.

General

BELDING, D. L.: *Textbook of Clinical Parasitology.* 2nd ed., New York, Appleton Century-Crofts, 1952.

COLE, C. R. *et al.*: Some Protozoan Diseases of Man and Animals: Anaplasmosis, Babesiosis and Toxoplasmosis, Ann. New York Acad. Sc. *64*:25–277, 1956.

HENNING, M. W.: *Animal Diseases in South Africa.* 3rd ed., Pretoria, South Africa, Central News Agency, 1957.

KUDO, R. R.: *Protozoology*, 5th Ed., Springfield, Charles C Thomas, 1966.

LEVINE, N. D.: *Protozooan Parasites of Domestic Animals and Man.* Minneapolis, Burgess Pub. Co., 1961.

SOULSBY, E. J. L.: *Helminths, Arthropods and Protozoa of Domesticated Animals (Mönnig).* 6th Ed., Baltimore, The Williams & Wilkins Co., 1968.

WEINMAN, D., and RISTIC, M.: *Infectious Blood Diseases of Man and Animals. Diseases Caused by Protista.* Vol. II. The Pathogens, the Infections and the Consequences. New York and London [Vol. 2], Academic Press, 1968.

COCCIDIOSIS

Coccidiosis is the name applied to the disease produced by protozoa of genera of the order Coccidida. Many species affect animals and birds, the tissues which are attacked depending upon the rather obligate preferences of each parasite. A few of the important coccidial parasites of animals are listed in Table 14–1.

Clinical Manifestations.—Coccidiosis affects the living host in many ways, depending upon the tissue preference of the particular parasite involved and the number of oöcysts in the initial infection. Most of these parasites attack the mucosa of the intestinal tract; therefore symptoms are predominantly enteric. Sudden onset of bloody diarrhea with fever, followed by dehydration, emaciation, and occasionally death are the expected manifestations but, more frequently,

Table 14–1.—*Examples of Tissue Localization of Coccidia*

Host	Coccidia	Tissues Affected
Chicken	*Eimeria tenella*	Ceca
Chicken	*Eimeria necatrix*	Small intestine, ceca
Chicken	*Eimeria brunetti*	Small intestine, ceca
Chicken	*Eimeria acervulina*	Small intestine, ceca
Dog and cat	*Isospora bigemina* and *Isospora felis*	Intestine
Dog and cat	*Eimeria canis* and *Eimeria felina*	Intestine
Rabbit	*Eimeria stiedae*	Intrahepatic bile ducts
Rabbit	*Eimeria magna*	Intestine
Rabbit	*Eimeria neoleporis*	Cecum
Cattle	*Eimeria zurnii*	Intestine
Sheep and goats	*Eimeria parva*	Intestine
Sheep and goats	*Eimeria intricata*	Intestine
Swine	*Eimeria scrofae*	Intestine
Swine	*Isospora suis*	Intestine
Geese	*Eimeria truncata*	Renal tubules
Equidae	*Klossiella equi*	Renal tubules
Mice	*Klossiella muris*	Renal tubules
Mice	*Eimeria falciformis*	Intestine
Rats	*Eimeria nieschulzi*	Small intestine
Rats	*Eimeria separata*	Cecum and colon
Rats	*Hepatozoon muris*	Schizogony-liver Gametocytes-leukocytes
Man	*Isospora hominus*	Intestine
Frogs	*Isospora lieberkuhni*	Renal tubules
Guinea pigs	*Klossiella cobayae*	Renal tubules

little or no evidence of infection is observed in the living animal. Hepatic coccidiosis in rabbits is rarely accompanied by diarrhea, and young animals may die suddenly without showing any obvious signs of disease, although jaundice and emaciation may be recognized in older animals.

Life Cycle.—The life cycles of coccidia are similar and must be understood in order to visualize their effects upon the host. The oöcysts are thick-walled, usually ovoid forms of the organism which resist drying and provide the means of transfer of infection from one host to another. The oöcysts of each species are distinctive morphologically but have essentially similar features. Within the genus *Eimeria*, each fully-matured oöcyst contains four sporocysts, each sporocyst

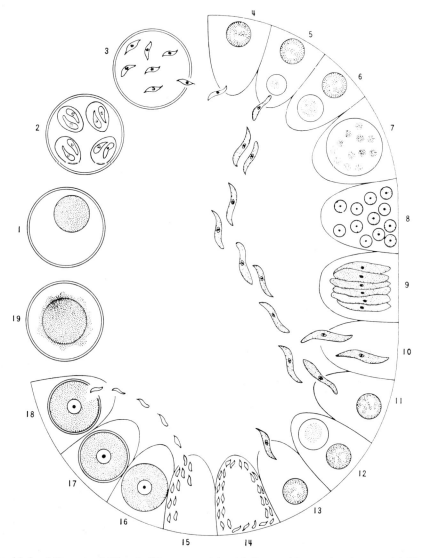

Fig. 14–1.—Life cycle of *Eimeria* (diagrammatic). (*1*) Oöcyst (*2*) sporulated oöcyst (*3*) liberation of sporozoites (*4*) sporozoites entering epithelial cells (*5–11*) schizogony: formation of schizonts and merozoites (*12*) sporogony: formation of macrogametocyte (*13–15*) sporogony: formation of microgametocytes (*16–17*) development of macrogametocyte (*18*) fertilization (*19*) formation of oöcyst.

bearing two sporozoites, a total of eight sporozoites to each oöcyst. Oöcysts of *Isospora* contain two sporocysts, each with four sporozoites; thus the total number of sporozoites is also eight. Each oöcyst has at one pole a tiny pore, the *micropyle*, which is sealed by a substance which, like the rest of the wall, is resistant to drying as well as to many chemical substances. When oöcysts are ingested and reach the small intestine the trypsin-kinase of the pancreatic juice digests the seal of the micropyle and through this opening the tiny sporozoites, now vigorously motile, escape from the oöcyst.

In hepatic coccidiosis of the rabbit, the sporozoites reach the intrahepatic bile ducts through the portal veins or lymphatics, not by way of the common bile duct. Intestinal infection is believed to take place by direct invasion of the intestinal epithelium. Each sporozoite enters a single epithelial cell where it undergoes asexual development known as **schizogony.** The sporozoite gradually increases in size and complexity, becoming first a trophozoite and finally a **schizont,** which literally fills the cytoplasm of the host cell, displacing the nucleus to one pole. Each mature schizont contains many elongated spores similar morphologically to sporozoites but known as **merozoites.** The schizont ruptures its own and the host's cell wall, liberating the merozoites, which infect other epithelial cells and continue this asexual life cycle.

At a certain stage, some of the merozoites enter into the sexual phase of the

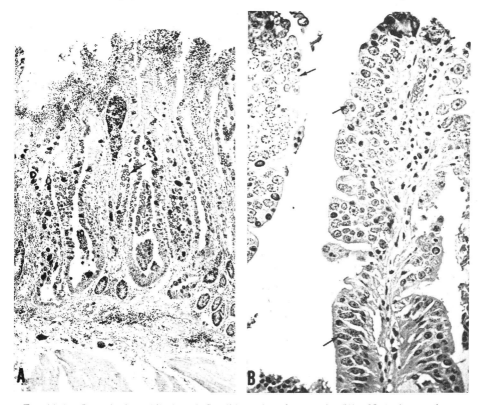

Fig. 14–2.—Intestinal coccidiosis. *A*, Small intestine of a goat (× 50). Note elongated crypts and villi lined with hyperplastic, tall columnar epithelial cells containing coccidia (arrow). Contributor: Dr. L. Z. Saunders. *B*, Small intestine of a mink (× 260). Many coccidia (arrows) in epithelial cells. (Courtesy of Armed Forces Institute of Pathology.) Contributor: Dr. C. L. Davis.

life cycle, known as **gametogenesis.** Each of these predestined merozoites develops within an individual host epithelial cell, into a female form, **macrogamete,** or its male counterpart, a microgametocyte, which eventually ruptures to release a large number of tiny motile **microgametes.** One of the microgametes unites with a single macrogamete, which, upon being so fertilized, soon becomes an oöcyst. Further development within the oöcyst, known as **sporogony,** requires oxygen and certain other conditions which are met outside the body of the host. When the oöcysts are taken in with food or water by a new host, the life cycle is repeated as described above.

Lesions.—Coccidia are obligate intracellular parasites whose development within the cytoplasm of epithelial cells results in the death of each cell which is parasitized. The total effect on the host depends upon (1) the magnitude of the initial infecting dose of oöcysts—which determines the number of cells invaded at the outset by sporozoites; and (2) the spread of infection during schizogony—which is affected to a great extent by immunity acquired by the host. As increasing numbers of organisms enter the sexual phase (gametogenesis), infection of new cells by merozoites diminishes and the disease gradually abates.

When many cells of the intestinal epithelium are parasitized at one time, the denuded mucosa may bleed freely and intense inflammation involves the lamina propria and sometimes the submucosa. As large numbers of epithelial cells are destroyed, the remaining epithelium is stimulated to replace that which was lost. This eventually causes hyperplasia of the intestinal epithelium, which is cast into

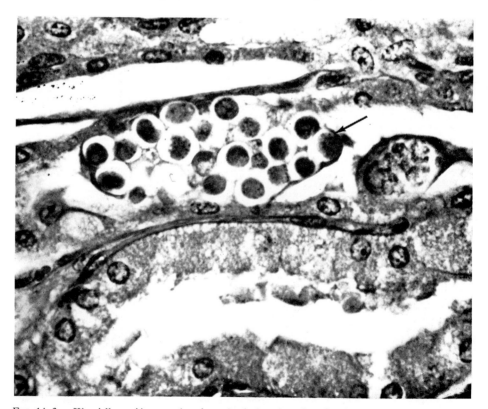

Fig. 14–3.—*Klossiella equi* in convoluted renal tubules of a zebra. Specimen courtesy of Dr. M. J. Eggert from case presented at 1961 Seminar of the American College of Veterinary Pathologists.

long papillary fronds as replacement of epithelial cells exceeds their loss. In lesions exhibiting this hyperplasia, coccidia in various stages of gametogenesis are most numerous. This is in contrast to the erosive, hemorrhagic stages in which organisms in various stages of schizogony are most common.

Hepatic coccidiosis in the rabbit, due to *Eimeria stiedae*, affects the intrahepatic biliary epithelium in somewhat the same manner that other species of coccidia affect the intestinal epithelium. The destruction of biliary epithelium dominates the picture in early lesions, but in those animals in which the course is somewhat longer, proliferation of this epithelium becomes the predominant feature. The bile ducts become enormously enlarged by proliferation of epithelium which is thrown up into papillary folds simulating adenomatous hyperplasia. These greatly enlarged segments of the bile ducts displace the adjacent liver parenchyma and appear grossly as irregularly shaped grayish areas which are seen as depressions in the surface of the capsule (Fig. 4–2).

The gross lesions of intestinal coccidiosis may be envisaged from the above account to appear as intensely congested, eroded and bleeding areas of certain segments of the small intestine, sometimes alternating with, or replaced, by areas in which the epithelium is thickened.

Certain coccidia localize in the convoluted tubules of the kidney. Among these parasites are: *Klossiella equi*, parasitic in horses, zebras and asses (Equidae); *Eimeria truncata* in the goose; *Klossiella muris* in the mouse and *Klossiella cobayae* in the guinea pig. Although these organisms destroy some renal epithelium, their total effect appears slight—no clinical signs are produced—the parasites are usually found incidentally at necropsy.

Diagnosis.—The clinical diagnosis is usually based upon the presence of oöcysts in fecal specimens, associated with sudden onset of typical bloody diarrhea. The microscopic lesions at necropsy are characteristic and are confirmed by demonstrating the organisms in tissue sections.

Coccidiosis

BIESTER, H. E., and MURRAY, C.: Studies in Infectious Enteritis of Swine. VIII. *Isospora suis* (N. Sp.) in Swine. J. Am. Vet. Med. Assn. *85*:207–219, 1934.

COSSEL, L.: Nierenbefunde beim Meerschweinchen bei Klossiellen-Infektion (*Klossiella cobayae*). (Zur Kenntnis der speziellen Pathologie der Versuchstiere.) Schweiz. allgem. Pathol. u. Bakteriol. *21*:62–73, 1958.

DAVIS, C. L., CHOW, T. L., and GORHAM, J. R.: Hepatic Coccidiosis in Mink. Vet. Med. *48*:371–373, 1953.

DAVIS, L. R. and BOWMAN, G. W.: The Endogenous Development of *Eimeria zurnii*, a Pathogenic Coccidium of Cattle. Am. J. Vet. Res. *18*:569–574, 1957.

GRÄFNER, G., GRAUBMANN, H.-D., and DOBBRINER, W.: Hepatic Coccidiosis in Mink Caused by a New Species, *Eimeria hiepei*. Mh. Vet. Med. *22*:696–700, 1967. V.B. *38*:2638, 1968.

HAMMOND, D. M., DAVIS, L. R., and BOWMAN, G. W.: Experimental Infections With *Eimeria bovis* in Calves. Am. J. Vet. Res. *5*:303–311, 1944.

HARTMAN, H. A.: The Protozoan Parasite, *Klossiella equi*, in the Mexican Burro. Am. J. Vet. Res. *22*:1126–1129, 1961.

HITCHCOCK, D. J.: The Life of *Isospora felis* in the Kitten. J. Parasitol. *41*:383–397, 1955.

LEE, C. D.: The Pathology of Coccidiosis in the Dog. J. Am. Vet. Med. Assn. *85*:760–781, 1934.

LEVINE, N. D., and IVENS, V.: Isospora Species in the Dog. J. Parasit. *51*:859–864, 1965.

LEVINE, P. P.· A New Coccidium Pathogenic for Chickens, *Eimeria brunetti*, N. Sp. (Protozoa: Eimeriidæ). Cornell Vet. *32*:430–439, 1942.

————: Subclinical Coccidial Infection in Chickens. Cornell Vet. *30*:127–132, 1940.

LOTZE, J. C.: The Pathogenicity of the Coccidian Parasite *Eimeria arloingi* in Domestic Sheep. Cornell Vet. *42*:510–517, 1952.

MUGERA, G. M.: Pathology of Coccidiosis in Kenya Goats. Bull. Epizoot. Dis. Afr. *16*: 101–106, 1968.

NEWBERNE, J. W., ROBINSON, V. B., and BOWEN, N. E.: Histological Aspects of *Klossiella equi* in the Kidney of a Zebra. Am. J. Vet. Res. *19*:304–307, 1958.

PIERCE, L.: Klossiella Infection of the Guinea Pig. J. Exp. Med. *23*:431–442, 1916.

POUT, D. D.: Review Article: Coccidiosis of Sheep. Vet. Bull. *39*:609–618, 1969.

SCHOLTYSECK, E.: (Electron Microscopy of Schizogony in *Eimeria perforans* and *E. stiedae*). Z. ParasitKde. *26*:50–62, 1965. V.B. *36*:515, 1966.

SEIBOLD, H. R. and THORSON, R. E.: *Klossiella equi*, N. S. P. (Protozoa-Klossiellidae) from the Kidney of an American Jack. J. Parasit. *41*:285–288, 1955.

SEIDELIN, H.: *Klossiella sp.* in the Kidney of a Guinea Pig. Ann. Trop. Med. and Parasitol. *8*: 553–564, 1941.

SHARMA DEORANI, V. P.: Histopathological Studies in Natural Infection of Goat Coccidiosis. Indian Vet. J. *43*:122–127, 1966.

SIVADAS, C. G., RAJAN, A., and NAIR, M. K.: Studies on Pathology of Coccidiosis in Goats. Indian Vet. J. *42*:474–479, 1965.

SMETANA, H.: Coccidiosis of the Liver in Rabbits. I. Experimental Study on the Excystation of Oocysts of *Eimeria stiedae*. Arch. Path. *15*:175–192, 1933.

—————: Coccidiosis of the Liver in Rabbits. II. Experimental Study on the Mode of Infection of the Liver by Sporozoites of *Eimeria stiedae*. Arch. Path. *15*:330–339, 1933.

—————: Coccidiosis of the Liver in Rabbits. III. Experimental Study of the Histogenesis of Coccidiosis of the Liver. Arch. Path. *15*:516–536, 1933.

SMITH, T. and JOHNSON, H. P.: On a Coccidium (*Klossiella muris*, ges. et. spec. Nov) Parasitic in the Renal Epithelium of the Mouse. J. Exp. Med. *6*:303–316, 1902.

SPINDLER, L. A.: Investigations on Coccidia of Sheep and Goats. Am. J. Vet. Res. *26*: 1068–1070, 1965.

VETTERLING, J. M.: Endogenous Cycle of the Swine Coccidium *Eimeria debliecki* Douwes, 1921. J. Protozool. *13*:290–300, 1966.

—————: Prevalence of Coccidia in Swine from Six Localities in the United States. Cornell Vet. *56*:155–166, 1966.

TOXOPLASMOSIS

Toxoplasma gondii, a small crescentic protozoön parasite, was first described in 1908, in material from a small rodent, the gondi, by Nicolle and Manceaux (1908) but its widespread distribution in the animal kingdom was not generally recognized until more than twenty years later. The organisms were rediscovered by Sabin and Olitsky in 1935 in the brains of guinea pigs that were being used to propagate encephalitis viruses. Shortly thereafter the incrimination of *Toxoplasma* as the cause of a diffuse encephalitis and chorioretinitis in a thirty-one-day old infant by Wolfe, Cowan and Paige (1939) stimulated great interest in toxoplasmosis.

Studies of Work and Hutchinson (1969) demonstrated an infective cyst in feces of cats experimentally infected with toxoplasma from mouse tissues. This cyst was identified by Frenkel, Dubey and Mullen (1969) as an oöcyst, typical of the genus *Isospora*, and associated with schizonts, micro- and macrogametocytes in the intestinal epithelium. The life cycle currently postulated assumes the cat to be the final host. The organism undergoes schizogeny in the cat's intestine to produce oöcysts which are resistant to environmental influences and are infective after sporogeny. The sporulated oöcysts can survive long periods and remain infective for mice or other intermediate hosts which may develop either chronic or acute infection. Transmission in mice may occur congenitally to fetuses, *in utero*, or to other carnivorous animals including cats who eat them. The cat may acquire infection by eating either trophozoites in acutely infected mice or or encysted cysts containing toxoplasmal merozoites in chronically-infected animals.

Thus *Toxoplasma gondii* at this writing appears to have the characteristics of Coccidida with schizogony and gametogony in the intestinal epithelium of cats resulting in oöcysts with two sporocysts and four sporozoites. Trophozoites multiply by endogeny in tissues of many species to produce acute or latent disease which will be discussed further.

The sexual states in the intestinal tract have been observed so far only in cats but the disease caused by the asexual parasites (trophozoites) is known to occur in man and nearly all wild and domesticated mammals and birds.

Clinical Manifestations.—In man, toxoplasmosis is recognized most frequently as a congenitally acquired infection of the newborn, manifested by encephalitis, chorioretinitis, microencephaly, macroencephaly, cerebral calcifications, convulsive disorders and mental retardation. In adults, chorioretinitis, lymphadenopathy, myocarditis, pneumonia, and meningoencephalitis have been associated with toxoplasma. In some instances, it appears that the concomitant presence of a virus or other deleterious influence makes it possible for toxoplasma to produce fatal infections.

In animals, such a wide diversity of manifestations have been attributed to toxoplasmosis that it is difficult to ascribe limits to the clinical signs of this infection. The organisms apparently can persist in the tissues of an animal for long periods, producing lesions and symptoms only under certain as yet incompletely understood circumstances. They most often affect the brain, myocardium, lymph nodes, lung, intestinal muscularis, pancreas, or liver, hence symptoms of toxo-

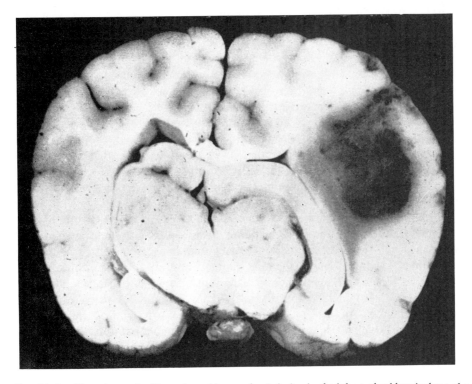

Fig. 14–4.—Toxoplasmosis. Necrotic and hemorrhagic lesion in the left cerebral hemisphere of a 4-year-old male poodle. Myriads of *Toxoplasma gondii* were demonstrated in microscopic sections of this lesion. (Courtesy of Angell Memorial Animal Hospital.)

plasmosis may be referable to involvement of any one or more of these organs. Several clinical laboratory tests have been developed which are of value in the diagnosis of toxoplasmosis in man and animals. Four such tests are in common use: First, the **Sabin-Feldman Dye Test,** in which toxoplasma are exposed to dilutions of suspected serum, then stained with alkaline methylene blue. In the presence of normal serum, both the cytoplasm and nucleus of the organism stain deeply, but antibody in the serum causes the nuclear endosome only to take the dye. Although this test has some technical hazards, it is of value in detecting significant antibody. A second test utilizes the complement-fixation reaction with antigens prepared from *Toxoplasma gondii* cultivated in mouse peritoneum or tissue cultures. A third test which is of much value is the isolation of organisms by intraperitoneal inoculation of mice. A fourth test, useful as a research tool, is a neutralization test using tissue cultures in which toxoplasma are grown. A hemagglutination test has also been developed for use in studying immunity in toxoplasmosis but is not yet available for widespread clinical usage. Organisms may be specifically stained with fluorescein-labeled antiglobulin which has an affinity for Toxoplasma antibody which may be bound to oöcyst and sporocyst walls in paraffin sections and sporozoites, schizonts and macrogametocytes in smears (Frenkel, Dubey and Miller, 1970).

Characteristics of Toxoplasma.—*Toxoplasma gondii* is believed to be the single species of this parasite which infects all varieties of animals and man. The organism is readily maintained in the laboratory by cultivation in the peritoneal cavity of the mouse or in tissue cultures. In these situations, the organism appears crescentic or arc-shaped with one end rounded and the other pointed. It measures 2 to 4 microns in width and 4 to 7 microns in length. It has a nucleus, most clearly demonstrated with Giemsa's stain, located near one pole of the cell. Its cytoplasm may contain chromatin and glycogen granules, but there is neither demonstrable centrosome nor kinetoplast (see trypanosomiasis). Electron microscope studies indicate that there is a truncated cone, "conoid," at the anterior end with several homogeneous fibrils called "toxonemes" extending from it toward the blunter end of the cell. The organisms are frequently found in parallel pairs, indicating that reproduction occurs by longitudinal division. These organisms, heretofore considered as the only form of *Toxoplasma*, now appear to be trophozoites which have the ability to multiply in animal tissues and form collections of organisms (schizonts) which under certain conditions (especially in the brain) may become encysted.

In tissue sections, trophozoites of *Toxoplasma* may be crescentic, but also occur in rounded and ovoid form. Presumably because of shrinkage in fixation, the organisms usually appear smaller in sections than in smears, about 2 microns wide and 4 microns long. They are most frequently found in the cytoplasm of cells but may be free. A large number of the organisms may be encountered in a single cell or may be contained by a thin, poorly defined membrane which is believed to be the remnant of the wall of a host cell by some, a product of the parasite by others. Those who consider this membrane to be the remnant of a tissue cell wall speak of the structure as a "pseudocyst," those who consider the wall to be formed by the parasite speak of it as a "cyst." It does appear that these encysted schizonts represent a resting stage of the parasite, because they are often seen in the absence of reaction in the adjacent host tissues and they are apparently more resistant to deleterious influences in this stage.

Electron photomicrographs and histochemical studies indicate that the cyst wall is actually formed by the organisms, thus the term "pseudocyst" is not valid.

Lesions.—From experimental evidence, infection with *Toxoplasma* is believed to result first in parasitemia, then in localization and multiplication of the organ-

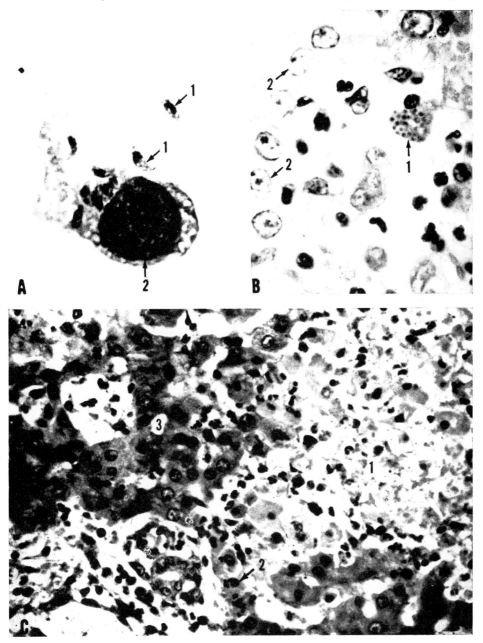

Fig. 14–5.—Toxoplasmosis. *A*, Trophozoites of *Toxoplasma gondii* (*1*) in mouse peritoneum, most organisms in macrophage (*2*). Contributor: Dr. W. B. Dublin. *B*, Trophozoites of *Toxoplasma gondii* (*1*) in lung of a cat. Note proliferation and cuboidal shape (*2*) of cells lining alveoli. Contributor: Dr. M. Zimmerman. *C*, Sharply demarcated necrotic lesion (*1*) in liver of a dog (× 500). Necrotic (*2*) and viable (*3*) liver cells are present. (Courtesy of Armed Forces Institute of Pathology.) Contributor: Angell Memorial Animal Hospital.

isms in various tissues. This localization may be followed by active lesions in the affected tissue or, for unknown reasons, by encystment of the *Toxoplasma*, in which form they remain viable for a long time. This occult infection is most likely to occur in the brain, where living organisms have been found several years following infection: after two years in dogs and rats and three years in pigeons. *Toxoplasma* trophozoites may therefore be demonstrable in microscopic sections of animal tissues in which the injury to the host may be intense, minimal or non-recognizable. The judgment of the pathologist may be severely tested in deciding just what influence, if any, *Toxoplasma* may have in a particular case. However, in active toxoplasmosis the microscopic findings in a particular organ are reasonably characteristic, hence will be considered under each organ.

In the **brain**, active infection is indicated by diffuse nonsuppurative infiltration of brain parenchyma, particularly adjacent to the meninges, which may be similarly infiltrated. Lymphocytic cells accumulate within the Robin-Virchow spaces and are scattered through the parenchyma. Vacuoles may occur in the white matter. *Toxoplasma* trophozoites may be found scattered singly or in pairs through the parenchyma or in aggregations (schizonts) containing up to 50 organisms. Necrotizing lesions have been observed in the basilar arteries in the cat, but their relationship to toxoplasmosis is not clearly established.

The liver in frank toxoplasmosis contains large, sharply delimited, microscopic-

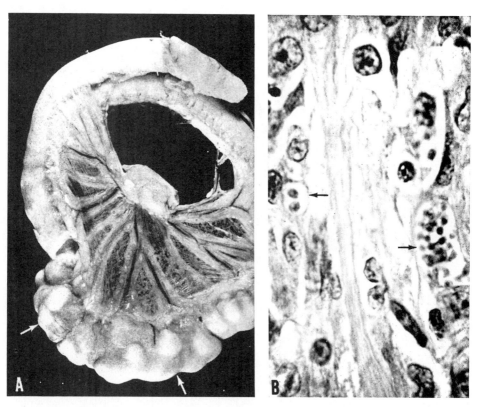

FIG. 14–6.—Toxoplasmosis. *A*, Nodular granulomatous lesion in the intestinal muscularis of a cat. *B*, Involved muscularis of intestine (× 1283). *Toxoplasma gondii* are in trophozoite pairs and larger groups (schizonts?) in smooth muscle cells (arrows). (Courtesy of Armed Forces Institute of Pathology.) Contributor: Dr. Leo L. Lieberman.

sized areas of coagulation necrosis, involving any part of the hepatic lobules. The necrotic areas, containing eosinophilic material and cell debris, are surrounded by apparently normal hepatic cells with little or no cellular reaction. Trophozoites may be found within liver or Kupffer cells, in cysts containing a large number of organisms, or singly or in pairs scattered sparsely in both the necrotic and viable tissues. Organisms may be few in number even when severe necrosis is present.

The **lung** exhibits rather striking changes, particularly in cats, although other species may show similar lesions. The changes are particularly evident in the alveolar walls whose lining becomes cuboidal or columnar and very rich in cells, suggesting in this respect the appearance of fetal lung (so-called "fetalization" of lung). This feature also has superficial resemblances to pulmonary adenomatosis. The alveoli are filled with large mononuclear cells and leukocytes with aggregations of *Toxoplasma* in the cells lining the alveoli. These lesions have a nodular distribution throughout the lung, appearing grossly as small, gray, tumor-like masses, scattered throughout one or all lobes.

The **lymph nodes,** particularly those contiguous to affected parenchymal organs, are commonly involved in active cases. They are usually enlarged to several times their normal size, are firm in consistency and densely congested. Extensive coagulation necrosis is seen microscopically, usually in sharply demarcated but irregular zones with slight leukocytic infiltration around the margins. Trophozoites may be found adjacent to these necrotic areas, particularly in endothelial cells of veins, but may be within the cytoplasm of monocytic cells or free in the tissues.

Ulcers in the **intestine,** presumably resulting from necrotic changes in submucosal lymph nodules, have been described in toxoplasmosis. Upon occasion, *Toxoplasma* invade the muscularis of the intestine where a chronic necrotizing lesion followed by production of granulation tissue results in large, grossly detectable granulomatous nodules which may replace the wall and impinge upon the lumen. The organisms are clearly demonstrable in small and large groups in the muscularis and the granulation tissue.

The **pancreas** may be a site of localization in toxoplasmosis, and here the acute necrotizing lesions arouse intense lymphocytic infiltration, edema and swelling.

The **eye** may be infected in human adults, and ocular infection has been reported in animals. The lesion is one of granulomatous chorioretinitis in which *Toxoplasma* are demonstrable.

The **myocardium** is frequently invaded by *Toxoplasma* which may be present in large or small groups within the cytoplasm of cardiac muscle cells. In some instances, severe lymphocytic inflammation is evoked, in others, the organisms are present with little associated inflammation.

Diagnosis.—The diagnosis of toxoplasmosis in the living animal is at present more of a problem than at necropsy. The complement fixation, neutralization, hemagglutination, mouse inoculation and Sabin-Feldman dye tests described above are of value. Isolation of the organisms is most decisive although concomitant infections must always be suspected. At necropsy, the demonstration of *Toxoplasma* in tissue sections in characteristic lesions should be supported by isolation of the organisms whenever possible. In tissue sections, the microscopic appearance of *Sarcocystis*, leishmanial forms of *Trypanosoma cruzi*, *Besnoitia besnoitia* and sporozoites of Coccidia must be differentiated from *Toxoplasma*. The size (about twice as large) and definite cyst wall around *Sarcocystis* are reliable points of differentiation. The leishmanial forms of *Trypanosoma cruzi* may be distinguished by their centrosome and kinetoplast which can be seen in some of the organisms. *Besnoitia* may be distinguished by the giant nuclei in the well-developed wall of the cyst in which the small organisms are found.

Toxoplasmosis

CAPEN, C. C., and COLE, C. R.: Pulmonary Lesions in Dogs with Experimental and Naturally Occurring Toxoplasmosis. Path. Vet. *3*:40–63, 1966.
CROWLEY, J. P.: Abortion and Prenatal Mortality in Sheep Associated with Toxoplasmosis. Irish J. Agric. Res. *3*:159–164, 1964.
FARRELL, R. L., DOCTON, F. L., CHAMBERLAIN, D. M., and COLE, C. R.: Toxoplasmosis. I. *Toxoplasma* Isolated From Swine. Am. J. Vet. Research *12*:181–185, 1952.
FELDMAN, H. A.: The Clinical Manifestations and Laboratory Diagnosis of Toxoplasmosis. Am. J. Trop. Med. & Hyg. *2*:420–428, 1953.
FRENKEL, J. K.: Ocular Lesions in Hamsters With Chronic *Toxoplasma* and *Besnoitia* Infection. Am. J. Ophth. *39*:203–225, 1955.
————: Host, Strain and Treatment Variation as Factors in Pathogenesis of Toxoplasmosis. Am. J. Trop. Med. & Hyg. *2*:390–415, 1953.
FRENKEL, J. K., DUBEY, J. P., and MILLER, N. L.: *Toxoplasma gondii*: Fecal Forms Separated from Eggs of the Nematode *Toxocara cati*. Science *164*:432–433, 1969.
————: *Toxoplasma gondii* in Cats: Fecal Stages Identified as Coccidian Oocysts. Science *167*:893–896, 1970.
GARNHAM, P. C. C., BAKER, J. R., and BIRD, R. G.: Fine Structure of Cystic Form of Toxoplasma gondii. Brit. Med. J. *83*:83–84, 1962. (VB 1462–62.)
GAVIN, M. A., WANKS, T., and JACOBS, L.: Electron Microscopic Studies of Reproducing and Interkinetic *Toxoplasma*. J. Prot. *9*:222–234, 1962.
GUSTAFSON, P. V., AGAR, H. D., and CRAMER, D. I.: An Electron Microscope Study of "*Toxoplasma*." Am. J. Trop. Med. & Hyg. *3*:1008–1022, 1954.
HARTLEY, W. J.: Some Investigations into the Epidemiology of Ovine Toxoplasmosis. N.Z. Vet. J. *14*:106–117, 1966.
HARTLEY, W. J., and MOYLE, G.: Observation on an Outbreak of Ovine Congenital Toxoplasmosis. Aust. Vet. J. *44*:105–107, 1968.
HARTLEY, W. J., LINDSAY, A. B., and MacKINNON, M. M.: Toxoplasma Meningioencephalomyelitis and Myositis in a Dog. N. Z. Vet. J. *6*:124–127, 1958.
HARTLEY, W. J. and KATER, J. C.: The Pathology of Toxoplasma Infection in the Pregnant Ewe. Res. Vet. Sci. *4*:326–332, 1963. (VB 2333–63.)
HIRTH, R. S., and NIELSEN, S. W.: Pathology of Feline Toxoplasmosis. J. Small Anim. Pract. *10*:213–221, 1969.
HULDT, G.: Experimental Toxoplasmosis: Studies of the Multiplication and Spread of Toxoplasma in Experimentally Infected Rabbits. Acta Path. microbiol. scand. *67*:401–423, 1966.
HUTCHISON, W. M., *et al.*: Coccidian-like Nature of *Toxoplasma gondii*. Brit. Med. J. *1*: 142–144, 1970.
JACOBS, L., MELTON, M. L., and COOK, M. K.: Observations in Toxoplasmosis in Dogs. J. Parasitol. *41*:353–361, 1955.
KATSUBE, Y., *et al.*: Studies on Toxoplasmosis. I. Isolation of Toxoplasma from Muscles of Humans, Dogs and Cats. Jap. J. Med. Sci. Biol. *20*:413–419, 1967.
KIRMSE, P.: *Toxoplasma gondii* Isolated from a Groundhog. Bull. Wildl. Dis. Assn. *1*:3–11, 1965.
KOESTNER, A. and COLE, C. R.: Neuropathology of canine toxoplasmosis. Am. J. Vet. Res. *21*:813–830, 1960.
————: Neuropathology of Porcine Toxoplasmosis. Cornell Vet. *50*:362–384, 1960.
LAINSON, R.: Observations on the Development of and Nature of Pseudocysts and Cysts of *Toxoplasma gondii*. Trans. R. Soc. Trop. Med. & Hyg. *52*:396–407, 1958.
McKISSICK, G. E., RATCLIFFE, H. L., and KOESTNER, A.: Enzootic Toxoplasmosis in Caged Squirrel Monkeys *Saimiri sciureus*. Path. Vet. *5*:538–560, 1968.
MEIER, H., HOLZWORTH, J., and GRIFFITHS, R. C.: Toxoplasmosis in the Cat, 14 Cases. J. Am. Vet. Med. Assn. *131*:395–414, 1957.
MOCSARI, E., and SZEMEREDI, G.: Diagnostical Value of the Complement Fixation Test and the Fluorescent Antibody Method in the Laboratory Diagnosis of Toxoplasmosis. Acta Vet. Hung. *19*:21–27, 1969.
MØLLER, T. and NIELSEN, S. W.: Toxoplasmosis in Distemper-susceptible Carnivora. Path. vet. *1*:189–203, 1964.

NAKABAYASHI, T., *et al.*: Studies on the Detection of *Toxoplasma gondii* with Mouse Inoculation Method and Fluorescent Antibody Technic in Slaughtered Pigs. Trop. Med. Nagasak *11*:16–26, 1969.

NICOLLE, C., and MANCEAUX, L.: Sur une infection à corps de Leishman (ou organismes voisins) du gondi. Compt. rend. Acad. d. sc. *147*:763–766, 1908.

NOBEL, T. A., NEUMAN, F., and KLOPFER, U.: An Outbreak of Toxoplasmosis in Hyrax (*Procavia capensis syriacus*). Refuah Vet. *22*:59–62, 1965.

OLAFSON, P., and MONLUX, W. S.: *Toxoplasma* Infection in Animals. Cornell Vet. *32*:176–190, 1942.

OVEDULVE, J. P.: The Probable Identity of Toxoplasma and Isospora and the Role of the Cat in the Transmission of Toxoplasmosis. Tijdschr. Diergeneesk. *95*:149–155, 1970.

PRIDHAM, T. J. and BELCHER, J.: Toxoplasmosis in Mink. Canad. J. Comp. Med. *22*:99–106, 1958.

SAXEN, E. and SAXEN, L.: The Histological Diagnosis of Glandular Toxoplasmosis. Lab. Invest. *8*:386–394, 1959.

SHEFFIELD, H. G., and MELTON, M. L.: *Toxoplasma gondii*: Transmission Through Feces in Absence of *Toxocara cati* Eggs. Science *164*:431–432, 1969.

————: *Toxoplasma gondii*: The Oocyst, Sporozoite, and Infection of Cultured Cells. Science *167*:892–893, 1970.

SHIMIZU, K., KITO, S., and SHIRAHATA, T.: Experiments on Mouse Passage of the Cyst Type Strain of *Toxoplasma gondii* for Enhancement of Virulence. Jap. J. Vet. Sci. *29*:71–78, 1967.

SIIM, J. C., HUTCHISON, W. M., and WORK, K.: Transmission of *Toxoplasma gondii*. Further Studies on the Morphology of the Cystic Form in Cat Faeces. Acta Path. Microbiol. Scand. *77*:756–757, 1969.

SMITH, C.: Staining of *Toxoplasma* in Histological Sections. Brit. J. Ophth. *37*:504–505, 1953.

TISSEUR, H., *et al.*: Histological Diagnosis of Toxoplasmosis in Animals. Recl. Med. Vet. *142*:15–23, 1966.

VAINISI, S. J., and CAMPBELL, L. H.: Ocular Toxoplasmosis in Cats. J. Am. Vet. Med. Assn. *154*:141–152, 1969.

WANKO, T., JACOBS, L., and GAVIN, M. A.: Electron Microscope Study of Toxoplasma Cysts in Mouse Brain. J. Prot. *9*:235–242, 1962.

WERNER, H., and EGGER, I.: Latent Toxoplasma Infection of the Uterus and Its Importance for Pregnancy. II. Influence on the Course of Pregnancy in Mice. Zentbl. Bakt. Parasit. I. *208*:122–135, 1968. V.B. *39*:1059, 1969.

WERNER, H., JANITSCHKE, K., and KÖHLER, H.: Über Beobachtungen an Marmoset-Affen *Saguinus (Oedipomidas) oedipus* nach oral und intraperitonealer Infektion mit verschiedenen zystenbildunden Toxoplasma—Stämmen unterschiedlicher Virulenz. Zentbl. Bakt. Parasit. I. *209*:553–569, 1969. V.B. *39*:4568, 1969.

WILDER, H. C.: *Toxoplasma* Chorioretinitis in Adults. Arch. Ophth. *48*:127–136, 1952.

WILDFÜHR, W.: Elektronenmikroskopische Untersuchungen zur Morphologie und Reproduction von *Toxoplasma gondii*. Zentbl. Bakt. Parasit *200*:525–547, 1966. V.B. *36*:4707, 1966.

WILSON, S. G., *et al.*: Toxoplasmosis in Pigs. An Experimental Study of Oral Infection and Infection Through the Skin. Vet. Rec. *81*:313–317, 1967.

WOLF, A., COWEN, D., and PAIGE, B.: Human Toxoplasmosis: Occurrence in Infants as an Encephalomyelitis. Verification by Transmission to Animals. Science *89*:226–227, 1939.

WORK, K., and HUTCHISON, W. M.: The New Cyst of Toxoplasma Gondii. Acta path. microbiol. scand. *77*:414–424, 1969.

ENCEPHALITOZOÖNOSIS

(Nosematosis)

Encephalitozoön cuniculi, a minute organism presently classified with the Protozoa, has been described as the cause of a paralytic and systemic disease of rabbits and has been encountered in brains of apparently normal laboratory rats, rabbits, mice and guinea pigs.

Findings by Nelson (1962) and Lainson *et al.* (1964) indicate that this organism at one point in its life cycle develops a capsule and extrudes a polar filament. Organisms maintained by intraperitoneal inoculation of mice also have a developmental cycle and fine structure typical of protozoa classified as Microsporidia, particularly in the family Nosematidae. It has consequently been suggested that the organism be named *Nosema cuniculi* (Levaditi *et al.*, 1923) and the disease, "nosematosis." However, further studies with the life cycles of these organisms (Cali, 1971) indicate that the species from mammals differs significantly from those which infect invertebrates and therefore should not be included in the genus, *Nosema.* The name *Encephalitozoon cuniculi* therefore appears to be valid for the mammalian parasite.

Of interest is the association of organisms of the family Nosematidae with diseases of bees, silkworms and other invertebrate species. *Nosema apis* is the cause of destructive "nosema-disease" of honey bees, *Apis mellifica*. The organisms infect the midgut wall and Malpighian tubules of the adult bees, especially the workers, although drones and queens are susceptible (Kudo, 1966).

Nosema bombycis may infect most cells of the silkworm, *Bombyx mori*, in any stage of development (embryo, larva, pupa, adult). Numerous tiny brownish-black foci are scattered over the body of the silkworm, giving rise to such names as "pebrine" and "Fleckenkrankheit." The organisms invade and multiply in the ova, infecting larvae before hatching and often causing their death before pupation.

Several other species of *Nosema* have been identified as parasites of mosquitoes, tapeworms, beetles, etc. (Kudo, 1966). *Encephalitozoon cuniculi* has been isolated from rabbit brain and cultivated on monolayer cell cultures from rabbit

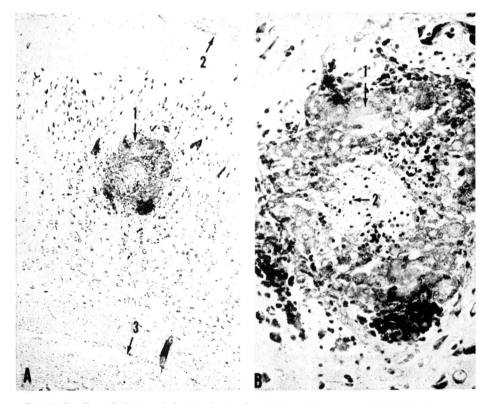

FIG. 14–7.—Encephalitozoon infection, brain of a rabbit. *A*, Low power ($\times$ 45) to show granuloma (*1*) in the cerebral cortex. Pia mater (*2*) and ependyma (*3*) of lateral ventricle. *B*, Higher magnification of granuloma. Large, foamy macrophages (*1*) surrounding necrotic center containing organisms (*2*). (Courtesy of Armed Forces Institute of Pathology.) Contributor: U.S. Army Environmental Health Laboratory.

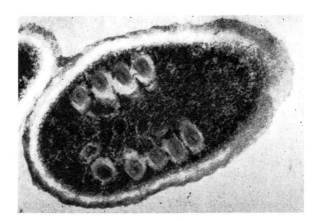

Fig. 14–8.—*Encephalitozoon cuniculi*, (× 36,800). Note cross sections of polar filament. (Courtesy of Dr. J. A. Shadduck, Ohio State University, and *Science*.)

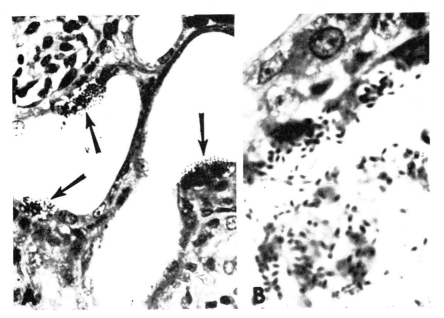

Fig. 14–9.—Encephalitozoonosis, rabbit. *A*, *Encephalitozoon* (*Nosema*) *cuniculi* (arrows) within renal tubular epithelial cells. *B*, Organisms being extruded from epithelial cells and free within tubular lumen.

choroid plexus by Shadduck (1969). The development of this method of pure culture, *in vitro*, of this organism will undoubtedly facilitate its study.

Subclinical infections and encephalitis in man have also been associated with this organism (Matsubayashi *et al.*, 1959). The possibility of transplacental passage of this organism has been proposed by Innes, *et al.* (1962).

The **lesions** associated with infection are most characteristic in rabbits. The usual experience is to find the lesions and the organisms incidentally in histological sections from rabbits which have shown no recognizable signs of infection, although in rare cases paralysis and death have been attributed to the parasite. In the brain, focal lesions are chiefly in the cerebral cortex but may occur anywhere. Microscopic-sized granulomas made up of epithelioid cells surrounding a tiny necrotic center are the common finding in these occult infections. Larger areas of necrosis may be seen in fatal cases and perivascular lymphocytic cuffing may be prominent. The organisms are demonstrable in the necrotic centers of the granulomas, usually appearing singly as short, plump rod-shaped bodies with rounded ends, measuring about 1 by 2 microns. They are stained intensely by silver impregnation methods (Warthin-Starry) and accept Giemsa's stain but are usually not visible in sections stained with hematoxylin and eosin.

In the mouse peritoneum, the organism may be demonstrated to extrude its polar filament and be actively motile. Electron micrographs reveal the polar filament when it is coiled within the body of the parasite and enveloped by membranes. Occasionally it may be seen in longitudinal array (Fig. 14-8). The spores are about 2 microns long and also contain a laminated structure known as the polaroplast.

Robinson (1954) has described a very prevalent, mild and chronic disease in laboratory rabbits which he associated with *Encephalitozoon* (*Nosema*). The lesions he found in the brain conform to those described above; the kidneys and myocardium also contained small focal scars, granulomas or lymphocytic infiltrations. The interstitial focal nephritis was often severe but did not seem to terminate in uremia and myocardial involvement was not severe enough to cause death. Further study is needed to clarify many questions about this organism and the lesions with which it is associated.

Encephalitozoönosis

BASSON, P. A., *et al.*: Nosematosis: Report of a Canine Case in the Republic of South Africa. J. S. Afr. Vet. Med. Assn. *37*:3–9, 1966.
INNES, J. R. M., *et al.*: "Occult, Endemic Encephalitozoonosis of the Central Nervous System of Mice." J. Neuropath. Exp. Neurol. *21* :519–533, 1962.
KOLLER, L. D.: Spontaneous *Nosema cuniculi* Infection in Laboratory Rabbits. J. Am. Vet. Med. Assn. *155*:1108–1114, 1969.
KUDO, R. R.: *Protozoology*, 5th Ed. Springfield, Charles C Thomas, 1966.
LAINSON, R., GARNHAM, P. C. C., KILLICK-KENDRICK, R., and BIRD, R. G.: Nosematosis, a Microsporidial Infection of Rodents and Other Animals, Including Man. Brit. Med. J. *2*:470–472, 1964.
L'ARRIVEE, J. C. M.: Tolerance of Honey Bees to Nosema Disease. J. Inv. Path. *7*:408–413, 1965.
MATSUBAYASHI, H. *et al.*: A Case of Encephalitozoon-like Body Infection in Man. Arch. Path. *67*:181–187, 1959.
NELSON, J. B.: An Intracellular Parasite Resembling a Microsporidian Associated with Ascites in Swiss Mice. Proc. Soc. Exper. Biol. & Med. *109*:714–717, 1962.
PERRIN, T. L.: Spontaneous and Experimental *Encephalitozoon* Infection in Laboratory Animals. Arch. Path. *36*:559–567, 1943.
————: *Toxoplasma* and *Encephalitozoon* in Spontaneous and in Experimental Infections of Animals. Arch. Path. *36*:568–578, 1943.
PETRI, M., and SCHIODT, T.: On the Ultrastructure of *Nosema cuniculi* in the Cells of the Yoshida Rat Ascites Sarcoma. Acta Path et Microbiol. Scand. *66*:437–446, 1966.
PLOWRIGHT, W.: An Encephalitis-Nephritis Syndrome in Dog Probably Due to Congenital *Encephalitozoon* Infection. J. Comp. Path. & Therap. *62*:83–92, 1952.
ROBINSON, J. J.: Common Infectious Disease of Laboratory Rabbits Questionably Attributed to *Encephalitozoon cuniculi*. A.M.A. Arch. Path. *58*:71–84, 1954.
SHADDUCK, J. A.: *Nosema cuniculi*: In Vitro Isolation. Science *166*:516–517, 1969.
WEISER, J.: *Nosema muris*, n.sp. a New Microsporidian Parasite of the White Mouse. (*Mus musculus. L.*). J. Protozool. *12*:78–83, 1965.

SARCOSPORIDIOSIS

Tiny tubular cysts filled with crescentic bodies are extremely common within skeletal and cardiac muscle fibers of some aquatic birds and most animals, particularly herbivora. Man, dog and other carnivores may also be infected upon

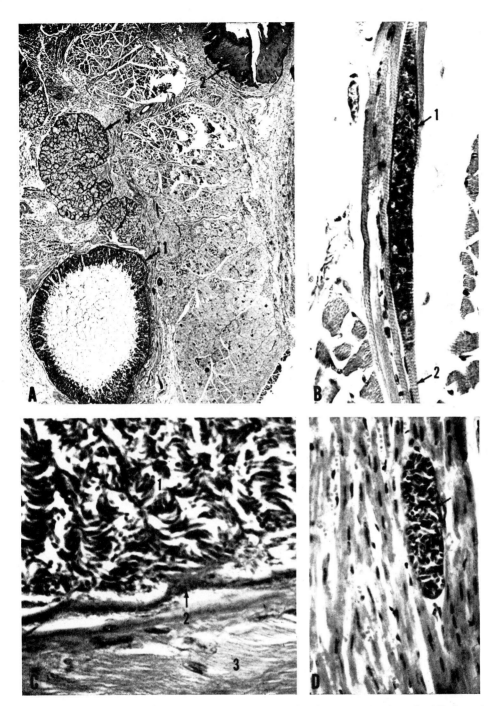

FIG. 14–10. —Sarcosporidiosis. *A*, *Balbiania gigantea* (*1*) in the tongue of a sheep (× 15), lingual epithelium (*2*) and lingual salivary glands (*3*). *B*, *Sarcocystis blanchardi* (*1*) in the tongue of a cow (× 330). Note the muscle bundle (*2*) contains the organism. *C*, Higher magnification of organisms in *A* (× 650). Note spores (*1*), cyst wall (*2*), and muscle fibers (*3*). (Courtesy of Armed Forces Institute of Pathology.) Contributor: Dr. C. L. Davis. *D*, *Sarcocystis blanchardi* in the myocardium of a cow (× 330).

rare occasions. These organisms, currently classified as Protozoa in the class Sporozoa and genus *Sarcocystis*, present an intriguing challenge to the pathologist and parasitologist. The veterinary pathologist encounters these structures with monotonous frequency, but he knows neither from whence they came, whither they will go, nor what significance they have to the host. Even their zoological classification is in doubt, some unconfirmed research claiming to have placed the organisms within the fungi, although most evidence favors their inclusion with the Protozoa. Miescher, in 1843, first described the organisms, later to be called "Miescher's bodies, sacs, or tubules," in the musculature of a house mouse. Today it is still not certain whether each host is infected by a separate species of *Sarcocystis* or whether one species may parasitize various hosts. Numerous species names of uncertain validity are in use at present within the genus *Sarcocystis* including such examples as: *Sarcocystis tenella* (sheep), *S. blanchardi* (cattle), *S. miescheriana* (swine), and *S. bertrami* (horses). Of special interest is another type found in the tongue, esophagus, and occasionally other muscles of the sheep. This type, *Balbiania gigantea*, forms quite large, grossly visible multinucleated saccules containing a fibrillar network within which myriads of crescentic spores, indistinguishable from *S. tenella*, are found. This may be a form of *S. tenella* or a separate species.

It is believed that the sporozoites of *Sarcocystis* are conveyed by the blood stream to the muscles and that a single motile parasite penetrates the sarcolemma to initiate the intracellular parasitism. The sporozoites within the sarcoplasm develop several rounded forms, sporoblasts, which become elongate and divide repeatedly by longitudinal fission to produce many ellipsoid or banana-shaped spores, each about 4 by 8 microns in size, enclosed in a clearly demonstrable cyst

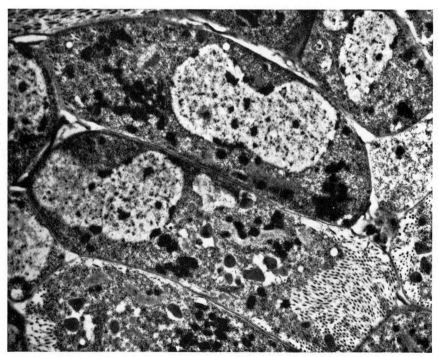

FIG. 14–11.—*Sarcocystis fusiformis.* Electron micrograph (× 18,000). (Courtesy of Dr. Charles F. Simpson and *The Journal of Parasitology.*)

taneous lesions are usually seen grossly as thickened, rugose, partially hairless areas of skin, particularly on legs, thighs and scrotum. The microscopic picture is dominated by the large spherical cysts which may occur in deeper areas and are frequently seen in the walls of small blood vessels. Invasion of the scrotum, epididymis and testis as well as upper gastrointestinal tract is common and may be accompanied by a severe granulomatous tissue reaction, particularly when numerous spores are released into the tissue. In contrast, the mature cysts with their wide, hyaline wall are usually surrounded by little other inflammatory tissue reaction.

The lesions in antelopes appear to be limited to the presence of the cysts in the cardiovascular system. The intima of veins, such as the jugular and peripheral veins of limbs, is the site of predilection for the cysts although some may be found in the muscularis or adventitia. In the impala, cysts are found especially in the walls of subcutaneous lymphatics. Some organisms may be found in the endocardium (McCully, *et al.*, 1966).

The **diagnosis** is based upon demonstration of the organisms in tissue sections.

Besnoitiosis

BIGALKE, R. D. and NAUDE, T. W.: The Diagnostic Value of Cysts in the Scleral Conjunctiva in Bovine Besnoitiosis. J. S. Afr. Vet. Med. Assn. *33*:21–27, 1962.
BIGALKE, R. D., *et al.*: The Relationship between Besnoitia of Antelopes and *Besnoitia Besnoiti* (Marotel, 1912) of Cattle. Bull. off. Int. Epizoot. *66*:903–905, 1966.
————: Studies on the Relationship between Besnoitia of Blue Wildebeest and Impala, and *Besnoitia besnoiti* of Cattle. Onderstepoort, J. Vet. Res. *34*:7–28, 1967.
BINNINGER, C. E., and McGUIRE, T. C.: Atypical Globidiosis in a Lamb. J. Am. Vet. Med. Assn. *151*:606–608, 1967.
BWANGAMOI, O.: Besnoitiosis and Other Skin Diseases of Cattle (*Bos indicus*) in Uganda. Amer. J. Vet. Res. *29*:737–743, 1968.
CAMPBELL, J. G.: Bangkok Haemorrhagic Disease of Chickens: An Unusual Condition Associated With an Organism of Uncertain Taxonomy. J. Path. & Bact. *68*:423–429, 1954.
FRENKEL, J. K.: Ocular Lesions in Hamsters With Chronic *Toxoplasma* and *Besnoitia* Infection. Am. J. Ophth. *39*:203–255, 1955.
HADWEN, S.: Cyst-forming Protozoa in Reindeer and Caribou, and a Sarcosporidian Parasite of the Seal (*Phoca richardi*). J. Am. Vet. Med. Assn. *61*:374–382, 1922.
JELLISON. W. L.: On the Nomenclature of *Besnoitia besnoiti*, a Protozoan Parasite. Ann. New York Acad. Sc. *64*:268–270, 1956.
JELLISON, W. L., FULLERTON, W. J., and PARKER, H.: Transmission of the Protozoan *Besnoitia jellisoni* by Ingestion. Ann. New York Acad. Sc. *64*:271–274, 1956.
McCULLY, R. M., *et al.*: Observations on Besnoitia Cysts in the Cardiovascular System of Some Wild Antelopes and Domestic Cattle. Ondestepoort J. Vet. Res. *33*:245–275, 1966.
NEUMAN, M.: An Outbreak of Besnoitiosis in Cattle. Refuah Vet. *19*:106–110, 1962.
POLS, J. W.: The Artificial Transmission of *Globidium besnoiti* Marotel, 1912, to Cattle and Rabbits. J. S. Afr. Vet. Med. Assn. *25*:37–44, 1954.
————: Studies on Bovine Besnoitiosis with Special Reference to the Aetiology. Onderstepoort J. Vet. Res. *28*:265–356, 1960. (VB 1426–61.)
————: Preliminary Notes on the Behavior of *Globidium besnoiti* Marotel, 1912, in the Rabbit. J. South African Vet. Med. Assn. *25*:45–48, 1954.
SCHULZ, K. C. A.: A Report on Naturally Acquired Besnoitiosis in Bovines with Special Reference to Its Pathology. J. S. Afr. Vet. Med. Assn. *31*:21–35, 1960. (VB 1427–61.)

AMEBIASIS

Parasitic protozoa classified within the Class Sarcodina—those with pseudopodia—are best known as pathogens of man but also of subhuman primates and less frequently other animals. These organisms usually inhabit the intestinal tract and may be present in the absence of recognizable effects. However,

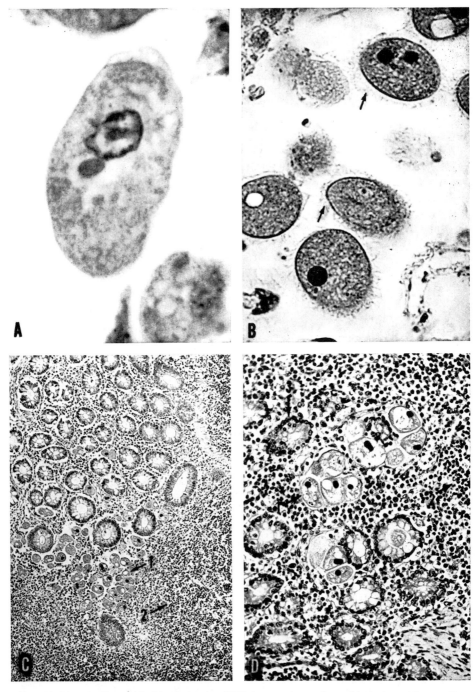

FIG. 14–14.—*A, Entamoeba histolytica* (× 1750) in experimental amebiasis in a kitten. Contributor: Dr. H. E. Melleney. *B, Balantidium coli* (× 600) from colon of an orangoutang. Note cilia (arrows). *C, Balantidium coli* (*1*) deep in the mucosa of the colon of an orangoutang (× 75). Note lymphocytes (*2*). Contributor: National Zoological Park. *D, Balantidium coli* (× 185) in mucosa of ileum of a pig (*1*), lymphocytes (*2*) and intestinal epithelium (*3*). (Courtesy of Armed Forces Institute of Pathology.) Contributor: Lt. Col. F. D. Maurer.

under some circumstances severe dysentery may result from their presence, the ameba may ulcerate and invade the intestinal wall, and possibly migrate to the liver or brain, resulting in "amebic" abscesses. The student will note that the diphthong (oe) is used in the names of some of these protozoa but, in the United States, is dropped in referring to the disease or organisms generally. Another point of possible confusion lies in the names of amebae of the genera *Entamoeba* and *Endamoeba*. At one time these organisms were considered in one genus, currently they are separated. *Entamoeba* includes pathogens of man and other mammals; *Endamoeba* are generally found in lower invertebrates.

The most important pathogen in this group appears to be *Entamoeba histolytica*, the cause of amebic dysentery in man, chimpanzee, rhesus monkey, dog, cat, rat and pig. The pathogenetic mechanisms of this organism are not fully understood although it requires bacteria to survive in the intestinal tract and lives in many cases without causing overt disease. Fully 10 per cent of normal people studied in some surveys (Soulsby, 1968) are shown to be carriers. The organism may be transmitted between hosts by contamination of food or water by food handlers who are carriers, by means of cysts borne by flies or cockroaches, or by consumption of contaminated water in which amebic cysts may survive for long periods.

Two forms have been recognized from the human intestinal tract: large and small. The larger, trophozoite, form is usually considered to be pathogenic because it is more often found in positions indicating tissue invasion. One view is that the two forms are separate races of *Entamoeba histolytica*, but this does not appear to be well established. The cystic form is agreed to be more resistant to deleterious influences and the form in which the organism survives outside a mammalian host. The trophozoites may be found deep in the wall of the colon, usually associated with a flask-shaped ulcer of the mucosa. The parasite is presumed to secrete a lytic enzyme under some as yet undetermined circumstances. Ulcerative colitis may lead to amebic abscesses in the liver or brain, at least in man, chimpanzee and rhesus monkey. One significant property of *E. histolytica* is its tendency to phagocytize erythrocytes.

The trophozoites of ameba are recognized in tissue sections as irregularly spherical organisms without cilia but often having pseudopodia. They have a distinct or indistinct nucleus, depending upon the species, and their abundant cytoplasm is often vacuolated and may contain phagocytized erythrocytes or tissue debris. Their over-all size is variable as they range from 10 to 60 microns in diameter. They may be seen in intestinal crypts, in necrotic foci in the submucosa or at the margins of sharply demarcated ulcers. The diagnosis may be made tentatively by identifying trophozoites of *E. histolytica* in the feces in the presence of dysentery and confirmed by demonstrating the organisms in ulcers or abscesses.

Amebiasis

BURROWS, R. B., and LILLIS, W. G.: Intestinal Protozoan Infection in Dogs. J. Amer. Vet. Met. Assn. *150*:880–883, 1967.

JORDAN, H. E.: Amebiasis (*Entamoeba histolytica*) in the Dog. Vet. Med., Small Anim. Clin. *62*:61–64, 1967.

MILLER, M. J., and BRAY, R. S.: *Entamoeba histolytica* Infections in the Chimpanzee (*Pan satyrus*). J. Parasit. *52*:386–388, 1966.

REES, C. W.: Pathogenesis of Intestinal Amoebiasis in Kittens. Arch. Path. *7*:1–26 1929.

SEBESTENY, A.: Pathogenicity of Intestinal Flagellates in Mice. Lab. Anim. *3*:71–77, 1969.

GIARDIASIS

Protozoa of the genus *Giardia* are pyriform in shape and bilaterally symmetrical. The anterior end is rounded and the posterior is elongated, nearly pointed. The convex ventral surface bears a large sucking disc. Each organism has four pair of flagella. These organisms are common inhabitants of the small intestine and colon of man and animals. The pathogenicity of these organisms is disputed, many contending that they produce no effect on the host, others stating that they may cause dysentery under some circumstances particularly in youug animals or children. One point made in support of this view is that removal of organisms from a host with dysentery has curative effects.

Several species of *Giardia* have been identified: *Giardia lamblia* (man), *G. conis* (dog), *G. cati* (cat), *G. chinchillae* (chinchilla) and *G. bovis* (cattle).

Giardiasis

BURROWS, R. B., and LILLIS, W. G.:　Intestinal Protozoan Infections in Dogs.　J. Am. Vet. Med. Assn. *150*:880-883, 1967.
KUDO, R. R.:　*Protozoology*, 5th Ed.　Springfield, Charles C Thomas, 1966.
SOULSBY, E. J. L.:　*Helminths, Arthropods and Protozoa of Domesticated Animals* (Mönnig). 6th Ed. Baltimore, The Williams & Wilkins Co., 1968.

PNEUMOCYSTOSIS

A protozoan organism of uncertain taxonomic classification, *Pneumocystis carinii*, is known to inhabit the pulmonary alveoli of man and animals and under certain conditions cause severe disruption of respiratory function.　Infants or children suffering from disorders of the lymphoreticular system or immune mechanisms, *e.g.*, agammaglobulinemia or who undergo adrenocorticosteroid therapy, may develop the disease.　Aged persons with malignant lymphoma or disease of bone marrow, especially if treated with corticosteroid, may contract the disease. Similar activation of latent infection has been reported in rats treated with cortisone acetate (Frenkel, Good and Shultz, 1966).　Although the organisms in human and rat lungs are morphologically indistinguishable, some evidence indicates that each may be specific for the respective species.　Failure to infect hamsters and rabbits with rat strains and absence of common complement-fixing antigens in human and rat strains supports this concept of species specificity. Infection with other organisms, particularly *Corynebacterium kutscheri* and *Aspergillus sp.* may complicate the disease in rats.

The organisms are located in alveoli adjacent to the surface of alveolar lining cells and may become numerous enough to entirely fill some alveoli.　Alveolar lining cells may become enlarged but inflammatory response to the organisms is usually minimal.　The organisms may be seen with the light microscope as spherical cysts about 4.5 microns in diameter, sometimes slightly wrinkled, cup-shaped or crescentic.　Some cysts contain intracystic bodies about 1 micron in diameter.　As many as eight of these bodies have been identified within a single cyst.　Gomori's methenamine silver stain is useful in delineating these organisms, some of which accept the silver stain.

Electron micrographs reveal thick- and thin-walled organisms containing intracystic bodies.　The thin-walled organisms have been interpreted to be trophozoites.　The thick-walled organisms contain 1 to 8 intracystic bodies which

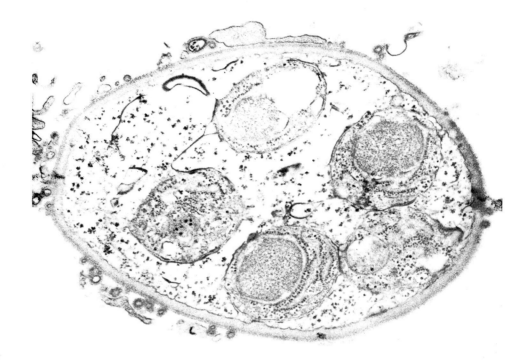

Fig. 14–15.—*Pneumocystis carinii*, from the lung of a rat following treatment with cortisone acetate. Electron micrograph (× 25,000) of thick-walled organism with five intracystic bodies. (Courtesy of Drs. Earl G. Barton, Jr., Wallace G. Campbell, Jr. and *The American Journal of Pathology*.)

are limited by a pellicle which is continuous with membranous structures in the cytoplasm of the cyst (Fig. 14–15). The completely developed intracystic body contains rough endoplasmic reticulum, a single mitochondrion, vacuoles and a nucleus containing a nucleolus. These bodies apparently escape from the cyst through defects in the cyst wall and grow to be trophozoites as large as 5 microns in diameter and contain particles resembling glycogen and lipid. Since liposomes, dense bodies, Golgi apparatus and cytosomes (p. 7) are not present, it is believed that these organisms do not utilize phagocytic processes and may metabolize substances of low molecular weight obtained from adjacent cells or intra-alveolar fluid (Barton and Campbell, 1969).

Pneumocystosis

BARTON, E. C., and CAMPBELL, W. G., JR.: *Pneumocystis carinii* in Lungs of Rats Treated with Cortisone Acetate. Ultrastructural Observations Relating to the Life Cycle. Amer. J. Path. *54*:209–236, 1969.
FRENKEL, J. K., GOOD, J. T., and SCHULTZ, J. A.: Latent Pneumocystis Infections of Rats, Relapse, and Chemotherapy. Lab. Invest. *15*:1559–1577, 1966.

HARTMANNELLOSIS

Certain protozoa in the class Sarcodina, order Amoebida have been incriminated as pathogenic in certain tissues of man and animals. These have been identified as belonging to one of two closely related and similar genera, *Hartmann-*

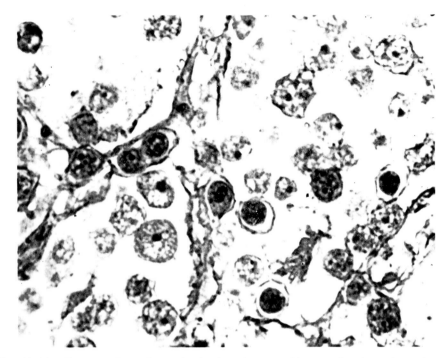

FIG. 14–16.—*Hartmannella sp.* from a bovine lung (× 900). Note trophozoite and cyst forms. (Courtesy of Col. F. N. Garner, V.C., Armed Forces Institute of Pathology.)

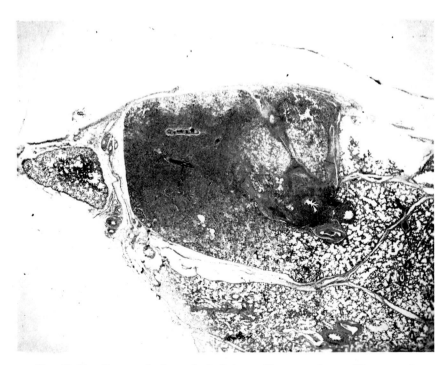

FIG. 14–17.—Pneumonia, lung of a bull due to *Hartmannella sp.* (Courtesy of Col. F. N. Garner, V.C., Armed Forces Institute of Pathology.)

ella or *Acanthamoeba*. A species name has not been applied but at the moment the genus *Hartmannella* is favored and the disease called hartmannellosis. Spontaneous cases of meningoencephalitis in man (Butt, 1966) have been attributed to this organism as has a case of gangrenous bronchopneumonia in a bull (McConnell, Garner and Kirk, 1968). Meningoencephalitis has also been reported in mice and monkeys following injections of material presumably contaminated with *Hartmannella sp.* (Culbertson, *et al.*, 1959).

The organisms are reportedly cultivatable without difficulty but also may be identified in tissue sections. They are usually present in large numbers in the lesions and are seen in two forms, with some intermediate types. In Ziegler's hematoxylin-eosin stain (Ziegler, 1944) the large form is about 9 to 12 microns in diameter, acidophilic, with a thin cell wall and one (occasionally two) central basophilic body, the karyosome. This karyosome serves to differentiate *Entamoeba histolytica* which does not have one. This form, considered the trophozoite, has a moderate affinity for Gomori's methenamine silver stain, and periodic acid Schiff (PAS) reaction and is blue to amphophylic with Giemsa's stain. The second form of *Hartmannella* is somewhat smaller (9 to 10 microns in diameter), more uniform in size and has a membranous capsule which is often separated from the central body by a clear halo. These cystic forms are more basophilic in H&E-stained sections. The PAS reaction is strongly positive and the organisms are quite argentophilic in Gomori's methenamine silver stain.

The diagnosis may be established by recovering and identifying the organisms in association with necrotizing lesions. The organisms may be identified in microscopic sections by their presence in typical lesions and their characteristic morphology and staining properties.

Hartmannellosis

BUTT, C. G.: Primary Amebic Meningoencephalitis. New Eng. J. Med. *274*:1473–1476, 1966.
CULBERTSON, C. G., *et al.*: Experimental Infection of Mice and Monkeys by *Acanthamoeba*. Amer. J. Path. *35*:185–197, 1959.
McCONNELL, E. E., GARNER, F. N., and KIRK, J. H.: Hartmannellosis in a Bull. Path. Vet. *5*:1–6, 1968.
ZIEGLER, E. E.: Hematoxylin-eosin Tissue Stain, an Improved and Uniform Technique. Arch. Path. *37*:68–69, 1944.

TRICHOMONIASIS

Protozoa in the Class Mastigophora include a Family, Trichomondidae, of flagellated organisms, some of which are pathogenic. Two genera are of special interest: *Tritrichomonas* (with three anterior flagella) and *Trichomonas* (with four anterior flagella). Organisms of the genus *Giardia* were discussed on page 704.

Tritrichomonas foetus is the cause of **bovine trichomoniasis,** an important genital infection in cattle. The organism is transmitted by coitus and results in vaginitis in the female and balanitis in the male. Infection of the uterus or placenta may result in endometritis or placentitis which terminates in early abortion and sometimes in sterility. Pyometra may result from uterine infection when the cervix is closed and the uterus fills with fluid teeming with trichomonads.

The diagnosis is established by demonstrating *Tritrichomonas foetus* in vaginal, uterine or preputial exudates in association with a herd history of decreased fertility, abortions, vaginitis, metritis and balanitis.

Tritrichomonas suis is found in the digestive and upper respiratory tracts of swine but its pathogenicity is not completely established. *Trichomonas gallinae* is the etiologic agent in **avian trichomoniasis,** a serious inflammation of the upper gastrointestinal tract of pigeons, turkeys, chickens and wild birds. *Trichomonas vaginalis* is found in the vagina, urethra and prostate of women and men. It may be carried without producing signs, especially in men, but also may result in vaginitis or urethritis. It is transmitted by coitus. Other species of trichomonads have been suspected in cases of gastrointestinal infection (Bennett and France, 1969) but it is difficult to prove that these organisms are pathogenic in the digestive tract where they may thrive in the absence of disease.

Trichomoniasis

BENNETT, S. P., and FRANCO, D. A.:   Equine Protozoan Diarrhea (Equine Intestinal Tricho-moniasis) at Trinidad Racetracks.   J. Am. Vet. Med. Assn. *154*:58–60, 1969.
SOULSBY, E. J. L.:   *Helminths, Arthropods and Protozoa of Domesticated Animals* (Mönnig). 6th Ed. Baltimore, The Williams & Wilkins Co., 1968.
TODOROVIC, R., and McNUTT, S. H.:   Diagnosis of *Trichomonas foetus* Infection in Bulls. Am. J. Vet. Res. *28*:1581–1590, 1967.

BALANTIDIASIS

The only member of the ciliated Protozoa, the Infusoria, which is of pathogenic significance (and this is questionable) is *Balantidium coli* (*B. suis*). This comparatively large single-celled organism is a natural inhabitant of the digestive tract of swine, man and sometimes other vertebrates, usually living in the lumen or between the villi and causing no recognizable effect on the host. Under some imperfectly understood circumstances, *Balantidium coli* will invade the intestinal mucosa, penetrating into the submucosa, localizing particularly in lymphoid nodules. Occasionally, it may reach the genital tract. This tissue penetration results in varying degrees of acute inflammation in the vicinity and may result in some manifestations of enteric disease. Since its pathogenicity is questioned and most certainly limited, *Balantidium coli* is of interest to the pathologist as an organism which might be present with frank pathogens but should not be mistakenly considered the cause of every disease with which it is associated.

TRYPANOSOMIASIS

Trypanosomiasis is often thought of as an exotic disease which occurs only in tropical Africa, India, and other far-off places. It is true that this disease is most serious in man and animals in certain regions of the world, but trypanosomes are distributed throughout all parts of the globe, often producing no recognizable disease in the host in which they reside. The disease in man with many names such as **African sleeping sickness, tsetse fly disease, maladie du sommeil, Schlaffkrankeit** and **doenca do sono,** has influenced the course of history, particularly in Africa, by denying people the use of certain lands and causing them to go to war over those areas relatively free of the disease. The disease in domesticated livestock has also played a similar historical role. Although urbanization and control measures have reduced the frequency of the disease, it still remains a serious problem in some areas of Africa and South America.

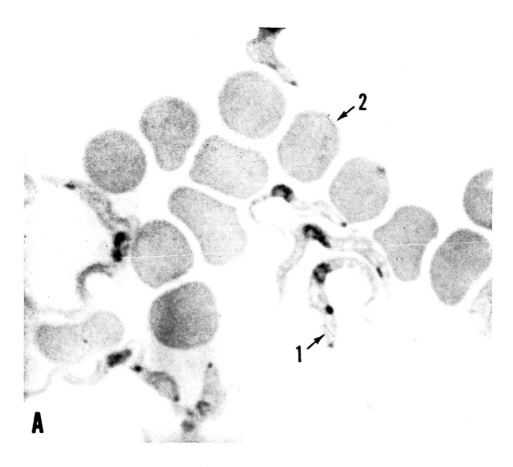

A

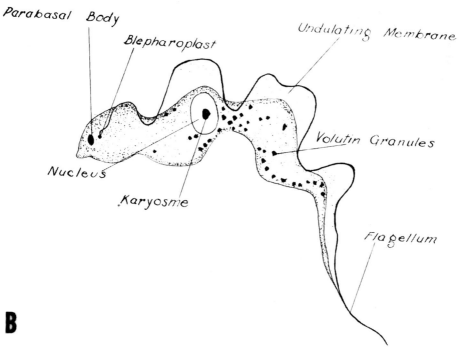

Parabasal Body

Blepharoplast

Undulating Membrane

Nucleus

Karyosme

Volutin Granules

Flagellum

B

FIG. 14–18.—Trypanosomiasis. *A, Trypanosoma equiperdum (1)* in the blood of a rat. Erythrocyte *(2).* (Courtesy of Armed Forces Institute of Pathology.) Contributor: Dr. Kent Davis. *B,* Diagram of the morphology of a trypanosome.

These protozoa are flagellated, motile parasites which frequent the blood of many vertebrate and invertebrate hosts and localize in tissues, sometimes in a non-flagellated form. Trypanosomes have certain common anatomic features, such as: an ovoid or rounded body in the non-flagellate stage and a slender, elongate body when it becomes flagellated; the flagellum arises from the dot-shaped blepharoplast and extends to or projects from the anterior pole of the organism; an undulating membrane extends along the border of the organism with the flagellum forming its margin; a spherical or rod-shaped structure, the parabasal body, together with the blepharoplast, makes up the kinetoplast. A relatively large round or ovoid nucleus containing a more deeply staining karyosome is usually located near the middle of the body.

Trypanosomes multiply by longitudinal fission, but the exact details of their division are unknown. They may be cultivated in noncellular media, tissue cultures or chick embryos but are commonly maintained by experimental infection of laboratory animals. The life cycle in nature involves both vertebrate and invertebrate hosts, the latter acting as vectors of the infection. Mechanical transmission of trypanosomes may be accomplished by certain biting flies (*Tabanus, Stomoxys*), but definite cyclic development occurs in the body of the true invertebrate hosts (*Glossina, Triatoma*). In these hosts, the trypanosomes multiply in various forms in the digestive tract and eventually migrate as infective forms to the salivary glands in preparation for infection of a new vertebrate host.

Trypanosomes usually can be identified by their morphologic features, such as size, shape, position, arrangement and development of the organelles, but no completely satisfactory classification scheme has yet been devised. Most species of trypanosomes do not produce serious effects upon their host but a few are important pathogens (Table 14–2).

The pathogenesis of trypanosomiasis in man or animals is not thoroughly understood. The mechanisms which induce disease or cause death are essentially unknown. According to Weinman (1968), death cannot be explained on the basis of terminal hypoglycemia, anoxia, acidosis or elevated potassium levels in the plasma. Some hepatic dysfunction is indicated by elevated serum levels of glutamic oxaloacetic and glutamic pyruvic transaminase. Except for *Trypanosoma cruzi* (p. 713), the organisms do not invade tissue cells and therefore do not produce effects by direct destruction of cells. No specific tissue response has been recognized although reticulo-endothelial proliferation has been described in spleen and liver.

Dourine.—A disease of Equidae, dourine has a cosmopolitan distribution but is now rare in the United States. In contrast to other trypanosomiases, the causative agent, *Trypanosoma equiperdum*, is transmitted by coitus, rarely by biting flies. The disease is manifest by edematous lesions in the genital tract and ventral body wall, persistent ulcerous plaques in the genitalia and skin and occasionally by anemia, incoordination and paralysis. The causative trypanosome is demonstrable in the lesions, particularly in those of the genitalia.

Nagana (Tsetse Fly Disease).—Nagana is most commonly used as a collective term for Africa trypanosomiasis of domesticated animals, particularly those infections caused by *Trypanosoma brucei* (Bruce, 1894), *T. congolense* (Broden, 1904) and *T. vivax* (Ziemann, 1905). The local term "Souma" is sometimes applied to infection with *T. vivax*. A large number and variety of wild animals may serve as reservoirs of infection, apparently with impunity to themselves.

Nagana occurs in all domesticated animals in tropical Africa, resulting in acute or chronic manifestations with irregular fever, anemia, emaciation, subcutaneous edema, weakness and sometimes photophobia. Death may occur following an acute illness or after a prolonged course during which gradual wasting is a dominant feature. Post-mortem examination usually discloses severe emaciation with edematous changes in all fatty tissues. The lymph nodes are swollen, edematous, occasionally with hemorrhage in the medulla; the liver is enlarged and congested. The spleen is either normal or atrophic with large prominent Malpighian corpuscles. Necrosis in the kidney and emphysema in the lungs have been described. Hemorrhages are common, particularly in subendocardial and epicardial locations. Pericardial fluid may be excessive. Congestion and hemorrhage may be a prominent feature in the gastrointestinal tract.

Surra.—The important trypanosomiasis of Asia occurs principally in Equidae, but dogs, elephants, and ruminants may be infected and wild ruminants can act as reservoirs. Camels are also quite susceptible. The causative organism, *Trypanosoma evansi* (Evans, 1880), is transmitted mechanically by the bite of horse flies (*Tabanus, Stomoxys*). The disease is recognized most frequently in a

Table 14–2.—*Important Trypanosomes of Man and Animals*

Species	Definitive Host	Intermediate Hosts (Vectors)	Geographic Distribution	Disease
T. lewisi	Rats	Fleas—several species	Cosmopolitan	None
T. theileri	Cattle	Tabanid flies	Cosmopolitan	None
T. melophagium	Sheep	Louse fly (Melophagus ovinus)	Temperate zones	None
T. theodori	Horses	Louse fly (Lipoptena caprina)	Palestine, Syria	None
T. cruzi	Man, armadillo, cat, opossum, dog	"Kissing bug" (Triatoma sp.)	S. America	Chagas' Disease South American Trypanosomiasis
T. evansi	Horse, mule, ass, cattle, buffalo	Horse flies (Tabanidae and Stomoxys)	Africa, Asia, S. America, Far East	Surra
T. equiperdum	Horse, ass	Trans. by coitus	Cosmopolitan	Dourine
T. vivax (uniforme)	Cattle, sheep, horse, goat, camel	Tsetse fly (Glossina sp.)	Central and S. America, Martinique, Guadaloupe, Mauritius and Africa	Souma
T. caprae	Horse, sheep, cattle	Tsetse fly	Tanganyika, Nyasaland	Trypanosomiasis
T. congolense, dimorphon	Cattle, horse, goat, sheep, ass, pig, dog, camel	Tsetse fly	Tropical Africa	Trypanosomiasis
T. simiae	Monkey, pig, horse, sheep	Tsetse fly	East Africa	Trypanosomiasis
T. brucei	Man, domestic and wild mammals, except goats	Tsetse fly	Tropical Africa	Nagana
T. rhodesiense	Man, antelope	Tsetse fly	East Africa	Acute "sleeping sickness"
T. gambiense	Man, antelope	Tsetse fly	Tropical Africa	Chronic "sleeping sickness"

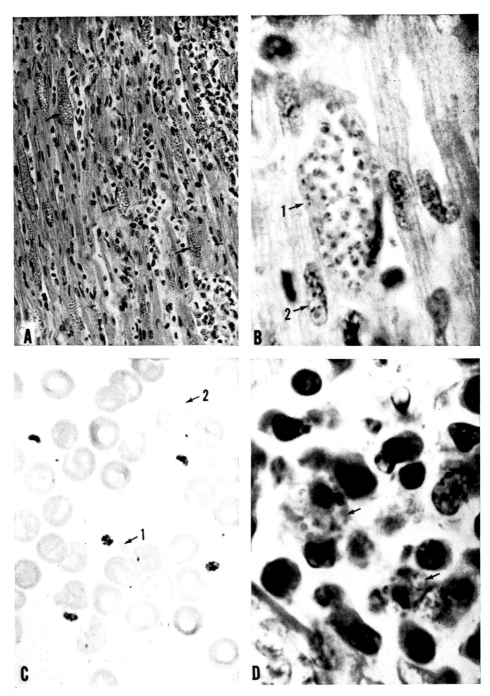

FIG. 14–19.—*A*, *Trypanosoma cruzi* (× 240) in the myocardium of a dog. *B*, Higher magnification (× 1240) showing leishmanial forms of *Tr. crusi* in the cytoplasm (*1*) of a cardiac muscle bundle. One nucleus of a cardiac muscle cell is indicated by (*2*). Contributor: Dr. Francisco Laranja. *C*, *Tr. cruzi* (*1*) in the blood of a rat. Erythrocytes (*2*). Contributor: Lt. Col. F. D. Maurer. *D*, Leishmaniasis, lymph node of dog (× 1780) organisms (arrows) are in cytoplasm of macrophages. (Courtesy of Armed Forces Institute of Pathology.) Contributor: Dr. W. S. Bailey.

severe form with paroxysms of intermittent fever associated with trypanosomes in the blood; gradual emaciation in spite of good appetite; serous nasal discharge; patchy alopecia; petechiae and ecchymoses of visible mucosae; weakness and incoordination; edema of the limbs and lower abdomen and thorax; icterus; progressive anemia and fatal termination.

Mal de Caderas.—This trypanosomiasis of tropical and subtropical South America which affects Equidae in particular is caused by *Trypanosoma equinum* (Voges, 1901). The disease is an acute infection quite similar to surra.

Murrina de Caderas (Derrengadera de caderas) occurs in Central America and is caused by *Trypanosoma hippicum*, first described by Darling in 1910. Horses and mules are particularly susceptible, cattle act as reservoirs of infection. The disease is essentially similar to surra, although a more prolonged course is described, weakness, emaciation, anemia, ecchymoses, edema, splenomegaly and paralysis being important features.

Chagas' Disease (South American Trypanosomiasis).—*Trypanosoma cruzi* was shown in 1909 by Chagas to be the cause of human trypanosomiasis in South America. The vectors were also proved by Chagas to be reduviid or "kissing" bugs (*Triatoma*). Dogs, cats, armadillos, monkeys, and small wild animals have been shown to harbor the infection and are believed to be subject to a disease quite similar to the human infection. *Trypanosoma cruzi* is of particular interest because it assumes the typical trypanosomal form in the blood and tissues of mammals, in cultures and in the intestine and rectum of insects, but also occurs in leishmanial forms in both mammalian cells and tissue cultures and develops transitional forms, typical of *Leptomonas* and *Crithidia*, intracellularly in mammals, in cultures and in intestines of insects. Thus, this trypanosome appears to be closely related to *Leishmania*, in fact, it demonstrates a relationship between the two genera. One classification (Weinman, 1968) places *Trypanosoma cruzi* in a new *genus Schizotrypanum*. It is further suggested that South American trypanosomiasis is no longer a specific name because a new trypanosome, *Trypanosoma rangelis* has been found to affect man in the Americas.

The **clinical manifestations** are significantly related to damage in the brain and myocardium, although in some species (man, mouse, dog) edema may be a prominent feature. These edematous swellings occur in the subcutaneous fasciae and muscles and elevate the skin. Congestive heart failure with ascites and passive congestive of liver and spleen may also occur. Nervous manifestations point toward brain involvement and cardiac collapse follows infection of the myocardium.

The **lesions** result in part from the growth and activity of *T. cruzi* in the blood but are most influenced by its intracellular activities. The initial lesion, seen in man following bite of a reduviid bug, is a hard, red, painful edematous mass occurring at the site of the bite. This soon subsides as the organisms spread. The lymph nodes may become enlarged, edematous, and show intense histiocytic proliferation and occasionally may contain microabscesses. Giant cells may form and contain leishmanial forms of *T. cruzi*. The heart is particularly affected. Myocardial fibers are penetrated by the organism which proliferates, filling and destroying muscle cells and resulting in severe myocarditis. The heart becomes enlarged, the myocardium mottled with yellow, and the pericardial sac distended with fluid. Large cystic collections of leishmanial forms are demonstrable microscopically in cardiac muscle cells. The experimental disease in mice often results in myocarditis, particularly in the right ventricle. The right ventricle becomes distended and the ventricular wall thin. Passive congestion of liver and spleen is an expected result.

Skeletal and smooth muscles may also be invaded by this organism. In man, infection of smooth muscles of esophagus and colon may result in megesophagus and megacolon. This finding has not been reported in animals.

In the brain, *T. cruzi* produces edema and congestion, particularly in the meninges, with some perivascular lymphocytic infiltration. Nodules of mononuclear and glial cells may occur throughout the brain. Within these areas the leishmanial forms of the trypanosomes are found in the cytoplasm of cells and free in the tissue.

The testicle may be severely invaded by *T. cruzi*; the germinal cells become laden with organisms and intense lymphocytic infiltration occurs in the interstitial stroma.

The **diagnosis** is dependent upon demonstration of *T. cruzi* in blood or tissues of infected animals.

Trypanosomiasis

CHAGAS, C.: Ueber eine neue Trypanosomiasis des Menschen. Mem. Inst. Oswaldo Cruz (Rio de Janeiro) *1*:159–218, 1909.

CROSS, R. F., REDMAN, D. R., and BOHL, E. H.: Trypanosomes Associated with Bovine Lymphocytosis. J. Am. Vet. Med. Assn. *153*:571–575, 1968.

EWING, S. A., and CARNAHAN, D. L.: Occurrence of *Trypanosoma theileri* in Bovine Peripheral Blood. J. Am. Vet. Med. Assn. *150*:1131–1132, 1967.

FERNANDEZ, D. B., RICO, F., and DUMAG, P. U.: Observations on an Outbreak of Surra Among Cattle. Philipp. J. Anim. Ind. *21*:221–224, 1965. V. B. *37*:517, 1967.

FIENNES, R. N. T. W., JONES, E. R., and LAWS, S. G.: The Course and Pathology of *Trypanosoma congolense* (Broden) Disease of Cattle, J. Comp. Path. & Therap. *56*:1–27, 1946.

GILL, B. S.: Studies of the Serological Diagnosis of *Trypanonosoma evansi*. J. Comp. Path. *75*:175–183, 1965.

GODFREY, D. G., et al.: Plasma Protein and Haemoglobin Levels in Zebu Cattle Infected with Trypanosomiasis in the Field. Bull. Epizoot. Dis. Afr. *16*:205–212, 1968.

HOARE, C. A.: Evolutionary Trends in Mammalian Trypanosomes. Adv. Parasit. *5*:47–91, 1967. V.B. *39*:2852, 1969.

—————: The Classification of Mammalian Trypanosomes. Ergebn. Mikrobiol. Immunitatsforsch. *39*:49–57, 1966. V.B. *36*:3868, 1966.

ISOUN, T. T.: The Pathology of *Trypanosoma simiae* Infection in Pigs. Ann. Trop. Med. Parasit. *62*:188–192, 1968. V. B. *39*:1532, 1969.

JOHNSON, C. M.: Cardiac Changes in Dogs Experimentally Infected With *Trypanosoma cruzi*. Am. J. Trop. Med. *18*:197–206, 1938.

KILLICK-KENDRICK, R.: The Diagnosis of Trypanosomiasis of Livestock; A Review of Current Techniques. V. B. *38*:191–197, 1968.

KUMAR, R., KLINE, I. K., and ABELMANN, W. H.: Experimental *Trypanosoma cruzi* myocarditis. Relative Effects upon the Right and Left Ventricles. Amer. J. Path. *57*:31–48, 1969.

LEHMANN, D. L.: Enzyme Content and Its Possible Relation to Infectivity of African Trypanosomes. Trans. R. Soc. Trop. Med. Hyg. *59*:297–299, 1965.

LUMSDEN, W. H. R., and WELLS, E. A.: Trypanosomiasis. Chapter 21 in *Infectious Blood Diseases of Man and Animals*. Vol. 2, New York, Academic Press, 1968.

MARSDEN, P. D., and HAGSTROM, J. W. C.: Trypanosoma cruzi in the Saliva of Beagle Puppies. Trans. R. Soc. Trop. Med. Hyg. *60*:189–191, 1966.

NELSON, B. D., and LINCICOME, D. R.: Serum Transaminases and Aldolase in Rats Inoculated with *Trypanosoma lewisi*. Proc. Soc. Exp. Biol. Med. *121*:566–569, 1966.

ORMEROD, W. E.: Taxonomy of the Sleeping Sickness Trypanosomes. J. Parasit. *53*:824–830, 1967. V.B. *38*:535, 1968.

PACKCHANIAN, A.: Studies on *Trypanosoma gambiense* Infection in Various Species of Experimental Animals. Tex. Rep. Biol. Med. *22*:707–715, 1964.

PAVLOV, P., and CHRISTOFOROV, L.: The Pathogenicity of *Trypanosoma equiperdum*. Proc. 1st Int. Congr. Parasit. Roma *1*:323–324, 1966. V. B. *37*:2050, 1967.

PETANA, W. B.:   American Trypanosomiasis in Br. Honduras.   V. Development of *Trypanosoma (Schizotrypanum) cruzi* in Animals Infected with Strains Isolated in the El Cayo District, and the Occurrence of Crithidia Forms in the Tissues.   Ann. Trop. Med. Parasit. *63*:39–45, 1969.

—————:   American Trypanosomiasis in British Honduras.   VI. A Natural Infection with *Trypanosoma (Schizotrypanum) cruzi* in the opossum, *Didelphis marsupialis* (Marsupialia, Didelphoidea), and Experimental Investigations of Different Wild-animal Species as Possible Reservoirs for the Parasite.   Ann. Trop. Med. Parasit. *63*:47–56, 1969.

—————:   American Trypanosomiasis in British Honduras.   VII. A Natural Infection in a Wild Cotton Rat (*Sigmodon hispidus*) (*Rodentia, Cricketidae*) with a Trypanosome Morphologically Resembling *Trypanosoma sigmodoni* Culbertson, 1941.   Ann. Trop. Med. Parasit. *63*:57–61, 1969.

REES, J. M., and CLARKSON, M. J.:   Serum Proteins in Trypanosomiasis of Sheep.   Trans. R. Soc. Trop. Med. Hyg. *61*:14, 1967.   V.B. *37*:2536, 1967.

SEN, H. G., MUKHERJEE, A. M., and RAY, H. N.:   Pathology of *Trypanosoma evansi* Infection in Rats.   Indian J. Vet. Sci. *29*:108–112, 1959.   (VB 1431–62.)

SOLTYS, M. A., and WOO, P.:   Multiplication of *Trypanosoma brucei* and *Trypanosoma congolense* in Vertebrate Hosts.   Trans. R. Soc. Trop. Med. Hyg. *63*:490–494, 1969.

SRIVASTAVA, R. V. N., MALHOTRA, M. N., and IYER, P. K. R.:   Pathology of Experimental *Trypanosoma evansi* Infection in Dogs.   Indian J. Anim. Sci. *39*:307–314, 1969.

VICKERMAN, K.:   Polymorphism and Transmissibility in Trypanosomes.   Parasitology *55*:16, 1966.   V. B. *36*:1335, 1966.

WEINMAN, D.:   The Human Trypanosomiases.   Chapter 17, in *Infectious Blood Diseases of Man and Animals*.   Ed. by Weinman, D., and Ristic, M.   New York, Academic Press, 1968.

LEISHMANIASIS

Infections of man and animals with protozoan organisms of the genus *Leishmania* have various local names but can be grouped together on the basis of their common characteristics.   Three species are recognized as important pathogens: *Leishmania donovani*, the cause of visceral leishmaniasis, kala azar, or dum dum fever; *L. tropica*, the agent of cutaneous leishmaniasis, Oriental sore or Delhi sore; and *L. braziliensis* which causes the entity called mucocutaneous or American leishmaniasis, espundia, or several other names.   The organisms are classified in the family Trypanosomidae which includes five parasitic genera: *Trypanosoma* (vertebrate and invertebrate hosts), *Leishmania* (vertebrates and invertebrates), *Leptomonas*, *Crithidia*, and *Herpetomonas* (parasites of invertebrate hosts).

Leishmania occur in vertebrate hosts in the leishmanial form, that is a small ovoid protozoan about 1 to 2 microns wide by 2 to 4.5 microns long which has neither flagellum nor undulating membrane.   In Romanovsky-stained preparations, it has pale blue cytoplasm containing, near the posterior end, a reddish nucleus with a deeper staining central karyosome.   Tangential and anterior to the nucleus is a deep violet, rod-shaped body, the kinetoplast, which contains the parabasal body and the dot-shaped blepharoplast.   In its invertebrate host (sandflies) or in cultures, the organisms assume shapes varying from the leishmanial to the leptomonad form, the latter being slender and spindle shaped, from 14 to 20 microns in length and 1.5 to 4 microns in width.   This form is motile by means of a flagellum which arises from the blepharoplast and projects from the anterior pole of the organism.

Leishmania reproduce in the vertebrate host by longitudinal binary fission, but the complete life cycle and maintenance of virulence depend upon an intermediate host or vector.   Many species of sandflies (*Phlebotomus*) are involved in the transmission of *Leishmania* and are necessary for their perpetuation, but certain flies, such as *Stomoxys calcitrans*, may mechanically transmit the infection.

Visceral leishmaniasis or kala azar (*L. donovani*) occurs naturally in man, dogs, cats, squirrels, cattle, horses and sheep, but many laboratory animals, especially hamsters and dogs, are susceptible to experimental infection. The disease has a wide geographic distribution but is most prevalent in countries bordering the Mediterranean, large areas of Africa, India and China. It also occurs in Argentina, Colombia, Brazil and Venezuela in South America, but cases reported in the United States originate elsewhere. Visceral leishmaniasis in animals usually is observed as a chronic debilitating disease with periods of fever and gradual weight loss with anemia appearing in the terminal stages. A history of persistent cutaneous ulcers which heal slowly may sometimes be obtained. In the United States, the disease should be suspected in animals imported from areas where the disease is known to occur. Splenomegaly, hepatomegaly and lymphadenopathy may be detected in dogs, and ascites occurs infrequently. The skin may become involved in late stages in a specific type of dermatitis.

Cutaneous leishmaniasis (*L. tropica*) occurs principally in those Southern European and North African countries bordering the Mediterranean. The reservoirs for human infections are various wild rodents, although dogs, mice, guinea pigs and monkeys are susceptible to experimental infection.

American or **mucocutaneous leishmaniasis** (*L. braziliensis*) occurs in Mexico and Central America, is particularly prevalent in Brazil, Venezuela, Colombia and Peru, but is unknown in Chile. Animals are not frequently found infected in nature, although ground squirrels, dogs, cats and monkeys are susceptible.

Lesions.—The organisms of visceral leishmaniasis stimulate the production of large numbers of huge macrophages with cytoplasm filled with leishmanial forms. The lymph nodes and spleen are particularly involved by reticulo-endothelial hyperplasia, although the liver, bone marrow, kidney and, less often, other viscera and skin may be infected. The gross findings at necropsy therefore consist of severe emaciation; enlarged lymph nodes, spleen and liver; sometimes pallor of mucosae and serous surfaces; soft red bone marrow and ulcers in the intestine. *Leishmania donovani* are found in histologic preparations of any of these organs, occurring in the cytoplasm of the enlarged macrophages. The lymph nodes may show moderate fibrosis as well as reticulo-endothelial hyperplasia. Macrophages also replace large areas in the spleen and infiltrate portal zones in the liver. The bone marrow may be hyperplastic or replaced largely with macrophages filled with *Leishmania*.

Diagnosis.—Other diseases which also cause proliferation of reticulo-endothelium present the most problems in differential diagnosis. These include histoplasmosis, toxoplasmosis (some cases), salmon disease, blastomycosis and epizoötic lymphangitis. Final determination must be based upon demonstration and identification of the causative organism in tissue sections, smears or cultures. Tissues taken by biopsy are most useful to demonstrate the organisms in a living animal or human patient.

Leishmaniasis

GALATI, P.: Reperto di Trombosi Multipla in cane con Leishmoniosi Viscerale. (Multiple thrombosis in a dog with visceral leishmaniasis) Atti. Soc. ital. Sci. Vet. *12*:508–512, 1958 (VB 3789–59)

RIOUX, J-A., GOLVAN, Y-J., and HOUIN, R.: Mixed *Hepatozoon canis* and *Leishmania canis* Infection in a Dog in the Sete Area, France. Annls. Parasit. Hum. Comp. *39*:131–135, 1964. V.B. 1302, 1965.

STAUBER, L. A.: Experimental Leishmaniasis in the Chinchilla. J. Parasitol. (abstract) *39*:11, 1953.

THORSON, R. E., BAILEY, W. S., HOERLEIN, B. F., and SEIBOLD, H. R.: A Report of a Case of Imported Visceral Leishmaniasis of a Dog in the United States. Am. J. Trop. Med. & Hyg. *4*:18–22, 1955.

MALARIA

Malaria has been recognized as an important disease of man in most recorded history and is still one of the most important infectious diseases in spite of great strides in eradication during the past two decades. The disease is thought of as especially prevalent in tropical and sub-tropical regions but is not unknown in temperate parts of the globe. It is especially deleterious to young children, often combining with hookworm, tuberculosis and other diseases to debilitate and kill. The name of the malady, *malaria*, comes from the Italian words *mala* (bad) and *aria* (air) in reference to the "miasmic vapors" which were believed to come from swamps.

One of the causative parasites was discovered by a French Army physician, Laveran, who in 1880 found what are now considered to be microgametocytes, probably of the organism now called *Plasmodium falciparum*. It was not until after the turn of the century that Sir Ronald Ross (1910) demonstrated mosquitoes to be the "miasmas" arising from swamps to spread the disease.

The causative protozoa, classified among the sporozoa, are currently all members of the genus *Plasmodium* which includes many pathogenic species. Man, birds and non-human primates are now known to be the vertebrate hosts for these organisms. Of particular interest is the recent discovery (Eyles, Coatney and Getz, 1960) that man is susceptible to certain of the simian plasmodia. Thus, simian malarias not only may serve as models for human malaria, but also may be a source for human infection (Manwell, 1968). Simian malaria is also encountered in monkeys imported into laboratories where it may interfere with the experimental data garnered from these animals. Thus malaria is now viewed as a group of diseases caused by different species of *Plasmodium*.

The life cycles of *Plasmodium*, as far as currently known, are quite similar. Two hosts are required: (1) vertebrates (man, other mammals, birds and reptiles), in which schizogony takes place in erythrocytes and other cells; and (2) invertebrate blood-sucking insects (mosquitoes). The cycle is started when a

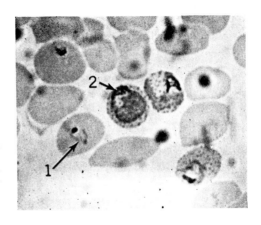

FIG. 14–20.—Malaria in a cynomologous monkey (*Macaca fascicularis*). Schizonts (*1*) and gametocytes (*2*) of *Plasmodium cynomologi* are present in erythrocytes. (Courtesy New England Regional Primate Research Center, Harvard Medical School.)

female mosquito penetrates the skin of the vertebrate host, introducing sporozoites into the peripheral circulation. After a few days of exoerythrocytic development in endothelial cells or hepatocytes, the parasites enter red blood cells.
Here they are called **schizonts**. Initially these schizonts appear as small rings
which grow and divide to develop into many (24 or more) **merozoites,** tiny
nucleated bodies which are released into the plasma as the cell disintegrates.
These merozoites may be phagocytized by leukocytes or infect other red blood
cells. This repeated schizogony, progressing geometrically, results in the paroxysmal recurrence of the signs of fever and anemia. Some of the merozoites
develop into **gametocytes** and remain in the blood as **macro-** and **micro-gameto-
cytes** until ingested by a mosquito or eliminated by phagocytosis as their life
span is completed.

The macro- and microgametocytes ingested by female mosquitoes (the males
do not ingest blood) undergo further development in the stomach of the mosquito—the macrogametocyte becomes one **macrogamete** and the microgametocyte
becomes 4 to 8 **microgametes.** Fusion of gametes results in a motile zygote called
oökinete which enters the gastric mucosa of the mosquito, becomes an oöcyst
which lies in the stroma adjacent to the gastric epithelium. Repeated nuclear
divisions result in many sporozoites which are set free by rupture into the
hemolymph, permitting migration to the salivary glands of the mosquito. From

Table 14–3.—Malarias

Organism	Vertebrate Hosts	Disease	Geographic Distribution
Plasmodium falciparum	Man	malignant tertian, falciparum, or sub-tertian malaria	Widely distributed in tropics, some in sub-tropics
P. malariae	Man, chimpanzee	quartan malaria	Philippine Islands, and India
P. ovale	Man,	mild tertian malaria	Africa, Philippines and India
P. vivax	Man, chimpanzee (experimental)	benign tertian or vivax malaria	Tropical, sub-tropical and some temperate regions, South and North America, England, Sweden, Argentina, Australia, Natal
P. knowlesi	Macaca fascicularis (Crab eater macaque) Man (experimental) M. nemestrina Presbytis melalophus	simian malaria	Malaya, Philippines
P. gallinaceum	Domestic fowl (other birds suscept. exper.)	avian malaria	India
P. relictum	Penguins, sparrows, many birds	avian malaria	U. S. A. (zoos)
P. brazilianum	Cebus apella (capuchin) Alouatta seniculus A. fusca (howler monkeys) Cacajo calvus (uakari) Chiropotes chiropotes (saki) Ateles paniscus p.	simian malaria (quartan type)	South and Central America

Table 14–3.—Malarias

Organism	Vertebrate Hosts	Disease	Geographic Distribution
	A. paniscus chamek (spider monkey) Lagothrix lagotricha L. cana (woolly monkeys) Brachyteles arachnoides (woolly spider monkey) Callicebus torquatus (titi) Saimiri sciureus (squirrel monkey) occasionally: man		
P. simium	Alouatta fusca (brown howler monkey) Brachyteles arachnoides (woolly spider monkey) occasionally: man	simian malaria (benign-tertian type)	Brazil
P. cynomolgi	Macaca fascicularis (crab eater macaque) M. nemestrina (pig-tailed macaque) M. cyclopis (Taiwan macaque) Cynopithecus niger, Presbytis sp.	simian malaria	Philippines, Taiwan Malaya, Java, Ceylon, India Cambodia, Pakistan
P. coatneyi	Macaca fascicularis (crab eater macaque)	simian malaria	Philippines, Malaya
P. inui	Macaca fascicularis M. mulatta (rhesus) M. radiata (bonnet monkey) M. nemestrina M. cyclopis, Cynopithecus niger, Presbytis sp.	simian malaria	Indochina, Philippines, etc. (Tropical Asia)
P. fieldi	M. nemestrina	simian malaria	Malaya
P. fragile	M. radiata, M. sinica	simian malaria	Ceylon
P. simiovale	M. sinica	simian malaria	Ceylon
P. pitheci	Pongo pigmaeus (orangutan)	simian malaria	Borneo
P. youngi	Hyalobates lar (gibbon)	simian malaria	Malaya
P. jefferyi	Hyalobates lar	simian malaria	Malaya
P. eylesi	Hyalobates lar	simian malaria	Malaya
P. hyalobates	Hyalobates lar	simian malaria	Java
P. gonderi	Cerocebus galeritus C. aterrimus C. atys, Mandrillus leucophaeus	simian malaria	West Africa
P. reichenowi	Gorilla gorilla (gorilla) Pan troglodytes (chimpanzee)	simian malaria	West and Central Africa
P. rhodhaini	Pan troglodytes	simian malaria	West and Central Africa
P. schwetzi	Gorilla gorilla Pan troglodytes	simian malaria	West and Central Africa
Hepatocystes (plasmodium) kochi (Hepatocystes simiae)	Cercopithecus sp Papio sp, etc.	simian malaria hepatocystis	Africa

this site, the **sporozoites** are available to infect a new vertebrate host when the female mosquito takes her blood meal.

The life cycle of *Plasmodium* closely resembles that of Coccidia (p. 680) in that an asexual stage (schizogony), passed in the tissue of the vertebrate host, is continued by a sexual stage with sporozoite formation. The differences are that Coccidia have a form which is spent outside any host (oöcyst) and the sexual stages develop in the vertebrate host: the sexual stages in *Plasmodium* occur in the alimentary tract of a blood-sucking arthropod and no form occurs which can survive outside the body of a host.

The signs in malaria are related to the numbers of parasites in the blood and appear five to fourteen or more days following infection; the incubation period depends to some extent upon the exoerythrocytic period of the parasites. Bouts of chills and fever appear at intervals roughly comparable to the periods of reproduction of the malaria parasite. The terms tertian (3rd) and *quartan* (4th) apply to the usual interval between paroxysms. After a forty-eight-hour cycle, as is the case in *Plasmodium vivax* and *P. falciparum* infection, the signs reappear on the third day (*tertian*). In the case of *quartan* malaria, the cycle of the parasite (*P. malariae*) is about seventy-six hours and the signs reappear each fourth day. Malaria due to *P. falciparum* may also have a cycle less than forty-eight hours (*subtertian*) due to presence of two broods of parasites. These features are covered in Table 14–3. Relapses often occur in human malaria, sometimes after long intervals, thus providing a carrier state. This state also appears to occur in other animals.

The pathologic effects of malaria vary to some extent with the organism involved but are similar in most vertebrate hosts. The destruction of parasitized erythrocytes results in hemolysis and anemia. Some effect on the bone marrow is postulated and possibly immunologic factors may contribute to the anemia. Splenomegaly is rather constant and rupture may occur. Hepatomegaly usually occurs and the liver has a dark color due to the presence of malaria pigment (hematin) in Kupffer cells. Hemorrhages in the brain may be associated with blood vessels occluded by parasitized red blood cells.

The **diagnosis** of malaria is usually established by demonstrating the organisms in erythrocytes in thin or thick smears stained with Giemsa's or Wright-Giemsa's stain.

Malaria

COATNEY, G. R.: Simian Malarias in Man: Facts, Implications, and Predictions. J. Trop. Med. Hyg. *17*:147–155, 1968.
CONTACOS, P. G., and COLLINS, W. E.: *Plasmodium malariae*: Transmission from Monkey to Man by Mosquito Bite. Science *165*:918–919, 1969.
DEANE, L. M.: Plasmodia of Monkeys and Malaria Eradication in Brazil. Rev. Lat. Amer. Microbiol. *11*:69–73, 1969.
EYLES, D. E., COATNEY, G. R., and GETZ, E.: Vivax Type Malaria Parasite of Macaques Transmissible to Man. Science *131*:1812–1813, 1960.
GARNHAM, P. C. C.: Malaria in Mammals Excluding Man. Adv. Parasit. *5*:139–204, 1967.
HELD, J. R.: Primate Malaria. Ann. New York Acad. Sci. *162*:587–593, 1969.
LAVERAN, C. L. A.: *Nature parasitaire des accidents de l'impaludisme; Description d'un nouveau parasite trouvé dans le sang des malades atteintes de fievre palustre*, Paris, Bailliere, 1881.
MANWELL, R. D.: "Malaria" pp. 25–29 in Weinman, D. and Ristic, M. (ed.). *Infectious Blood Diseases of Man and Animals*. Vol. II. New York, Academic Press, 1968.
MILLER, L. H.: Distribution of Mature Trophozoites and Schizonts of *Plasmodium falciparum* in the Organs of *Aotus trivirgatus*, the Night Monkey. Amer. J. Trop. Med. *18*:860–865, 1969.

RIGDON, R. H.: Hemoglobinuria (Blackwater Fever) in Monkeys. A Consideration of the Disease in Man. Amer. J. Path. *25*:195–209, 1949.

Ross, R.: *The Prevention of Malaria.* London, Murray, 1910.

HEPATOCYSTES

Hepatocystes (or *Hepatocystis*) *kochi* is a protozoan organism until recently named *Plasmodium kochi*, which is parasitic in many species of non-human primates. The organism is found in primates in the genera *Cercopithecus*, *Papio*, *Hyalobates* and *Macaca*. Other species, such as leaf-nosed bats (*Hipposideros armiger armiger*) and red-bellied tree squirrels (*Callosciurus sciurus*), have been reported to be infected. One vector is reported to be *Culicoides adersi*.

One distinguishing feature of this parasite is its production of grossly visible cysts in the liver of vertebrate hosts. This cyst, called a **merocyst,** starts by invasion of a single hepatic cell by a merozoite which grows within the hepatocyte causing it to undergo hypertrophy as the parasite grows. Continued growth of the organism eventually results in a many-celled structure as large as 2 mm. in diameter with a central fluid-filled space. The outer wall is occupied by myriads of tiny **merozoites** which are released when the cyst ruptures. These merozoites then parasitize erythrocytes, producing ring forms and eventually gametocytes. Gametogony is believed to take place in the invertebrate host, *Culicoides adersi*.

This merocyst initially destroys a single hepatic cell and displaces others as the organism grows. Varying degrees of tissue reaction result, presumably depending

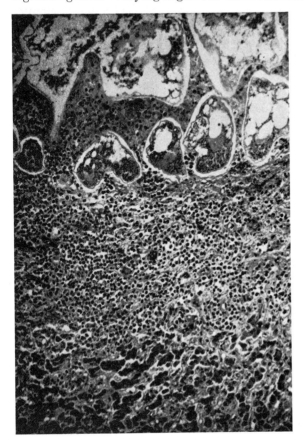

FIG. 14–21.—*Hepatocystis kochi*, liver of a baboon. The section includes part of the cyst (top), a zone of reaction, and liver cells (bottom).

upon immunologic factors (p. 307). The host may react by surrounding the cyst with epithelioid granulation tissue and multinucleated giant cells, finally by fibrous connective tissue. Recently ruptured cysts may be surrounded by hemorrhage. A fibrous scar eventually results.

Hepatocystes

DESOWITZ, R. S.: *Hepatocystis sp.* from a Gibbon. Trans. Roy. Soc. Trop. Med. Hyg. *62*:4, 1968.
GARNHAM, P. C. C.: Exoerythrocytic Schizogony in *Plasmodium kochi*, Laveran. A Preliminary Note. Trans. Roy. Soc. Trop. Med. & Hyg. *40*:719–722, 1947.
————: The Developmental Cycle of *Hepatocystes (Plasmodium) kochi* in the Monkey Host. Trans. Roy. Soc. Trop. Med. & Hyg. *41*:601–616, 1948.
MANWELL, R. D., and KUNTZ, R. E.: Hepatocystis in Formosan Mammals with a Description of a New Species. J. Protozool. *13*:670–672, 1966.
SHIROISHI, T., DAVIS, J., and WARREN, M.: *Hepatocystis* in White-cheeked Gibbon, *Hylobates concolor*. J. Parasit. *54*:168, 1968.
VICKERS, J. H.: *Hepatocystis kochi* in Cercopithecus Monkeys. J. Am. Vet. Med. Assn. *149*: 906–908, 1966.
WARREN, McW., SHIROISHI, T., and DAVIS, J.: A Hepatocystis-like Parasite of the Gibbon. Trans. Roy. Soc. Trop. Med. & Hyg. *62*:4, 1968.

HEPATOZOON INFECTIONS

Organisms of the genus *Hepatozoon* are placed in the Class Sporozoa of the Protozoa and contain several pathogenic species. Schizogony occurs in endothelial cells of the liver and gametocytes may be found in erythrocytes or leukocytes of the vertebrate host, depending upon the species of the protozoa. Sporogony occurs in blood-sucking arthropods.

Hepatozoon canis infects dogs, cats, hyenas and jackals in the Middle East, North Africa, Italy and the Far East. The developmental cycle of the organism involves the brown dog tick, *Rhipicephalus sanguineus*, which, when infected, carries sporocysts in its body cavity. Ingestion of the infected vector tick by the vertebrate host results in release of **sporozoites** which penetrate the intestinal wall to reach the spleen, liver and bone marrow via the blood stream. The parasites enter tissue cells to become **schizonts,** reproducing several generations in these cells. Eventually **merozoites** are produced which penetrate or are engulfed by leukocytes and become **gametocytes, or gamonts.** These gametocytes become differentiated into macro- and microgametocytes in the body of the vector tick, sexual union results in a motile zygote, the **oökinete.** This oökinete migrates to the hemocoel of the tick where it grows to a large oöcyst, 100 microns in diameter, in which large numbers of sporozoites are formed within sporocysts. The sporozoites are released from the oöcyst after the tick is ingested by the vertebrate host.

The **signs** of this infection consist of fever, anemia, splenomegaly, progressive emaciation and sometimes paralysis. Death may occur four to eight weeks following outset of clinical signs. The **lesions** are related to the anemia insofar as is known but have not been studied adequately. The **diagnosis** is based on demonstration of the organisms—gametocytes in leukocytes in blood smears—or schizonts in biopsy or necropsy specimens of liver, spleen or bone marrow.

Several other organisms of this genus are known to infect vertebrates, some of them are: *Hepatozoon cuniculi* (host: rabbit in Europe); *H. muris* (brown rat, *Rattus norvegicus*, or black rat, *Rattus rattus*—the vector is the rat mite, *Echinolaelaps echidminus*); *H. procyonis* (raccoon); *Hepatozoon sp.* (impala in South Africa); *H. musculi* (white mouse in England).

Hepatozoon

BASSON, P. A., *et al.*: Observations on a Hepatozoon-like Parasite in the Impala. J. S. Afr. Vet. Med. Assn. *38*:12–14, 1967. V.B. *37*:4651, 1967.

SCHNEIDER, C. R.: *Hepatozoon procyonis* Richards, 1961, in a Panamanian Raccoon, *Procyon cancrivorus panamensis* (Goldman). Rev. Biol. Trop. *15*:123–135, 1968.

SOULSBY, E. J. L.: *Helminths, Arthropods and Protozoa of Domesticated Animals (Mönnig)* 6th Ed. Baltimore, The Williams & Wilkins Co., 1968.

BABESIOSIS

(Piroplasmosis, Tick Fever, "Red Water")

Organisms of the genus *Babesia*, Protozoa of the Order Sporozoa, parasitize the erythrocytes of a wide variety of vertebrate hosts, multiplying in the erythrocytes by means of binary fission, giving rise to two or four daughter individuals. Ticks act as intermediate host-vectors in which the parasites reproduce, sometimes penetrating the egg to infect the young tick. Bovine babesiosis (piroplasmosis, Texas or tick fever) was the first infection of any kind to be shown to be transmitted by an arthropod vector (Smith and Kilborne, 1893); this was a major scientific achievement and milestone in the conquest of disease. Dogs, cattle, horses, sheep and swine are susceptible to one or more separate species of *Babesia*, but the general features of the disease are similar in all hosts.

The **clinical manifestations** of babesiosis are so capriciously variable that they are of little help in diagnosis. The signs common to most cases include fever, malaise and listlessness, anorexia and anemia. Icterus, hemoglobinuria and ascites may appear during late stages and progressive debility terminates in death.

Babesia are found in the circulating erythrocytes of mammals as pyriform or ovoid bodies, usually in pairs, and measure approximately 3 microns in length. They are particularly well demonstrated by Romanovsky-type stains. The important pathogens of domestic animals are listed in Table 14–3. Several other species of Babesia are apparently tolerated by animals with little ill effect.

Bovine Babesiosis (Texas Fever, Tick Fever, Piroplasmosis).—This disease of cattle is of historical interest because it has now been virtually eliminated from the Southern United States where it was once very prevalent. Its eradication was accomplished by elimination of the tick vector, *Boöphilus annulatus*. Babesiosis is still present in many other parts of the world.

The gross **lesions** of this bovine disease are of interest. Necropsy of the emaciated carcass of animals dead of the disease discloses the blood to be thin and watery and the plasma is red-tinged. The subcutaneous, subserous and intramuscular connective tissue is edematous and yellow and the fat is similarly affected. Gastroenteritis is indicated by swelling and patchy reddening of the abomasal and intestinal mucosa. Icteric discoloration is clearly recognizable in all viscera. The spleen is constantly enlarged 4 to 5 times normal size and its parenchyma is soft and dark red. The splenic corpuscles are usually prominent. The liver is enlarged and yellow-brown with the gallbladder distended with dark green bile. The lungs are slightly edematous and the urinary bladder usually contains red-colored urine.

The microscopic findings are characteristic of severe hemolytic anemia. *Babesia* may be demonstrable in large numbers in capillaries in the brain and optic choroid even though they cannot be found elsewhere. The organisms in these sites are described as being both free in the lumen and in packed erythrocytes.

Table 14–4.—Babesia Infections

Organism	Animals Affected	Geographic Distribution	Tick Vectors
B. bigemina . . .	cattle, zebu, water buffalo, deer	Central and South America, Africa, Australia and Southern Europe	Boophilus annulatus B. microplus B. australis B. calcaratus B. decolaratus Rhipicephalus evertsi Rh. bursa Rh. appendiculatus Haemaphysalis punctata
B. bovis . . .	cattle, roe deer stag	Southern Europe Africa, Asia	Ixodes ricinus I. persulcatus B. calcaratus Rh. bursa
B. argentina . . .	cattle	Central and South America, Australia	B. microplus
B. divergens . . .	cattle	Northern Europe	I. ricinus Dermacentor reticulatus
B. canis	dog, wolf, jackal	Asia, Africa, Southern Europe, United States, Central and South America, Soviet Union	Rh. sanguineus D. reticulatus D. marginatus H. leachi Hyalomma plumbeum Ha. bispinosa
B. gibsoni	dog, wolf, fox, jackal	India, Ceylon, China, Turkestan, North Africa	Rh. sanguineus
B. equi	horse, mule, donkey, zebra	Asia, Africa, United States, Europe, South America, Soviet Union	D. reticulatus D. marginatus Rh. bursa Rh. sanguineus Rh. evertsi Hyalomma excavatum Hy. plumbeum Hy. dromedarii
B. caballi	horses, donkey, mule	Southern Europe, Asia, Soviet Union, Africa, Panama, United States	D. marginatus D. silvarum D. nitens Hy. excavatum Hy. dromedarii Hy. scupense Rh. bursa Rh. sanguineus D. reticulatus
B. motasi	sheep, goats	Southern Europe, Middle East, Soviet Union, Asia, Africa	D. silvarum Ha. punctata Rh. bursa
B. ovis	sheep, goats	Tropics, Southern Europe, Soviet Union	Rh. bursa
B. trautmanni . . .	pig, wart hog, bush pig	Southern Europe, Soviet Union, Congo, Tanganyika	Rh. turanicus Rh. sanguineus B. decoloratus D. reticulatus
B. felis	domestic cat, wildcat, lion, leopard, puma, American lynx	Sudan, South Africa, U. S. (Zoos)	unknown

Equine Babesiosis (Piroplasmosis).—Recently recognized for the first time in the United States, this disease is arousing some concern. Two species of *Babesia* are responsible for the disease in equine hosts but are not infective for other mammals. This genus-specificity is characteristic of these hemoprotozoan parasites. *Babesia caballi* affects horses, mules and donkeys as does *B. equi* which has also been found in zebras. *B. caballi* may be distinguished by their appearance in erythrocytes where they occur as paired pyriform bodies, 2.5 × 4.0 microns in maximum dimensions, with their pointed ends meeting at an acute angle. *B. equi* may be distinguished by their occurrence in erythrocytes in groups of four with pointed ends meeting to form a Maltese cross. The trophozoites are smaller (seldom exceeding 2.0 microns in length) and more pleomorphic with round, oval, and ring forms. Groups of four are common because of their tendency to divide into four daughter trophozoites. *B. equi* is considered to be more pathogenic than *B. caballi.*

The clinical signs are variable and are related for the most part to the destruction of erythrocytes: fever, anemia, icterus, weakness, occasionally hemoglobinuria and subcutaneous edema around the head. Respiratory signs may result from the anemia and be intensified by pneumonia. The findings at post mortem also indicate destruction of erythrocytes and the secondary effects of anemia. Hyperplasia of hematopoietic tissues in spleen, bone marrow, and liver may be evident plus centrilobular necrosis in the liver as a consequence of anoxia. Excessive fluid in peritoneal, pericardial and pleural sacs may be a feature.

Canine Babesiosis.—This disease is distributed world-wide and two causative organisms have been identified: *B. canis* in the Western Hemisphere, Africa, Europe, parts of Asia and the Soviet Union; *B. gibsoni* in India, Ceylon, China, Turkestan and North Africa. Cases have been reported from several of the United States and considering the ubiquitous distribution of the vector brown dog tick, *Rhipicephalus sanguineus*, the disease should be anticipated to occur in any part of the Western Hemisphere. Natural infection with *B. canis* (and other *Babesia*) has been demonstrated in splenectomized men. Experimental splenectomy of rhesus monkeys has been shown to render them susceptible to the disease.

The signs in the early acute case start with high fever which may undergo remission and exacerbation, enlarged spleen, ataxia, bilateral chemosis and anemia often with fewer than three million erythrocytes per cu. mm. of blood. Organisms may be demonstrated in large numbers in circulating erythrocytes at this time. As the disease progresses, fever abates, anemia continues, icterus appears and conjugated as well as unconjugated bilirubin is excreted in the urine. The excretion of conjugated bilirubin indicates injury to the liver as well as hemolysis in severe, prolonged cases. Injury to the kidney is indicated by anuria and elevated urea nitrogen in blood, proteinuria, plus cellular and granular casts in urine. Damage to the liver is indicated by elevated glutamic pyruvic transaminase in serum and by prolonged clearance time for bromsulfothalein. Alkaline phosphatase levels in serum may also be elevated.

Brown (cited by Malherbe, 1956) has noticed involvement of masseter muscle in dogs with babesiosis. This results in inability to open the mouth and in manifestations of severe pain if the jaw is forcibly opened. The outcome of this muscular involvement is not reported but the clinical similarity to so-called "eosinophilic myositis" of dogs is noteworthy (p. 1053).

The trophozoites of *Babesia canis* are usually very numerous in erythrocytes in the early stages but may become difficult to find later, although the anemia persists. It has been suggested that an immunologic basis for the anemia may be present in the later stages. On occasion, dogs may harbor organisms for months without manifesting severe disease (Ewing, 1965).

The lesions are related to the anemia and possibly to the occlusion of small blood vessels by heavily parasitized, clumped erythrocytes. Thrombosis of ophthalmic veins have been reported and may explain the severe chemosis noted in many cases (Basson and Pienaar, 1965). Large numbers of organisms in clumps of erythrocytes have been seen in capillaries in the brain, and in some instances frank thrombosis is evident. These tend to be distributed in the brain in a bilaterally symmetrical manner, producing grossly visible hemorrhages. Hypoxia, due to the anemia, also appears to be a possible factor in the induction of lesions, particularly in the brain and liver. Similar vascular lesions appear to be the basis for focal edema and necrosis of skeletal muscle, liver, spleen and lymph nodes.

Diagnosis.—The diagnosis is confirmed by identification of *Babesia* in blood smears, but all clinical manifestations must be judiciously weighed because of their variety and the occurrence of non-pathogenic *Babesia* in animals which may be ill from other causes. The organisms may be identified by their morphology and their stimulation of specific antibodies in the serum of infected animals. These antibodies may be detected by hemagglutination, complement fixation and bentonite agglutination tests.

Babesiosis

Basson, P. A., and Pienaar, J. G.: Canine Babesiosis: A Report on the Pathology of Three Cases with Special Reference to the "Cerebral" Form. J. S. Afr. Vet. Med. Assn. *36*:333–341, 1965.

Brown, J. M. M., cited by Malherbe, W. D.: The Manifestations and Diagnosis of *Babesia* Infections. Ann. New York Acad. Sci. *64*:128–146, 1956.

Callow, L. L. and Johnston, L. A. Y.: *Babesia spp.* in the Brains of Clinically Normal Cattle and Their Detection by a Brain Smear Technique. Aust. Vet. J. *39*:25–31, 1963.

Curnow, J. A., and Curnow, B. A.: An Indirect Haemagglutination Test for the Diagnosis of *Babesia argentina* Infection in Cattle. Aust. Vet. J. *43*:286–290, 1967.

Dennig, H. K.: Influence of Splenectomy on Latent Piroplasmosis in Horses. Berl. Munch. tierarztl. Wschr. *78*:204–209, 1965.

Dorner, J. L.: A Hematologic Study of Babesiosis of the Dog. Amer. J. Vet. Clin. Path. *1*:67–75, 1967.

Ewing, S. A.: Observations on Leukocytic Inclusion Bodies from Dogs Infected with *Babesia canis*. J. Am. Vet. Med. Assn. *143*:503–506, 1963.

—————: Observations on the Persistence and Recurrence of *Babesia canis* Infections in Dogs. Vet. Med. Small Anim. Clin. *60*:741–744, 1965.

—————: Method of Reproduction of *Babesia canis* in Erythrocytes. Am. J. Vet. Res. *26*:727–733, 1965.

—————: Evaluation of Methods Used to Detect *Babesia canis* Infections in Dogs. Cornell Vet. *56*:211–220, 1966.

Frerichs, W. M., Holbrook, A. A., and Johnson, A. J.: Equine Piroplasmosis: Complement-fixation Titers of Horses Infected with *Babesia caballi*. Am. J. Vet. Res. *30*:697–702, 1969.

Garnham, P. C. C., and Voller, A.: Experimental Studies on *Babesia divergens* in Rhesus Monkeys with Special Reference to Its Diagnosis by Serological Methods. Acta Prot. Warszwa *3*:183–187, 1965.

Hirsh, D. C., *et al.*: An Epizootic of Babesiosis in Dogs Used for Medical Research. Lab. Anim. Care *19*:205–208, 1969.

Maegraith, B., Gilles, H. M., and Devakul, K.: Pathological Processes in *Babesia canis* Infections. G. Tropenmed. u. Parasit. *8*:485–514, 1957. (V.B. 369–59)

Mahoney, D. F.: Circulating Antigens in Cattle Infected with *Babesia bigemina* or *B. argentina*. Nature (Lond.) *211*:422–428, 1966.

MALHERBE, W. D.: The Manifestations and Diagnosis of *Babesia* Infections. Ann. New York Acad. Sc. *64*:128–146, 1956.

————: Clinico-pathological Studies of *Babesia canis* Infection in Dogs. I. The Influence of the Infection on Bromsulphalein Retention in the Blood. J. S. Afr. Vet. Med. Assn. *36*:25–30, 1965.

————: Clinico-pathological Studies of *Babesia canis* Infection in Dogs. II. The Influence of the Infection on Plasma Transaminase Activity. III. The Influence of the Infection on Plasma Alkaline Phosphatase Activity. J. S. Afr. Vet. Med. Assn. *36*:173–176, 179–182, 173–182, 1965.

————: Clinico-pathological Studies of *Babesia canis* Infection in Dogs. V. The Influence of the Infection on Kidney Function. J. S. Afr. Vet. Med. Assn. *37*:261–264, 1966.

MAURER, F. D.: Equine Piroplasmosis—Another Emerging Disease. J. Am. Vet. M. A. *141*:699–702, 1962.

MENDONCA, H. S. C. and RIBEIRO, A. M.: Um caso de piroplasmose por *Babesia caballi* (Nuttall, 1910). Rev. Ciencias Vet. (Lisbon). *56*:248–257, 1961.

NEITZ, W. O.: Classification, Transmission and Biology of Piroplasms of Domestic Animals. Ann. New York Acad. Sc. *64*:56–111, 1956.

RIEK, R. F.: *Infectious Blood Diseases of Man and Animals:* Edited by D. Wienman and and M. Ristic. New York, Academic Press, 1968, pp. 219–268.

SCHOLTENS, R. G., *et al.*: A Case of Babesiosis in Man in the United States. Amer. J. Trop. Med. Hyg. *17*:810–813, 1968.

SCHROEDER, W. F., COX, H. W., and RISTIC, M.: Anaemia, Parasitaemia, Erythrophagocytosis, and Haemagglutinins in *Babesia rodhaini* Infection. Ann. Trop. Med. Parasit. *60*: 31–38, 1966.

SENEVIRATNA, P.: The Pathology of *Babesia gibsoni* (Patton, 1910) Infection in the Dog. Ceylon Vet. J. *13*:107–110, 1965.

————: Studies of *Babesia gibsoni* Infections of Dogs in Ceylon. Ceylon Vet. J. *13*: 1–6, 1965.

SIBINOVIC, S., SIBINOVIC, K. H., and RISTIC, M.: Equine Babesiosis: Diagnosis by Bentonite Agglutination and Passive Hemagglutination Tests. Am. J. Vet. Res. *30*:691–695, 1969.

SIMPSON, C. F., KIRKHAM, W. W., and KLING, J. M.: Comparative Morphologic Features of *Babesia caballi* and *Babesia equi*. Am. J. Vet. Res. *28*:1693–1697, 1967.

SIPPEL, W. L. *et al.*: Equine Piroplasmosis in the United States. J. Am. Vet. Med. A. *141*: 694–698, 1962.

THEILERIASIS

Protozoan parasites of the genus *Theileria*, like *Babesia*, are found in the erythrocytes but reproduce by schizogony in lymphocytes or histiocytes, and are classified in the Family Theileriidae. Two related genera are *Gonderi*, whose members reproduce by schizogony in lymphocytes and by fission in erythrocytes, and *Cytauxzoön*, which multiply by schizogony in histiocytic cells and by fission in erythrocytes. Table 14–5 indicates the important pathogenic *Theileria*.

Theileria parva, the cause of East Coast fever, a disease of cattle of much importance in Africa, is transmitted by several species of ticks, most of them in the genus *Rhipicephalus* and *Hyalomma*. *Theileria parva* appears in the erythrocytes of affected cattle as tiny rod-, comma- or ring-shaped organisms somewhat smaller than *Babesia*. Young forms also occur in the circulating lymphocytes as even smaller rod or coccoid organisms which fill the cytoplasm. These forms are also found in the cytoplasm of lymphocytes and histiocytes in lymph nodes, spleen, liver and other organs. Called **Koch's bodies,** after their discoverer, these cytoplasmic aggregations of *Theileria* are considered characteristic of the disease.

Unlike babesiosis, recovery from East Coast fever not only results in solid immunity, but the organisms disappear from the body and hence are not in position to cause relapses or result in a carrier state.

The **clinical manifestations** start with fever which appears about fifteen days following exposure by the bite of infected ticks. Several days after *Theileria*

Table 14–5.—Theileriases

Organism	Animals Affected	Geographic Distribution	Tick Vector
Theileria parva.	cattle, African buffalo Indian water buffalo	Africa	*Rhipicephalus appendiculatus*
Th. annulata	cattle, zebu, water buffalo	North Africa, Middle & Far East, Southern Europe, Soviet Union	*Hyalomma detritum* *H. dromedarii* *H. excavatum* *H. turanicum* *H. savignyi* *H. plumbeum* *H. scupense*
Th. mutans	cattle, deer	Africa, Asia, Australia, Soviet Union, United States, England	*Rhicephalus appendiculatus* *Rh. evertsi* *Haemaphysalis bispinosa* *H. punctata*
Th. hirci	sheep, goats	North & East Africa, Iraq, Turkey, Soviet Union, Greece	*Rhipicephalus bursa* (?)
Th. ovis	sheep, goats	Africa, Asia, India, Soviet Union, Europe	*Rhipicephalus bursa* *Rh. evertsi* *Dermacentor sylvarum* *Haemaphysalis sulcata* *Ornithodorous lahorensis*
Th. cervi	white tailed deer	United States	unknown

becomes demonstrable in the blood, the appetite is gradually lost, rumination ceases and milk secretion decreases. The superficial lymph nodes become noticeably enlarged, the muzzle dry, the hair coat rough, and salivation as well as lacrimation becomes excessive. Respiratory distress may follow pulmonary edema and death may result from asphyxia. In some cases, death follows gradual emaciation, delirium and coma.

The most constant **lesions** found at necropsy consist of generalized enlargement of lymph nodes, pulmonary edema and emphysema, subcutaneous and intramuscular edema. The spleen is of normal size. Excessive pericardial and pleural fluid may be present and the liver is generally enlarged, yellowish, and frequently mottled. White foci of various sizes may be seen in the renal cortex.

The principal microscopic finding is proliferation of lymphocytic cells in lymph nodes, spleen, Peyer's patches and elsewhere. Koch's bodies may be found in tissue sections. The effects of anemia will also be evident in the bone marrow.

The **diagnosis** of theileriasis is dependent upon demonstration of the organisms in erythrocytes and in lymphocytes (Koch's bodies). Babesiosis is the most important disease from which it must be differentiated.

Theileriasis

BARNETT, S. F.: In *Infectious Blood Diseases of Man and Animals* edited by D. Wienman and M. Ristic. New York, Academic Press, 1969, pp. 269–328.
JARETT, W. F. H., and BROCKLESBY, D. W.: Preliminary Electron Microscopic Studies on East Coast Fever. Parasit. *55*:13, 1965.

—————: A Preliminary Electron Microscopic Study of East Coast Fever (*Theileria parva* Infection). J. Protozool. *13*:301–310, 1966.

KRIER, J. P., RISTIC, M., and WATRACH, A. M.: *Theileria sp.* in a Deer in the United States. Am. J. Vet. Res. *23*:657–663, 1962.

MATSON, B. A.: Theileriosis Due to *Theileria parva, T. lawrencei* and *T. mutans.* Bibliography 1897–1966. Weybridge: Commonwealth Bureau of Animal Health, pp. 44, 1967.

RAFYI, A., MAGHAMI, G., and HOUSHMAND, P.: (The Virulence of *Theileria annulata* and Premunition Against Bovine Theileriosis in Iran.) Bull. Off. Int. Epizoot. *64*:431–446, 1965. V.B. *37*:854, 1967.

SOULSBY, E. J. L.: *Helminths, Arthropods and Protozoa of Domesticated Animals.* (Mönnig.) 6th Ed. Baltimore, The Williams & Wilkins Co., 1968.

SPLITTER, C. J.: *Theileria mutans* Associated with Bovine Anaplasmosis. J. Am. Vet. Med. Assn. *117*:134–135, 1950.

STECK, W.: Histologic Studies on East Coast Fever. South Africa, Onderstepoort 13th & 14th Reports. Part 1, 1928, pp. 243–282.

WILDE, J. K. H.: East Coast Fever. Adv. Vet. Sci. *11*:207–259, 1967.

24

15

Diseases Caused by Parasitic Helminths and Arthropods

PARASITIC HELMINTHS

Parasitic helminths, or worms, are important incitants of disease in all species of animals. Although these parasites in many instances produce little serious damage to the host, they are never beneficial and in some instances can produce severe and even fatal disease. The effect of various helminths upon animal hosts is given chief consideration in this chapter. Life cycles, host range, immunity and infectivity will be discussed only in so far as they influence the lesions resulting from parasitism. The reader is referred to standard texts and the selected references at the end of this chapter for more detailed information on the many other important aspects of helminthic parasitism (*helminthiasis*).

The parasitic helminths to be considered in this chapter are classified by the International Code of Zoological Nomenclature in three phyla, as follows:

Phylum Platyhelminthes, including the **trematodes** or **flukes,** and the **cestodes** or **tapeworms;**

Phylum Nemathelminthes, including the **nematodes** or **roundworms,** which infect a wide variety of hosts including animals, man and plants; and

Phylum Acanthocephala, including the **thorny-headed worms,** a few of which are important parasites of animals.

Effects of Helminthic Parasites Upon the Host.—Helminthic parasites produce deleterious effects upon their hosts in a wide variety of ways. These can be outlined as follows:

1. Mechanically interfere with function:
    a. Obstruct blood or lymph channels:—
       Right ventricle and pulmonary artery—*Dirofilaria immitis* (dog)
       Carotid arteries—*Elaeophora schneideri* (sheep)
          Lymphatic channels—*Dracunculus insignis* (dog)
       Mesenteric arteries—*Strongylus vulgaris* (horse)
       Aorta—*Spirocerca lupi* (dog); *Strongylus vulgaris* (horse)
       Vena cava—*Schistosoma bovis*; *S. hematobium*
    b. Obstruct ducts or tracts:—
          Bile duct—liver flukes, ascarids, fringed tapeworms
          Esophagus—*Spirocerca lupi* (dog)
       Intestinal lumen—ascarids, tapeworms
       Respiratory tract—*Filaroides osleri, Metastrongylus apri*
       Urinary tract—*Dioctophyma renale*

    c. Attach to or utilize functional tissue:
> Stomach mucosa—*Trichostrongylus axei* (sheep & cattle), *Draschia megastoma* (horses)
>
> Small intestine—hookworms
>
> Cecum and large intestine—strongyles (horses), cecal worms (turkeys, dogs)

    d. Act as foreign bodies, with resultant tissue reactions displacing normal structures:
> Schistosome ova (flukes)
>
> Dead larvae of many nematodes—*Toxocara canis*, *Dirofilaria immitis*

2. Invade and displace cells and tissues, producing necrosis and loss of function:
   a. Skin—hookworm larvae, *Habronema* larvae, *Rhabditis sp.*, *Onchocerca* larvae, *Elaeophora schneideri* larvae, *Stephanofilaria stilesi*
   b. Liver—giant liver flukes, kidney worm larvae, cysticercus, ecchinococcus and coenurus cysts, ascarid larvae, *Capillaria hepatica* (rat, man)
   c. Intestinal wall—nodular worms (*Œsophagostomum sp.*), larvae of strongyles (horses)
   d. Brain and spinal cord—coenurus, echinococcus, filaria—other helminth larvae
   e. Lung—lungworms, ascarid larvae, hookworms
   f. Musculature—trichinae, cysticerci

3. Devour blood and thereby cause anemia:
   a. Hookworms (dogs, cattle)
   b. Strongyles (horses)
   c. Stomach worms (cattle and sheep)

4. Utilize food needed by the host:
   a. Tapeworms
   b. Ascarids

5. Induce or predispose to neoplasia:
   a. Esophagus—*Spirocerca lupi* (dog)
   b. Liver—*Cysticercus fasciolaris* (rat)
   c. Urinary bladder—*Schistosoma hematobium* (man)

6. Introduce bacterial or other infection into tissues of the host:
   a. Lungs—lungworms, ascarid larvae
   b. Intestinal wall—hookworms, nodule worms, salmon flukes (dog)
   c. Cecum—cecal worms (histomonads of turkeys)
   d. Perirenal tissues—*Stephanurus dentatus*

7. Devour tissues of host:
   a. Ascarids
   b. Stomach worms

8. Secrete toxic products (hemolysins, histolysins, anticoagulants):
   a. Hookworms, nodule worms
   b. Stomach worms
   c. Strongyles

IDENTIFICATION OF HELMINTHS IN TISSUES

The discovery of one or more fragments of a helminth in histologic sections of tissue presents a challenge to the pathologist. In order to evaluate fully the significance of such a finding, he must know the potentialities of the parasite; whence it came; where it was going when trapped by the fixative; and what its total effect upon the host might be. The identification of the parasite is therefore critical. Complete, well-preserved specimens should be secured for referral to a parasitologist whenever possible. However, presumptive identification of the parasite can often be made from fragments of the organism in tissues, or it may be possible to tease parasites in recognizable form from fixed gross tissues. Although far from complete, the information concerning the appearance of helminths in tissue sections is even now sufficient to permit the recognition of many species.

In determining the identity of a parasite in tissues, several factors may be utilized to narrow the field of consideration: the host and its usual parasites, the anatomic location of the parasite, the nature of the tissue reaction, and, most important, the morphologic features of the parasite itself. Nematodes, for example, have an external cuticle supported by a thin membrane, the hypodermis, within which is a muscular wall surrounding the body cavity. They have an alimentary canal and the sexes are separate. All of these features can be detected in cross sections of the adults and, in some cases, of the larvae. Further, the midsomatic muscular wall of the nematodes has some distinguishing features. The muscle cells are arranged longitudinally in a single layer just within the hypodermis and, in cross section of helminths of most species, are seen to be divided into four groups by cords of cells (chords) of the hypodermis, which project toward the center. Thus, one dorsal, one ventral and two lateral chords are formed by the hypodermis. These cells in many species are also distinctive, varying in size and number. Nematodes are said to have a **polymyarian** somatic musculature (*Ascaris, Filaria,* and *Dracunculus*), when numerous long slender muscle cells extending toward the body cavity are divided into four longitudinal units by dorsal, ventral and lateral chords made up of a single row of cells (Fig. 15–6). Those nematodes with closely packed, somewhat flattened muscle cells in units containing three or four cells are classified as **meromyarian,** and include such genera as *Enterobius, Ancylostoma,* and *Necator.* In a third group of nematodes the muscle cells, although closely packed, are not divided by chords but encircle the body cavity completely. This group is classified as **holomyarian** and includes the genus *Trichuris.*

The eggs or larvae can be used as a guide in the identification of some adult parasites in tissues. Sections are often made through the ovary or uterus of adult worms in which numerous ova or larvae are present. The size, shape and shell of many ova are distinctive for the species; for example, the ovoid egg with double-contoured shell of *Strongylus,* the single polar eminence of ova of *Oxyuris,* and the double polar eminence of ova of *Capillaria* (Fig. 15–21). Some nematodes are viviparous, the ova embryonating and hatching in the uterus, the larvae escaping as free forms (*Dirofilaria*); others are ovoviviparous and produce ova which are embryonated, but the larvae are still within the egg shell when they are expelled from the parasite (*Spirocerca*).

Trematodes and cestodes generally can be differentiated from nematodes in tissue sections. They do not have a body cavity, although some of the larval forms may be suspended in a bladder (see Cysticerci). Most of them are hermaphroditic, hence male and female sex organs can often be seen in tissue sections of a single parasite. Nematodes may or may not have a spiny cuticle, but cestodes generally do not. The anatomic site in which cestodes and trematodes are found, the nature of the tissue reaction they evoke, and their structural form are often guides to the tentative identification of these parasites in tissues. Familiarity with their life cycle, host range, and morphology is thus an asset to the pathologist.

The cestodes possess a specialized proglottid, the scolex, which can often be detected in larval forms as well as in the adult in tissue sections. The scolex may bear two or more elongated suctorial grooves, or may have cup-shaped sucking discs, and a proboscis. In some species, the proboscis is armed with characteristic hooklets (Fig. 15–29). An external cuticle surrounding a germinal layer from which scolices or brood capsules containing scolices may arise also serves to identify cestodes in tissue sections.

The presence of some trematodes in the body may be determined by the identification of the ova of the parasite, even though the adult is not found. This is of particular value in schistosomiasis, in which many ova are carried by the blood stream to various organs where they become embedded in small granulomas. Some of the filarid worms are seldom seen in adult form in the tissues, but their larval forms are sufficient for diagnosis. Microfilaria of *Dirofilaria immitis*, for example, may be recognized in sections in glomerular tufts or other capillaries, even though adult worms are not found in the right heart. However, it is possible that microfilaria seen in sections of canine tissues may be either *Dirofilaria* or *Dipetalonema* species (p. 749).

Immunity to Parasites.—Delayed or cellular hypersensitivity (p. 311) has been demonstrated specifically in the course of infections by several parasites— namely, *Trichinella spiralis*, *Trichostrongylus colubriformis*, *Ancylostomum caninum*, *Fasciola hepatica* and *Hymenolepis nana* (Larsh, 1967).

General

BELDING, D. L.: *Textbook of Clinical Parasitology*. 3rd ed., New York, Appleton-Century-Crofts, Inc., 1965

BENBROOK, E. A.: *Outline of Parasites Reported for Domesticated Animals in North America*. 6th Ed., Ames, Iowa State Univ. Press, 1963.

BENBROOK, E. A., and SLOSS, M. W.: *Veterinary Clinical Parasitology*, 3rd Ed., Ames, Iowa State Univ. Press, 1961.

DIKMANS, G.: Check List of the Internal and External Animal Parasites of Domestic Animals in North America (United States and Possessions, and Canada). Am. J. Vet. Research 7:211–241, 1945.

HABERMAN, R. T., WILLIAMS, F. P., and THORP, W. T. S.: Identification of Some Internal Parasites of Laboratory Animals. U. S. Public Health Ser. Pub., 343, pp. 1–29, 1954.

HERMS, W. B.: *Medical Entomology*, 6th Ed., New York, The Macmillan Co., 1969.

JARRETT, W. F. H., MILLER, H. R. P., and MURRAY, M.: The Relationship between Mast Cells and Globule Leucocytes in Parasitic Infections. Vet. Rec. *80*:505–506, 1967.

LARSH, J. E., JR.: Delayed (Cellular) Hypersensitivity in Parasitic Infections. Amer. J. Trop. Med. Hyg. *16*:735–745, 1967.

MORGAN, B. B., and HAWKINS, P. A.: *Veterinary Helminthology*, Minneapolis, Burgess Publishing Co., 1949.

POYNTER, D.: Some Tissue Reactions to the Nematode Parasites of Animals. Adv. Parasit. *4*:321–383, 1966.

SOULSBY, E. J. L.: *Helminths, Arthropods and Protozoa of Domesticated Animals* (Mönnig), 6th Ed., Baltimore, The Williams & Wilkins Co., 1968.

WHITLOCK, J. H.: *Diagnosis of Veterinary Parasitisms*. Philadelphia, Lea & Febiger, 1960.

WHUR, P.: Relationship of Globule Leucocytes to Gastrointestinal Nematodes in the Sheep, and *Nippostrongylus brasiliensis* and *Hymenolepis nana* Infections in Rats. J. Comp. Path. *76*: 57–65, 1966.

ASCARIASIS

(Common Roundworm Infection, Ascarid Worm Infection)

Ascarids (Phylum: Nemathelminthes; Family: Ascaridae) are extremely common roundworms whose adult forms are found in abundance in the gastrointestinal tract of birds and mammals throughout the world. Ascarids occur not only in great numbers but in many varieties, most of them being host-specific. Certain ascarids that are morphologically indistinguishable, such as those which infect man and swine, are host-specific and rarely develop to maturity in other than the true host.

The adults are usually large robust worms which are found in the small intestine, the cecal worms of chickens being an exception. The eggs are thick-shelled and unsegmented when laid, and a period of incubation and two molts within the shell are required before the embryo becomes infective. The eggs are resistant to desiccation, low temperatures and many chemical agents. Young animals are particularly susceptible to infection with ascarids; many adults lose their ascarid parasites spontaneously.

A few representative species are listed below by the name currently preferred:

Species of Ascarid	Definitive Hosts
Ascaris lumbricoides	Man, swine (var. suis)
Toxocara canis	Dog, man (rarely)
Toxocara cati	Cat, dog, wildcat, lion, leopard, man (rarely)
Toxascaris leonina	Dog, cat, lion, tiger, fox
Neoascaris vitulorum	Cattle
Parascaris equorum	Horse
Ascaridia galli	Chickens, turkeys

In the evolutionary extension of their range of final hosts to include birds, terrestrial and aquatic mammals, the life cycle of the ascarid and the migratory behavior of their larvae have been modified in many ways. The larvae or the eggs of some species are ingested by an intermediate host (insect larvae, amphibia, rodents or insectivora) in whose tissues they usually remain and develop until they gain access to the definitive host. This phenomenon has been demonstrated in several ascarids of veterinary importance—namely, *Ascaris columnaris*, *Toxocara canis*, *Toxocara cati* and *Toxascaris leonina*. Other helminths of this group do not utilize an intermediate host (none require it); the embryonated eggs are ingested by the host, the infective larvae escape from the egg and invade the host tissues, and then development to the adult form is completed at the end of their migration through the tissues. The lesions produced are determined by the migratory pattern the specific larvae follow, which are of three principal types.

(1) Infective larvae penetrate the intestinal wall, pass through the liver to the lungs, break through into the alveoli, gain the bronchi, ascend the trachea, are swallowed, and then develop into adults in the intestinal lumen. This "tracheal migration" of larvae is characteristic of *Ascaris lumbricoides* (man), *A. lumbricoides* var. *suis* (swine), *Parascaris equorum* (horses) and *Toxocara canis* (dogs).

(2) Larvae migrate not only through the liver and lungs, but also through the somatic tissues, sometimes causing prenatal infection of the fetus. This has been demonstrated with *Toxocara canis* (dogs) and *Neoascaris vitulorum* (cattle).

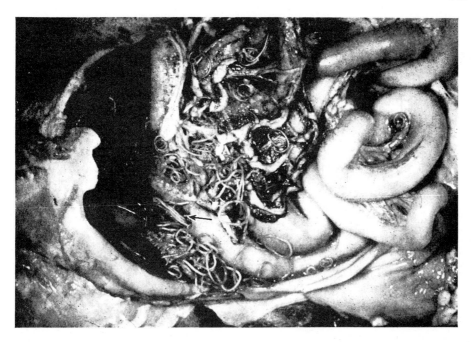

FIG. 15–1.—Ascariasis. Unusually severe infection of a seven-week-old Collie puppy with *Toxocara canis*, resulted in rupture of duodenum (arrow) and death. (Photo courtesy of Angell Memorial Animal Hospital.)

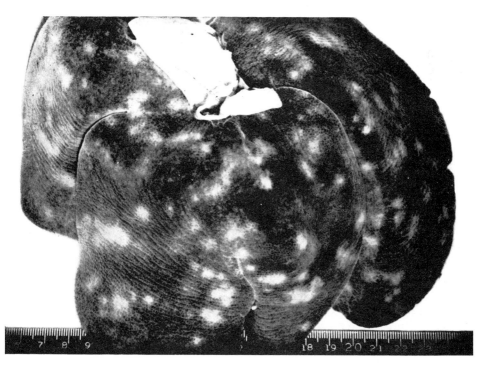

FIG. 15–2. Ascariasis, liver of a young pig. Gray, fibrous areas are caused by migration of ascaris larvae.

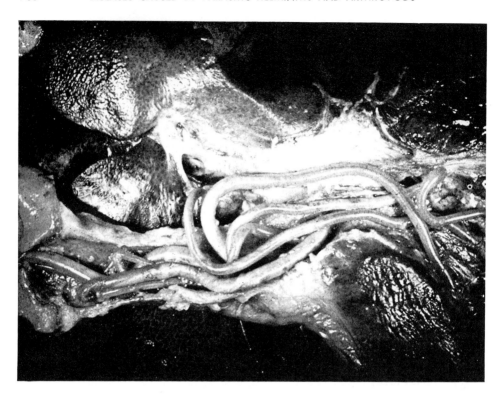

FIG. 15–3. *Ascaris lumbricoides, var. suis* in bile ducts of a pig.
Photograph courtesy of Dr. C. L. Davis.

(3) Larvae penetrate the wall of the intestine, where they develop without involving other somatic or visceral tissues; then return to the intestinal lumen to become adults. This pattern is followed by *Toxascaris leonina* and *Toxocara cati.*

It is readily apparent that ascarid larvae can penetrate various tissues of the host, where they may remain for some time and produce tissue damage. While the intestinal wall, the liver and the lungs are the common routes for larval migration, any tissue of the body could be invaded. The interval between ingestion of infective forms and the appearance of eggs in the feces of the final host is called the **prepatent period.** Obviously this is a period during which the host can sustain serious damage from the migration and development of larvae in the tissues. The prepatent period for different species of worms varies; it may be relatively long, for example, eighty to ninety days for *A. lumbricoides.*

Lesions.—Adult ascarids ordinarily live free in the lumen of the small intestine. They feed on the intestinal contents, occasionally gnaw on the mucosa, and, by a swimming movement, maintain their position in the tract in spite of peristaltic action. Their motility may be enhanced by several factors, among which are increased temperature (fever in the host) and starvation. On the other hand, they may be unable to maintain their position against the exaggerated peristalsis that occurs in diarrhea or after purging, and be swept out of the intestine. When their motility increases, it is not uncommon for ascarids to move into the stomach, the hepatic or pancreatic ducts. In the bile ducts, they may produce obstruction, with icterus a prominent manifestation. Jaundice of this origin is a fairly common reason for condemnation of hog carcasses inspected in abattoirs. Adult ascarids remaining in their usual location may become so numerous as to cause obstruction of the intestinal lumen, which may be fatal, particularly in young animals. On occasion, penetration of the intestinal wall has produced peritonitis in the host. Inanition in the host and retardation of growth of the young animal are the most common effects produced by ascarids, for they deprive the host of food and interfere with its digestive processes.

The lesions produced by the infective larvae during their migration and development in the tissues of the host range from minimal to severe. As the larvae migrate, tissues along the route are damaged and reparative processes become part of the pathologic picture. Larvae that penetrate the intestinal mucosa may carry bacteria into the tissues. In the liver, heavy infection with larvae often produces rather intense inflammation, with edema, neutrophils, eosinophils and lymphocytes as components of the inflammatory reaction. Larvae may be identified in a central mass of characteristic caseous necrosis surrounded by epithelioid cells, eosinophils, lymphocytes, and neutrophils. The portal areas are most severely involved, but subsequent fibrosis may obliterate entire lobules. However, in the average case as seen at necropsy, tissue changes are negligible. In swine, a diffuse, subcapsular fibrosis is considered to mark the sites of previous larval invasion of the liver. Larval migration through the lungs sets up considerable inflammatory reaction which may result in mild to severe respiratory involvement, which usually heals with few residual lesions.

Hemorrhages occur as the larvae break out of the pulmonary capillaries to enter the alveoli, and in heavy infections loss of bronchiolar epithelium and infiltration of leukocytes may be additional features. Ascarid larvae may wander throughout the body and produce granulomatous nodules in many sites. Invasion of the eye by nematode larvae has been demonstrated in children by Wilder (1950); Beautyman and Woolf (1951) have reported them in the brain of a child. The larvae of ascarids, such as *Toxocara canis*, are also responsible for *"visceral larval migrans,"* a disease of young children, puppies and calves. (See also cerebrospinal nematodiasis.)

Diagnosis.—Clinical diagnosis of ascariasis is established by demonstration of ova or adults in the feces and the correlation of these findings with the clinical symptoms. During the prepatent period, ova will not be found in the feces, although immature forms may be present in the tissues or intestinal lumen. Ascarid larvae may be identified in tissue sections and their relationship to lesion clearly demonstrated. Occlusion of hepatic ducts by adult ascarids may occur and is usually recognized at necropsy.

Ascariasis

BARRON, C. N., and SAUNDERS, L. Z.: Visceral Larva Migrans in the Dog. Path. Vet. *3*: 315–330, 1966.
BARRY, J. M., and O'ROURKE, F. J.: Ascariasis in Pig and Man. Scient. Proc. R. Dubl. Soc. Ser. *A3*: No. 4, 39–55, 1967.
BEAUTYMAN, W., and WOOLF, A. L.: An Ascaris Larva in the Brain in Association with Acute Anterior Poliomyelitis. J. Path. & Bact. *63*:635–647, 1951.

DUBEY, J. P.:   *Toxocara cati* and Other Intestinal Parasites of Cats.   Vet. Rec. *79*:506–508, 1966.

FITZGERALD, P. R., and MANSFIELD, M. E.:   Visceral Larva Migrans (*Toxocara canis*) in Calves.   Am. J. Vet. Res. *31*:561–566, 1970.

KOUTZ, F. R., GROVES, H. F., and SCOTHORN, M. W.:   The Prenatal Migration of *Toxocara canis* Larvae and Their Relationship to Infection in Pregnant Bitches and in Pups.   Am. J. Vet. Res. *27*:789–795, 1966.

MATOFF, K.:   Hypotheses Concerning the Migration Routes of Ascarid Larvae.   Z. Parasit-Kde. *31*:137–154, 1968.   V.B. *39*:2995, 1969.

MATOFF, K., and KOMANDAREY, S.:   Comparative Studies on the Migration of the Larvae of *Toxascaris leonina* and *Toxascaris transfuga*.   Z. ParasitKde. *25*:538–555, 1965.

MITCHELL, J. R.:   Detection of *Toxocara canis* Antibodies with the Fluorescent Antibody Technique.   Proc. Soc. Exp. Biol. N.Y. *117*:267–270, 1964.

MONCOL, D. J., and BATTE, E. F.:   Peripheral Blood Eosinophilia in Porcine Ascariasis.   Cornell Vet. *57*:96–107, 1967.

MORROW, D. A.:   Pneumonia in Cattle Due to Migrating *Ascaris lumbriocoides* Larvae.   J. Am. Vet. Med. Assn. *153*:184–189, 1968.

OKOSHI, S., and USUI, M.:   Experimental Studies on *Toxascari leonina*. VI. Experimental Infection of Mice, Chickens and Earthworms with *Toxascaris leonina*, *Toxocara canis* and *Toxocara cati*.   Jap. J. Vet. Sci. *30*:151–166, 1968.

RUBIN, L. F., and SAUNDERS, L. Z.:   Intraocular Larva Migrans in Dogs.   Path. Vet. 2: 566–573, 1965.

SCHWARTZ, B.:   Experimental Infection of Pigs with *Ascaris suum*.   Am. J. Vet. Res. *20*:7–13, 1959.

SCOTHORN, M. W., KOUTZ, F. R., and GROVES, H. F.:   Prenatal *Toxocara canis* Infection in Pups.   J. Am. Vet. Med. Assn. *146*:45–58, 1965.

SHALKOP, W. T. *et al.*:   Report on Investigations of Icterus in Swine.   North Am. Vet. *34*:257–262, 1953.

SPRENT, J. F. A.:   The Life Cycles of Nematodes in the Family Ascaridae, Blanchard, 1896.   J. Parasitol. *40*:608–617, 1954.

UECKERT, B.:   Larva Migrans, A Review.   Southwestern Vet. *15*:223–230, 1962.

WEIDE, K. D. and TWIEHAUS, M. J.:   Hematological Studies of Normal, Ascarid Infected and Hog Cholera Vaccinated Swine.   Am. J. Vet. Res. *20*:562–567, 1959.

WILDER, H. C.:   Nematode Endophthalmitis.   Tr. Amer. Acad. Ophth. (Oct):99–108, 1950.

WISEMAN, R. A.:   Toxocariasis in Man and Animals.   Vet. Rec. *84*:214–216, 1969.

ANCYLOSTOMIASIS

(Hookworm Disease)

Hookworms (Family: Ancylostomidae) are important parasites of animals and in some parts of the world produce widespread disease in man.   These parasites are cosmopolitan in distribution, although limited to certain areas by environmental conditions such as moisture and temperature.   One or more species of hookworm occur in every domestic animal, with the singular exception of the horse.   Hookworms as a group have several characteristics that influence their pathologic effects and therefore merit brief mention: (1) they have well-developed buccal cavities containing tooth-like structures, and all suck blood from the host; (2) adults normally inhabit the small intestine, eggs are passed in the feces, hatch under suitable conditions into rhabditiform larvae, which after two molts become filariform and may infect another host by penetration of the skin or through ingestion; (3) infective larvae that penetrate the skin migrate to the lungs and gain access to the intestine via the tracheal route; (4) although most hookworm species are host-specific, many can penetrate the epidermis of aberrant hosts, producing a specific dermatitis (*creeping eruption*); (5) larvae of at least one species (*Ancylostoma caninum*) appear in the milk to infect suckling young but infection *in utero* does not occur.

A few important hookworms are listed under the names currently in use:

Hookworm	Definitive Host
Ancylostoma duodenale	Man
Necator americanus	Man
Ancylostoma caninum	Dog, cat
Ancylostoma braziliense	Dog, cat
Uncinaria stenocephala	Dog, fox
Bunostomum phlebotomum	Cattle
Bunostomum trigonocephalum	Sheep, goats
Globocephalus urosubulatus	Swine

Signs produced in the host by hookworms depend upon the effects of both the adults and the infective larvae. The third stage (infective) larvae penetrate the intact skin, producing ancylostome dermatitis in the natural host (in man, "ground itch," "coolie's itch" or "water itch"). In aberrant hosts, e.g., Ancylostoma braziliense in man, infective larvae penetrate the epidermis and migrate for short distances in the dermis, producing indurated reddish papules from which linear serpiginous tunnels, 1 to 2 mm. in diameter, extend for a few centimeters. This lesion is known as "creeping eruption." In their natural host, the infective larvae, after penetrating the skin, invade the lungs. The usual symptoms are cough and, in severe cases, pneumonia.

The adult hookworms which attach themselves to the mucosa of the small intestine may produce symptoms of anemia (usually microcytic, hypochromic) in the host. These include pallor of the mucosae, hypoproteinemia, weakness, diarrhea, and progressive emaciation, with cardiac failure and death resulting in some cases.

Lesions.—Infective larvae may excite severe dermatitis during their migration through the skin of sensitized animals. The tissue reaction is usually limited to the vicinity of the migratory path of the larvae and is not distinctive, although lymphocytes, eosinophils and macrophages predominate in the exudate that infiltrates the dermis. These larvae may also breach the placenta and cause prenatal infection in the young. The most severe effects of the larval invasion are seen in the lung. As the larvae break into the alveoli from the pulmonary capillaries, hemorrhage occurs and in heavy infections may be severe. Leukocytic infiltration follows, sometimes of such severity as to amount to lobular pneumonia. Secondary bacterial infection is believed to contribute to this lesion in many instances. Fibrosis of affected lung parenchyma is a common sequel. From the alveoli the larvae invade the bronchial tree, are coughed up and then swallowed to reach the small intestine of the host.

The adult hookworms have buccal tooth-like structures and a powerful esophagus which permits them to draw bits of intestinal mucosa into their buccal cavity. In addition, they secrete an anticoagulant which promotes the sucking of blood at a rapid rate; in some instances intact erythrocytes are passed through the digestive tract of the parasite. Worms may change position, leaving a lesion denuded of epithelium from which blood continues to flow and through which bacteria can enter the tissues. The destructive effect upon the mucosa gives rise to enteritis, and the loss of blood to anemia. It is now believed that in most instances the anemia of hookworm disease is entirely attributable to loss of blood. Anemia may be very severe, the erythrocyte content of the blood dropping to 25 per cent of normal in some cases. The blood loss usually results in hyperplasia of the hematopoietic elements of the bone marrow, which may be accompanied by myeloid metaplasia in the spleen.

Diagnosis.—The diagnosis can be confirmed clinically by demonstration of hookworm ova in the feces. At necropsy, adult worms may be found attached to the mucosa of the small intestine. Larvae may be demonstrable microscopically in tissue sections, but this is a matter of chance.

Ancylostomiasis

MAYHEW, R. L.: Studies on Bovine Gastro-intestinal Parasites. I. The Mode of Infection of the Hookworm and Nodularworm. Cornell Vet. *29*:367–376, 1939.
————: Studies on Bovine Gastro-intestinal Parasites. IX. The Effects of Nematode Infections During the Larval Period. Cornell Vet. *34*:299–307, 1944.
MILLER, T. A.: Blood Loss During Hookworm Infection, Determined by Erythrocyte Labeling with Radioactive Chromium. I. Infection of Dogs with Normal and with X-irradiated *Ancylostoma caninum*. J. Parasit. *52*:844–855, 1966.
————: Blood Loss During Hookworm Infection, Determined by Erythrocyte Labeling with Radioactive [51]Chromium. II. Pathogenesis of *Ancylostunun braziliense* Infection in Dogs and Cats. J. Parasit. *52*:856–865, 1966.
PACENOVSKY, J., and BREZANSKA, M.: Penetration of *Bunostomum phlebotomum* Larvae into the Body of Cattle. Vet. Med. Praha *13*:277–383, 1968. V.B. *39*:2583, 1969.
SOULSBY, E. J. L., VENN, J. A. J., and GREEN, K. N.: Hookworm Disease in British Cattle. Vet. Record *67*:1124–1125, 1955.
STONE, W. M., and GIRARDEAU, M.: Transmammary Passage of *Ancylostoma caninum* Larvae in Dogs. J. Parasit. *54*:426–429, 1968.

TRICHOSTRONGYLOSIS

The Superfamily Trichostrongyloidea includes several helminths that are important parasites of cattle and sheep. Trichostrongyles of a number of species may infect the hosts simultaneously, producing severe damage which is manifested by anemia, cachexia, diarrhea, debility and sometimes death (particularly in lambs and calves). For this reason, trichostrongylosis may be considered an entity, although the parasitic genera involved in the clinical syndrome may differ in individual cases.

Helminths of the Superfamily Trichostrongyloidea are small, slender worms in which the buccal cavity is absent or rudimentary, without leaf crowns and usually toothless; their spicules are usually long and filiform or short and stout with protuberances. Their life cycle is direct; ellipsoidal ova pass to the ground in the feces of the host, hatch into filariform larvae, develop through larval stages in the soil, and produce infection in a new host when they are ingested with fresh grass. There is no migratory stage and the adults are found in the abomasum or small intestine, where they molt to the fourth stage.

One of the best known of these helminths is *Haemonchus contortus* ("barber pole worm," "twisted stomach worm" or "common stomach worm") which is the largest of the group. Infective third stage larvae, after they are ingested, reach the abomasum, molt to the fourth stage and attach themselves to the mucosa. After feeding on the host's blood for about eighteen days, they reach sexual maturity. Eggs appear in the feces of the host nineteen to twenty-one days after ingestion of the filiform larvae. The adult worms live free in the lumen but feed by piercing the mucosa with their pharyngeal lancets to suck blood. Not only do they rob the host of large quantities of blood, but they leave lacerations on the mucosa which predispose to gastritis.

The small trichostrongyles include helminths of the genera *Ostertagia* (*O. ostertagi*, the brown stomach worm), *Trichostrongylus* (*T. axei*—hairlike stomach worm), *Cooperia* and *Nematodirus*. Each of these genera includes several species beside those mentioned. The life cycle of these worms is similar to that of *Haemonchus contortus*, except that their embryonated eggs are highly resistant to drying and may accumulate on the ground during the dry season, then produce overwhelming infections when all larvae hatch at the same time, as the rainy season starts. These parasites also differ from *Haemonchus* in that they penetrate the tissues of the host. The infective larvae of *Trichostrongylus axei* burrow into the mucosa of the abomasum; other species of *Trichostrongylus* and *Cooperia* invade the mucosa of the small intestine. Larvae of *Ostertagia* also penetrate the mucosa of the abomasum but burrow deeper, remain longer and generally cause more damage to the gastric wall. The parasites develop to maturity in small nodules; the adults may emerge completely or may be seen partially projecting from the nodules in the mucosa.

Kates and Turner (1955) have studied the life cycle of *Nematodirus spathiger*, which is parasitic in the intestines of sheep and other ruminants, and have compared this parasite with others of this genus which have a similar life cycle. Many of the trichostrongylids of this genus, *Nematodirus*, produce infective larvae which invade the lamina propria of the mucosa of the small intestine, and thereby produce superficial erosions and sloughing of the mucosa. This characteristic of the parasite may produce severe effects on the host, including death in heavy infections. Several species of *Nematodirus* have been identified from sheep in the United States by Bechlund and Walker (1967), namely—*N. spathiger*, *abnormalis, filicollis, lanceolatus, helvetianus* and *davtiani*.

Stomach Worms in Swine— *Hyostrongylus rubidus* has been reported in at least one severe infection in which the lesions were diphtheritic gastritis. The gastric mucosa was covered with a yellowish membrane, beneath which large numbers of the worms were visible (Nicholson and Gordon, 1959). The submucosa was of gelatinous appearance because of edema. This sow was emaciated but active when she was sacrificed. The feces contained 1200 eggs per gram.

Signs.—The signs of trichostrongylosis are most severe in young or malnourished animals and may appear rather suddenly after rains which have broken a dry season. Anemia is the most outstanding symptom in acute infections, due to *Haemonchus*; lambs, in particular, may die from loss of blood without warning. In more prolonged infections, anemia is associated with edematous swellings under the jaw and sometimes the ventral abdomen (p. 134). The body fat is replaced by gelatinous tissue (see Mucoid Degeneration, p. 52), hence emaciation is seldom apparent. Affected animals grow progressively weaker, their gait becomes staggering; death follows after prolonged illness. In cases in which the small trichostrongyles predominate, diarrhea with thin, fetid, black-colored feces may be noted in addition to anemia and cachexia.

Lesions.—Necropsy findings are dominated by the severe anemia in acute cases, the mucous membranes as well as the viscera appearing extremely pale or chalk-white, the blood thin and watery. In cases of longer standing, anemia is also in evidence, but edematous swellings in the subcutis under the jaw and abdomen may be seen as well. Excessive amounts of fluid are usually present in the thoracic, pericardial and peritoneal cavities. The body fat undergoes mucoid degeneration (p. 52) and becomes highly edematous. The liver is light brown and friable, and contains areas of fatty change. The abomasum may contain large numbers of worms which remain actively motile as long as the body is warm. Shallow ulcers or many small red bite marks may be present in the mucosa as a result of the feeding habits of *Haemonchus contortus*. Small, round nodules, 1 to 2 mm. in diameter, in the abomasal mucosa mark the points at which parasites of the *Ostertagia* species have penetrated the walls.

Microscopically, evidence of anemia is seen in the overactive bone marrow; fatty change may be present in the liver; edematous replacement (mucoid atrophy, p. 52) of fat cells may be detected, and some worms may be demonstrated in the wall of the abomasum or small intestine.

Diagnosis.—Although demonstration of ova in the feces will identify some infections, fatal trichostrongylosis can occur during the prepatent period. For this reason, when herd problems are encountered, it may be necessary to sacrifice an animal or two to establish the presence of this disease conclusively. The finding of helminths in large numbers in the abomasum and small intestine of animals which have been anemic and the demonstration of characteristic gross changes at necropsy are considered sufficient for diagnosis in most situations. Worms of the genera *Trichostrongylus, Ostertagia* and *Cooperia* are so small some usually competent veterinarians miss finding them even in fatal cases. Washings from which the coarser ingesta have been removed by a sieve should be examined with a hand lens or dissecting microscope.

Trichostrongylosis

BECKLUND, W. W., and WALKER, M. L.: Nematodirus of Domestic Sheep, *Ovis aries*, in the United States with a Key to the Species. J. Parasit. *53*:777–781, 1967.

DODD, D. C.: Hyostrongylosis and Gastric Ulceration in the Pig. N. Z. Vet. J. *8*:100–103, 1960.

FOURIE, P. J. J.: The Haematology and Pathology of Haemonchosis in Sheep. 17th Report of the Director of Veterinary Services An Ind, Union of So. Africa, Aug., 1931.

GARDINER, M. R.: Pathological Changes and Vitamin B$_{12}$ Metabolism in Sheep Parasitised by *Haemonchus contortus, Ostertagia spp.* and *Trichostrongylus colubriformis*. J. Helminth. *40*:63–67, 1966.

HOTSON, I. K.: *Ostertagiosis in Cattle.* Aus. Vet. J. *43*:383–388, 1967.

JENNINGS, F. W., et al.: Experimental *Ostertagia ostertagi* Infections in Calves: Studies with Abomasal Cannulas. Am. J. Vet. Res. *27*:1249–1257, 1966.

KATES, K. C., and TURNER, J. H.: Observations on the Life Cycle of *Nematodirus spathiger*, a Nematode Parasitic in the Intestine of Sheep and Other Ruminants. Am. J. Vet. Res. *16*: 105–115, 1955.

KENDALL, S. B., THURLEY, D. C., and PEIRCE, M. A.: The Biology of *Hyostrongylus rubidus*. I. Primary Infection in Young Pigs. J. Comp. Path. *79*:87–95, 1969.

MARTIN, W. B., THOMAS, B. A. C., and URQUHART, G. M.: Chronic Diarrhea in Housed Cattle Due to Atypical Parasitic Gastritis. Vet. Rec. *69*:736–739, 1957.

MICHEL, J. F.: Morphological Changes in a Parasitic Nematode Due to Acquired Resistance of the Host. Nature (Lond.) *215*:520–521, 1967.

NICHOLSON, T. B., and GORDON, J. G.: An Outbreak of Helminthiasis Associated with *Hyostrongylus rubidus*. Vet. Rec. *71*:133, 1959.

OSBORNE, J. C., BATTE, E. G., and BELL, R. R. The Pathology Following Single Infections of *Ostertagia ostertagi* in Calves. Cornell Vet. *50*:223–224, 1960.

RITCHIE, D. S., ANDERSON, M., and ARMOUR, J.: The Pathology of Lesions Seen in Bovine Ostertagiasis. Proc. 1st Int. Congr. Parasit. Roma *2*:851–852, 1966.

RITCHIE, J. D. S., et al.: Experimental *Ostertagia ostertagi* Infections in Calves: Parasitology and Pathogenesis of a Single Infection. Am. J. Vet. Res. *27*:659–667, 1966.

ROSS, J. G., and TODD, J. R.: Biochemical, Serological and Haematological Changes Associated with Infections of Calves with the Nematode Parasite, *Ostertagia ostertagi*. Brit. Vet. J. *121*:55–64, 1965.

ROSS, J. G., and DOW, C.: The Course and Development of the Abomasal Lesion in Calves Experimentally Infected with the Nematode Parasite *Ostertagia ostertagi*. Brit. Vet. J. *121*:228–233, 1965.

Ross, J. G., Purcell, A., Dow, C., and Todd, J. R.: Experimental Infections of Calves with *Trichostrongylus axei*: Observations on Lethal Infections. Res. Vet. Sci. *9*:314–318, 1968.

Sharma, K. M. L.: Studies on Total Serum Proteins and Serum Proteins in Calves Experimentally Infected with *Ostertagia ostertagi*. Indian J. Anim. Hlth. 7:93–96, 1968. V.B. *39*: 1184, 1969.

Sinclair, I. J.: An Investigation into the Serology of Calves Infected with Parasitic Nematodes. I. The Complement-fixation Test. Immuno. 7:557–566, 1964.

OESOPHAGOSTOMIASIS

(Nodule Worm Disease)

An important parasitic disease is produced in cattle, sheep, and goats in many parts of the world by the nodule worms, *Oesophagostomum radiatium* and *Oe. columbianum*. Similar species also infect swine and subhuman primates. The parasite is a small slender nematode which has a direct life cycle. Adults in the large intestinal lumen produce ova which pass out in the feces and, after a period outside the host, develop into infective larvae. These larvae upon ingestion by another host penetrate the intestinal mucosa, become encysted and molt in the submucosa, and eventually return to the lumen where they reach maturity.

Signs are most often observed in young animals; profuse diarrhea is the most constant and apparently is more intense when the larvae are returning from the submucosa to the intestinal lumen. Heavy infections of long standing usually result in chronic diarrhea, emaciation, cachexia, prostration and death. Even though symptoms are mild, lesions may be found at postmortem inspection.

Lesions.—The exudation of mucus and inflammatory cells from the intestinal mucosa of the host is believed to be the response to irritation caused by substances secreted by the adult parasite, perhaps from its cephalic or esophageal glands.

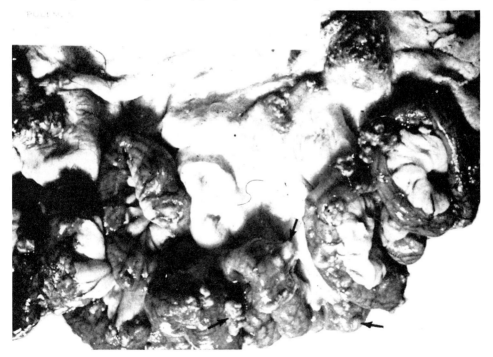

Fig. 15–4. Oesophagostomiasis, small intestine of a sheep. Subserosal nodules are indicated by arrows. Photograph courtesy of Dr. C. L. Davis.

It is thought that this exudate is the chief source of food for the worms, for they are not blood suckers, neither do they attach themselves to the mucosa or cause obstruction of the lumen, hence their deleterious effect is limited.

The larvae, on the other hand, produce severe and striking lesions (Fig. 15-4). They penetrate the mucosa at any point from the pylorus to the anus in order to reach the deeper parts of the submucosa where they encyst and undergo a molt. Some may encyst in the lamina propria on the superficial face of the muscularis mucosae, but most of them are found in the submucosa on the deeper side of the muscularis mucosae. In initial infections, the larvae shed a striated skin and return to the intestinal lumen in five or six days, having produced only transitory inflammation in the mucosa and submucosa. In contrast, local tissue sensitivity develops in animals repeatedly exposed to these parasites, and the subsequent entry of larvae into the submucosa evokes an intense tissue reaction. Large numbers of eosinophils, lymphocytes, macrophages and foreign body giant cells surround the larvae and infiltrate the adjacent submucosa and mucosa. The center of these lesions becomes caseated, often calcified, and is surrounded by a dense capsule which preserves the nodular character of the lesions. A few larvae survive and escape by wandering through the muscularis, but most of them die without finding their way back to the lumen.

The nodules may become infected and enlarged and displace the muscularis to serve as a nidus for local or generalized peritonitis, but usually they remain as calcified, encapsulated nodules. These lesions give the intestine a nodular appearance as they thicken the wall and project from the serosal surface. When present in large numbers, these nodules sometimes interfere with peristalsis and intestinal absorption.

Diagnosis.—Clinical diagnosis may be made by finding eggs or fourth stage larvae in fecal specimens. At necropsy the lesions are recognized by their characteristic gross and microscopic features, for which the popular term, nodule disease, is an especially graphic summation.

Oesophagostomiasis

ANDREWS, J. S., and MALDONADO, J. F.: Intestinal Pathology in Experimental Bovine Esophagostomiasis. Am. J. Vet. Research *3*:17–27, 1942.
BERGER, H., and RIBELIN, W. E.: Pathology of the Swine Nodular Worm, *Oesophagostomum dentatum* in Rabbits. J. Parasit. *55*:1099–1101, 1969.
DOBSON, C.: Globule Leucocytes, Mucin and Mucin Cells in Relation to *Oesophagostomum columbianum* Infections in Sheep. Aust. J. Sci. *28*:434, 1966.
————: Pathological Changes Associated with *Oesophagostomum columbianum* Infestations in Sheep: Haematological Observations on Control Worm-free and Experimentally Infested Sheep. Aust. J. Agric. Res. *18*:523–538, 1967.
ELEK, P., and DURIE, P. H.: The Histopathology of the Reactions of Calves to Experimental Infection with the Nodular Worm, *Oesophagostomum radiatum* (Rudolphi, 1803). II. Reaction of the Susceptible Host to Infection with a Single Dose of Larvae. Aust. J. Agric. Res. *18*:549–559, 1967.
FOURIE, P. J. J.: A Contribution to the Study of the Pathology of Oesophagostomiasis in Sheep. Onderstepoort J. of Vet. Sc. & Animal Ind. *7*:277–350, 1936.
FRANDSEN, J. C.: The Nonenzymic Histochemistry of Early Oesophagostomiasis and Ostertagiasis in Cattle. J. Parasit. *51*:175–179, 1965.
ROBERTS, F. H. S., ELEK, P., and KEITH, R. K.: Studies on Resistance in Calves to Experimental Infections with the Nodular Worm *Œsophagostomum radiatum* (Rudolphi, 1803), Railliet, 1898. Aust. J. Agric. Res. *13*:551–573, 1962. (VB 3219–63.)
SKELTON, G. C., and GRIFFITHS, H. J.: *Oesophagostomum columbianum*: Experimental Infection in Lambs. Effects of Different Types of Exposure in the Intestinal Lesions. Path. Vet. *4*:413–434, 1967.

DIROFILARIASIS

(Canine Filariasis, "Heart Worm Disease")

Infection with the "heart worm," *Dirofilaria immitis*, is not uncommon, particularly in the southern and eastern coastal regions of the United States. Dogs, cats, foxes, wolves and muskrats and rarely—man, have been reported to be infected. Adult worms of a closely related species, *Dirofilaria tenuis*, have been reported in the subcutis of raccoons (*Procyon lotor*) in Florida and Louisiana (Orihel & Beaver, 1965). This species has also been found in the subcutis of man. *Dirofilaria conjunctivae* has also been reported from man. The disease in its earliest stages may give rise to few signs, but severely affected animals will exhibit shortness of breath, weakness, cardiac enlargement, hepatomegaly, ascites, occasionally hypertrophic pulmonary osteoarthropathy (p. 1069) and may die with failure of the right heart. In a few instances, fatal outcome may be the result of pulmonary embolism by adult *Dirofilaria*, which die and are swept into the smaller branches of the pulmonary artery. In one case, we have observed dead worms lodged in the pulmonary artery, resulting in a thrombus and aneurysm in the branch of this artery supplying the diaphragmatic lobe. Subsequent rupture of the aneurysm into the adjacent bronchus resulted in severe hemoptysis and exsanguination in a few minutes.

The adult worms are slender, almost thread-like, filarial parasites. Males, 12 to 30 cm., and females, 25 to 31 cm. in length, are found in the right ventricle of the heart, less often in the right auricle or the pulmonary arteries. The males and females copulate in these sites; the viviparous female releases highly motile microfilariae which circulate with the blood. These microfilariae are taken up from the cutaneous circulation by certain biting insects (mosquitoes, fleas) in whose bodies they undergo stages of development. The infective filariae then gain access to the tissues of a new host through the bite of the intermediate host. These filarial larvae undergo further development in muscles, subcutaneous and adipose tissues of the new host. When they reach a length of about 5 cm. they enter veins and are carried to the right heart (Kume, 1953). The cycle is complete when adult filariae start reproduction in the right ventricle of the host.

Lesions.—The principal effects of *Dirofilaria immitis* are produced by the adult worms which interfere with circulation through the right heart. It is assumed that mechanical interference applied over rather long periods produces compensatory hypertrophy and enlargement of the right ventricle; insufficiency of the right heart results in passive congestion of the lungs, liver and spleen, as well as ascites. Occasional adults die and are transported through the pulmonary artery to the lungs where they produce pulmonary embolism. This complication is relatively infrequent, except in dogs treated with certain filaricidal drugs. Changes in the pulmonary arterial system of infected dogs have been described (Adcock, 1961, Porter, 1951). They include the formation of longitudinally arranged rows of villous projections of the intima into the lumen (Fig. 15–7) of the pulmonary arteries, with diffuse thickening of the subintima; severe endothelial proliferation in small pulmonary arterioles, sometimes with almost complete obliteration of the lumen; and medial hypertrophy of certain of the larger pulmonary arterioles. The cause of these lesions is unknown, nor has their relation to the parasites been clearly established. Von Lichtenberg, Jackson and Otto, 1962, demonstrated the occurrence during life of *D. immitis* in the venae cavae of heavily infected dogs.

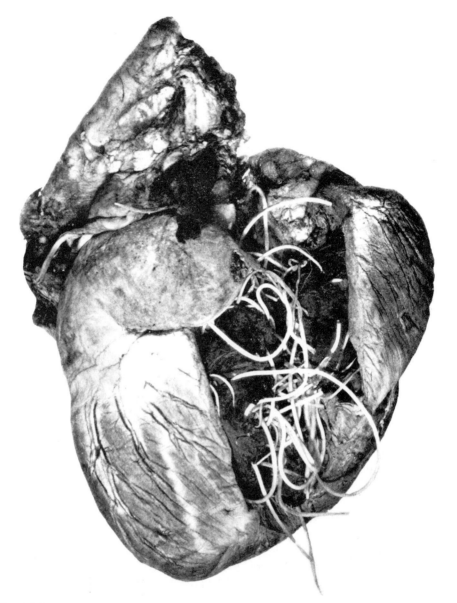

FIG. 15–5. Dirofilariasis. Many adult *Dirofilaria immitis* in right ventricle (opened) of a dog. (Courtesy of Armed Forces Institute of Pathology.) Contributor: Col. Wm. P. Hill, V.C.

In these animals, phlebosclerosis of the vena cava was often noted and the collecting tributaries of the hepatic veins also appear thickened. Chronic passive congestion was evident in the liver. Microscopically, cavernous dilatation of the hepatic veins was a significant feature, with a large number of dilated vessels replacing the centrolobular venule. In longitudinally cut veins, multiple saccular dilatations along their course gave them a haustrated appearance. Usually all traces of these centrolobular veins were lost and the site became occupied by multiple cavernous channels. It is presumed that these lesions are the end result of chronic passive congestion due to the presence of the worms in the vena cava,

It has been suggested that the occurrence of immature forms of *Strongylus vulgaris* in the anterior mesenteric artery is merely the result of accidental localization of wandering larvae.   One of the writers (Jones) holds the view that this localization is not fortuitous, but a definite and necessary stage in the development of the parasite.   The presence of nearly mature worms in the arterial lesions and the extremely high incidence of the lesions in young and adult equines are evidence in support of this opinion.

The strongyle larvae burrow into the intimal stroma of the artery and evoke proliferation of intima and endothelium, sometimes associated with hemorrhage and necrosis.   Fibrin and cellular debris accumulate over the roughened intimal areas, extend out into the lumen and occasionally cause occlusion.   In reasonably long-standing cases, the wall of the artery becomes greatly thickened by the proliferation of both intimal and adventitial fibrous tissue.   Collections of lymphocytes often gather in the thickened wall of the artery.   This is the most common lesion and is appropriately regarded as **verminous arteritis.**   To produce a less common lesion, the arterial wall becomes both thickened and sacculated, forming a dilated segment with a relatively smooth lining.   This is properly considered a **verminous aneurysm.**   Rupture of such aneurysms is almost unknown, although in some encountered at necropsy the wall is extremely thin at certain points.

Strongylus equinus, the triple-toothed strongyle, sclerostome or bloodworm, is found in its adult form in the cecum and rarely in the colon of equines.   It is usually attached to the mucosa and engorged with blood.   The male is about 35 mm. long, the female up to 55 mm.   The life cycle of *S. equinus* is known to be direct, but the migratory path of the immature worm has not been fully traced. The larvae that have been ingested are believed to penetrate the intestine, enter

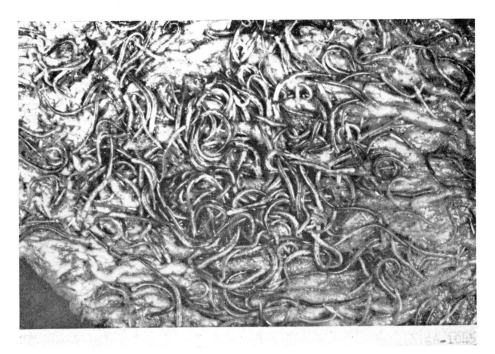

Fig. 15–9.—Equine strongylidosis. Adult *Strongylus equinus* in the cecum of a two-year-old gelding. (Courtesy of Dr. C. R. Cole, Ohio State University.)

the blood stream, and migrate through the liver, heart and lungs; thence, after being coughed up, they are swallowed to reach the large intestine. However, numbers of nearly mature worms may be found in the intestine, tissues of the pancreas, spleen, lungs and liver, and frequently in the abdominal fat just under the parietal peritoneum. It seems reasonable that this parasite's migration through the tissues may be more purposeful than is generally conceded.

Strongylus edentatus, the toothless strongyle, occurs in adult form in the cecum and colon of equines, usually attached to the mucosa. The males are about 28 mm., the females as much as 44 mm. in length. The life cycle is direct; infective larvae ingested with grass are believed to penetrate the wall of the ventral colon and to encyst in the abdominal wall for three or four months. The larvae, by the same route, perhaps through the mesentery, reach the serosa of the small intestine, particularly the jejunum and ileum, then burrow in the subserosa. Here the larvae produce elevated subserous masses about 3 mm. high, 5 mm. wide, and one to several centimeters long. These lesions, when fresh, are bright red from recent hemorrhage; later they turn to shades of yellow and brown as the blood cells disintegrate to release blood pigment which remains as hematoidin or hemosiderin. Microscopically, these subserosal lesions are seen to be made up of edema, connective tissue, free red blood cells, leukocytes, macrophages, blood pigment and, in some sections, a central fragment of caseous necrotic debris. It is difficult to find larvae in the subserosal lesions, but occasionally a tract can be followed through the muscularis into the submucosa. Occasionally, the offending larvae may be cut in cross section in histologic preparations. It is assumed that larvae reaching the submucosa undergo further development before breaking into the intestinal lumen.

The parasitic nodules (called "haemomelasma ilei" by Cohrs, 1954) may be very numerous in the subserosa of the small intestine, presenting a striking appearance at necropsy. These lesions, in spite of their florid appearance, seem to have little effect upon the host, hence their proper evaluation is of importance (Fig. 15–20*B*).

Another member of the Family Strongylidae which closely resembles equine strongyles, is *Chabertia ovina,* which inhabits the colon of sheep, goats, cattle and wild ruminants. The males of the species measure up to 14 mm. long; females as much as 20 mm. They have a large buccal capsule on the anterior end which they use to attach to the mucosa of the colon. They draw in a piece of mucosal epithelium, digest it with their esophageal secretions, and may ingest blood. Hemorrhages and loss of blood to the parasite may terminate in anemia and death. A deleterious effect upon the growth of wool has also been ascribed to this parasite.

Diagnosis.—Quantitative determinations of the strongyle ova in the feces are used to estimate the parasitic burden in the living animal. This is necessary because these parasites are so common that a few ova in a fecal specimen have no diagnostic significance. The diagnosis of equine strongylidosis must be based upon mature evaluation of all symptoms and ova counts. Verminous arteritis and lesions due to migration of the parasite are usually recognized at necropsy.

Strongylidosis

Cohrs, P.: *Lehrbuch der Speziellen Pathologischen Anatomie der Haustiere.* 3rd ed., Jena. Fischer, p. 299, 1954.
Foster, A. O., and Clark, H. C.: Verminous Aneurysm in Equines of Panama. Am. J. Trop. Med. *17*:85–99, 1937.

HERD, R. P., and ARUNDEL, J. H.: Life Cycle, Pathogenicity and Immunogenicity of *Chabertia ovina*. Vet. Rec. *84*:487–488, 1969.

POHLENZ, J., SCHULZE, D., and ECKERT, J.: (Spinal Infection with *Strongylus vulgaris* in a Pony.) Dt. tierarztl. Wschr. *72*:510–511, 1965. V.B. *36*:1472, 1966.

ROSS, J. G., and TODD, J. R.: The Pathogenicity of *Chabertia ovina* in Calves. Vet. Rec. *83*: 682–683, 1968.

SEGAL, M.: "Mal seco", enfermedad de equinos, contribución al conociniento de su etio-patogenia, observaciones y experiencia en Junín de los Andes (Nequen) Rev. Vet. Milit. Buenos Aires 7:3–10, 66–68, 70–74, 106, 108–116, 1959. (VB 752–60.)

SPIROCERCOSIS

Infection with the spiruroid worm, *Spirocerca lupi* (*Spirocerca sanguinolenta, Spiroptera sanguinolenta, Filaria sanguinolenta*, esophageal worm) is particularly common in certain of the southern United States, but it has also been reported from many parts of the world. The adult worms, which are usually bright red, have been found coiled in nodules in the walls of the esophagus, aorta, stomach and other organs of the dog, fox, wolf and cat. The males measure 30 to 54 mm. in length, the females 54 to 80 mm.; the eggs are thick-walled, about 37 by 15 microns in maximum dimensions, and contain larvae when deposited.

The life cycle of this helminth is complex. The embryonated eggs are passed in the feces and do not hatch until ingested by certain coprophagous beetles. In these intermediate hosts, the larvae develop into the infective (third) stage, then encyst. If eaten by an abnormal host, such as a frog, snake, lizard or any one of many birds and mammals, the larvae burrow into the mesentery where they remain in a viable state for some time. If infected beetles or other transport hosts are eaten by one of the final hosts (dog, fox, wolf, cat), the larvae penetrate the stomach wall and by following the course of the arteries, migrating through adventitia and media, they reach the wall of the aorta and localize in the adventitia, usually of the upper thoracic portion. After a period of development at this site, the parasites move to the adjacent esophagus and burrow into its wall, where they develop to adults in cystic nodules. Their eggs reach the esophageal lumen through a small opening in the nodule.

Signs may be absent in mild infections, or persistent vomiting may be caused by esophageal obstruction. Sudden death from hemorrhage from aortic lesions has been reported.

Lesions.—The principal lesions in this disease are produced by the adult worms as a result of their localization in the adventitia of the aorta and the submucosa of the esophagus. The worms become the center of a tumor-like nodule in the aortic wall which may initiate the formation of aneurysm with possible rupture and fatal hemorrhage. In microscopic sections of active lesions in the aorta, worms may be found in areas of the adventitia and media where normal tissue is destroyed and replaced by leukocytes and debris. Sometimes the worms are seen burrowing into the media, with necrotic tracts leading to the intima. The intimal stroma undergoes considerable proliferation. In most instances, however, it appears that the worm eventually departs from the aortic media or adventitia for the esophagus, leaving a lesion in the wall of the aorta. It is not uncommon to observe well-developed worm-containing nodules in the esophagus of the same animal in which there is evidence of previous localization in the aorta. On the intimal surface, these lesions appear as roughened, slightly elevated plaques of various sizes or as depressed aneurysmal scars.

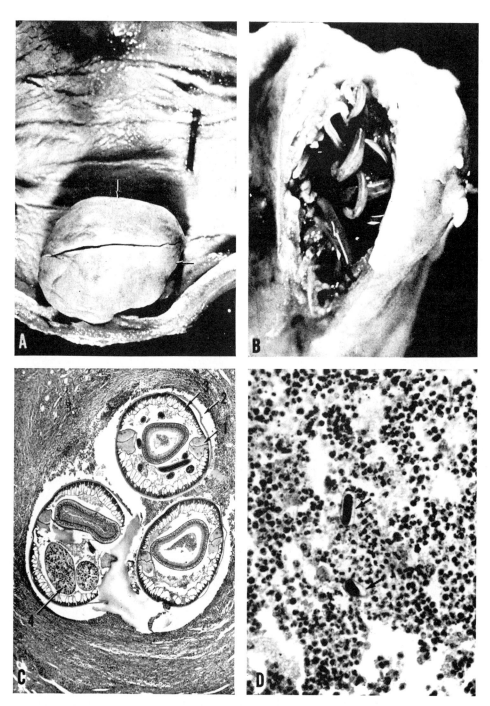

FIG. 15–10.—Spirocercosis. *A*, Nodule (arrows) in thoracic esophagus of a dog. *B*, A nodule opened to show the coiled nematodes within. Photographs courtesy of Major C. N. Barron. *C*, Section through a nodule (× 48) containing adult worms. Note lateral chord cells (*1*) cuticula (*2*), muscle cells (*3*) and uterus filled with ova (*4*). Contributor: Major C. N. Barron. *D*, Ova of *Spirocerca lupi* (× 300) surrounded by pus in an esophageal nodule. (Courtesy of Armed Forces Institute of Pathology.) Contributor: Major C. N. Barron.

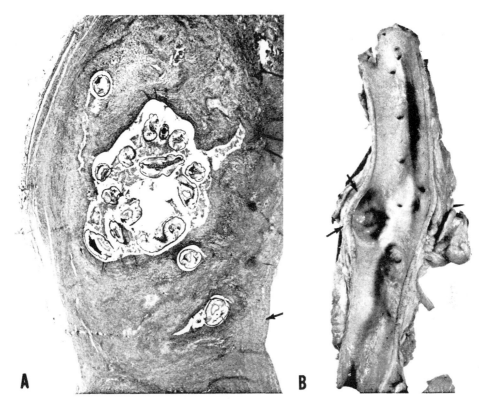

Fig. 15–11.—Spirocercosis. *A*, Section of aorta (× 12) with a large worm-filled nodule in the adventitia. The intima is indicated by an arrow. Contributor: Dr. H. R. Seibold. *B*, A large sacculate lesion (arrows) in the aorta resulting from spirocercosis. (Courtesy of Armed Forces Institute of Pathology.) Contributor: Major C. N. Barron.

The esophageal lesions are most common near its terminus, usually a few centimeters from the cardia of the stomach. Grossly, one or several nodules are seen on the luminal surface, elevating the epithelium a centimeter or more. One or several worms may be embedded in each nodule, with parts of the worms protruding from a small orifice. Cross section of one of the nodules usually reveals a thick fibrous wall partially covered by epithelium, enclosing a cavity containing worms and yellowish pus. Microscopically, the worms form the center for a mass of neutrophils surrounded by a thick wall of connective tissue infiltrated with macrophages, lymphocytes and plasma cells. Strangely, eosinophils are usually absent. The adult worms have a thick cuticle surrounding a meromyarian muscle wall, interrupted by a double row of very large specialized muscle cells arranged along each side of the body cavity. Ova within the gravid uterus are flattened and ovoid, and are embryonated before they are discharged through the genital pore.

Seibold *et al.* (1955) have described a "deformative ossifying spondylitis" in the thoracic vertebrae of the host, which they believe is related to the migration and encystment of *Spirocerca lupi*. This lesion is characterized by irregular coarse exostoses of the ventral surfaces of the bodies of certain of the thoracic vertebrae. These writers also described osteosarcomas or fibrosarcomas (p. 194) originating in the wall of the esophagus in intimate relation to the lesions of *Spirocerca lupi*.

While it has not been established that the parasite is the cause of the neoplasms, their close association suggests such a relationship. Additional significance to this relationship has been provided by the work of Ribelin and Bailey (1958) (p. 279). Also described by Seibold *et al.* was the frequent manifestation of hypertrophic pulmonary osteoarthropathy (p. 1069) in dogs with large esophageal tumors, some of which had metastasized to the lungs and other viscera.

Diagnosis.—Infection with *Spirocerca lupi* in the living animal can be confirmed by the identification of embryonated ova in the feces. Post-mortem diagnosis is easily made by demonstration of characteristic lesions in the aorta, esophagus, or ventral face of thoracic vertebrae in association with the adult parasites.

Spirocercosis

ANANTARAMAN, M., and SE, K.: Experimental Spirocercosis in Dogs with Larvae from a Paratenic Host, *Calotes versicolor*, the Common Garden Lizard in Madras. J. Parasit. *52*: 911–912, 1966.

BWANGAMOI, O.: Spirocercosis in Uganda and Its Association with Fibrosarcoma in a Dog. J. Small Anim. Pract. *8*:395–398, 1967.

CHOWDHURY, N., and PANDE, B. P.: The Development of the Infective Larvae of the Canine Oesophageal Tumour Worm *Spirocerca lupi* in Rabbits and Its Histopathology. Z. ParasitKde. *32*:1–10, 1969.

DIXON, K. G., and McCUE, J. F.: Further Observations on the Epidemiology of *Spirocerca lupi* in the Southern United States. J. Parasit. *53*:1074–1075, 1967.

MURRAY, M.: Incidence and Pathology of *Spirocerca lupi* in Kenya. J. Comp. Path. *78*: 401–405, 1968.

MURRAY, M., CAMPBELL, H., and JARRETT, W. H. F.: *Spirocerca lupi* in a Cheetah. E. Afr. Wildl. J. *2*:164, 1964.

RESSANG, A. A., and HONG, L. Y.: The Occurrence of *Spirocerca lupi* in the Indonesian Dog and Its Relation to Neoplasm Formation. Commun. Vet., Bogor 7:9–17 (Ind.). 1963. (VB 281–64.)

RIBELIN, W. E., and BAILEY, W. S.: Esophageal Sarcomas Associated with *Spirocerca lupi* Infection in the Dog. Cancer *2*:1242–1246, 1958.

SEIBOLD, H. R. *et al.*: Observations on the Possible Relation of Malignant Esophageal Tumors and *Spirocerca lupi* Lesions in the Dog. Am. J. Vet. Research *16*:5–14, 1955.

CEREBROSPINAL NEMATODIASIS

(Neurofilariasis, Setariosis)

The accidental wandering of nematode larvae into the brain or spinal cord is not difficult to envisage on the basis of what is known of their meanderings through other tissues. However, the selective affinity of certain nematodes for the central nervous system is also a possibility and may be the explanation for important paralytic diseases of animals. For many years obscure neuroparalytic symptoms of unknown cause have been observed seasonally in animals in the Far East, particularly in Japan, Korea, India and Ceylon. In sheep and goats, such a clinical entity has been known as "lumbar paralysis," while a similar disease in horses has been called "kumri" (Hindustani for "weakness of the loin"). The observations of Innes (1953) have done much to characterize these diseases pathologically and to explain both their symptomatology and etiology. Most of the studies in the Far East have been conducted by Japanese workers (Innes, 1951). The presence of nematodes in the central nervous system in animals with obscure paralytic signs has also been reported in sheep in New York State by Kennedy *et al.* (1952) and in moose in Minnesota by Fenstermacher (1934). Tiner (1953) observed death of mice, squirrels and guinea pigs preceded by nervous symptoms which developed after exposure to infective larvae of certain

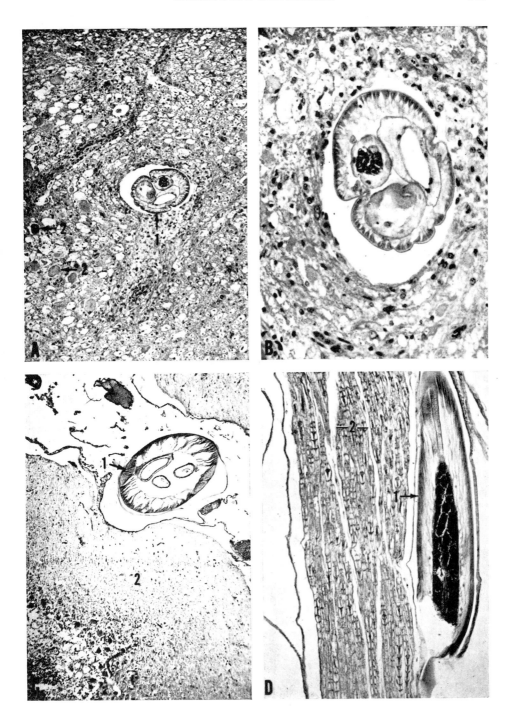

FIG. 15–12.—Cerebrospinal nematodiasis. *A*, Nematode (*1*) in the spinal cord (× 77) of a sheep. Note swollen axones (*2*). *B*, Higher magnification (× 215) to show the parasite in greater detail. Contributor: Dr. Peter Olafson. *C*, Nematode (*1*) in the pia mater (× 53) of a horse. Cerebellar cortex (*2*). *D*, Another larva (*1*) in the longitudinal section (× 100) in a spinal nerve (*2*) from the same horse as *C*. (Courtesy of Armed Forces Institute of Pathology.) Contributor: 406th Medical General Laboratory.

Ascaris species, especially ascarids from raccoons. Unfortunately, he did not study the lesions in the central nervous system in these animals. One of us (Jones) has observed several larval nematodes in the spinal nerves, meninges and cerebral cortex of a Korean horse from which the Japanese B encephalitis virus reportedly was isolated. It is established, therefore, that nematodes can and do invade the central nervous system.

Several nematode species appear to have an affinity for the brain and spinal cord, but identification of individual worms in lesions is often difficult. Japanese workers have identified *Setaria digitata*, a natural parasite of the bovine, in the central nervous system of sheep and goats, while Kennedy *et al.* (1952) and Whitlock˙ (1959) ascribe the lesions they observed in sheep to a metastrongyle currently named *Pneumostrongylus* (*Elaphostrongylus* or *Odocoileostrongylus*) *tenuis*. This parasite is now known to cause disease by invading the nervous system of moose (*Alces alces*) (Anderson, 1964). White-tailed deer (*Odocoileus virginianus*) are apparently the normal host for this parasite but it nevertheless invades the central nervous system of this host as well. *Pneumostrongylus tenuis* is also pathogenic for sheep, goats and guinea pigs under experimental conditions, causing neurological signs but not developing to maturity in sheep or guinea pigs. Other cervids (wapiti-elk *Cervus canadensis nelsoni*; and mule deer *Odocoileus hemionus hemionus*) are also quite susceptible to invasion of the nervous system by *P. tenuis* following experimental exposure (Anderson, Lankester and Strelive, 1966). Other species now known to be neurotropic include: *Angiostrongylus cantonensis* (parasite of rats—larvae causing "eosinophilic meningitis" of man) and *Guretia paralysans* (a filarid usually found in veins of Felidae in South America). Similar diseases due to unidentified helminths have been described in beaver (*Castor canadensis*) and groundhogs (*Marmota monax*) by Kelly and Innes (1966) and Richter and Kradel (1964). The reports of Beautyman and Woolf (1951), Sprent (1955), and Tiner (1953) indicate that ascarid larvae can also invade the brain or spinal cord; thus it appears that more than one species of nematode can be incriminated. This fact makes the name "cerebrospinal nematodiasis" suggested by Innes (1953) preferable for the disease.

The seasonal appearance (late summer and autumn) of cerebrospinal nematodiasis in the Far East has been correlated by Japanese workers with the presence of mosquito vectors (*Anopheles hyrcanus sinensis, Armigeres obturbans, Aëdes togoi*, etc.) which transport microfilariae of filarid worms such as *Setaria digitata*. These microfilariae mature in infected mosquitoes about two weeks after a blood meal from an infected host (*i.e.*, cattle). Sheep and goats bitten by such mosquitoes, after a latent period of about a month, exhibit the earliest neurologic manifestations, presumably as the result of invasion of the central nervous system by filarid larvae. Young and adult animals may be infected, but the disease is unknown in newborn lambs, kids or foals.

Signs.—Manifestations of cerebrospinal nematodiasis are extremely varied as might be expected from the lesions to be described. Mildly affected animals may show only motor weakness, incoordination or slight loss of balance. Animals with severe lesions may exhibit paresis of one or all limbs, the hind legs being most frequently and severely affected. The onset may be dramatically sudden in some cases, more insidious in others; death may intervene within a few days, or recovery may follow, with or without residual nervous manifestations such as drooping of eyelid or ear, weakness or impaired gait.

Lesions.—Grossly visible lesions are unusual except in those infrequent instances in which hemorrhage occurs in the primary malacic focus caused by the migration of the parasites. Meticulous microscopic study of the brain and spinal cord is usually necessary to uncover the areas affected. The primary foci may be single or multiple and occur in any part of the central nervous system, although the spinal cord and thalamus appear to be favored sites. The lesions are usually asymmetrical, each appearing as a solitary, raggedly bounded focus of cavitation, rarely containing hemorrhage. Under low magnification, these foci appear as cracks, crevices, or spongy areas, and, in some, tracts leading from the nearby meninges can be detected. Under higher magnification, it will be seen that nervous tissue is partially or completely lost in the center of the affected zone. Around this axis cylinders in cross section appear as large, irregularly shaped, rounded bodies, which are stained darkly eosinophilic in hematoxylin and eosin preparations and are heavily impregnated when the Bodian method is employed. Longitudinal sections of these axis cylinders show that they are irregularly enlarged, tortuous and fragmented. Axons similarly affected are seen in ascending and descending tracts extending above and below the primary malacic locus. Axonal damage is associated with swelling and distortion of myelin sheaths and, in long-standing cases, with glial proliferation. This secondary (wallerian) degeneration is no different from that observed as a frequent consequence of injuries to the central nervous system (p. 1381). The degenerative lesion in nerve fiber tracts may lead to the primary lesion, if sufficient numbers of serial sections are prepared and examined.

Cellular infiltration composed of lymphocytes, neutrophils or occasionally eosinophils is frequently observed in the pia mater near the primary malacic foci. These cells may also be seen in irregular nests in the pia arachnoid, in subdural and epidural locations, and sometimes extending along the spinal nerve roots. Perivascular lymphocytic cuffing may be prominent adjacent to primary malacic foci.

The offending helminths will be seen in tissue sections only fortuitously, unless a diligent search of serial sections through characteristic lesions is made. It is assumed that migratory larvae not only can invade nervous tissue, but can also wander out again. In some cases it is possible to demonstrate the parasites only by filtration of the spinal fluid, although evidence of their invasion of nervous tissue may be readily found.

Diagnosis.—Definitive diagnosis can be made only after meticulous microscopic examination of the central nervous system. Typical lesions must be found and some should contain the causative nematodes. Clinical diagnosis is made in geographic regions in which the disease is enzoötic, but at present can be based only upon presumptive evidence.

Cerebrospinal Nematodiasis

ANDERSON, R. C.: Neurological Disease in Moose Infected Experimentally with *Pneumostrongylus tenuis* from White-Tailed Deer. Path. Vet. *1*:289–322, 1964.

————: The Development of *Pneumostrongylus tenuis* in the Central Nervous System of White-tailed Deer. Path. Vet. *2*:360–379, 1965.

————: The Pathogenesis and Transmission of Neurotropic and Accidental Nematode Parasites of the Central Nervous System of Mammals and Birds. Helminth. Abstr. *37*:191–210, 1968.

ANDERSON, R. C., *et al.*: Further Experimental Studies of *Pneumostrongylus tenuis* in Cervids. Canad. J. Zool. *44*:851–861, 1966.

ANDERSON, R. C., and STRELIVE, U. R.: The Transmission of *Pneumostrongylus tenuis* to Guinea Pigs. Canad. J. Zool. *44*:533–540, 1966.
————: Experimental Cerebrospinal Nematodiasis (*Pneumostrongylus tenuis*) in Sheep. Canad. J. Zool. *44*:889–893, 1966.
————: The Penetration of *Pneumostrongylus tenuis* into the Tissues of White-tailed Deer. Canad. J. Zool. *45*:285–289, 1967.
————: The Effect of *Pneumostrongylus tenuis* (Nematoda: Metastrongyloidea) on Kids. Canad. J. Comp. Med. *33*:280–286, 1969.
BEAUTYMAN, W., and WOOLF, A. L.: An Ascaris Larva in the Brain in Association with Acute Anterior Poliomyelitis. J. Path. & Bact. *63*:635–647, 1951.
FENSTERMACHER, R.: Further Studies of Diseases Affecting Moose. Univ. Minnesota Agric. Exper. Sta. Bull. 308, 1934.
INNES, J. R. M.: Necrotising Encephalomyelitis (or Encephalomyelomalacia) of Unknown Aetiology in Goats in Ceylon with Similarities to Setariasis of Sheep, Horses and Goats in Japan. (Including a brief review of nervous diseases of goats.) Brit. Vet. J. *107*:187–203, 1951.
INNES, J. R. M., and SHOHO, C.: Cerebrospinal Nematodiasis. Focal Encephalomyelomalacia of Animals Caused by Nematodes (*Setaria digitata*). A Disease Which May Occur in Man. A.M.A. Arch. Neurol. & Psychiat. *70*:325–349, 1953.
INNES, J. R. M., and PILLAI, C. P.: Kumri—so-called Lumbar Paralysis—of Horses in Ceylon (India and Burma), and its Identification with Cerebrospinal Nematodiasis. Brit. Vet. J. *111*:223–235, 1955.
KELLY, W. R., and INNES, J. R. M.: Cerebrospinal Nematodiasis with Focal Encephalomalacia as a Cause of Paralysis of Beavers (*Castor canadensis*) in the Dublin Zoological Gardens. Brit. Vet. J. *122*:285–287, 1966.
KENNEDY, P. C., WHITLOCK, J. H., and ROBERTS, S. J.: Neurofilariosis, a Paralytic Disease of Sheep. I. Introduction, Symptomatology, Pathology. Cornell Vet. *42*:118–124, 1952.
KURTZ, H. J., LOKEN, K., and SCHLOTTHAUER, J. C.: Histopathologic Studies on Cerebrospinal Nematodiasis of Moose in Minnesota Naturally Infected with *Pneumostrongylus tenuis*. Am. J. Vet. Res. *27*:548–557, 1966.
LOKEN, K. I., *et al.*: *Pneumostrongylus tenuis* in Minnesota Moose (*Alces alces*). Bull. Wildl. Dis. Assn. *1*:7, 1965.
RICHTER, C. B., and KRADEL, D. C.: Cerebrospinal Nematodosis in Pennsylvania Groundhogs ((*Marmota monax*). Am. J. Vet. Res. *25*:1230–1235, 1964.
SHOHO, C., and TANAKA, T.: Further Observations on Cerebrospinal Nematodosis in Animals. II. The Problems of Reinfection by Nematodes and Clinically-silent Cases. Brit. Vet. J. *111*:102–111, 1955.
SMITH, H. J., and ARCHIBALD, R. McG.: Moose Infected with the Common Cervine Parasite, *Elaphostrongylus tenuis*. Canad. Vet. J. *8*:173–177, 1967.
SPRENT, J. F. A.: On the Invasion of the Central Nervous System by Nematodes. I. The Incidence and Pathological Significance of Nematodes in the Central Nervous System. Parasitology. *45*:31–40, 1955.
————: On the Invasion of the Central Nervous System by Nematodes. II. Invasion of the Nervous System by Ascariasis. Parasitology. *45*:41–55, 1955.
TINER, J. D.: The Migration, Distribution in the Brain and Growth of Ascarid Larvae in Rodents. J. Infect. Dis. *92*:105–113, 1953.
————: Fatalities in Rodents Caused by Larval *Ascaris* in the Central Nervous System. J. Mammol. *34*:153–167, 1953.
WHITLOCK, J. H.: *Elaphostrongylus*, the proper designation of *Neurofilaria*. Cornell Vet. *49*:3–27, 1959.
WILDER, H. C.: Nematode Endophthalmitis. Tr. Am. Acad. Ophth. (Oct):99–108, 1950.

TRICHINOSIS

(Trichiniasis, Trichinelliasis)

Although animals are seldom observed to be seriously affected by trichinosis, they are the source of infection for man, in whom the disease may be debilitating or fatal. The causative agent is a tiny, slender nematode which spends its adult life in the mucosa of the small intestine of a wide variety of animals, including man, domestic and wild swine, rats, bears, dogs and cats. The female is 3 to 4 mm. in length and the male about half as long. The females are viviparous, producing larvae which are the principal excitants of symptoms and lesions because they burrow through tissues and encyst in striated muscles. The causative parasite, *Trichinella spiralis*, is classified among the Nematoda under the family Trichinellidae and is the chief pathogen in this family.

Completion of the **life cycle** of *Trichinella spiralis* is dependent upon consumption by the host of raw or undercooked flesh containing encysted larvae. The infective larvae are released from the ingested muscle by the action of digestive juices; then, in rapid succession, undergo four molts and mature into adults. After copulation the male dies, but the female burrows into the lamina propria of the intestinal villi and deposits large numbers of larvae in the lymphatic spaces. Some larvae may escape into the intestinal lumen, but most of them are carried to the blood stream and reach the musculature. The larvae invade the muscle bundles, where they encyst and remain throughout the life of the host. Further development of the parasite follows upon ingestion of the infected muscle by another host. The fetuses of rats, mice and rabbits may become infected *in utero* under experimental conditions (Hartmannova and Chroust, 1968).

The **symptoms** and **signs** of trichinosis, rarely observed in animals, are varied and often nonspecific in man. Even in man, small numbers of trichina larvae undoubtedly can reach the muscles without provoking detectable symptoms, but in large numbers they produce muscular pain, nausea, vomiting, diarrhea, fever, edema of the face, increased respiratory rate and urticarial skin manifestations. Invasion of cardiac muscle by the larvae may result in feeble or dicrotic pulse, muffled heart sounds, systolic murmur or palpitation. When larvae invade the central nervous system, a plethora of signs may appear, including disorientation, apathy, stupor, delirium, paralysis and coma. The most significant clinical laboratory evidence of the infection is in the blood cell count. Leukocytosis with eosinophilia, which in extreme cases may reach 90 per cent, is characteristic. Although fluctuating within wide limits, this circulating eosinophilia may persist for months or even years. Identification of adult trichinae in the stools, or demonstration of larvae in biopsy specimens of muscle, is decisive in confirming the clinical diagnosis of trichinosis.

Lesions.—Except for transitory catarrhal enteritis provoked by the activities of the adults, the lesions of trichinosis are confined to the skeletal and, to a much smaller extent, the cardiac musculature and are the result of invasion and encystment of the larvae. In man, the muscles most frequently and heavily parasitized are the diaphragmatic, intercostal, masseteric, laryngeal, lingual and ocular. The heart muscle may be invaded by young larvae during the time that they are being liberated in the intestinal villi, but encysted larvae are rarely found in cardiac muscle. The larvae penetrate the skeletal muscle bundles, most frequently near the tendinous portion, eliciting some inflammatory reaction in the adjacent stroma. This inflammation, which is evidenced by the presence of edema, neutrophils, lymphocytes and eosinophils, soon subsides as each larva becomes encased in a muscle bundle. The sarcoplasm is replaced at the site of invasion by the encapsulated worm, and adjacent parts of the muscle bundle may undergo some degenerative changes. The sarcolemma is distorted by the parasite, the nuclei are increased in size and number; the sarcoplasm may be granular and its cross striations lost. Droplets of fatty material collect in the sarcolemma near the poles of the cyst containing the parasite. Often after a period of time calcium salts are deposited, first in the thick hyaline capsule around the parasite, now

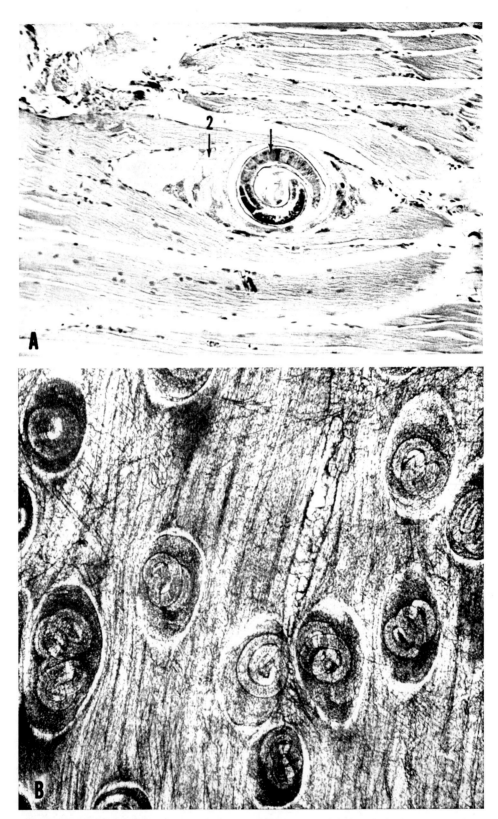

Fig. 15–13.—Trichinosis.   *A*, *Trichinella spiralis* larva (*1*) encysted in a skeletal muscle bundle of a rat.   Note capsule (*2*) around nematode (×80).   (Courtesy of Armed Forces Institute of Pathology.)   Contributor: Dr. J. C. Swartz.   *B*, Crush preparation of skeletal muscle containing *Trichinella spiralis* larvae.

dead or dying, and later in the parasite itself. Fully calcified lesions, appearing as short chalk-colored streaks in skeletal muscle, can occasionally be detected by examination with the naked eye.

Diagnosis.—Histologic demonstration of the trichina larvae in the muscles of animals is sufficient to establish the nature of the parasitism, but not enough to prove that the larvae were the cause of any clinical symptoms. This is a somewhat academic problem in animals, although of more importance in man. Trichina larvae can be demonstrated by digestion of muscle and collection of the parasites in a Baermann apparatus.

A European meat inspection practice utilizes bits of fresh skeletal muscle (usually diaphragm) which are compressed between two heavy glass plates and examined under low magnification. Larvae are readily recognized in these preparations, but in mild infections this method may not disclose any larvae. Routine histologic sections will also reveal the encysted larvae coiled within a hyaline membrane inside a muscle bundle (Fig. 15–13*A*).

Trichinosis

GELLER, E. H., and ZAIMAN, H.: Incidence of Infection with *Trichinella spiralis* in Dogs. J. Am. Vet. Med. Assn. *147*:253–254, 1965.
HARTMANNOVA, B., and CHROUST, K.: Congenital Trichinellosis. Acta Univ. Agric. Fac. Vet. Brno. *37*:93–103, 1968. V.B. *39*:1198, 1969.
HUNT, G. R.: *Trichinella spiralis* in Dogs and Cats. Parasitology *53*:659, 1967.
SADUN, E. H., ANDERSON, R. I., and WILLIAMS, J. S.: Fluorescent Antibody Test for the Serological Diagnosis of Trichinosis. Exp. Parasitol. *12*:423–433, 1962. (VB 2041–63.)
STRAFUSS, A. C., and ZIMMERMANN, W. J.: Hematologic Changes and Clinical Signs of Trichinosis in Pigs. Am. J. Vet. Res. *28*:833–838, 1967.
SULZER, A. J.: Indirect Fluorescent Antibody Tests for Parasitic Diseases. I. Preparation of a Stable Antigen from Larvae of *Trichinella spiralis*. J. Parasit. *51*:717–721, 1965.

PULMONARY NEMATODIASIS

(Lungworm Disease, Dictyocauliasis, Dictyocaulosis, Metastrongylidosis, Verminous Pneumonia)

Certain thread-like worms are distinguished by their parasitic habitat: the respiratory passages (trachea, bronchi, alveoli) of numerous domesticated and wild animals. These lungworms often produce disease which may lead to death, but surprisingly often they live in the lungs with little apparent effect upon the host. Usually each host has its specific lungworm, but a few related animals (deer and sheep, sheep and cattle) may share the same parasite.

The life cycle of each worm in this group is essentially similar to the others, differing only in detail. The adults live embedded in the mucosa of the trachea or in the lumen of the trachea, bronchi or bronchioles. Copulation occurs here and eggs are laid in these sites. They are either coughed up and swallowed, the larvae developing in the digestive tract, or, more commonly, remain in the alveoli until they have undergone embryonation. The larvae that hatch in the alveoli are coughed up, swallowed and eliminated with the feces. The life cycle of lungworms of the genera *Dictyocaulus* and *Capillaria* is direct, but for other genera, *Metastrongylus, Protostrongylus, Muellerius, Cystocaulus, Bronchostrongylus, Angiostrongylus, Crenosoma, Aelurostrongylus*, an intermediate host is necessary.

Signs.—The signs of lungworm disease may be barely recognizable or so severe

Table 15–1.—Common Lungworms

Host	Parasite	Site of Adult Parasite
Cattle, deer, mouse, reindeer and pig	Dictyocaulus viviparus (cattle lungworm)	Trachea and bronchi
Cat	Aelurostrongylus abstrusus (cat lungworm)	Right ventricle and pulmonary artery
Deer, sheep, goat, cattle and other ruminants	Dictyocaulus filaria (Thread lungworm, sheep lungworm)	Bronchioles
	Protostrongylus rufescens	Bronchioles
	Protostrongylus brevispiculum	Bronchioles
Dog	Filaroides osleri	Mucosa of trachea and bronchi
Dog	Filaroides milksi	Bronchi, bronchioles, alveoli
Fox, dog, wolf, cat	Capillaria aerophila (fox lungworm)	Trachea, bronchi, bronchioles
Horse, donkey, tapir	Dictyocaulus arnfieldi (horse lungworm)	Bronchi and bronchioles
Sheep and goats	Muellerius capillaris (minutissimus) (hair lungworm)	Alveoli
	Cystocaulus ocreatus	Alveoli
Swine	Metastrongylus apri	Trachea, bronchi, bronchioles
	Metastrongylus pudendotectus	Trachea, bronchi, bronchioles
	Metastrongylus salmi	Trachea, bronchi, bronchioles
Rabbits, wild	Protostrongylus boughtoni (rabbit lungworm)	Bronchi and bronchioles
Foxes, dogs, cats	Crenosoma vulpis	Bronchi, trachea
Skunks	Crenosoma canadensis	Bronchi, bronchioles
Cat, leopard, tiger	Bronchostrongylus subcrenatus	
Dog, fox	Angiostrongylus vasorum	Pulmonary artery
Rat, fox	Angiostrongylus cantonensis	Pulmonary artery

that death results. Severe infection is limited almost exclusively to young animals. The presence of a few lungworms usually causes only a hacking cough. Heavy infections, however, may result in labored respiration, anorexia, diarrhea and stunted growth. Occasionally, death may follow pulmonary consolidation caused by secondary bacterial infection of occluded bronchioles and alveoli.

Lesions.—As the infective larvae break through the capillary and alveolar walls, they cause some hemorrhage into the lumens of alveoli. This hemorrhage and the reparative process that follows may result in consolidation of alveoli, but usually this is transitory and involves only a fraction of the lung. In animals sensitized by previous exposure, the inflammatory reaction to infective larvae is more intense. Entire lobules may become filled with leukocytes, among which eosinophils predominate. As the lungworms grow to maturity, they move toward the alveolar ducts from the alveoli, establishing their adult abode in the bronchioles or bronchi. Their presence in this part of the respiratory tract produces some irritation which attracts leukocytes and an excessive amount of mucus. This exudate often occludes the bronchioles and leads to atelectasis or consolidation of the related alveoli. Most lungworm adults, feeding head down upon mucus and cellular detritus in the bronchial tree, deposit ova which lodge in the alveoli

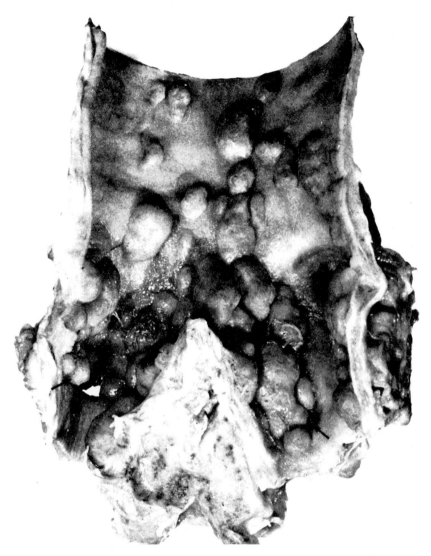

Fig. 15-14.—Pulmonary nematodiasis. Nodules containing adult *Filaroides osleri* in the tracheal mucosa near the bifurcation. Note that the nodules produce partial stenosis of the lumen of the bronchi (arrows). (Courtesy of Armed Forces Institute of Pathology.) Contributor: Dr. F. D. Gentry.

where they embryonate to become larvae. These embryonating ova act as foreign bodies, provoking inflammation that results in consolidation of viable lung. Secondary bacterial infection may intervene at any time, with purulent pneumonia the usual sequel. Emphysema is common in unconsolidated parts of the lungs.

The lesions produced by certain other lungworms differ in important respects from these described. The adults of the dog lungworm, *Filaroides osleri*, for example, are found in nodules in the mucosa of the trachea or bronchi, occasionally in sufficient numbers to occlude the respiratory passage and produce death from asphyxia. The life cycle and mode of infection of this parasite are unknown. The cat lungworm, *Aelurostrongylus abstrusus*, has been the subject of some dispute. The habitat of the adults is in small branches of the pulmonary arteries or the right ventricle, where they produce ova which break through capillary walls into alveoli. Larvae developing from the ova move into alveolar ducts and bronchioles, are coughed up and swallowed to pass out with the feces. These ova and larvae may cause considerable loss of air space in sharply circumscribed parts of the lung, but apparently only very heavy parasitism will result in death of the host. The larvae which reach the outside must, according to present opinion, be ingested by certain molluscs (snails and slugs) in order to continue their life cycle. A dissenting opinion indicates that mice may act as the first intermediate host. Transport hosts, such as frogs, toads, lizards, snakes and birds, may ingest the molluscs containing the third stage infective larvae. The final host, the cat, becomes infected by eating a transport host or the true intermediate host.

Evidence has accumulated to associate infection by *Aelurostrongylus abstrusus* and *Toxocara cati* with characteristic lesions in the wall of branches of the pulmonary artery (Fig. 22–13C) of cats. The lesion consists of hyperplasia of the media and fibrosis of the intima which nearly obliterates the lumen. The effect of this change is to produce a sharply-demarcated stenosis of the artery which decreases the blood supply to varying-sized segments of the lung. The exact mechanism which results in this lesion is not understood, but the effect is clearly demonstrable

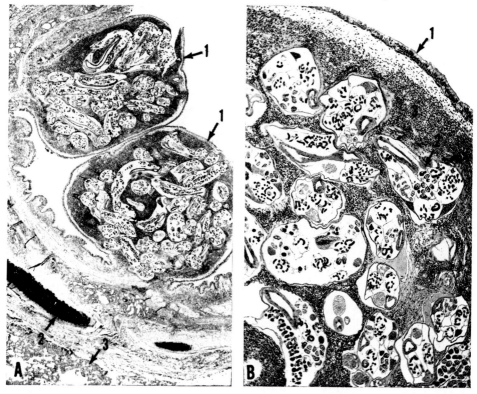

FIG. 15–15.—Pulmonary nematodiasis. *A*, Two nodules filled with adult *Filaroides osleri* in the bronchial mucosa of a dog (× 13). The epithelium (*1*) is elevated. Bronchial cartilage (*2*) and lung parenchyma (*3*). *B*, Enlarged view (× 50) of one of the nodules in *A*. Bronchial epithelium (*1*), adult worms containing larvae (*2*), lymphocytic inflammatory reaction (*3*). (Courtesy of Armed Forces Institute of Pathology.) Contributor: Dr. F. D. Gentry.

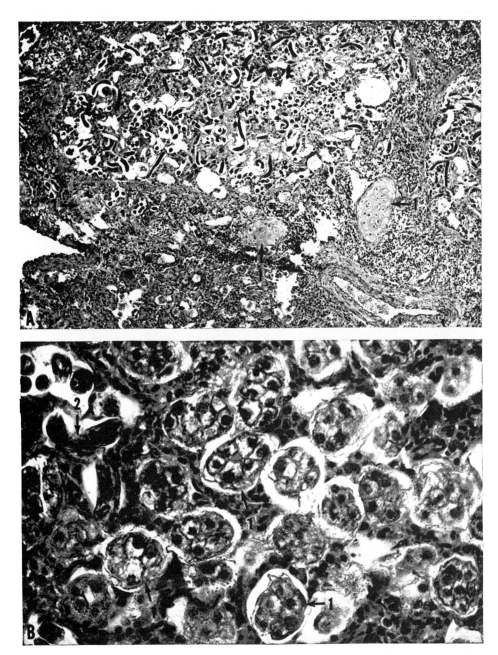

FIG. 15–16.—Pulmonary nematodiasis. *Aelurostrongylus abstrusus* in the lung of a cat. *A*, Larvae filling a small bronchus outlined by its cartilage (*1*) (× 83). *B*, Another area in the same lung with embryonating ova (*1*) in alveoli and larvae in alveolar duct (*2*) (× 385). (Courtesy of Armed Forces Institute of Pathology.) Contributor: Dr. W. S. Bailey.

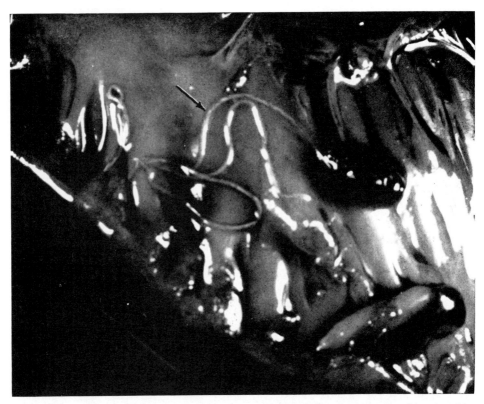

FIG. 15–17.—*Aelurostrongylus abstrusus* (adults) in right ventricle of a four-year-old male tabby and white cat.   (Courtesy of Angell Memorial Animal Hospital.)

by experimental infection with either of these parasites (Hamilton, 1966; Jonas, Swerczek and Downing, 1970).

Diagnosis.—The diagnosis of lungworm disease can be suspected from the signs and confirmed by identifying lungworm larvae in the feces of the living animal.   Demonstration of adult lungworms in the bronchi or bronchioles and ova and larvae in the lung parenchyma at necropsy is often necessary to establish the nature of a herd infection.   Careful examination with the naked eye and use of the hand lens are advisable, especially when searching for the smaller lungworms, and histopathologic examination is recommended.

Pulmonary Nematodiasis

ALLEN, G. W.: Acute Atypical Bovine Pneumonia Caused by *Ascaris lumbricoides*. Canad. J. Comp. Med. *26*:241–243, 1962. (VB 2878–63.)

BERESFORD-JONES, W. P.: Observations on *Muellerius capillaris* (Muller, 1889), Cameron 1927. II. Experimental Infection of Mice, Guinea-pigs, and Rabbits with Third Stage Larvae. Res. Vet. Sci. *7*:287–291, 1966.

CAMERON, T. W. M.: Observations on the Life History of *Aelurostrongylus abstrusus* (Railliet) the Lungworm of the Cat. J. Helminthol. *5*:55–66, 1927.

DORRINGTON, J. E.:   Preliminary Report on the Transmission of *Filaroides osleri* (Cobbold, 1879) in Dogs. J. S. Afr. Vet. Med. Assn. *36*:389, 1965. V.B. *36*:3563, 1966.

———: *Filaroides osleri*: (Cobbold, 1879) Infestation in the Dog. J. S. Afr. Vet. Med. Assn. *38*:91, 1967. V.B. *38*:1942, 1968.

———: Studies on *Filaroides osleri* Infestation in Dogs. Onderstepoort. J. Vet. Res. *35*:225–285, 1968. V.B. *39*:1684, 1969.

DUBEY, J. P., BEVERLEY, J. K. A., and CRANE, W. A. J.: Lung Changes and *Aelurostrongylus abstrusus* Infestation in English Cats. Vet. Rec. *83*:191–194, 1968.

GERICHTER, C. B.: Studies on the Nematodes Parasitic in the Lungs of Felidæ in Palestine. Parasitology. *39*:251–262, 1949.

HAMILTON, J. M.: The Number of *Aelurostrongylus abstrusus* Larvae Required to Produce Pulmonary Disease in the Cat. J. Comp. Path. 77:343–346, 1967.

————: Parental Infection of the Cat by Larvae of *Aelurostrongylus abstrusus*. J. Helminth. *43*:31–34, 1969.

————: Experimental Lungworm Disease of the Cat. Association of the Condition with Lesions of the Pulmonary Artery. J. Comp. Path. 76:147–157, 1966.

HAMILTON, J. M., and McCAW, A. W.: I. The Role of the Mouse in the Life Cycle of *Aelurostrongylus abstrusus*. II. An Investigation into the Longevity of First Stage Larvae of *Aelurostrongylus abstrusus*. J. Helminth. *41*:309–312 and 313–320, 1967.

HOBMAIER, M.: Newer Aspects of the Lungworm (*Crenosoma*) in Foxes. Am. J. Vet. Research *2*:352–354, 1941.

JARRETT, W. F. H., McINTYRE, W. I. M., and URQUHART, G. M.: The Pathology of Experimental Bovine Parasitic Bronchitis. J. Path. and Bact. *73*:183–193, 1957.

JINDRAK, K.: The Pathology of Radicular Involvement in Angiostrongylosis as Observed in Experimentally Infected Calves and Pigs. Virchows. Arch. Path. Anat. *345*:228–237, 1968.

JINDRAK, K., and ALICATA, J. E.: Comparative Pathology in Experimental Infection of Pigs and Calves with Larvae of *Angiostrongylus cantonensis*. J. Comp. Path. *78*:371–382, 1968.

————: Experimentally Induced *Angiostrongylus cantonensis* Infection in Dogs. Am. J. Vet. Res. *31*:449–456, 1970.

JONAS, A. M., SWERCZEK, T. W., and DOWNING, S. E.: Vaso-occlusive Pulmonary Hypertension. A Feline Model System. Lab. Invest. *22*:502, 1970.

JUBB, K. V.: The Lesions Caused by *Filaroides milksi* in a Dog. Cornell Vet. *50*:319–325, 1960.

KERSTEN, E., and BECHT, H.: Ein Beitrag zer Pathologie der Lungenwurminfektionen. Deutsche tieräztl Wchnschr. *67*:173–177, 1960. (Metastrongylus larvæ in guinea pigs)

MICHEL, J. F., and MACKENZIE, A.: Duration of the Acquired Resistance of Calves to Infection with *Dictyocaulus viviparus*. Res. Vet. Sci. *6*:344–395, 1965.

MILLS, J. H. L., and NIELSEN, S. W.: Canine *Filaroides osleri* and *Filaroides milksi* Infection. J. Am. Vet. Med. Assn. *149*:56–63, 1966.

NAYAK, D. P., KELLEY, G. W., and UNDERDAHL, N. R.: The Enhancing Effect of Swine Lungworms on Swine Influenza Infections. Cornell Vet. *54*:160–175, 1964.

PORTER, D. A., and CAUTHEN, G. E.: Experiments on the Life History of the Cattle Lungworm, *Dictyocaulus viviparus*. Am. J. Vet. Res. *3*:395–400, 1942.

POYNTER, D., and SELWAY, S.: Diseases Caused by Lungworms. Vet. Bull. *36*:539–554, 1966.

ROSEN, L., ASH, L. R., and WALLACE, G. D.: Life History of the Canine Lungworm *Angiostrongylus vasorum* (Baillet). Am. J. Vet. Res. *31*:131–143, 1970.

SHARMA, K. M. L.: Observations Made on Haematological and Electrophoretic Analysis of Serum Protein from Heifers Naturally Infected with Lung Worm (*Dictyocaulus viviparus*). Indian Vet. J. *44*:489–493, 1967.

SHOHO, C.: Observations on Rats and Rabbits Infected with *Angiostrongylus cantonensis* (Chen). Brit. Vet. J. *122*:251–258, 1966.

SIMPSON, C. F. *et al.*: Pathological Changes Associated with *Dictyocaulus viviparus* (Block) Infection in Calves. Am. J. Vet. Res. *18*:747–755, 1957.

SUBRAMANIAM, T., D'SOUZA, B. A., and VICTOR, D. A.: Broncho-pneumonia in Baby Pigs Due to *Metastrongylus apri*. Indian Vet. J. *44*:121–127, 1967.

TAFFS, L. F.: Lungworm Infection in Swine. Vet. Rec. *80*:554, 1967.

WILSON, G. I.: Investigations on the Pathogenicity and Immunology of *Dictyocaulus filaria* in Sheep and Goats. Diss. Abstr. *26*:5612–5613, 1966. V.B. *37*:619 1967.

RENAL DIOCTOPHYMOSIS

The giant kidney worm *Dioctophyma renale* (*Eustrongylus gigas*, *Ascaris renalis*) is an uncommon parasite of the dog and mink, and rarely of man. The adult worms are found in the renal pelvis, occasionally in the intestinal lumen and the peritoneal cavity. The female is a surprisingly large, cylindrical nematode, reddish in color and 20 to 100 cm. in length. The male is smaller, 14 to 40 cm. long. According to Woodhead (1950), eggs from these worms in the kidneys of wild mink pass out with the urine and hatch when swallowed by an annelid worm, *Cambarincola chirocephala*. This worm is parasitic on crayfish and the first stage larvae of *D. renale* encyst in the crayfish. This intermediate host is eaten by a bullhead fish, *Ameirus melas*. The parasitic larvae pass through the third into the fourth stage and encyst in the liver and mesentery. Mink, and presumably dogs, become infected with *D. renale* by eating the fish. Apparently, other species of fish may also carry the infective larvae. The clinical diagnosis is confirmed by the presence of the brownish yellow ova with their thick, pitted shells and bipolar caps in the urine.

The adult worms with their habitat in the renal pelvis produce hydronephrosis (p. 1283) which eventually destroys all the functional kidney. The contralateral kidney undergoes compensatory hypertrophy in the usual case, but bilateral renal involvement is obviously fatal.

Renal Dioctophymosis

COOPERRIDER, D. E., ROBINSON, V. B., and STATON, L. B.: *Dioctophyma renale* in a Dog. J. Am. Vet. Med. Assn. *124*:381–383, 1954.
DE ALENCAR, R. A., JR.: Renal Dioctophymosis in a Dog. Biologico. *32*:34–36, 1966. V.B. *36*:4403, 1966.
EUBANKS, J. W., and PICK, J. R.: *Dioctophyma renale* Infection in a Dog. J. Am. Vet. Med. Assn. *143*:164–169, 1963.
HALLBERG, C. W.: *Dioctophyma renale* (Goetze, 1782). A Study of the Migration Routes to the Kidneys of Mammals and Resultant Pathology. Amer. Microscop. Soc. *72*:351–363, 1953.
McLEOD, J. A.: *Dioctophyma renale* Infections in Manitoba. Canad. J. Zool. *45*:505–508, 1967.
McNEIL, C. W.: Pathological Changes in the Kidney of Mink Due to Infection with *Dioctophyma renale* (Goetze, 1782), the Giant Kidney Worm of Mammals. Amer. Microscop. Soc. *67*:257–261, 1948.
WOODHEAD, A. E.: Life History Cycle of the Giant Kidney Worm, *Dioctophyma renale* (Nematoda), of Man and Many Other Mammals. Tr. Amer. Microscop. Soc. *69*:21–46, 1950.

HABRONEMIASIS

The stomach worms of horses are of three species: *Habronema muscae, Habronema majus (Habronema microstoma)* and *Draschia megastoma (Habronema megastoma)*. The adult nematodes are small and slender and are found in nodules in the submucosa of the stomach. Severe infections may interfere with gastric function, but a few parasites rarely have any significant clinical effect. The life cycle of each of these three parasites is similar in that eggs and larvae passed in the feces are ingested by larvae (maggots) of the housefly (*Musca domestica*) or in the case of *H. majus* by the larvae of the stable fly. The larvae undergo further development in the pupae of the fly and migrate as infective larvae into the proboscis of the adult fly. The infective larvae are believed to be deposited on the lips of horses and eventually swallowed to develop into adults in the stomach. The occurrence of the helminth larvae in lesions of the skin suggests that they may gain access to the host through the epidermis and migrate to the stomach.

According to de Jesus (1963), *H. muscae* is associated with diffuse gastritis; *H. microstoma* with gastric ulcers and *H. megastoma* with granulomatous gastritis.

Cutaneous habronemiasis (summer sores), a persistent disease of the skin of equines, results from the activity of larvae of stomach worms, especially *Draschia megastoma*. The larvae are deposited on the skin by the housefly, which is attracted to some pre-existing ulceration or wound in the skin. Lesions are particularly

by a pustular dermatitis, larvae being demonstrable in microscopic sections of hair follicles. The larvae were found in large numbers in the moist rice hulls used as bedding for these animals.

Rhabditis dermatitis

CHITWOOD, B. G.: The Association of *Rhabditis strongyloides* with Dermatitis in Dogs. North Amer. Vet. *13*:35–40, 1932.
JIBBO, J. M. C.: Bovine Parasitic Otitis. Bull. Epizoot. Dis. Afr. *14*:59–63, 1966.
RHODE, E. A., *et al.*: The Occurrence of *Rhabditis* in Cattle. North Amer. Vet. *34*:634–637, 1953.
SCHLOTTHAUER, C. F., and ZOLLMAN, P. E.: The Occurrence of *Rhabditis strongyloides* in Association with Dermatitis in a Dog. J. Am. Vet. Med. Assn. *127*:510–511, 1955.

STEPHANOFILARIASIS

Nematode dermatitis occurring in cattle in widely scattered parts of the world is caused by several related filarial worms. *Stephanofilaria stilesi*, originally recognized by Stiles and described by Dikmans (1948), has been reported in skin lesions of cattle in most of the western and midwestern states, as well as Louisiana. This filarid causes a circumscribed dermatitis usually located on the abdomen near the midline. *S. dedoesi* has been reported from Java, Sumatra, Celebes and Indonesia; it produces lesions on the sides of the neck, withers, dewlap, shoulders

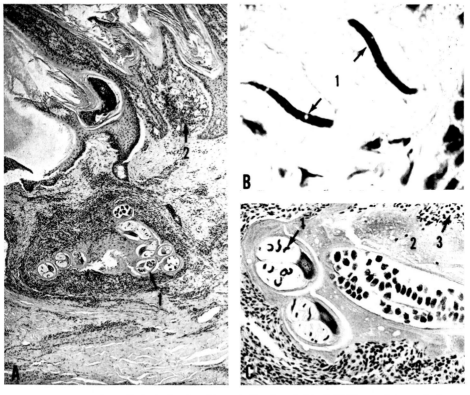

FIG. 15–23.—Stephanofilariasis, bovine skin. *A*, Section of skin (× 75) containing coiled adult *Stephanofilaria stilesi* (1) deep in a hair follicle and larvae in the dermal papillae (2). Note acanthosis and hyperkeratosis. *B*, Larvae (1) (× 900) in papilla. *C*, Adult (× 150) worm with larvae in uterus (1), hyaline material (2) surrounding it, and zone of inflammation (3). (Courtesy of Armed Forces Institute of Pathology.) Material courtesy of Dr. C. L. Davis.

and around the eyes. *S. assamensis*, occurring in Assam and other parts of India, causes a chronic dermatitis in Zebu cattle, known as "hump sore." In Malaya, a fourth species, *S. kaeli*, is reported to produce "filarial sores" on the lower legs of cattle. An apparently new species of *Stephanofilaria* has been identified (Kono, 1965) in the Ryukyu Islands as the cause of pruritic lesions on the muzzle of cattle. These lesions result in erosion of the epidermis over zones of infiltration of papillary and reticular layers of the dermis by lymphocytes, plasma cells, macrophages and eosinophils in relation to adult nematodes. In the United States, Hibler (1966) has shown that the horn fly, *Haematobia irritans*, is an intermediate host for *Stephanofilaria stilesi*. Other flies may have a similar role for *Stephanofilaria* in other parts of the world.

The adult forms of *Stephanofilaria stilesi* are found either in small cysts with epithelial linings in the base of hair follicles or in the dermis near the epidermis (Fig. 15–23). In either site, the worms are surrounded by a zone of inflammation containing eosinophils, lymphocytes, some neutrophils and histiocytes, and often a layer of connective tissue. The microfilariae are found a short distance from the adults in spaces in the dermal papillae. The adults and microfilariae can often be seen in the same field when the low power of the microscope is used (Fig. 15–23). Hyperkeratosis and parakeratosis may be noted in the epidermis of parasitized areas and crusts of exuded serum and detritus may collect on the surface. Death of the parasites and sensitization of the host result in a rather severe dermatitis. The diagnosis may be established by the demonstration of adults and microfilariae in biopsy or necropsy specimens of affected skin. The parasites can also be collected by deep scrapings of skin and identified by microscopic examination.

Stephanofilariasis

Hibler, C. P.:   Development of *Stephanofilaria stilesi* in the horn fly. J. Parasit. *52*:890–898, 1966.

Kono, I., and Fukuyoshi, S.:   Leucoderma of the Muzzle of Cattle Induced by a New Species of *Stephanofilaria*. II. Jap. J. Vet. Sci. *29*:301–313, 1967. V.B. *38*:4627, 1968.

Levine, N. D., and Morrill, C. C.:   Bovine Stephanofilarial Dermatitis in Illinois. J. Am. Vet. Med. Assn. *127*:528–530, 1955.

Loke, Y. W., and Ramachandran, C. P.:   Histopathology of *Stephanofilaria kaeli* Lesions in Cattle. Med. J. Malaya *20*:348–353, 1966. V.B. *37*:931, 1967.

Mia, A. S., and Haque, A.:   Skin Diseases in Cattle. Pakist. J. Vet. Sci. *1*:76–83, 1967. V.B. *39*:1271, 1969.

Ramachandran, C. P., Loke, Y. W., and Nagendram, C.:   Studies on *Stephanofilaria kaeli* in Cattle. Med. J. Malaya *20*:344–347, 1966.

Sharma Deorani, V. P.:   Studies on the Pathology of Stephanofilariasis Assamensis in Cattle. Curr. Sci. *34*:410–411, 1965.

THELAZIASIS

"Eye worms" have been reported from the conjunctival sac, tear duct, the bulbar and tarsal conjunctiva and membrana nictitans of animals. Several species are of interest: *Thelazia californiensis* has been reported in the United States from sheep, dogs, deer and rarely cats and man. *T. callipaeda* occurs in Asia in the membrana nictitans of the dog, less frequently in the rabbit and man. *T. gulosa* occurs in cattle (France and Sumatra); *T. alfortensis* in cattle (France); *T. skrjabini* in calves and *T. lacrymalis* in the horse. *T. rhodesii* has been reported from Asia, Africa and Europe in the conjunctival sac of buffaloes, cattle, goats and sheep.

The life cycle (Soulsby, 1968) of these spiruroid worms depends upon flies as intermediate hosts and vectors. The larvae move from the gut to develop first in the ovary of the fly where they penetrate and develop in ovarian follicles. They spend their second and third stages in the ovary then as third stage, infective, larvae migrate to the mouth parts of the fly ready to be transferred to the conjunctivae of cattle.

The intermediate hosts are as follows: For *T. rhodesii*: *Musca larvipara*, *M. convexifrons*; for *T. skrjabini*: probably *M. amica*; for *T. gulosi*: *M. amica* and *M. larvipara*. The intermediate hosts and vectors for *T. californiensis*, *T. callipaeda*, *T. alfortensis* and *T. lacrymalis* are at present unknown.

Their presence in the conjunctival sac results in considerable photophobia and excessive lacrimation; if not removed, they are reported to cause blindness, presumably through production of corneal opacity. The diagnosis is made by finding and identifying the parasites in the conjunctiva.

Thelaziasis

FITZSIMMONS, W. M.: Verminous Ophthalmia in a Cow in Berkshire—A Review of Thelazia Infections as a Veterinary Problem. Vet. Rec. 75:1024–1027, 1963.
SOULSBY, E. J. L.: *Helminths, Arthropods and Protozoa of Domesticated Animals* (Mönnig). 6th Ed., Baltimore, The Williams & Wilkins Co., 1968, pp. 274–276.

STEPHANURIASIS (KIDNEY WORM DISEASE)

The swine kidney worm, *Stephanurus dentatus*, is a stout parasitic nematode, 20 to 40 mm. in length, found principally in the perirenal fat and adjacent tissues. It is especially common in the southern United States. These worms form cystic cavities which communicate with the lumen of the ureter and permit the discharge of ova with the urine. The larvae hatch only in moist, shaded soil and remain infective for some time unless exposed to direct sunlight and desiccation. The infective larvae may be ingested by the host or penetrate the mud-caked skin. The larvae lose their sheaths to reach the fourth stage in one of two sites, depending upon the route of entry. Orally ingested worms molt in the wall of the stomach, while those which penetrate the skin undergo this change in the abdominal muscles. The fourth stage larvae soon migrate to the liver where they remain for two or three months, their movements exciting severe tissue reaction. Eventually the larvae break out of the liver into the peritoneal cavity and wander extensively, most of them eventually reaching the perirenal fat. Here the successful adults copulate and the female lays her eggs in a cyst which empties into the ureter. This life cycle requires about six months. Infected swine are commonly emaciated in spite of a good appetite, and ascites is frequent as a result of liver damage. Death may occur following secondary infection, extensive tissue destruction, or urinary obstruction. The condemnation of livers and carcasses of infected animals slaughtered for food makes the disease an important economic problem.

Lesions.—Both the larvae and the adult forms of this nematode produce severe effects upon the host. Nodules and edema in the subcutis and transitory enlargement of superficial lymph nodes are produced by the passage of larvae, but their most serious effect is upon the liver. Not only do these worms burrow into the liver, but during their relatively long stay they move about aggressively. This restive sojourn in the liver eventually results in extensive portal fibrosis, which may spread to obliterate many liver lobules. The fibrotic change is accompanied by intense tissue eosinophilia, foci of coagulation necrosis and infiltration by other leukocytes. The lesions are often so severe as to render the liver totally unfit for human food.

This parasite, to a greater extent than most others, wanders through the host's tissues, producing widespread damage. Although the successful worms find their way to the vicinity of the ureters, many wander to other sites where they excite a local purulent tissue reaction. *S. dentatus* has been found in the kidney, lumbar muscles, myocardium, lungs, pleural cavity, spleen and even the spinal canal. Paralysis may result from destruction of the lumbar spinal cord by the migrations of these worms.

Diagnosis.—The diagnosis may be made by demonstrating the ova in the urine or by finding the worms at necropsy. Leukocytic infiltration and fibrosis in the liver are usually much more intense and extensive than the changes in this organ caused by other larvae (*e.g.* ascarids), a point which may be used in histologic differentiation.

Stephanuriasis

BATTE, E. G., MONCOL, D. J., and BARBER, C. W.: Prenatal Infection with the Swine Kidney Worm (*Stephanurus dentatus*) and Associated Lesions. J. Am. Vet. Med. Assn. *149*:758–765, 1966.

PENEYRA, R. S., and NAUI, V. C.: Observations on the Incidence and Pathology of Kidney-worm Infection in Swine (Slaughterhouse Material). Philipp. J. Vet. Med. *4*:129–140, 1967.

GONGYLONEMIASIS

These tiny worms are of interest because of their habitat in the stratified squamous epithelium of the esophagus, the rumen and stomach. They are often encountered in histologic sections of these organs, coiled in the epithelium (Fig.

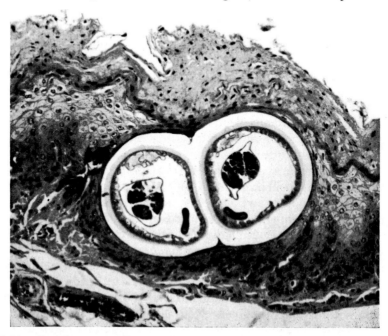

FIG. 15–24.—*Gongylonema sp.* Cross sections of a parasite embedded in the epithelium of the tongue of a rhesus monkey (*Macaca mulatta*). (Courtesy New England Regional Primate Research Center, Harvard Medical School.)

15–24) apparently inciting little or no host reaction. *Gongylonema pulchrum* occurs in sheep, cattle, goats, pigs, buffalo, and occasionally the horse, camel, wild boar and donkey. It has been reported in man. *G. verrucosum* inhabits the rumen of sheep, goats, cattle, deer and zebu. It is known in the United States, India and South Africa. *G. monnig* infects sheep and goats in South Africa. Other species infect the rat (*G. neoplasticum*) and non-human primates (Fig. 15–24).

Gongylonemiasis

SOULSBY, E. J. L.: *Helminths, Arthropods and Protozoa of Domesticated Animals* (Mönnig). 6th Ed., Baltimore, The Williams & Wilkins Co., 1968.

ACANTHOCEPHALAN INFECTIONS

Acanthocephalan or thorny-headed worms have important pathogenic effects upon their host because of their tendency to burrow into and attach to the intestinal wall. These worms are classified in a separate phylum (*Acanthocephala*) and have parasitic representatives in many species of mammals, birds and fishes. They invariably attach to the intestinal wall of the host and in the host have somewhat flattened bodies which tend to round up after removal. The arrangement and number of "thorns" on the head parts are used to identify individual species. *Macracanthorhynchus hirudinaceus* is the thorny-headed worm which infects domestic swine and incidentally provides young veterinary students with a "jawbreaker" name which, when mastered in pronunciation and spelling, somehow makes it easier to cope with other scientific names.

Prosthenorchis elegans (Figs. 15–25 and 26) is found in the small intestine and colon of South American monkeys, such as the squirrel monkey (*Saimiri sciureus*) and marmosets (*Tamarinus, Saguinus, Cebuella*). One of its intermediate hosts is the cockroach. *Acanthocephus jacksoni* is known to parasitize several species of fresh-water fish in New England.

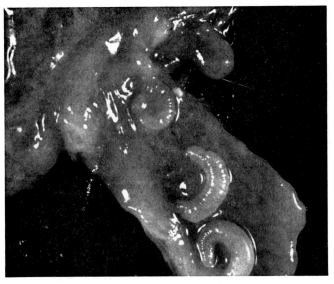

FIG. 15–25.—*Prosthenorchis elegans*, marmoset (*Saguinus oedipus*). These acanthocephalids characteristically embed their thorny heads in the mucosa of the terminal ileum. (Courtesy New England Regional Primate Research Center, Harvard Medical School.)

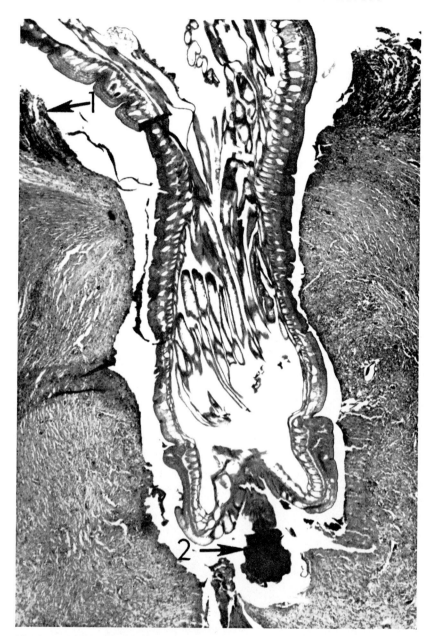

FIG. 15–26.—Acanthocephalid in a marmoset (*Saguinus oedipus*). *Prosthenorchis elegans* which has penetrated through the mucosa of the ileum (*1*) assisted by its thorny proboscis (*2*). (Courtesy New England Regional Primate Research Center, Harvard Medical School.)

Acanthocephalan Infections

BULLOCK, W. L.: Intestinal Histology of Some Salmonid Fishes with Particular Reference to Histopathology of Acanthocephalan Infections. J. Morphol. *112*:23–44, 1963.

CHAICHARN, A., and BULLOCK, W. L.: The Histopathology of Acanthocephalan Infections in Suckers with Observations on the Intestinal Histology of Two Species of Catostomid Fishes. Acta Zool. *48*:19–42, 1967.

DUNN, F. L.: Acanthocephalans and Cestodes of South American Monkeys and Marmosets. J. Parasit. *49*:717–722, 1963.

RICHART, R., and BENIRSCHKE, K.: Causes of Death in a Colony of Marmoset Monkeys. J. Path. & Bact. *86*:221–223, 1963.

TAKOS, M. J., and THOMAS, L. J.: The Pathology and Pathogenesis of Fetal Infections Due to an Acanthocephalid Parasite of Marmoset Monkeys. Amer. J. Trop. Med. & Hyg. 7:90–94, 1958.

VAN CLEAVE, H. J.: "Acanthocephala of North American Mammals." Illinois Biol. Monograph *23*:(1–2):1–179, 1953.

CESTODIASIS

(Tapeworm Disease, Taeniasis)

Cestodes, or tapeworms (Phylum: Platyhelminthes, Class: Cestoda), are common parasites of all vertebrate animals, including man. An exception occurs in the United States at least, where the pig seems to be singularly free of tapeworms. The adult forms in the intestinal tract of the definitive host are flat worms made up of a chain of independent, hermaphroditic segments (proglottides), fastened together, and usually attached to the intestinal mucosa by a specialized segment (scolex) at the anterior end. Each proglottis contains male and female genitalia and is complete in other respects; hence the tapeworm is in reality a colony of individuals attached to one another in a tape-like chain. As proglottides of most tapeworms mature, those at the caudal end are shed and are expelled from the body with the feces, to release their innumerable ova.

All tapeworms have one or more larval stages through which they pass in various intermediate hosts, including insects and mammals; some tapeworms require more than one intermediate host. Only one tapeworm, *Hymenolepis nana*, a parasite of rodents, has a direct life cycle, the definitive host serving also for the stages of development usually completed within the intermediate host. These larval forms invade animal tissues and by replacing vital cells can produce serious effects upon the host. Certain tapeworm larvae were recognized for a long time before their connection with the adult form was appreciated. For this reason the larval form may have a separate, well-established name—for example, *Cysticercus cellulosae*, the bladderworm of "measly pork," is the larval form of *Taenia solium*, a tapeworm of man.

The class Cestoda is usually divided into eleven orders, nine of these include parasites of fishes, annelids, reptiles or amphibia and two, Pseudophyllidea and Cyclophyllidea, in which are classified all tapeworms which are parasitic for man and other mammals. The Pseudophyllidea are largely parasites of fish, the adult of only one species, *Diphyllobothrium latum*, is parasitic in mammals. Species of this order have a scolex which has no hooks and narrow, deep grooves, *bothria*, instead of suckers. The eggs are usually operculated, resembling those of trematodes. All of the rest of the species of tapeworms parasitic for mammals are classified in the order Cyclophyllidea.

The adult tapeworms apparently produce little serious effect upon the host except in very heavy infections in which they interfere with digestion or cause partial obstruction. The parasites in their intermediate stages produce much more important effects upon the host. The pathologist may encounter these intermediate stages of tapeworms in animal tissues; therefore the identifying features of the different types are of diagnostic significance. The larvae usually develop in one of two possible ways to become (1) solid larvae and (2) bladder larvae. In the first (solid), the ovoid, operculate ovum is passed out of the uterus to hatch into a ciliated motile embryo, the **coracidium,** which escapes through the operculum and becomes free-living. The coracidium is ingested by a fresh-water crustacean in whose tissues it develops into an elongated form, the **pro-cercoid** larva. Development of this larva continues after the arthropod is swallowed by a second intermediate host (often a fish) until it becomes an elongated solid larva (**plerocercoid**) with a head resembling that of the mature tapeworm. The broad fish tapeworm (*Diphyllobothrium latum*) provides an ex-ample of larval development of this type.

In development of the second type, the bladder larvae arise from eggs, which are usually round or nearly square, released from the uterus by disintegration of the proglottis, or by discharge through one or more uterine pores by those species which have them. These eggs are fully developed when they escape from the uterus in that they contain a larva, the **onchosphere,** or **hexacanth embryo,** sur-rounded by a dense membrane. In the intestine of the intermediate host, the onchosphere is released to migrate into the tissues, where it becomes transformed into a bladder-shaped structure with one or more inverted scolices in an invag-inated portion of the wall. If the larva has a solid caudal portion and a bladder-like proximal portion, it is called a **cysticercus.** Modifications of the cysticercus include the **strobilocercus,** with an invaginated scolex attached to a small bladder by a segmented portion; the **coenurus** or **multiceps,** with a germinal layer capable of producing scolices beneath the bladder wall; and **echinococcus** or **hydatid cyst,** with a germinal layer that produces brood capsules within which scolices develop. **Cysticercoid,** a form which usually is found in invertebrates, consists of a small vesicle with a tiny cavity and one scolex. The scolices in all of these larval stages possess suckers and (in armed species) hooklets identical to those of the adult stage. When ingested by the definitive host, the scolex evaginates and attaches itself to the intestinal mucosa; growth of the tapeworm then proceeds by prolif-eration of segments at the posterior extremity.

Some of the features of important tapeworms of domestic animals are outlined in Table 15–2.

Cysticercosis.—The presence of larvae of certain tapeworms in the tissues of man or animals results in a disease known as **cysticercosis** (beef or pork "measles," bladderworm disease). The effect upon the host depends largely upon the organs involved and the degree of parasitism. In some sites, such as peritoneum and subcutis, the cysticerci are tolerated with little reaction, but those species which invade and displace tissue in critical organs (liver, heart, brain) may produce grave signs or death.

Cysticercus bovis (larva of *Taenia saginata*, beef bladderworm), which may be found in muscle, liver, heart, lungs, diaphragm, lymph nodes, and other parts of the body of cattle, is of importance because the bovine parasite is the intermediate stage of a human tapeworm. Few symptoms are produced in cattle, but in some cases of massive infection death may occur following a febrile course. The cysti-cerci are usually found on post-mortem inspection as small cysts, up to 9 mm. in diameter, in musculature or (in the heart) partly embedded and partly projecting from the surface. The cysts are white or gray, with a small yellowish spot representing the scolex which is unarmed (without hooklets). As a rule, the principal tissue change is displacement of normal cells, with little inflammatory reaction surrounding the viable bladderworm. In long-standing cases, however, death of the parasite is followed by dense encapsulation with eventual formation

Table 15–2.—Outline of Features of Some Important Tapeworms

Name of Tapeworm	Adult Host	Intermediate Stage		
		Anatomic Site	Type of Larva	Intermediate Hosts
Taenia saginata	Man	Heart, skeletal muscle	Cysticercus (bovis)	Cattle
Taenia solium	Man	Muscle, heart, viscera	Cysticercus (cellulosæ)	Swine, cattle
Echinococcus granulosus	Man, dog, fox, wolf, jackal	Liver, lungs, and other viscera	Echinococcus (granulosus)	Man, cattle, swine, sheep, deer, horse, moose, etc.
Echinococcus multilocularis	Man, dog, fox, wolf, jackal	Liver, lungs, and other viscera	Echinococcus (multilocu- laris)	Man, cattle, swine, sheep, deer, horse, moose, etc.
Taenia hydatigena	Dog	Liver, mesentery, etc.	Cysticercus (tenuicollis)	Squirrels, cattle, wild ruminants, sheep, goats, swine
Taenia ovis	Dog, fox, wolf, coyote	Muscles	Cysticercus (ovis)	Sheep
Taenia pisiformis	Dog, cat, fox, wolf	Liver capsule and peritoneum	Cysticerus	Rabbit, squirrel and other small rodents
Taenia taeniaeformis syn.: *T. crassicollis*	Cat, dog, fox	Liver	Cysticercus (fasciolaris)	Rats, mice, rabbits
Multiceps multiceps	Dog	Brain and spinal cord	Coenurus (cerebralis)	Sheep and goats
Multiceps serialis	Dog and other carnivores	Subcutis	Coenurus serialis	Rabbit
Diphyllobothrium latum	Man, bear, dog, cat, pig, fox	Muscles	Procercoid and plerocercoid	Microcrustacean and fresh water fish
Dipylidium caninum	Dog, cat		Cysticercoid	Dog flea and biting lice
Moniezia expansa	Sheep, goats, cattle	—	Cysticercoid	Mites: *Galumna*, *Scheloribates*, and *Scutovertex minutus*
Moniezia benedeni	Sheep, goats, cattle	—	Cysticercoid	*Scutovertex minutus*
Anoplocephala magna	Equines	—	Cysticercoid	Mites of family *Oribatidæ*
Anoplocephala perfoliata	Equines	—	Cysticercoid	*Oribatidæ*
Paranoplocephala mammillana	Equines	—	Cysticercoid	*Oribatidæ*
Thysanosoma actinioides	Sheep, cattle, goats and deer	—	Cysticercoid	*Orbatidæ*

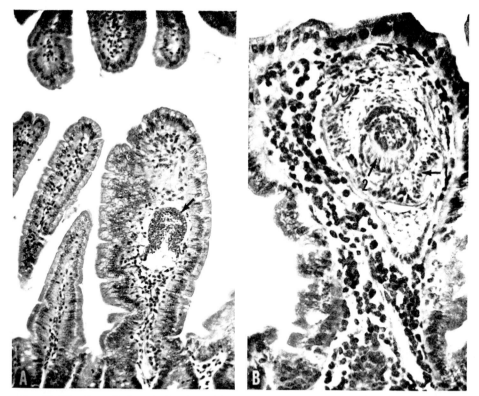

FIG. 15–27.—Cestodiasis. *A*, Cysticercoid larva (arrow) of *Hymenolepis nana* (× 45) in intestinal villus of a mouse. *B*, Later stage in larval development (× 395). Note sucker (*1*) and hooklets (*2*) of the larva encysted in the lamina propria of the intestinal villus. (Courtesy of Armed Forces Institute of Pathology.) Contributor: Dr. W. S. Bailey.

of a scar. Microscopic sections through the lesion may disclose the thin bladder wall and the invaginated scolex of the cysticercus.

Cysticercus cellulosae, the pork bladderworm, or worm of "pork measles," is the intermediate stage of *Taenia solium*, the adult which occurs in the small intestine of man. In some instances this bladderworm has been found in cattle, sheep, deer and man. The cysticerci are most frequent in striated muscles, particularly of the neck, cheek, shoulder and tongue, but the heart, abdominal wall, liver, lungs, brain and eye may be involved. This bladderworm is very like *Cysticercus bovis*, except that the scolex bears a double row of hooklets. This tapeworm is of serious import in man because of the possibility of autoinfection, with cysticerci developing in the tissues. Diagnosis in man is often possible by radiography because of the frequent calcification of mature cysts.

Cysticercus ovis, the intermediate stage of *Taenia ovis*, a tapeworm of dogs, foxes, wolves, coyotes, and other carnivores, is the cause of sheep "measles," or ovine cysticercosis. The bladderworms are found in the connective tissue of the heart, voluntary muscles, esophagus, and rarely the lungs of sheep and goats. The effect of this parasite on its intermediate host is similar to that of the other cysticerci that invade the same tissues. Experimental feeding of large numbers of gravid proglottides of *Taenia ovis* has caused death in sheep. Heavy infections are also the cause of condemnation of animals slaughtered for food.

Coenurus cerebralis, the larval stage of a dog tapeworm, *Multiceps multiceps*, is the causative agent of a rather uncommon disease of the central nervous system of sheep, known as "gid" or "sturdy," and may also infect other herbivorous animals. Symptoms indicating central nervous involvement depend upon localization of the bladderworms in the brain or spinal cord and vary from incoordination to paralysis. The larvae wander through the body before localizing in nervous tissue in the form of cysts which reach a diameter of 50 mm. or more. Each cyst is filled with clear fluid and contains as many as 500 scolices, visible through the thin walls of the cyst as small white foci. The **coenurus** is a modified cysticercus with a germinal layer and the ability to produce many scolices.

Cysticercus tenuicollis, the intermediate stage of a tapeworm of dogs and other carnivores, *Taenia hydatigena*, is found chiefly in the liver, mesentery and omentum of squirrels, cattle, wild ruminants, sheep and swine. The cysticerci may be large, often attaining a diameter of 80 mm., but they contain only a single scolex armed with a double row of hooklets. The effect upon the intermediate host may not be obvious, the cysticerci merely being noted during post-mortem examination.

Other cysticerci that may be encountered by the veterinary pathologist include *Cysticercus pisiformis*, which occurs on the peritoneum and liver capsule of rabbits, squirrels and other small rodents. The adult stage of this parasite (*Taenia pisiformis*) is attained in the small intestine of the dog, cat, fox, wolf and other carnivores. A similar parasite, *Cysticercus fasciolaris* (or *crassicollis*), is found embedded in the liver of rats, mice and other rodents; the adult form (*Taenia taeniaeformis*) being a tapeworm of the cat, less often of the dog, fox and other carnivores. *Cysticercus fasciolaris* is of particular interest because of the undifferentiated sarcoma which often develops in the rat liver adjacent to the parasites. A bladderworm found in the subcutis of rabbits is known as *Coenurus serialis* and is the intermediate stage of *Multiceps serialis*, a tapeworm of the dog and closely related carnivores.

Sparganosis is a term used to designate infection with the larva (**sparganum**) of certain Pseudophyllidea; the adults occur in mammals. The sparganum is an elongated, solid larva (**plerocercoid**) which may increase in number by transverse division. The first intermediate hosts are species of *Cyclopidae* and the second are frogs, snakes and mammals. In some, the sparganum is recognized but the adult form has not been identified. *Sparganum proliferum* occurs in the muscles and connective tissues of man in Taiwan and Japan and the adult stage is thought to be *Spirometra ranarum*, parasitic in frogs. *Spirometra mansoni*, found in dogs and cats in Asia, produces spargana which are found in the connective tissues of frogs and snakes. This *Sparganum mansoni* may infect the eye of man through the practice of applying the flesh of frogs to treat eye disease or by the consumption of infected *Cyclops sp.* or frogs or snakes.

Spirometra mansonoides parasitizes the cat, bobcat and dog in North America. Larvae (*procercoids*) infect various *Cyclops* species (*C. leukarti, C. bicuspidatus* and *C. viridis*) and the second intermediate hosts are wild mice, rats and snakes. Experimental infection of man has been demonstrated.

Spirometra erinacei has been found in the intestine of foxes and cats in Asia and Australia.

Wild pigs infected with spargana have been found in the same habitat and are believed to have acquired them from infected crustaceans or frogs. The precise association and identification of the larvae and adult forms of these parasites are not clearly established.

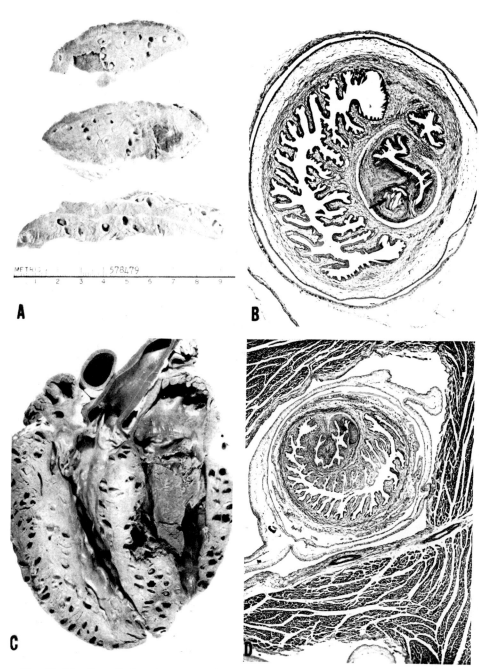

FIG. 15–28.—Cestodiasis. An unusual bovine infection with the pork tapeworm *Cysticercus cellulosae* (*Taenia solium*). *A*, Skeletal muscles containing cysticerci. *B*, A single inverted scolex (× 38). Note hooklets (arrow) which distinguish this larva from that of the more common beef tapeworm, *Cysticercus bovis* (*Taenia saginata*). *C*, Cysticerci in the myocardium. *D*, A single cysticercus (× 21) in the heart muscle. (Courtesy of Armed Forces Institute of Pathology.) Contributor: Major C. N. Barron.

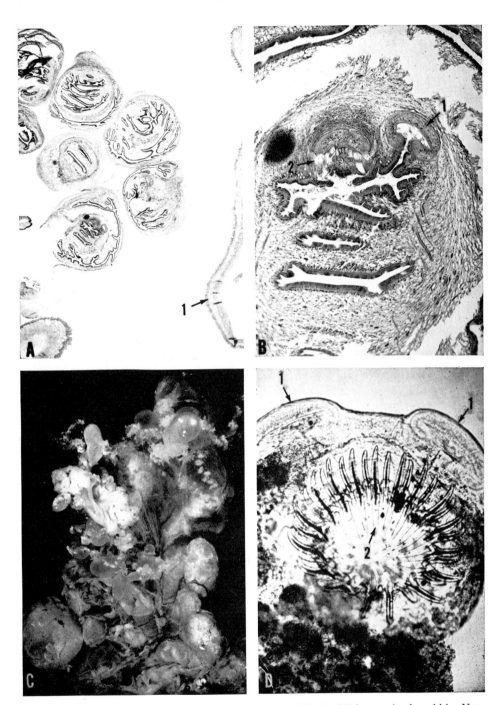

FIG. 15–29.—Cestodiasis. *A*, Coenurus of *Multiceps serialis* (× 12) in muscle of a rabbit. Note several scolices and wall of cyst (*1*). *B*, A single inverted scolex of *M. serialis* (× 50). Note sucker (*1*) and hooklets (*2*). Contributor: Capt. Morris Schneider, V.C. *C*, *Multiceps serialis*, larvae from the subcutis of a monkey. Contributor: National Zoological Park. *D*, Everted scolex (× 150) of *Taenia pisiformis*, larva from the peritoneum of a deer. Note suckers (*1*) and hooklets (*2*). (Courtesy of Armed Forces Institute of Pathology.) Contributor: Capt. James R. Prine.

Cysticercosis, Coenuriasis, Sparganosis

BANERJEE, D., and SINGH, K. S.: Studies on *Cysticercus fasciolaris*. III. Histopathology and Histochemistry of Rat Liver in Cysticerciasis. Indian J. Anim. Sci. *39*:242–249, 1969.

CLARK, J. D.: Coenurosis in a Gelada Baboon (*Theropithecus gelada*). J. Am. Vet. Med. Assn. *155*:1258–1263, 1969.

CORKUM, K. C.: Sparganosis in Some Vertebrates of Louisiana and Observations on Human Infection. J. Parasit. *52*:444–448, 1966.

DEWHIRST, L. W., and CRAMER, J. D.: Serum Enzyme Levels in Cattle Infected with Cysticerci of *Taenia saginata*. J. Parasit. *51*:40, 1965.

DINNIK, J. A., and SACHS, R.: Cysticercosis, Echinococcosis and Sparganosis in Wild Herbivores in East Africa. Vet. Med. Rev. Leverkusen, No. 2. 104–114, 1969.

DUGUID, J. B., and SHEPPARD, E. M.: A Diphyllobothrium Epidemic in Trout. J. Path. & Bact. *56*:73–80, 1944.

GEORGI, J. R., DE LAHUNTA, A., and PERCY, D. H.: Cerebral Coenurosis in a Cat. Report of a Case. Cornell Vet. *59*:127–134, 1969.

GREVE, J. H., and TYLER, D. E.: *Cysticercus pisiformis* (Cestoda: Taenidae) in the Liver of a Dog. J. Parasit. *50*:712–716, 1964.

IRFAN, M., and HATCH, C.: The Pathology of *Taenia hydatigena* Infection in Irish Lambs. Irish Vet. J. *23*:62–66, 1969.

IVENS, V., CONROY, J. D., and LEVINE, M. D.: *Taenia pisiformis* Cysticerci in a Dog in Illinois. Am. J. Vet. Res. *30*:2017–2020, 1969.

KASSAI, T., and MAHUNKA, S.: Vectors of *Moniezia*. Magy. Allatorv. Lap. *19*:531–538, 1964. V.B. *35*:4282, 1965.

LARSH, J. E., JR., RACE, G. J., and ESCH, G. W.: A Histopathologic Study of Mice Infected with the Larval Stage of *Multiceps serialis*. J. Parasit. *51*:45–52, 1965.

LLOYDS, T. S.: Hepatitis Cysticercosa Causing Sudden Death in a Pig. Vet. Rec. *76*:1080, 1964.

McINTOSH, A., and MILLER, D.: Bovine Cysticercosis, with Special Reference to the Early Developmental Stages of *Taenia saginata*. Am. J. Vet. Res. *21*:169–177, 1960.

MARAZZA, V. and PERSIANI, G.: Indagine Cisticercopsia in Luce di Wood su Carni Bovine Nazionali ed estere Ammesse al Libero Consume. Arch. Vet. Ital. *12*:201–226, 1961. (VB 187–62.)

NORMAN, L., SADUM, E. H., and ALLAIN, D. S.: A Bentonite Flocculation Test for the Diagnosis of Hydrated Disease in Man and Animals. Am. J. Trop. Med. & Hyg. *8*:46–50, 1959.

REES, G.: Pathogenesis of Adult Cestodes. Helminth Abstr. *36*:1–23, 1967.

SCHIEFER, B.: Sudden Death of Pigs Caused by *Cysticercus tenuicollis*. Tierarztl. Umsch *21*:276–278, and 281, 1966. V.B. *36*:4819, 1966.

SHARMA DEORANI, V. P.: Histopathological Studies on Hepatitis-cysticercosa Lesions in Sheep and a Deer. Indian Vet. J. *44*:939–942, 1967.

SHUL'TS, R. S., *et al.*: Pathological and Immunological Changes During Prolonged Repeated Infection with Helminths. Izv. Akad. Nauk. kazakh. SSR, Ser. biol. Nauk No. 5, 19–29, 1968. V.B. *39*:2572, 1969.

SILVERMAN, P. H. and HULLAND, T. J.: Histological Observations on Bovine Cysticercosis. Res. Vet. Sci. *2*:248–252, 1961. (VB 4022–61.)

TAZIEVA, A. KH.: Histological Differences Between Cysticerci of Small Ruminants. Parazity sel'skokhoz zhivotnykh Kazakhstan *3*:7–29, 1964. V.B. *35*:975, 1965.

THOMPSON, J. E.: Some Observations on the European Broad Fish Tapeworm *Diphyllobothrium latum*. J. Am. Vet. Med. Assn. *89*:77–86, 1936.

TROPLO, J.: *Cysticercus pisiformis* and *Fasciola hepatica* Infection in Hares. Medycyna wet. *20*:592–594, 1964. V.B. *35*:1388, 1965.

VICKERS, J. H., and PENNER, L. R.: Cysticercosis in Four Rhesus Brains. J. Am. Vet. Med. Assn. *153*:868–871, 1968.

VOGE, M., and BERNTZEN, A. K.: Asexual Multiplication of Larval Tapeworms as the Cause of Fatal Parasitic Ascites in Dogs. J. Parasit. *49*:983–988, 1963.

WARDLE, R. A., and McLEOD, J. A.: *The Zoology of Tapeworms*, Minneapolis, University of Minnesota Press, 1952.

Echinococcosis.—The intermediate stage of *Echinococcus granulosus*, a tapeworm of dogs, foxes, wolves and other carnivores, is of importance because of the effects of the larvae upon their intermediate hosts, which include sheep, goats, cattle, horses, deer, moose, swine, monkeys and man. In man, **echinococcosis or hydatid disease** is particularly serious because the cysts may reach any part of the

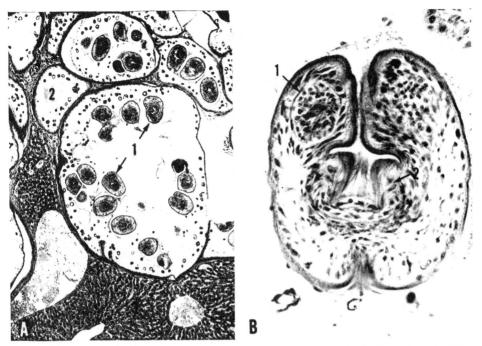

FIG. 15–30.—Echinococcosis. *A, Echinococcus multilocularis* ($\times$ 50) in the liver of a vole. Note many inverted scolices (*1*), some surrounded by a thin, brood capsule. Some daughter cysts (*2*) do not yet contain fully developed scolices. Liver parenchyma (*3*) is displaced by the cysts. *B*, A single scolex ($\times$ 525). Note part of inverted sucker (*1*) and hooklets (*2*). (Courtesy of Armed Forces Institute of Pathology.) Contributor: Dr. Robert Rausch.

body, especially the liver and lung, but also the brain, where their large size (up to 200 mm. diameter) and tendency to produce endogenous daughter cysts may displace vital tissues. The cysts grow slowly, often being encapsulated by dense fibrous tissue of the host. The larva has an outer dense laminated wall without nuclei, which encloses a germinal layer. From this layer numerous spherical brood capsules arise, which may be attached by a short stalk or may be free in the bladder. Each brood capsule contains germinal epithelium from which as many as 40 scolices arise. Each scolex is ovoid and bears a crown of 32 to 40 hooklets, 21 to 29 microns in length. In addition to producing brood capsules, the germinal epithelium of the larva may give rise to daughter cysts, which may remain free within the parent cyst or grow outside the parent cyst. The ability to form exogenous daughter cysts is limited to *Echinococcus multilocularis (alveolaris)*, according to the work of Rausch (1954). His observations indicate that the "alveolar form" of the disease is caused by *E. multilocularis*, a distinct species with a separate but overlapping host and geographic distribution. Daughter cysts may produce additional brood capsules containing scolices. Individual scolices also may arise within the brood capsules or directly from the germinal layers of parent or daughter cysts. It is readily apparent that the potential of the intermediate stage of either *Echinococcus granulosus* or *multilocularis* for growth and reproduction is considerable. The effect upon the intermediate host is therefore dependent upon the organ parasitized and the size attained by the hydatid cysts. In some parts of the world hydatidosis is a major problem in public health.

Several subspecies of *E. granulosa* have been described from South Africa (Verster, 1965). The host range of these parasites has not been defined. They have been named as follows: *Echinococcus granulosus, E. g. africanus, E. g. felidus, E. g. lycaontis,* and *E. g. ortleppi.*

Diagnosis.—The presence of the adult worm in the intestinal tract can be verified by the demonstration of segments and ova in the feces, but the intermediate stage presents more difficulties. The hydatid cysts may be identified by pathologic examination of tissue removed at exploratory laparotomy or at necropsy. A complement fixation test is known.

Echinococcosis

CROSBY, W. H., *et al.*:   Echinococcus Cysts in the Savannah Baboon.   Lab. Anim. Care *18*: 395–397, 1968.

DENT, C. H. R.:   Cerebral Hydatids in a Cow.   Aust. Vet. J. *42*:28–30, 1966.

HEALY, G. R., and HAYES, N. R.:   Hydatid Disease in Rhesus Monkeys.   J. Parasit. *49*:837, 1963.

HUTCHISON, W. F.:   "Studies on *Echinococcus Granulosus*. III. The Rhesus Monkey (*Macaca mulatta*) as a Laboratory Host for the Larval Stage."   J. Parasit. *52*:416, 1966.

ILIEVSKI, V., and ESBER, H.:   Hydatid Disease in a Rhesus Monkey.   Lab. Anim. Care *19*: 199–204, 1969.

KOSTYAK, J., and ADAM, T.:   Experimental Echinococcosis in Pigs.   Magy. Allatorv. Lap. *20*:166–169, 1965.   V.B. *36*:1861, 1966.

LEIBY, P. D.:   Cestode in North Dakota: Echinococcus in Field Mice.   Science *150*:763, 1965.

LEIBY, P. D., and OLSEN, O. W.:   The Cestode *Echinococcus multilocularis* in Foxes in North Dakota.   Science *145*:1066, 1964.

MATOFF, K., and YANCHEV, Y.:   The Fox as Definitive Host of *Echinococcus granulosus*. Acta Vet. Hung. *15*:155–160, 1965.   V.B. *36*:640–1966.

MYERS, B. J., KUNTZ, R. E., and VICE, T. E.:   Hydatid Disease in Captive Primates (*Colobus* and *Papio*).   J. Parasit. *51*: (Suppl.) 22, 1965.

POWERS, R. D., PRICE, R. A., HOUK, R. P., and MATTLIN, R. H.:   Echinococcosis in a Drill Baboon.   J. Am. Vet. Med. Assn. *149*:902–905, 1966.

RAUSCH, R.:   Studies on the Helminth Fauna of Alaska.   XX. The Histogenesis of the Alveolar Larvae of *Echinococcus* Species.   J. Infect. Dis. *94*:178–186, 1954.

RAUSCH, R., and SCHILLER, E. L.:   Studies on the Helminth Fauna of Alaska.   XXIV. *Echinococcus sibiricensis* N. Sp. from St. Lawrence Island.   J. Parasitol. *40*:659–662, 1954.

SIMITCH, T.:   (*Echinococcus multilocularis* and *E. granulous:* World Incidence and Distribution.)   Bull. Off. Int. Epizoot. *62*:1031–1061, 1964.

SMYTH, J. D., and SMYTH, M. M.:   Some Aspects of Host Specificity in *Echinococcus granulosus*.   Helminthologia *9*:519–529, 1968.

VERSTER, A. J. M.:   Review of Echinococcus Species in South Africa.   Onderstepoort J. Vet. Res. *32*:7–118, 1965.

WARD, J. W.:   Additional Records of *Echinococcus granulosus* from Dogs in the Lower Mississippi Region.   J. Parasit. *51*:552–553, 1965.

DISTOMIASIS

(Fascioliasis, Liver Fluke Disease, Liver Rot, Fascioloidiasis, Dicrocoeliasis)

The liver flukes recognized as significant pathogens in domestic animals are presently classified within the order Digenea under the class Trematoda and are limited to two families, Fasciolidae and Dicrocoeliidae. Four species are of particular importance as the cause of distomiasis in animals: *Fasciola hepatica* (common liver fluke), *Fasciola gigantica* (large Africa liver fluke), *Fascioloides magna* (large liver fluke), and *Dicrocoelium dendriticum* (lancet fluke).

Fasciola hepatica in its adult form is found in the liver, bile ducts and gallbladder of cattle and sheep, but it may also parasitize the horse, goat, dog,

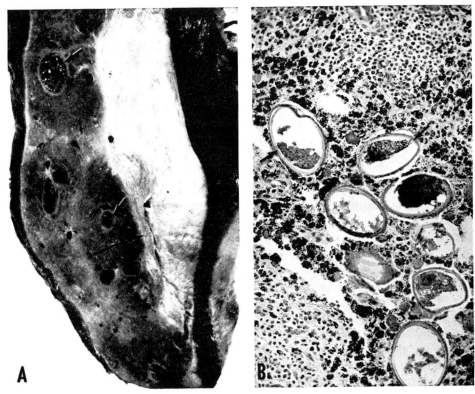

FIG. 15–31.—Distomiasis. *A*, Liver of a sheep with distended, thick-walled bile ducts (arrows) containing *Dicrocoelium dendriticum.* Contributor: Dr. G. Dikmans. *B*, Ova of *Fascioloides magna* (arrows) in a bovine liver (× 150). Note black granular pigment interspersed among the ova. (Courtesy of Armed Forces Institute of Pathology.) Contributor: Dr. Henry J. Griffiths.

rabbit, guinea pig, squirrel, deer, beaver, pig and man. The adult fluke is 20 to 30 mm. long and about 13 mm. wide, flattened and leaf-like, and usually reddish-brown. It is hermaphroditic and reproduces by depositing ova in the biliary passages, through which they reach the intestine and are expelled with the feces. Each ovum produces a free-living form, a miracidium, which penetrates the body of one of several varieties of snails where encystment and asexual reproduction take place through several stages, the parasites finally emerging from the snail in motile forms known as cercariae which usually encyst on plants or other vegetation. In this form, called **metacercariae**, the parasites are ingested by cattle or other hosts; when they reach the intestines they excyst, penetrate the wall and migrate to the liver, eventually developing to maturity in the biliary passages.

Fasciola gigantica resembles *Fasciola hepatica* but is larger, the adult measures up to 75 mm. in length and is about 12 mm. wide. The eggs measure 156 to 197 microns by 90 to 104 microns. These flukes are common parasites of cattle and sheep in Africa and are reported to occur in India, Taiwan, Hawaii and the Philippines. The intermediate hosts (Kendall and Parfitt, 1965) are different races of the snail *Lymnaea auricularia.* The effects of this trematode on the adult host are similar to those caused by *Fasciola hepatica.*

The **signs** of distomiasis are hardly specific, since they consist of weakness, **anemia,** emaciation and, at times, icterus. Diarrhea and constipation have been observed.   Severe infection, particularly of calves, may result in prostration and death.

The **lesions** produced by the common liver fluke are most constant and important in the liver, although occasional parasites may wander into the lungs or other tissues, where they are usually found within abscesses.   Infective metacercariae of *Fasciola hepatica*, upon ingestion by a definitive host, pass through the intestinal wall into the peritoneal cavity, thence migrating into the liver parenchyma.   The immature flukes spend about six weeks in the liver parenchyma, starting to reach the bile ducts during the seventh week.   As the larvae migrate through the liver parenchyma they result in damage to the liver which is dependent upon the number of parasites, their survival at death at this site and the tissue reaction of the host.   After the initial penetration of the liver parenchyma by the flukes, hepatic cells are destroyed and the larvae lie in a pool of blood, fibrin and cellular debris.   As some larvae die and the host apparently develops sensitivity to the parasite, neutrophils, eosinophils and lymphocytes become part of the infiltrate.   Macrophages and epithelioid cells become increasingly numerous in older lesions and particularly around dead larvae.

This migration of metacercariae through the liver results in interference with liver function which may be manifest by icterus, changes in liver function tests, loss of weight and in severe infections, death.   These changes are described in detail by Dow, Ross and Todd (1967 and 1968) in calves and sheep.   Changes in serum enzymes are reported by Thorpe and Ford (1969).

The flukes which reach the bile ducts start producing eggs by the tenth week following oral infection.   The presence of these parasites in the biliary passages excites considerable tissue reaction.   The biliary epithelium is stimulated to excessive growth in some places and is eroded in others.   Partial or complete occlusion of bile ducts is a frequent effect.   The walls of involved bile ducts even-

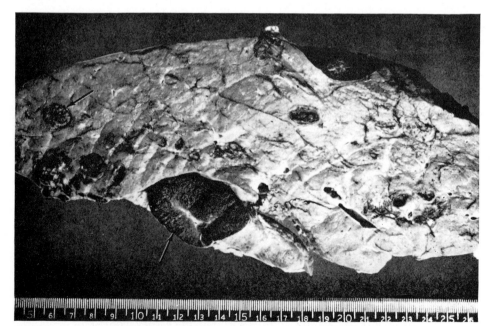

FIG. 15–32.—Circumscribed zones of black pigment in the liver of a deer infected with *Fascioloides magna*, the large liver fluke.   The adjacent lymph nodes contained similar pigment.

tually become greatly thickened from fibrous proliferation, and calcification may take place in the fibrotic areas. The scarring around bile ducts often extends deep into the hepatic lobules, producing severe fibrosis in the perilobular connective tissue. Scarring and calcification may affect large parts of the liver. In long-standing infections, fibrosis and occasional occlusion of bile ducts interferes with liver function, leading to weight loss or failure to gain normally. A normocytic, normochromic anemia may result in this chronic phase of the infection. This anemia is not due to blood-sucking by the parasites because they have been shown to feed on hepatic and ductal tissue, not blood. One postulated explanation is that the presence of the flukes interferes with the absorption of vitamin B_{12} or in some other way depresses hematopoiesis.

Fascioloides magna, the large liver fluke, occurs in the liver of cattle, deer, sheep, moose, horses, wapiti, yak and bison, and has also been reported in the lungs of some of these hosts. Rabbits and guinea pigs are susceptible to experimental infection. This fluke is similar in appearance to the common liver fluke except that it is larger, 30 by 80 mm. in greatest dimensions, and has more rounded ends. It is hermaphroditic and its life cycle is similar to that of *Fasciola hepatica*, snails being required as intermediate hosts. The infective forms penetrate the intestinal wall and wander around in the peritoneal cavity before invading the liver. Within the liver parenchyma, the migrations of this fluke produce severe damage in some hosts, less in others. In the "true" hosts (deer, wapiti, moose), the parasite is reasonably well tolerated. Although it soon becomes encysted, the cyst wall is thin and its lumen communicates with bile ducts. Thus, ova of the fluke escape with its excreta into the intestinal lumen of the host, a factor which favors the completion of the life cycle of the parasite.

In **Bovidae** (cattle, bison, yak), however, the flukes wander briefly through the liver parenchyma, destroying tissue and eliciting a reaction of the host which encapsulates the parasites. A cyst soon forms, but its lumen rarely communicates with the bile ducts; hence, excreta and ova accumulate around the fluke. Black granular pigment collects in the cyst and is phagocytized by the macrophages of the host. This distinctive pigment is believed to be part of the excrement of the fluke, because similar material can be found within its alimentary tract. The black, sooty pigment is often grossly visible in affected liver. The failure of the fluke to establish and maintain continuity with the bile ducts in these hosts prevents the ova from escaping. For this reason, cattle and bison are unfavorable hosts for the propagation of the parasite.

In **sheep**, the migration of this large liver fluke through the liver is almost entirely unchecked; hence, severe tissue destruction and marked clinical disease result. A severe neutrophilic tissue reaction with little attempt at encapsulation is the rule in the liver of infected sheep. Even a few flukes may, by their wanderings through the liver, produce severe symptoms and death in sheep. The death of this host brings to a halt the life cycle of the parasite; therefore the sheep is not considered a true host for *Fascioloides magna*.

Dicrocoelium dendriticum, the Old World, or lancet, fluke, is known to be capable of infecting cattle, sheep, goats, horses, camels, deer, elk, pigs, rabbits and man. This parasite, smaller than the other flukes, is from 5 to 12 mm. long and about 1 mm. wide. It is slender, flat and lancet-shaped, with pointed ends.

The life cycle of the lancet fluke has been elucidated by the work of Krull and Mapes (1953), who found that this parasite requires not only a snail as intermediate host, but also an ant (*Formica fusca*) as a second intermediate host. The final hosts are infected by the ingestion of ants containing encysted metacercariae. A fascinating bit of biological knowledge lies in the report of Anokhin (1966) who confirmed Hohorst's observation that encysted metacercariae in the brains of ants (*Formica nigricans*) cause the ants to remain on herbage after normal ants return to their nest. This presumably increases the possibility that infected ants will be ingested by a grazing cow or sheep. The adult flukes are found in the bile ducts of the definitive host. Their effect is similar to that of *Fasciola hepatica*, but, being smaller, they may be found in smaller bile ducts. The walls of the bile ducts are thickened, and general periportal fibrosis may be produced by the parasite. There is little tendency for destruction of liver parenchyma.

Diagnosis.—Distomiasis can be recognized in the living host by the identification of characteristic ova in the feces (Fig. 15–31). At necropsy, or biopsy of the liver, the lesions in the liver are typical and the parasite can usually be found in the liver parenchyma or affected biliary system.

Distomiasis

ANOKHIN, I. A.: The Diurnal Rhythm of Ants Invaded by *Dicrocoelium lanceatum* Metacercariae. Dokl. Akad. Nauk. SSSR *166*:757–759, 1966.

ASHIZAWA, H.: Pathological Studies on Fascioliasis. I. The Liver of Goats. II. The Liver of Sheep. III. The Liver of Cattle. IV. The Liver of Experimentally Infected Goats, Rabbits and Guinea Pigs. Bull. Fac. Agric. Univ. Miyazaki *9*:1–44 & 143–191; *10*:1–40 & 189–221, 1963/65. V.B. *35*:3886, 1965.

————: Pathological Studies on Fascioliasis. V. Parasitic Bronchiectasis in Cattle Caused by *Fasciola sp.* Bull. Fac. Agric. Univ. Miyazaki *12*:1–57, 1966. V.B. *37*:4779, 1967.

BAILENGER, J., *et al.*: Hares and Rabbits as Reservoirs of *Fasciola hepatica* and *Dicrocoelium dendriticum*. Annls. Parasit. Hum. Comp. *40*:51–54, 1965. V.B. *35*:4644, 1965.

BAKER, D. W., and NELSON, S. K.: *Dicrocoelium dendriticum* Infections in New York State Cattle. Cornell Vet. *33*:250–256, 1943.

BASCH, P. F.: Completion of the Life Cycle of *Eurytrema pancreaticum* (Trematoda: Dicrocoeliidae.) J. Parasit. *51*:350–355, 1965.

BENGTSSON, E., *et al.*: Infestation with *Dicrocoelium dendriticum*—the Small Liver Fluke—in Animals and Human Individuals in Sweden. Acta Path. Microbiol. Scand. *74*:85–92, 1968.

COSGROVE, G. E.: The Trematodes of Laboratory Primates. Lab. Anim. Care *16*:23–39, 1966.

DOW, C., ROSS, J. G., and TODD, J. R.: The Pathology of Experimental Fascioliasis in Calves. J. Comp. Path. *77*:377–385, 1967.

————: The Histopathology of *Fasciola hepatica* Infections in Sheep. Parasitology *58*:129–135, 1968.

HATCH, C.: *Fasciola hepatica* Infection in Donkeys. Irish Vet. J. *20*:130, 1966.

HOLMES, P. H., *et al.*: Albumin and Globulin Turnover in Chronic Ovine Fascioliasis. Vet. Rec. *83*:227–228, 1968.

KECK, G., and SUPPERER, R.: Studies on the Large Liver Fluke. I. The X-ray Picture of Isolated Ox Livers. II. The Course of Infection of the Bovine Liver. Wien. tierarztl. Mschr. *53*:29–33, & 328–331, 1966. V.B. *36*:3548, 1966.

KENDALL, S. B.: Host Specificity as Evidenced by Species of *Fasciola*. Helminthologia *8*:223–233, 1968.

KENDALL, S. B., and PARFITT, J. W.: The Life-history of Some Vectors of *Fasciola gigantica* under Laboratory Conditions. Ann. Trop. Med. Parasit. *59*:10–16, 1965.

KONRAD, J.: The Biochemical Picture of Bovine Hepatic Cirrhosis Due to Fascioliasis. Tier-arztl. Umsch. *23*:369–372, & 375–376, 1968. V.B. *39*:215, 1969.

KRULL, W. H., and MAPES, C. R.: Studies on the Biology of *Dicrocoelium dendriticum* (Rudolphi, 1819) Looss 1899 — Including its Relation to the Intermediate Host, *Cionella lubrica* (Müller). III. Observations on the Slimeballs of *Dicrocoelium dendriticum*. Cornell Vet. *42*:253–276, 1952.

————: Studies on the Biology of *Dicrocoelium dendriticum* (Rudolphi, 1819) Looss 1899 — Including its Relation to the Intermediate Host, *Cionella lubrica* (Müller). IV. Infection Experiments Involving Definitive Hosts. Cornell Vet. *42*:277–285, 1952.

————: Studies on the Biology of *Dicrocoelium dendriticum* (Rudolphi, 1819) Looss 1899 — Including its Relation to the Intermediate Host *Cionella lubrica*. IX. Notes on the Cyst, Metacercaria, and Infection in the Ant, *Formica fusca*. Cornell Vet. *43*:389–410, 1953.

MACLEAN, J., *et al.*: Pathophysiology of *Fasciola hepatica* Infections. In *"Isotopes and Radiation In Parasitology,"* 117–123, Vienna, Internat. Atomic Energy Agency, 1968.

MORRILL, P. R., and SHAW, J. N.: Studies of Pathology in Cattle Produced by Liver Fluke (*Fasciola hepatica*). Oregon State Coll. Exper. Sta. Bull. 408, p. 30, 1942.

NANSEN, P., *et al.*: Chronic Fascioliasis in Sheep. II. Metabolism of ^{131}I-labelled Albumin and ^{125}I-labelled Immunoglobulin-G. Nord. Vet. Med. *20*:651–656, 1968.

PINKIEWICZ, E., and MADEJ, E.: Changes in the Peripheral Blood of Ca, P, K, Na, Mg and AP in the Course of Experimental Fascioliasis in Sheep. Acta Parasit. Polon. *15*:225–229, 1967. V.B. *39*:217, 1969.

POLJAKOVA-KRUSTEVA, O., *et al.*: The Morphogenesis of Experimental Fascioliasis. J. Helminth. *42*:367–372, 1968.

RAHKO, T.: The Pathology of Natural *Fasciola hepatica* Infection in Cattle. Path. Vet. *6*: 244–256, 1969.

ROBINSON, V. B. and EHRENFORD, F. A.: Hepatic Lesions Associated with Liver Fluke (*Platynosomum fastosum*) Infection in a Cat. Am. J. Vet. Res. *23*:1300–1303, 1962.

ROSS, J. G., DOW, C., and TODD, J. R.: A Study of *Fasciola hepatica* Infections in Sheep. Vet. Rec. *80*:543–546, 1967.

————: The Pathology of *Fasciola hepatica* Infection in Pigs. A Comparison of the Infection in Pigs and Other Hosts. Brit. Vet. J. *123*:317–322, 1967.

ROSS, J. G.: Experimental Infections of Cattle with *Fasciola hepatica*: A Comparison of Low and High Infection Rates. Nature (Lond.) *208*:907, 1965.

————: Studies of Immunity to *Fasciola hepatica*. Naturally Acquired Immunity in Rabbits. Brit. Vet. J. *122*:209–211, 1966.

ROSS, J. G., and DOW, C.: The Problem of Acute Fascioliasis in Cattle. Vet. Rec. *78*:670, 1966.

ROSSOW, N., *et al.*: The Liver in Bovine Fascioliasis: Biopsy and Function Tests. Arch. Exp. Vet. Med. *20*:307–321, 1966. V.B. *37*:602, 1967.

ROTHENBACHER, H. and LINDQUIST, W. D.: Liver Cirrhosis and Pancreatitis in a Cat Infected with *Amphimerus pseudofelineus* (a fluke). J. Am. Vet. Med. Assn. *143*:1099–1102, 1963.

RUBAJ, B., and FURMAGA, S.: Pathomorphological and Histochemical Studies of Livers of Sheep Experimentally Infected with the Liver Fluke. Acta Parasit. Polon. *16*:77–81, 1969. V.B. *39*:5048, 1969.

SEWELL, M. M. H.: The Immunology of Fascioliasis. II. Qualitative Studies on the Precipitin Reaction. Immunology *7*:671–680, 1964.

————: The Pathogenesis of Fascioliasis. Vet. Rec. *78*:98–105, 1966.

————: Serum Enzyme Activities in Acute Ovine Fascioliasis. Vet. Rec. *80*:577–578, 1967.

SIMESEN, M. G., *et al.*: Chronic Fascioliasis in Sheep. I. Clinical, Clinical-pathological and Histological Studies. Nord. Vet. Med. *20*:638–650, 1968. V.B. *39*:2100, 1969.

SINCLAIR, K. B.: Iron Metabolism in Ovine Fascioliasis. Brit. Vet. J. *121*:451–461, 1965.

————: The Effect of Splenectomy on the Pathogenicity of *Fasciola hepatica* in the Sheep. Brit. Vet. J. *126*:15–29, 1970.

SOFRENOVIC, D. *et al.*: Pathology, Incidence and Diagnosis of Liver Flukes in Pigs. In Serbian. Acta Vet., Belgrade. *11*:31–40, 1961. (VB 186–62.)

STEMMERMANN, G. N.: Human Infestation with *Fasciola gigantica*. Am. J. Path. *29*:731–753, 1953.

STRAUSS, J. M., and HEYNEMAN, D.: Fatal Ectopic Fascioliasis in a Guinea Pig Breeding Colony from Malacca. J. Parasit. *52*:413, 1966.

SWALES, W. E.: The Life Cycle of *Fascioloides magna* (Bassi, 1875). The Large Liver Fluke of Ruminants in Canada. Canad. J. Research. *12*:177–215, 1935.

————: Further Studies on *Fascioloides magna* (Bassi, 1875), Ward 1917, as a Parasite of Ruminants. Canad. J. Research *14*:83–95, 1936.

SYMONS, L. E. A., and BORAY, J. C.: The Anaemia of Acute and Chronic Ovine Fascioliasis. Z. Tropenmed. Parasit. *19*:451–472, 1968. V.B. *39*:1648, 1969.

THORNBERRY, H.: *Dicrocoelium dendriticum* in Sheep. Irish Vet. J. *18*:213–214, 1964.

THORPE, E.: An Immunocytochemical Study with *Fasciola hepatica*. Parasitology *55*: 209–214, 1965.

————: A Histochemical Study with *Fasciola hepatica*. Res. Vet. Sci. *8*:27–36, 1967.

————: Comparative Enzyme Histochemistry of Immature and Mature Stages of *Fasciola hepatica*. Expl. Parasit. *22*:150–159, 1968.

THORPE, E., and FORD, E. J. H.: Serum Enzyme and Hepatic Changes in Sheep Infested with *Fasciola hepatica*. J. Path. *97*:619–629, 1969.

TSVETAEVA, N. P., and GUMEN'SHCHIKOVA, V. P.: Pathology and Histochemistry of the Liver of Sheep with Acute or Chronic Fascioliasis Following Single Infection, Superinfection and Reinfection. Mater. Konf. Vses. Obshch. Gel'mint. *2*:255–259, 1965. V.B. *37*:2693, 1967.

SCHISTOSOMIASIS

Studies of ancient Egyptian records and mummies indicate that since the pre-Christian era the people of the Middle East have been subject to a disease in which hematuria, dysentry and cirrhosis were prominent features. It was not until 1851 that Bilharz observed adult flukes in the veins of an Egyptian, and even later before he demonstrated the relation of the organisms to this prevalent and historic disease. Many more years elapsed before Leiper, in 1918, demonstrated experimentally that two separate parasites were responsible for the human disease and that snails were necessary intermediate hosts for the blood flukes.

Although schistosomiasis is today an important parasitic disease in man and animals in many parts of the world, it is not prevalent in the United States, except for some infection of wild birds.

These worms are small trematodes which live in the blood vessels of their hosts; their ova, which circulate as emboli and lodge in tissue as foreign bodies, produce the principal pathologic changes in the host. The females are slender round worms, 1.4 to 2.0 cm. in length; the distinctive feature of the slightly shorter male is a long gynecophoric canal, a canoe-shaped structure in which the female is

Table 15–3.—Schistosomiasis

Species	Natural Definitive Hosts	Anatomic Site of Adult Fluke	Geographic Distribution
Schistosoma japonicum	Man, dog, cat, rat, cattle, sheept, water buffalo, goat, horse, swine.	Mesenteric veins, hemorrhoidal plexus.	China, Japan, Taiwan, Celebes, Philippines.
S. hematobium	Man, monkey.	Pelvic veins, esp. vesical and mesenteric, vesico-prostatic, pubic and uterine plexus.	Africa, Western Asia, Southern Europe and Australia.
S. mansoni	Man, monkey.	Mesenteric veins, hemorrhoidal plexus.	Africa, South America, West Indies.
S. bovis	Cattle, sheep, goat, horse, mule, antelope and baboon.	Portal and mesenteric veins.	Africa, Southern Asia, Sardinia.
S. spindale	Cattle, sheep, goat, horse, antelope, water buffalo.	Mesenteric veins.	India, Sumatra, Africa.
Schistosomatium douthitti	Meadow mouse, muskrat.	Mesenteric veins.	North America.
Trichobilharzia ocellata	Wild and domesticated ducks.	Mesenteric veins.	Europe and North America.
T. stagnicolae	Canaries, other birds (?).	Mesenteric veins.	North America.
T. physellae	Ducks and teal.	Mesenteric veins.	North America.
Heterobilharzia americana	Dog, raccoon, bobcat, rabbit, nutria.	Mesenteric veins.	North America.
Orientobilharzia harinasutai	Water buffalo.	Portal and mesenteric veins.	Thailand.
Schistosoma hippopotami	Hippopotamus.	Cardiovascular system generally.	South Africa.
Schistosoma incognitum	Dog, pig.	Mesenteric and portal veins.	India.

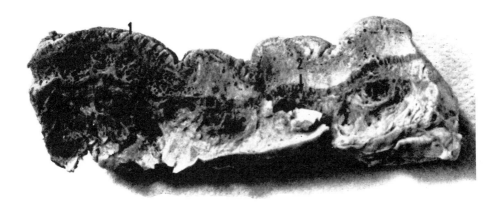

A

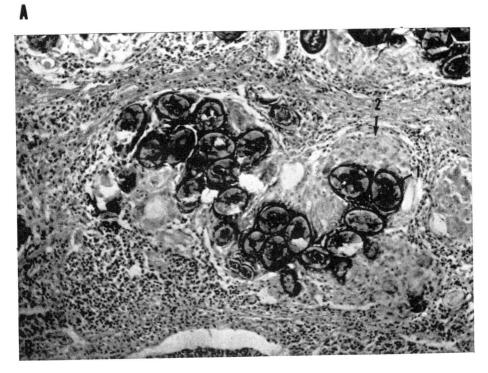

FIG. 15-33.—Schistosomiasis. *A*, Small intestine of a dog, with thickened submucosa (*1*) and muscularis. The inner part of the muscularis is marked (*2*). *B*, Ova of *Schistosoma japonicum* in a lymph node (× 135) of a dog. The ova (*1*) are surrounded by epithelioid cells (*2*) and fibrous stroma. (Courtesy of Armed Forces Institute of Pathology.) Contributor: 36th Evacuation Hospital.

held during coitus. The blood flukes are classified as Trematoda within the suborder Strigeata, with the parasites of birds and mammals grouped in the family Schistosomatidae. Table 15–3 summarizes certain characteristics of important blood flukes of man and animals.

Life Cycle.—All the blood flukes have similar life cycles. The adult female, after copulation with the male within the lumen of a vein, moves against the venous blood stream into small venules where she deposits the ova. Schistosomes that live in the mesenteric veins (*S. bovis, S. japonicum, Heterobilharzia americana* and *S. mansoni*) deposit their ova in venules of the intestine, while those that dwell in the vesical and other pelvic veins (*S. hematobium* and occasionally *S. mansoni*) utilize venules of the urinary bladder. The ova so deposited secrete cytolytic fluid through pores of the egg shell, which, assisted by the movement of the host's tissues, permits them to rupture the capillary walls and move through the tissues toward the lumen of the intestine or the urinary bladder. The successful ova leave the body of the host with the feces (*S. japonicum, S. bovis, H. american* and *S. mansoni*) or the urine, (*S. hematobium, S. mansoni*). Unsuccessful ova may remain in any tissue through which they are unable to pass, or they may be transported via the blood stream to other organs where they produce lesions. Fertile ova will not hatch in the tissues of the host, but upon reaching a favorable external environment, a single, ovoid ciliated organism, a **miracidium,** quickly escapes from the ovum. The miracidium swims about in water until it finds a suitable intermediate host, a snail, whose body it penetrates by a head-on boring action with the aid of proteolytic enzymes secreted by its cephalic glands.

Each schistosome has an affinity for one or more species of snail which it utilizes as an intermediate host. The availability of suitable gastropod hosts thus influences the geographic distribution of schistosomiasis.

Within the body of the snail, the miracidium soon becomes a thin-walled saccular sporocyst which reproduces several daughter sporocysts. Each of these secondary sporocysts releases thousands of tiny fork-tailed organisms, **cercariae,** which wander through the tissues of the snail, occasionally killing it, and finally emerge into the surrounding water. These cercariae must find a suitable definitive host in order to carry their life cycle further. Upon meeting with such a host, the cercariae penetrate the skin, usually between the hair follicles, undergo certain structural changes, become **metacercariae** and enter small peripheral veins. The metacercariae are carried by the venous circulation to the lungs, where, it is believed they either break through the lung parenchyma, migrating directly to the liver, or reach the arterial system to be carried to the liver. Within the intrahepatic portal system the flukes grow in size, then eventually migrate to the portal, mesenteric or pelvic veins, depending upon the species, where they attain their adult form and continue the reproductive cycle.

Lesions.—It is obvious from the life cycle of parasites of this group that injury to the definitive host can result from the presence of (1) adults in the veins, (2) ova in veins or tissues, (3) cercariae as they penetrate the skin, or (4) metacercariae as they migrate through the tissues.

The adult blood flukes living within the veins may produce some phlebitis with intimal proliferation and occasionally venous thrombosis. Vascular lesions are most likely to be severe when the adult worms die or are trapped in unusual sites. The adult schistosomes also consume erythrocytes and discharge blood pigment, which is engulfed by macrophages and may be found in reticulo-endothelial tissues in the liver and spleen. This pigment appears in the cytoplasm of macrophages as black granules, not unlike that seen in association with certain liver flukes (p. 799).

The ova of the blood flukes are the most important factors in the production of lesions. The ova deposited in the venules reach venous capillaries, adhere to and become embedded within the endothelium, then rupture the basement membrane by means of enzymes secreted through the pores of the egg shell by the miracidium within, and escape into the tissues. Pressure added to endothelial and subendothelial inflammation appears to assist in this movement. Within the tissues, the ovum also stimulates considerable inflammatory reaction upon the part of the host. A micro-abscess containing neutrophils and eosinophils may surround the ovum at the outset, but if it remains long at the site, endothelioid granulation tissue with foreign body giant cells soon replaces the abscess. This granuloma, or "pseudotubercle," is a characteristic feature of the microscopic findings in schistosomiasis. In sections, ova can be seen within these granulomas, often engulfed by large foreign body giant cells. These schistosome eggs are ovoid with a thick, hyaline, unstained or yellow wall. Sometimes a single spine may be seen protruding from this wall. The spine is located along the lateral surface in ova of *S. mansoni*, at one terminal pole in *S. hematobium*, and is lateral, small and inconspicuous on the ova of *S. japonicum*. The nature and location of the spine can be utilized in identifying the type of infection in some cases. Microscopic sections of ova may contain recognizable parts of the miracidium, but in older lesions only the egg shell may be left. It is often ruptured in such situations and only a fragment may be present, but the tissue reaction and microscopic appearance of the egg shell are characteristic.

As the disease progresses, fibrosis around the granulomas leads to further destruction of tissue and interference with function. Ova in the submucosa or lamina propria of the intestine or the submucosa of the urinary bladder may be assumed to be on their way out of the body of the host. However, many ova are not successful in continuing the life cycle, because they gain access to the blood stream and are circulated widely throughout the body. These ova may cause endarteritis, periarteritis or phlebitis, or become entrapped in capillaries which they rupture to escape into the tissues and produce the typical foreign-body granulomas. These embolic ova may reach the liver, spleen, lungs, lymph nodes, skin, testes, brain, or any other organ of the body. In the liver, the cirrhosis in long-standing cases is the result of periportal fibrosis which follows formation of granulomas around embolic ova brought to this site by the portal radicles.

Cutaneous lesions develop in man and animals as a result of penetration of the skin by the cercariae of schistosomes. The intensity of the tissue reaction depends to some extent upon the sensitivity and resistance of the host to the parasite. As the cercariae reach the dermis, a leukocytic reaction of varying intensity is elicited, including neutrophils, lymphocytes and eosinophils. This is accompanied by urticaria, itching and formation of tiny nodules which elevate the epidermis. In sensitized animals or man, a severe tissue reaction is provoked, and death of the parasite in the dermis may set up a prolonged local tissue reaction. Cercariae have the ability to penetrate the epidermis of hosts in which complete development of the fluke does not occur, the cercariae dying in the dermis. This is the basis of cercarial dermatitis ("swimmer's itch," "collector's itch," "swamp itch"), a problem to individuals exposed to infested waters (agricultural workers, swimmers, etc.). Numerous schistosomes of birds and mammals have been demonstrated to cause cercarial dermatitis, but the most important appear to be *Trichobilharzia stagnicolae*, a blood fluke of canaries; *Trichobilharzia ocellata*, a parasite of ducks; *Trichobilharzia physellae* (wild ducks and teal), *Schistosomatium douthitti* (meadow mouse, muskrat) and *Schistosoma spindale* (cattle, sheep, goat, horse, antelope and water buffalo).

A schistosome of some importance in parts of Southern United States is *Heterobilharzia americana*. This parasite, reported for the first time by Malek *et al.*, 1961, to be a parasite of the dog, usually has other definitive hosts: bobcat (*Lynx rufus*), rabbit (*Sylvilagus aquaticus*), raccoon (*Procyon lotor*) and the nutria (*Myocastor coypus*). The life cycle of this schistosome is essentially the same as others described previously. The free-swimming miracidium is released from an ovum to penetrate a snail (*Lymnaea cubensis* or *Pseudosuccinea columella*) in whose digestive gland it undergoes development to a mature cercaria which in turn penetrates the skin of its mammalian host. After periods of maturation in the lung and liver, the adults move to the mesenteric veins and undergo copulation. Ova reach the intestine, liver and other viscera and incite the tissue reaction described above for *S. japonicum* and *S. mansoni*. Ova appear in the feces about 68 days after cercariae penetrate the skin (the prepatent period).

Diagnosis.—The clinical diagnosis of schistosomiasis can be confirmed by demonstration of schistosome ova in the feces or by histologic examination of biopsy specimens of rectal mucosa, liver or other affected organs. The adult parasite may be found in veins at necropsy, and the typical ova in granulomas are demonstrable by histologic examination of specimens collected at necropsy or biopsy.

Schistosomiasis

AHLUWALIA, S. S.: Studies on Blood Flukes of Domestic Animals. II. Observations on Natural Infection in Pig with *Schistosoma incognitum*, Chandler, 1926. Indian J. Vet. Sci. *29*:40–48, 1959. (VB 1556–62.)

BARBOSA, F. S., BARBOSA, I., and MAGALAES-FILHO, M. A.: Natural Infection of Cattle with *Schistosoma mansoni*. Proc. 1st Int. Congr. Parasit. Roma, *2*:703–710, 1964. V.B. *37*: 2689, 1967.

BRACHETT, S.: Pathology of Schistosome Dermatitis. Arch. Dermat. & Syph. *42*:410–418, 1940.

DINNIK, J. A., and DINNIK, N. N.: The Schistosomes of Domestic Ruminants in Eastern Africa. Bull. Epizoot. Dis. Afr. *13*:341–359, 1965. V.B. *36*:3138, 1966.

DOMINGO, E. D., and WARREN, K. S.: Endogenous Desensitization: Changing Host Granulomatous Response to Schistosome Eggs at Different States of Infection with *Schistosoma mansoni*. Amer. J. Path. *52*:369–379, 1968.

FENWICK, A.: "Baboons as Reservoir Hosts of *Schistosoma mansoni*." Tr. R. Soc. Trop. Med. Hyg. *63*:557–567, 1969.

HSU, H. F., HSU, S. Y. L., and OSBORNE, J. W.: Immunization against *Schistosoma japonicum* in Rhesus Monkeys. Nature, Lond. *206*:1338–1340, 1965.

HSU, H. F., DAVIS, J. R., and HSU, S. Y. L.: Histopathological Lesions of Rhesus Monkeys and Chimpanzees Infected with *Schistosoma japonicum*. Z. Tropenmed. Parasit. *20*:184–205, 1969.

KRUATRACHUE, M., BHAIBULAYA, M., and HARINASUTA, C.: *Orientobilharizia harinasutai sp. nov.*, a Mammalian Blood-fluke, Its Morphology and Life-cycle. Ann. Trop. Med. Parasit. *59*:181–188, 1965.

MACHATTIE, C., and CHADWICK, C. R.: *Schistosoma bovis* and *S. mattheei* in Iraq with Notes on Development of Eggs of *S. haematobium* Pattern. Tr. Roy. Soc. Trop. Med. & Hyg. *26*:147–156, 1932.

MACHATTIE, C., MILLS, E. A., and CHADWICK, C. R.: Can Sheep and Cattle Act as Reservoirs of Human Schistosomiasis? Tr. Roy. Soc. Trop. Med. & Hyg. *27*:173–184, 1933.

MALEK, E. A., ASH, L. R., LEE, H. F., and LITTLE, M. D.: *Heterobilhartzia* Infection in the Dog and other Mammals in Louisiana. J. Parasitol. *47*:619–623, 1961.

McCULLY, R. M., VAN NIEKERK, and KRUGER, S. P.: Observations on the Pathology of Bilharziasis and other Parasitic Infestations of *Hyppopotamus amphibius* Linnaeus, 1758, from the Kruger National Park. Onderstepoort J. Vet. Res. *34*:563–618, 1967.

MUKHERJEE, R. P. and DORANI, V. P. S.: Massive Infection of Sheep with *Amphistomes* and the Histopathology of the Parasitized Rumen. Indian Vet. J. *39*:668–670, 1962. (VB 2443–63.)

OLIVIER, L., and WEINSTEIN, P. P.: Experimental Schistosome Dermatitis in Rabbits. J. Parasitol. *39*:280–291, 1953.

PENNER, L. R.: Possibilities of Systemic Infection with Dermatitis—Producing Schistosomes. Science *93*:327–328, 1941.

PERROTO, J. L., and WARREN, K. S.: Inhibition of Granuloma Formation around *Schistosoma mansoni* Eggs. IV. X-irradiation. Amer. J. Path. *56*:279–292, 1969.

PIERCE, K. R.: *Heterobilharzia americana* Infection in a Dog. J. Am. Vet. Med. Assn. *143*: 496–499, 1963.

PRICE, H. F.: Life History of *Schistosomatium douthitti* (Cort). Am. J. Hyg. *13*:685–727, 1931.

SAEED, A. A., NELSON, G. S., and HUSSEIN, M. F.: Experimental Infections of Calves with Schistosomes. Trans. R. Soc. Trop. Med. Hyg. *63*:15, 1969.

SOBRERO, R.: Alterazioni del Fegato nella Schistosomiasi dei Bovini Somali (Liver lesions due to schistosomiasis in Somali cattle). Riv. Parassit. *19*:113–116, 1958. (VB 1455–59.)

TEWARI, H. C., DUTT, S. C., and IYER, P. K. R.: Observations on the Pathogenicity of Experimental Infection of *Schistosoma incognitum* Chandler (1962) in Dogs. Indian J. Vet. Sci. *36*:227–231, 1966.

THRASHER, J. P.: Canine Schistosomiasis. J. Am. Vet. Med. Assn. *144*:1119–1126, 1964.

VON LICHTENBERG, F., and RASLAVICIUS, P.: Host Response to Eggs of *Schistosoma mansoni*. V. Reactions to Purified Miracidia and Egg Shells and to Viable and Heat-killed Whole Eggs. Lab. Invest. *16*:892–904, 1967.

WARREN, K. S.: Inhibition of Granuloma Formation Around *Schistosoma mansoni* Eggs. V. "Hodgkins-like Lesion in SJL/J Mice. Amer. J. Path. *56*:293–304, 1969.

WU, K.: Cattle as Reservoir Hosts of *Schistosoma japonicum* in China. Am. J. Hyg. *27*:290–297, 1938.

PARAGONIMIASIS

Small reddish-brown, egg-shaped flukes of the genus *Paragonimus* are important parasites of man and animals. These flukes are 8 to 12 mm. long, 4 to 6 mm. in diameter, hermaphroditic and have a spiny cuticle. They are currently classified in the family Troglotrematidae, which includes the intestinal fluke of salmon-poisoning *Nanophyetus (Troglotrema) salmincola* (see page 537). Two species are of particular interest: *Paragonimus westermani*, parasitic in man, and *P. kellicotti* whose adult host may be mink, dog, cat, pig, muskrat or opposum.

The adult flukes, *P. kellicotti*, are found in cysts in the lung where their presence may result in cough, blood-stained sputum (man), mild anemia and slight fever. The hermaphroditic flukes produce ova which escape from ruptured cysts in the lung parenchyma to reach the bronchi or to enter the circulation and thereby reach the spleen, liver, brain, urinary system, intestinal wall muscles, or other tissues. In these tissue sites, the thick-walled, anisotropic, yellowish-brown ova, which measure 80 to 118 microns in length and 48 to 60 microns in width, incite the production of characteristic epithelioid granulation tissue. The resulting lesion is very similar in microscopic appearance to the lesion caused by ova of liver flukes or schistosomes (pages 798 and 805).

The **life cycle** of *P. kellicotti* is rather complex. Ova which reach the bronchi are coughed up, swallowed and reach the exterior with the feces. Under most conditions *miracidia* develop slowly in these ova, hatch into water and then burrow into the tissues of various snails. In the United States, the fresh-water snail, *Pomatiopsis lapidaria* is most frequently this first intermediate host. Within the snail, the miracidia change into sporocysts which each produce about

12 first generation *rediae* which in turn produce a similar number of second generation rediae. These result in 30 to 40 fully developed *cercariae* about seventy-eight days after infestation of the snail. The cercariae creep or float with the current until contact is made with the second intermediate host. On the North American continent these hosts are usually species of crayfish of the genus *Cambarus*, which live in small sluggish streams. In China, Japan, and the Philippines, fresh water crabs are the usual second intermediate hosts but in Korea, crayfish may play this role.

The fully developed *cercariae* pierce the cuticle of the crayfish and make their way to the heart or pericardium where they encyst and in six weeks or more develop into infective *metacercariae*. If ingested with uncooked crayfish (or crab), the young flukes bore through the wall of the duodenum of their adult host, wander about in the peritoneal sac, then penetrate the diaphragm and lung. The tissue reaction to the fluke in the lung parenchyma results in the formation of a cyst.

Paragonimiasis

AMEEL, D. J.: Paragonimiasis, its Life History and Distribution in North America and its Taxonomy. Am. J. Hyg. *19*:279–317, 1934.
COMFORT, C. F. and AXELSON, R. D.: Two Reports of Unusual Parasites Diagnosed in Dogs. Canad. Vet. J. *3*:22–24, 1962.
GREVE, J. H., *et al.*: Paragonimiasis in Iowa. Iowa State Univ. Vet. *26*:21–28, 1963–64. (No. 1.)
HERMAN, L. H., and HELLAND, D. R.: Paragonimiasis in a Cat. J. Am. Vet. Med. Assn. *149*:753–757, 1966.
LaRUE, G. R. and AMEEL, D. J.: The Distribution of *Paragonimus*. J. Parasit. *23*:382–388, 1937.
NIELSON, S. W.: Canine Paragonimiasis. N. Amer. Vet. *36*:657–662, 1955.
SEED, J. R., SOGANDARES-BERNAL, F., and MILLS, R. R.: Studies on American Paragonimiasis. II. Serological Observations of Infected Cats. J. Parasit. *52*:358–362, 1966.

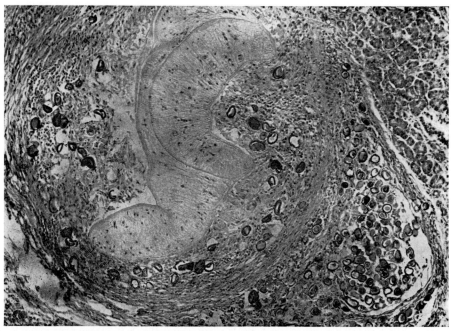

FIG. 15–34.—A fluke, *Eurytrema pancreaticum*, in the pancreatic duct of a Brazilian cow. Note the large numbers of ova, and the inflammation in the duct. Contributor: Dr. A. V. Machado, University of Munas Gervais.

OTHER FLUKES

A small red fluke, *Eurytrema pancreaticum,* is found in the pancreatic duct of sheep, goats, cattle and buffalo in Eastern Asia and Brazil. These flukes are only about 1 cm. in length but when present in large numbers may result in fibrosis of the duct and the acinar tissue as well. See page 1240 and Figure 15–34.

PARASITIC ARTHROPODS

Veterinary entomology is generally regarded as the science that deals with all parasitic arthropods of animals, although many members of this phylum are not insects. The phylum **Arthropoda** is in general made up of organisms characterized by bilateral symmetry, metameric segmentation, the presence of jointed append-ages and a hardened exoskeleton. It is divided into five classes as follows:

Crustacea: Crabs, crayfish, shrimp, copepods
Onychophora: *Peripatus*
Myriapoda: Centipedes and millipedes
Insecta: Six-legged insects (mosquitoes, flies, etc.)
Arachnida: Spiders, scorpions, ticks and mites

The classes **Insecta** and **Arachnida** contain most of the parasitic species and the vectors of disease-producing viruses, protozoa, nematodes, rickettsia and spiro-chetes. Each of these insect vectors is considered briefly in the part of this text devoted to the disease which it transmits. In the class **Insecta** there are many orders, some of which contain species that are parasitic to animals, but those of most interest are the Diptera (flies), Hemiptera (bugs), Siphonaptera (fleas) and suborders anoplura and mallophaga (lice). Other orders contain species of less interest which may act as vectors of disease, but these will not be discussed here. Fleas, lice and bugs, although vexing and sometimes injurious parasites, do not often have a serious portent from the pathologist's viewpoint; hence, will not be considered further. Flies, however, do incite specific and severe pathologic changes, thus are pathogens in their own right.

MYIASIS

Myiasis results from the invasion of living tissues of animals by the larval stage of flies of the order **Diptera.** The sites of invasion of these larvae provide a basis for their clinical classification: (1) cutaneous—the larvae live in or under the skin *e.g.,* ox warble; (2) intestinal—in the stomach or intestines *e.g.,* horse "bots"; (3) atrial—in the oral, nasal, ocular, sinusal, vaginal and urethral cavities —for example, *Oestrus ovis*; (4) wound invading—"screw-worm larvae" and (5) external—bloodsucking larvae. Some fly larvae occupy more than one of these sites during the course of development in the host. Many fly larvae are specific parasites of a certain host; others are accidental or nonspecific parasites in that they are deposited in or near diseased or wounded tissues in which they find a favorable environment.

Botflies.—The genus *Gasterophilus* contains three species whose larvae are parasitic for equines in the United States. *Gasterophilus intestinalis* (syn. *G. equi*), De Geer, 1776, the most common botfly in the United States, is a brown fly which deposits its eggs on hair of horse's fetlocks or forelegs—occasionally also in the scapular region. The female fly darts in quickly and attaches her pale yellow eggs to the hair with a tenacious material. These eggs are ready to hatch in five to ten

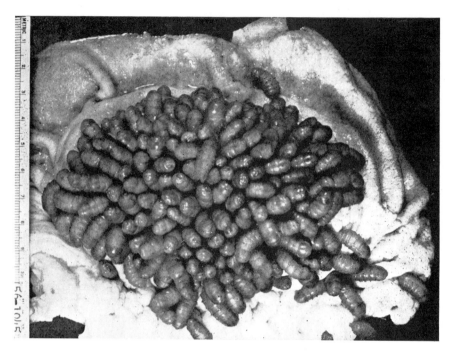

Fig. 15–35.—Larvae of *Gasterophilus intestinalis*, "bots," attached to the stomach of a two-year-old gelding. (Courtesy of Dr. C. R. Cole, Ohio State University.)

days, but actual hatching requires licking or rubbing by the horse. This action also helps the larvae to reach the animal's mouth, where they penetrate the mucosa and wander beneath it as far as the pharynx. The developing larvae remain in the cheek or tongue for twenty-one to twenty-eight days then migrate to the stomach and with their mouth parts attach to the mucosa in its cardiac portion. These bot larvae at this stage have a reddish color and are quite selective in their location, only rarely are they found attached to the fundic or pyloric portion of the stomach. Each larva causes a small umbilicated ulcer at its site of attachment. Large numbers of bots obviously interfere with function in the affected part of the stomach but only occasionally do they produce general debility in the host. Surprisingly often they are tolerated without recognizable effect. The larvae remain attached to the mucosa, living on blood and tissue, for ten to twelve months. After this period, they loosen their hold and pass out with the feces the larvae pupate in soil for three to five weeks and then emerge as adults.

Gasterophilus hemorrhoidalis, Linne, 1761, the "nose botfly," is a small red-tailed fly which lays its eggs on hairs around the mouth, nose and cheeks of horses. The eggs of this species are dark brown or black in color, elongated and pointed at one end with an operculum at the other. The larvae hatch from these eggs then pierce the skin of the face and wander into the mouth. The young red-colored larvae are sometimes found in the pharynx but eventually become attached at the cardia of the stomach. Here they have a similar effect to that of *G. intestinalis*, and remain for ten to twelve months at this site before passing to the rectum where they again attach for a few days before passing out with the feces. The rest of their life cycle is similar to that of *G. intestinalis*.

Gasterophilus nasalis, Clark, 1897, (Synonym: *G. veterinus*, Linne, 1761), the "chin" or "throat" fly, lays its eggs on hairs in the intermandibular region of horses. The larvae are pale yellow and migrate to eventually become attached to the mucosa of the pylorus and duodenum. Otherwise, their life cycle and effect upon the host are similar to that of *G. intestinalis*.

Gasterophilus pecorum, Fabricus, 1794, is a botfly found in Europe, but not in the United States. The female fly deposits her eggs on the hoofs of horses and on inanimate objects such as food and other materials. The eggs are dark colored and must be rubbed or licked by the host before the larvae can emerge. The larvae penetrate the mucosa of the cheeks and soon assume a blood-red color. The third stage larvae attach to the stomach mucosa and before leaving the host in the spring attach to the rectal mucosa for a few days.

Gasterophilus inermis, Braurer, 1858, is principally a botfly of Europe but has been observed in North America. The adult fly deposits her eggs on hairs around the mouth and cheeks. The larvae may penetrate the skin and leave tracks as they wander toward the mucosa. The third stage larvae attach to the mucosa of the rectum. Otherwise the life history is similar to that of *G. intestinalis*.

Oestrus ovis, the botfly or "head grub" of sheep, deposits its larvae in the nose of sheep; the larvae migrate into the nasal cavity and nasal sinuses, where they attach and undergo further development. Growth and migration of these larvae in these sites result in serious damage to the tissues and may cause death. The successful larvae eventually drop to the ground, where they pupate and later emerge as adult flies.

Heel Flies.—The genus *Hypoderma* contains two species of interest, *H. bovis*, and *H. lineatum*, the hairy yellow, and black "warble," or heel flies of cattle, which occasionally attack horses and, rarely, man. The female fly deposits her eggs on the hairs of the legs, flanks or dewlap of cattle, producing much irritation and excitement in their victims while so doing. The larvae from these eggs hatch and penetrate the skin, migrate through the tissues into the thoracic and abdominal cavities, and eventually reach the subcutaneous tissues of the back. Occasionally these larvae invade the central nervous system and cause death. Surprisingly enough, the migration pathway of these larvae is usually sterile, even though there is considerable tissue destruction along the way. The larvae remain in an encapsulated nodule in the subcutis of the back during the winter months. In the spring, they gradually produce a large hole in the epidermis, through which the grub eventually emerges. Heavy infestation leaves holes in the skin which make the hide unfit for use. The larvae pupate after reaching the ground, emerging as adult flies forty to fifty days later.

In some parts of the United States the **"screw-worm" fly**, *Callitroga* (*Cochliomyia*) *americana*, can be a very important problem in animal agriculture and may also cause a serious disease in man. The pathogenic effects of this fly are produced by the larvae which feed upon living tissues and thereby may produce serious effects upon their hapless host. In man, very deleterious effects have been produced by the maggots' invasion of the nasopharynx (nasopharyngeal myiasis). In animals, the larvae attack any wounds in which they can gain entrance. In sheep and lambs "needle" grass may produce wounds which the maggots can invade, although cuts in the skin made by shearing can also be very troublesome. In cattle, the "screw-worm" larvae may invade the umbilicus of the newborn calf or the vagina of its mother. Dehorning and castration may also provide wounds which invite the assault of this parasite.

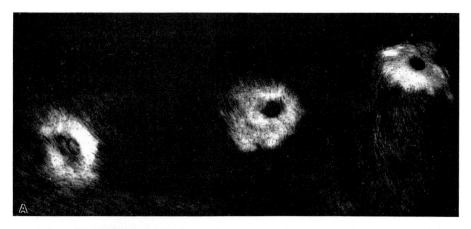

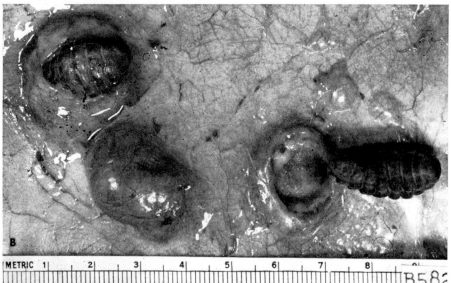

FIG. 15–36.—*Hypoderma bovis,* "ox warble," in the bovine skin. *A,* Three holes viewed from the external surface of the skin. The larvae lie under these holes which eventually enlarge to permit escape of the larvae. *B, H. bovis* larvae from the deep surface of the bovine skin. (Courtesy of Dr. C. R. Cole, Ohio State University.)

The adult fly has a dark greenish-blue metallic abdomen with an orange or reddish face and three stripes on the surface of the thorax. The female deposits her eggs in large numbers near wounds and after eleven to twenty-one hours, the larvae emerge to feed voraciously for three to five days. A prepupal stage lasts from a few hours to three days, and the pupal stage about seven days. The entire cycle from egg to adult is completed in about eleven days.

Cutaneous myiasis may also be caused by larvae of flies of the subfamily Cuterebrinae. Two genera are of particular interest: *Dermatobia* and *Cuterebra*. *Dermatobia hominis* may infect man, cattle, dogs, sheep, cats, rabbits and other animals, particularly in tropical America. The adults do not feed, surviving on food stores obtained during the larval period. The adult female, about 12 mm. long with a dark blue thorax and short broad abdomen with a brilliant blue color glues her ova to the abdomen of a mosquito or blood-sucking fly. The larvae hatch on this transport host, penetrate the skin of a warm-blooded host upon which the transport host feeds. The larvae of *D. hominis* develop in the subcutis, producing a painful enlargement with a pore opening to the surface. The larvae require up to ten weeks to mature to about 25 mm. in length with rows of strong spines on their surface. The larvae escape from the skin to the ground where they pupate to produce the mature fly.

The genus *Cuterebra* is made up of large flies with bee-like bodies, 20 mm. or more in length. The adult flies oviposit near the mouths of burrows of rodents and rabbits. Larvae hatch to penetrate the skin of the host, mature in about a month and produce large subcutaneous lesions. The larvae pupate on the ground and also are covered with bands of characteristic spines. *Cuterebra buccata, C. americana,* and *C. lepivora* are usually parasitic in rabbits but may also infect dogs, cats and man. Another species, *C. emasculator,* usually parasitizes mice and chipmunks but may also involve other species. Larvae may invade the brain or scrotum as well as the subcutis (Hatziolos, 1967).

Myiasis

BEESLEY, W. N.: Recent Work on the Ox Warble Flies (*Hypoderma*). Vet. Bull. *35*:1–6, 1965.
————: Further Observations on the Development of *Hypoderma lineatum* de Villiers and *Hypoderma bovis*, Degeer (*Diptera, Oestridae*) in the Bovine Host. Brit. Vet. J. *122*:91–98, 1966.
DAVIS, C. L., and LEADBETTER, W. A.: Fatal Brain Hemorrhage in a Bull Caused by the Cattle Grub (*Hypoderma bovis*). North Am. Vet. *33*:703–705, 1952.
GREVE, J. H., and CASSIDY, D. R.: Aberrant *Hypoderma bovis* Infection in a Cow. J. Am. Vet. Med. Assn. *150*:627–628, 1967.
HATZIOLOS, B. C.: Cuterebra Larva in the Brain of a Cat. J. Am. Vet. Med. Assn. *148*: 787–793, 1966.
————: Cuterebra Larva Causing Paralysis in a Dog. Cornell Vet. *57*:129–145, 1967.
OLANDER, H. J.: The Migration of *Hypoderma lineatum* in the Brain of a Horse. A Case Report and Review. Path. Vet. *4*:477–483, 1967.
ROBERTS, I. H. and COLBENSON, H. P.: Larvae of *Oestrus ovis* in the Ears of Sheep. Am. J. Vet. Res. *24*:628–630, 1963.
SIMMONS, S. W.: Some Histopathological Changes Caused by *Hypoderma* Larvae in the Esophagus of Cattle. J. Parasitol. *23*:376–381, 1937.
ZUMPT, F.: *Myiasis in Man and Animals,* 1965, Butterworth, London.

ACARIASIS

Within the class Arachnida, the order Acarina includes the ticks and mites, both of which are at times parasitic in their relation to animals. Ticks are particularly important as vectors of disease-producing agents, but except when present in large numbers or in particular sites, as in the ears, do not produce any immediate or serious effect upon the host. An important exception is **tick paralysis, a** dramatic paralytic disease observed in man, cattle and bison. The paralytic symptoms, which occur when one or more *Dermacentor andersoni* (wood ticks) are attached to the skin of the host, disappear dramatically when the offending ticks are removed. Death occurs in animals and man when the ticks are not detected and removed in time. The symptoms are believed to be the result of a neuroparalytic toxin secreted by the tick; the lesions have not been described.

In Australia, *Ixodes holocyclus* is the one tick that causes tick paralysis in sheep and cattle (with violent retching, drooling of saliva, complete flaccid paralysis, extreme dehydration). An effective immune serum made from hyperimmunized dogs is available. Cats and children have the disease but are more resistant. Removal of the tick does not necessarily cure the disease nor relieve the symptoms. The tick usually has to be on the patient for four days before symptoms appear. The bandicoot is the natural host for this tick.

The tissue-burrowing habits of mites cause them to produce more obvious lesions in animals than do ticks. Common mites which are pathogenic for animals are listed in Table 15–4. These mites may be appropriately considered in groups arranged in accord with the body system which they attack, *i.e.*, pulmonary, cutaneous, intestinal and urinary.

Pulmonary Acariasis.—The frequent occurrence of pulmonary lesions caused by a lung mite, *Pneumonyssus simicola*, in monkeys is of some interest in connection with the experimental use of these animals. According to Innes *et al.*, (1954) nearly all imported rhesus monkeys are infected with lung mites whose presence in the bronchiolar system incites rather characteristic lesions. Clinical manifestations are not usually observed, but the possible effect of these parasites upon the course of infections, such as tuberculosis, has not been explored. Neither the life cycle nor the mode of dissemination of these mites is known.

Table 15–4.—*Acarid (Mite) Parasites of Animals*

Name	Anatomic Site	Disease	Hosts
Demodex folliculorum (demodectic mange mite)	Hair follicles and sebaceous glands	Demodectic or "red" mange	Dog, cat, man, swine, sheep, cattle
Demodex phylloides	Hair follicles and sebaceous glands	Demodectic mange	Swine
Sarcoptes scabiei var. suis, bovis, etc. (sarcoptic mange mite)	Epidermis generally	Scabies, sarcoptic mange	Cattle, sheep, dog, man, swine, horse
Notoedres sp.	Epidermis, especially of neck	Notoedric mange	Cat and others
Psoroptes communis var. equi, ovis, etc.	Epidermis of ears and generally	Psoroptic mange, sheep scab	Sheep, cattle, horse, rabbit
Chorioptes sp.	Epidermis, feet and base of tail	Chorioptic mange	Cattle, sheep, horse, goat
Cytoleichus nudus (air sac mite)	Air sacs, respiratory tract	Air sac mite infection	Bird
Pneumonyssus caninum	Paranasal sinuses	Mite infection	Dog
Pneumonyssus simicola	Bronchioles, alveoli of lung	Pulmonary acariasis	Macaca mulatta
Dermanyssus gallinae (common red mite)	Epidermis generally	Anemia, mite dermatitis	Poultry
Cnemidocoptes mutans (Scaly leg mite)	Scales of legs	Scaly leg disease	Chicken
Cnemidocoptes gallinae (feather mite)	Feather follicles	Depluming mite infestation	Chicken
Linguatula serrata (tongue "worm," pentastoma worm)	Nasal and respiratory passages	Pentastomiasis or linguatuliasis	Dog, fox, wolf, man, horse, goat, sheep
Tyroglyphus sp. (cereal mite)	Urinary and intestinal tract	"Grocer's itch"	Man, dog
Psorergates simplex	Epidermal cysts in skin	"Mouse mange"	Mice
Psorergates ovis	Same	Mange	Sheep
Cheyletiella parasitivorax	Epidermis	"Mange"	Dog, rabbit, cat

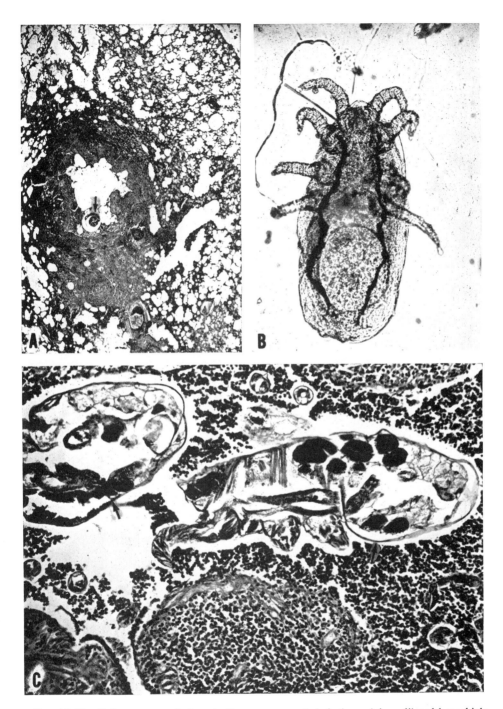

Fig. 15–37.—Pulmonary acariasis. *A, Pneumonyssus simicola* (arrow) in a dilated bronchiole with thickened wall, lung of a rhesus monkey *Macaca mulatta*. *B*, A female, egg-bearing mite teased from a lesion. *C*, Section of two mites in a bronchiole. Photographs courtesy of Dr. J. R. M. Innes.

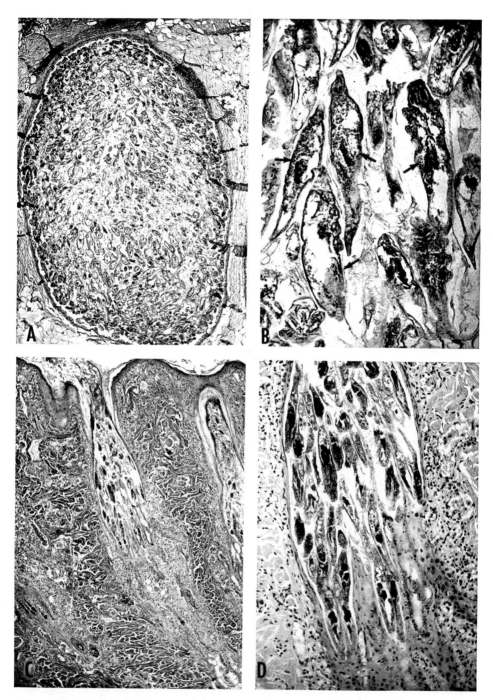

FIG. 15–38.—Cutaneous acariasis. *A*, Demodectic mange in the skin of a pig (× 35). Large dilated hair follicle filled with *Demodex phylloides*. *B*, Higher magnification (× 210) of *A*, to show detail of sections of mites (arrows). Contributor: Dr. C. L. Davis. *C*, Demodectic mange, skin of a dog (× 35). Note the acanthosis and prominent, distended hair follicles. *D*, A single follicle (× 115) from *C*, containing many *Demodex folliculorum*. (Courtesy of Armed Forces Institute of Pathology.) Contributor: Dr. R. D. Turk.

little harm but can cause serious lesions in another. Such a mite is *Demodex folliculorum*, a cigar-shaped mite, commonly demonstrable in normal human hair follicles, where it survives with no visible effect upon the host. Morphologically identical parasites are the cause of **demodectic** or **red mange** in dogs, a persistent and disfiguring skin disease in that species. These mites burrow into the hair follicles of the canine skin, producing intense itching accompanied by alopecia and scaling of the epidermis. The itching causes the animal to rub the affected part, accentuating the symptoms and promoting exudation of serum and scab formation on the denuded surface. The mites may burrow into sebaceous or sweat glands or to the depths of hair follicles, causing proliferation and then necrosis of the epithelium, followed by intense inflammation of the underlying dermis. In some cases, the mites migrate even deeper and may reach lymph nodes. Secondary pyogenic infections can result in death. The deep folliculitis and dermatitis can be readily recognized in tissue sections and the offending parasites easily demonstrated. Deep scrapings of affected skin may also be examined microscopically for the mites.

A similar, but morphologically distinguishable mite, *Demodex phylloides*, occasionally causes lesions in the hair follicles and sebaceous glands of the skin of swine. It is common for the parasite to produce dilatation of the skin adnexa with the formation of epithelial-lined cysts filled with the mites. These lesions have somewhat the same effect as an epidermal inclusion cyst, exciting little inflammation unless it ruptures and causes a reaction of foreign-body type. It is possible for *Demodex* mites to be present in hair follicles or sebaceous glands in the skin, particularly in man and the dog, without exciting any inflammation. The factors which make these mites pathogenic are unknown.

Sarcoptic mange is caused by a specific mite, *Sarcoptes scabiei* (sarcoptic mange mite) which may attack many species, including cattle, sheep, dogs, swine, horses and man. Morphologically indistinguishable varieties of *S. scabiei* (*bovis, suis*, etc.) are found in each host species, each variety of mite having its definite host preference; cross infection of heterologous species rarely occurs. The sarcoptic mange mite burrows in the deeper parts of the strateum corneum or the superficial layers of the stratum malpighii of the skin, and rarely goes deeper. Even in this superficial position, however, the mites cause severe itching, hyperkeratosis and acanthosis, with resultant loss of hair or wool. The intense pruritus results in rubbing of the skin, which in turn causes loss of epithelium and secondary infection of the dermis. In dogs at least, the pruritus is much more intense in sarcoptic than in demodectic mange.

Species of other genera, *Notoedres*, *Psoroptes* and *Chorioptes*, produce similar lesions but with slightly different host range and anatomic site of preference. The diseases caused by these mites are known, respectively, as **notoedric, psoroptic** or **chorioptic mange**. The offending mites can be seen in tissue sections, but it is necessary to tease them out and mount them under a cover slip in order to identify them. This can be done as readily with fixed specimens of skin as with fresh skin scrapings.

Of particular interest to laboratory investigators is the rabbit ear mite, *Psoroptes communis* var. *cuniculi* which lives in the external auditory meatus of rabbits, where it produces severe lesions which may lead to middle or inner ear infection and death. The mites tunnel into the superficial layers of the stratum malpighii, producing hyperkeratosis and exfoliation of keratin and debris which

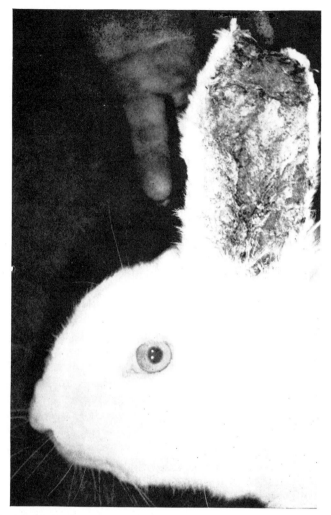

FIG. 15–43.—Lesions of ear mites (*Psoroptes communis* v. *cunuliculi*) in the ear of a New Zealand white rabbit.

accumulates in the ear canal. The ear mite of the domestic cat, *Felis catus*, is also of interest here as it produces similar lesions. The usual parasite is *Notoedres cati*.

Intestinal and Urinary Acariasis.—Certain mites live normally in cereal products and are not pathogenic but may produce dermatitis ("grocer's itch"), enteritis or urethritis in man or animals if they gain access to these structures. Of interest are the cereal mites, *Tyroglyphus sp.*, which have been reported in feces of dogs fed infested cereal products. Few symptoms are produced and the mites do not multiply in the intestinal tract, but their close resemblance to mange mites may at times be confusing when they are encountered upon microscopic examination of fecal specimens.

Acariasis (Mite Infestation)

BAKER, E. W., EVANS, T. M., GOULD, D. J., HULL, W. B., and KEEGAN, H. L.: *A Manual of Parasitic Mites of Medical or Economic Importance.* New York, National Pest Control Assn., Inc., 1956.

BAKER, D. W., and NUTTING, W. B.: Demodectic Mange in New York State Sheep. Cornell Vet. *40*:140–142, 1940.

BAKER, K. P.: The Histopathology and Pathogenesis of Demodecosis of the Dog. J. Comp. Path. *79*:321–327, 1969.

BAKER, K. P.: Infestation of Domestic Animals with the Mite *Cheyletiella parasitivorax*. Vet. Rec. *84*:561, 1969.

BERESFORD-JONES, W. P.: Occurrence of the Mite *Psorergates simplex* in Mice. Aust. Vet. J. *41*:289–290, 1965.

CARTER, H. B.: A Skin Disease of Sheep Due to an Ectoparasitic Mite, *Psorergates ovis*, Womersley, 1941. Australia Vet. J. *17*:193–201, 1941.

CHALLIER, A., GIDEL, R., and TRAORE, S.: Porocephalosis Caused by *Armillifer (Nettorhynchus) armillatus*, Wyman 1847, in a Bull and Pig. Revue Elev. Med. Vet. Pays Trop. *20*:255–259, 1967.

DANILOV, I.: Lethal Infestation of Goats with Juvenile Forms of *Linguatula serrata*. Vet. Sbir. *56*:24–25, 1959. (VB 3513–59.)

DE TOIT, R., and SUTHERLAND, R. J.: *Armillifer armillatus* (Wyman) (Order: Pentastomida) from Slaughter Stock. J. S. Afr. Vet. Med. Assn. *39*:77–79, 1968.

EWING, S. A., MOSIER, J. E., and FOXX, T. S.: Occurrence of *Cheyletiella spp.* on Dogs with Skin Lesions. J. Am. Vet. Med. Assn. *151*:64–67, 1967.

FLYNN, R. J., and JAROSLOW, B. N.: Nidification of a Mite (*Psorergates simplex*, Tyrrell, 1883: Myobiidae) in the Skin of Mice. J. Parasitol. *42*:49–52, 1956.

FOXX, T. S., and EWING, S. A.: Morphologic Features, Behavior, and Life History of *Cheyletiella yasguri*. Am. J. Vet. Res. *30*:269–285, 1969.

FRENCH, F. E.: *Demodex canis* in Canine Tissues. Cornell Vet. *54*:271–290, 1964.

GRIFFIN, C. A., and DEAN, D. J.: Demodectic Mange in Goats. Cornell Vet. *34*:308–311, 1944.

GRONO, L. R.: Studies of the Ear Mite, *Otodectes cynotis*. Vet. Rec. *85*:6–8, 1969.

INNES, J. R. M., COLTON, M. W., YEVICH, P. P., and SMITH, C. L.: Pulmonary Acariasis as an Enzootic Disease Caused by *Pneumonyssus simicola* in Imported Monkeys. Am. J. Path. *30*:813–835, 1954.

KHALIL, G. M., and SCHACHER, J. F.: *Linguatula serrata* in Relation to Halzoun and the Marrara Syndrome. Amer. J. Trop. Med. Hyg. *14*:736–746, 1965.

KIRKWOOD, A., and KENDALL, S. B.: Demodectic Mange in Cattle. Vet. Rec. *78*:33–34, 1966.

LEERHOY, J., and JENSEN, H. S.: Sarcoptic Mange in a Shipment of Cynomolgus Monkeys. Nord. Vet. Med. *19*:128–130, 1967.

MARTIN, H. M., and DEUBLER, M. J.: Acariasis (*Pneumonyssus sp.*) of the Upper Respiratory Tract of the Dog. Univ. of Pa. Bull. *43*:21–27, 1943.

MILLER, J. K., TOMPKINS, V. N., and SIERACKI, J. C.: Pathology of Colorado Tick Fever in Experimental Animals. Arch. Path. *72*:149–157, 1961.

NELSON, W. A. and BAINBOROUGH, A. R.: Development in Sheep of Resistance to the Ked, *Melophagus ovinus* (L.). III. Histopathology of Sheep Skin as a Clue to the Nature of Resistance. Exp. Parasitol. *13*:118–127, 1963. (VB 3570–63.)

NEMESERI, L. and SZEKY, A.: Demodecicosis in Cattle. Zctz. Vet. Acad. Sci. Hung. *11*:209–221, 1961. (VB 493–62.)

————————: Demodicosis in Sheep. Acta Vet. Hung. *16*:53–63, 1966. V.B. *36*:4809, 1966.

————————: Demodicosis of Swine. Acta Vet. Hung. *16*:251–261, 1966. V.B. *37*:1720, 1967.

SAVOV, N.: Death of a Heifer Caused by Massive Infestation with Juvenile Forms of *Linguatula serrata*. Vet. Sbir. *56*:22–24, 1959. (VB 3512–1959.)

SCHAFFER, M. H., BAKER, N. F., and KENNEDY, P. C.: Parasitism by *Cheyletiella parasitivorax*. A Case Report of the Infestation in a Female Dog and Its Litter. Cornell Vet. *48*:440–447, 1958.

SCHNELLE, G. B., and JONES, T. C.: Occurrence of the Cereal Mite in War Dogs. J. Am. Vet. Med. Assn. *104*:213–214, 1944.

SHARMA DEORANI, V. P., and CHAUDHURI, R. P.: On the Histopathology of the Skin Lesion of Goats Affected by Sarcoptic Mange. Indian J. Vet. Sci. *35*:150–156, 1965.

SLOAN, C. A.: Mortality in Sheep Due to *Ixodes species*. Aust. Vet. J. *44*:527–528, 1968.

SMITH, D. B., and CLAYPOOLE, T. F.: Canine Scabies in Dogs and in Humans. J. Am. Med. Assn. *199*:59–64, 1967.

YASGUR, I.: Parasitism of Kennel Puppies with the Mite *Cheyletiella parasitivorax*. Cornell Vet. *54*:406–407, 1964.

16
Pathologic Effects of Ionizing Radiations

The injurious properties of radioactive substances were recognized, after bitter experience, by early workers with radium and x-ray, but the potential hazard has been magnified tremendously during the past decade by the development of nuclear energy as a source of explosive and controlled power. Radioactive substances produced in huge quantities in the explosion of a nuclear bomb may be scattered widely by blast and wind, with possible hazard to man and animals downwind from the point of detonation. The operation of increasing numbers of nuclear power reactors and atomic "piles," as well as high voltage x-ray machines, also results in greatly increased radioactivity which presents a potential threat to health. It is important, therefore, to study the biologic effects of radiation from these sources in order to develop fuller understanding of its potential.

Radiation of the type to be considered, which exists both in wave and particulate form, gives up its energy and in general produces its effect upon tissues by the production of ion pairs (ionization). This property, the ionization of matter, also provides the usual means for detection of radiation of this type; thus the term **ionizing radiation** is appropriate and useful to differentiate it from radiation of other types (heat, light, ultraviolet) which also produce biologic effects.

DEFINITIONS

Volumes of information in atomic physics lie outside the scope of this book, but some of the nomenclature of the physicist must be used in studying the lesions produced by ionizing radiations. A few terms necessary to an understanding of the effects of ionizing radiation are defined as follows:

Types of Ionizing Radiations.—The *alpha particle* (α) is a helium nucleus consisting of two protons and two neutrons with a double positive charge and having a definite mass. A stream of alpha particles (so-called alpha ray) has high ionizing but very low penetrating properties and short range, since a thin sheet of paper, the keratin layer of the skin or other material of comparable thickness will prevent its passage. It has little biologic effect except when alpha-emitting isotopes (such as radium) are deposited in bone, where prolonged effects are produced on hematopoietic and osteogenic cells.

The *beta particle* (β) is a charged particle emitted from the nucleus of an atom; its mass and charge are equal in magnitude to those of the electron. Depending somewhat on its energy, it has a longer range and deeper penetration than the alpha particle but causes only medium degrees of ionization. Radio-active isotopes which emit beta particles ("beta emitters") may produce lesions in the skin upon continued contact and may be particulary dangerous when concentrated in bone (as in radioactive isotopes which are deposited in bone; *i.e.* "bone seekers").

Gamma rays (γ) are electromagnetic radiations of short wavelengths emitted from the nucleus of radioisotopes. They are essentially similar to x rays but usually are of higher energy, and generally come from different sources. Gamma rays have long range and deep penetration in tissues but low ionization per unit of matter penetrated. These rays may penetrate deep into the body and produce an effect upon the entire body (total body effect).

X rays or *Roentgen rays* are penetrating electromagnetic radiations having wave lengths less than those of visible light. Although similar to gamma rays, they usually are of much lower energy and are produced by the bombardment of a metallic target by fast moving electrons in a high vacuum. Their biologic effects are similar to those of gamma rays.

Neutrons (n) are elementary nuclear particles that bear no electrical charge and have a mass approximately the same as that of hydrogen atoms. Neutrons have very long range, deep penetration and may induce radioactivity.

Positrons (β^+) are particles equal in mass to the electron and having an equal but opposite (positive) charge. Their biologic properties are similar to those of the beta particle.

Cosmic rays are complex radiation phenomena that originate in outer space and are largely absorbed by the earth's atmosphere. Some constituents of cosmic rays are capable of extremely deep penetration, even in dense matter such as rock.

Measurement of Radiation.—The *roentgen* (r) is a unit of x or gamma radiation used, as a rule, in measuring dosage. It is defined as that quantity of x or gamma radiation which is of such magnitude that its associated corpuscular emission per 0.001293 gram of air produces in air ions carrying one electrostatic unit of electricity of either sign. The intensity of the roentgen (r) is measured in air, hence is not an accurate indication of radioactivity absorbed by the tissues. In order to overcome this discrepancy, a unit of measurement of absorbed dosage of radiation, the *RAD*, was adopted by the International Commission on Radiologic Units at the Seventh International Congress of Radiology, Copenhagen, in 1953. The *RAD* is a measure of the energy (100 ergs per gram) imparted to matter by ionizing particles per unit mass of unit material at the place of interest. In biologic systems, the matter irradiated is usually stated as a specific tissue.

The *curie* (c) is that quantity of radioactive material having associated with it 3.7×10^{10} disintegrations per second. It is therefore a measure of radioactivity and is most commonly used in biology as millicurie (mc) units.

The *half life* of a radioactive substance is the length of time (in seconds, hours, days or years) required for the substance to lose 50 per cent of its radioactivity by decay. The *biological half life* of a substance is the time required for the body to eliminate one-half of an administered dose of the substance by the usual processes of elimination.

The *Median Lethal Dose* (MLD) is the dosage of radiation required to kill, within a specified period, 50 per cent of individuals in a group of animals or organisms in a specified time. The *lethal dose* (LD) is more common and practical, since it will indicate accurately varying percentages of lethality in a specified

27

time. Thus, LD 50/30 is the dosage of radiation required to kill 50 per cent of a group of animals in thirty days.

An *Electron Volt* (ev) is a unit of energy equivalent to the amount of energy gained by an electron passing through a potential difference of one volt. Large multiples of this unit are commonly used, *viz.:* *kev* (thousand electron volts), *mev* (million electron volts) and *bev* (billion electron volts).

Linear energy transfer (LET) is a term used to express the quality of radiation. It concerns the spatial distributions of energy transfers which occur along and within the tracks of particles as they penetrate matter. These energy transfers influence the effectiveness of an irradiation in producing physical, chemical or biological changes and are independent of other physical factors such as *total energy dissipated, absorbed dose, absorbed dose rate* and *absorbed dose fractionation.* The precise, technical definition of these terms may be found in the report of the International Commission on Radiation Units and Measurements (1970).

Radioisotopes.—An isotope of an element is one of several nuclides of that element having the same number of protons in their nuclei, hence the same atomic number, but differing in the number of neutrons and consequently in mass number. Isotopes of a particular element have almost identical chemical properties, but some are unstable, undergo radioactive decay, and are therefore called *radioactive isotopes* or *radioisotopes.* Only a few radioisotopes occur in nature and generally these do not constitute a large source of radioactivity. The fission reaction in the atomic bomb or the neutron bombardment of stable isotopes in a nuclear reactor can produce large quantities of artificial radioisotopes which have wide use in science, industry and medicine. Isotopes are usually designated by their chemical symbol and mass number; thus, radium-223 (^{223}Ra), potassium-40 (^{40}K), uranium-238 (^{238}U) are naturally occurring radioisotopes; iodine-131 (^{131}I), and phosphorus-32 (^{32}P) are artificially produced radioisotopes; while potassium-39 (^{39}K), carbon-13 (^{13}C) and oxygen-16 (^{16}O) are stable isotopes. These symbols may be written with left (^{32}P) or right (P^{32}) superscripts. The convention using the left superscript for the mass number and a left subscript for the atomic number of the element may also be encountered—*i.e.*; $^{1}_{1}$H for hydrogen and $^{2}_{1}$H for heavy hydrogen (deuterium). The student is referred to the texts listed under references for further information on this vitally important subject.

Definitions

International Commission on Radiation Units and Measurements (ICRU). *Linear Energy Transfer*, ICRU Report No. 16, 1970. Washington, D.C.
LAPP, R. E., and ANDREWS, H. L.: *Nuclear Radiation Physics.* 2nd Ed., New York, Prentice-Hall, 1954.
National Council on Radiation Protection and Measurements. *Radiation Protection in Veterinary Medicine.* NCRP Report No. 36, 15 August 1970, Washington, D.C.
UPTON, A. C.: *Radiation Injury*, Chicago, Univ. Chicago Press, 1969.

EFFECTS OF RADIATION ON BIOLOGIC SYSTEMS

Direct.—Direct effects of radiation may be explained on the basis of the target theory; particularly in relation to viruses, genes and chromosomes (Florey, 1970). The target is visualized as one of relatively large molecular dimensions and the effect is attributed to a single ionization, or a small number of ionizations, anywhere within the structure. It is presumed that a chemical change is produced in a molecule when ionization occurs directly within it. A larger molecule is more likely to be hit than a smaller one, thus the dose required to change a quantity of a substance by radiation will be inversely proportional to its molecular weight. A method based upon this principle has been used to determine the molecular weight of some proteins.

Quantitation of direct effects depends upon the target size, type of radiation and intensity of radiation dosage.

Indirect.—Indirect action of radiation is particularly applicable in aqueous solution and depends upon ionization which produces free radicals which in turn may react chemically. These free radicals, for example, hydroxyl (OH^-) and perhydroxyl (HO_2) radicals, are highly reactive and may become responsible for chemical changes in other molecules in the solution. This indirect effect upon molecules would be dependent upon the number of free radicals released and not upon molecular size or concentration. If a single substance in solution is radiated, changes in that solute will increase linearly with the dose of radiation. If two or more substances are present in the irradiated solution, one may have a protective effect by competing for the free radicals.

Enzymes and Enzyme Systems.—The inactivation of vital enzymes or enzyme systems in cells has been postulated as one of the possible means by which radiant energy could injure cells. Purified enzymes, such as ribonuclease, in the solid state may be partially inactivated by x radiation if very large doses are used (*i.e.* 20×10^6 rads). This appears to be due to direct effect of the radiation. In dilute aqueous solution, a purified enzyme is inactivated more readily but increased concentrations appear to be protective, suggesting an indirect effect of the radiation. Many compounds, particularly those such as cysteine and glutathione which have an affinity for reaction with oxidizing radicals, exert a protective effect upon enzymes radiated in solution. Oxidative phosphorylation in biological systems results in the generation of adenosine triphosphate (ATP) from adenosine diphosphate (ADP) or monophosphate (AMP). This generation of ATP in cells is accomplished principally in the mitochondria (p. 5). Radiation of isolated mitochondria, *in vitro*, has little effect on their phosphorylation potential, unless very high doses are used (10,000 rads). On the other hand, mitochondria from spleen or thymus of irradiated rats (700 rads), have decreased phosphorylating capacity. Isolated calf thymic nuclei, *in vitro*, have phosphorylating activity which can be inactivated by radiation. Phosphorylation of nuclear histone is also depressed by gamma irradiation. Synthesis of deoxyribonucleic acid (DNA) (p. 317) is also inhibited in plant cells following irradiation, particularly if done prior to the onset of mitosis.

Viruses.—The direct effect of radiation on viruses appears to be most significant in purified, dry or concentrated solution, or in the presence of protective substances. The mean lethal dose may be correlated with the size of some plant and phage viruses. However, with the larger vaccinia virus, the target volume appears to be smaller than the virus itself, perhaps indicating a more radiosensitive component of the virus complex.

Bacteria.—The survival of bacteria has been studied following ionizing radiation in the dry state or suspended in water or nutrient media. Curves prepared of the logarithmic numbers of surviving bacteria usually indicate an exponential relationship to dose but in some instances an increasing percentage of bacteria are killed by each increment of radiation dosage before this exponential relationship is reached. In some conditions, bacteria are protected from the lethal effects of radiant energy by freezing or by the presence of reducing agents in the solution.

Mammalian Cells.—The radiosensitivity of cells, *in vitro*, has been demonstrated for many types of neoplastic and normal animal cells. Many neoplastic murine cells (lymphoma, Ehrlich ascites, sarcoma, mammary carcinoma and squamous cell carcinoma) have been exposed, *in vitro*, to x ray or gamma rays under varying experimental conditions. Of interest is the observation that most of these tumor cells are much more radiosensitive in the oxygenated as compared to the anoxic state. The sensitivity of these cells also varies widely in relation to the stage of the mitotic cycle in which they are irradiated. Certain tumor cells (human "HeLa" cell strain) are quite radiosensitive during mitosis, then are resistant for a period, until the start of DNA synthesis. After completion of DNA synthesis, these cells remain radioresistant until mitosis again is resumed.

Some heritable changes have been demonstrated to occur in cultures of irradiated mammalian cells (Abraham and Barry, 1970). The nucleus of most cells is clearly more sensitive to radiation than the cytoplasm. Although most cells irreparably injured by radiation are unable to reproduce subsequently, many functions of the cell are not impaired until the cell actually undergoes necrosis. A few cells, particularly oocytes and lymphocytes, are quite sensitive in interphase, undergoing necrosis shortly after receiving a small dose.

Non-lethal doses of radiant energy may produce lesions in **chromosomes** which are of particular interest. Modern cytogenetic techniques (p. 322) make it possible to examine chromosomes in metaphase and to detect anomalies in number and morphology. These effects have been observed in human patients who were irradiated for treatment of one of various disorders and in radiation workers whose circulating lymphocytes were subsequently studied by cytogenetic methods (Court-Brown, Buckton and McLean, 1965). These abnormalities have also been seen in many animal karyotypes. Certain lesions in chromosomes are considered unstable in that they are usually lost as the cell undergoes mitosis. These include: chromatid breaks (fracture of one arm of the chromosome), acentric fragments (bits of chromosome with no centromere, resulting from fracture), dicentric chromosomes (with two centromeres, resulting from fracture and rejoining at centromere), tricentric chromosomes (three centromeres) and aneuploidy (more or less than the normal diploid number). Stable, or permanent, lesions include: reciprocal translocations (exchange transfer of parts of chromatids between two chromosomes), ring chromosomes (breaks with fusion of telomeric ends of chromosomes) and aneuploidy (trisomy especially, may also be unstable).

Lesions in chromosomes have been shown to occur in increased numbers in lymphocytes of patients and experimental animals following x-ray treatment. Similar breaks occur in unirradiated subjects, but usually in less than 1 per cent of the cells examined. Following irradiation, these may constitute as much as 37 per cent of the cells karyotyped. These defects undoubtedly change the metabolism of the affected cells but have not been shown to affect germ cells and thus influence the genetic makeup of offspring.

Genes.—The rearrangement, loss or addition of parts of a chromosome doubtlessly has an effect upon the metabolism and progeny of the affected cell. It is also possible for radiant energy to cause chemical alteration in the DNA of cells, resulting in **mutation.** The mutagenic effect of ionizing radiation has been clearly demonstrated in such organisms as the bread mold, *Neurospora*, and fruit fly, *Drosophila*. The evidence for such mutagenic effects in mammals such as mice, is not as convincing. It is possible that mutagenic effects do occur in mammalian germ cells but resulting gametes are less viable, resulting in fewer zygotes carrying the mutant gene.

Carcinogenesis.—Several clear-cut examples exist to indicate that some forms of neoplasia appear with increased frequency in animals and man following exposure to ionizing radiation. (See Neoplasia, page 277.) The possible interaction of certain oncogenic viruses in some neoplasms is yet to be explained. Leukemia in Japanese people who were exposed to irradiation at Hiroshima or Nagasaki clearly became more frequent than in their unirradiated countrymen. Irradiated mice also have significant increased frequency of lymphoma (so-called leukemia). The appearance of squamous cell carcinomas on the hands of radiologists and veterinarians following x-ray injury also is acceptable evidence. Clearly, ionizing radiation may be an antecedent event in certain types of malignant disease, although the precise etiologic relationship and pathogenic mechanisms are not yet established.

Environmental Pollution.—Some forms of radioactivity, particularly resulting from atomic explosions, may become concentrated by biologic processes and therefore represent a special kind of pollutant. Radioiodine is one example, the ^{131}I is concentrated in the thyroid of animals after consumption of contaminated forage. Radiostrontium is more important in this respect because it is metabolized as a chemical analogue of calcium and is concentrated by aquatic plants and animals. Here it becomes part of the food chain of animals and man and therefore a hazard. Radiostrontium (^{90}Sr) is stored in bones of animals and excreted in milk. However, specific biologic discrimination by the cow (*i.e.* intestinal absorption of only part of the ^{90}Sr, deposit of some of it in bone and subsequent urinary excretion with calcium) makes milk one of the safest sources of calcium in an area contaminated by radioactive fallout. In other words, foods directly contaminated would provide relatively more ^{90}Sr to be absorbed and metabolized as calcium (Comar, 1965).

Effects on Biological Systems

ABRAHAM, E. P., and BERRY, R. J.: Some Biological Effects of Radiant Energy. Chapters 25 and 26 in Florey, H. W., *General Pathology*, 4th Ed., Philadelphia, W. B. Saunders Co., 1970.
BENDER, M. A., and GOOCH, P. C.: Persistent Chromosome Aberrations in Irradiated Human Subjects. Radiation Res. *16*:44–53, 1962.
BRILL, A. B., and FORGOTSON, E. H.: Radiation and Congenital Malformations. Amer. J. Obstet. Gynecol. *90*:1149–68, 1964.
COMAR, C. L.: *Radioisotopes in Biology and Agriculture*. New York, McGraw-Hill, 1955.
COURT-BROWN, W. M., BUCKTON, K. E., and McLEAN, A. S.: Quantitative Studies of Chromosome Aberrations in Man Following Acute and Chronic Exposure to X Rays and Gamma Rays. Lancet *1*:1239–1241, 1965.
CHEESEMAN, E. A., and WALBY, A. L.: Intrauterine Irradiation and Iris Heterochromia. Ann. Human Genet. (Lond.) *27*:23–29, 1963.
HOLLAENDER, A.: *Radiation Biology*. New York, McGraw-Hill, 1954.
HUGON, J., and BORGERS, M.: Fine Structure of the Nuclei of Duodenal Crypt Cells after X-irradiation. Amer. J. Path. *52*:701–723, 1968.
LINDOP, P. J., and SACHER, G. A. (Eds.): *Radiation and Ageing*, London, Taylor & Francis Ltd., 1966.
LOUTIT, J. F.: *Irradiation of Mice and Men*. Univ. Chicago Press, Chicago, 1962.
MACLEOD, J., HOTCHKISS, R. S., and SITTERSON, B. W.: Recovery of Male Fertility after Sterilization by Nuclear Radiation. J. Amer. Med. Assn. *187*:637–641, 1964.

MOORE, W., JR., and GILLESPIE, L. J.:   Persistence of Chromosomal Damage Following *In Utero* Irradiation of the Dog. Amer. J. Vet. Res. *28*:890–891, 1967.

MURPHREE, R. L., WHITAKER, W. M., WILDING, J. L., and RUST, J. H.:   Effects of Whole Body Exposure to Irradiation upon Subsequent Fertility of Male Rabbits. Science *115*:709–711, 1952.

NILSSON, A.:   "Effects of Radiostrontium on the Blood and Hematopoietic Tissues of Mice." Acta vet. scand. *3*:1–24, 1962.

RIGGSBY, W. S., JONES, N. D., and GODDEN, W. R.:   Effects of Radiation on Some Serum Enzymes and Trace Elements in Large Animals. p. 36, Air Force Weapons Lab., Kirtland Air Force Base, New Mexico. Tech. Rept. No. AFWL-TR-65-112, 1966.

RUSSELL, W. L.:   The Effect of Radiation Dose Rate and Fractionation on Mutation in Mice in *Repair from Genetic Radiation Damage*, ed. F. H. Sobels, pp. 205–217, Oxford, Pergamon Press, 1963.

SPALDING, J. F., BROOKS, M. R., and ARCHULETA, R. F.:   Genetic Effects of X-irradiation of 10, 15 and 20 Generations of Male Mice. Health Phys. *10*:293–296, 1964.

TARICHENKO, I. I., BUZADZHI, M. I., and BUZADZHI, A. V.:   (Influence of Small Doses of Ionizing Radiation on Some Biochemical Values of the Blood of Calves.) Dokl. vses. Akad. sel'khoz. Nauk No. *7*:35–36, 1966. V.B. *37*:1866, 1967.

WARREN, S.:   *Neoplasms in Pathology*, W. A. D. Anderson, St. Louis, C. V. Mosby Co., 1957, pp. 417–442.

WOLFF, S.:   Some Postirradiation Phenomena that Affect the Induction of Chromosome Aberrations. J. Cell Comp. Physiol. *58*: (Supp. 1) 151–162, 1961.

RADIOSENSITIVITY OF TISSUES

The susceptibility of tissues to radiation varies widely even in the same species. In general, those tissues undergoing the most rapid growth are most susceptible to the injurious effects of ionizing radiation; conversely, cells that have a slower rate of reproduction are most resistant. Thus, cells may be listed in order of their susceptibility to radiation:

1. Lymphoid cells (most susceptible)
2. Epithelial cells of small intestine
3. Hematopoietic cells
4. Germinal cells
5. Epithelial cells of skin
6. Connective tissue cells
7. Cartilage and growing bone cells
8. Cells of brain and spinal cord
9. Cells of skeletal muscle and mature bone

SUSCEPTIBILITY OF DIFFERENT SPECIES

The susceptibility of various animal species to ionizing radiation differs within wide limits. In large animals, the LD 50/30 is also influenced by the source of the radiation and the dosage rate, Rust, *et al.* (1954). The following list from Bond, Fliedner and Archambeau, 1965, indicates the approximate Lethal Dose (LD 50/30) of x or gamma radiation given in one dose over the total body:

Species	rad	Species	rad
Sheep	200–300	Guinea pig	400–500
Swine	200–300	Rhesus monkey	500–600
Dog	240–320	Mouse	525–775
Goat	250–300	Rabbit	700–800
Burro	250–300	Rat	700–820

Simpler forms of life are, in general, much more resistant to the lethal effects of radiation. For example, 750,000 r are required to kill all bacteria in milk; sporulating bacteria may require as much as 500,000 r to kill all spores; tobacco mosaic virus is killed by 1,800,000 r, and although some enzyme systems show measurable effects after this large amount of radiation, many times this dose is required to destroy all enzyme systems in tissues.

Susceptibility of Different Species

BOND, V. P., FLIEDNER, T. M., and ARCHAMBEAU, J. O.: *Mammalian Radiation Lethality: A Disturbance in Cellular Kinetics*, New York, Academic Press, 1965.

GLEISER, C. A.: The Determination of the Lethal Dose 50/30 of Total Body X-radiation for Dogs. Am. J. Vet. Res. *14*:284–286, 1953.

RUST, J. H., WILDING, J. L., TRUM, B. F., SIMONS, C. S., KIMBALL, A. W., and COMAR, C. L.: The Lethal Dose of Whole-Body Tantalum Gamma Irradiation for the Burro (Equus asinus asinus). Radiology *60*:579–582, 1953.

RUST, J. H., TRUM, B. F., and KUHN, U. S. G., III: Physiological Aberrations Following Total Body Irradiation of Domestic Animals with Large Doses of Gamma Rays. Vet. Med. *49*:318, 1954.

WHOLE BODY RADIATION

In contrast to radiation delivered to a specific part of the body (as in radium or x-ray therapy), whole body radiation is the exposure of the entire surface of the body so as to give a uniform dose of ionizing radiation to all parts of the body. This type of radiation injury may be produced experimentally by x and gamma rays and may occur following the detonation of an atomic blast. If dosages are sufficiently high, several systems of the body will be affected, resulting in the syndrome of **radiation sickness.**

The **clinicopathologic changes** in animals exposed to whole body radiation will include immediate and severe lymphopenia with a slow recovery in surviving animals. Within a few days the polymorphonuclear cells in the circulating blood decrease. Thrombocytes in the blood are progressively reduced and return very slowly to the circulation. This thrombocytopenia undoubtedly underlies the hemorrhagic phenomena that follow. Anemia slowly becomes evident, probably due to the reduction of the red cell precursors; blood clot retraction is delayed, and blood levels of alkaline phosphatase are reduced. The iodine uptake by the thyroid may be decreased, the respiratory quotient is reduced, and urea excretion is slightly increased.

The **signs** observed in animals exposed to lethal doses of ionizing radiation depend to some extent upon the dose as well as the dose rate. A few dogs which receive twice a 100 per cent lethal dose ($2 \times$ LD 100/30) of total body radiation may die suddenly within seventy-two hours without manifesting significant symptoms. Diarrhea may develop in some animals, and after a time the stools may become tarry or bloody. Other animals receiving similar doses may not show symptoms for seven to nine days following radiation; then hemorrhages may be observed in visible mucosae, septicemia follows the severe agranulocytosis, and death soon supervenes. Animals exposed to a very high dosage may suddenly exhibit severe disturbances of locomotion and die within seventy-two hours. The symptoms which may be observed, therefore, are not specific and easily could be mistakenly attributed to any one of several causes.

Gross Lesions.—The most prominent gross changes in animals dying after lethal doses of whole body radiation are hemorrhages, which may occur anywhere in the body but most frequently involve the heart, the gastrointestinal and the genitourinary systems. In early stages, congestion of small blood vessels of heart, brain, lungs, mesentery, intestine and subcutis may be the only findings, but later, scattered petechiae also may be found in these organs. The hemorrhages observed in severely affected animals vary from small petechiae to extensive extravasations with occasional hematomas. In goats and pigs, petechiae have been described in the renal cortices and pelves, with large blood clots in the pelves.

Hemorrhages may be seen in the musculature of the back, abdomen, legs, thorax and diaphragm. This is particularly common in guinea pigs, rare in rats, and occasionally seen in goats and pigs. The lymph nodes and tonsils are characteristically hemorrhagic, edematous, enlarged and dark red in color; on cut surfaces hemolytic areas are interspersed with gray, moist-appearing lymphoid tissue. Hemorrhages and ulcerations are the predominant lesions in the gastrointestinal tract. The ulcers are most common in the large intestine and are superficial. Fibrinous membranes, stained with feces, may be removed from the mucosal surface with difficulty, leaving raw, eroded areas in the underlying mucosa. The bone marrow usually loses its deep red color and appears pale and often gelatinous with a yellowish tint.

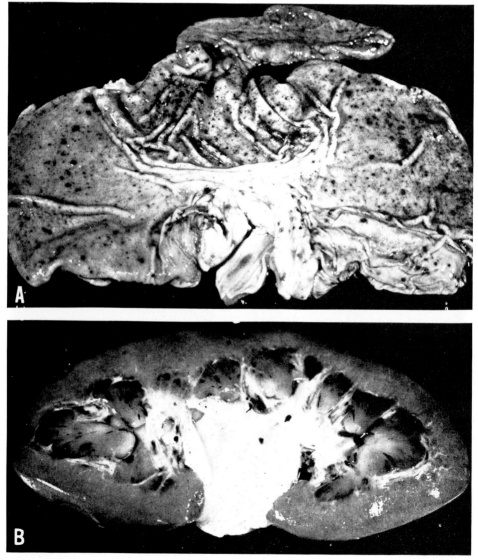

FIG. 16-1.—A, Whole body radiation. Hemorrhages in the stomach of a pig. B, Whole body radiation. Hemorrhages in the renal medulla, kidney of a pig. Contributor: Medical Section, Joint Task Force No. 1, Operation Crossroads. (Courtesy of Armed Forces Institute of Pathology.)

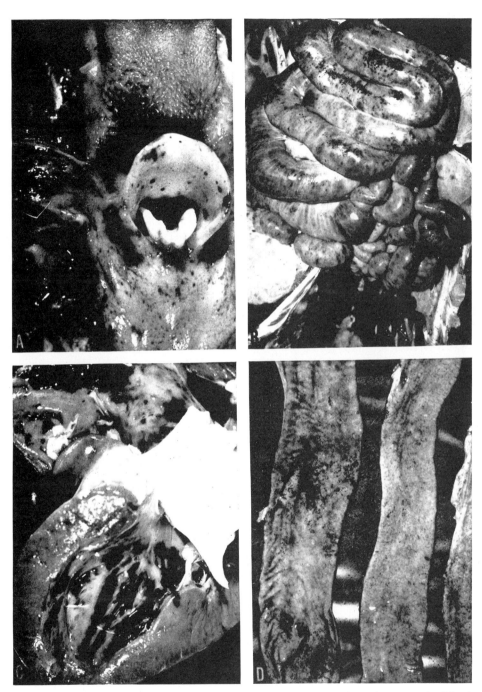

FIG. 16–2.—*A*, Whole body radiation. Hemorrhages in the mucosa of the pharynx and epiglottis of a pig. *B*, Whole body radiation. Hemorrhages in the intestinal serosa of a pig. *C*, Whole body radiation. Subendocardial hemorrhages, heart of a pig. *D*, Whole body radiation. Hemorrhages in the intestinal wall of a pig. Contributor: Medical Section, Joint Task Force No. 1, Operation Crossroads. (Courtesy of Armed Forces Institute of Pathology.)

Microscopic Lesions.—The microscopic findings in lethal whole body radiation generally can be correlated with the gross as well as the clinical manifestations. The degree of injury to tissues depends to some extent upon dosage, but to a greater extent upon the radiosensitivity of the tissue. Lymphoid cells, being most susceptible, will manifest the most severe changes, while mature bone will be least affected.

Lymphoid tissues, such as lymph nodes, spleen, thymus and tonsils, are affected promptly and this is reflected in the microscopic alterations. Necrosis of lymphocytes as evidenced by pyknosis, karyorrhexis and karyolysis of nuclei is the earliest and most significant finding. As a result the germinal centers soon appear "washed out," leaving only the reticulo-endothelial cells. The sinuses are dilated and filled with macrophages, some of which have engulfed erythrocytes as well as tissue debris. Recent hemorrhages may be evident, and, in cases of longer duration, collections of blood pigment. Secondary changes due to abscesses, ulcers, hemorrhages or other lesions in the organs drained by a particular lymph node may occur in cases with prolonged survival time.

Bone Marrow.—Microscopically, detectable lesions occur in the bone marrow within a few hours after heavy doses of radiation. Necrosis of hematopoietic cells, particularly the most immature, occurs very early. The myelocytes appear most susceptible, the megakaryocytes and erythrocytes less so, and the reticular cells quite resistant. The sinuses become dilated with plasma or red blood cells. Within a week or two, most radiosensitive elements disappear from the bone marrow, leaving aplastic, acellular marrow which contains only fat cells, reticular cells, edema and hemorrhage. Secondary infection may be the means by which colonies of fungi or bacteria are transplanted in the marrow, where they grow, usually without apparent inflammatory reaction to their presence. Bloom (1948) has described a change in irradiated small animals in which the bony trabeculae on the diaphyseal side of the epiphyseal cartilage disappear and are replaced by fibrillar stroma. The resulting separation of the epiphyseal cartilage from the spongy bone on the diaphyseal side has been referred to as "severance" of the epiphyseal plate.

Digestive System.—Shallow ulcers with little or no underlying leukocytic infiltration are common in the oral and pharyngeal mucous membranes, especially along the margins of the tongue and adjacent to the tonsillar crypts. These shallow ulcers have a necrotic base, but only if the animal is beginning to recover from agranulocytosis do leukocytes appear. The mucous membrane of the digestive tract from the esophagus to the anus is severely affected by whole body radiation. Edema of the submucosa and subserosa is common throughout the tract, and is usually associated with necrosis of the mucosal epithelium and frequent hemorrhages in all parts of the wall. The necrosis of the epithelium rarely extends deeper than the submucosa, and perforation seldom occurs. Blood vessels of the lamina propria and submucosa adjacent to ulcers may be dilated and contain fibrin thrombi. Individual epithelial cells may be seen to have undergone several changes; namely, vacuolization of cytoplasm or nuclei, and distortion in size and shape. Hyaline changes in the submucosal stroma may occur late in association with formation of bizarre fibroblasts and fibrocytes.

Genital System.—The germinal cells of the testis and ovary are among the more radiosensitive cells of the animal body, hence are readily destroyed by radiation. In the acute stage, hemorrhage and edema may be seen, but the most specific effect is the destruction of spermatogonia as well as spermatocytes, with little effect upon spermatozoa. It should be pointed out that whole body radiation in sufficient dosage to destroy germinal cells would be enough to kill the animal, hence sterility would be an academic problem. If the same dosage were applied only to the gonads, the whole body effect would be nil, but sterility of temporary or permanent duration would result.

Other Systems.—The microscopic lesions in the lungs, skin, urinary system, liver and gallbladder, brain, bone and muscle, except for involvement by widely distributed hemorrhages, are either inadequately studied or are generally believed to be inconstant and not specific.

Whole Body Radiation

BEHRENS, C. F.: *Atomic Medicine*, New York, Thomas Nelson & Sons, 1949.
GLEISER, C. A.: A Review of Some Basic Concepts of the Biology and Pathogenesis of Acute Ionizing Body Radiation. J. Am. Vet. Med. Assn. *124*:220–224, 1954.
—————: The Pathology of Total Body Radiation in Dogs Which Died Following Exposure to a Lethal Dose. Am. J. Vet. Res. *15*:329–335, 1954.
GUTTMAN, P. H., and KOHN, H. I.: Progressive Intercapillary Glomerulosclerosis in the Mouse, Rat and Chinese Hamster, Associated with Aging and X-ray Exposure. Amer. J. Path. *37*:293–307, 1960.
HALEY, T. J., McCULLOH, E. F., McCORMICK, W. G., TRUM, B. F., and RUST, J. H.: Response of the Burro to 100 r Fractional Whole Body Gamma Ray Irradiation. Am. J. Physiol. *180*: 403–407, 1955.
HALEY, T. J., CARTWRIGHT, F. D., and BROWN, D. G.: Plasma Minerals in Normal and Neutron Irradiated Burros. Nature, Lond. *212*:820–821, 1966.
LANE, J. J., PAYSINGER, J. R., MURPHREE, R. L., RUST, J. H., and TRUM, B. F.: Effect of Total Body Irradiation on Rabbit Pituitary as Measured by Gonadotropin Response in Chicks. Proc. Soc. Exper. Biol. & Med. *86*:36–38, 1954.
LEIBOW, A. A., WARREN, S., and DeCOURSEY, E.: Pathology of Atomic Bomb Casualties. Am. J. Path. *25*, 853–1027, 1949.
MAYHEW, C. J., KUHN, U. S. G., III, RUST, J. H., TRUM, B. F., and WOODWARD, J. M.: Bacterial Permeation of the Gut Wall in Irradiated Burros. Am. J. Vet. Res. *16*:525–528, 1955.
McLEAN, F. C., RUST, J. H., and BUDY, A. M.: Extension to Man of Experimental Whole-Body Irradiation Studies; Some Military and Civil Defense Considerations. Mil. Surg. *112*: 174–182, 1953.
MEWISSEN, D. J., COMAR, C. L., TRUM, B. F., and RUST, J. H.: A Formula for Chronic Radiation Dosage Versus Shortening of Life Span: Application to a Large Mammal. Radiation Res. *6*:450–459, 1957.
OLSEN, R. E.: The Effects of Wholebody Gamma-irradiation on Some Blood Constituents and Hemopoietic Organs of the Calf. Diss. Abstr. *26*:7266, 1966.
RUST, J. H., FOLMAR, G. D., JR., LANE, J. J., and TRUM, B. F.: The Lethal Dose of Total Body Cobalt-60 Gamma Radiation for the Rabbit. Am. J. Roentgen. *74*:135–138, 1955.
RUST, J. H., TRUM, B. F., HEGLIN, J., McCULLOH, E., and HALEY, T. J.: Effect of 200 Roentgens Fractional Whole Body Irradiation in the Burro. Proc. Soc. Exper. Biology & Med. *85*:258–261, 1954.
RUST, J. H., TRUM, B. F., LANE, J. J., KUHN, U. S. G., III, PAYSINGER, J. R., and HALEY, T. J.: Effects of 50 Roentgens and 25 Roentgens Fractional Daily Rotal-Body r-Irradiation in the Burro. Radiation Research *2*:475–482, 1955.
RUST, J. H., TRUM, B. F., WILDING, J. L., SIMONS, C. S., and COMAR, C. L.: Lethal Dose Studies with Burros and Swine Exposed to Whole Body Cobalt-60 Irradiation. Radiology *62*: 569–574, 1954.
SNIDER, R. S., and RAPER, J. R.: Histopathological Effects of Single Doses of Total-Surface Beta Radiation of Mice, in Zirkle, R. E. (Ed.): *Effects of External Beta Radiation*. New York, McGraw-Hill, 1951, chap. 9, pp. 152–178.
TESSMER, C. F., and HORAVA, A.: Spleen Cytology Studies in Swine Exposed to Nuclear Radiation. Lab. Invest. *10*:411–434, 1961.
TRUM, B. F., HALEY, T. J., BASSIN, M., HEGLIN, J., and RUST, J. H.: Effect of 400 Fractional Whole Body X-Irradiation in the Burro (Equus asinus asinus). Am. J. Physiol. *174*:57–60, 1953.

Trum, B. F., Rust, J. H., and Wilding, J. L.: Clinical Observations Upon the Response of the Burro to Large Doses of External Whole Body Gamma Irradiation. The Auburn Veterinarian 8:131–136, 1952.
Warren, S.: Effects of Radiation on Normal Tissues. Arch Path. 34:443–450, 917–1084, (with C. E. Dunlap) 562–608, (with N. B. Friedman) 749–88, 1942.
————: The Histopathology of Radiation Lesions. Physiol. Rev. 24:225–238, 1944.

RADIOACTIVE FALLOUT

The explosion of a thermonuclear weapon releases not only vast quantities of energy in the form of heat, light and blast, but also great amounts of radioactivity. Part of this radioactivity is released instantaneously in the form of neutrons and gamma rays which can produce radiation effects within their range. This range, or distance through which these radiations travel and thus produce biological effects, is dependent upon the energy of the explosion but is not great even in the most powerful explosions. However, fast-moving neutrons can penetrate deeply into matter and induce radioactivity in otherwise stable substances. This **induced**, or **secondary**, radioactivity, under certain circumstances, can be an important source of ionizing radiation.

Of far greater significance in an explosive fission reaction is the release of radioactive substances in particulate form. These particles consist of radioactive fission products, matter (sea water, air, soil) in which radioactivity has been induced and, perhaps, remnants of the original fissionable material. The explosive power of the bomb may send great quantities of these radioactive

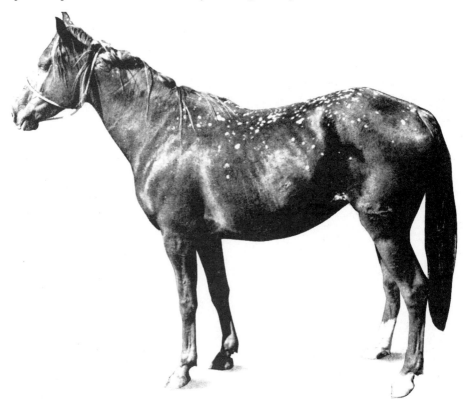

Fig. 16–3.—Effect of radioactive fallout. The lesions are discrete and located on the dorsal portions of the body of this horse. Photograph courtesy of Lt. Col. B. F. Trum, V.C.

materials high into the earth's atmosphere, wind currents move them as clouds over great distances, then rain or other atmospheric conditions cause the particulate matter to fall back to the earth. This **fallout** may constitute serious hazard to man, plants and animals in areas downwind from the point of detonation. The areas of serious radioactivity would vary in size according to such factors as yield and height of burst, the nature of the surface over which the burst occurs, and the meteorological conditions present. The radioactive material may lodge on the skin of the backs of animals which are out in the open, or may fall on pasture or animal feed where it may be ingested and cause **internal radiation,** a condition which will be discussed later.

The **fallout** of radioactive materials may occur as a shower of dry flaky material or as minute invisible particles, perhaps accompanied by rain. The fact that radioactivity is associated with particles has an important influence upon skin lesions resulting from contact with this material. The chemical nature of material in radioactive fallout will depend upon the composition of the bomb as well as the medium in which it was exploded (air, sea, underground). Most radioisotopes of importance in such radioactive clouds decay by emission of *beta particles* and *gamma rays*. *Alpha particle* emitters are a possibility, but because of their low penetrability would have little effect upon the skin.

The effect of radioisotopes on the skin depends upon (1) their energy and type of emission, (2) duration of their contact with the skin, (3) their radioactive half-life, (4) any irritating effect due to their chemical nature.

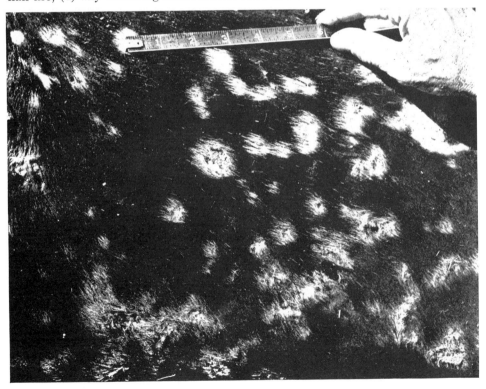

Fig. 16–4.—Radioactive fallout. Lesions in the skin of the back of a horse. Depigmentation of hair in sharply circumscribed areas with alopecia and ulceration in the center of some of them. Photograph courtesy of Lt. Col. B. F. Trum. V.C.

Lesions will develop in the skin of animals exposed to radioactive fallout, provided the material is in contact with the skin for a sufficient length of time. As indicated previously, alpha particles do not penetrate the keratin layer, hence produce no effect upon the skin; gamma rays penetrate deeply but have low specific ionization in the superficial layers, therefore produce little direct effect upon the skin; beta particles, on the other hand, penetrate most layers of the skin, have high specific ionization and produce severe effects. The skin lesions caused by beta particles have been called "beta burns," but they are not strictly burns since no heat is involved.

The sequence of changes resulting from contact with beta-emitting radio-isotopes has been studied by Moritz and Henriques (1952) who placed beta-emitting plaques in contact with the skin of swine. These workers used radioisotopes of different energies, sulfur-35 (0.17 mev), cobalt-60 (0.31 mev), cesium-137 (0.55 mev), yttrium-91 (1.53 mev) and strontium-yttrium-90 (0.61 and 2.2 mev), to demonstrate the relationships between the energy of the isotope and the surface, or transepidermal, dose to the resultant radiation injury. These studies provide information on the development of changes following radiation of this type; some of these changes have been observed in "field" cases of injury due to radioactive fallout. The remarks that follow are based on the reports of Moritz and Henriques.

The first observable change in swine skin following exposure to these radio-active isotopes is **erythema,** which may appear within twenty-four hours. If erythema persists seventy-two hours or more, it is indicative of injury severe enough to result in chronic radiation dermatitis. Edema of dermal papillae, if recognizable within forty-eight hours following irradiation, will be followed by transepidermal necrosis. Death of cells in the basal and deeper malpighian layers of the epidermis, demonstrated by increase in staining intensity of their nuclei, occurs within twenty-four hours following high dosage, but with lower dosage may not appear for ten to fourteen days. **Epidermal atrophy,** one of the least severe changes, is recognized in microscopic sections only and is seen one to two weeks following radiation. This change is evidenced by thinning of the rete, presumably as a result of depression of cell division in the basal layer plus continued desquamation of surface layers. It persists for two to four weeks and appears to be completely reversible, since there are no residua. **Exfoliation** and crust formation follow more severe injury, begin during the second week, and may be precursors of chronic radiation dermatitis. A scaling brown crust is shed for weeks or months, apparently because of accelerated maturation of malpighian cells without loss of their nuclei, thus resulting in **parakeratosis.** Death of individual cells in the deeper parts of the epidermis may continue for many weeks after irradiation.

Epidermal necrosis and exfoliation follow higher dosages of radiation. The first indication of probable irreversible injury is swelling and vacuolation of cytoplasm of epidermal cells which may appear ragged or coagulated into round, acidophilic hyaline masses. There is also disorganization of the basal and malpighian layers with vesicles appearing at the dermal-epidermal interface. **Transepidermal necrosis** with ulceration of the entire target area follows still higher dosage and may be complete within forty-eight hours. With lower dosage, several weeks may elapse before necrosis of the epidermis is complete. Radiation of lower energy (sulfur-35, 0.17 mev) produces shallow ulcers with little damage to the dermis, while higher energy beta radiation—from strontium-yttrium-90

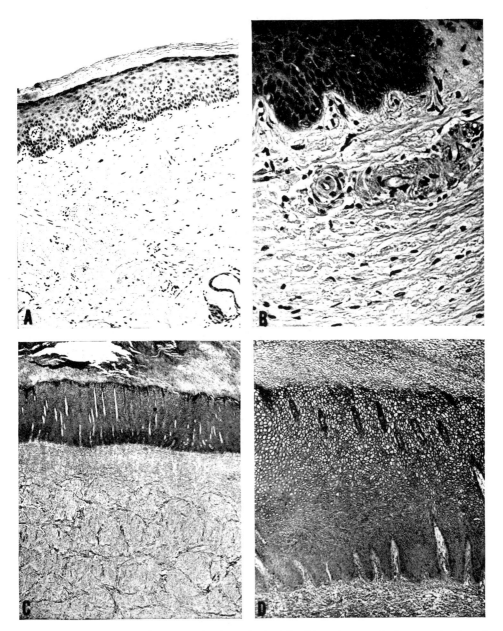

FIG. 16–5.—A, Radioactive fallout, bovine skin (× 75). Note absence of sebaceous glands and remnant of sweat gland in dermis. B, Radioactive fallout, bovine skin (× 250). Thickened hyaline wall in capillary of dermis. Specimen taken several years after exposure. C, Radioactive fallout, bovine skin (× 11). Several years after exposure. Severe hyperkeratosis, acanthosis and loss of adnexa. D, Higher magnification of C (× 48), illustrating acanthosis and part of the layer of hyperkeratosis. (Courtesy of Armed Forces Institute of Pathology.) Contributor: Dr. Cyril Comar.

(0.61 and 2.2 mev), cobalt-60 (0.31 mev), and cesium-137 (0.55 mev) — results in deep injury to the dermis and is followed by chronic radiation dermatitis.

Changes in the **dermis** and **subcutis** are observed only if the epidermis is damaged. The earliest lesion is hyperemia of the capillaries in the dermal papillae, followed by edema, asteroid swelling of fibrocytes and exudation of lymphocytes and neutrophils in relation to the ulceration of epidermis. Edema, capillary ectasia and degenerative changes in arterioles may persist after regeneration of epithelium, but the dermis in this state apparently cannot support the growth of epithelium, therefore ulceration recurs.

Epilation takes place when the dosage of higher energy beta particles is sufficient to produce recognizable injury in the epidermis; lower energy beta radiation from sulfur-35, however, does not produce epilation. When dermal papillae receive sufficient radiation to cause loss of hair, they become atrophic and contracted, particularly in length. Atrophy occurs in epithelial cells of the hair matrix, including the inner root sheath, and may or may not be associated with swelling and squamous metaplasia. Sometimes columns of cells from hair follicles may persist, but they undergo central dissolution, producing epithelial-lined cysts, which may or may not communicate with the surface. In severe injury, hair follicles are permanently destroyed.

Other **skin adnexa,** sebaceous and sweat glands, may disappear without a trace after high energy beta radiation in sufficient dosage to destroy the epidermis. These structures are not replaced. Less severely affected tubular glands may become atrophic and be surrounded by a dense hyaline membrane.

In **chronic radiation dermatitis,** characterized clinically by persistent exfoliation with crust formation of one to three months' duration, the microscopic findings are parakeratosis, with atrophy (or less often, hyperplasia) of the epidermis associated with chronic inflammation in the dermis. In some instances, there is proliferation and downward growth of the epithelium with pleomorphism, loss of polarity and increased numbers of mitotic figures. This change suggests a trend toward neoplasia.

The skin of cattle studied several years after exposure to severe doses of radiation from fallout presented irregular areas of scarring, surrounded by zones of epilation and white hair. The scarred areas were partially covered by dense layers of tough horny material several centimeters in thickness. Microscopically, these scarred areas were covered by thick stratified squamous epithelium with an overlying dense layer of keratin. The rete pegs, hair follicles, sebaceous and sweat glands were absent under the affected epithelium but occasionally were present, although atrophic, at the edges of lesions (Fig. 16–5).

In horses exposed to radioactive fallout, focal areas of ulceration surrounded by a wide zone of white hair (Fig. 16–4) have been reported. Because radioactivity emitted from particulate fallout usually arises from a point source and is given off nearly equally in all directions, the volume of skin affected will be roughly hemispherical in depth, while the surface lesion will be round.

Radioactive Fallout

ARCHAMBEAU, J. O., FAIRCHILD, R. G., and COMMERFORD, S. L.: Response of Skin of Swine to Increasing Exposures of 250 KVP X-Ray. *In* Bustad, L. K. & McClellan, R. O. *Swine in Biomedical Research*, 463–489, Richland, Wn, Battelle Memorial Institute, 1966.
BROWN, D. G., REYNOLDS, R. A., and JOHNSON, D. F.: Late Effects in Cattle Exposed to Radioactive Fallout. Am. J. Vet. Res. 27:1509–1514, 1966.

COMAR, C. L.: Movement of Fallout Radionuclides through the Biosphere and Man. Ann. Rev. Nucl. Sci. *15*:175–206, 1965.

GEORGE, L. A., and BUSTAD, L. K.: Comparative Effects of Beta Irradiation of Swine, Sheep and Rabbit Skin. *In* Bustad and McClellan *Swine in Biomedical Research*, 491–500, Richland, Wn., Battelle Memorial Institute, 1966.

HENRIQUES, F. W., JR.: Effect of Beta Rays on the Skin as a Function of the Energy Intensity and Duration of Radiation. I. Physical Considerations. Preparation and Calibration of Beta-emitting Plaques. Lab. Invest. *1*:153–166, 1952.

MORITZ, A. R., and HENRIQUES, F. W., JR.: Effect of Beta Rays on the Skin as a Function of the Energy, Intensity and Duration of Radiation. II. Animal Experiments. Lab. Invest. *1*:167–185, 1952.

TESSMER, C. F.: Radioactive Fallout Effects on Skin. I. Effects of Radioactive Fallout on Skin of Almagordo Cattle. Arch. Path. *72*:175–190, 1961.

TESSMER, C. F., and BROWN, D. G.: Carcinoma of Skin and Bovine Exposed to Radioactive Fallout. J. Amer. Med. Assn. *179*:210–214, 1962.

TULLIS, J. L., and WARREN, S.: Gross Autopsy Observation in the Animals Exposed at Bikini; Preliminary Report. J. Amer. Med. Assn. *134*:1155–1158, 1947.

TULLIS, J. L., LAWSON, B. C., and MADDEN, S. C.: Pathology of Swine Exposed to Total Body Gamma Radiation from an Atomic Bomb Source. Amer. J. Path. *31*:41–51, 1955.

INTERNAL RADIATION

Radioactive isotopes may gain access to the human or animal body by inhalation, ingestion, parenteral injection, or absorption through wounds in the skin. The effect produced by these isotopes depends upon many factors, the most important of which are: the quantity, specific ionization and energy of radioactivity taken into the body; its deposition in critical or radiosensitive tissues; the biological half-life of the isotope, and the size and importance to life of the organ in which the isotope is deposited. Internal radiation is, except in the immediate region of an explosion and close-in areas of fallout, a much greater hazard than external radiation, since the isotope is in contact with the animal tissues for longer periods of time, and, even if of low energy, may be deposited in critical tissues (bone, thyroid) in intimate enough contact to cause serious damage. Sources of radioactivity which possibly could become internal radiation hazards to animals include fallout following explosions of atomic weapons with contamination of animal feeds, water or pastures; contamination of feed or water by inadequate disposal of radioactive wastes from atomic "piles," power reactors or industrial and medical facilities in which radioisotopes are used.

Radioactive isotopes are metabolized in the body in exactly the same manner as are nonradioactive isotopes of the same element. Therefore, radioiodine (^{131}I) is rapidly concentrated in the thyroid exactly as is stable iodine (^{127}I). Radiocalcium (^{45}Ca) is deposited in bone as are its nonradioactive isotopes (^{40,42}Ca, etc.)

FIG. 16–6.—Positive print of an autoradiograph of the femur of a dog which had received strontium-90. Photograph courtesy of Dr. Arthur Lindenbaum, Argonne National Laboratory.

and is eliminated not only in feces and urine but in milk. Radiosodium (^{24}Na) is distributed more widely through the tissues and is eliminated rather rapidly, hence is not as great a hazard as ^{131}I or ^{45}Ca.

Many radioisotopes are not ordinarily metabolized by the body but are deposited in tissues in much the same way as are similar chemical elements. The most important of these are the **"bone seekers"** which include strontium-90, radium-226, uranium, radioactive rare earths and plutonium.

Bone-seeking radioisotopes are deposited in growing bone, at first most heavily concentrated in the metaphysis, particularly adjacent to the epiphyseal line where they remain in greatest concentration. After a time, radioactivity can be demonstrated also in the diaphyses of the long bones by radioautographs (Fig. 16–6), prepared by placing slabs of affected bone in contact with photographic film for a period of time, then developing the film. Radioactive components darken the film, indicating their site of deposition in the tissue.

The deposition of radioactivity in the bones may destroy the hematopoietic elements, thus producing aplastic anemia, and may adversely affect the growing bone, predisposing to osteogenic sarcoma. Aside from these effects upon the individual, radioactive bones in meat-producing animals could become a food hazard to man or to other animals.

Radioiodine (^{131}I) in sufficient dosage can cause enough destruction of thyroid tissue to interfere seriously with the function of the gland. Internal radiation from these isotopes has especially deleterious effects on young animals.

Internal Radiation

BLOOM, W.: *Histopathology of Irradiation from External and Internal Sources.* New York, McGraw-Hill Book Co., 1948.
KRUMHOLZ, L. A., and RUST, J. H.: Osteogenic Sarcoma in a Muskrat from an Area of High Environmental Radiostrontium. A.M.A. Archives of Pathology 57:270–278, 1954.
PROSSER, C. L., et al.: Plutonium Project; Clinical Sequence of Physiological Effects of Ionizing Radiation in Animals. Radiology 49:299–312, 1947.
SOBELLS, F. H.: *Repair from Genetic Radiation Damage,* Oxford, Pergamon Press, 1963.

17

Diseases Due to Extraneous Poisons

Some poisons are produced by pathogenic microorganisms in the course of an infection, a few are generated by disorders of body metabolism, but the majority are formed outside the body, which they enter via the digestive canal, by inhalation, through the skin or occasionally by other routes.

Poisons entering the body produce their evil effects in a variety of ways. (1) Many poisons, when in sufficient concentration, kill the tissues with which they come in contact (necrosis) or, if the action is milder, injure the tissues and initiate an acute inflammatory reaction. Poisons in this category are those which have a strong chemical action on organic matter, the strong acids, strong alkalies or compounds with a highly active ion such as fluorine. If the poison has been ingested, it is the alimentary mucous membranes which suffer the necrosis or inflammation. The most powerful ones such as lye destroy the lining of the mouth or esophagus as they are swallowed and then carry their effect to the stomach. Others pass through the stomach with little damage and cause superficial necrosis and inflammation in the upper or lower intestine, presumably because they remain longer in contact with the injured part. In speaking of the intestine, it may be interjected here that some poisons (such as mercury) after absorption into the blood are excreted into the large intestine, producing inflammation as they pass through the mucous membrane.

(2) Poisons of a second and very important group have little or no immediate action but, after absorption from the alimentary mucosa, other mucous membrane or the skin, produce their effect upon the delicate epithelial cells of such parenchymatous organs as the liver or kidneys, which they reach via the blood stream. This group includes most of the poisons of the first group when diluted sufficiently that they do not kill by direct local destruction. It also includes most of the plant poisons as well as bacterial toxins.

(3) Other poisons owe their effect to interference with some vital nervous function and often leave no visible pathological change to betray their harmful handiwork. Strychnine is an example.

(4) Certain poisons owe their effects to, or at least reveal their presence by, numerous petechiae or ecchymoses, the result of injury to the endothelium of capillaries. (5) Some hemolyze the circulating erythrocytes; (6) a few destroy the hematopoietic powers of the bone marrow. (7) Certain ones produce their effects by blocking vital enzyme systems, usually without any identifying lesions. Many combine several of the above and other actions.

It is hoped here to summarize such information as is available concerning the tissue changes resulting from those poisons commonly involving domestic animals. Unfortunately, many of the poisons have not been adequately studied from the standpoint of their pathological effects, diagnosis being, therefore, unnecessarily difficult.

Having ourselves been pupils at one time (and still being students), we suspect considerable effort may be necessary, if the reader is to keep clearly in mind the characteristic symptoms and lesions which go with each of the poisonings requiring description in this chapter. With a view to facilitating this somewhat painful process we have undertaken to group the various poisons in accordance with some outstanding lesion which, upon being encountered, might be expected to afford a clue to the diagnosis. To effect such a grouping is by no means easy, not only because the manifestations of a given poisoning vary in different individuals, but more so because many of the poisons attack the patient by several of the mechanisms outlined above and produce a number of lesions, no one of which is salient among the others. It thus becomes most difficult to decide to which pathological family a particular poison belongs. Nevertheless, we venture to hope that a grouping of this nature may facilitate fixing in mind at least one important pathological feature of each poison, thus providing a bit of assistance in problems of differentiation. Obviously reference must be had to each description for a complete picture of what may be expected in a case of poisoning by each agent.

Whenever it is possible to use pathologic and clinical features to decrease the number of suspected etiologic agents, further investigation is simplified. Chemical identification of the poison or clear demonstration of its ingestion or contact should always be attempted when the situation permits. In only a few poisonings are lesions characteristic enough to permit definitive diagnosis. As with infectious diseases, it is important to demonstrate the etiologic agent in association with the lesions that it is expected to cause.

Many poisonous plants will be referred to in this chapter by their common and scientific names. No further effort is made to identify the plants. This identification is admirably accomplished by John M. Kingsbury in his book, *Poisonous Plants of the United States and Canada*, Prentice-Hall, 1964.

Extraneous poisons will be taken up in the following sequence:

Group A. (p. 845) POISONS WHICH PRODUCE LOCAL INJURY.

| Venoms | Phenol | Lewisite | Mustard gas |

Group B. (p. 848) POISONS WHICH CAUSE GASTROENTERITIS AS A PROMINENT FEATURE.

Arsenic	Ground glass	Castor beans	Oaks
Salt	Dynamite	Locusts	Oleander
Petroleum	Urea	Tung oil tree	Lantana
Sodium fluoro-	Nicotine	Fluorensia cernua	Milk weeds
acetate	Nightshades		Red squill

Group C. (p. 864) HEPATOTOXIC POISONS. OFTEN ALSO NEPHROTOXIC.

Phosphorus	Phenothiazine	Senecios	Mushrooms
Phosphates	Phenanthridinium	Tarweed	Heliotrope
Copper	Clay pigeons, Pitch	Sacahuiste	Lupines
Tannic acid	Hydrogen sulfide	Drymaria	Vetch
Carbon tetrachlo-	Gossypol	Lechugilla	Algae
ride	Cocklebur	Phyllanthrus	Moldy Feeds
Tetrachloroethylene			Aflatoxin

Group D. (p. 893) POISONS WHICH ARE PREDOMINANTLY NEPHROTOXIC.

| Turpentine | Sulfonamides | Oxalates | Broomweed |
| | Chloroform | | Chinese Tallow Tree |

Group E. (p. 901)   POISONS CAUSING DEATH THROUGH CARDIAC INSUFFICIENCY.

Selenium   Death camas   Aconite   Baileya   Jimson weed

Group F. (p. 906)   POISONS CAUSING EXTENSIVE HEMORRHAGES.

Dicoumarin   Bracken fern   Crotalaria   Trichloroethylene-extracted
                                                  soybean meal

Group G. (p. 916)   POISONS CAUSING HEMOLYTIC ANEMIA.

Molybdenum   Naphthalene   Onions

Group H. (p. 917)   POISONS CAUSING PRODUCTION OF METHEMOGLOBIN AND CHOCOLATE-COLORED
BLOOD.

Nitrates   Nitrites   Chlorates

Group I. (p. 920)   POISONS CAUSING PRODUCTION OF CARBOXYHEMOGLOBIN AND CHERRY RED
BLOOD.

                    Carbon monoxide   Cyanides

Group J. (p. 922)   POISONS CAUSING MARKED AND CONSPICUOUS EDEMA.

Alpha-naphthyl Thiourea (ANTU)   Toxic fat

Group K. (p. 925)   A POISON CAUSING MARKED AND CONSPICUOUS PULMONARY EMPHYSEMA.

                    Rape, Kale

Group L. (p. 927)   POISONS CAUSING GANGRENE OF THE EXTREMITIES.

                    Ergot   Fescue grass

Group M. (p. 928)   A POISON CAUSING UNUSUAL LESIONS OF BONE AND TEETH.

                    Fluorine

Group N. (p. 935)   POISONS CAUSING LOSS OF HAIR OR WOOL.

                    Thallium   Jumbay tree

Group O. (p. 938)   A POISON CAUSING EPITHELIAL HYPERPLASIA.

                    Chlorinated naphthalenes

Group P. (p. 942)   POISONS CAUSING NERVOUS MALFUNCTION.

Strychnine   Atropine   Yellow Star Thistle   Mercury
Nitrogen trichloride Equisetum   Botulinus   Chlorinated hydro-
                                                            carbons

Loco   Hemlocks   Anguina   Organic phos-
Vetch-like Astragali Lathyrus   Carbon disulfide   phates
                                     Ortho-tricresyl
                                     Phosphate
Claviceps paspali   Larkspur   Lead   Cycada

Group Q. (p. 968)   POISONS CAUSING DEGENERATION OF CARDIAC AND SKELETAL MUSCLES.
Coffee senna   Coytillo   Hairy vetch (p. 885)

Group R. (p. 971)   POISONS CAUSING TERATOGENIC OR OTHER EFFECTS ON THE EMBRYO OR FETUS.
Veratrum californicum   Lupin (p. 882)
Thalidomide   Selenium (p. 901)
                                               Lathyrus (p. 951)

Group S. (p. 975)   MISCELLANEOUS OR UNCLASSIFIED POISONS.
Smallhead sneezewood   Yew   Nitrogen dioxide
Box   Phalaris grass   Cobalt
Grasstree   Sorghum   Hexachlorophene
Stinkwood   Sesbania   Chloroquine
Pokeweed   Estrogen   Zinc

*   *   *   *   *

Group A: **Poisons which produce local injury** (necrosis and inflammation) to the tissues with which they come in contact. Obviously an appropriate degree of concentration is essential to the production of this effect. As mentioned earlier, strong acids and alkalies fall in this group but only the following will be accorded specific headings.

Venoms   **Phenol**   **Lewisite**   **Mustard gas**

VENOMS OF SNAKES AND OTHER CREATURES

Snake bites, at least those of the North American rattlesnakes, copperheads and moccasins, promptly cause an extremely rapid, though weakening heartbeat, but their most spectacular effect is tremendous local swelling, which is well under way within minutes after the bite is inflicted. The swelling is the result of inflammatory edema, or more precisely, of serous inflammatory exudation. Within three or four hours the maximum is reached and, if the bite is on the nose, as it usually is in horses and may be in the case of dogs and cattle, suffocation may ensue from closing of the nostrils or glottis. If the animal survives, the swelling subsides in from four to seven days, but the toxic injury is sometimes so severe that necrosis and sloughing of a large mass of tissue may supervene. Hemolysis is another effect of the venom, perhaps to the extent that hemoglobinuria and hemolytic icterus may be noticeable. There is also interference with clotting of the blood. Post-mortem findings include the above changes plus extreme passive congestion of all organs and hemorrhages in the region of the bite. Local gas gangrene or tetanus occasionally supervenes, initiated by the bacterial contamination of the serpent's mouth.

The **stings of bees** and various other insects are similar to snake bites in causing an extreme degree of serous exudation. This fluid in either type of poisoning exerts a valuable protective effect by diluting the poison and causing so much local pressure that circulation of the blood and the consequent dissemination of the poison are inhibited. The severity of the reaction to the stings of bees and scorpions and the bites of ants varies greatly in different individuals of any species, apparently on an allergic basis. Even horses have died from multiple bee stings, methemoglobinemia and bilirubinemia being noted.

The **black widow spider** (*Latrodectus mactans*), according to Pritchard (1940), requires careful consideration in the diagnosis of sudden canine illnesses in practically all parts of the United States and many other countries. While some dogs appear to be entirely immune (whether from a previous exposure is unknown) the bite of this black spider with the red "hour-glass" spot on its abdomen may well be fatal to a dog or, presumably, to a cat. The period of illness may be terminated fatally in two hours or it may continue for two or three days with recovery or death. Early symptoms commence with pain at the site of the bite, which may be very severe. Edema (serous inflammatory exudate) also develops around the bite. The whole integument becomes painful and hypersensitive to slight pressure; the abdominal wall becomes rigid through reflex contraction of the muscles. In some cases, hyperesthesia which appears to reside in the articular surfaces causes fleeting but pronounced pain which, in a matter of minutes, may shift from one limb to another. If the intoxication persists, a gradually increasing paralysis may appear on the second or third day and become so extensive as to produce death, the pain, meanwhile, having subsided. Post mortem, there is little to be seen but venous congestion.

Venoms of Snakes and Other Creatures

BAERG, W. J.: The Black Widow: Its Life History and the Effects of the Poison. Scient. Monthly *17*:535–547, 1923.
COMSTOCK, J. H.: *The Spider Book*. Ithaca, New York, Comstock Pub. Co., Inc. 1948.
CRIMMINS, M. L.: Facts about Texas Snakes and Their Poisons. J. Am. Vet. Med. Assn. *71*:704–712, 1927.

Ditmars, R. L.: Snake Bites among Domestic Animals. J. Am. Vet. Med. Assn. *94*:383–388, 1939.

McNellis, R.: Rattlesnake Bite. J. Am. Vet. Med. Assn. *114*:145–146, 1949.

Nighbert, E. M.: Effects of Bites of Poisonous Snakes on Dogs. North Am. Vet. *24*:363–364, 1943.

Parrish, H. M., Scatterday, J. E., and Pollard, C. B.: The Clinical Management of Snake Venom Poisoning in Domestic Animals. J. Am. Vet. Med. Assn. *130*:548–551, 1957. (Includes pathology.)

Pritchard, C. W.: Black Widow Spider and Snake Venom in Small Animals. J. Am. Vet. Med. Assn. *96*:356–358, 1940.

Schöll, G.: Todlicher Kreuzotterbiss bei einem Dackel (Necropsy Findings in a Dachshund Bitten by a Common Viper.) Die Kleintierpraxis, *13*:113–115, 1968.

Stahnke, H. L.: Scorpions. Tempe, Ariz., Poisonous Animals Research Lab., Ariz. State College.

Wirth, D.: Bienenstichvergiftung beim Pferd. [Bee Sting Poisoning in Horses.] Wien. tierärztl. Monatschr. *30*:129–134, 1943.

PHENOL

Phenol, or carbolic acid, is used in medicine much less than formerly, but poisoning through accidental ingestion or by absorption through the skin is still occasionally seen. In general, symptoms are those of nervous shock and nervous depression, paralysis and coma. The salient lesion results from the action of all but high dilutions of phenol as a potent tissue fixative. Mucous membranes (mouth, stomach) with which it comes in contact promptly become firm and white, a state of coagulative necrosis. Microscopically, the white, coagulated tissue is found to be perfectly preserved, while adjoining areas may show postmortem autolysis in keeping with the time between death and preservation of the tissue.

LEWISITE

This war gas, chlorovinyldichloroarsine or a mixture of closely related compounds, is vesicant and necrotizing on the skin or other tissues with which it comes in contact. The eyes and air-passages suffer severely when the gas is inhaled; the mouth and whole gastrointestinal tract, when it is ingested. There is also absorption of the material with the result that the blood-borne poison produces the usual changes of acute toxic hepatitis (p. 1223) and a less severe toxic nephrosis (p. 1266). The epithelium of the bile ducts and gallbladder may suffer necrosis as the result of elimination of some of the poison in the bile. Shock, comparable to that which results from ordinary burns, may develop after a few days, with a fatal termination.

Lewisite

Cameron, G. R., Carlton, H. M., and Short, R. H. D.: Pathological Changes Induced by Lewisite and Allied Compounds. J. Path. and Bact. *58*:411–422, 1946.

MUSTARD GAS

Animals have been poisoned by eating forage or pasturage contaminated with this deadly war gas, which chemically is B, B^1-dichloroethyl sulfide. The symptoms described are profuse salivation, lacrimation and conjunctivitis, mucous rhinitis, refusal to eat, pain in the mouth and pharynx, nausea, and rapid pulse and respiration. Lesions are chiefly due to the local irritant and necrotizing action upon the mucous membranes of the mouth, esophagus, and stomach. These could lead to confusion with "mucosal disease" (p. 492), or, in sheep, with contagious ecthyma (p. 413) or possibly with other viral infections. Hemorrhages and focal pre-necrotic degeneration are reported in the myocardium. Burns can, of course, occur on the skin when the poisonous liquid or vapor comes in contact with it. Coagulative necrosis is the fundamental change with ulceration supervening. In fatal cases death, after several days, is partly attributable to secondary infection of the ulcerated surfaces.

Mustard Gas

KOSCHNICK, H.: Gelbkreuz-(Lost-)vergiftungen bei Pferden. Z. Veterinärk. 55:57–63, 1943.
PULLINGER, B. D.: Some Characters of Coagulation Necrosis Due to Mustard Gas. J. Path. and Bact. 59:255–259, 1947.
WATSON, J. F.: Mustard Gas Poisoning in the Horse. Vet. Rec. 55:338, 1943.
YOUNG, L.: Effects of Mustard Gas on the Rat. Canad. J. Research, Sect. E, 25:141–151, 1947.

Group B: Poisons which cause gastroenteritis as a prominent feature.

Arsenic	Ground glass	Castor beans	Oaks
Salt	Dynamite	Locusts	Oleander
Petroleum	Urea	Tung oil tree	Lantana
Sodium fluoro- acetate	Nicotine	Flourensia	Milk weeds
	Nightshades	cernua	Red squill

ARSENIC

Animals rather frequently acquire arsenic in poisonous quantities through the accidental ingestion of such compounds as lead arsenate and Paris green, which are kept on the farm for use as insecticidal sprays, and lead arsenite, which is used as a cutaneous parasiticide (dips) for ticks and mites. Another frequent accident consists in animals eating plants and weeds which have been sprayed with arsenicals intentionally (to kill the plants) or inadvertently while the spray was being applied to fruit trees. Poisoning occurs readily through cutaneous absorption if animals are dipped in a solution which is too concentrated. Occasional poisoning results from excessive administration of arsenical medicaments such as Fowler's solution or neoarsphenamine. Chronic poisoning also occurs in animals grazing on land subject to precipitated fumes from smelters and blast furnaces using arsenic-containing ores. Arsenous acid, in the experience of one of the authors (Jones), has accidentally contaminated commercial dog food, with numerous fatalities. Arsanilic acid is currently used in poultry and swine feeds as a stimulant to growth. It is also occasionally used to control dysentery in swine. These practices have added to the possibility of causing arsenic poisoning by error in compounding feed or by contamination of feeds intended for other species.

Harding, *et al.* (1968) have experimentally induced poisoning in pigs by adding arsanilic acid to the feed at the rate of 611, 1,000 or 2,000 grams arsanilic acid to each (English) ton of feed. The usual recommended dose as a growth stimulant is 100 grams per ton or for treatment of dysentery, 250 grams per ton. At all dose levels, signs of intoxication were produced. Clinical signs appeared earlier

Terminally there are dilated pupils and muscular incoordination. Some animals recover in a few days.

Post-mortem lesions include acute enteritis with marked enteric edema, renal hyperemia, perhaps with hemorrhages, and acute cystitis. Pulmonary congestion and edema are prominent in case the oil contained much volatile material. **Kerosene** is occasionally administered accidentally and more often is given by the laity for some supposed medicinal effect. Not all of the victims die, but in those that do, pneumonia is usually an outstanding lesion, presumably because of inhalation of irritant fumes. It is sometimes applied externally (for lice, etc.) and has caused loss of hair in the horse. In cattle severe dermatitis and hematuria have been reported.

Petroleum

BOTTARELLI A.: Grave forma di intossicazione da sabbie petrolifere in un allevamento suino. [Poisoning of Pigs by Crude Oil-bearing Sand from an Oil Well.] Atti. Soc. ital. sci. vet. *5*:208–212, 1951.
FOLEY, J. C., *et al.*: Kerosene Poisoning in Young Children. Radiology *62*:817–829, 1954.
GIBSON, E. A., and LINZELL, J. L.: Diesel Oil Poisoning in Cattle. Vet. Rec. *60*:60–61, 1948.
MCCONNELL, W. C.: Salt Water and Oil Pollution and Its Relation to Livestock Losses. North Am. Vet. *26*:600–601, 1945.
PARKER, W. H., and WILLIAMSON, T. F.: Paraffin [Crude Petroleum] Poisoning in Cattle. Vet. Rec. *63*:430–432, 1951.
RICHARDSON, J. A., and PRATT-THOMAS, H. R.: Toxic Effects of Varying Doses of Kerosene Administered by Different Routes. Am. J. Med. Sci. *221*:531–536, 1951.
STROBER, M.: Toxicity for Cattle of Crude and Heating Oil. Dtsch. tierarztl. Wschr. *69*:386–390, 1962.

SODIUM FLUOROACETATE

This compound of fluorine, sometimes sold as "Formula 1080," is used as a poison for destroying rats. It is sometimes accidentally eaten by dogs when it is placed in meat as a bait and by cattle which may ingest contaminated forage or grain. Signs include increasing weakness and rapidity of the heart, which eventually becomes exhausted. Signs of severe abdominal pain and nausea are prominent in dogs and swine (experimentally). Nervous disturbances terminate in opisthotonos and convulsions with death in a few or several hours after ingestion of the poison. It is said that the prognosis is hopeless once symptoms have appeared. Lesions are few, but there is ordinarily severe inflammation of the small intestine. As a result of cardiac failure and anoxia, the blood is dark and there are subepicardial and subendocardial petechiae. Studies of the nervous tissues have not been reported.

Sodium Fluoroacetate

JENSEN, R., TOBISKA, J. W., and WARD, J. C.: Sodium Fluoroacetate Poisoning in Sheep Am. J. Vet. Research. *9*:370–372, 1948.
NICHOLS, H. C. *et al.*: Poisoning of Two Dogs with 1080 Rat Poison (Sodium Fluoroacetate). J. Am. Vet. Med. Assn. *115*:355–356, 1949.
OELRICHS, P. B. and MCEWAN, T.: Isolation of the Toxic Principle in *Acacia georginae*. Nature, London. *190*:808–809, 1961.
SCHNAUTZ, J. O.: Sodium Fluoroacetate Poisoning in Cattle. J. Am. Vet. Med. Assn. *114*:435, 1949.
SCHWARTE, L. H.: Toxicity of Sodium Monofluoroacetate for Swine and Chickens. J. Am. Vet. Med. Assn. *111*:301–303, 1947.

GROUND GLASS

More or less finely shattered glass is administered from time to time to man or animals with felonious intent. In a majority of cases, no effects are noticed. In some instances, there is transient abdominal discomfort, diarrhea and mild gastroenteritis.

Ground Glass

MAYO, N. S.: Effect of Ground Glass on the Gastro-intestinal Tract of Dogs. J. Am. Vet. Med. Assn. *55*:202–203, 1919.
SIMMONS, J. S., and VON GLAHN, W. C.: Effect of Ground Glass on the Gastro-intestinal Tract of Dogs. J. Am. Med. Assn. *71*:2127, 1918.

DYNAMITE

Incredible as it may seem, cattle are sometimes poisoned by eating dynamite or the wrappings thereof. One suspects that the native bovine curiosity which is sometimes manifested in most incongruous ways has more to do with the animal's eating a substance of this kind than has the actual appetite. Nitroglycerine is, of course, available as a drug and would have the same effect as dynamite if ingested in excessive amounts.

Signs are polyuria and polydipsia, nausea and colic, and perhaps coma. In fatal cases, death comes in from twenty-four to thirty-six hours. Post-mortem lesions are acute gastroenteritis, acute toxic tubular nephritis (p. 1266), dark or chocolate-colored blood due to the formation of methemoglobin, and often petechiae due to terminal anoxia.

Dynamite

BUFFINGTON, R. M.: Nitroglycerine (Dynamite) Poisoning in Cattle. Vet. Bull. *21*:197–198, 1928.
HOLM, L. W. *et al.*: Experimental Poisoning of Cattle and Sheep with Dynamite. Cornell Vet. *42*:91–96, 1952.
KINNELL, G. N.: Dynamite Poisoning. Am. Vet. Rev. *17*:554–556, 1894.

UREA

Since the practice has developed of feeding to cattle and other ruminants artificially concocted feeds containing urea as a substitute for protein, deaths attributed to poisoning by this substance have ceased to be rare. It appears that 2 or 3 per cent of the total ration (dry-weight basis) can safely be urea, but that larger amounts are likely to produce poisoning. Urea is much better tolerated when mixed with plentiful amounts of other feeds than when, for any reason, it enters the digestive tract less well diluted; hence, the occurrence of poisoning is erratic.

Poisoning is due to the local and generalized effects of ammonia or ammonium carbamate released by decomposition of the urea. Symptoms arise suddenly and may lead to death in one or two hours or less. However, illness does not necessarily develop at the first ingestion of the urea-containing feed but apparently occurs whenever, through intestinal inactivity or other functional irregularity, a sufficient amount of ammonia is released at one time and (judging from experimental administration via the stomach tube [Dinning, *et al.*, 1948]) in the same region of the digestive canal. Signs are attributable to the effect of ammonia on the nerve centers and include twitching of eyelids, lips and tail, ataxia in locomotion and convulsions. Salivation may be prominent, with frothing at the mouth. Pulse and respirations become progressively slower and death follows. The resemblance to strychnine poisoning is often marked. Blood-urea nitrogen, as well as ammonia-nitrogen in the rumen, are elevated. The pH of the blood and urine are abnormally high.

Post-mortem lesions are not extensive. There is usually a rather severe acute catarrhal or, at times, hemorrhagic enteritis. In the experience of some the inflammation has been found in the stomach (abomasum); in the experience of one of the writers (Smith), there has always been severe inflammation in the last one-third of the small intestine. Mild toxic hepatitis (p. 1223) and toxic tubular nephrosis (p. 1266) accompany the enteric injury. In the lungs, there may be hemorrhages, either peribronchial or intra-alveolar, as well as mild acute catarrhal bronchitis. The central nervous lesions, consisting of neuronal degenerations (p. 1379), pial hemorrhages and congestion, are probably attributable to the direct effects of ammonia.

Urea

CLARK, R., OYAERT, W., and QUINN, J. I.: The Toxicity of Urea to Sheep Under Different Conditions. Onderstepoort J. Vet. Sci. *25*:73–78, 1951.

DAVIS, G. K. and ROBERTS, H. F.: Urea Toxicity in Cattle. Bul. Fla. Agric. Expt. Sta., No. 611, pp. 16, 1959.

DINNING, J. S. *et al.*: Effect of Orally Administered Urea. Am. J. Physiol. *153*:41–46, 1948.

ENGELS, O.: Ist Handelsdünger Gift für die Tiere? Ztschr. f. Schafzucht. *31*:137–138, 1942.

FUJIMOTO, Y., and TAJIMA, M.: Pathological Studies on Urea Poisoning. Jap. J. Vet. Sci. *15*:125–134, 1953. (English summary.) Abstr. Vet. Bull. No. 1769, 1955. (In Japanese. Original title not reproducible.)

GREEN, D. F.: Urea Feeding. North Am. Vet. *36*:733–736 and 827–833, 1955.

HALE, W. H., and KING, R. P.: Possible Mechanism of Urea Toxicity in Ruminants. Proc. Soc. Exper. Biol. and Med. *89*:112–114, 1955. Abstr. Vet. Bull. No. 4104, 1955.

KOVAL, M. P., and VAS'KO, I. V.: (Poisoning of cows with Carbamide [urea]). Veterinariya (Moscow) *41*:49–50, 1964.

OSEBOLD, J. W.: Urea Poisoning in Cattle. North Am. Vet. *28*:89–91, 1947.

NICOTINE

Poisoning by nicotine occurs in animals almost exclusively from the improper use of insecticidal solutions on the skin or of nicotine sulfate as an anthelmintic internally. One of the most deadly poisons known, nicotine is promptly absorbed from mucous membrane or skin and acts rapidly, producing at first nervous stimulation and then depression. If swallowed, there is local pain in the throat and stomach. Muscular tremors and weakness cause the animal to fall. Convulsions are followed in a matter of minutes by loss of voluntary movement so that the patient lies quietly. Concurrently with vomiting and purging, the pulse and respiration become weaker and slower with death from respiratory failure and collapse, all within two or three hours. A case of a dog being poisoned by eating cigarette stubs (equivalent of 15 to 20 cigarettes per day) is on record (Boissière, 1938). Depression and polyuria were followed by vomition and then by diarrhea lasting four days. Another reported fatality, in a three-month-old puppy, resulted from eating a pack of cigarettes (Kaplan, 1968).

As would be expected from the rapidity of the poisonous action, lesions are

minimal. Acute inflammation of the stomach (abomasum) and intestines is
likely to be pronounced, even when the mode of entry is by cutaneous absorption.
Mesenteric vessels are severely hyperemic, the blood being bright red.

Nicotine

Boissière: Intoxication du chien par le tabac. Rec. méd. vét. *114*:35, 1938.
Crawshaw, H. A.: Nicotine Poisoning in Lambs. Vet. Rec. *56*:276–277, 1944.
Fincher, M. G.: Blackleaf 40 Poisoning. Cornell Vet. *24*:86, 1934.
Kaplan, B.: Acute Nicotine Poisoning in a Dog. Vet. Med. Sml. Anim. Clin. *63*:1033–1034, 1968.

NIGHTSHADES

Genus *Solanum*

For the pathology of Deadly Nightshade, see Belladonna, page 949.

In the genus *Solanum* are included the common or black nightshade, *S. nigrum*,
the "bitter apple," *S. incanum*, a plant very similar in appearance to the common
tomato, its close relative, the "apple of Sodom," *S. panduraeforme*, the "Jerusalem
berry," *S. pseudocapsicum*, the white "horse nettle," *S. eleagnifolium*, and the
"buffalo bur," *S. rostratum*, not to mention the common potato, *S. tuberosum*. All
of these and various other, less toxic species contain the poisonous glycoalkaloid,
solanin, either constantly or transiently, in the whole or certain parts of the
plant, their poisonous actions being similar. In the case of potatoes, the growing
sprouts on stored tubers are more or less poisonous, as is also the skin of a tuber
which has grown partly exposed at the surface of the ground so that its skin
becomes thickened and green. Gastrointestinal signs, salivation, stomatitis,
vomiting, tympanites and diarrhea, are usually overshadowed by nervous
depression, apathy, narcosis and paralysis. A mild degree of poisoning may exhibit only an exanthematous form. Lesions in the digestive tract are acute
catarrhal or hemorrhagic gastritis and enteritis, sometimes accompanied by ulcers
which extend to or through the muscularis propria. There is rarely desquamation
of patches of buccal mucosa. Tissue changes accounting for the nervous symptoms have not been described and apparently histopathological studies of the
brain have not been made. Since the poison usually acts within a matter of
hours, such studies possibly would yield little. In the exanthematous form,
which is relatively chronic and benign, the more tender areas of skin show vesicles
and hyperemia. Conjunctivitis is a frequent accompaniment. The degree of
toxicity of these plants varies greatly from time to time.

Nightshades

Andrade, S. O.: Estudos sobre a Toxicidade de *Sessea brasiliensis* (*Solanaceæ*). Arq. Inst.
Biol. S. Paulo. *27*:191–196, 1960.
Casselberry, N. H.: Nightshade Poisoning of Swine. Vet. Med. *34*:444–445, 1939.
Eckell, O. A.: Acción Toxica del *Solanum glaucum*, Dun (Duraznillo blanco). An. Fac.
Med. Vet. Univ. La Plata. *5*:9–91, 1942.
Koslowski, B.: Wyprysk u prosiat ssacych-wyowlany karmieniem macior niedojrzlymi
ziemniakami. [Dermatitis in Unweaned Pigs from Feeding Green Potatoes to the Sows.]
Méd. vét., Varsovie. *9*:505, 1953. Abstr. Vet. Bull. No. 3290, 1954.
Simic, W. J.: Solanine Poisoning in Swine. Vet. Med. *38*:353–354, 1943.
Steyn, D. G.: *Toxicology of Plants in South Africa*. 1934, Johannesburg, The Central
News Agency, Ltd.

CASTOR BEANS

The meal remaining after the extraction of oil from castor beans contains ricin, an extremely potent poison, which is water-soluble, hence not found in the castor oil. Ricin resembles bacterial exotoxins in that an animal can be hyper-immunized to it so that the serum has high antitoxic properties. As in the case of bacterial toxins, heat (about 56° C.) destroys a toxic fraction (toxophore) and leaves an immunizing fraction (haptophore). Boiling the meal or the whole seeds definitely renders them non-poisonous.

Signs appear a few hours after ingestion of small amounts of meal or of the whole seeds. They consist chiefly in vomiting, violent diarrhea, signs of severe abdominal pain (grinding of teeth, humping of back), tumultuous heart action, slightly elevated temperature and collapse. In horses, there is profuse sweating, and tetanic spasms have occurred. Lesions are severe acute gastritis (abomasitis in ruminants) with the reddening and edema continuing into the upper small intestine, where they are accompanied by petechiation. Free blood may be found in the bowel. Microscopically, the epithelium of the affected gastrointestinal areas is necrotic although sometimes still present. The liver shows hydropic degeneration, fatty change and areas of necrosis (acute toxic hepatitis). The renal epithelium displays a less severe fatty degeneration and necrosis (acute toxic nephritis). There is a striking destruction of lymphocytes in the lymphoid organs (possibly simulating that seen in rinderpest and in irradiation). Necrosis has been demonstrated in the brain. In horses, severe edema is reported in the lungs, with a less severe degree in bronchial, mesenteric and hepatic nodes and elsewhere. There is much fluid in the inflamed digestive tract. Treatment is symptomatic unless serum from a previously hyperimmunized animal should be available.

Castor Beans

CLARKE, E. G. C.: Poisoning by Castor Seed. Vet. J. *103*:273–278, 1947.
GEARY, T.: Castor Bean Poisoning. Vet. Rec. *62*:472–473, 1950.
McCUNN, J., ANDREW, H., and CLOUGH, G. W.: Castor-bean Poisoning in Horses. Vet. J. *101*:136–138, 1945.

LOCUSTS

The seeds, leaves, bark and roots of the black locust tree (*Robinia pseudoacacia*) have long been known to be poisonous, several different alkaloidal or glucosidal poisonous principles having been described. The clammy locust (*Robinia viscosa*) is also known to be poisonous and presumably the same is true of other locusts. Horses and also humans have been poisoned by chewing the bark of young trees; chickens, by eating leaves and young sprouts.

Signs appear several hours after the poisonous material is ingested and include extreme muscular weakness, mental depression and maximum dilatation of the pupils There is serious cardiac depression with slowness or, at any rate, no marked acceleration. The beat may be weak, but in the terminal stages it is frequently reported as being characterized by a very loud thump, audible for some distance. There may be signs of abdominal pain and humans report nausea, but rarely, if ever, is there purgation. Salivation and bleeding from the mouth have been described in the horse. Many patients, man and animal, after a few days recover and gradually regain their strength.

28

Necropsy, in those that die, shows a mucous inflammation of the gastro-intestinal tract and occasionally a more severe gastroenteritis. Gardiner (1903) found that the "stomach and intestine contained nearly all the fluids of the body." There is venous congestion and some have described a yellowish dis-coloration of the mucous membranes "similar to" icterus.

Some experimental evidence indicates that the toxicity is seasonal (early and mid-summer) or at least that the locust trees are not constantly poisonous (Barnes, 1921).

Locusts

BARNES, M. F.: Black Locust Poisoning of Chickens. J. Am. Vet. Med. Assn. *59*:370–372, 1921.
GARDINER, W. W.: Locust-tree Bark Poisoning. Am. Vet. Rev. *27*:599–600, 1903.
PAMMEL, L. H.: The Toxicity of Black Locust. North Am. Vet. *8*:41–43, 1927.
WALDRON, C. A.: Poisoning from Locust Bark. Am. Vet. Rev. *33*:456–459, 1908.

TUNG OIL TREE

The tung tree (*Aleurites fordi*) is cultivated in warm countries for the produc-tion of its oil, which is valuable in paints and varnishes. Poisoning of farm animals, including chickens, has resulted from attempts to feed the meal which remains after extraction of the oil from the tung nuts and from ingestion of foliage, not from the tree directly, but in the form of cut leaves and branches, which have considerable palatability to cattle.

Profuse watery or bloody diarrhea occurs after an interval of a few days and is the chief symptom. Illness lasts from one to three weeks before terminating fatally. Lesions are severe hemorrhagic gastroenteritis, severe congestion of the splanchnic organs and early toxic changes in the liver.

Tung Oil Tree

DAVIS, G. K. *et al.*: Tung Meal in Rations for Growing Chicks. Poult. Sci. *25*:74–79, 1946.
EMMEL, M. W. *et al.*: Toxicity of Foliage of *Aleurites fordi* for Cattle. J. Am. Vet. Med. Assn. *101*:136–137, 1942.
HURST, E.: *The Poison Plants of New South Wales.* 1942. Univ. of Sydney and N.S.W. Dept. Agric., Sydney.

FLOURENSIA CERNUA

Known popularly as **blackbush** or **tarbrush,** this plant is indigenous to the arid areas of the Southwestern United States and Mexico. Poisoning is almost exclusively in sheep and goats which eat the berry-like fruit, sometimes merely in the course of being driven through an infested area.

Symptoms are salivation, grinding of teeth and signs of severe abdominal pain such as groaning, and arching of the back. Muscular twitchings are not infre-quent. If the animal lives for some time, there is likely to be mucous rhinitis. Death frequently occurs in twenty-four to forty-eight hours; animals that sur-vive five days usually recover. Lesions are severe inflammation of the abomasum and duodenum. In cases of some standing, the inflammatory infiltration of fluid and leukocytes extends into the muscularis.

Flourensia Cernua

MATHEWS, F. P.: Toxicity of the Ripe Fruit of Blackbrush, or Tarbrush (*Flourensis cernua*). Exp. Sta. Bull. 644, 1944. Texas A. & M. College, College Station.

OAKS

Several hundred species of oak trees or shrubs are known, and poisoning by members of this genus (*Quercus*) has been recognized for a long time but is not fully understood. Since oak bark is a principal source of tannic acid, it was natural to try to explain oak poisoning of cattle, sheep and horses as tannic-acid poisoning. No doubt some deleterious effects such as constipation and indigestion can result from this substance and, coupled with malnutrition and semi-starvation, are able to cause death. But the usual form of oak poisoning is of a different nature. It occurs at the time the young leaf-buds and flowers are making their annual springtime appearance and accordingly is often called "oak-bud poisoning." The usual outbreaks of the disease result from the ingestion of the buds and young leaves of certain small shrub-like species known as shin-oak or shinnery oak, *Quercus havardi*, indigenous to the Southwestern United States, and it may well be that this species is more poisonous than others. However, typical oak-bud poisoning has occurred when budding branches of large oak trees have been made accessible to cattle or sheep in the course of lumbering operations. To what extent some or all oaks are more poisonous during the budding and early leafing stage, and to what extent the occurrence of poisoning at that time may be related to the contemporary shortage of other green feed and an appetite for the oaks are questions which have not been answered. At any rate, oak-bud poisoning is a definite and recognizable disease-entity of considerable importance in many areas.

Signs of oak-bud poisoning are chiefly alimentary and urinary in nature. While a few cases have diarrhea from the outset, the great majority have severe constipation with tenesmus. The frequent efforts at defecation produce small, hard balls of mucus-covered feces, to which blood is sometimes adherent. After several days, in those animals still living, the constipation commonly gives way to a fetid and hemorrhagic diarrhea. A blood-stained nasal exudate is a frequent sign that should be mentioned. Ventral edema of renal origin (p. 134) is also characteristic, especially in sheep. The severe injury to the kidneys, which appears to be always a part of the syndrome, is evidenced by polydipsia and polyuria, clear urine of low specific gravity being voided at frequent intervals. The illness may terminate fatally in twenty-four hours, after several days, or may yield to slow recovery in two or three weeks. New cases may appear for approximately a week after the herd or flock has been removed from access to the budding oaks.

The lesions are those which would be predicted from the signs. Mucous enteritis involves the last half of the digestive canal and becomes partly or eventually almost entirely hemorrhagic. The mesenteric lymph nodes are edematous. In addition to the subcutaneous edema already mentioned, there are usually hydropericardium and hydroperitoneum. The liver is congested and shows a moderate degree of acute toxic hepatitis (p. 1223). The gallbladder is distended with viscid, brownish bile (p. 1237). The kidneys are of the large, pale type (p. 1267) but rather uniformly sprinkled with petechiae 2 or 3 mm. in diameter

(Fig. 17–11*B*). The medulla is congested. The microscopic renal picture comes near being pathognomonic (Fig. 17–12). Numerous proximal convoluted tubules contain dense casts of albumin, their pink color being stained with brown, doubtless from bile pigment and possibly also from hemoglobin. The necrotic epithelial lining cells are usually so intimately mixed with the proteinaceous contents of the lumen that the whole forms a dense, homogeneous mass limited by the basement membrane and interstitial tissue. Adjacent to such a tubule are others which appear quite uninjured. The glomeruli show little change and the medulla remains of nearly normal appearance except for congestion. In our experience, this type of tubular damage has not been duplicated in any other disease.

Oaks

BEGOVIC, S., *et al.*: [Poisoning of Cattle by Oak Leaves.] Vet. Glasn. *11*:673–679, 1957. (In Croat. Ger. summary.) Abstr. Vet. Bull. No. 3725, 1958.
BOUGHTON, I. B., and HARDY, W. T.: Oak Poisoning in Range Cattle and Sheep. J. Am. Vet. Med. Assn. *89*:157–162, 1936.
KINGREY, B. W., RICHTER, W. R., and DINGEL, R. M.: Acorn Poisoning in Cattle. Iowa State Univ. Vet. *22*(No. 1):30–31, 1959.
MARSH, C. D., CLAWSON, A. B., and MARSH, H.: Oak-leaf Poisoning of Domestic Animals. U. S. Dept. Agric. Bull. 767, 1919.
SMITH, H. A : The Pathology of Oak Poisoning. Southwestern Vet. *13*:343–349, 1959.

OLEANDER

The oleander (*Nerium oleander*), native to most of the warmer parts of the world and grown as an ornamental plant in the Southern United States, has been known for its extreme toxicity since ancient times. Humans have been fatally poisoned not only by eating a few leaves, but even when oleander twigs were used as skewers in meat (Hurst, 1942). Horses, cattle and sheep do not usually eat it; most cases of poisoning occur when cuttings from a garden are thoughtlessly thrown into a dry lot, especially where animals are accustomed to having forkfuls of hay placed before them.

Signs are abdominal pain, nausea, vomiting, diarrhea and tenesmus, plus a digitalis-like stimulation of the heart and constriction of vessels. As a result, extremities are cold, while the general body temperature is raised and the pulse rapid. Respirations are augmented both in rate and depth. Tremors and tetanic stiffness give way to paralysis and death usually without convulsions. The duration of symptoms is usually less than twenty-four hours.

Lesions are chiefly those of severe catarrhal or hemorrhagic gastroenteritis, the irritation even beginning in the pharynx in some cases. Terminal petechial and ecchymotic hemorrhages are common on the heart, serous and mucous membranes, including the gallbladder and the meninges. Blood-stained or clear fluid is frequent in the serous cavities. In a case studied by one of the writers (Smith), there were petechiae in the renal cortex and hematuria. The case also showed early toxic hepatitis (p. 1223) and toxic tubular nephrosis. The cortical tubules were largely in a state of coagulative necrosis and contained casts of hemoglobin-stained albumin.

Oleander

HURST, E.: *The Poison Plants of New South Wales.* 1942. Univ. of Sydney and N.S.W. Dept. Agric., Sydney.

Nausea, vomiting and abdominal pain then appear and are succeeded by fever, polydipsia and polyuria. The appearance of jaundice is followed by delirium, convulsions and coma, the whole illness lasting usually from two to five days.

At autopsy, there may be mild inflammation of parts of the gastrointestinal tract but the principal lesions consist of degenerative changes in the liver and kidneys. Icterus is prominent and is said to be due in many cases to obstructive swelling of the bile duct. However, the outstanding change is fatty change (p. 34), for which phosphorus poisoning is one of the classical causes. In the liver, the great majority of the cells are filled with fat droplets, centrilobular necrosis supervening if the patient lives for a while. Fatty change of the kidney and heart is pronounced and smaller amounts can be demonstrated in other tissues. In the kidney of the dog, at least, most of the fat is in the epithelium of the ascending loops of Henle in the medullary rays. The distal convoluted tubules are second in the fatty deposition; other structures of the kidney may have slight amounts. The accumulation of lipids appears to be due to interference with oxidative processes, phosphorus being a most readily oxidizable substance. Hydropic degeneration is marked in the proximal convoluted tubules. The spleen is regularly small and atrophic. Hydrothorax and more or less generalized edema occur in some cases, doubtless because of gradual failure of the degenerating heart muscle. One of the writers (Smith) has seen very severe hemorrhagic enteritis, cholecystitis and urinary cystitis in an experimental dog. Ecchymotic hemorrhages sometimes occur in the heart and elsewhere.

There is a very chronic form of phosphorus poisoning in humans characterized by a necrotizing purulent osteomyelitis of the mandible and maxilla, with multiple draining sinuses and deformity. This usually results from inhalation of phosphorus-containing fumes in industrial plants, to which animals are unlikely to be exposed.

PHOSPHATES

Cattle are poisoned rarely by eating commercial fertilizers which are usually mixtures of phosphates, nitrates, potassium and ammonium. It appears, however, that these poisonings are chiefly attributable to nitrates or potassium rather than to phosphates. Ammonium nitrate has been shown to be surprisingly harmless; nitrates are considered on page 917 and potassium on page 1007. Chickens and other birds have been poisoned by zinc phosphate, used as a treatment for seed-wheat. Characteristic features were dullness, anorexia, thirst and terminal nervous symptoms, ending fatally a few hours after ingestion. A garlic-like odor of $Zn_3(PO_4)_2$ was noted in the contents of the crop. (See also, Organic Phosphates, p. 966.)

Phosphates

ADUTSKEVICH, V. A., and ZAITSEVA, A. G.: Ob otravlenii domashnikh zhivotnykh i ptits zheltym fosforom i ego proizvodnymi. [Phosphorus Poisoning in Animals and Birds.] Veterinariya, Moscow. *8* and *9*:40–43, 1944. Abstr. Vet. Bull. No. 1653, 1948.

BUBIEN, Z., and MIEDZOBRODZKI, K.: [Zinc phosphate poisoning in birds.] Méd. Vét., Varsovie. *13*:422–425, 1957. Abstr. Vet. Bull. No. 887, 1958.

SMITH, H. A.: Renal Lipidosis. Thesis, University of Michigan, Ann Arbor, 1949. (Three phosphorus experiments.)

SWAN, J. B., and McINTOSH, I. G.: Toxicity of North African Phosphate and Superphosphate to Milking Cows. Proc. New Zealand Soc. Animal Prod. *12*:83–88, 1952.

COPPER

While ingestion or cutaneous absorption of adequate amounts of copper salts is able to produce acute gastroenteric poisoning with greenish tinged, fluid feces, the usual poisoning in domestic animals is a chronic disorder which terminates precipitously in acute symptoms when copper stored in the liver reaches a critical level. Herbivorous animals, especially sheep, become poisoned by eating herbage growing on soils too rich in copper. Included are soils naturally so afflicted and those of old orchards, which have been contaminated by heavy spraying (Bordeaux mixture, etc.). Poisoning has occurred where copper sulfate has been used in wet pastures to control the snails which are one of the hosts for liver flukes. Contamination from mines and smelters has also been responsible. More often it has resulted from misapplication of copper medication, especially when copper sulfate was mixed with the animals' salt for anthelmintic purposes, also when solutions used in treating "foot-rot" were ingested. Vaginal bougies containing copper sulfate have also been incriminated.

Signs last twenty-four to forty-eight hours and include weakness and exhaustion (trembling), arching of the back (renal pain), icterus and hemoglobinuria. The last two are so constant and pronounced that the disease was known as **ictero-hemoglobinuria** before its cause was discovered. At autopsy, the icterus proves to be both toxic and hemolytic. The liver is yellow and friable grossly, with centrilobular fatty change and necrosis and possible increase of reticuloendothelial cells (acute toxic hepatitis). There is terminally a pronounced hemolytic anemia with counts as low as 2,000,000 per cmm. and erythrocytic changes characteristic of hemolytic destruction and myeloid regeneration (Allen and Harding, 1962). The kidneys show toxic degenerative changes (acute toxic nephrosis) plus blocking of the tubules by erythrocytes and hemoglobin. Severe hemorrhagic nephritis has been described (p. 1293). The spleen is markedly enlarged and crowded with whole or fragmented erythrocytes. Grossly, it is often a "blackberry-jam" spleen resembling that of anthrax. Analysis of the liver shows a high content of copper, above 500 parts per million. The amount of copper in the blood is also high when symptoms appear, for example, 250 p.p.m.

Salts of molybdenum appear to have a certain protective action against excessive copper.

The abnormal accumulation of copper in the tissues and blood is a point of similarity with a disease of man known as **hepatolenticular** or **hepatocerebral degeneration** or **Wilson's disease.** This disease is believed to be inherited as an autosomal recessive trait but is characterized by excessive deposition of copper in the liver, basal ganglia, cerebral cortex, kidney and cornea. Lesions and functional changes are produced in each of these organs. Hepatic cirrhosis with nodular regeneration in the liver is accompanied by icterus and decreased liver function. Neurologic abnormalities appear to result from injury to the basal ganglia and cerebrum where cavitation, increase in size and number of astrocytes and decrease in neurons occur. Deposits of copper-bearing pigment in the renal tubular epithelium is often accompanied by glycosuria, aminoaciduria, phosphaturia and uricosuria. A characteristic brown or gray-green precipitation at the limbus of the cornea is considered specific and is called the **Kayser-Fleischer Ring** (Robbins, 1967).

The mechanisms involved in hepatolenticular degeneration are not understood. Two theoretical possibilities are current: The first postulates a defect in the synthesis of ceruloplasmin, a copper-containing alpha globulin, which is demonstrably low in such patients. As a result, copper is combined loosely with albumin rather than with alpha-2-globulin and this poor binding with protein presumably results in its deposition in abnormal sites. The second theory proposes a defect in protein metabolism in which abnormal polypeptides with high avidity for copper are formed. These proteins, with their copper content, are presumed to be deposited in the sites affected.

Ultrastructural lesions have been observed in hepatocytes of rats poisoned with copper (Barka, *et al.*, 1964) which closely resemble the changes in human patients with Wilson's disease. Electron dense structures corresponding to copper-bearing lipofuscin pigment appears to be specific. Other changes were observed in mitochondria, endoplasmic reticulum, sinusoidal borders and golgi apparatus. The pigment formation, changes in histochemical distribution of acid phosphatase and mobilization of Kupffer cells are common features of Wilson's disease and experimental copper intoxication.

Lesions described as spongy transformation in myelinated tracts in the midbrain, pons and cerebellum of sheep poisoned by long-term feeding of a diet containing 80 parts per million of copper have been described by Doherty, *et al.* (1969). This is of interest in comparison with hepatolenticular degeneration of man. According to Gardiner (1967) high levels of dietary copper appear to increase the susceptibility of sheep to lupinosis (p. 883).

Copper

ALLEN, M. M. and HARDING, J. D. J.: Experimental Copper Poisoning in Pigs. Vet. Rec. 74:173–179, 216, 248, 277, 306 and 304, 1962.
BARKA, T., SCHEUER, P. J., SCHAFFNER, F., and POPPER, H.: Structural Changes of Liver Cells in Copper Intoxication. Arch. Path. 78:331–349, 1964.
BOUGHTON, I. B., and HARDY, W. T.: Chronic Copper Poisoning in Sheep. Bull. 499. Division of Vet. Science, Texas Agric. Exper. Sta., 1934.
BULL, L. B.: Chronic Copper Poisoning in Grazing Sheep in Australia. Rept. 14th Internat. Vet. Congr. 3:39–42, 1952.
CUNNINGHAM, I. J.: The Toxicity of Copper to Bovines. New Zealand J. Sci. Tech. (Sec. A). 27:372–376, 1946.
CUNNINGHAM, I. J., HOGAN, K. G., and LAWSON, B. M.: The Effect of Sulphate and Molybdenum on Copper Metabolism in Cattle. N. Z. J. Agric. Res. 2:145–152, 134–144, 1959.
DOHERTY, P. C., BARLOW, R. M., and ANGUS, K. W.: Spongy Changes in the Brains of Sheep Poisoned by Excess Dietary Copper. Res. Vet. Sci. 10:303–304, 1969.
FINCHAM, I. H.: Copper Poisoning in Sheep. Vet. Rec. 57:581, 1945.
GARDINER, M. R.: The Role of Copper in the Pathogenesis of Subacute and Chronic Lupinosis of Sheep. Aust. Vet. J. 43:243–248, 1967.
MUTH, O. H.: Chronic Copper Poisoning in Sheep. J. Am. Vet. Med. Assn. 120:148–149, 1952.
O'HARA, P. J., NEWMAN, A. P., and JACKSON, R.: Parakeratosis and Copper Poisoning in Pigs Fed a Copper Supplement. Austr. Vet. J. 36:225–229, 1960.
PIERSON, R. E., and AANES, W. A.: Treatment of Chronic Copper Poisoning in Sheep. J. Am. Vet. Med. Assn. 133:307–311, 1958. (Includes pathology, experimental.)
ROBBINS, S. L.: *Pathology*, 3rd Ed., Philadelphia, W. B. Saunders Co., 1967.
ST. GEORGE-GRAMBAUER, T. D. and RAC, R.: Hepatogenous Chronic Copper Poisoning in Sheep in South Australia due to Consumption of *Echium plantagineum* L. Austr. Vet. J. 38:288–293, 1962.
SUTTER, M. D., *et al.*: Chronic Copper Toxicosis in Sheep. Am. J. Vet. Res. 19:890–892, 1958.
TODD, J. R., and THOMPSON, R. H.: Studies on Chronic Copper Poisoning. III. Effects of Copper Acetate Injected into the Blood Stream of Sheep. J. Comp. Path. 74:542–551, 1964.

——————: Studies on Chronic Copper Poisoning. IV. Biochemistry of the Toxic Syndrome in the Calf. Brit. Vet. J. *121*:90–97, 1965.

WEISS, E., BAUR, P., and PLANK, P.: Chronic Copper Poisoning in Calves. Vet. Med. Nachr. 35–51, 1967. No. 1. V.B. *38*:301, 1968.

WOLFF, S. M.: Copper Deposition in the Rat. Arch. Path. *69*:217–223, 1960.

WYSSMANN, E.: Rüekblick auf Vergiftungsfälle bei Teiren. (Copper poisoning in domestic animals.) Schweiz. Arch. Tierheilk. *87*:142–154 and 222–233, 1945.

TANNIC ACID

The astringent action of tannic acid interferes so much with absorption from the digestive mucosa that poisoning by this route is quite unlikely and is even difficult to produce experimentally. The same cannot be said when the substance is introduced into the animal body parenterally. The usual form of poisoning by tannic acid appeared contemporaneously with the use of this drug in the treatment of burns, and results from applying it over too large an area, whence it is extensively absorbed. There is one outstanding lesion, namely, acute toxic hepatitis with centrilobular necrosis. Several days are usually required to produce death, during which there are symptoms of depression, inappetence and other signs traceable to hepatic impairment. Liver-function tests usually show decreased hepatic function. There are also experimental indications that tannic acid leads to "increased permeability of capillaries" and loss of fluid from the blood. This contributes to the anhydremia and shock (p. 140) which are often very serious complications developing approximately three days after severe burns. However, this syndrome is not infrequent in burns without treatment with tannic acid; toxic hepatitis is not usual from the burn alone.

While oak trees contain tannic acid, being used in making the well-known oak-tanned leather, oak-bud or oak poisoning is not due to tannic acid.

Tannic Acid

BARNES, J. M., and ROSSITER, R. J.: Toxicity of Tannic Acid. Lancet *245*:218–222, 1943.

CAMERON, G. R., MILTON, R. F., and ALLEN, J. W.: Toxicity of Tannic Acid, an Experimental Investigation. Lancet *245*:179–186, 1943.

CLARK, E. J., and ROSSITER, R. J.: Liver Function in Rabbits after Injection of Tannic Acid. Lancet *245*:222–223, 1943.

HANDLER, P., and BAKER, R. D.: Toxicity of Orally Administered Tannic Acid. Science *99*:393, 1944.

CARBON TETRACHLORIDE AND TETRACHLORETHYLENE

Humans become poisoned on carbon tetrachloride through inhalation of its vapor, as in the clothes-cleaning industry. In animals, poisoning is not altogether infrequent as the result of the use of this substance as an anthelmintic. Such poisoning is ordinarily acute. Symptoms include loss of appetite, gastro-intestinal pain, diarrhea (after a few hours) and blood-stained feces. Icterus is often but not always present. Collapse and death come in about twenty-four hours.

Lesions are acute catarrhal or hemorrhagic gastritis and enteritis, and acute toxic changes in the liver and kidneys. The hepatic changes are those usually found in acute toxic hepatitis (p. 1223), namely hydropic degeneration, fatty change and necrosis with cellular infiltrations if the animal lives long enough. Often there is little but necrosis at the time of death. The necrosis tends to be central but often becomes massive, involving whole groups of lobules in their entirety. In the kidney, the changes are often less pronounced but consist principally of fatty change and necrosis of the epithelium of the tubules. Nevertheless in some cases, death must be attributed to renal failure. Petechial hemorrhages, said to be due to thrombocytopenia, may be present in various organs and tissues. In chronic cases, which are unusual, the acute toxic hepatitis becomes chronic toxic hepatitis, in other words, cirrhosis.

Tetrachlorethylene is considerably less toxic than carbon tetrachloride, hence more desirable as an anthelmintic, but the two have similar actions. Gallagher and Simmonds (1959) found a preventive effect in nicotinic acid or tryptophane. These substances are precursors of the respiratory co-factors, pyridine nucleotides.

Animal species vary a great deal in susceptibility to carbon tetrachloride. Poisonings have been reported in several rather unique situations. One of the most interesting is the high sensitivity of male mice of certain inbred strains. A minute amount of carbon tetrachloride, released into an animal room, may cause the death of many adult male mice (Meshorer and Benhar, 1966). Male mice of the inbred strains Bal b/c, A/He, C_3H and Swiss are susceptible in that order. Inbred strains C58, DBA/2, SJL, AKR and RF are apparently quite as resistant as all females and young. This sensitivity in mice is quite similar to that observed with chloroform (p. 900).

Carbon tetrachloride is often used to poison laboratory animals experimentally in order to produce a model of hepatic necrosis. The literature contains reports of such studies. The observations of Hase (1968) on intoxication of rats with carbon tetrachloride caused him to conclude that four stages toward the development of cirrhosis were recognizable. These are: (1) Diffuse centrilobular necrosis; (2) Regeneration of hepatic venous radicles in circulatory periphery of sinusoids and formation of hepatohepatic venous anastomoses; (3) Extension of hepatic venous radicles to portal canals and formation of portahepatic venous shunts; and (4) Cirrhosis.

Muth (1960) suggests that selenium deficiency may cause sheep to be more susceptible to carbon tetrachloride poisoning. Robinson and Harper (1967) exposed dogs, monkeys, rats and mice to carbon tetrachloride vapor under varying simulated altitudes and concluded that the higher altitudes (with 100 per cent oxygen) had an additive effect upon the toxicity of carbon tetrachloride on these species.

Carbon Tetrachloride and Tetrachlorethylene

CHANDLER, A. C., and CHOPRA, R. N.: The Toxicity of Carbon Tetrachloride for Cats. North Am. Vet. 7:49, 1926.

FAIRFAX, R. E.: *Carbon Tetrachloride Poisoning of Sheep.* New South Wales, Yearb. Inst. Insp. Lvstk, 1948, p. 73.

GALLAGHER, C. H., and SIMMONDS, R. A.: Prophylaxis of Poisoning by Carbon Tetrachloride. Nature, Lond. *184*, Suppl. No. *18*:1707–1708, 1959.

HARPER, D. T., JR., and ROBINSON, F. R.: Comparative Pathology of Animals Exposed to Carbon Tetrachloride in Oxygen at 238mm. HG and in Ambient Air. Aerospace Med. *38*: 784–788, 1967.

HARRIS, F. H.: Acute Carbon Tetrachloride Poisoning. U. S. Armed Forces Med. J. *3*:1023–1028, 1952.

HASE, T.: Development of Portahepatic Venous Shunts and Cirrhosis in Carbon Tetrachloride Poisoning in Rats. Amer. J. Path. *53*:83–98, 1968.

KONDOS, A. C., and McCLYMONT, G. L.: Enhanced Toxicity of Carbon Tetrachloride in Sheep on High Protein Intakes. Aust. Vet. J. *41*:349–351, 1965.

LEVINE, S.: A Case of Tetrachlorethylene Poisoning in an English Setter. Vet. Med. *33*:171–172, 1938.

MESHORER, A., and BENHAR, E.: Accidental Poisoning in Inbred Male Mice by Carbon Tetrachloride. Lab. An. Care 16:198–201, 1966.

MUTH, O. H.: Carbon Tetrachloride Poisoning of Ewes on a Low Selenium Ration. Am. J. Vet. Res. 21:86–87, 1960.

SETCHELL, B. P.: Poisoning of Sheep with Anthelmintic Doses of Carbon Tetrachloride. Chemical Pathology. Austr. Vet. J. 38:580–582, 1962.

SHERMAN, S. R., and BINDER, C. F.: Hazards of Carbon Tetrachloride in Present-day Use. U. S. Naval Med. Bull. 43:590–599, 1944.

WIRTSCHAFTER, Z. T., and DeMERITT, M. G: Reticulo-Endothelial Response to Carbon Tetrachloride. Arch. Path. 67:146–158, 1959.

WOODS, W. W.: The Changes in the Kidneys in Carbon Tetrachloride Poisoning, and Their Resemblance to the "Crush Syndrome." J. Path. and Bact. 58·767–777, 1946.

PHENOTHIAZINE

This important anthelmintic drug produces highly variable toxic effects, principally in horses. There appear to be two important factors that determine whether poisoning will result from a dose of given size. The first and most crucial is the diet and nutritional state of the patient. As is the case with many hepatotoxic drugs, a well-nourished animal on a high protein diet with ample stores of glycogen in the liver is much less apt to suffer ill effects than an animal in the opposite condition. The second factor is the degree of refinement of the phenothiazine and the presence or absence of diphenylamine, which is a contaminant of the crude drug. Poisoned animals show more or less severe anemia which reaches its height a few days after the drug is ingested. This is an hemolytic anemia and it is occasionally rapid enough to cause hemoglobinuria. There are also acute toxic hepatitis (p. 1223) and nephrosis (p. 1266) of varying degrees of severity. The hepatic injury is of such a nature that photosensitization (p. 77) occasionally arises. Symptoms include depression, dullness, weakness and coma, in addition to the derangements directly traceable to the pathological changes. Many animals recover from the depressive symptoms after some hours, from the anemia and hepato-renal symptoms after several days.

Cattle may also be poisoned by phenothiazine with similar effects. Jha and Iyer (1967) report the following in calves exposed to lethal doses of phenothiazine: oligocythemia, reduced hemoglobin, neutrocytosis with left shift, lymphopenia and eosinopenia, plus albuminuria and glycosuria in some animals.

Phenothiazine is also a cause of primary photosensitizational dermatitis which is described in Chapter 3 (p. 77).

Phenothiazine

BISWAL, G. and PATNAIK, B.: Photosensitized Keratitis in Calves and Kids Following Administration of Phenothiazine. Indian Vet. J. 38:400–403, 1961.

BOLTON, J.: A Case of Phenothiazine Poisoning in Young Bovines. Vet. Rec. 60:479, 1948.

BRITTON, J. W.: Phenothiazine Poisoning in Pigs. Cornell Vet. 33:368–369, 1943.

EICHELBERGER, L., and ROMA, M.: Phenothiazine Poisoning in a Farm Dog. Vet. Med. 42:302–303, 1947.

HEBDEN, S. P. and SETCHELL, B. P.: Phenothiazine Toxicosis. Austr. Vet. J. 38:399, 1962.

JHA, G. J., and IYER, P. K. R.: Pathology of Phenothiazine Intoxication in Cattle—Clinical Pathology. Indian Vet. J. 44:457–466, 1967.

————: Pathology of Phenothiazine Intoxication in Cattle and Sheep—Changes in Endocrine Organs. Indian J. Vet. Sci. 37:165–171, 1967.

McSHERRY, B. J., ROE, C. K., and MILNE, F. J.: The Hematology of Phenothiazine Poisoning in Horses. Can. Vet. J. 7:3–12, 1966.

MITROVIC, M.: Due casi di avvelenamento ad esito letale in cavalli trattati con dosi terapeutiche di fecondita. Zootec. Vet., Milan, 3:157–160, 1948. (English summary.)

WESTERMARCK, H.: Doseringens inverkan paa phentiazinets toxiska och antiparasitära effekt, särskilt med hänsyn till detta ämnes inverkan paa blodets bilirubin-, hemoglobinoch Protrombinspegel. (Toxicity of phenothiazine for horses.) Suom. Eläinlääkäril. *54*:43–72, 1948. (English summary.)

WISE, G. H., JAMES, C. A., and ANDERSON, G. W.: Toxicity of Phenothiazine Derivatives Excreted in the Milk of Dairy Cows Treated with Massive Doses of the Drug. J. Dairy Sci. *30*:55–59, 1947.

WOOLF, F. P., and SIMMS, B. T.: Studies of the Toxicology of Phenothiazine in Horses and Mules. North Am. Vet. *24*:595–599, 1943.

PHENANTHRIDINIUM AND OTHER TRYPANOCIDAL DRUGS

Certain compounds of phenanthridinium, especially 2:7-diamino-9-phenyl-10 methyl phenanthridinium bromide, commonly called dimidium bromide, and ethidium bromide, which is identical except that it has an ethyl group instead of the methyl radical, are currently used parenterally to free animals of trypanosomal infections. Quinapyramine sulfate and chloride, usually in a mixture bearing the common name of antrycide, have the same therapeutic use. While toxicity of these drugs is not so great as to nullify their usefulness, poisoning may occur when the amount administered is too great or too frequently repeated. The effects of a single or repeated dose are commonly delayed for five to seven weeks, during which the animal, usually a bovine, loses weight severely. The van den Bergh reaction and other tests show impaired hepatic function. The principal lesion is an acute toxic hepatitis beginning with hydropic or vacuolar degeneration of the hepatic cells at the periphery of the lobule. This is followed by fatty change, which spreads toward the center of the lobule. Photosensitization (p. 77) follows in some individuals, especially if the dose is later repeated. In the case of antrycide, toxic tubular nephritis is more severe than the hepatitis and is accompanied by anemia. Many animals recover from the toxicity of either drug.

Phenanthridinium and Other Trypanocidal Drugs

BURDIN, M. L., and PLOWRIGHT, W.: Toxic Effects of Four Trypanocidal Substances for East African Type of Zebu Cattle. Vet. Rec. *64*:635–639, 1952.

GRETILLAT, E. H.: Observations sur le accidents toxiques survenus a la suite du traitement de la trypanosomiase bovine par le bromure de dimidium dans quelques troupeaux du Kwango. Bull. Agric. Congo belge. *44*:787–812, 1953.

PLOWRIGHT, W., BURDIN, M. L., and THOROLD, P. W.: Delayed Toxicity Due to Dimidium Bromide. J. Comp. Path. & Therap. *62*:136–140 and 178–195, 1952.

"CLAY-PIGEON" POISONING—COAL-TAR PITCH

It has happened more than once that a club of trap-shooters has rented a small piece of ground for the site of their shooting contests and then turned it back to the farmer. The "clay pigeons" which are used as targets to be shattered in the air by the marksman are constructed of an amalgam held together by a kind of pitch derived from coal tar, a heterogeneous and variable mixture in which a number of poisonous chemical compounds have been identified. The fragments remain in the soil and are tasty to pigs which may be pastured on the contaminated ground. At least a few days are required for illness to develop, depending on the amount of the material consumed. There are usually only a few hours of nonspecific symptoms.

The principal post-mortem lesion consists in very severe centrilobular necrosis of the liver with blood replacing the lost cells and filling the center of the lobule. The supporting reticular tissue of the lobule appears to remain intact. Since involvement of the liver tends to be patchy, the organ is grossly spotted with reddish and yellowish areas. There may be a limited fibrinous or adhesive peri-hepatitis. Other lesions include a well-marked anemia with erythrocyte counts and hemoglobin often approximating half the normal, jaundice, edema of lymph nodes and ascites. Blood glucose is also reduced prior to death and thymol turbidity, serum chloride and phosphorus are increased, according to Davis and Libke (1968). White cell counts, sedimentation rate, serum protein, calcium and creatinine are not changed.

"Clay-Pigeon" Poisoning—Coal-Tar Pitch

DAVIS, J. W., and LIBKE, K. G.:   Hematologic Studies in Pigs Fed Clay Pigeon Targets. J. Am. Vet. Med. Assn. *152*:382–384, 1968.
GRAHAM, R., HESTER, H. R., and HENDERSON, J. A.:   Coal-tar Pitch Poisoning in Pigs. J. Am. Vet. Med. Assn. *96*:135–140, 1940.
GIFFEE, J. W.:   Clay Pigeon Poisoning in Swine.   Vet. Med. *40*:97, 1945.
RUMMLER, H. J.:   Pigsty Flooring Materials Containing Tar and Bitumen. Mh. Vet. Med. *17*:482–487, 1962.

HYDROGEN SULFIDE

Animals have been poisoned by the inhalation of H_2S in the atmosphere of stables so constructed that the gases from manure pits could enter them.   (In some cold countries the excreta are collected and stored in underground pits, where decomposition processes reduce it to a semi-liquid mass, very useful as fertilizer.)   A concentration of as much as 0.03 per cent in the air is dangerous. While harmless in medicinal amounts, the accidental feeding of a large quantity of sulfur has resulted in a similar type of poisoning, H_2S being formed as a decomposition product.

Signs, which may last for a few hours, are dyspnea, cyanosis, mucous exudate from the upper respiratory passages, depression and apathy or, in some species, convulsions. Lesions include severe pulmonary edema, hyperemia and catarrhal inflammation of the air passages, acute toxic hepatitis (p. 1223) and nephrosis (p. 1266) and subendocardial and other hemorrhages. The tissues of the gastro-intestinal tract are edematous but not congested. There is also edema of the brain. The blood does not clot properly, sulfhemoglobin being formed.

Hydrogen Sulfide

BLASER, E.:   Ein Beitrag zur Kenntnis der Schwefelwasserstoffvergiftung beim Tier durch Jauchegase.   Schweiz. Arch. f, Tierheilk. *88*:401–413 and 433–446, 1946.
COGHLIN, C. L.:   Hydrogen Sulphide Poisoning in Cattle.   Canad. J. Comp. Med. *8*:111–113, 1944.
DOUGHERTY, R. W., WONG, R., and CHRISTENSEN, B. E.:   Studies on Hydrogen-Sulfide Poisoning.   Am. J. Vet. Res. *4*:254–256, 1943.
O'DONOGHUE, J. G.:   Hydrogen Sulphide Poisoning in Swine.   Canad. J. Comp. Med. *25*: 217–219, 1961.
SKRYPNIK, E. I.:   (Poisoning of Cattle by Water Containing H_2S, Chlorine, and Chlorides.) Veterinariya, Moscow *10*:42–44, 1945.   (In Russian.   Original title not reproducible.)

GOSSYPOL

A by-product of the cotton industry, cottonseed meal is a valuable protein concentrate for cattle and other farm animals. A small amount of a poisonous substance, gossypol, remains in the meal which is made from the seeds after cottonseed oil has been extracted from them. The processor endeavors to keep the gossypol at a level approximating 0.02 to 0.04 per cent but, owing to variations in temperature with the hydraulic-press process and to undesirable solvents in other processes, this amount may be greatly exceeded.

Swine are much more susceptible to poisoning than other species, and it is usually recommended that cottonseed meal not exceed 9 per cent of the total ration of these animals. Signs commonly develop after pigs have been fed from one to three months on rations containing excessive amounts of gossypol. They consist principally of dyspnea, panting, weakness, and anorexia and last commonly for several, rarely for many, days before death occurs.

The **lesions** account readily for the signs. Most conspicuous are hydrothorax, hydropericardium, hydroperitoneum, edema of the lungs, of many or all lymph nodes and often of the subcutaneous tissues. Edema of the wall and attachments of the gallbladder is conspicuous in half the cases. Passive congestion is prominent in the lungs, liver and kidneys. All this is readily explained as cardiac edema (p. 139) and congestive heart failure when the heart is examined.

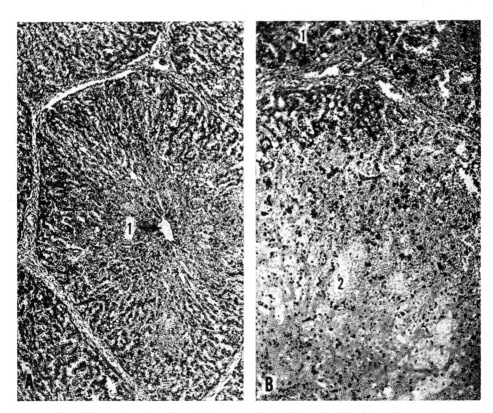

Fig. 17–3.—Liver of a pig poisoned by gossypol. *A*, Necrosis of hepatic cells around central vein (*1*) (× 60). *B*, Same liver (× 100). Portal area (*1*) is relatively unaffected but necrosis and hemorrhage are extensive in the center of the lobule (*2*).

Dilatation of the ventricles is readily demonstrable in nearly all cases, with well-marked hypertrophy in the more prolonged ones. "White muscles," a definite paleness of various skeletal muscles (p. 1049), exist in two-thirds of the affected individuals. Icterus is noticeable in a minority of cases. The livers are most often redder than normally, because of the congestion, but some, containing less blood, show the paleness indicative of necrosis and other changes. In either case, the lobular architecture is more distinct even than that which is normal for the pig, so that the experienced prosector has little doubt grossly of the existence of some form of toxic hepatitis (p. 1223).

Microscopic changes are in accord with what is seen grossly, those in the liver and heart requiring especial mention. The fundamental hepatic lesion is centrilobular necrosis. The space left by the lost parenchymal cells is filled with blood, the scanty reticulum of Kupffer cells remaining, at least for a time. In 80 per cent of the livers, the necrosis in practically all lobules is so extensive that hepatic cells remain in only a narrow peripheral zone, perhaps only three or four cells wide, the rest of the lobule being filled with blood. This condition is obviously responsible for the red color of these livers grossly. In a minority of livers, a limited zone of cells in a state of fatty degeneration exists between the peripheral living zone and the blood-filled central area. Whether the centrilobular necrosis should be attributed to direct toxic injury of the gossypol or to anoxia resulting from cardiac insufficiency, it is difficult to prove. Both conditions are present, but the extent of necrosis is greater than that which usually results from cardiac disease alone. Microscopic examination of the heart reveals necrosis or degeneration of numerous myocardial fibers; some are without the normal number of nuclei; in some there are large and poorly outlined vacuoles in the cytoplasmic areas; some are greatly atrophied. Except in the hearts of pigs that die early, fibers showing compensatory hypertrophy mingle with those that have degenerated. The hypertrophy is evidenced by a limited increase in the size of the fiber, but more especially by a marked increase in both the size and the number of nuclei in the hypertrophic fiber.

Diagnosis can be made with considerable assurance on the basis of the combination of cardiac changes, the marked edema and the hepatic changes, the clinical history being important if available. (It is usually inconclusive as to the amount of gossypol consumed.) Poisoning by coal-tar pitch (p. 871) occurs in swine and produces comparable hepatic changes, but in the experience of one of the writers (Smith), the destroyed centrilobular areas have never been as large as they have been in gossypol poisoning. A similar form of hepatic destruction has also been described as due to dietary disorders, but the involvement of lobules seems to be less universal. At any rate, cardiac injury and edema have not been described in either the dietary disorder or the pitch poisoning.

Gossypol

DINWIDDIE, R. R., and SHORT, A. K.: Cottonseed Poisoning of Livestock. Exp. Sta. Bull. 108, Univ. Arkansas, Fayetteville, 1911, pp. 395–410.

HOVE, E. L., and SEIBOLD, H. R.: Liver Necrosis and Altered Fat Composition in Vitamin E-Deficient Swine. J. Nutrition. 56:173–186, 1955.

LAMBERT, R. A., and ALLISON, B. R.: Types of Lesion in Chronic Passive Congestion of the Liver. Bull. Johns Hopkins Hosp., 27:350–356, 1916.

OBEL, A. L.: Studies on the Morphology and Etiology of So-called Toxic Liver Dystrophy (Hepatosis Diaetetica) in Swine. Acta path. et microbiol. Scandinav. Supp. 94, 1953, pp. 1–87.

Smith, H. A.: Pathology of Gossypol Poisoning. Am. J. Path., *33*:353–365, 1957.

West, J. L.: Lesions of Gossypol Poisoning in the Dog. J. Am. Vet. Med. Assn. *96*:74–76, 1940.

Withers, W. A., and Carruth, F. E.: Gossypol, the Toxic Substance in Cottonseed Meal. J. Agric. Res. *5*:261–288, 1916.

COCKLEBUR

Cockleburs (*Xanthium italicum et spp.*) are most poisonous, as well as least unpalatable, at or shortly after the two-leaf, seedling stage. Pigs are more often poisoned than other species, but cattle and sheep have also suffered. Symptoms appear several hours after ingestion of the plants and are those of gastrointestinal pain and irritation and of cardiac and muscular weakness. There are also opis-thotonos and convulsions. The failing heart, with weak and rapid pulse, is responsible for death after an illness of a few hours. Lesions include subepicardial and other subserous hemorrhages, a moderate degree of gastritis and enteritis, but toxic injury to the liver, kidneys and heart is more important. The liver shows the usual changes of acute toxic hepatitis (p. 1223) with fatty change pre-dominant in some individuals, necrosis in others. The necrosis is preceded by acute cellular swelling and narrowing of the hepatic cords; it is centrilobular at first but may extend throughout all but the most peripheral parts of the lobule. Fatty change, of a patchy distribution and demonstrable only by fat stains, is present in various parts of the myocardium. In the kidney, fat is prominent in the ascending loops of Henle and incipient necrosis of the proximal convoluted tubules is usually present. The lower tubules often contain albuminous casts. Changes in the central nervous system appear not to have been investigated.

Xanthium pungens, the Novgoora bur, causes a very similar form of poisoning in Australia.

Cocklebur

Forrest, G. P.: Cocklebur Poisoning. J. Am. Vet. Med. Assn. *93*:42–43, 1938.

Kenny, G. C., Everist, S. L., and Sutherland, A. K.: Noagoora Bur Poisoning of Cattle. Queensland Agric. J. *70*:172–177, 1950.

Pribicevic, S., and Sevkovic, N.: Experimental Study of Poisoning by *Xanthium sacchar-atum* in Pigs. Acta Vet. Belgrade *4*:58–64, 1954. Abstract from English summary, Vet. Bull. No. 3371, 1955.

SENECIOS

Plants of the genus *Senecio* are of almost world-wide distribution. Character istically they are woody herbs with terminal clusters of yellow flowers, bushy in form and commonly reaching a height between 20 and 50 cm. Like most poison-ous plants, they are eaten only when more palatable pasturage is not available. Certain species are popularly known in many localities as ragworts or groundsels. In Europe, South Africa, New Zealand or the plains region of the United States and Canada, at least the following species are known to be poisonous, *S. aquaticus, burchelli, ilicifolius, integerrimus, jacobaea, longilobus, plattensis, riddellii* and *scleratus*. Chemically it has been shown that pyrrolizidine alkaloids or their N-oxides are the chemical compounds responsible for the toxicity.

Poisoning involves horses and cattle chiefly, sheep being much less susceptible. In earlier times what is now known to be poisoning by Senecios was described

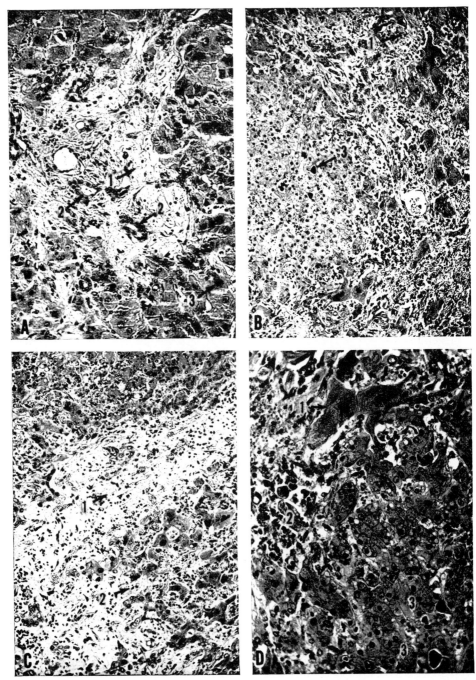

FIG. 17–4.—*A*, Bovine liver (× 150) in Senecio poisoning. Periportal fibrosis (*1*), hyperplasia of bile ducts (*2*) and hyperchromatism in hepatic nuclei (*3*). Photograph courtesy of Dr. C. L. Davis. *B*, Equine liver in crotalaria poisoning (× 100). Periportal fibrosis (*1*), regenerating liver cells (*2*), and distended bile canaliculi (*3*). *C*, Another field, equine liver in *B* (× 100). Note portal fibrosis (*1*) which extends into the lobule (*2*). *D*, Equine liver (same as *B* and *C*) (× 210). Regenerating liver cells (*1*), leukocytes in portal region area (*2*), and distended bile canaliculi (*3*). Photographs courtesy of Dr. H. R. Seibold.

as several different diseases before their true nature was recognized. Of these, the principal ones were **Molteno disease** (Chase, 1904) of cattle in Cape Colony (Africa), **Winton disease** (Gilruth, 1905) of horses and cattle in New Zealand, **Pictou disease** (Pethick, 1906) of cattle in Canada and **Van Es' walking disease** (Van Es *et al.*, 1929) of horses in Nebraska (U.S.A.). **Zd'ar disease** of horses in Bohemia and probably **Schweinsberger disease** in Bavaria have recently been shown to belong in this list (Vanek, 1959).

Signs appear after the animal has consumed varying amounts of the plant for a number of days or as long as three weeks. There is a disturbance of consciousness which causes the animal to walk aimlessly but stubbornly, and to press the head continually against an object with which it collides. In the later stages of the illness, which usually lasts a few days, there may be mania. The semi-domesticated cattle of the western ranges, especially, may become dangerously belligerent, with a behavior suggestive of rabies but without the terminal paralysis which characterizes the latter disease. In addition, there is jaundice and severe intestinal irritation which results in frequent watery defecations with marked tenesmus and even eversion of the rectum.

Senecios can be classed among the stronger hepatotoxic poisons. **Post-mortem** lesions are those of a chronic toxic hepatitis (p. 1225) with actively acute inflammation usually still in progress, and the jaundice and abdominal edema incident thereto. Hepatic changes vary from fatty change and necrosis of the hepatic cells to full-fledged portal cirrhosis (p. 1227), depending on the duration of the disease, its severity and the rapidity of its progress. The fibrous tissue tends to spread into the lobule in an irregular fashion, differing in this respect from the typical portal, or atrophic, cirrhosis. Proliferation of new bile ducts is prominent in many areas, perhaps somewhat more so than in the usual examples of portal cirrhosis. With the necrosis of the hepatic parenchymatous cells, there are frequently conspicuous attempts at regeneration. Such areas are recognized by the unusually large size of the cells and their nuclei and the relative frequency of cells with more than one nucleus. As a result of the architectural derangement, the bile canaliculi are occluded in various areas. Such areas show considerable deposits of bile pigment (p. 73) microscopically; grossly, there is the greenish-brown discoloration of icteric liver tissue. Since there is also considerable congestion in the less fibrotic areas, the typical liver shows a totally irregular mottling grossly and is unduly hard in proportion to the amount of cirrhosis (p. 1225). The hepatic lymph nodes may be enlarged due to reticulo-endothelial proliferation (Mathews, 1933).

The generalized toxic jaundice (p. 74) is usually of conspicuous severity and is stated by Mathews (1933) to be invariably present. The abdominal edema is widely diffused in the subserosa of the intestines and often of the stomach. The mesenteries are often markedly thickened with fluid. The gallbladder not only has a highly edematous wall, but also is distended with unused bile, sometimes to enormous proportions. The bile is stated to be of normal quality, hence, the condition is presumed to represent a combination of edema based upon intra-hepatic obstruction and of the usual accumulation of bile which occurs in the absence of cholecystikinetic stimuli from the intestine (p. 1237). There is commonly considerable edema in the mucosa and submucosa of the stomach and intestines. Since this is not proportional to the subserosal edema and since a certain degree of catarrhal enteritis is demonstrable on the basis of hyperemia and other changes, the submucous fluid should doubtless be considered as inflammatory (p. 136). While the toxic action of the senecio plants is mainly upon the liver, there is also a noticeable degree of toxic tubular nephrosis (p. 1266). Petechial and ecchymotic hemorrhages are rather prominent on the heart, mesentery and omentum and are doubtless attributable to toxic injury of capillaries.

There appear to be no extensive studies of the brain which would determine whether the manic symptoms are based upon cerebral lesions or merely upon the tendency for nervous hyperirritability which so frequently accompanies hepatic diseases (p. 1241). The violent behavior has been reported chiefly by Mathews and to those familiar with the untamed range cattle with which he worked, their belligerency is rather understandable merely as an expression of the bodily discomfort which they undoubtedly felt. Even these cattle, Mathews points out, commonly showed no bellicose symptoms when, during the course of experimental studies, they were fed the plants while confined in a small pen.

Diagnosis must be based upon a combination of presence of the plant, symptoms and lesions. There are no specific tests, neither are there many other equally hepatotoxic substances which are likely to be encountered under circumstances where senecio plants would be ingested.

Senecios

CHASE, W. H.: The Molteno Cattle Disease. Agric. J. of Cape of Good Hope 25:675–678 1904.

CRAWFORD, M.: Mycotoxicosis in Veterinary Medicine. Vet. Bul. 32:415–420, 1962.

DIENER, U. L. et al.: Toxin-producing Aspergillus Isolated from Domestic Peanuts. Science 142:1491–1942, 1963.

EVANS, W. C.: Poisoning of Farm Animals by the Marsh Ragwort. Nature (London). 164:30–31, 1949.

GILRUTH, J. A.: Hepatic Cirrhosis or Winton Disease. Thirteenth Rept. Dept. of Agriculture, New Zealand, 1905, p. 178. (Cited by Mathews.)

HARDING, J. D. J., et al.: Experimental Poisoning by Senecio jacobaea in Pigs. Path. Vet. 1:204–220, 1964.

MATHEWS, F. P.: Poisoning of Cattle by Species of Groundsel. Exp. Sta. Bull. 481, Texas A. & M. College, College Station, Texas, 1933.

PETHICK, W. H.: Special Report on Pictou Cattle Disease. Canadian Dept. Agriculture, No. 8, 1906. (Cited by Mathews.)

SELZER, G., and PARKER, R. G. F.: Senecio Poisoning Exhibiting as Chiari's Syndrome. Am. J. Path. 27:885–907, 1951.

VANEK, J.: Vergiftung mit Kreuzkraut (Senecio) als Ursache der Zdárer Pferdeseuche. (Poisoning with Senecio erraticus as the cause of Zd'ár disease of horses.) Schweiz. Z. Allg. Path. 21:821–848, 1959. Abstr. Vet. Bull. No. 3724, 1958.

VAN ES, L., CANTWELL, L. R., MARTIN, H. M., and KRAMER, J.: Nature and Cause of the "Walking Disease" of Northwestern Nebraska. Exp. Sta. Bull. No. 43, Univ. of Nebraska, Lincoln, 1929.

TARWEED

Tarweed, *Amsinckia intermedia,* is a weed which often seriously contaminates the wheat fields of the Pacific region of the United States and occasionally other areas. The rather small seeds are harvested with the crop and are separated from the wheat at the flour mill, going into the cull portion known as "screenings." The latter are commonly returned to the farm to be used as feed for animals, chiefly swine. After a few or many weeks on a diet containing considerable amounts of the seeds, icterus and other signs of toxic hepatitis appear. As evidence of alimentary irritation and disturbance, small ulcers often appear in the mouth. Mild ataxia and the central nervous disturbances characteristic of many hepatic disorders (p. 1241) appear in the later stages. The behavior of horses is comparable to what is seen in Van Es' walking disease, in other words, senecio poisoning (p. 875). Swine often reach marketable age with no more conspicuous disturbance than general unthriftiness and at slaughter are found to be victims of "hard-liver disease." As the reader has already surmised, the lesions are those of acute or chronic toxic hepatitis or, most often, of both together.

Tarweed

McCULLOCH, E. C.: Hepatic Cirrhosis of Horses, Swine and Cattle Due to Ingestion of Seeds of the Tarweed, *Amsinckia intermedia*. J. Am. Vet. Med. Assn. *96*:5–17, 1940.
————: Use of Grain Containing Tarweed Seed as Poultry Feed. J. Am. Vet. Med. Assn. *101*:481–483, 1942.
WOOLSEY, J. H., JASPER, D. E., CORDY, D. R., and CHRISTENSEN, J. F.: Two Outbreaks of Hepatic Cirrhosis in Swine in California, with Evidence Incriminating Tarweed. Vet. Med. *47*:55–58, 1952.

SACAHUISTE

Sacahuiste, sacahuista, or beargrass (*Nolina texana*) is a perennial plant which grows in the moderately arid parts of the Southwestern United States, principally in central and western Texas. Because of its extremely long, blade-like leaves (60 to 160 cm. long, 2 to 5 mm. wide), which rise to a height of 50 to 75 cm., then bend and droop on all sides, the plant resembles a very large tuft of grass. In early spring, it sends up flowering stems which bear panicles of fine flowers of inconspicuous grayish color. Only the flowering panicles and the buds are poisonous, according to the experimental work of Mathews (1940). Sheep and goats more frequently eat poisonous amounts than cattle.

This is one of the photosensitizing plants, and if the animal at the same time eats adequate amounts of chlorophyll-containing material and is exposed to sunlight, the usual edema and necrosis of the unpigmented skin result. These changes are most prominent in the face and ears. The ears of sheep may swell to a thickness of 2 or 3 cm., drooping because of the added weight. Dermatitis is frequently characterized by severe pruritus. Necrosis of areas of skin may or may not supervene, depending on the severity of this phase of the disease. Passing over the photosensitization, which has been treated in detail elsewhere (p. 77), the outstanding signs of poisoning by sacahuiste include icterus, which appears within a day or two after the first loss of appetite, a discharge of tenacious, yellow exudate from the nostrils and a copious conjunctival exudate which is serous at first and later purulent. The urine is dark yellow or sometimes reddish. The latter discoloration appears to be due to hemoglobin; at least there is no hematuria. A band of purplish discoloration encircling the hoof just below the coronary band is thought by Mathews to represent an aspect of the photosensitization. Poisoned animals usually live a week or more after the appearance of symptoms, seeking water and shade meanwhile. A few recover.

The lesions are those of acute toxic hepatitis (p. 1223) with a greenish paleness and greasy feeling of the liver grossly. Upon incision, greenish casts of inspissated bile can be expressed from the severed ducts. Microscopically, the hepatic changes are cloudy swelling, disorganization of the hepatic cords, fatty change, chiefly centrilobular, biliary casts containing cholesterol clefts (p. 26) and a minimal amount of necrosis. The other principal changes are those of toxic tubular nephrosis, the large, pale kidney grossly (p. 1267), hydropic degeneration and fatty change being most prominent microscopically. As in the liver, actual necrosis is minimal. Albuminous casts (p. 1292) are numerous and may extend into Bowman's capsules. Bile pigment tends to produce a greenish-brown discoloration macroscopically, which is carried over into the microscopic sections to temper the usual staining reactions of the cells.

In diagnosis, the absence of marked changes in the gallbladder and the frequent presence of photosensitization help to differentiate this poisoning from that caused by senecios and possibly from those due to some other plants having the same geographical habitat. It is doubtful that any of the chemical poisons produce exactly this combination of changes.

Sacahuiste

MATHEWS, F. P.: Poisoning in Sheep and Goats by Sacahuiste (*Nolina texana*) Buds and Blooms. Exp. Sta. Bull. 585. Texas A. & M. College, College Station, Texas, 1940.

DRYMARIA PACHYPHYLLA

This plant, found on the arid ranges of the Southwestern United States, has been shown by Mathews (1933) to be highly poisonous to sheep and somewhat less so to cattle and goats. A member of the "chickenweed" group, it grows flat on the ground, reaching a width of as much as 40 cm. Its rather sparse, trailing branches bear ovate leaves about a centimer in length, which are thick and juicy. (*Pachyphylla* means thick-leaved.) Its fruits and seeds are quite tiny and are borne where the short leaf-stalks come off from the branches.

Signs appear in a little less than twenty-four hours after ingestion of the plant (experimentally) and may be followed by death in two hours or possibly by recovery in about two days. They consist of diarrhea and evidence of mild abdominal pain. Lethargy, coma and death tend to follow rapidly, depending on the severity of the poisoning. Pulse and respiration remain practically normal.

Lesions include hemorrhagic inflammation at least of the ileum and at times of higher portions of the intestine. This is accompanied by severe serous and often hemorrhagic cholecystitis with edematous pericholecystitis and pericholangitis. Ecchymotic hemorrhages are described as numerous in the diaphragm, epicardium and outer myocardium. The liver and spleen are markedly congested. The liver also undergoes centrilobular necrosis, usually coagulative in type with markedly acidophilic staining of the cytoplasm. More peripherally there is fatty change. Toxic changes in the kidneys are much more limited and without casts.

Diagnosis is not likely to be possible on the basis of lesions alone, but should become reasonably certain if the availability of the plant and the unavailability of normal and palatable forage are known to exist. The poison may be classified, in summary, as enteritis-producing and hepatotoxic.

Drymaria Pachyphylla

MATHEWS, F. P.: The Toxicity of *Drymaria pachyphylla* for Cattle, Sheep and Goats. J. Am. Vet. Med. Assn. *83*:255–260, 1933.

vetch," are raised, like certain lupines (p. 882), as proteinaceous forage or as nitrogen-fixing soil-builders. The seeds of this and some other species contain poisonous amounts of prussic acid, especially before maturity. However, the toxic effects of the vetches in hay or forage are in most cases of a different nature, resembling those of lupinosis. The illness, which usually extends over several days or longer, is characterized especially by vague digestive disturbances and icterus. In more acute forms, there are muscular twitchings and definite signs of gastroenteritis. In the case of *Vicia faba*, the "broad bean" or "horse bean," hemolytic anemia and hemoglobinuria are also symptoms. Lesions are those of acute toxic hepatitis (p. 1223) with or without gastroenteritis.

A syndrome in cattle has been associated with feeding upon pastures containing hairy vetch (*Vicia villosa*) by Panciera, Johnson and Osburn (1966). This disease differs in several ways from that usually associated with other vetch poisoning and deserves mention. The disease was observed in 13 herds in which dermatitis, conjunctivitis, and diarrhea were the principal signs of illness. Approximately 800 cattle were observed, about 7 per cent of them were sick and about half of these sick cattle died. The affected skin became thickened, folded and in places denuded of hair. The lesions occurred in pigmented as well as non-pigmented areas of the skin. A few pregnant cows aborted.

The lesions in fatal cases were distributed through the myocardium, kidney, adrenal, lymph nodes, and thyroid and appeared grossly as focal or confluent grayish infiltrations, usually moderately firm and sharply demarcated from the

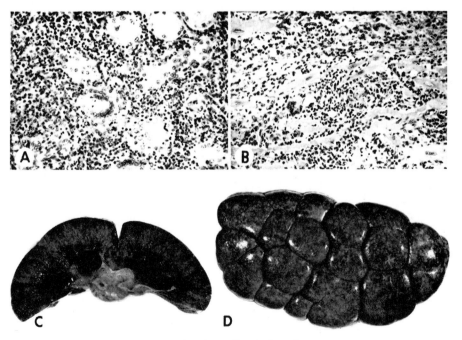

FIG. 17–6.—Poisoning by hairy vetch (*Vicia villosa*) of cattle.

A, Kidney. Distortion of tubules and leukocytic infiltration.

B, Myocardium. Necrosis and calcification of muscle fibers, proliferation of sarcolemma, regeneration of muscle cells and leukocytic infiltration.

C, Cross section of kidney. Grayish, infiltration of cortex.

D, Kidney. Grayish foci disseminated through cortex. (Courtesy of Dr. Roger J. Panciera and Journal of the American Veterinary Medical Association.)

adjacent tissue. Microscopically, these focal lesions were formed by necrosis of parenchyma and infiltration by macrophages, multinucleated giant cells, eosinpohils and lymphocytes. Myocardial fibers were necrotic, sometimes mineralized (Fig. 17–6), and the sarcoplasma often absent, leaving sarcolemmal nuclei and many giant cells. Necrosis of renal tubules was also observed in this syndrome, accompanied by replication of tubular epithelial cells, intense infiltration by leukocytes, principally lymphocytes, and peculiar membranous thickening of the glomerular tufts (Fig. 17–6).

A specific hemolytic anemia, **favism,** in certain human subjects is dependent upon a genetic factor and the ingestion of the broad bean, *Vicia faba.* The inherited defect in susceptible human patients results in a deficiency of the enzyme glucose-6-phosphate dehydrogenase. Deficiency of this enzyme (G-6-PD) is reflected in reduced glutathione in the red blood cells. Extracts of beans of *Vicia faba* have been shown to have a destructive effect upon the erythrocytes of susceptible individuals, *in vitro*, and it is therefore believed that the beans may act similarly on the susceptible red blood cells, *in vivo*, resulting in hemolytic anemia.

Vetch

Bowman, J. E., and Walker, D. G.: Action of *Vicia faba* on Erythrocytes: Possible Relation to Favism. Nature *189*:555–556, 1961.
Panciera, R. J., Johnson, L., and Osburn, B. I.: A Disease of Cattle Grazing Hairy Vetch Pasture. J. Am. Vet. Med. Assn. *148*:804–808, 1966.
Steyn, D. G.: *Toxicology of Plants in South Africa.* Johannesburg, The Central News Agency, 1934.

ALGAE

Certain kinds of green or blue-green algae, usually not identified as to species, some of which grow beneath, rather than on the surface of waters of lakes and rivers, are at times extremely poisonous to all species of animals which drink the water. Poisoning has usually occurred when winds have blown much of this material to the shore at which cattle drink, especially during mid-summer.

Death occurs suddenly within approximately an hour or two after drinking the water. Symptoms are acute prostration followed by convulsions, or else rapidly developing general paralysis. Post-mortem lesions are usually stated to be absent excepting possibly the presence of hydroperitoneum. On the other hand, subacute and chronic cases are reported in South Africa. In the former, there is acute toxic hepatitis with icterus, the liver being yellow and friable. There are bloody or yellowish fluid in the serous cavities, acute swelling of the spleen and sometimes hemorrhagic enteritis. In a few chronic cases, the liver is described as hard, presumably cirrhotic. In cattle which have recovered, severe cutaneous lesions characteristic of photosensitization (p. 77) have developed. Toxicity of the water can be demonstrated in experimental animals orally or parenterally, but toxic conditions in the lakes may change very quickly through the "water-bloom" being blown elsewhere or by other means.

Algae

Brandenburg, T. O., and Shigley, F. M.: "Water Bloom" as a Cause of Poisoning in Livestock in North Dakota. J. Am. Vet. Med. Assn. *110*:384–385, 1947.
Deem, A. W., and Thorp, F. Jr.: Toxic Algæ in Colorado. J. Am. Vet. Med. Assn. *95*:542–544, 1939.

FITCH, C. P., BISHOP, L. M., and BOYD, W. L.: "Water Bloom" as a Cause of Poisoning in Domestic Animals. Cornell Vet. *24*:30–38, 1934.

FRANCIS, G.: Poisonous Australian Lake. Nature *18*:11–12, 1878.

GORHAM, P. R.: Toxic Waterblooms of Blue-Green Algae. Canad. Vet. J. *1*:235–245, 1960.

MOLDY FEEDS

The term mold is a rather indefinite designation for practically any of the hundreds of species of filamentous fungi. The word is seldom applied to pathogenic fungi, practically all molds being saprophytes. Following the usual concept that a pathogen grows and multiplies in the tissues, we have discussed fungi having that ability in connection with the specific infectious disease produced by each. There remain to be considered a large number of instances where illness or death is more or less clearly attributable to the ingestion of molds or their products in or on the animal's feed. A large number of species in various genera of fungi have been suspected or accused of being causative in outbreaks of animal disease. Among these are some of our commonest *Aspergilli* and *Penicillia*, which under most circumstances are certainly harmless. Efforts to reproduce the disease experimentally frequently fail completely. In some instances (Sippel, *et al.*, 1953), it has been possible to produce the disease with mold-contaminated feed, but it is not certain that the original disease has ever been reproduced by oral administration merely of cultures of the suspected organisms. The problem thus becomes most elusive. Previous to the discovery in 1930 of the virus causing equine encephalomyelitis, horses were the frequent victims of **"forage poisoning"** supposedly caused by moldy hay or grain. The great majority of these cases have now been clearly resolved as examples of the virus-caused equine encephalomyelitis (p. 356).

There remains, however, "moldy corn poisoning" in the horse, which is an encephalomalacia (p. 1380) rather than an encephalitis. The experimental work of Schwarte, Biester and Murray (1937) appears to be conclusive both as to the causative status of the moldy corn (both the stalks or the unripe ears were moldy and both were fed) and as to the lesions, which were softening and liquefactive necrosis chiefly of the white matter of the cerebrum, with edema and congestion but no inflammatory reaction. Attempts to reproduce the disease with cultures of any of the molds encountered were entirely unsuccessful.

Sippel, Burnside and Atwood (1953) had similar experience with a mold poisoning which affected cattle and swine. The principal lesions in these animals, when acutely affected, were variously located petechiae, ecchymoses and massive hemorrhages, together with acute toxic hepatitis and toxic tubular nephrosis. These animals died after an illness of one or two days characterized by great weakness, staggering and early jaundice. In cases of longer duration, the hemorrhages were minimal, and the toxic changes in liver and kidneys of increasing extent and importance. Centrilobular necrosis was sometimes so severe as to lead to replacement of almost the whole lobule with blood as is the case with gossypol poisoning (p. 873). The kidneys showed, in addition to hydropic degeneration and necrosis of the cortical tubules and fatty change in the medullary rays, generalized dilation of the tubules and atrophy of the glomeruli. This disease was reproducible by the artificial feeding of the moldy corn but not by cultures of any of the molds isolated. However, Carll, in discussing Sippel's work, brought to light the production of very similar lesions by feeding calves cultures of *Aspergillus glaucus* and *A. clavatus* and, in mice, *Penicillium regulosum*.

The reports cited may be taken as examples of a considerable number which are on record. As is readily seen, quite different disease syndromes appear to arise from moldy feeds under different circumstances and in various species of animals. There is no uniformity as to the species of mold incriminated. Unequivocal proof of the directly poisonous qualities of any of these molds cannot be said to exist. Symbiosis of the fungus and the growing plant may be essential, and it may be that the requisite synergistic chemical combination can occur only at certain stages of growth of either the thallophyte or the spermatophyte, or perhaps only under rather closely restricted environmental conditions. The problem is most elusive and, with the possible exception of the encephalomalacia of horses, the diagnosis of mold poisoning must be made with great caution.

For the toxin of *Aspergillus flavus*, see Aflatoxin, page 888. For *Pithomyces chartarum* (*Sporodesmium bakeri*), see Photosensitization, page 77.

Moldy Feeds

ALBRIGHT, J. L. *et al.*: Moldy Corn Toxicosis in Cattle. J. Am. Vet. Med. Assn. *144*:1013–1019, 1964.

BAILEY, W. S., and GROTH, A. H., JR.: The Relationship of Hepatitis-X of Dogs and Moldy Corn Poisoning of Swine. J. Am. Med. Assn. *134*:514–516, 1959.

BERTHELON, M., LADRAT, J., and BOUICHOU, A.: Toxicité du blé carié pour les animaux. Rev. méd. vét. Lyon et Toulouse *96*:52–59, 1945. (*Tilletia tritici*, a smut, not poisonous.)

DO REGO CHAVES, L.: Doença de sintomatologia nervosa causada por intoxicaçã pelo milho. Rev. milit. remonta vet. *10*:199–215, 1950.

HORI, M. *et al.*: A Fungus Isolated from Malt Root Feed Causing Mass Death in Cows. J. Jap. Vet. Med. Assn. *7*:56–63, 1954. (In Japanese. Original title not reproducible.) Abstr. Vet. Bull. No. 2533, 1955. (*Penicillium urticariæ*.)

LAPCEVIC, E., PRIBICEVIC, S., and KOZIC, L.: Trovanje konja prouzrokovacem crne rde—*Puccinia graminis*. (Poisoning in horses with the wheat rust fungus, *Puccinia graminis*.) Vet. Glasn. *7*:268–271, 1953. (In Croat. German summary.)

MUHRER, M. E., and GENTRY, R. F.: A Hemorrhagic Factor in Mouldy Lespedeza Hay (*Lespedeza stipulacea*). Exper. Sta. Research Bull. 429, Univ. Missouri, Columbia, 1948.

OKSAMITNYI, N. K., and VLASOV, A. T.: [Mass Poisoning of Pigs with Ustilaginous Fungi.] Veterinariya, Moscow. *35*:(10)83, 1958. Abstr. Vet. Bull. No. 1904, 1959.

SCHWARTE, L. H., BIESTER, H. E., and MURRAY, C.: A Disease of Horses Caused by Feeding Moldy Corn. J. Am. Vet. Med. Assn. *90*:76–85, 1937.

SIPPEL, W. L., BURNSIDE, J. E., and ATWOOD, M. B.: A Disease of Swine and Cattle Caused by Eating Moldy Corn. Proc. Am. Vet. Med. Assn., 1953, pp. 174–181.

AFLATOXINS

Mycotoxin, Aflatoxicosis, Groundnut poisoning, toxin of *Aspergillus spp.*

Historically, mycotoxins (p. 887) have been suggested as a cause of morbidity in animals since 1901 (Buckley and MacCallum, 1901) but the existence of aflatoxin appears to have been first indicated by the natural occurrence of an animal disease following much the same pattern which led to the discovery of dicoumarin (p. 906). Seibold and Bailey, 1952, described an epizootic toxic hepatitis ("hepatitis X") in dogs which was later demonstrated by Newberne, Bailey and Seibold, 1955, to be the result of feeding commercial dog foods which contained contaminated peanut meal. The presence of mycotoxins in mouldy feedstuff was further supported by the report of Burnside, *et al.*, 1957, of a disease of cattle and swine; toxin-producing strains of moulds were isolated from the suspected feeds and subsequently used to induce a toxic disease in animals. The chemical isolation of aflatoxins was first achieved (DeJongh *et al.*, 1962) in the course of searching for the toxic principle in groundnut meal known to be poisonous for turkeys (Blount, 1961, DeJongh *et al.*, 1962).   It now appears that all domestic species thus far tested and fish are susceptible to poisoning by aflatoxins; furthermore aflatoxins are suspected as etiologic agents of liver disease in man.   The literature is now voluminous on the subject.

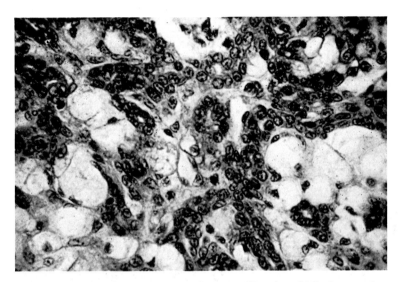

FIG. 17–7.—Poisoning due to aflatoxin. Liver of rat, proliferation of bile ducts and vacuoles in hepatocytes. (Courtesy of Dr. Paul M. Newberne.)

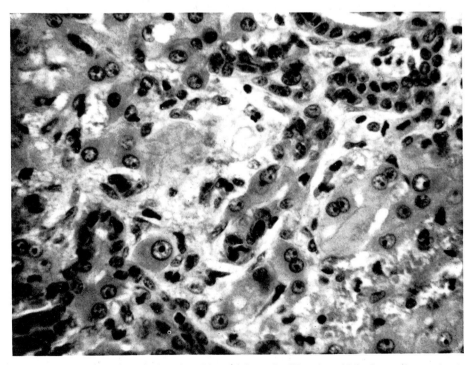

FIG. 17–8.—Poisoning due to aflatoxin. Liver of dog. Proliferation of bile ducts, disorganization of hepatocytes. (Courtesy of Dr. Paul M. Newberne.)

Currently, several aflatoxin fractions have been isolated and differentiated from one another by their fluorescence, R_F values on thin-layer chromatography and by structural identification and synthesis. These have been designated as aflatoxins B_1, B_2, G_1, G_2, M_1, B_{2a} (Newberne, Butler, 1969, and Kraybill, 1969) mainly by their fluorescence and R_F characteristics. These toxins are produced by the growth in cereal grains, nuts and seed products of certain molds, including *Aspergillus flavus*, *A. ochraceus*, *A. versicolor*, *A. parasiticus* and *Penicillium rubrum*.

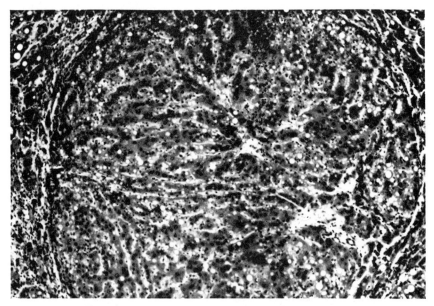

FIG. 17–9.—Poisoning by aflatoxin. Hepatoma of rat.
(Courtesy of Dr. Paul M. Newberne.)

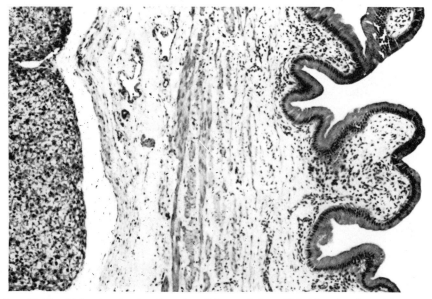

FIG. 17–10.—Poisoning due to aflatoxin. Edema of the gallbladder of a dog. (Courtesy of Dr. Paul M. Newberne.)

The **clinical signs** in acute cases in dogs appear in two to fourteen days (average five days) and consist of anorexia, icterus, bile-stained urine, prostration, occasional blood in feces, vomition (sometimes bloody), epistaxis and rarely convulsions. Chronic cases after one to two months may exhibit icterus, ascites, loss of weight, occasional edema of the legs, elevated blood urea nitrogen (BUN), and prolonged clearance time for bromosulfalein; fever is rarely observed. The signs in other species are similar when recognized, and for the most part are related to the interference with liver function. The susceptibility to aflatoxin B_1 as measured by LD_{50}, has been determined experimentally to vary among different species. The following animals are listed in approximate order of decreasing susceptibility: duckling, rabbit, turkey, chicken, neonatal rat, cat, pig, dog, trout, guinea pig, rhesus monkey, adult rat, cattle and sheep. However, the strain of animal and its nutritional status can have a profound effect on the response.

The clinical-pathologic features of aflatoxin poisoning have been most clearly demonstrated in experimentally-poisoned swine (Gumbmann and Williams, 1969; Cysewski et al., 1968; and Sisk, Carlton and Curtin, 1968). Biochemical changes are dependent upon hepatic injury and their time of occurrence is related to the dose administered. Doses adequate to produce death within seventy-two hours will result in detectable liver damage within three hours and several alterations in liver function within six hours. The serum levels of glutamic oxaloacetic transaminase (GOT), ornithine carbamyl transferase (OCT), alkaline phosphatase (APase) and isocitric dehydrogenase (IDH) are markedly elevated. These enzymes are concomitantly lost from the damaged liver. Expectedly, the serum levels of the following are reduced: albumin, albumin-globulin ratio, non-protein nitrogen (NPN), urea nitrogen (UN) and adenine nucleotides (AN). Leukocyte counts and prothrombin times are usually elevated within twenty-four hours of such lethal poisoning. Chromatographic demonstration of metabolites of aflatoxins in urine plus clinical-pathologic or histologic demonstration of liver damage are considered adequate for definitive diagnosis.

The principal **lesions** occur in the liver and may be classified as toxic hepatitis (p. 1223). Natural cases usually result from repeated ingestion of toxin and therefore the hepatic lesions are seen in various stages but it should be pointed out that lesions are not necessarily specific. Single, non-lethal or lethal doses have been given to many different animals under experimental conditions, revealing variation in response among different species (Newberne and Butler, 1969). One of the most constant responses to aflatoxin B_1 is proliferation of small bile ductules at the periphery of hepatic lobules. This appears in all species tested so far. Changes in hepatocytes (vacuolization, fatty change, loss of parenchyma, pyknosis) leading to necrosis are usually localized in one part of the hepatic lobule, depending on the species. These effects are **periportal** in ducklings, cats, adult rats, turkey, chickens and rhesus monkeys; **midzonal** in rabbits and **centrilobular** in the pig, dog, guinea pig and cattle. Diffuse necroses are seen in neonatal rats and trout with hemorrhage a conspicuous feature in the latter.

Edema of the gallbladder has been noted frequently in the dog and pig.

Nodular regeneration of hepatic lobules has been observed in the duckling, pig, trout, guinea pig, turkey, chicken and rhesus monkey. Fibrosis or cirrhosis has been reported in the duckling, pig, guinea pig, turkey, chicken, rhesus monkey and cow but occurrence of true cirrhosis is still under debate. Occlusive lesions in hepatic venules have also been reported in cattle.

The carcinogenic activity of aflatoxin is well established although the exact conditions under which neoplasia develops are not completely understood. Hepatic neoplasms, hepatomas and hepatic cell carcinomas, have been produced by feeding aflatoxin to: ducklings, guinea pigs, turkeys, chickens, trout, swine, neonate, young or adult rats and one sheep.

Aflatoxins

Buckly, S. S., and MacCallum, W. G.: Acute Haemorrhagic Encephalitis Prevalent Among Horses in Maryland. Amer. Vet. Rev. *25*:99–102, 1901.

Burnside, J. E., *et al.*: A Disease of Swine and Cattle Caused by Eating Mouldy Corn. II. Experimental Production with Pure Cultures of Mould. Amer. J. Vet. Res. *18*:817–824, 1957.

Butler, W. H., and Barnes, J. M.: Carcinoma of the Glandular Stomach in Rats Given Diets Containing Aflatoxin. Nature, Lond. *209*:90, 1966.

Carnaghan, R. B. A., *et al.*: Biochemical and Pathological Aspects of Groundnut Poisoning in Chickens. Path. Vet. *3*:601–615, 1966.

Cysewski, S. J., *et al.*: Clinical Pathologic Features of Acute Aflatoxicosis of Swine. Am. J. Vet. Res. *29*:1577–1590, 1968.

De Jongh, H., *et al.*: Investigation of the Factor in Groundnut Meal Responsible for "Turkey X Disease." Biochem. Biophys. Acta *65*:548–551, 1962.

Ellis, J., and DiPaolo, J. A.: Aflatoxin B₁ Induction of Malformations. Arch. Path. *83*:53–57, 1967.

Gagné, W. E., Dungworth, D. L., and Moulton, J. E.: Pathologic Effects of Aflatoxin in Pigs. Path. Vet. *5*:370–384, 1968.

Gumbmann, M. R., and Williams, S. N.: Biochemical Effects of Aflatoxin in Pigs. Toxic. Appl. Pharmacol. *15*:393–404, 1969.

Harding, J. D. J., *et al.*: Experimental Groundnut Poisoning in Pigs. Res. Vet. Sci. *4*:217–229, 1963.

Hodges, F. A., *et al.*: Mycotoxins: Aflatoxin Isolated from *Penicillium puberulum.* Science *145*:1439, 1964.

Kraybill, H. F.: The Toxicology and Epidemiology of Mycotoxins. Trop. Geogr. Med. *21*:1–18, 1969.

Legator, M. S.: Mutagenic Effects of Aflatoxin. J. Am. Vet. Med. Assn. *155*:2080–2083, 1969.

Madhavan, T. V., Tulpule, P. G., and Gopalan, C.: Aflatoxin-induced Hepatic Fibrosis in Rhesus Monkeys. Pathological Features. Arch. Path. *79*:466–469, 1965.

Newberne, J. W., Bailey, W. S., and Seibold, H. R.: Notes on a Recent Outbreak and Experimental Reproduction of Hepatitis X in Dogs. J. Am. Vet. Med. Assn. *27*:59–62, 1955.

Newberne, P. M., Carlton, W. W., and Wogan, G. N.: Hepatomas in Rats and Hepatorenal Injury in Ducklings Fed Peanut Meal or *Aspergillus flavus* Extract. Path. Vet. *1*:105–132, 1964.

Newberne, P. M., *et al.*: Histopathologic Lesions in Ducklings Caused by *Aspergillus flavus* Cultures, Culture Extracts and Crystalline Aflatoxins. Toxic. Appl. Pharmacol. *6*:542–556, 1964.

Newberne, P. M., Russo, R., and Wogan, G. N.: Acute Toxicity of Aflatoxin B₁ in the Dog. Path. Vet. *3*:331–340, 1966.

Newberne, P. M., Harrington, D. H., and Wogan, G. N.: Effects of Cirrhosis and Other Liver Insults on Induction of Liver Tumors by Aflatoxin in Rats. Lab. Invest. *15*:962–969, 1966.

Newberne, P. M., Rogers, A. E., and Wogan, G. N.: Hepatorenal Lesions in Rats Fed a Low Lipotrope Diet Exposed to Aflatoxin. J. Nutr. *94*:331–343, 1968.

Newberne, P. M., and Rogers, A. E.: Carcinoma, Thymidine Uptake, and Mitosis in the Liver of Rats Exposed to Aflatoxin. New Zeal. Med. J. *67*:8–17, 1968.

Newberne, P. M., and Wogan, G. N.: Sequential Morphologic Changes in Aflatoxin B₁ Carcinogenesis in the Rat. Cancer Res. *28*:770–781, 1968.

Newberne, P. M., and Butler, W. H.: Acute and Chronic Effects of Aflatoxin on the Liver of Domestic and Laboratory Animals: A Review. Cancer Res. *29*:236–250, 1969.

Rogers, A. E., and Newberne, P. M.: The Effects of Aflatoxin B₁ and Dimethylsulfoxide on Thymidine-3H Uptake and Mitosis in Rat Liver. Cancer Res. *27*:855–864, 1967.

Seibold, H. R., and Bailey, W. S.: An Epizootic of Hepatitis in the Dog. J. Amer. Vet. Med. Assn. *121*:201–206, 1952.

Sisk, D. B., Carlton, W. W., and Curtin, T. M.: Experimental Aflatoxicosis in Young Swine. Amer. J. Vet. Res. *29*:1591–1602, 1968.

SPORN, M. B., *et al.*: Aflatoxin B: Binding to DNA *In Vitro* and Alterations of RNA Metabolism *In Vivo*. Science *151*:1539–1542, 1966.

SVOBDA, D., GRADY, H. J., and HIGGINSON, J.: Aflatoxin B$_1$ Injury in Rat and Monkey Liver. Amer. J. Path. *49*:1023–1051, 1966.

TULPULE, P. G., MADHAVAN, T. V., and GOPALAN, C.: Effect of Feeding Aflatoxin to Young Monkeys. Lancet, May 2nd, 962–963, 1964.

WILSON, B. J., *et al.*: Relationship of Aflatoxin to Epizootics of Toxic Hepatitis Among Animals in Southern U. S. Am. J. Vet. Res. *28*:1217–1230, 1967.

WOGAN, G. N., and NEWBERNE, P. M.: Dose-response Characteristcis of Aflatoxin B$_1$ Carcinogenesis in the Rat. Cancer Res. *27*:2370–2376, 1967.

WRAGG, J. B., ROSS, V. C., and LEGATOR, M. S.: Effect of Aflatoxin B$_1$ on the Deoxyribonucleic Acid Polymerase of *Escherichia coli*. Proc. Soc. Exp. Biol. Med. *125*:1052–1055, 1967.

* * * * *

Group D: Poisons which are predominantly nephrotoxic.

Turpentine	Sulfonamides	Oxalates	Broomweed
Chloroform		Chinese Tallow Tree	

TURPENTINE

Turpentine is a local as well as a diffusible irritant. Skin is readily blistered within one or two hours after a single topical application. Ingested without adequate dilution, turpentine causes severe gastroenteritis, in addition to stomatitis and esophagitis. When it is inhaled, the result is bronchopneumonia. A considerable amount, however, is tolerated in the digestive tract if properly diluted. Fatalities, if they occur, result from the acute toxic tubular nephrosis (p. 1266) which develops within a few days. Most cases of poisoning result from attempts by stockmen to use the substance for therapeutic purposes. An unusual case of fatal nephritic poisoning came to the attention of one of us (Smith) when a dog walked upon a freshly painted floor and the owner used turpentine to wash the animal's feet. Giffee (1939) reports sudden fatal poisoning when turpentine was applied to castration wounds in little pigs. Symptoms of acute peritonitis appeared within minutes and death of several came within an hour or two.

Turpentine

GIFFEE, J. W.: Turpentine Poisoning in Pigs. J. Am. Vet. Med. Assn. *95*:509, 1939.

SULFONAMIDES

The usual toxic effects of the sulfonamide drugs, as seen in domestic animals, depend upon obstruction of renal tubules by precipitated crystals of the sulfonamide in question. With the unaided eye, masses of the yellowish crystals can often be seen in the renal papillae and pelvis, or even forming pale radial lines which mark distended medullary tubules. It is said that their amount is sometimes so great as to act as obstructive calculi in the ureter. Microscopically, the crystals in the papillae are seen to lie within the ducts of Bellini and collecting tubules, which they commonly obstruct and whose lining their sharp points mechanically irritate. Fatalities appear to be possible from these effects alone, but in some instances the obstructive changes may be accompanied by the formation of albuminous casts, suggesting a more subtle renal injury. This is accom-

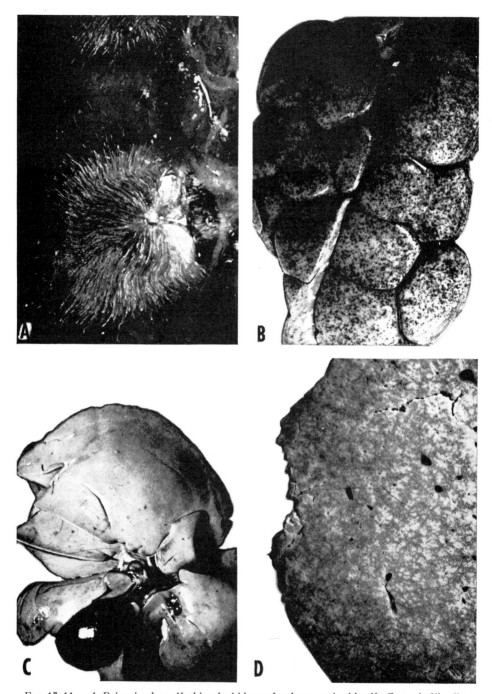

Fig. 17–11.—*A*, Poisoning by sulfathiazole, kidney of a three-week-old calf. Crystals fill collecting tubules. Case at Texas Sch. Vet. Med. *B*, Kidney of a Brahman heifer poisoned by eating oak buds. Case at Texas Sch. Vet. Med. *C*, Liver of a dog which survived three days after being poisoned by phosphorus. The liver was pale yellowish in color. Case at Iowa Sch. Vet. Med. *D*, Liver of a horse with toxic hepatitis, probably due to crotalaria poisoning.

panied by mild degenerative changes in the cells of the proximal convoluted tubules.

In humans, the kidneys often contain foci of necrosis in and around which there has been a heavy accumulation of reticulo-endothelial and other inflammatory cells so extensive as to amount to a granulomatous reaction. This is the so-called nephrotoxic reaction; it is considered to be an allergic process, supposedly depending on previous sensitization. The rarity or nonexistence of this phenomenon in animals might be thought to be attributable to the infrequency with which an animal patient has a first, and later a second, illness, both treated by sulfonamides. However, when one considers the alacrity and nonchalance with which stockmen administered sulfonamide drugs (until antibiotics replaced them) for illness of all sorts, such an explanation seems doubtful.

Other disorders which have been noted as a result of administration of sulfonamides include temporary nervous dysfunctions, such as blindness, failure of optical adaptation and accommodation, hyperesthesia, incoordination, ataxia and convulsions. These usually follow a single excessive dose of the drug. Demyelinization of nerves has also resulted, and serious or fatal results have attended the application of sulfonamide medications where they came into contact with central or peripheral nervous tissue.

The therapeutic administration of sulfonamides occasionally leads to detectable porphyrinuria in human patients. We do not find reports of accompanying photosensitization, but the situation might well be different in case a farm animal, normally exposed to much sunlight, were to suffer the provocative hepatic damage. Experimentally, in rats, sulfonamides administered to the pregnant mother have inhibited ossification of the bones of the fetus. In young chickens, as little as 0.06 per cent of sodium sulfaquinoxaline in the drinking water for four days has produced a hemorrhagic syndrome of serious import.

In spite of the several dangerous possibilities, however, the sulfonamides remain highly useful therapeutic agents. Crystallization in the renal tubules as the glomerular filtrate is concentrated into urine, the most likely catastrophe, is rendered improbable by promoting alkalinity in those species having an acid urine and even more by a copious intake of water.

Sulfonamides

BENESCH, R., CHANCE, M. R. A., and GLYNN, L. E.: Inhibition of Bone Calcification by Sulphonamides. Nature. London *155*:203–204, 1945.

DAVIES, S. F. M.: Sulphonamide Poisoning in Chickens Treated for Coccidiosis. Papers Presented to Tenth World's Poultry Congr., Edinburgh, 1954, pp. 275–278.

DELAPLANE, J. P., and MILLIFF, J. H.: Gross and Micropathology of Sulfaquinoxaline Poisoning in Chickens. Am. J. Vet. Research *9*:92–96, 1948.

FIGGE, H., CAREY, T. N., and WEILAND, G. S.: Porphyrin-excretion by a Patient Treated with Sulfadiazine and Later with Sulfanilamide. J. Lab. and Clin. Med. *31*:752–756, 1946.

FRENCH, A. J.: Hypersensitivity in the Pathogenesis of Histopathologic Changes Associated with Sulfonamide Chemotherapy. Am. J. Path. *22*:679–701, 1946.

JONES, L. M., SMITH, H. A., and ROEPKE, M. H.: Effects of Large Doses of Various Sulfonamides Injected in Dairy Cattle. Am. J. Vet. Research. *10*:318–326, 1949.

MOORE, R. H., McMILLAN, G. C., and DUFF, G. L.: Pathology of Sulfonamide Allergy in Man. Am. J. Path. *22*:703–735, 1946.

OXALATE-BEARING PLANTS AND ETHYLENE GLYCOL

This poison, usually in the form of oxalates, is important as a toxic constituent of certain plants which may be eaten by animals. Ordinary garden rhubarb

(*Rheum rhaponticum*) is one of these, but of more significance in causing losses of livestock are halogeton (*Halogeton glomeratus*) and greasewood (*Sarcobatus vermiculatus*), both of which grow in the Rocky Mountain region of the United States. In dry weather, halogeton has been known to contain oxalates, largely sodium and potassium oxalate, equivalent to 19 per cent of anhydrous oxalic acid. Soursob (*Oxalis cernua*), indigenous to South Australia, is another plant which owes its poisonous qualities to its content of oxalates, as is also the common sorrel, *Rumex acetosa*.

Another plant demonstrated by analysis (Marshall, Buck and Bell, 1967) to contain high levels of oxalate is *Amaranthus retroflexus*, pigweed, redroot or careless weed. The leaves of this plant may contain as much as 30 per cent of total oxalate on a dried weight basis. This plant is believed to be one of the causes of an entity called *perirenal edema disease* of swine. This syndrome has been observed (Buck, *et al.*, 1966) in swine given access to pastures bearing heavy growth of common pig lot weeds, such as *Amaranthus retroflexus* or the weed called lambs' quarters (*Chenopodium album*). Other weeds, such as black nightshade (*Solanum nigrum*), buffalo burr (*Solanum rostratum*) and Jimson weed (*Datura stramonium*) have also been suspected as causative.

The signs in this perirenal edema syndrome are trembling, weakness, incoordination, sternal recumbency and coma, followed by death. The characteristic post-mortem lesion is the presence of a large amount of edema surrounding the kidney between the renal capsule and the perirenal peritoneum. Sometimes this edema fluid is tinged with blood but the affected kidneys are usually pale and normal in size. Edema in the wall of the abdomen, around the rectum, and in the wall of the stomach may also be present. Clear, transparent or straw-colored fluid may distend the peritoneal and pleural cavities. The renal capsule is not usually affected although the edema may extend into the renal parenchyma. Microscopic evidence of toxic tubular nephrosis (p. 1266) with interstitial edema in the renal cortex has been described.

The lesions are not typical of oxalate poisoning, oxalate crystals are not readily identifiable in tissue sections, hence the exact mechanisms are not settled. The possibility of nitrate as a factor is still open because it is known that *D. retroflexus* may contain elevated levels of nitrate. Feeding of this plant appears to have produced this entity in swine (Bennett, 1964).

Oxalates are used routinely in hematology laboratories to prevent the clotting of blood samples, which they do by forming insoluble calcium oxalate and thereby removing the soluble calcium, which is essential to the clotting mechanism. This is presumably the same reaction which causes acute poisoning when oxalates are ingested in large amounts at one time. The signs of poisoning in sheep are observed two to four hours after the ingestion of toxic amounts of halogeton (Shupe and Jones, 1969). These signs consist of depression, anorexia, slight to moderate bloating, weakness, incoordination, restlessness, frequent attempts to urinate, occasional reddish-brown urine and brownish-black feces, blood-tinged nasal exudate, coma, followed by death.

Hypocalcemia has been demonstrated in sheep, the plasma level of calcium may be reduced from a normal mean of 9.3 to 5.1 mg. per 100 ml. of plasma. Blood urea nitrogen expectedly is increased due to reduced renal function.

Calcium oxalate is precipitated in the renal tubules during the process of elimination, and a fatal outcome may occur from renal insufficiency and uremia

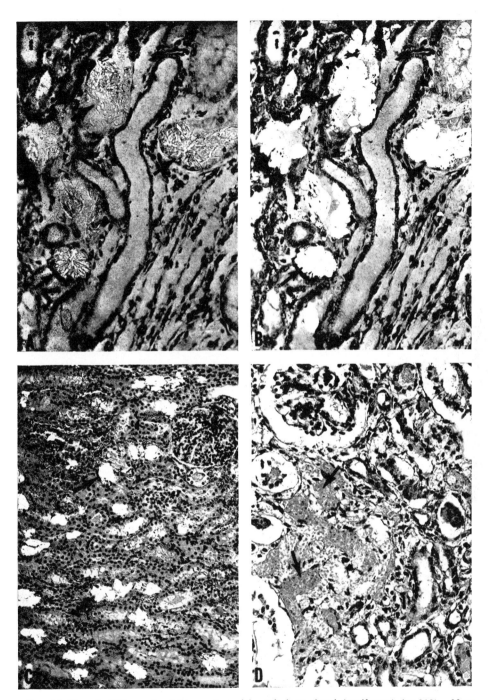

FIG. 17–12.—*A*, Kidney of a kitten poisoned by ethylene glycol (antifreeze) (× 210). Note oxalate crystals (arrows) in tubules. *B*, Same section as *A*, photographed under polarized light. Note brilliance of oxalate crystals (arrows). Courtesy of Dr. Wm. J. Hadlow. *C*, Kidney of a sheep poisoned by eating Halogeton plants (× 125). Note oxalate crystals (arrows), photographed under polarized light. Courtesy of Dr. Wayne C. Anderson. *D*, Kidney of a steer poisoned by eating buds of an oak tree (× 210). Necrosis (arrows) of certain convoluted tubules.

after the earlier symptoms have abated. Recovery, on the other hand, is possible, with blood urea levels slowly subsiding after about a month. Cystitis and urethritis may be a part of this syndrome. Post-mortem diagnosis can usually be made in these cases by the presence of numerous nearly transparent crystals in the renal tubules. Visible when the light is sharply reduced, these may be single, irregularly rhomboidal in shape and some 30 or 40 microns in length. Often, however, the crystals lie closely packed in a radial arrangement, the whole rosette-like structure more than filling the lumen of the tubule and occupying space at the expense of the epithelial cells (Fig. 17–12). The latter eventually become necrotic, although the extent of cellular damage depends upon whether death occurred early or late. There is also severe congestion of all parts of the kidney, moderate increase in cellularity of the glomeruli and marked albuminous precipitate in the tubules. Those epithelial cells not directly affected by the crystals show but little toxic injury.

The widespread hemorrhages and edema, particularly in the rumen of sheep poisoned by halogeton, found at post mortem, are associated with deposits of calcium oxalate in the walls of blood vessels. The presence of the oxalate at these sites appears to damage the blood vessel wall.

The poisonous effects of calcium oxalates are also produced in some species (man, dog, cat) by the ingestion of toxic amounts of **ethylene glycol.** This colorless, odorless, slightly viscous, dihydric alcohol has a sweetish taste and is widely used as a solvent in manufacturing (Kersting and Nielsen, 1965). Its common use as a nonvolatile antifreeze makes it available in many households and its taste appeals to some people, cats and dogs. Ethylene glycol is metabolized in the liver by **alcohol dehydrogenase** which results in the formation of oxalates. This enzyme is also necessary for the degradation of ethyl alcohol. The simultaneous administration of ethyl alcohol competes for this enzyme in the liver and decreases the formation of oxalate. This fact is utilized in the treatment of ethylene glycol poisoning (Wacker, *et al.*, 1965).

Experimental poisoning of dogs (Kersting and Nielsen, 1966) results in the rapid development of ataxia, polydipsia, depression, miosis, tachycardia, tachypnea, hyperpnea, bradycardia and coma. Convulsions and vomiting are infrequent. Death follows, in most cases, administration of doses of 6.6 ml./per kg. of body weight, or more.

The diagnosis is usually established, post mortem, by the demonstration of characteristic birefringent crystals in renal tubules and cerebral blood vessels (Fig. 17–12). Non-fatal doses do not appear to produce permanent damage to renal tubules.

Studies (Roberts and Seibold, 1969) of the toxicity of ethylene glycol administered to three species of Old World monkeys (*Macaca mulatta, M. fascicularis,* and *M. radiata*) reveal lesions similar to those described in other species. The toxic dose in these species is believed to be similar to that in man, 1.6 ml. per kg. of body weight.

Oxalates

BENNETT, P. C.: Edema Disease. In *Diseases of Swine*, H. W. Dunn, Ed., Ames, Iowa State University Press, 1964.
BENNETT, B. and ROSENBLUM, C.: Identification of Calcium Oxalate Crystals in Patients with Uremia. Lab. Investig. *10*:947–955, 1961.

BUCK, W. B., *et al.*: Perirenal Edema in Swine: A Disease Caused by Common Weeds. J. Am. Vet. Med. Assn. *148*:1525–1531, 1966.

DODSON, M. E.: Oxalate Ingestion Studies in the Sheep. Austr. Vet. J. *35*:225–233, 1959.

DUNN, J. S., HAWORTH, A., and JONES, N. A.: Urea Retention in Oxalate Nephritis. J. Path. and Bact. *27*:377–400, 1924.

DURRELL, L. W., JENSEN, R., and KLINGER, B.: Poisonous Plants in Colorado. Exp. Sta. Bull. 445 Colorado A. & M. College, Fort Collins.

HADLOW, W. J.: Acute Ethylene Glycol Poisoning in a Cat. J. Am. Vet. Med. Assn. *130*: 296–297, 1957.

JAMES, L. F.: Serum Electrolyte, Acidbase Balance, and Enzyme Changes in Acute *Halogeton glomeratus* Poisoning in Sheep. Can. J. Comp. Med. *32*:539–543, 1968.

JEGHERS, H., and MURPHY, R.: Practical Aspects of Oxalate Metabolism. New England J. Med. *233*:208–215, and 238–246, 1945.

JONSSON, L., and RUBARTH, S.: Ethylene Glycol Poisoning in Dogs and Cats. Nord. Vet. Med. *19*:265–276, 1967.

KERSTING, E. J., and NIELSEN, S. W.: Ethylene Glycol Poisoning in Small Animals. J. Am. Vet. Med. Assn. *146*:113–118, 1965.

————: Experimental Ethylene Glycol Poisoning in the Dog. Am. J. Vet. Res. *27*: 574–582, 1966.

MARSHALL, V. L., BUCK, W. B., and BELL, G. L.: Pigweed (*Amaranthus retroflexus*); an Oxalate-containing Plant. Am. J. Vet. Res. *28*:888–889, 1967.

MAYMONE, B. *et al.*: Oxalic Acid Metabolism in Ruminants on Prolonged Diet of *Oxalis cernua* Thunb. 8th Int. Congr. Anim. Prod. Hamburg *2*:54–55, 1961.

ROBERTS, J. A., and SEIBOLD, H. R.: Ethylene Glycol Toxicity in the Monkey. Toxicol. Appl. Pharmacol. *15*:624–631, 1969.

SHUPE, J. L., and JAMES, L. F.: Additional Physiopathologic Changes in *Halogeton glomeratus* (Oxalate) Poisoning in Sheep. Cornell Vet. *59*:41–55, 1969.

SMITH, W. S.: Soursob Poisoning in Sheep. J. Dept. Agric. S. Australia *54*:377–378, 1951.

THOMAS R. M., and PRIER, J. E.: An Experimental Case of Urinary Calculus in a Steer. J. Am. Vet. Med. Assn. *120*:85–86, 1952.

WACKER, W. E. C., *et al.*: Treatment of Ethylene Glycol Poisoning with Ethyl Alcohol. J.A.M.A. *194*:1231–1233, 1965.

WATTS, P. S.: Effects of Oxalic Ingestion by Sheep. I. Small Doses to Chaff-Fed Sheep. II. Large Doses to Sheep on Different Diets. J. Agric. Sci. *52*:244–255, 1959.

WILSON, B. J. and WILSON, C. H.: Oxalate Formation in Mouldy Feedstuffs as a Possible Factor in Livestock Toxic Disease. Am. J. Vet. Res. *22*:961–969, 1961.

BROOMWEED

The broomweeds (*Xanthocephalum*, or *Gutierrezia spp.*) are plants that grow on the arid ranges of the Western United States, are eaten by cattle and sheep under stress of necessity and are commonly but, judging by experimental results, not always poisonous. It is probable that the different degrees of toxicity may be related to variations in growing conditions, although they do not appear to depend upon the stage of maturity of the plant. The plant is a somewhat herbaceous perennial which makes a very bushy growth to a height of about 1 foot (30 cm.). It has very fine foliage, covered with a sticky exudate, and large numbers of tiny yellow flowers.

Signs appear after an animal has been eating appreciable amounts of the plant for at least a few days and begin with anorexia, listlessness, arched back and drooping head. There is a noticeable degree of icterus. Appropriate tests reveal a well-marked uremia and in severe acute cases, there is also hematuria. Abortion often occurs in pregnant sheep or cattle.

The lesions can be summarized as those of acute toxic tubular nephrosis (p. 1266) and a rather unusual form of toxic hepatitis. The proximal and distal convoluted tubules and the ascending loops of Henle suffer from hydropic degeneration and disintegration of the cytoplasm of their epithelial cells with ultimate necrosis if the animal lives long enough. In the more acute cases, there are hemorrhages into the Bowman's capsules and the tubules, as well as into the intertubular tissue, while in animals with a more prolonged course (one to two weeks), there is a considerable degree of lymphocytic infiltration. The hepatic changes consist successively of hydropic degeneration, an hydropic condition of the cytoplasm and finally necrosis, all being diffusely distributed without regard to any particular zone in the lobule. While there are many diseases characterized by toxic nephrosis and hepatitis, it would seem that the hemorrhages into the nephron and the hydropic degeneration of the liver cells would serve to distinguish broomweed poisoning from many of the nephrotoxic and hepatotoxic poisonings.

The toxic principle in broomweed appears to be saponin which produces the clinical signs, including abortion, when administered orally to pregnant rabbits, cows and goats (Dollahite, Shaver and Camp, 1962). This saponin isolated from broomweed has no estrogenic properties but stimulates contractions of isolated uterine muscle (Shaver, Camp and Dollahite, 1964) under laboratory conditions.

Broomweed

DOLLAHITE, J. W., and ANTHONY, W. V.: Poisoning of Cattle with *Guttierrezia microcephala*, a Perennial Broomweed. J. Am. Vet. Med. Assn. *130*:525–530, 1957.
DOLLAHITE, J. W., SHAVER, T., and CAMP, B. J.: Injected Saponins as Abortifacients. Am. J. Vet. Res. *23*:1261–1263, 1962.
MATHEWS, F. P.: Toxicity of Broomweed (*Gutierrezia microcephala*) for Sheep, Cattle and Goats. J. Am. Vet. Med. Assn. *88*:55–61, 1936.
SHAVER, T. N., CAMP, B. J., and DOLLAHITE, J. W.: The Chemistry of a Toxic Constituent of *Xanthocephalum* species. Ann. New York Acad. Sci. *111*:737–743, 1964.

CHLOROFORM

Chloroform toxicity serves to emphasize specific sexual dimorphisms and genetically determined sensitivity in certain inbred strains of laboratory mice. Experience has taught laboratory workers to avoid opening a bottle of chloroform in a room in which inbred mice are kept. Even a slight exposure to chloroform vapor will cause the death of male mice. The following inbred strains are particularly susceptible: CBA-p, DBA, C₃H,A, and HR. Immature males, adult females and castrated males are relatively insusceptible. Castrated males become sensitive after administration of testosterone.

Inhalation of chloroform vapor by these susceptible mice results in necrosis of liver cells, glomeruli and proximal convoluted tubules. Animals which survive sub-lethal doses may later be demonstrated to have many calcified deposits in glomeruli and tubules in the renal cortex (Dunn, 1965).

Chloroform

BENNET, R. A., and WHIGHAM, A.: Chloroform Sensitivity of Mice. Nature (Lond.) *204*: 1328, 1964.
CHRISTENSEN, L. R., *et al.*: Accidental Chloroform Poisoning of Balb/c AnNIer Mice. Zschr Versuchstierk *2*:135–140, 1963.
DERINGER, M. K., DUNN, T. B., and HESTON, W. E.: Results of Exposure of Strain C₃H Mice to Chloroform. Proc. Soc. Exp. Biol. Med. *83*:474–479, 1953.
DUNN, T. B.: Spontaneous Lesions of Mice. pp. 303–329 in *The Pathology of Laboratory Animals*. Ribelin, W. E. and McCoy, J. R., Eds., Springfield, Charles C Thomas, 1965.
ESCHENBRENNER, A. B., and MILLER, E.: Induction of Hepatomas in Mice by Repeated Oral Administration of Chloroform, with Observations on Sex Differences. J. Nat. Cancer Inst. *5*: 251–255, 1945.
————: Sex Difference in Kidney Morphology and Chloroform Necrosis. Science *102*: 302–303, 1945.

HEWITT, H. B.: Renal Necrosis in Mice After Accidental Exposure to Chloroform. Brit. J. Exp. Path. *37*:32–39, 1956.

JACOBSEN, L., ANDERSEN, E., and THORBORG, J. V.: Accidental Chloroform Nephrosis in Mice. Acta Path. Microbiol. Scand. *61*:503–513, 1964.

SHUBIK, P., and RITCHIE, A. C.: Sensitivity of Male dba Mice to the Toxicity of Chloroform as a Laboratory Hazard. Science *117*:285, 1953.

CHINESE TALLOW TREE

The Chinese tallow tree (*Sapium sebiferum, Croton sebiferum,* or *Stillingia sebifera*), originally imported from China, is grown in the United States as an ornamental plant. It is quite abundant along the Atlantic coast from South Carolina to Florida and along the Gulf Coast west to Texas and Oklahoma and is suspected to cause poisoning in cattle. Leaves and fruit from these trees have been shown experimentally to be toxic to cattle but less so for sheep and goats (Russell, Schwartz and Dollahite, 1969). Administration of material from this tree to cattle was followed by severe diarrhea, weakness and dehydration within twelve hours. Usual hematologic values (packed cell volume, hemoglobin) were not affected nor were total serum protein or serum glutamic oxaloacetic transaminase changes. Blood urea nitrogen and serum creatinine phosphokinase levels were elevated in some animals.

Gross lesions were found in the intestines which were thickened and irregularly hyperemic. The kidneys were slightly swollen and one liver had a yellow oily appearance. The principal lesion appeared to be toxic tubular nephrosis.

The Chinese tallow tree does appear to have a potential for poisoning cattle although differing conditions of growth may affect its toxic properties.

Chinese Tallow Tree

RUSSELL, L. H., SCHWARTZ, W. L., and DOLLAHITE, J. W.: Toxicity of Chinese Tallow Tree (*Sapium sebiferum*) for Ruminants. Am. J. Vet. Res. *30*:1233–1238, 1969.

*   *   *   *   *

GROUP E: **Poisons causing death through cardiac insufficiency, with consequent venous congestion, anoxia,** and the petechiae and other changes commonly attendant upon anoxic processes (p. 119). Many more poisons have this effect than appear in the group for the reason that, if the poison also had characteristics entitling it to a place in some other group, we felt that it would be more readily recognized in the latter position.

Selenium   Death camas   Aconite   Baileya multiradiata   Jimson weed

SELENIUM

The rare element selenium exists in appreciable concentrations in the soil of certain areas in the arid western part of North America and in similar situations in other parts of the world. All plants able to grow in such soils tend to incorporate the element into their tissues. This amounts to 20 or 30 parts per million in the case of most of the common cereal and forage plants, but certain uncultivated plants which thrive in selenium areas commonly harbor as much as 5000 to 15,000 parts per million. In the latter group are species of the genus *Astragalus*, including the common loco weed and milk vetch (*A. bisulcatus*) as well as the woody aster (*Aster parryi*) and saltbush (*Atriplex nuttallii*). (This is not to imply that loco poisoning, p. 944, is due to selenium.) Appreciable amounts of selenium in plants can be detected by a sulfurous odor when the plants are crushed in the hand.

Acute selenium poisoning occurs in herbivorous animals as the result of eating one or several meals of some of the strongly seleniferous weeds, such as those mentioned. Another source of acute poisoning is the administration of overdoses of selenium in the therapeutic or preventative treatment of animals suspected of being deficient in selenium (p. 1010). As little as 10 mg. of sodium selenite given orally to young lambs has resulted in fatalities (Morrow, 1968). Differences in susceptibility between species may be considerable and many other factors such as nature of the diet, chemical form of the selenium and rate of administration have been shown to modify the toxic effects (Muth and Binns, 1964). This form of poisoning is largely an acute congestive and enteric disease with gastrointestinal symptoms and collapse from respiratory and myocardial failure in a few hours or a day or two. Post-mortem lesions include hemorrhagic enteritis and proctitis, passive congestion of the lungs and abdominal viscera, early toxic changes in the liver and kidneys (acute toxic hepatitis, p. 1223, and toxic tubular nephrosis, p. 1266) and terminal anoxic hemorrhages in the epicardium and elsewhere. Mucosae of both the bladder and gallbladder, as well as that of the folds of the omasum are commonly inflamed, probably because the poisonous substance is eliminated through them.

Chronic selenium poisoning has been described under two rather distinct syndromes, "blind staggers" and "alkali disease."

A rather violent termination of slow, cumulative poisoning is picturesquely, though inaccurately, designated by the name, **blind staggers.** This is a reversion to the layman's terminology of a century ago when mad staggers meant violently painful spasmodic colic, blind staggers any of the toxic or infectious nervous disturbances characterized by a desire to press forward, and staggers, in general, suggested the antics of a horse in severe abdominal pain. This form of selenium poisoning has, however, been seen most commonly in cattle. Somewhat as in Van Es' "walking disease" of horses, which is simply toxic hepatitis caused by senecio poisoning (p. 875), the animal is impelled to seek relief from constant abdominal discomfort by continuous walking; as the condition worsens there is actual nervous impairment of vision, as well as of other functions and the animal tries to walk through obstacles which he would normally avoid. He frequently stands pressing his forehead against some solid object, possibly gaining some relief thereby. Great weakness and paralysis supervene, being most severe in the forelimbs, and dyspnea, cyanosis and death follow as the result of respiratory failure.

The form of chronic selenium poisoning known as **alkali disease** was at one time attributed to excessive ingestion of soil alkali (sodium carbonate, sulfate, etc.), which is commonly very plentiful in the same arid areas where selenium is concentrated. It is now known to result from consumption of mildly seleniferous plants over a period of weeks or months. It is characterized by falling of hair, especially of the mane and tail **(bob-tail disease)** and a related malnutrition of the hoofs. The latter develop deep encircling grooves parallel to the coronary band which are more pronounced than those of laminitis. In the more severe cases, the groove may become a painful crack which causes partial separation of the hoof. Occasionally, one or more hoofs become detached from the sensitive laminae and slough off. More often the distorted hoof remains attached and, with the amount of wear reduced by painful locomotion, the toe grows to an inordinate length which deforms it with an anterior concavity. This applies to the hoofs of either cattle or horses. Eroded joints also make walking difficult and the animal may die from inability to get food and water.

The **lesions** are basically similar in the two clinical syndromes of chronic selenium poisoning. Myocardial insufficiency accounts for chronic passive congestion of the lungs and splanchnic viscera, and is itself based upon focal necroses in the heart muscle and a reaction that has been described as sero-fibrinous and as spreading into the muscle from the endocardium. Lymphocytic infiltrations accompany these changes in advanced cases. Edema of the pericardial, thoracic and peritoneal cavities and of the brain and lymph nodes is doubtless traceable to a cardiac (p. 139) origin as well.

Petechiae and ecchymoses on the external and internal cardiac surfaces and in various other organs are apparently attributable to a direct toxic origin, as are the comparatively mild toxic changes in the liver (p. 1223) and kidneys (p. 1266). In the liver, these are described as hydropic degeneration and necrosis with eventual fibrous scarring.

In sheep, the hepatic damage may attain the status of acute yellow atrophy (p. 1222); in the slowly developing alkali disease of cattle, some livers become truly cirrhotic (p. 1225). In the kidney, there are cloudy swelling of the renal epithelium and hyaline changes and hyaline casts in the convoluted tubules.

The gastrointestinal mucosa suffers from rather mild inflammatory changes in the omasum and upper intestine which become less conspicuous in proportion to the duration of the illness. Apparently due to a depressant action on smooth muscle, there is nearly always impaction of a dilated rumen and even of the omasum. The accumulation of hemosiderin in the spleen in the most chronic (alkali disease) cases probably rests entirely upon the chronic passive congestion, although the possibility of an hemolytic action seems not to have been investigated.

The malnourished and deformed hoofs have been described. As a further cause of lameness, there are very commonly erosions of the articular surfaces of the long bones, especially of the distal end of the tibia and the proximal end of the metatarsus.

The fetus shares in the deposition of selenium and malformations are common (another example of non-genetic developmental anomalies). Eggs from selenium-fed hens show a constant and severe impairment of hatchability which is directly proportional to the amount of selenium ingested. Those chicks which do hatch have little vitality.

Selenium

GARDINER, M. R.: Chronic Selenium Toxicity Studies in Sheep. Aust. Vet. J. *42*:442–448, 1966.
GLENN, M. W., JENSEN, R., and GRINER, L. A.: Sodium Selenate Toxicosis: The Effects of Extended Oral Administration of Sodium Selenate on Mortality, Clinical Signs, Fertility and Early Embryonic Development in Sheep. Am. J. Vet. Res. *25*:1479–1485, 1964.
————: Sodium Selenate Toxicosis: Pathology and Pathogenesis of Sodium Selenate Toxicosis in Sheep. Am. J. Vet. Res. *25*:1486–1494, 1964.
GLENN, M. W., MARTIN, J. L., and CUMMINS, L. M.: Sodium Selenate Toxicosis: The Distribution of Selenium Within the Body After Prolonged Feeding of Toxic Quantitites of Sodium Selenate to Sheep. Am. J. Vet. Res .*25*:1495–1499, 1964.

JACOBSSON, S. O., and OKSANEN, H. E.:   The Placental Transmission of Selenium in Sheep. Acta vet. Scand. 7:66–76, 1966.

MORROW, D. A.:   Acute Selenite Toxicosis in Lambs.   J. Am. Vet. Med. Assn. *152*:1625–1629, 1968.

MUTH, O. H., and BINNS, W.:   Selenium Toxicity in Domestic Animals.   Ann. New York Acad. Sci. *111*:583–590, 1964.

NEETHLING, L. P., BROWN, J. M. M., and DE WET, P. J.:   The Toxicology and Metabolic Fate of Selenium in Sheep.   J. S. Afr. Vet. Med. Assn. *39*:25–33, 1968.

ROSENFELD, I., and BEATH, O. A.:   *Selenium: Geobotany, Biochemistry, Toxicity and Nutrition.*   New York, Academic Press, 1964.

DEATH CAMAS

Zygadenus gramineus, Z. nuttallii and other closely related species are known by the name of death camas or by the very descriptive synonym of wild onion. These are among the most poisonous of plants, toxic to all species but eaten most often by sheep. Symptoms usually do not appear for several hours after the plant is eaten. They consist of nausea and salivation, failing heart and respiration and great weakness and nervous depression. Terminal coma may be of several hours' duration. Post-mortem lesions are usually limited to the congestions of anoxic heart failure and to very early changes of acute toxic hepatitis (p. 1223) and tubular nephrosis (p. 1266), demonstrable microscopically.

Death Camas

MARSH, C. D., CLAWSON, A. B., and MARSH, H.:   Zygadenus, or Death Camas.   U.S. Dept. Agric. Bull. 125, 1915.

MORRIS, M. D.:   Nuttall Death Camas Poisoning in Horses.   Vet. Med. *39*:462, 1944.

NIEMAN, K. W.:   Death Camas Poisoning in Fowls.   J. Am. Vet. Med. Assn. *73*:627–631, 1928.

ACONITE

Aconitum columbianum, a flowering and ornamental plant known either as monkshood or aconite, is similar to, and often confused with, larkspur. Animals are occasionally poisoned by it either on the ranges or through contact with garden plants. Therapeutically, the drug is used to slow the heart. In poisonous doses, it not only slows, but weakens the cardiac action. Symptoms are those of restlessness and anxiety, nausea, salivation, abdominal pain, increasing weakness and prostration, a weakening and terminally rapid heart and final asphyxia. Of special diagnostic significance are continual swallowing movements, due to a peculiar irritation of the throat, and a pronounced risus sardonicus, the lips being maximally retracted and displaying the foam-covered teeth as the horse or other animal lies helpless on the ground. Cats and rabbits jump vertically into the air, topple over backwards and go into convulsions. Death is seldom delayed more than an hour or two, so that few lesions can be expected beyond the hemorrhages and congestions incident to asphyxia.

BAILEYA MULTIRADIATA

This is a plant of the arid Southwest, from Texas to California, which sheep eat reluctantly with poisonous results. Its many slender stalks reach a height of 50 or 60 cm., bear elongated, tongue-shaped leaves on their lower parts, and terminate, each, in a single yellow flower-head at the top.

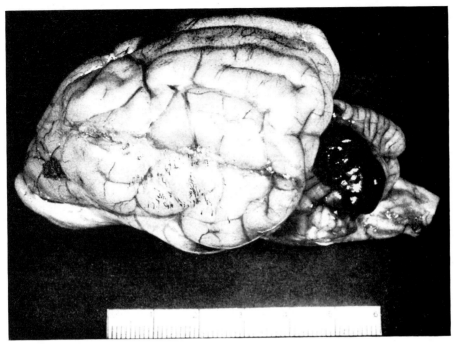

Fig. 17–13.—Hemorrhage in the leptomeninges due to Warfarin (dicoumarin) poisoning in a fifteen-year-old male mongrel collie. (Courtesy of Angell Memorial Animal Hospital.)

Signs include the usual arched back, loss of weight and disinclination to move. Excessive salivation appears early. If the animal is forced to exercise, cardiac embarrassment, which is the fundamental disturbance, is revealed by a rapid, pounding heart action audible at a distance of several feet.

The lesions are those of congestive heart failure, including venous congestion of the liver, spleen, kidneys and other abdominal viscera. Zenker's necrosis and preliminary degenerative changes proceed in the myocardium, commonly involving muscle cells individually here and there. Pursuant to the congestive and anoxemic state, the parenchymatous cells of the liver and renal cortical tubules undergo hydropic degeneration and fatty change. If the illness continues for several days, acute dilatation of the damaged ventricles develops. On the other hand, if the cardiac failure brings a more sudden anoxic death, widespread hemorrhages over the epicardium, diaphragm and other areas result, as is usual in terminal anoxia.

A considerable proportion of animals slowly recover after several days during which all food is refused.

Baileya

Mathews, F. P.: Toxicity of *Baileya multiradiata* for Sheep and Goats. J. Am. Vet. Med. Assn. *83*:673–679, 1933.

JIMSON WEED, THORNAPPLE

Datura stromonium and a few other closely related species are known by the names given in the title or as mad apple, stinkweed, stinkwort, Jamestown lily and some other names and are of world-wide distribution. While ordinarily unpalatable, the plant, if eaten, has a very considerable toxicity, which is due to the powerful alkaloids, atropine and hyoscyamine. The domesticated herbivora, birds and humans are sometimes poisoned.

Signs are chiefly nervous, with excitement which may deepen into insane delirium somewhat suggestive of rabies, and which is usually followed by inco-ordination, coma and death. Dilated pupils are of considerable diagnostic significance. Inhibition of salivary and related secretions leads to extreme thirst with consequent polyuria. The heart-beat, no longer restrained by the paralyzed vagus, becomes rapid and weak and death is from anoxia. Symptoms commence within minutes or after only a few hours. Recovery, if it occurs, requires several days. Lesions include marked congestion and edema of the lungs, hydrothorax, congestion of the meninges and dilation of the ventricles. Hemorrhages characteristic of asphyxia occur, as well as petechiae in the brain and the stomach and upper intestine. Recognizable fragments of the large leaves or of the "thorn-apples" may be found in the stomach or forestomachs.

Jimson Weed

BEHRENS, H. and HORN, M.: Tolerance of Pigs to Datura Stramonium Seeds (TT). Prakt Tierarzt. No. 2:43–44, 1962.
KING, E. D., JR.: Jimson Weed Poisoning. J. Am. Vet. Med. Assn. *64*:98–99, 1923.

* * * * *

Group F: **Poisons causing extensive hemorrhages.**

| Dicoumarin | Bracken fern | Crotalaria | Trichloroethylene-extracted soybean meal |

DICOUMARIN

Sweet clover hay (not pasturage) contains a substance called coumarin which not infrequently undergoes change into a related compound, dicoumarin, coumarin, or Dicumarol. This substance is such a potent anticoagulant for the blood that it has been adopted as a drug for use when reduced coagulability of the blood is desired and has been utilized as a rat-poison in the commercial product called Warfarin. The anticoagulant action depends on disruption of the action of prothrombin in a manner not completely understood. Vitamin-K inhibits the anticoagulant effect but apparently is not a complete antidote for the poisoning (Collentine and Quick, 1951). Horses are not affected by this hay. Rabbits are very susceptible and may be used to test the safety of a given supply of hay since they die from hemorrhages in a much shorter time than cattle (six to twelve days). Warfarin is poisonous to dogs and doubtless to all species.

Historically, the development of dicoumarin as an important anticoagulant drug started with the studies of Schofield (1924), on a new disease of cattle. This disease was described by Schofield to be manifest by large hemorrhages which occurred in animals recently fed on hay made from sweet clover. Schofield aptly named the disease sweet clover poisoning and correctly ascribed the signs and lesions to the anticoagulant effect of something in the sweet clover. Roderick (1931) demonstrated that this substance was water-soluble and easily extracted from sweet clover hay. Campbell and Link (1941) eventually isolated, crystallized and identified the active ingredient as dicoumarin.

Signs arise after cattle have consumed the poisonous hay for about a month, and consist of uncontrollable hemorrhage from accidental or operative wounds and slow internal hemorrhages as the result of bruises and minor injuries. Post-mortem lesions take the form of "hematomas" in the subcutis, between the muscles or beneath the capsules of organs. Ecchymotic hemorrhages occur in many places, commonly beneath the endocardium. The liver lobule is likely to contain petechiae and may show lipidosis or hydropic degeneration. Necrosis and hyaline-droplet degeneration involve the renal tubules; scattered small foci of necrosis may be found in the heart.

Newborn calves may be affected, because dicoumarin crosses the placenta, even though their dams do not manifest clinical signs at the time of parturition. This apparently results from a transient hypoprothrombinemia in calves which is intensified by the transplacental passage of dicoumarin. Cows which produce such calves may be shown to be feeding on sweet clover hay and the clotting time of their blood is prolonged.

Dicoumarin

BROMAN, U.: The Post-mortem Findings in Dicoumarol Poisoning in Dogs and Cats. Nord. Vet. Med. *13*:604–611, 1961.
CAMPBELL, H. A., *et al.*: Studies on the Hemorrhagic Sweet Clover Disease. I. The Preparation of Hemorrhagic Concentrates. J. Biol. Chem. *136*:47–55, 1940.
CAMPBELL, H. A., and LINK, K. P.: Studies on the Hemorrhagic Sweet Clover Disease. IV. The Isolation and Crystallization of the Hemorrhagic Agent. J. Biol. Chem. *138*:21–33, 1941.
CAMPBELL, H. A., *et al.*: Studies on the Hemorrhagic Sweet Clover Disease. II. The Bioassay of Hemorrhagic Concentrates by Following the Prothrombin Level in the Plasma of Rabbit Blood. J. Biol. Chem. *138*:1–20, 1941.
CLARK, W. T. and HALLIWELL, R. E. W.: The Treatment with Vitamin K Preparations of Warfarin Poisoning in Dogs. Vet. Rec. *75*:1210–1213, 1963.
COLLENTINE, G. E. and QUICK, A. J.: The Interrelationship of Vitamin K and Dicoumarin. Am. J. Med. Sci. *222*:7–12, 1951.
FRASER, C. M. and NELSON, J.: Sweet Clover Poisoning in Newborn Calves. J. Am. Vet. Med. Assn. *135*:283–286, 1959.
PRIER, R. F. and DERSE, P. H.: Evaluation of the Hazard of Secondary Poisoning by Warfarin-Poisoned Rodents. J. Am. Vet. Med. Assn. *140*:351–354, 1962.
RODERICK, L. M.: Sweet Clover Disease. J. Am. Vet. Med. Assn. *74*:314–324, 1929.
STAHMANN, M. A., HUEBNER, C. F., and LINK, K. P.: Studies on the Sweet Clover Disease. V. Identification and Synthesis of the Hemorrhagic Agent. J. Biol. Chem. *138*:513–527, 1941.
SCHOFIELD, F. W.: Damaged Sweet Clover: The Cause of a New Disease in Cattle Simulating Hemorrhagic Septicemia and Blackleg. J. Am. Vet. Med. Assn. *64*:553–575, 1924.
WIGNELL, W. N.: Dicoumarol Poisoning of Cattle and Sheep in South Australia. Austr. Vet. J. *37*:456–459, 1961.

BRACKEN FERN

This common fern, *Pteris aquilina* (*Adlerfarn*, German), grows in most humid parts of the world. Poisoning of cattle has been reported from the Eastern and far Northwestern United States, Central Europe, Great Britain, Central and South America, the Middle East, Southern India, Java and the Philippines. Illness appears after the plant has been consumed in quantity for several months. Under experimental conditions as long as fifteen months may be required. An acute, usually terminal episode may occur weeks after removal from access to the plant. Some reports indicate that hematuria may precede the acute attack but this might escape observation. The illness may start suddenly with high fever, hemorrhages from any and often several body openings, delayed clotting time, thrombocytopenia, neutropenia, anemia and death in one to three days. Diarrhea or upper respiratory inflammation may be noted.

Experimental evidence now available (Rosenberger, 1960) supports the idea that **bovine enzootic hematuria** (p. 1298) is a part of the syndrome resulting from poisoning by bracken fern. Although the active principle is not yet clearly established, prolonged feeding of bracken fern to cattle is followed by lesions in the bladder and the generalized hemorrhagic syndrome.

Autopsy lesions include widespread petechiae and ecchymoses, especially on the heart and other serous surfaces, on mucous membranes and in muscles and the subscutaneous tissues. Abomasal ecchymoses in cattle may lead to ulceration. The large bowel often contains clotted blood. Necrotic areas in the liver have been described by some. Thrombocytopenia is marked and is the cause of the hemorrhages. Neutropenia and terminal anemia accompany the thrombocytopenia and are due to destruction of the early myeloid cells. Megakaryocytes disappear.

The lesions in the urinary system most often involve the bladder, but may also occur in the ureters or renal pelvis, and appear to represent a chronic but violently hyperplastic and hemorrhagic inflammation which leads to frank neoplasia. The transitional epithelium undergoes localized proliferation with metaplasia to mucinous columnar or stratified squamous types or a mixture of the two (Fig. 17–14). In many cases, the hyperplastic epithelium acquires neoplastic properties, developing into a squamous cell or adenocarcinoma which is locally invasive and may metastasize to the regional lymph nodes and lungs. The capillaries of the inflammatory lesion also participate in the hyperplasia, sometimes to the extent of forming hemangiomas in the stroma or projecting from the mucosal surface. These hemangiomas may be the source of much of the hemorrhage into the urine and are capable of developing malignant qualities.

Additional evidence of the carcinogenic properties of bracken fern arises from feeding it to rats which subsequently develop adenocarcinomas in the small intestine (Evans and Mason, 1965).

In differential diagnosis, it is to be noted that in sweet clover poisoning the hemorrhages are very large with hematomas often forming in the tissues, and there is no fever. Blood transfusions are promptly curative in sweet clover poisoning. In crotalaria poisoning, the hemorrhages may show no differential features, but the liver usually shows considerable fibrosis, the gallbladder is distended, and there is often edema of the abomasal and duodenal tissues. In poisoning by trichloroethylene-extracted soybean meal, hemorrhages and anemia are the principal lesions, and differentiation may depend on the history. Anaplasmosis has to be considered but can usually be distinguished by the large spleen and by finding the causative organism in the erythrocytes. Leptospirosis causes fever and hemorrhages, but the latter are much less extensive. Icterus should be present with both these infections. Demonstration of a high serological titer or of the leptospirae in the kidney or liver by silver techniques is decisive. In none of the above conditions except at one stage of leptospirosis is there a neutropenia comparable to that of bracken poisoning.

In horses and in experimental rats, the usual bracken poisoning is cured by administration of thiamine (Cordy, 1952), but this is not so in cattle. Thiaminase appears to be one of the active toxic principles. Presumably cattle synthesize adequate thiamine and other B-vitamins, and develop illness only when more

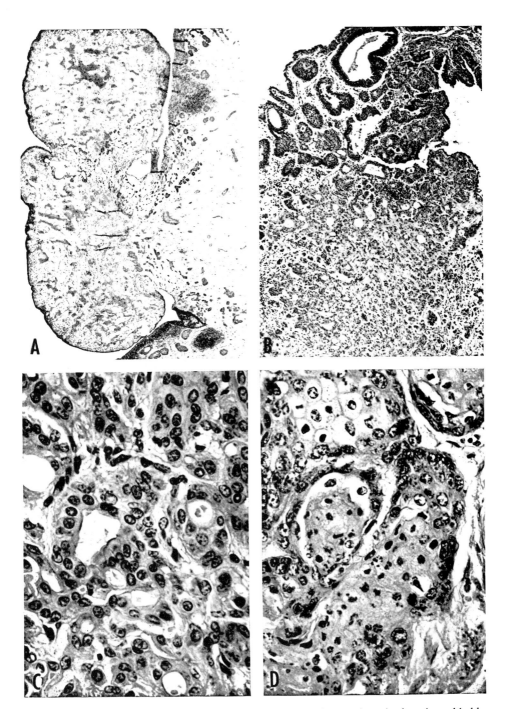

F<small>IG</small>. 17–14.—Bovine enzootic hematuria. *A*, Papillomatous hemangioma in the urinary bladder (× 24). *B*, Neoplastic transformation in the urinary bladder (× 50) with transitional cell carcinoma and adenocarcinoma in juxtaposition. *C*, Adenocarcinoma (× 350), higher magnification of *B*. *D*, Squamous cell carcinoma (× 350) in bovine urinary bladder. (*A*, *C* and *D* courtesy of Armed Forces Institute of Pathology.) Contributor: Dr. Sati Baran.

fundamental and irreversible toxic changes have taken place. Beyond this, no satisfactory treatment is known, although a few bovine patients recover. Bracken poisoning has been identified in sheep in Great Britain by Parker and McCrea (1965). The disease is infrequently recognized in sheep, presumably due to their reluctance to eat the plant and the long period before toxicity is manifest. Otherwise the disease appears to be similar to acute bracken poisoning in cattle.

Bracken Fern

BERAN, G. W.: Bovine Cystic Hematuria in the Philippines: A Report on an Enzootic Area. J. Am. Vet. Med. Assn. *149*:1686–1690, 1966.

BRYAN, G. T., BROWN, R. R., and PRICE, J. M.: Studies on the Etiology of Bovine Bladder Cancer. Ann. New York Acad. Sci. *108*:924–937, 1963.

CORDY, D. R.: The Pathology of Experimental Bracken Poisoning in Rats. Cornell Vet. *42*:108–117, 1952.

DÖBEREINER, J., *et al.*: Metabolites in Urine of Cattle with Experimental Bladder Lesions and Fed Bracken Fern. Pesquisa agropec. bras. *1*:189–199, 1966. V.B. *38*:1133, 1968.

DZUVIC, A.: Bovine Chronic Haematuria: Histopathology of the Bladder in Spontaneous and Experimental Cases. Deutsch. tierarztl. Wschr. *76*:260–263, 1969. V.B. *39*:4763, 1969.

EVANS, I. A., and MASON, J.: Carcinogenic Activity of Bracken. Nature *208*:913–914, 1965.

EVANS, I. A., *et al.*: Studies on Bracken Poisoning in Cattle. Part V. Brit. Vet. J. *114*:253–267, 1958.

GEORGIEV, R., and ANTONOV, S.: Aetiology of Chronic Bovine Haematuria. II. The Presence of Carcinogenic Metabolites in the Urine of a Healthy Cow Fed on Hay from a Haematuria Region. Vet. Med. Nauki. Sofia *1*:29–32, 1964. V.B. *35*:293, 1965.

GEORGIEV, R., *et al.*: Aetiology of Bovine Chronic Hematuria. I. Its Cancerous Nature. Vet. Med. Nauki, Sofia *1*:21–35, 1964. V.B. *35*:292, 1965.

GORISEK, J., and MARZAN, B.: Changes in Blood Picture and Blood Coagulation in Calves with Bracken Poisoning. Wien. tierarztl. Mschr. *52*:530–538, 1965. V.B. *36*:744, 1966.

GUILHON, J., *et al.*: Étude histologique des lésions du syndrome hémorrhagique des bovidés bretons. Bull. acad. vét française *23*:181–184, 1950.

HAGAN, W. A.: Bracken Poisoning of Cattle. Cornell Vet. *15*:326–332, 1925.

HOWELL, R. M., and EVANS, L. S.: Chromatographic Characteristics of Fibrinogen and Seromucoid in Bovine Bracken Poisoning. J. Comp. Path. *77*:117–128, 1967.

NANDI, S. N.: Histopathology of Enzootic Bovine Haematuria in the Darjeeling District of India. Br. Vet. J. *125*:587–590, 1969.

PAMUKCU, A. M., OLSON, C., and GOKSOY, S. K.: Influence of a Papilloma Vaccine on Chronic Bovine Enzootic Haematuria. Cancer Res. *27*:2197–2200, 1967.

PARKER, W. H., and McCREA, C. T.: Bracken (*Pteris aquilina*) Poisoning of Sheep in the North York Moors. Vet. Rec. *77*:861–866, 1965.

PARODI, A.: Lesions in Idiopathic Haematuria of Cattle. Revue Path. Comp. *66*:589–591, 1966. V.B. *37*:4867, 1967.

ROSENBERGER, G.: Uber die Ursache der Haematuria Vesicalis Bovis. Proc. 17th World Vet. Congr. Hanover, *2*:1167–1170, 1963.

ROSENBERGER, G.: Prolonged Feeding of Bracken (*Pteris aquilina*), as Cause of Bovine Chronic Haematuria. Wien. tierarztl. Mschr. *52*:415–421, 1965. V.B. *36*:743, 1966.

ROSENBERGER, G., and HEESCHEN, W.: Adlerfarn (*Pteris aquilina*)—die ursache des sog. Stallrotes der Rinder (*Haematuria vesicalis bovis chronica.*) Deutsch. Tierarztl. Wschr. *67*:201–208, 1960.

ROSENBERGER, G.: Prolonged Feeding of Bracken (*Pteris aquilina*) as Cause of Bovine Chronic Haematuria. Wien. tierarztl. Wschr. *52*:415–421, 1965. V. B. *36*:743, 1966.

SIPPEL, W. L.: Bracken Fern Poisoning. J. Am. Vet. Med. Assn. *121*:9–13, 1952.

STAMATOVIC, S., BRATANOVIC, U., and SOFRENOVIC, D.: The Clinical Picture of Haematuria in Cattle, Experimentally Produced by Feeding of Bracken (*Pteris aquilina*). Wien. tierarztl. Mschr. *52*:589–596, 1965. V.B. *36*:321, 1966.

CROTALARIA

The *Crotalaria* genus includes several leguminous plants which are used as soil-building cover crops or, in some cases, to provide hay or forage of rather questionable value. Some species are weeds in other parts of the world, particularly

South Africa and Australia. *Crotalaria spectabilis* is probably the most poisonous species. With certain other, less toxic species, it is grown rather extensively in the Southeastern United States. All species of farm animals are susceptible, including chickens and turkeys.

In general, there are acute and chronic forms. In the former the period of illness is at most a few days, although the poison has usually been accumulating as the result of repeated ingestion over weeks or months. Symptoms are those of gastrointestinal disturbance accompanied by salivation, weakness and relatively non-violent nervous malfunction, such as staggering, incoordination and ultimate inability to stand. Diarrhea with severe tenesmus and partial eversion of the rectum have been prominent in bovines. In the more chronic cases, the illness persists for a few weeks or several months, with anorexia, inactivity and terminal emaciation. In horses, there may be pressing against solid objects, the so-called "blind staggers" (p. 1241). Icterus is noticeable in chronic cases, especially. Emphysema, pulmonary and later subcutaneous, is characteristic.

In North America, the outstanding post-mortem lesion is hemorrhage which appears in the form of petechiae or large ecchymoses. These hemorrhages, characterized by as yet unexplained bright red color, involve serous and mucous surfaces. All organs are congested, many are edematous, especially the abomasum, omasum and gallbladder. The severely congested liver in the acute case may progress to cirrhosis if the poisoning is prolonged. In the lungs, emphysema alternates with atelectasis and hemorrhages. Liver injury, as described in other countries, does appear in cases with prolonged course.

In South Africa, *Crotalaria dura* and *C. globifera*, both known as wild lucerne, cause chronic poisoning having many of the features outlined above but also affect horses and sheep, with repeated febrile episodes of pulmonary disease and eventually fatal termination. Early in the course of the disease, pulmonary

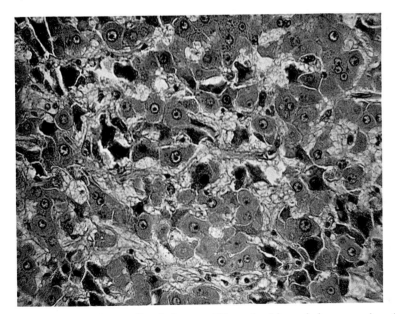

FIG. 17–15.—Poisoning due to *Crotalaria spectabilis* seed. Liver of rhesus monkey (*Macaca mulatta*). Variation in cell size, staining of nuclei and distortion of nuclei. (Courtesy of Dr. J. R. Allen and American Journal of Veterinary Research.)

emphysema, alveolar and interstitial, is the salient feature. Spreading from the lungs via the hilus, air appears in the mediastinal tissues and ultimately in the subcutaneous tissues of the neck. Terminally, the lungs undergo a chronic proliferative process involving all parts. The proliferated cells are largely epithelioid, probably originating from the alveolar walls. There are also gland-like proliferations of the bronchial epithelium resembling the "jaagsiekte" discussed on page 1113 and, indeed, sometimes called by that name.

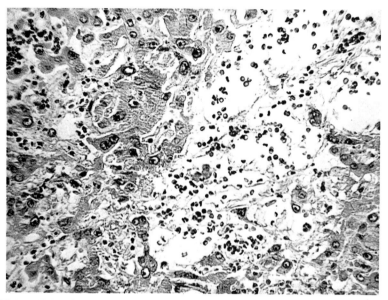

FIG. 17–16.—Poisoning due to *Crotalaria spectabilis* seed. Liver of *Macaca mulatta*. Focal necrosis with loss of hepatocytes. (Courtesy of Dr. J. R. Allen and American Journal of Veterinary Research.)

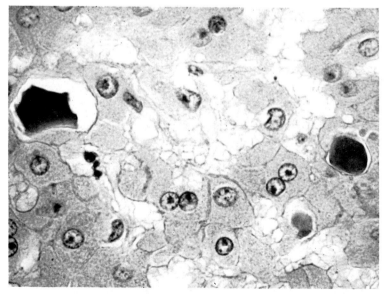

FIG. 17–17.—Poisoning due to *Crotalaria spectabilis*. Liver of *Macaca mulatta*. Vacuoles in hepatocytes and bile stasis. (Courtesy of Dr. J. R. Allen and American Journal of Veterinary Research.)

and Apt, 1949). While symptoms include anorexia and nausea, the principal effect is the destruction within a few days of a majority of the erythrocytes with hemoglobinuria and hemolytic jaundice. The liver and kidneys develop toxic degenerative changes. The contrast with the pathological effects of the *chlorinated* naphthalenes is interesting.

Naphthalene

ABELSON, S. M., and HENDERSON, A. T.: Moth Ball Poisoning. U.S. Armed Forces Med. J. *2*:491–493, 1951.

ZUELZER, W. W., and APT, L.: Acute Hemolytic Anemia Due to Naphthalene Poisoning. J. Am. Med. Assn. *141*:185–190, 1949.

ONIONS

In onion-growing districts, it is not unusual for cattle and sheep to be given cull or unsalable onions (*Allium cepa*) as a major part of their diet. Even when somewhat decomposed, onions appear to be palatable and commonly harmless. Nevertheless, poisoning, often fatal, does occur unexpectedly in these animals and in horses, and in dogs experimentally.

Both symptoms and lesions can be summarized as hemolytic anemia, hemolytic icterus and hemoglobinuria. The symptoms may arise with a few days of the onion diet; the anemia, as estimated by hemoglobin determinations, may be extreme, but clinical recovery occurs in a very few days if the animal, not yet moribund, is given a change in diet. The breath, urine and tissues have a strong odor of onions, making diagnosis easy. Wild onions, of which there are several species, have the same propensities, but animals are not likely to get sufficient quantities to do more than flavor the milk, in the case of dairy cows. Experimental feeding of one species of wild onion (*Allium validum*) to pregnant ewes resulted in loss of appetite and weight plus depression of erythropoietic tissues but no effect on fetal development (James and Binns, 1966).

Onions

GOLDSMITH, W. W.: Onion Poisoning in Cattle. J. Comp. Path. and Therap. *22*:151, 1909.

JAMES, L. F., and BINNS, W.: Effect of Feeding Wild Onions (*Allium validum*) to Bred Ewes. J. Am. Vet. Med. Assn. *149*:512–514, 1966.

KOGER, L. M.: Onion Poisoning in Cattle. J. Am. Vet. Med. Assn. *129*:75, 1956.

SEBRELL, W. H.: Anemia of Dogs Produced by Feeding Onions. Pub. Health Rep. *45*:1175–1191, 1930.

THORP, F., JR., and HARSHFIELD, G. S.: Onion Poisoning in Horses. J. Am. Vet. Med. Assn. *94*:52–53, 1939.

* * * * *

Group H: **Poisons causing production of methemoglobin and chocolate-colored blood.**

| Nitrates | Nitrites | Chlorates |

NITRATES AND NITRITES

Humans, as well as animals, have been poisoned by drinking or ingesting with the food, water containing nitrates in solution. Such water always comes from shallow, surface wells (or possibly from ponds or pools). Waters causing poisoning usually have contained between 1000 and 3000 parts per million of nitrate; however, since the presence of nitrates indicates organic pollution, water containing any amount of nitrate is undesirable even if within the limits of chemical safety. Another possible source of poisoning is the swallowing of lubricating oil to which nitrites have been added by the manufacturer. This has happened in a human being. Herbivorous animals will also lick or eat commercial fertilizers left in their way and are poisoned by the nitrates contained therein. Sheep are especially prone to eat such salty-tasting compounds, even when adequately supplied with sodium chloride. "Salting the range" was the spreading of saltpetre (potassium nitrate) in places where sheep would eat it, a practice which our pioneer cattlemen are said to have used in an effort to drive sheep-raisers and their flocks from an area of free range in the public domain of the then unsettled western United States.

But the usual source of nitrate and nitrite poisoning in veterinary practice is in plants, growing or cured, which have derived a large amount of nitrate, chiefly KNO_3, from a soil excessively rich in that substance. Among the plants which have been found at one time or another to contain poisonous amounts of nitrates are oats, either green, as hay, straw or stubble, barley, wheat, millets, flax, cornstalks (maize), sorghums, sugarbeet leaves, and a number of weeds, including pigweed (*Amaranthus retroflexus*) and variegated (or "bull") thistle (*Silybum marianum*). The application of weed killers such as "2, 4-D," 2, 4-dichlorophenoxyacetic acid, sometimes causes a marked increase in the nitrate content of some plants, such as sugar-beets, the leaves of which after harvesting are a standard feed for ruminants. The sorghums are, of course, noted for the development of hydrocyanic acid (p. 921) but occasionally appear to have been poisonous through an excessive content of nitrate. To what extent the rather frequent "corn-stalk poisoning" has been poisoning by nitrates is a difficult question, but evidence indicates that some of the outbreaks may be explainable on this basis.

Nitrates are irritants to the kidneys and urinary tract; potassium nitrate was at one time used as a diuretic. Poisoning by ingestion of excessive amounts of this chemical results in severe hemolytic anemia (p. 126) despite active hematopoiesis, as well as toxic injury to the renal parenchyma (Whitehead, 1953). There is localized gastroenteritis and, probably because of sensations originating in the gastrointestinal disorder, dogs show mental disturbances and depression. Decomposition of the nitrate into the nitrite is insignificant and consequently methemoglobinemia is minimal or absent.

Quite the opposite is true of the nitrates contained in the tissues of plants. In the presence of moisture and possibly with the aid of bacteria, the phytogenous nitrates are rather easily reduced to nitrites (and eventually to ammonia). This occurs either in the stomach, and especially the rumen, or externally, as in stacks of hay that have become wet from rain or snow. In the experiments of Riggs (1945), the process (in oat hay) reaches a maximum in twenty hours after the application of moisture. Poisoning from excessive nitrates in the various plants, hay and straw, then, is poisoning by nitrites, the principal effect of which is the formation of methemoglobin (p. 69), sometimes from more than half of the total hemoglobin. The process involves transformation of the Fe atom from the ferrous to the ferric state, and hemoglobin so deranged has no oxygen-carrying capacity. Nitrites also markedly dilate the arterioles, thereby lowering blood pressure and accelerating the pulse.

The lethality of ingested nitrates is influenced by the manner and rate of administration. The LD_{50} for nitrate fed to cattle with forage is about 45 grams per 100 pounds of body weight. About a third of this amount would produce lethality when administered in a drench (Crawford, *et al.*, 1966).

Signs of nitrite poisoning which have attracted most attention include cyanosis, dyspnea, extremely rapid pulse (150 per minute), great weakness and recumbency, diarrhea and the voiding of colorless urine every few minutes. Some mention terminal convulsions, but coma seems to be more usual.

The outstanding lesion is the dark, brownish color of the blood, the effect of methemoglobin. It is commonly described as chocolate-colored, but this must not be taken too literally. Clotting remains approximately normal. The mucous membranes are cyanotic, except those of the stomach and intestines, which show more or less hyperemia and inflammation. There may be a few petechiae, as in most anoxemias. Blood-stained pericardial fluid is a frequent finding. The discoloration of the blood should be diagnostic but tests for methemoglobin can be performed remembering that small amounts are demonstrable in healthy cattle (Householder, *et al.*, 1966).

Nitrates and Nitrites

ANDERSEN, H. K.: Methaemoglobinaemia in Pigs Due to Drinking Nitrite-Containing Water that Condensed in Ventilating Shafts in Piggeries (TT). Nord. Vet. Med. *14*:16–28, 1962.

ASBURY, A. C. and RHODE, E. A.: Nitrite Intoxication in Cattle: The Effects of Lethal Doses of Nitrite on Blood Pressure. Am. J. Vet. Res. *25*:1010–1013, 1964.

BODANSKY, O.: Methemoglobinemia and Methemoglobin-Producing Compounds. Pharmacol. Rev. *3*:144–196, 1951.

CAMPBELL, J. B., DAVIS, A. N., and MYHR, P. J.: Methemoglobinemia of Livestock Caused by High Nitrate Contents of Well Water. Canad. J. Comp. Med. *18*:93–101, 1954.

CAMPBELL, D. J., and WETHERELL, G. D.: Parasitic Bronchitis in Adult Cattle. J. Am. Vet. Med. Assn. *131*:273–275, 1957.

CRAWFORD, R. F., KENNEDY, W. K., and DAVISON, K. L.: Factors Influencing the Toxicity of Forages that Contain Nitrate When Fed to Cattle. Cornell Vet. *56*:3–17, 1966.

DIVEN, R. H., REED, R. E., and PISTOR, W. J.: The Physiology of Nitrite Poisoning in Sheep. Ann. New York Acad. Sci. *111*:638–643, 1964.

DIVEN, R. H. *et al.*: The Determination of Serum or Plasma Nitrate and Nitrite. Am. J. Vet. Res. *23*:497–499, 1962.

DOBAI, A. A.: Investigations and Observations on Pigs Concerning Methemoglobinemia. Proc. XVIth Int. Vet. Congr. Madrid. *2*:251–252, 1959.

HOUSEHOLDER, G. T., DOLLAHITE, J. W., and HULSE, R.: Diphenylamine for the Diagnosis of Nitrate Intoxication. J. Am. Vet. Med. Assn. *148*:662–665, 1966.

JAINUDEEN, M. R., HANSEL, W., and DAVISON, K. L.: Nitrate Toxicity in Dairy Heifers. 3. Endocrine Responses to Nitrate Ingestion During Pregnancy. J. Dairy Sci. *48*:217–221, 1965.

JENSEN, C. W., and ANDERSON, H. D.: Rate of Formation and Disappearance of Methemoglobin Following Oral Administration or Injection of Sodium Nitrite. Proc. S. Dakota Acad. Sci. *21*:37–40, 1941.

KENDRICK, J. W., TUCKER, J., and PEOPLES, S. A.: Nitrate Poisoning in Cattle Due to Ingestion of Variegated Thistle, *Silybum Marianum*. J. Am. Vet. Med. Assn. *126*:53–56, 1955.

LEWIS, D.: The Reduction of Nitrate in the Rumen of the Sheep. Biochem. J. *48*:175–180, 1951.

LI CHUAN WANG, GARCIA-RIVERA, J., and BURRIS, R. H.: Metabolism of Nitrate by Cattle. Biochem. J. *81*:237–242, 1961.

MICHEL, J. F., and SHAND, A.: A Study of the Epidemiology and Clinical Manifestations of Parasitic Bronchitis in Adult Cattle. Vet. Rec. *67*:249, 1955.

RIGGS, C. W.: Nitrite Poisoning from Ingestion of Plants High in Nitrate. Am. J. Vet. Research *6*:194–197, 1945.

RUBIN, R., and LUCKER, J. T.: The Course and Pathogenicity of Initial Infections with *Dictyocaulus viviparus*, the Lungworm of Cattle. Am. J. Vet. Res. *17*:217–226, 1956.

SEERLEY, R. W., *et al.*: Effect of Nitrate or Nitrite Administered Continuously in Drinking Water for Swine and Sheep. J. Anim. Sci. *24*:1014–1019, 1965.

SINCLAIR, B. K., and JONES, D. I. H.: Nitrate Toxicity in Sheep. J. Sci. Fd. Agric. *15*: 717–721, 1964.

STAHLER, L. M., and WHITEHEAD, E. I.: Effect of 2, 4-D on Potassium Nitrate Levels in Leaves of Sugar Beets. Science *112*:749–751, 1950.

TAYLOR, E. R.: Parasitic Bronchitis in Cattle. Vet. Rec. *63*:859–873, 1951.

WHITEHEAD, J. E.: Potassium Nitrate Poisoning in a Dog. J. Am. Vet. Med. Assn. *123*: 232–233, 1953.

WINTER, A. J. and HOKANSON, J. F.: Effects of Long-Term Feeding of Nitrate, Nitrite, or Hydroxylamine on Pregnant Dairy Heifers. Am. J. Vet. Res. *25*:353–361, 1964.

CHLORATES

Sodium chlorate, a strong oxidizing agent, is used to kill noxious weeds, being sprayed on the foliage and on the ground in a concentration amounting to 4 pounds per square rod (72 grams per square meter). Trials indicate that animals are not poisoned by eating any ordinary amount of sprayed foliage, especially if a few days have elapsed since the spraying, nor from the soil, but poisoning has occurred when animals accidentally gained access to supplies of the chemical, which is palatable because of its salty taste. The minimum lethal dose for sheep and probably for other farm mammals approximates 2 or 3 grams per kilogram of body weight, death coming in six to forty-eight hours.

Signs are somnolence and dyspnea, the temperature being normal. If small, sublethal amounts are ingested over a period of time, icterus and a dark or brownish discoloration of the conjunctivae can be expected. Post-mortem lesions are those of methemoglobinemia, ably described for sheep and cattle by McCulloch and Murer, 1939. The musculature is dark or almost black, cut surfaces becoming somewhat lighter on exposure to air. The blood is very dark or blackish but clots readily. The liver is almost black; the lungs have the color of normal liver. The heart is flabby and dark. The spleen is dark but not enlarged. The abomasum contains ulcerated areas which are very black; all other parts of the alimentary tract were without lesions in the experience of these writers. Concentrations of the chemical in ingesta or blood are too slight to respond to the ordinary chemical tests. There is no satisfactory treatment.

Chlorates

FITCH, C. P., BOYD, W. L., and HEWITT, E. A.: Toxicity of Sodium Chlorate (NaClO₃) for Cattle. Cornell Vet. *19*:373–375, 1929.

HOLZER, F. J., and STÖHR, R.: Eine Massenvergiftung von Schafen durch das Unkraut-vertilgungsmittel Natriumchlorat. Schweiz. Arch. f. Tierheilk. *92*:339–354, 1950.

JOUBERT, L., MAGAT, A., and OUDAR, J.: Intoxication pseudo-charbonneuse par ingestion de cheddite (chlorate de soude et trinitrotoluene) chez le Mouton. Bul. Soc. Sci. Vet. Lyon. *63*:327–332, 1961.

McCULLOCH, E. C., and MURER, H. K.: Sodium Chlorate Poisoning. J. Am. Vet. Med. Assn. *95*:675–682, 1939.

MOORE, G. R.: Sodium Chlorate Poisoning in Cattle. J. Am. Vet. Med. Assn. *99*:50–52, 1941.

SEDDON, H. R., and McGRATH, T. T.: Toxicity of Sodium Chlorate. Agric. Gaz. of New South Wales *41*:765–766, 1930.

SKJERVEN, O.: Natriumklorat-forgiftning. [Sodium Chlorate Poisoning in Cattle.] Norsk. vet. tidsskr. *56*:274–276, 1944.

* * * * *

Group I: **Poisons causing production of carboxyhemoglobin and cherry-red blood.**

Carbon monoxide   Cyanides

CARBON MONOXIDE

An important form of poisoning in humans, carbon monoxide poisoning, in veterinary practice, is ordinarily limited to pet animals which may chance to be confined in houses or basements where defective heating equipment may permit accidental accumulation of the gas. We have seen it, however, where the owner deliberately "helped the dog commit suicide" by means of an automobile exhaust.

Signs include incoordination and ataxia, vomiting, involuntary urination and defecation and unconsciousness. In humans, the fatal drowsiness often overcomes the victim so stealthily that he is unaware of the danger from which he could at first easily remove himself The one salient and usually diagnostic lesion is the bright cherry-red color of the blood and tissues This color is due to the formation of carboxyhemoglobin (p. 69). The CO radical replaces the O of hemoglobin, which has greater affinity for CO. Inability of the blood to transport oxygen leads to fatal asphyxia. Some cases survive a few days; in these there is loss of neurons in various parts of the brain.

Carbon Monoxide

BARONDES, R. DE R.: Carbon Monoxide Poisoning in a Dog. Vet. Med. *34*:105, 1939.
FINCK, P. A.: Exposure to Carbon Monoxide: Review of the Literature and 567 Autopsies. Mil. Med. *131*:1513–1539, 1966.
POPPENHOUSE, G. C.: Carbon Monoxide Poisoning in a Dog. Vet. Med. *34*:324–325, 1939.
STERLING, J. R.: Acute Carbon Monoxide Poisoning in a Dog. Vet. Med. *33*:66–68, 1938.

CYANIDES

While accidents with chemical preparations of cyanides are possible, the usual cause of cyanide poisoning in animals is ingestion of cyanogenic plants such as sorghums of all kinds, Sudan, Johnson, arrow and velvet grasses, African, or giant star grass (*Cynodon plectostachyum*), a plant of Australia and certain southern parts of Africa, flax, suckleya (*Suckleya suckleyana*), reed sweetgrass (*Poa aquatica*), hydrangea and wild or domesticated members of the cherry family (including cherry pits by chickens).

Death may be instantaneous, but usually symptoms last for some minutes or an hour. The animal falls, with convulsions, frothing at the mouth, unconsciousness and infrequent gasping respirations. Pupils are dilated and involuntary defecation and micturition occur. Respiration ceases while the heart still beats. Acute cases are without lesions in the organs, but a bright red, arterial color of the venous blood is a diagnostic change. It is seen best by putting a small amount of blood over a dark background; the bright red persists for several hours despite drying. The proverbial odor of almonds or cherry pits is seldom detectable. There is seldom any erosion or inflammation of the alimentary mucosa. Repeated minute doses over a period of time have produced multiple foci of necrosis in the brain.

The poison acts by preventing the intracellular oxidative process, although the blood does not lack for oxygen. This action is the reason for the bright red blood which is prevented from losing its oxygen to the tissues. A test for cyanides which is practicable with minimal laboratory equipment is as follows: Prepare "picrate paper" by wetting filter paper with a solution of 5 gm. of sodium carbonate and 0.5 gm. of picric acid in 100 ml. of distilled water. The solution keeps indefinitely and the papers, after drying, retain their strength for a few days. Crush or shred some of the suspected plant material or rumen contents and place in water in a test-tube. Add a few drops of chloroform to hasten autolysis. Suspend (as by the cork) a piece of the picrate paper, slightly moistened, at the top of the tube and maintain the tube upright at a temperature approximating 30 or 35° C. The appearance of a brick-red color in the previously yellow picrate paper indicates the presence of hydrocyanic acid. A mild reaction appearing after one or several hours indicates what are probably nontoxic amounts of cyanogenetic substance. A well-marked red color appearing in a few minutes is definitely significant (Henrici, 1926).

Cyanides

HADLEY, F. B.: Sudan Grass Poisoning Problem. Canad. J. Comp. Med. 2(6):169–170, 1938.

HAYMAKER, W., GINZLER, A. M., and FERGUSON, R. L.: Residual Neuropathological Effects of Cyanide Poisoning. (A Study of the Central Nervous System of 23 Dogs Exposed to Cyanide Compounds.) Military Surg. 3:231–246, 1952.

HENRICI, M.: Occurrence of HCN in the Grasses of Bechuanaland. 11th and 12th Rept. Director Vet. Ed. and Research, U. of So. Africa. 1926. pp. 495–498.

LEVINE, S., and GEIB, L. W.: Leukoencephalopathy in a Cat Due to Accidental Cyanide Poisoning. Path. Vet. 3:190–195, 1966.

MANGES, J. D.: Cyanide Poisoning. Vet. Med. 30:347–349, 1935.

MATHEWS, F. P.: Johnson Grass (*Sorghum halepense*) Poisoning. J. Am. Vet. Med. Assn. 81:663–666, 1932.

PETERS, A. T., SLADE, H. B., and AVERY, S.: Poisoning of Cattle by Common Sorghum and Kafir Corn (*Sorghum vulgare*). Expt. Sta. Bull. 77, Univ. Nebr., Lincoln. 1903.

REBER, K.: Hydrocyanic Acid Content of Flaxseed. (Abstr. from Schweiz. Apoth. Ztg. 76:229, 1938.) J. Am. Pharm. Assn. 5:82–83, 1939.

ROSE, C. L., et al.: Cobalt Salts in Acute Cyanide Poisoning. Proc. Soc. Exp. Biol. Med. 120:780–783, 1965.

SCHUBEL, E. C. W.: Poisoning by Hydrocyanic Acid. J. Am. Vet. Med. Assn. 95:371–373, 1939.

SHARMAN, J. R.: Cyanide Poisoning of Cattle Grazing "Reed Sweet-grass." N. Z. Vet. J. 15:7–8, 1967.

TIMSON, S. D.: Prussic Acid Content of the Giant Star Grasses (*Cynodon plectostachyum*) and of Kavirondo Sorghum. Rhod. Agric. J. 40:371–373, 1943.

*   *   *   *   *

Group J: Poisons causing marked and conspicuous edema.

Alpha-naphthyl Thiourea   Toxic fat

ALPHA-NAPHTHYL THIOUREA (ANTU)

This compound is popular for killing rats, usually mixed with meat or grain for that purpose. It was originally heralded as not dangerous to dogs because it was thought they would rid themselves of the substance by vomiting. Experience has proved otherwise in spite of the fact that vomition does occur. Symptoms include cardiac and respiratory embarrassment with imperceptible but rapid pulse and rapid, shallow respiration. Vomitus is frothy and may become bloody. Diarrhea is severe, becoming bloody. Weak and comatose, the dog commonly dies in the sternal recumbent position, fluid from the lungs often running out from his mouth. The temperature becomes markedly subnormal before death. All this transpires and death occurs in from one to four hours after the ANTU is eaten, as a rule.

Post-mortem lesions of poisoning by alpha-naphthyl thiourea are practically diagnostic. Marked hydrothorax is present in nearly all cases. If the thorax is opened carefully and without contaminating hemorrhage from the vessels, it is found to be full to overflowing with clear watery fluid. Extremely severe edema of the lungs occurs almost without exception, fluid often running out the trachea, if the thoracic organs are raised posteriorly. The lungs also show severe congestion with diapedesis of erythrocytes into numerous alveoli. In the stomach, the fundic mucosa is severely inflamed and reddened in more than half the cases, moderately so in most of the remainder. Microscopically, the stomach shows considerable mucous exudate, as well as hyperemia. The surface epithelium is intact, but the chief cells are inconspicuous in appearance and numbers as compared to the parietal cells. This catarrhal inflammation continues into the small intestine and subsides gradually in the large bowel. Considerable amounts of bile are found in the upper intestine, although the gallbladder is not completely emptied. The kidneys are severely congested, often deep red. In the cortex and some of the medullary rays fatty change of the epithelial cells is demonstrable. In the liver, the light color of vacuolization and central necrosis alternates in spots with the red of acute congestion. Fatty change, however, is absent. The spleen is small and empty of blood.

Poisoning by alpha-naphthyl thiourea has also occurred in horses through the accidental ingestion of poison bait.

Alpha-naphthyl thiourea

ANDERSON, W. A., and RICHTER, C. P.: Toxicity of Alpha Naphthyl Thiourea for Chickens and Pigs. Vet. Med. *41*:302–303, 1946.
FRICK, E. J., and FORTENBERRY, J. D., Equine ANTU Poisoning. Vet. Med. *43*:107–108, 1948.
JONES, L. M., SMITH, D. A., and SMITH, H. A.: Alpha-naphthyl (ANTU) Thiourea Poisoning in Dogs. Am. J. Vet. Research *10*:160–167, 1949.
HESSE, F. E., and LOOSLI, C. G.: The Lining of the Alveoli in Mice, Rats, Dogs, and Frogs Following Acute Pulmonary Edema Produced by ANTU Poisoning. Anat. Rec. *105*: 299–324, 1949.
LATTA, H.: Pulmonary Edema and Pleural Effusion Produced by Acute Alpha-Naphthyl Thiourea Poisoning in Rats and Dogs. Bull. Johns Hopkins Hosp. *80*:181–197, 1947.
LOPES, A. C.: Pathology and Histology of Experimental Poisoning of Dogs with ANTU, Alpha-naphthyl Thiourea. Pesquisa agropec. bras. *2*:287–291, 1967. V.B. *39*:334, 1969.

TOXIC FAT

The occurrence of a toxic factor in the unsaponifiable fraction of certain fats was first indicated by the sudden appearance of a disease in chickens fed diets containing these fats. The disease in poultry was named "hydropericardium," "edema disease," "water belly" and "ascitic disease" by poultrymen and veterinarians, indicating the common post-mortem findings. Certain lots of broilers were first reported (Schmittle, *et al.*, 1958) to undergo 90 per cent mortality in a short time. These losses were soon associated with certain lots of poultry feed. The problem has been studied by several groups (Simpson, *et al.*, 1959, Allen, 1964, Allen and Carstens, 1966). The toxic factor is also found in the fat of affected birds and has been demonstrated (Allen and Carstens, 1967) to be poisonous to rhesus monkeys (*Macaca mulatta*) as well.

The experimental disease in monkeys is of particular interest in mammalian pathology. Allen and Carstens have proposed that the toxic fat extends its effect upon the hepatocytes, endothelium and myocardium with the development of anasarca (p. 135). Monkeys fed upon this material in doses from 0.125 to 10 per cent of the diet, developed signs and lesions at time intervals inversely related to the dosages. The skin was first affected, with alopecia and edema starting in the eyelids and lips, then extending to the ventral trunk, extremities, scrotum and prepuce. Some interference with micturition was evident in severely edematous animals. Loss of body weight was a constant feature and about 75 per cent of the animals evidenced diarrhea. As the disease progressed, serum albumin was decreased, particularly as death approached. The packed cell volume was similarly reduced gradually and hemoglobin levels became as low as 6.0 gm./100 ml. blood. Red and white blood cell counts were also depressed severely during the last month of life. Prothrombin time, serum bilirubin, serum electrolytes, blood urea nitrogen and cholesterol levels in blood remained unchanged.

The gross lesions at necropsy consisted of generalized subcutaneous edema, dilation of the heart with myocardial hypertrophy; small, firm moderately yellow liver; isolated areas of atelectasis, congestion, edema and fibrosis of the lungs; small spleen; tan and edematous lymph nodes; fatty bone marrow; pale and edematous skeletal muscles; hypertrophy of gastric mucosa in fundic and pyloric regions and normal-appearing testes.

Light microscopic findings were for the most part related to the gross lesions. Edema was evident in subcutis, skeletal muscles and myocardium. Individual myocardial cells were often hypertrophic with enlarged, distorted and hyperchromic nuclei. The architecture of the liver was moderately distorted. Some hepatocytes were enlarged, multinucleated and poorly stained, others were small and hyperchromic. Focal necroses in centrilobular locations were frequent, with vacuolization and fatty change in adjacent hepatic cells. Small areas of periportal fibrosis were evident. The reduced size of the spleen appeared to be due to the loss of lymphocytes. In the mesenteric lymph nodes narrow bands of lymphocytes surrounded the germinal centers, protein filled sinusoids and the medullary cords were indistinct. The sternal marrow was hypoplastic, much of it fatty, but the few erythroid and myeloid cells present were about equal in numbers. The testes were moderately edematous and contained no spermatids or spermatozoa. The hyperplastic gastric epithelium contained numerous ulcers between large folds of epithelium.

Allen and Carstens (1967) also described the ultrastructural changes in liver cells of monkeys poisoned with toxic fat. An early change was the disruption of the orderly arrangement of the granular endoplasmic reticulum, dilation of cysternae spaces and loss of ribosomes—giving an apparent increase in smooth endoplasmic reticulum. Mitochondria were swollen and a few cytosomes were present in the cytoplasm. Fat vacuoles were abundant. Some cells were apparently shrunken and more dense in the electron micrographs. These dark cells contrasted markedly with other hepatocytes whose organelles were widely dispersed and more easily visualized. Epithelial cells of bile ducts were often electron-dense and as a result microvilli on the luminal surface of the plasmalemmae seemed thin and elongated. In the myocardium, intercellular spaces were dilated in the affected monkeys and the myofibrils widely separated from one another. Cytosomes were more abundant than in controls and mitochondria were often swollen. Many endothelial cells were also shrunken and more dense in electron micrographs and many contained myelin bodies. Further details may be found in the original reference (Allen and Carstens, 1967).

Norback and Allen, 1969, have described concentric membrane arrays in hepatocytes of rats poisoned with this toxic fat.

Toxic Fat

ALLEN, J. R.: The Role of "Toxic Fat" in the Production of Hydropericardium and Ascites in Chickens. Am. J. Vet. Res. *25*:1210–1219, 1964.

ALLEN, J. R., and CARSTENS, L. A.: Electron Microscopic Observations in the Liver of Chickens Fed Toxic Fat. Lab. Invest. *15*:970–979, 1966.

——————: Light and Electron Microscopic Observations in *Macaca mulatta* Monkeys Fed Toxic Fat. Am. J. Vet. Res. *28*:1513–1526, 1967.

CANTRELL, J. S., WEBB, N. C., and MABIS, A. J.: The Identification and Crystal Structure of a Hydroperitoneum-producing Factor: 1,2,3,7,8,9-Hexachlorodibenzo-p-dioxin. Act. Cryst. B*25*:150–155, 1969.

NORBACK, D. H., and ALLEN, J. R.: Morphogenesis of Toxic Fat-induced Concentric Membrane Arrays in Rat Hepatocytes. Lab. Invest. *20*:338–346, 1969.

SCHMITTLE, S. C., EDWARDS, H. M., and MORRIS, D.: A Disorder of Chickens Probably Due to a Toxic Feed—Preliminary Report. J. Am. Vet. Med. Assn. *132*:216–219, 1958.

SIMPSON, C. F., PRITCHARD, W. R., and HARMS, R. H.: An Endotheliosis in Chickens and Turkeys Caused by an Unidentified Dietary Factor. J. Am. Vet. Med. Assn. *134*:410–416, 1959.

*   *   *   *   *

Group K: **A poison causing marked and conspicuous pulmonary emphysema.**

RAPE, KALE

and other Plants of Genus Brassica

The disease recognized as rape poisoning commonly makes its appearance in a herd in from seven to ten days after the cattle or sheep have been placed in a pasture of this kind. Luxuriant growth, wet weather, and, possibly, frosting, appear to increase the danger. In Schofield's experience, it is more likely to occur on certain farms than on others (1948).

Signs include (1) more or less digestive disturbance, usually absence of peristalsis and constipation, occasionally the reverse with fetid diarrhea; (2) respiratory difficulties including dyspnea with open mouth and a thumping sound at each respiration; (3) gradually increasing anemia, usually with hemoglobinuria and mild icterus, thus a hemolytic anemia. Whether the icterus is hemolytic or toxic (p. 75) has not been made clear. The anemia has been described as hyperchromic and macrocytic (Rosenberger, 1943). Weakness, ataxia and nervous abnormalities, as well as blindness, are also described. If the cow is recently postparturient, the condition has been found to be indistinguishable from the poorly understood disorder called puerperal hemoglobinuria.

Of the lesions, a severe and destructive pulmonary emphysema, accompanied by congestion and edema and involving all parts of both lungs, is the most spectacular in the experience of Schofield and other Canadian investigators. Microscopically, rupture of the pulmonary alveoli is uniformly widespread and both the emphysema and edema also involve the interlobular septa. Emphysema of the mediastinal and even of subcutaneous tissues also develops in some cases when the pulmonary emphysema has existed for a few days. There may be hemorrhages in the trachea and bronchi; it is not clear whether bronchiectasis is also present. There is moderate acute toxic hepatitis, shown chiefly by centrilobular necrosis. The gallbladder regularly shows the distention with viscid bile which is characteristic of alimentary inactivity (p. 1237).

The pathogenetic mechanisms have been the subject of considerable speculation and study. Some suspect that the condition has an allergic basis. Schofield has found in a number of instances a heavy invasion of the contents of the alimentary canal by *Clostridium perfringens*, with evidence of toxin similar to that of the enterotoxemia (p. 1211) which develops under other circumstances and is characterized by other species of Clostridia. The concept of a specific poisonous substance is supported, not only by the variety of lesions produced, but, to some extent, by the fact that rape seed has been found poisonous to fowls. Wild cabbage (*Brassica oleracea*) has been reported as poisoning cattle when in the seed stage only (Angelo, 1951). Rape-seed cake has been found to have a locally irritant action with the production of vesicles. But see also the Pulmonary Emphysema-Adenomatosis Syndrome (p. 1124).

Feeding of kale to cattle (Grant, *et al.*, 1968) has been shown to reduce the hemoglobin and packed cell volume of experimental groups in comparison with controls. No significant changes were observed in the following values: *in vitro* uptake of ^{131}I triiodothyronine by erythrocytes, total serum protein, serum calcium, inorganic phosphorus, magnesium, serum glutamic-oxaloacetic acid transaminase, or serum ornithine-carbamyl-transferase.

The feeding of kale to sheep (Grant, *et al.*, 1968, Tucker, 1969) was demonstrated to result in a relatively severe anemia and the production of hemoglobin C by sheep with hemoglobin genotype AB and AA. Also observed was a decrease in red cell mean corpuscular hemoglobin concentration (p. 123) and the appearance of increased numbers of Heinz bodies in the red blood cells of sheep with hemoglobin genotypes BB, AB and AA.

Rape, Kale

ANGELO, M.: Anemia emolitica emologobinurica da cavoli fioriti in bovine lattifere. [Anaemia and Hemoglobinuria in Dairy Cattle Caused by Wild Cabbage (*Brassica oleracea*) Gone to Seed.] Zooprofilassi. *6*:361–363, 1951.

CLEGG, F. G. and EVANS, R. K.: Haemoglobinemia of Cattle Associated with the Feeding of Brassica Species. Vet. Rec. *74*:1169–1176, 1962.

COTE, F. T.: Rape Poisoning in Cattle. Canad. J. Comp. Med. *8*:38–41, 1944.

CRAWSHAW, H. A.: Rape Blindness. Vet. Rec. *65*:254, 1953; and DALTON, P. J.: *Ibid.* p. 298.

EVANS, E. T. R.: Kale and Rape Poisoning in Cattle. Vet. Rec. *63*:348–349, 1951.

GORISEK, J.: Metabolic Disorders in Cows Related to the Feeding of Sugar-Beet Leaves (TT). Proc. 17th World Vet. Congr., Hanover *2*:1343–1344 (G.e.f.sp.) 1963.

GRANT, C. A., *et al.*: Kale Anaemia in Ruminants. I. Survey of the Literature and Experimental Induction of Kale Anaemia in Lactating Cows. Acta vet. scand. *9*:126–140, 1968.

GRANT, C. A., *et al.*: Kale Anaemia in Ruminants. II. Observations on Kale Fed Sheep. Acta vet. scand. *9*:141–150, 1968.

GREENHALGH, J. F. D., SHARMAN, G. A. M., and AITKEN, J. N.: Kale Anaemia . I. The Toxicity to Various Species of Animal of Three Types of Kale. Res. vet. Sci. *10*:64–72, 1969.

PATRIZI, F., and MORICONI, M.: Morte di 10 bovine per avvelenamento da colza. [Deaths of Cattle from Rape Seed Cake Poisoning.] Atti Soc. ital. sci. vet. *5*:225–227, 1951.

PENNY, R. H. C., DAVID, J. S. E., and WRIGHT, A. I.: Observations on the Blood Picture of Cattle, Sheep, and Rabbits Fed on Kale. Vet. Rec. *76*:1053–1059, 1964.

ROSENBERGER, G.: Kohlanämie des Rindes. Deutsch. tierärztl. Wchnschr. *51*:63–67, 1943.

SCHOFIELD, F. W.: Acute Pulmonary Emphysema of Cattle. J. Am. Vet. Med. Assn. *112*:254–259, 1948.

STAMP, J. T., and STEWART, J.: Haemolytic Anemia with Jaundice in Sheep. J. Comp. Path. and Therap. *63*:48–52, 1953.

TUCKER, E. M.: The Onset of Anaemia and the Production of Haemoglobin C in Sheep Fed on Kale. Brit. Vet. J. *125*:472–479, 1969.

*　*　*　*　*

Group L:　**Poisons causing gangrene of the extremities.**

Ergot   Fescue grass

ERGOT

Most of the agricultural "small grains" and many different grasses are parasitized by the ascomycetic fungus, *Claviceps purpurea*. Each sclerotium of the fungus is a hard, black, elongated body which destroys and replaces a grain or seed of the maturing plant, being usually somewhat larger than the neighboring grains. These sclerotia constitute the substance known as ergot, which is used as a drug and whose poisonous properties have long been familiar. As late as the early nineteenth century humans were not infrequently poisoned by contaminated flour. In animals, including birds, poisoning may occur through the feeding of contaminated grain, but in herbivora, it results more frequently from the use of hay or straw containing a considerable proportion of parasitized plants.

In general, the action of ergot is to stimulate smooth muscle. This action upon the uterine musculature is responsible for its use as an oxytocic. Long continued contraction of the vascular musculature is the principal basis for its poisonous effects. The usual manifestation of chronic poisoning by ergot, which is known as ergotism, consists in dry gangrene (p. 26) of the limbs, tail and ears, so that after several weeks of ingestion of small amounts the most distal parts of the extremities may drop off. The early stages are characterized by lameness, irregular gait and evidence of pain in the feet, the posterior extremities being chiefly affected. Palpation of the parts involved shows them to be cold and insensitive. These signs may begin as early as a week after the first consumption of contaminated material. Occasionally, the gangrene has been moist instead of dry, at least in the feet and phalanges. As would be expected, there is usually a clear line of demarcation and an inflammatory zone just proximal to it. In birds, the parts which become gangrenous are the comb, tongue and beak. Less noticeable signs based upon involvement of the gastrointestinal musculature may precede or accompany those arising in the extremities. They include indigestion, colic, vomiting and either diarrhea or constipation. Pregnant animals often abort.

The above-described signs mark the usual "gangrenous form." In the rare "spasmodic form," there are tonic contractions of the flexors of the limbs, trembling of the muscles, opisthotonos, tetanic spasms of the whole body, convulsions, delirium and death. This type of reaction is presumed to be related to failing blood supply in the central nervous system.

The post-mortem lesions are obvious in the gangrenous cases. In addition, congestion is described in the visceral organs and, occasionally, hemorrhages. Another related fungus, *Claviceps paspali*, produces different effects on animals and is therefore considered separately (p. 948).

Ergot

DILLON, B. E.: Acute Ergot Poisoning in Cattle. J. Am. Vet. Med. Assn. *126*:136, 1955.
DOLLAHITE, J. W.: Ergotism Produced by Feeding *Claviceps Cinera* Growings on Tobosagrass (*Hilaria Mutica*) and Galletagrass (*Hilaria Jamesii*). SW. Vet. *16*:295–296, 1963.
LUMB, J. W.: Ergotism of Cattle in Kansas. J. Am. Vet. Med. Assn. *81*:812–816, 1932.
MANTLE, P. G., and GUNNER, D. E.: Abortions Associated with Ergotised Pastures. Vet. Rec. *77*:885–886, 1965.
SALIKOV, M. I.: Novo kormovoe zabolevanie loshadei i kropnovo rogatovo skota. [New form of food poisoning in horses and cattle (due to the fungus *Claviceps paspali*).] Veterinariya, Moscow. No. 2–3, pp. 41–43, 1944. Abstr. Vet. Bull. No. 143, 1946.
SZEWCZYKOWSKI, J., *et al.*: Effects of Ergot Alkaloids (Hydergine) on Cerebral Hemodynamics and Oxygen Consumption in Monkeys. J. Neurol. Sci. *10*:25–31, 1970.
WOODS, A. J., JONES, J. B., and MANTLE, P. G.: An Outbreak of Gangrenous Ergotism in Cattle. Vet. Rec. *78*:742–749, 1966.

FESCUE GRASS

In Australia and in the United States, there has been reported a poisoning of cattle characterized by gangrene of the extremities which is entirely comparable to the usual case of ergotism. Commencing within two weeks after the animals start eating this grass there are lameness, local heat, swelling and severe pain involving a digit and extending upward to a line of demarcation in the phalanges or at or above the fetlock joint. The dried and shriveled extremity may then separate at this line.

The causative grass is a kind known as fescue grass, usually tall fescue, *Festuca arundinacea*, but a shorter, improved variety was incriminated in one instance. The toxic principle has not been identified but apparently it is a vasoconstrictive substance which becomes concentrated in the grass as it dries. Cows appear to be most susceptible when they graze on dry fescue meadows and receive no supplemental feed or protection from the cold weather.

The signs and lesions are similar and must be differentiated from those of ergotism, selenium poisoning or cold injury.

Fescue Grass

CUNNINGHAM. I. J.: A Note on the Cause of Tall Fescue Lameness in Cattle. Austr. Vet. J. *25*:27–28, 1949.
GOODMAN, A. A.: Fescue Foot in Cattle in Colorado. J. Am. Vet. Med. Assn. *121*:289–290, 1952.
JACOBSON, D. R. and MILLER, W. M.: Fescue Toxicity. J. Anim. Sci. *20*:960–961, 1961.
PULSFORD, M. F.: A Note on Lameness in Cattle Grazing on Tall Meadow Fescue (*Festuca arundinacea*) in South Australia. Australian Vet. J. *26*:87–88, 1950.
STEARNS, T. J.: Fescot Foot or Ergot-like Disease in Cattle in Kentucky. J. Am. Vet. Med. Assn. *122*:388–389, 1953.
WILLIAMS, G. F.: Epidemiology of Fescue Toxicity. J. Dairy Sci. *48*:1135, 1965.

Group M: **A poison causing unusual lesions of bones and teeth.**

FLUORINE

Chronic fluorosis occurs in animals receiving more than a minute amount of fluorine in the diet over a long period of time. The minimum amount of fluorine in the form of soluble fluorides required to produce evidence of injury in cattle and other farm animals lies between 1 and 2 mg. per kilogram of body weight per day or between 12 and 27 p.p.m. of the diet. As a partially soluble contaminant of rock phosphate, a somewhat larger amount may possibly be harmless. In humans, the amount tolerated without lesions (in the teeth) is said to be much less. Chronic poisoning of this nature occurs in animals eating pasturage or forage contaminated by air-borne residues from aluminum manufactories, phosphate refineries and similar industrial installations, or drinking well-water containing soluble fluorides to the extent of 10 or more parts per million. When, as is commonly the case, both water and forage contain considerable amounts of fluorine, the safe level for the water alone is less than the figure given.

The clinical signs of chronic fluorine poisoning in cattle according to Shupe, *et al.* (1964) include (1) mottling and abrasion of teeth, (2) intermittent lameness, (3) periosteal hyperostosis, demonstrable radiographically, and (4) demonstration of more than 6 p.p.m. of fluorine in the urine. In fluorosis as much as 30 p.p.m. of fluorine may be present in the urine, depending upon the age of the animal, specific gravity of the urine and length of time the animal has ingested fluorine.

The pathognomonic lesions of chronic fluorine poisoning involve the teeth, the bones, and possibly the kidneys. The principal changes in the teeth are (1) "chalky" areas, (2) "mottling," (3) excessive attrition, and (4) hypoplastic pitting of the enamel. The chalky areas have received this description because the enamel has lost its shiny, translucent appearance and has assumed the dull, white opacity characteristic of chalk. Slight degrees of this condition are best

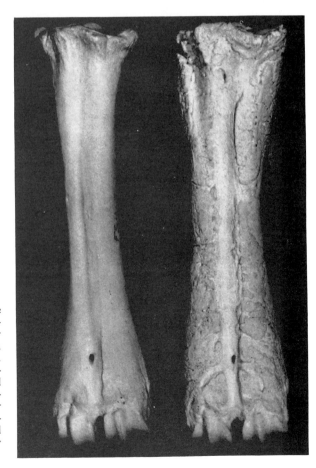

FIG. 17–18.—Chronic bovine fluorosis. Left: normal metatarsal bone of a dairy cow after ingesting 12 p.p.m. fluorine in the diet for about 7 years. Right: Hyperostosis and roughened periosteum of metatarsal bone of a dairy cow after consuming 93 p.p.m. fluorine for approximately 7 years. (Courtesy of Dr. J. L. Shupe and American Journal of Veterinary Research.)

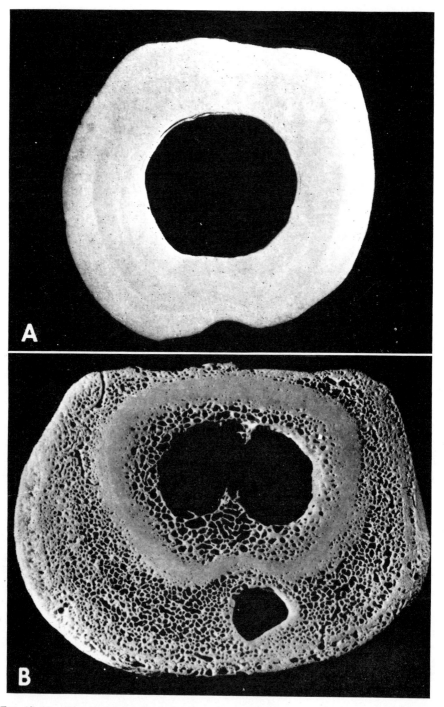

Fig. 17–19.—Chronic bovine fluorosis, ground cross sections of metatarsus. *A*, Osteosclerosis, of a cow which received slightly elevated levels of fluorine for several years. *B*, Osteoporosis, with periosteal hyperostosis and endosteal resorption, bone from a cow which received high levels of fluorine in its diet for several years. (Courtesy of Dr. J. L. Shupe and Annals of New York Academy of Sciences.)

detected by placing a light behind the tooth. The mottling consists in spots of yellow, brown or greenish black. The pigmentation is in the enamel and cannot be removed from it but may tend to be accentuated at the site of hypoplastic defects. The excessive attrition results from an abnormal softness of the enamel and perhaps also of the dentine. Affected teeth are short because of rapid wear, which may reduce them to the level of the gums in the worst cases. The *pitting* consists in punctate or linear depressions on the side of the tooth due to deficient deposition of enamel at those places. The distribution of the hypoplastic "pits" may follow a horizontal pattern considered to represent a chronological period in the development of the tooth. It is to be noted that these dental lesions develop only in case the fluorosis is present and active during the time when the tooth is being formed. Once the tooth is fully formed, it is not affected by fluorosis. For this reason, the deciduous teeth do not develop lesions, and the permanent teeth which are formed earliest in life show the least damage. The more lateral incisors, as well as the later arriving molars and premolars, having been subjected to the fluorine over a longer period in most naturally occurring cases, are more worn and discolored than the older teeth, a situation quite the contrary to the wear of normal teeth.

The bony changes are most pronounced in the metacarpals, metatarsals and mandible, although all bones, like the teeth, store considerable amounts of fluoride and suffer from it. The bones become thicker and heavier than normal, the marrow cavity often being diminished in size and the periosteal layer, in severe cases, is thickened. Microscopically, the bony trabeculae are thickened at the expense of the intertrabecular marrow spaces. The trabeculae have a dense appearance, with sharp, heavy outlines. However, it has been claimed that osteopetrotic changes, such as these, are due to calcium fluoride but that sodium fluoride causes the opposite condition of osteoporosis (p. 1057). Another view (Shupe, *et al.*, 1964) is that osteosclerosis occurs in animals receiving low doses of fluorine over a long time. Osteoporosis, with endosteal resorption and periosteal hyperostosis, on the other hand, is believed to result in animals receiving high doses of fluorine over a similarly prolonged period. The periosteal proliferation

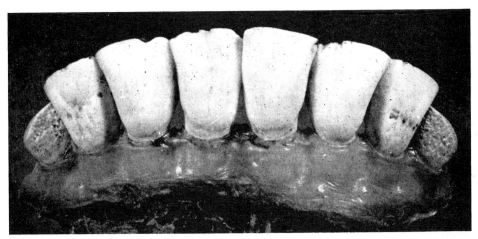

Fig. 17-20.—Incisor teeth of a Holstein cow fed sodium fluoride at a level of 2.5 mg. of fluorine per kg. of body weight per day for 4 years. The first two pairs of incisors had already erupted when the experiment began. Molars were not affected. (Courtesy of Stanford Research Institute.)

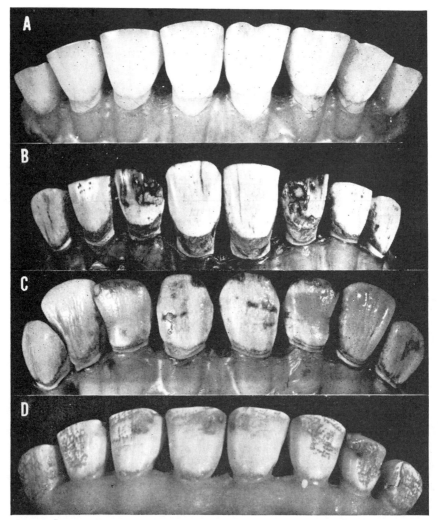

FIG. 17–21.—Teeth in chronic bovine fluorosis. *A*, Normal incisors. *B–D*, Varying degrees of mottling of enamel of incisor teeth. (Courtesy of Dr. J. L. Shupe.)

may result in microscopically demonstrable subperiosteal thickening and often, in the more severely affected individuals, is accompanied by the formation of sessile exostoses, seldom more than $\frac{1}{2}$ cm. in height. These may or may not be detectable clinically but, in company with the general periosteal disturbance, result in stiffness and lameness. Chemically the bones of appreciably poisoned animals contain fluorine to the extent of 4000 to 15,000 parts per million (1.5 per cent). This concentration has been developed slowly over a period of years and could conceivably represent absorption of fluorine from environmental sources no longer present; the same, of course, is true of the dental changes.

In the kidneys of experimental rats, degenerations and disintegration of the tubular epithelium, slight glomerular changes, thickened arterioles and terminal fibrosis are described. The fibrotic areas are radially arranged and are devoid of alkaline phosphatase. Polydipsia, polyuria and poorly concentrated urine are concomitant signs.

The general health of the animal is not necessarily affected when mild dental changes are the only sign of fluorosis, but in more severe cases there are lameness, anorexia, loss of weight, decreased production of milk, general unthriftiness and perhaps intermittent diarrhea. Fluorine passes through the placenta and may accumulate in the bones of the fetus but no significant direct effect upon fertility has been demonstrated.

The exact mechanisms involved in chronic fluorosis are unknown. One hypothesis is that fluoride ions replace hydroxyl radicals in the apatite crystal and that

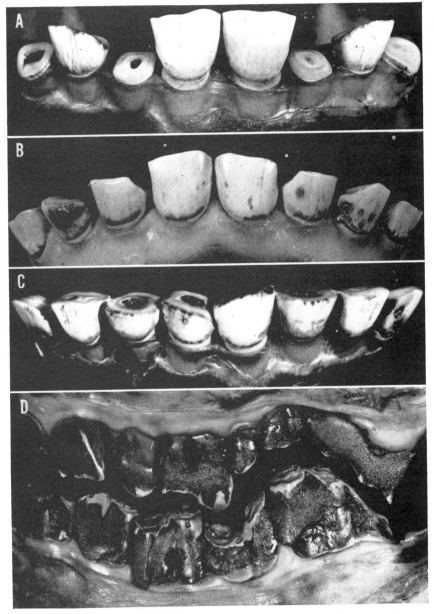

Fig. 17–22.—Teeth in chronic bovine fluorosis. *A*, Irregular wear of incisors. *B*, Irregular mottling of incisors. *C*, Excessive wear of incisors. *D*, Irregular wear and stained enamel of molar teeth. (Courtesy of Dr. J. L. Shupe.)

this in some way results in abnormal osteoid. This in turn is thought to be responsible for the poor bony matrix which is defective and irregularly mineralized. It is evident that osteoblastic activity is abnormal, as judged by the defective new bone and dentine.

Chronic fluorosis in the guinea pig has been identified by Hard and Atkinson (1967) as the underlying factor in a syndrome referred to in Australia as "slobbers." This descriptive name comes from the characteristic excessive salivation which results from abnormal teeth. The teeth grow irregularly, become elongated or wear excessively and the enamel is eroded and often encrusted with tartar. The irregularly shaped teeth are thought to interfere with swallowing, resulting in drooling of saliva. Affected animals eventually die unless the diet is corrected. At necropsy, lesions in the teeth are most significant. Elevated levels of fluorine in bones of naturally and experimentally affected animals corroborate the diagnosis. Levels of up to 6700 p.p.m. in naturally affected guinea pigs and over 5700 p.p.m. in experimentally poisoned animals have been recorded, in contrast to levels of not over 160 p.p.m. of fluorine in normal animals.

One source of fluorine in guinea pig feed appears to have been rock phosphate of high content used as a component of pelleted feed.

Acute Fluorine Poisoning.—This results from accidents or the improper use of sodium fluoride, which is employed as a vermifuge in swine and externally for lice in poultry. It also occurs in dogs which eat dead rats poisoned by the rodenticide, **sodium monofluoroacetate** ("compound 1080"), or when a domestic animal eats the bait itself. Lasting a few hours or a day or two, the symptoms are extreme abdominal pain, convulsions and frenzy alternating with weakness and lethargy. Diarrhea develops shortly. Collapse is followed by death from respiratory and myocardial arrest. The post-mortem lesions are those of acute gastroenteritis.

Fluorine

ATKINSON, F. F. W., and HARD, G. C.: Chronic Fluorosis in the Guinea-pig. Nature (Lond.) *211*:429–430, 1966.

BECMEUR, LAMOTTE, MASSOTTE and ROUSSON: Darmous et fluoroses. Maroc. méd. *30*:490–496, 1951.

BOND, A. M., and MURRAY, M. M.: Kidney Functions and Structure in Chronic Fluorosis. Brit. J. Exper. Path. *33*:168–176, 1952.

FACCINI, J. M., and CARE, A. D.: Effect of Sodium Fluoride on the Ultrastructure of the Parathyroid Glands of the Sheep. Nature (Lond.) *207*:1399–1401, 1965.

GARLICK, N. L.: Dental Fluorosis. Am. J. Vet. Research *16*:38–44, 1955.

HARD, G. C., and ATKINSON, F. F. V.: "Slobbers" in Laboratory Guinea Pigs as a Form of Chronic Fluorosis. J. Path. Bact. *94*:95–102, 1967.

————: The Aetiology of "Slobbers" (Chronic Fluorosis) in the Guinea Pig. J. Path. Bact. *94*:103–112, 1967.

HOOGSTRATTEN, B., *et al.*: Effect of Fluorides on Hematopoietic System, Liver and Thyroid Gland in Cattle. J. Am. Med. Assn. *192*:26–32, 1965.

JENSEN, R. ,TOBISKA, J. W., and WARD, J. C.: Sodium Fluoroacetate Poisoning in a Sheep. Am. J. Vet. Research *9*:370–372, 1948.

NAROZNY, J.: Dental Fluorosis in Cattle. Vet. Med. Praha *7*:421–424, 1965. V.B. *36*:273, 1966.

NEELEY, K. L., and HARBAUGH, F. G.: Effects of Fluoride Ingestion on a Herd of Dairy Cattle in the Lubbock, Texas, Area. J. Am. Vet. Med. Assn. *124*:344–350, 1954.

NEWELL, G. W., and SCHMIDT, H. J.: The Effects of Feeding Fluorine, as Sodium Fluoride, to Dairy Cattle. Am. J. Vet. Res. *19*:363–376, 1958.

NICHOLS, H. C., THOMAS, E. F., BRAWNER, W. R., and LEWIS, R. Y.: Poisoning of Two Dogs with 1080 Rat Poison (Sodium Fluoroacetate). J. Am. Vet. Med. Assn. *115*:355–356, 1949.

RAND, W. E., and SCHMIDT, H. J.: The Effect upon Cattle of Arizona Waters of High Fluoride Content. Am. J. Vet. Research *13*:50–61, 1952.

REINHARD, H.: Die Fluorschaden im unteren Fricktal. Schweiz. Arch. Tierheilk. *101*:1–14, 1959.

SCHMIDT, H. J., and RAND, W. E.: A Critical Study of the Literature on Fluoride Toxicology with Respect to Cattle Damage. Am. J. Vet. Research *13*:38–49, 1952.

SCHMIDT, H. J., NEWELL, G. W., and RAND, W. E.: The Controlled Feeding of Fluorine, as Sodium Fluoride, to Dairy Cattle. Am. J. Vet. Research *15*:232–239, 1954.

SHUPE, J. L., *et al.*: Relative Effects of Feeding Hay Atmospherically Contaminated by Fluoride Residue, Normal Hay Plus Calcium Fluoride, and Normal Hay Plus Sodium Fluoride to Dairy Heifers. Am. J. Vet. Res. *23*:777–787, 1962.

—————: The Effect of Fluorine on Dairy Cattle. V. Fluorine in the Urine as an Estimator of Fluorine Intake. Am. J. Vet. Res. *24*:300–306, 1963.

—————: The Effect of Fluorine on Dairy Cattle. II. Clinical and Pathologic Effects. Am. J.. Vet. Res. *24*:964–979, 1963.

SHUPE, J. L., MINER, M. L., and GREENWOOD, D. A.: Clinical and Pathological Aspects of Fluorine Toxicosis in Cattle. Ann. New York Acad. Sci. *111*:618–637, 1964.

SUTTIE, J. W.: Vertebral Biopsies in the Diagnosis of Bovine Fluoride Toxicosis. Am. J. Vet. Res. *28*:709–712, 1967.

WEATHERELL, J. A., and WEIDMANN, S. M.: The Skeletal Changes of Chronic Experimental Fluorosis. J. Path. Bact. *78*:233–241, 243–255, 1959.

ZIPKIN, I., EANES, E. D., and SHUPE, J. L.: Effect of Prolonged Exposure to Fluoride on the Ash, Fluoride, Citrate, and Crystallinity of Bovine Bone. Am. J. Vet. Res. *25*:1595–1597, 1964.

Group N: **Poisons causing loss of hair or wool.**

Thallium   Jumbay tree

THALLIUM

A heavy metal with toxic effects and atomic weight similar to lead and mercury, thallium may be involved in poisonings of man and animals. The thallous form, particularly thallous sulfate, is most active pharmacologically and is odorless, colorless and tasteless; each of these characteristics favors its use as a pesticide. Although banned by Federal law from sale to the general public for household use, accidental poisonings of children, dogs and cats still occur. Cattle and sheep have also been reported to have eaten poisoned bait. Poisonings from industrial wastes and use of thallium as a depilatory seem to be decreasing.

The clinical signs reflect involvement of several body systems and depend to some extent on the amount of thallium ingested. According to Zook and Gilmore (1967) dogs exhibit these signs in order of frequency: vomiting, cutaneous alterations, depression, anorexia, nervous signs, diarrhea, respiratory distress, conjunctivitis, dehydration and esophageal paralysis. The cutaneous lesions first appear as localized areas of erythema from the third to seventh day after poisoning. Serum oozes from these lesions and in a few days they become covered with thick crusty material. Hair may be plucked easily in early stages, later it may fall readily from large areas of skin. Necrosis and sloughing of skin may eventually occur.

Clinical laboratory findings in dogs, in order of frequency, include: lymphopenia, neutrophilia, eosinopenia, left shift of neutrophils, hemoconcentration and circulating immature red blood cells. Blood urea nitrogen often is elevated. Serum glutamic pyruvic transaminase may be elevated and serum glutamic oxaloacetic transaminase is usually elevated. Proteinuria and bilirubinuria may be present. Elevated specific gravity is characteristic of the urine, presumably due

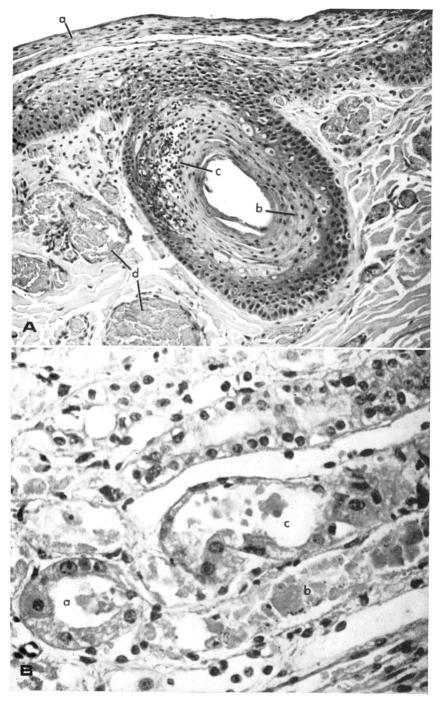

FIG. 17–23.—Thallium poisoning. *A*, Thallium poisoning in a one-year-old male Scottish terrier. Note: (*a*) parakeratosis and acanthosis in the epidermis and the hair follicle (*b*); intraepithelial abscess (*c*) and congestion of capillaries (*d*). *B*, Kidney of a two-year-old castrated male collie which died of thallium poisoning. Note: (*a*) renal tubule with slightly affected cells (cytoplasm swollen, cells partially individualized); tubule with completely necrotic epithelium (*b*) and part of one with some of its cells necrotic (*c*). (Courtesy of Angell Memorial Animal Hospital.)

to dehydration. Glycosuria may be evident and granular casts, erythrocytes, leukocytes and epithelial cells are usually excessive in the urine sediment.

The **microscopic lesions** of thallotoxicosis are found in most systems of the body. The changes in the skin are striking and characteristic (Fig. 17–23A), consisting of severe acanthosis and parakeratosis involving epidermis and hair follicles, occasional intraepithelial abscesses and congestion of epidermal capillaries. Necrosis of isolated renal convoluted tubules is also typical (Fig. 17–23B) with proteinaceous material in some Bowman's spaces. In later stages some leukocytic infiltration may occur, completing the picture of toxic tubular nephrosis (p. 1266). Edema of the lungs is usual and purulent bronchopneumonia may be found in about a third of the cases. Disseminated focal necroses of skeletal and cardiac muscle fibers are constant, with the expected leukocytic infiltration at the sites of necrosis. Spleens and lymph nodes are often edematous and enlarged with hyperplasia of reticuloendothelial elements. Some myelinated nerves may be demonstrated to have some degenerated axons with enlarged, empty myelin sheaths. Aspermatogenesis with formation of multinucleated masses of spermatids is evident in the testes. Ulceration of the esophagus with focal necrosis in nearby muscle fibers is a constant finding. Hepatic lesions are usually limited to early toxic hepatitis with necrosis and distention of sinusoids near central veins. In the brain, lesions may be found in animals in which neurologic involvement is indicated by the clinical signs. These consist of disseminated early necrotic lesions (with chromatolysis and neuronophagia) and edema throughout the cerebellum and cerebrum.

The **gross lesions,** as may be judged from the clinical signs and microscopic findings, consist of: patchy or diffuse areas of cutaneous erythema, alopecia or dermatitis, cardiac hypertrophy, subendocardial hemorrhages, severe congestion of the kidneys, edema and consolidations of the lungs, edema and enlargement of lymph nodes, enlargement of the spleen and dilation, erosion or ulceration of the esophagus.

The pathologic diagnosis is established by the microscopic lesions, particularly those in the skin, and by the chemical demonstration of thallium in urine or tissues.

Thallium

EGYED, M.: Distribution of Thallium in the Body Fluids and Organs of Experimentally Poisoned Sheep. Refuah vet. *25*:81–82, and 108–110, 1968. V.B. *39*:824, 1969.

GABRIEL, K. L. and DUBIN, S.: A Method for the Detection of Thallium in Canine Urine. J. Am. Vet. Med. Assn. *143*:722–724, 1963.

NEWSOM, I. E., LOFTUS, J. B., and WARD, J. C.: The Toxicity of Thallium Sulphate for Sheep. J. Am. Vet. Med. Assn. *76*:826–832, 1930.

PILE, C. H.: Thallium Poisoning in Domestic Felines. Austr. Vet. J. *32*:18–20, 1956.

SCHULTE, F.: Thalliumvergiftung beim Hund. Dtsch. tierarztl. Wschr. *57*:92–93, 1950.

SCHWARTZMAN, R. M. and KIRSCHBAUM, J. O.: The Cutaneous Histopathology of Thallium Poisoning. J. Investig. Dermatology *39*:169–173, 1962.

SKELLEY, J. F., and GABRIEL, K. L.: Thallium Intoxication in the Dog. Ann. New York Acad. Sci. *111*:612–617, 1964.

VACIRCA, G., and AGOSTI, M.: (Thallium Poisoning in Dogs). Veterinaria, Milano *16*: 171–196, 1967. V.B. *37*:4897, 1967.

VISMARA, E.: Reperti dell'avvelenamento spontaneo da tallio nel cane. Atti. Soc. Ital. Sci. Vet. *15*:523–530, 1961.

WENGER, P. and RUSCONI, I.: A New Specific Reaction for the Identification of Thallium. Helv. Chim. Acta. *26*:2263–2264, 1943.

WILLSON, J. E.: Thallotoxicosis (Thallium Poisoning). J. Am. Vet. Med. Assn. *139*:1116–1119, 1961.

ZOOK, B. C., and GILMORE, C. E.: Thallium Poisoning in Dogs. J. Am. Vet. Med. Assn. *151*:206–217, 1967.

ZOOK, B. C., HOLZWORTH, J., and THORNTON, G. W.: Thallium Poisoning in Cats. J. Am. Vet. Med. Assn. *153*:285–299, 1968.

JUMBAY TREE

Leucaena glauca

A chronic poisoning of horses in the Bahamian Islands has been reported by Mullenax. It is due to the consumption for several weeks of the leaves and twigs of a small leguminous tree, *Leucaena glauca*, commonly known as the jumbay. *Leucaena glauca* is known as "Ipil-Ipil" in the Philippines, as "Lamtoro" in Indonesia, "Cow Bush" in Australia. In Hawaii, where it is culti- vated extensively, it is called "Kao Haole," or "Ekoa" or "White Popinac." It is able to grow in the worst kinds of soil and with little water, has good value as forage, may contain up to 30 per cent protein (dry weight) and twice as much carotene as alfalfa. Toxicity is due to an unbound amino acid called mimosine (the plant belongs to the Family Mimosaceae). Horses and pigs are most fre- quently affected; ruminants are less susceptible than monogastric animals. The most striking symptom is partial to complete loss of the long hair of the mane, tail and forelock; if the case is severe a patchy loss above and below the knees and hocks and in the flanks and neck occurs. Experimental feeding of high levels have produced severe stomatitis, hemorrhagic enteritis, proctitis, edema of the hind legs and genitals and chronic laminitis with rings in the hoof. Recovery occurs after feeding is discontinued and possibly some tolerance develops.

Jumbay Tree

MULLENAX, C. H.: A Dietary Cause of Hair Loss in Bahamian Livestock. J. Am. Vet. Med. Assn. *131*:302, 1957.

——————: Observations on *Leucaena glauca*. Aust. Vet. J. *39*:88–91, 1963.

* * * * *

Group O: **A poison causing epithelial hyperplasia.**

CHLORINATED NAPHTHALENES

A well-marked disease entity, known as **hyperkeratosis** previous to the dis- covery of its etiology, has been traced to the presence of highly chlorinated naphthalenes (five or more Cl ions, probably) which gain access to the animal metabolism either through ingestion or cutaneous absorption. While the disease was first described in connection with a wood preservative used on stables in which cattle were kept, a more common source of the naphthalene compounds has been lubricating oils. Such compounds have been found to improve the lubricating properties of the oil, but minute amounts have contaminated com- mercially produced feeds, especially those made into pellets, from the bearings of machines used in the process. Animals have also absorbed the poison through contact with farm machinery so lubricated. Cattle are ordinarily involved, al- though sheep have been poisoned experimentally.

Signs include lacrimation, which may develop within a week after the first contact with the poison, often salivation, afebrile depression, anorexia, emaciation, terminal diarrhea and death after several weeks.

Lesions can be summarized as an overgrowth of epithelium. This includes marked increase of the cornified layer (hyperkeratosis) on those surfaces where the epithelium is already stratified squamous, and squamous metaplasia in many places where it is normally of the columnar type. This results in marked thickening of the skin, especially over the neck and withers, with coarse, deep wrinkling, scaliness and loss of hair. Microscopically, there is some degree of acanthosis with deepening of the rete pegs, but most of the increased thickness is in the cornified layer. The keratohyalin of this layer extends deep into the hair follicles, compressing the surrounding zone of cellular epithelium. The corium commonly shows a noticeable infiltration with lymphocytes.

On the mucosa of the mouth and lips and especially on the tongue, there are likely to be raised "plaques" of thickened, hyperkeratotic epithelium. These average a centimeter or more in diameter. Judging from early experimental cases, they apparently are preceded by shallow ulcers. Similar but smaller nodular proliferations are likely to be found in the esophagus. The same tendency toward nodular increase of epithelium extends through the digestive tract, where thickened spots or areas occasionally develop through hyperplasia of the columnar epithelium, forming cysts filled with mucus and cell debris. This general tendency is more likely to be seen in the gallbladder and in the extrahepatic and intrahepatic bile ducts. The latter often develop thickenings characterized by irregular epithelial-lined cysts which vary from microscopic size up to a diameter of a centimeter. Within the liver, such ducts are encircled by increased fibrous tissue. In a few instances, the changes approach those of biliary cirrhosis (p. 1227). The ducts of the salivary glands and pancreas sometimes show metaplastic changes similar to those in the bile ducts.

In the kidneys, the same tendency toward epithelial hyperplasia reveals itself in enlargement and dilatation of tubules, chiefly the collecting tubules of the medullary rays. The epithelium of these tubules is not compressed but hyperplastic, even to the extent that small papillary projections extend into the lumen. A certain amount of fibrosis accompanies these tubular changes if they are marked.

Squamous metaplasia and cornification are likely to be found in the tubular and glandular organs of the male genitalia, especially in the seminal vesicles.

In sheep, similar squamous metaplasia has been found in the endometrial lining and glands. The epithelium of the cervix may be hyperplastic in both cattle and sheep.

It is not to be expected that all of the above lesions will be found in the same animal. Usually any of them, if unequivocally developed, are sufficient for a diagnosis.

A milder degree of epithelial hyperplasia and hyperkeratosis is characteristic of avitaminosis-A. Investigations have shown that in poisoning by chlorinated naphthalenes the amount of vitamin-A in the blood declines sharply within five days after the first ingestion of the poison. It falls as low as 25 micrograms per 100 ml. but does not reach zero as it almost does in experimental deprivation of the vitamin (p. 981). This anti-vitamin-A effect persists for at least a month after ingestion of the poison has ceased. Feeding five times the normal require-

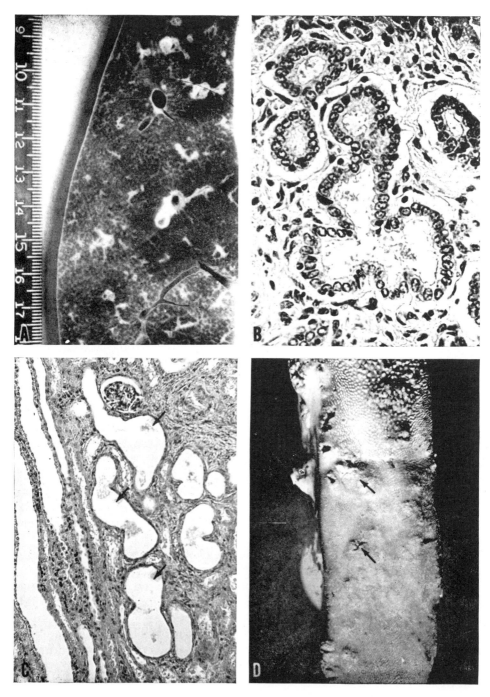

FIG. 17–24.—Poisoning caused by chlorinated naphthalene (bovine hyperkeratosis). *A*, Bovine liver with prominent biliary system. *B*, Hyperplasia of bile ducts ($\times$ 485) in portal region. Contributor: Dr. J. F. Ryff. *C*, Hyperplasia and dilatation of renal tubules (arrows) in a bovine kidney ($\times$ 100). (Courtesy of Armed Forces Institute of Pathology.) Contributors: Drs. Kenneth McEntee and Peter Olafson. *D*, Tongue of an affected cow. Note elevated lesions in epithelium (arrows). Case at Iowa Sch. Vet. Med.

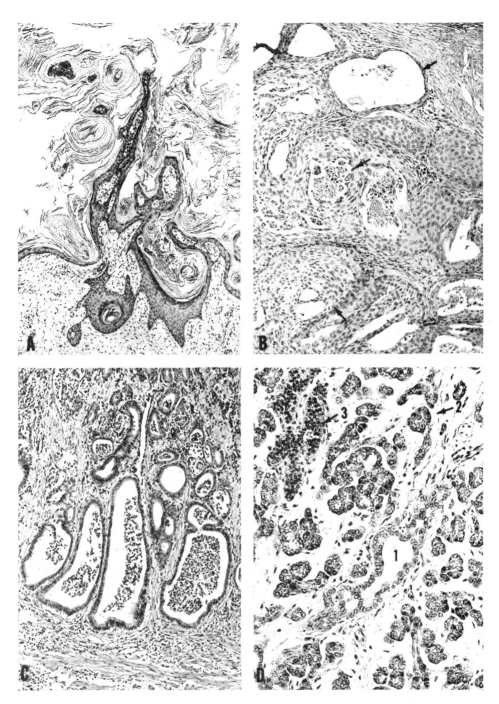

Fig. 17–25.—Poisoning from chlorinated naphthalene (bovine hyperkeratosis). A, Severe hyperkeratosis in bovine skin (× 56). Contributor: Dr. J. F. Ryff. B, Squamous metaplasia of tubular epithelium (arrows) of epididymis (× 100). Contributors: Drs. Kenneth McEntee and Peter Olafson. C, Hyperplasia and cystic dilatation of epithelium in crypts of small intestine (× 70). Contributor: Dr. J. F. Ryff. D, Hyperplasia of ductal epithelium, bovine pancreas (× 195). Duct (1), stroma (2) and island of Langerhans (3). This is more severe than usual. (Courtesy of Armed Forces Institute of Pathology.) Contributor: Dr. J. F. Ryff.

ment of vitamin-A (5 × 5000 I.U. vitamin-A per 100 pounds of body weight per day) maintains a satisfactory amount of the vitamin in both blood and liver against a limited amount of the toxic feed, but this effect is transient and it does not appear that larger amounts of the vitamin are able to keep pace with increases of the poison. If administration of the vitamin is continued adequately beyond the period of ingestion of the poison, some animals recover and some do not. The question of just how the chlorinated naphthalene neutralizes the effect of vitamin-A has baffled investigators. There is evidence that it interferes with conversion of carotene to vitamin-A, doubtless through impairment of the liver, but this is by no means the only toxic action, nor is it possible to duplicate the lesions by deprivation of the vitamin, no matter how complete.

Since the epithelial hyperplasia of this disease sometimes reaches such proportions as to be suggestive of neoplasia, the question arises as to whether chlorinated naphthalenes could possibly have carcinogenic actions. The answer, to date, is entirely in the negative and is supported by extensive experimentation. To the question whether any other substances can have the same effects as chlorinated naphthalenes, the answer is possibly less certain but apparently this also is in the negative.

Chlorinated Naphthalenes

HANSEL, W., McENTEE, K., and OLAFSON, P.: The Effects of Two Causative Agents of Experimental Hyperkeratosis on Vitamin-A Metabolism. Cornell Vet. *41*:367–376, 1951.
HOEKSTRA, W. G., HALL, R. E., and PHILLIPS, P. H.: Relationship of Vitamin-A to the Development of Hyperkeratosis (X Disease) in Calves. Am. J. Vet. Research *15*:41–46, 1954.
KNOCKE, K. W.: Hyperakeratose in einem Rinderbestand 13 Jahre nach Anwendung eines Holzschutmittels. Dtsch. tierärztl. *68*:701–703, 1961.
OLAFSON, P.: Hyperkeratosis (X Disease) of Cattle. Cornell Vet. *37*:279–291, 1947.
PALLASKE, G.: Zur pathologischen Anatomie der Chlornaphthalinvergiftung der Rinder. Monatsheft f. Veterinärmed *11*:677–678, 1956.
SCHMIDT, H. and FRANKLIN, T. E.: Hyperakeratosis Investigations in Texas, 1946–56. Bul. MP-316, Texas Agric. Exp. Sta., 1958.
SIKES, D., and BRIDGES, M. E.: Experimental Production of Hyperkeratosis ("X Disease") of Cattle with a Chlorinated Naphthalene. Science *116*:506–507, 1952.
TEUSCHER, R.: Ein seltener klinischer Fall von zweimaliger Vergiftung unes Rinderbestandes durch chloriente naphthaline. Monatsheft. f. Veterinärmed. *11*:675–677, 1956.
WAGENER. K.: Hyperkeratosis of Cattle in Germany. J. Am. Vet. Med. Assn. *119*:133–137, 1951.

*　*　*　*　*

Group P:　**Poisons causing nervous malfunction** with or without demonstrable lesions in the tissues. Those at the first of the list are characterized by hyperirritability; those at the last, by nervous depression, paralysis or coma. In the case of some of these, diagnosis is better made from the symptoms than from the lesions, although both forms of abnormality should be carefully considered.

Strychnine	Claviceps paspali	Lathyrus	Carbon disulfide
Nitrogen trichloride	Deadly nightshade	Larkspur	Ortho-tricresyl
Loco	Equisetum	Yellow Star Thistle	Phosphate
Vetch-like Astragali	Hemlocks	Botulinus	Lead
		Anguina	Mercury
			Chlorinated hydrocarbons
			Organic phosphates
			Cycada

STRYCHNINE

The intermittent tonic spasms, initiated by noises or other external stimuli, provide a well-known symptomatology which is practically diagnostic. Their physiological basis is stated to be hyperirritability and lack of normal inhibitory restraint in the spinal part of the spinal reflex arc. There are no post-mortem lesions, except possibly petechiae resulting from the anoxia incident to arrest of respiration during the spasms. The very absence of lesions often has diagnostic significance when associated with typical symptoms. The drug can be identified by chemical procedures or by microscopic identification of typical crystals, but both methods are complicated and expensive. If a frog is available, an infusion of suspected ingesta or urine can be inoculated either into the dorsal lymph space or the peritoneum with the result that the frog shows the characteristic tonic spasms when irritated by touch. This should occur within twenty minutes. The test is regarded as highly sensitive; the urine of any dog fatally poisoned is stated to contain sufficient strychnine at death for a positive test. In addition to malicious poisoning, accidents in the use of strychnine-containing rodent and grasshopper poisons afford instances of poisoning.

Strychnine

Cox, D. H.: Isolation and Identification of Strychnine and Other Alkaloids in Veterinary Toxicology. Am. J. Vet. Res. *18*:929–931, 1957.

Thienpont, D. and Vandervelden, M.: Dichapetalum michelsonii Hauman, Nouvelle Plante Toxique pour le Betail du Ruanda-Burundi. Rev. Elev. *14*:209–211, 1961.

NITROGEN TRICHLORIDE

Under the trade name of **Agene,** nitrogen trichloride, NCl_3, has been used extensively as a bleaching agent in the production of white flour from wheat. At least as early as the 1920's, dogs have been afflicted with a nervous disorder called **fright disease, hysteria** or **running fits.** Some dogs become sullen, but a larger number have spells when they suddenly appear frightened. With a wild and unnatural expression, the dog may run off for a very considerable distance, returning after five to thirty minutes in an exhausted and depressed condition. This may be repeated on subsequent occasions, and before many days incoordination and ataxia become prominent. Such a "running fit" may begin and quickly terminate in convulsions of one or two minutes' duration. Ultimately death may ensue.

The observation made in Europe that this syndrome appeared to be restricted to dogs fed biscuits made from certain flours imported from the United States during the years immediately following World War II led to the discovery that the cause was the toxic effect of this bleaching agent in the flour. Nitrogen trichloride has been found toxic to dogs, ferrets and rabbits but not to guinea pigs, cats, monkeys and humans. Several nontoxic bleaching agents, particularly chlorine dioxide, ClO_2, have now largely replaced the earlier product. The lesions have been studied by Lewey (1950) and found to consist chiefly of patchy necrosis in the deeper parts of the cerebral cortex with beginning liquefaction and rather similar changes in the hippocampus. The nerve cells show the usual changes of necrosis, shrinking, distortion, loss of structure and eventual disappearance. These changes are not obvious grossly.

Nitrogen Trichloride

IMPEY, S. G., MOORE, T., and SHARMAN, I. M.: Effect of Flour Treatment on the Suitability of Bread as Food for Dogs. J. Sci. Fd. Ag. *12*:729–732, 1961.
LEWEY, F. H.: Neuropathological Changes in Nitrogen Trichloride Intoxication of Dogs. J. Neuropath. and Exper. Neurol. *9*:396–405, 1950.

LOCO

A nervous disorder (*loco*, Spanish for madness) related to consumption of certain plants (loco weeds) was first recognized in the horses of De Soto and other Spanish Conquistadores during their explorations of the New World. The offending plants grow particularly in the Western United States and are classified in the genus *Astragalus*, such as *A. earlei*, *A. mollissimus* (purple woolly loco), *A. pubentissimus* and *A. lentiginosus* or in the genus *Oxytropis*, such as, *O. sericea* and *O. lambertii*. In Australia, plants, such as *Swainsona luteola*, *S. greyana* and *S. galegifolia*, are known as the cause of a similar disease ("pea struck") in sheep (Kater, 1965) which has been reproduced experimentally in guinea pigs (Huxtable, 1969). The active principle in all loco weeds appears to be **locoine.**

Teratogenic effects have been observed in nature and reproduced experimentally in sheep (James, Keeler and Binns, 1969). Feeding of *Astragalus pubentissimus* to pregnant sheep results in frequent occurrence of congenital anomalies in the offspring. The type of anomaly appears to be dependent upon the stage of pregnancy during which the loco weed is eaten. If this loco weed is consumed by the ewes during the twenty-fifth to the forty-ninth days of pregnancy, aplasia of the lower jaw is the dominant congenital anomaly in the lambs. Ingestion of *A. pubentissimus* between the fortieth to sixtieth days of pregnancy often results in hypermobility of the hock and stifle joints in affected lambs. Feeding the plant between the sixtieth and ninetieth days of gestation results in offspring with flexures of carpal joints. Lambs born of ewes which ingested loco between the one hundredth and one hundred twentieth days of pregnancy, are apt to have relaxed pastern joints. Abortions are common and some ewes die from this plant poisoning. *Oxytropis sericea* has also been fed to ewes between the eighty-second and one hundred second days of gestation, leading to contracted flexor tendons (or muscles) in the offspring. A few cases of arthrogryposis (see lupines, p. 884) have been associated with loco weed poisoning.

Experimental feeding of rams on loco weeds has been shown by Shupe, *et al.* (1968) to result in loss of weight of the body and testes, but to produce no effect on libido or sperm counts. Clinical laboratory findings have been reported by James and Binns (1967) to consist of elevated levels of serum glutamic oxaloacetic transaminase and serum glutamic pyruvic transaminase; increased retention of sulfobromophthalein administered as a dye test; slight increase in blood urea nitrogen and an increase in blood proteins, particularly the gamma and alpha 2 globulin fractions. No changes were observed in red and white blood cell counts, blood glucose, serum vitamin A, serum phosphorus, cholinesterase in red blood cells, hemoglobin or red blood cell volume.

The disease develops slowly in cattle; consumption over a period of sixty days of an amount equal to 90 per cent of the body weight is necessary to produce symptoms; ninety-eight days and 3.2 times the animal's weight are the minimum likely to cause death. In the horse, however, consumption equivalent to only 30 per cent of the animal's weight during a period of forty-nine days has

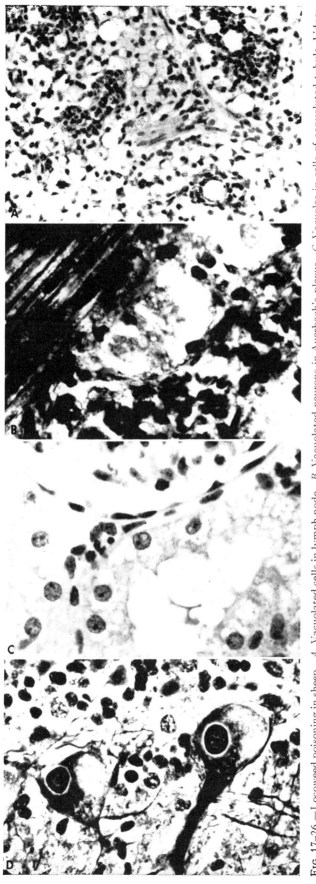

Fig. 17–26.—Locoweed poisoning in sheep. *A*, Vacuolated cells in lymph node. *B*, Vacuolated neurons in Auerbach's plexus. *C*, Vacuoles in cells of convoluted tubule, kidney. *D*, Cytoplasmic vacuolation in Purkinje cells. (Courtesy of Dr. Kent R. Van Kampen and *Pathologia Veterinaria*.)

been fatal experimentally (Mathews, 1946). In the horse, hyperexcitability, fright and violent reactions to slight stimuli are the early signs of loco poisoning. Much of this may be due, however, to inability to see clearly. The same impaired vision and disordered judgment cause a cow to perform all the movements of drinking while her mouth is 6 inches above the water. The sensory and motor derangements increase until the animal is unable to get food for itself. A slowly increasing ataxia of the limbs has by this time become an ascending paralysis, so that death results from a combination of nervous failure and starvation. Sheep are depressed from the start; goats suffer from posterior paresis and ascending paralysis beginning in the initial stages, with opisthotonos at the last. In all species, the terminal aspects are similar.

The **microscopic lesions,** described in detail by Van Kampen and James (1969) in sheep experimentally poisoned with *Oxytropis sericea, Astragalas pubentissimus* or *A. lentigimosus*, tend to explain the clinical signs. The principal lesion is the result of accumulation of vacuoles in the cytoplasm of cells of various tissues. The nature of this cytoplasmic lesion has not been determined but the accumulated material which imparts the vacuolated appearance in sections seen by light microscopy is not lipid or glycoprotein as indicated by negative reactions to oil-red-O and PAS stains. The material does accumulate in the cytoplasm, displacing the nucleus to one side and eventually, at least in neurons, leads to necrosis.

Damage to neurons is most significant and may be found in any part of the central and peripheral nervous systems, including those in Meissner's and Auerbach's plexuses in the gastrointestinal tract.

In late stages, karyolysis, karyorrhexis or cytolysis leads to loss of neurons or mineralization of the necrotic remnants. Axonal degeneration may be found but myelin is not significantly altered. Gliosis and neuronophagic nodules are not conspicuous. Perivascular edema is usually evident throughout the central nervous system.

Accumulations of material similar to that noted in neurons have been described in many other organs, including the follicular epithelium of the thyroid, chief cells of parathyroid, adrenal cortical cells, serous cells of salivary glands, hepatocytes, reticulo-endothelial cells of lymph nodes and spleen, epithelial cells of renal convoluted tubules and transitional epithelium of the urinary tract. The vacuolated, sometimes foamy appearance of affected cells has been compared to some lipid storage diseases of man but of course the cytoplasmic material is not the same. Perhaps further studies with electron microscopy or histochemistry will reveal the precise nature of this lesion and give a clue to the exact effect of the toxin on cells.

Nearly identical vacuolar lesions in neurons, and renal epithelium were encountered by Laws and Anson (1968) in sheep poisoned naturally and experimentally by eating *Swainsona luteola* and *S. galegifolia*. James, Van Kampen and Hartley, 1970, compared the toxic effects on pregnant ewes of *Swainsonia galegifolia, Astragalus pubentissimus* and *A. lentiginosus* and concluded that the active poisonous principle in each of these plants may be the same.

The **gross lesions** are not diagnostic but enlargement of thyroids, emaciation, golden color of liver and renal cortex, generalized edema, and focal erosions in the mucosa of the abomasum near the pyloris have been described. In pregnant cows, the severe edema may resemble **hydrops amnii** (p. 1322). Similarities in clinical signs and chemical interrelationships have suggested that some of the toxins in locoweeds are related to those of lathyrus (p. 951).

Loco

FRAPS, G. S., and CARLYLE, E. C.: Locoine, the Poisonous Principle of Loco Weed. Exper. Sta. Bull. 537, 1936. Texas A. & M. College, College Station.

HUXTABLE, C. R.: Experimental Reproduction and Histo-pathology of *Swainsona galegifolia* Poisoning in the Guinea-pig. Aust. J. Exp. Biol. Med. Sci. *47*:339–347, 1969.

JAMES, L. F., and BINNS, W.: Blood Changes Associated with Locoweed Poisoning. Am. J. Vet. Res. *28*:1107–1110, 1967.

JAMES, L. F., KEELER, R. F., and BINNS, W.: Sequence in the Abortive and Teratogenic Effects of Locoweed Fed to Sheep. Am. J. Vet. Res. *30*:377–380, 1969.

JAMES, L. F., VAN KAMPEN, K. R., and HARTLEY, W. J.: Comparative Pathology of *Astragalus* (Locoweed) and *Swainsonia* Poisoning in Sheep. Path. Vet. *7*:116–125, 1970.

KATER, J. C.: Some Observations on the Pathology of Swainsona Poisoning in Sheep, and Possible Lines of Further Investigation. Vet. Insp. N. S. W. *28*:58–59, 1964.

LAWS, L., and ANSON, R. B.: Neuropathology in Sheep Fed *Swainsona luteola* and *Swainsona galegifolia*. Aust. Vet. J. *44*:447–452, 1968.

MATHEWS, F. P.: The Poisonous Astragali. The Veterinary Student. Fall, 1946. pp. 26–30. Iowa State College, Ames, Iowa.

NOCKOLDS, C.: Poisoning by Loco Weed. Am. Vet. Rev. *20*:569–571, 1896.

SCHWARTZKOPF, D.: Effects of "Loco Weed." Am. Vet. Rev. *12*:160–163, 1888.

SHUPE, J. L., *et al.*: The Effect of Loco Plant on Libido and Fertility in Rams. Cornell Vet. *58*:59–66, 1968.

VAN KAMPEN, K. R., and JAMES, L. F.: Pathology of Locoweed Poisoning in Sheep. Path. Vet. *6*:413–423, 1969.

VETCH-LIKE ASTRAGALI

A number of small leguminous plants which resemble the true vetches and sometimes receive that designation produce poisoning on the ranges of the Rocky Mountain region of the United States. They are classified, however, in the genus *Astragalus*, which is notable because of the loco weeds (above) which are also included in it. The form of poisoning produced, like loco, involves the nervous system principally and does not resemble the hepatotoxic effects of the true vetches.

Under the name of timber milkvetch, we may include *Astragalus decembens*, *A. convallarius*, *A. hylophilus* and *A. compestris*, which are very similar or identical species. The *red-stemmed peavine*, *A. emoryanus*, is a similar plant; it grows in the more southern regions, whereas the timber milkvetch reaches north into Canada.

Another classification of these plants (Williams, Van Kampen and Norris, 1969) places several varieties in a single genus, *Astragalus miser*. These are : *A. miser var oblongifolius, serotinus, hylophilus, miser, tenuifolius, praeteritus, decumbens* and *crispatus*. The first three have been incriminated in poisoning of livestock. Cattle appear to be most susceptible, sheep much less so, rabbits and chickens may be poisoned experimentally. The basic sign is nervous weakness and incoordination involving the hind limbs. When mild, this may be shown only by a momentary sinking of the hindquarters at the start of a forward movement. Later there is distinct incoordination such as crossing of the legs and weakness shown by "knuckling over" of the fetlock joints. Ultimately, the animal falls frequently and rises with difficulty. In the cattle poisoned by milkvetch, the metatarsal and phalangeal joints are abnormally relaxed and poorly controlled so that in walking the dewclaws (first metatarsal rudiments) strike the hoofs with a flapping sound. This has resulted in the nickname of "cracker-heel" for the disease. In sheep, another prominent, and at times primary, symptom is dyspnea accompanied by a loud rasping noise at inspiration and a cough frequently at expiration. The morphological basis for this seems not to have been determined. It may be presumed that complete microscopic studies of the nervous system would reveal degenerative changes which would account for the posterior weakness. On the other hand, the fact that a considerable number of victims die suddenly from acute dilatation of the heart, while the usual difficulties are yet at an early stage, raises the suspicion of interference with the metabolic processes of muscle. It should be noted that, while the posterior weakness and paraplegia are much like the corresponding effects of the closely related locoweeds (*Astragalus mollissimus et spp.*), there are no disturbances of sensation or of the sensorium in the presently considered poisonings.

One toxic agent has been identified as miserotoxin, the β glucoside of 3-nitro-1-propanol. This toxin is catabolized *in vivo* to two toxic fractions, inorganic nitrite and a 3-carbon nitro side chain (Williams, Van Kampen and Norris, 1969). Nitrite (NO_2) produces methemoglobinemia (p. 69) particularly in rabbits.

Vetch-like Astragali

MATHEWS, F. P.: Toxicity of Red-Stemmed Peavine for Cattle, Sheep and Goats. J. Am. Vet. Med. Assn. *97*:125–134, 1940.
NEWSOM, I. E. *et al.*: Timber Milk Vetch as a Poisonous Plant. Exper. Sta. Bull. 425, 1936. Colorado State College, Fort Collins.
WILLIAMS, M. C., VAN KAMPEN, K. R., and NORRIS, F. A.: Timber Milkvetch Poisoning in Chickens, Rabbits, and Cattle. Am. J. Vet. Res. *30*:2185–2190, 1969.

CLAVICEPS PASPALI

A so-called ergot, *Claviceps paspali*, grows upon Dallis grass (*Paspalum dilatatum*), a pasture plant of the Southern United States and produces what is known as Dallis-grass poisoning. This ergot (sclerotium), like the seed it replaces, is much smaller than that of *Claviceps purpurea* and often of a brownish color. Symptoms of **Dallis-grass poisoning** appear after cattle have had access to parasitized seedheads of the grass for a few or several days. They are essentially nervous in character and manifest themselves in (1) nervous hyperirritability, excitability and even belligerency, and (2) muscular incoordination. The latter is worse when the cow or horse is excited and results, as it grows worse, in frequent falling and eventual inability to stand. Many recover with a change in feed. Gross lesions are minimal and microscopic studies appear to have been neglected. However, some have attributed certain forms of dermatitis to this fungus.

A symptomatically similar disease has occurred in certain years among cattle on the "bunch grass" ranges of the northern Rocky Mountain regions (Columbia basin of the state of Washington), and an ergot on the grass has been suspected. A more or less identical disease terminating in complete paralysis has been traced to *Claviceps paspali* in Southern Russia. Information is not available as to the species of grass involved. (The term ergotism [p. 927], as commonly understood, applies only to the disease caused by *C. purpurea*.)

Claviceps paspali

PEREK, M.: *Claviceps paspali* in Pasture as a Cause of Poisoning in Cattle in Israel. Refuah. Vet. *12*:106–110, 1955.

PEREK, M. Ergot and Ergot-Like Fungi as the Cause of Vesicular Dermatitis (Sod Disease) in Chickens. J. Am. Vet. Med. Assn. *132*:529–533, 1958.

SIMMS, B. T.: Dallis Grass Poisoning. Auburn Veterinarian. Summer, 1945.

TATRISHVILI, P. S. [Pathology of Experimental *Claviceps paspali* Poisoning in Livestock.] Trud. vsesoyuz. Inst. eksp. Vet. *20*:226–237, 1957. Abstr. Vet. Bull. No. 3383, 1958.

ATROPINE

Deadly Nightshade, Belladonna

The foliage and the unripe berries of the belladonna plant (*Atropa belladonna*) poison swine and rarely other animals by virtue of the atropine (and other alkaloids) which they contain. Symptoms are largely those of loss of nervous control with incoordination shortly followed by convulsions and death, usually within twelve hours after the plant is eaten. There are typically mydriasis, falling temperature and a failing heart. Post-mortem lesions are not diagnostic but may include subserous sero-fibrinous exudations, perhaps tinged with blood, especially around the kidneys and gallbladder. Of prime importance in diagnosis is the mydriatic action of belladonna. Not only are the patient's pupils dilated, but instillation of a small amount of the patient's urine into the conjunctival sac of a small experimental animal, particularly a cat, dog or rabbit, should dilate the pupil within a few minutes.

Belladonna

SMITH, H. C., TAUSSIG, R. A., and PETERSON, P. C.: Deadly Nightshade Poisoning in Swine. J. Am. Vet. Med. Assn. *129*:116–117, 1956.

EQUISETUM

Known by such names as **horsetail,** mare's tail and jointed rush, several species of equisetum, of which *E. arvense* is the most common, are poisonous, chiefly to horses. Signs are those of nervous disorder and muscular weakness, the latter probably related to faulty innervation. Incoordination gradually increases until there are staggering, reeling and ultimately inability to stand. Progressive muscular rigidity reaches the point where the animal can only lie on its side with the four limbs stiffly outstretched. Constipation and tenesmus are marked. Large amounts of watery urine are voided. The pupils are dilated; the animal's expression and actions reveal a state of apprehension which deepens into fright as the result of noises or other stimuli. In a recumbent state, the horse continues to live for several days, maintaining a good appetite until too weak to eat.

Lesions found post mortem include a pale and flabby state of the skeletal musculature, frequently hydroperitoneum and marked congestion and inflammatory edema (serous exudate, p. 153) of the cerebellar and spinal meninges. Microscopic studies are needed, especially of the nervous tissues and of the kidneys, which appear from the polyuria to be damaged.

It is found that poisoning by equisetum is prevented and usually cured by the administration of large amounts of thiamine (vitamin-B₁) but not by other components of the B-complex. From this it is inferred that equisetum owes its toxicity to a powerful opponent of thiamine; indeed an extract of the plant has been shown to neutralize thiamine *in vitro*. Biochemical studies by Forenbacher have shown that carbohydrate metabolism was impaired in equisetum poisoning in the same way that it is in thiamine deficiency. Glycolysis by the blood *in vitro* was diminished. Glucose tolerance in the living animal was depressed, as were the amounts of glycogen in liver and muscle. The pyruvic acid in the blood rose to 1.52 mg. per 100 ml., with oxalic acid behaving similarly; phosphates reached levels of 13 mg. and potassium 50 mg. The levels of alkaline phosphatase and cholesterinase also rose. (See thiaminase, p. 985 and polioencephalomalacia, p. 1409.)

Equisetum

FORENBACHER, S.: Otrovanje konja preslicom (Equisetum L.) i kompleks vitamina B. [Equisetum Poisoning of Horses and the Vitamin B Complex.] Vet. Arhiv. *20*:405–471, 1950, and *21*:497–547, 1951. (English summary.) Abstr. Vet. Bull. No. 2671, 1953; also in Schweiz. Arch. f. Tierheilk. *94*:153–171, 1952.
HENDERSON, J. A. *et al.*: The Antithiamine Action of Equisetum. J. Am. Vet. Med. Assn. *120*:375–378, 1952.
LOTT, D. G.: The Use of Thiamin in Mare's Tail Poisoning of Horses. Canad. J. Comp. Med. *15*:274–276, 1951.
RICH, F. A.: Equisetum Poisoning. Am. Vet. Rev. *26*:944–954, 1903.

HEMLOCKS

Poisoning by Deadly Hemlock, *Conium maculatum*, has been recognized since the dawn of history. Ancient Greeks compelled condemned prisoners (Socrates the most famous) to drink an infusion of this plant, causing a relatively painless death. Herbivorous animals, including swine, occasionally eat the plant in spite of unpalatability and an offensive odor which it releases when bruised. After a mild and very transient stimulation, the plant acts as a nerve depressant and it is upon this nervous depression that the signs are based. While varying somewhat in different species, they involve loss of muscular strength and gradual loss of the power of locomotion, the hind limbs, as is usual in nervous and paralytic disorders, being the most severely affected. In some cases, there are tremors and rarely generalized trembling, but more often the animal's activities quietly subside into a sort of coma in which consciousness appears to be greatly depressed but not disordered. Death may come in an hour or thereabouts, but many animals remain comatose for one or several hours and then quietly recover. In cattle, lacrimation, salivation, dyspnea and fetid or bloody diarrhea have been described. Signs usually commence within an hour or two after the plants are eaten and last for several hours or a day or two.

The post-mortem lesions are based upon the cardiac depressant action of the poison, which is an alkaloid called coniine. As a consequence of the slow cardiac failure there is widespread passive congestion, most noticeable in the lungs and liver and the vessels which nourish the heart muscle. It would appear from descriptions of "watery blood" that there is probably hemolysis or decreased clotting power, or both, but opportunities for systematic studies have seldom arisen. Severe localized catarrhal or hemorrhagic enteritis have been described in cattle. Recognizable fragments of leaves or stems may be found in the fore-stomachs of ruminants and true stomachs of other species, constituting a valuable aid in diagnosis.

There is also a very similar plant, *Cicuta douglasii et spp.*, which grows in wet places in the Rocky Mountain region of the United States, and which is known as Hemlock, **Water Hemlock** or Poison Hemlock.   Its large, chambered primary stem and the adjoining roots are especially poisonous.   It differs from *Conium maculatum* in causing convulsions of the greatest violence, which are almost always fatal.

Also of interest are the Poisonous Quails of North Africa, which in both biblical and modern times have poisoned people who ate their flesh.   Evidence indicates that the meat of the quails contained the poisonous principle of hemlock plants which the birds had eaten.   The much greater resistance of birds to many poisons than that possessed by mammals is a well-known phenomenon.

Hemlocks

AGGIO, C.: Two Interesting Outbreaks of Vegetable Poisoning. Am. Vet. Rev. *32*:368–369, 1907.

BUCKINGHAM, J. L.: Poisoning in a Pig by Hemlock (*Conium maculatum*). Vet. J. *92*:301–302, 1936.

DURREL, L. W. *et al.*: Poisonous and Injurious Plants in Colorado. Exper. Sta. Bull. 412-A, Colorado A. & M. College, Fort Collins.

GUNN, A.: Cattle Poisoned by Hemlock. Vet. J. and Ann. Comp. Path. *13*:233–235, 1881.

MACDONALD, H.: Hemlock Poisoning in Horses. Vet. Rec. *49*:1211–1212, 1937.

SERGENT, E.: Les cailles empoisonneuses dans la Bible, et an Algérie de nos jours. Aperçu historique et recherches expérimentales. Arch. Inst. Pasteur D'Algérie *19*:161–192, 1941.

————: Les cailles empoisonneuses en france. (Toxicity of flesh after ingestion of seeds of *Conium maculatum* or *Oenanthe crocata*.) Arch. Inst. Pasteur D'Algérie *26*:249–252, 1948.

LATHYRUS

Although there are several other closely related toxic species, the principal one is *Lathyrus sativus*.   Several common names are in use, including Indian pea, dogtooth pea, flat pea and Singletary pea.   *Lathyrus odoratus* is the common sweet pea grown in flower gardens for its fragrance.   *L. sativus* is also known in some English-speaking countries as "chickling vetch" but it is not to be confused with the usual vetchcs, which belong to a different genus, although they are, indeed, leguminous plants of generally similar appearance.   *Lathyrus sativus*, frequently in mixture with the closely related *L. cicera* and *L. clymenum*, are grown as forage plants especially in Mediterranean countries and India, and the seeds are a frequent article of human food.   Under the name of "lathyrism," poisoning from excessive consumption of the seeds is well known in humans and domestic animals, especially horses.   Since, in limited amounts, it is a nutritious legume, rich in protein, and because of its hardiness, it has been introduced into the agricultural regions of Africa, Canada and the mountainous ranges of the United States.

Poisoning only occurs when large amounts of seeds are eaten over a period of at least a few weeks, more often months.   In man and animals, the one outstanding symptom is gradually increasing paralysis of the posterior (inferior) limbs.   This is said to depend upon degeneration and disappearance of neurons in the spinal cord accompanied by gliosis and ultimate atrophy of the cord. Since many well-established cases, human and animal, recover, it is difficult to believe that irreversible changes occur until the late stages of illness.   Some refer to the changes in the cord as inflammatory rather than degenerative.   Paralysis of the recurrent laryngeal nerve with the production of "roaring" has been noted several times in horses.   In cattle, blindness, torticollis and anesthesia of the skin are additional symptoms that have been recorded. In any species, the pulse becomes rapid and weak because of incipient vagal paralysis. Constipation and mild digestive disturbances occur occasionally. Death is from respiratory paralysis.

In addition to the lesions of the spinal cord, there are mild chronic enteritis, perhaps with cecal or other impactions, terminal subepicardial hemorrhages (asphyxiative) and pulmonary congestion. The work of Lee and of Huang *et al.* appears to have excluded anti-oxidant, anti-enzymic or anti-vitaminic processes, formerly suspected, as the fundamental pathogenetic mechanisms.

Ground sweet pea seeds (*Lathyrus odoratus*) fed to growing rats result in striking skeletal deformities and changes in other mesodermal tissues. Periosteal new bone formation, kyphoscoliosis and dissecting aneurysms of the aorta occurred, presumably as a result of severe disturbance of the growth of cartilage, bone or elastic tissues. Paralysis in these rats appeared to result either from pressure upon segments of the spinal cord, as a consequence of the severe scoliosis, or from specific destruction of neurons in the cord. The effect upon bone, cartilage and tendons is considered by Levene (1962) to be the result of impairment of cross-linkage of collagen molecules. The active principles are often referred to as osteolathyrogens or neurolathyrogens, depending upon their effects. Some evidence has accrued (Mennin and Thomas, 1970) that some of these compounds may affect both bone and nervous tissue. The principal lathyrogenic compounds now known are: aminoacetonitrile, a,r-diaminobutyric acid, B-aminopropionitrile, B-cyanoalanine, B-N-oxalyl-L-2,3 diaminopropionic acid, r-glutamyl-B-cyanoalanine and r-glutamyl-B-aminopropionitrile.

Poisoning of pregnant animals, particularly sheep, has been shown by Keeler, *et al.* (1967) to result in abortions, intrauterine death, contracted tendons and aplasia of the lower jaw in the offspring. Thus this group of plant toxins has a teratogenic potential (p. 971).

In turkeys, lathyrism is associated with dissecting aneurysms of the aorta.

Lathyrus

BACHAUBER, T. E., and LALICK, J. J.: "The Effect of Sweet Pea Meal on the Rat Aorta." Arch. Path. *59*:247–253, 1955.

BACHHUBER, T. E. *et al.*: Lathyrus-Factor Activity of Beta-aminoproprionitrile and Related Compounds. Proc. Soc. Exper. Biol. and Med. *89*:294–297, 1955.

CAMERON, J. M.: Lathyrism-like Changes in Chicks. J. Path. Bact. *82*:519–521, 1961.

CLEARY, E. G.: Lathyrism in Swine. Aust. J. Exp. Biol. Med. Sci. *46*:8–9, 1968.

HUANG, T. C., CUNHA, T. J., and HAM, W. E.: Deleterious Effects of Flat Pea Seeds for Rats. Am. J. Vet. Res. *11*:217–220, 1950.

KEELER, R. F., *et al.*: An Apparent Relationship between Locoism and Lathyrism. Canad. J. Comp. Med. *31*:334–341, 1967.

LEE, J. G.: Experimental Lathryism Produced by Feeding Singletary Pea (*Lathyrus Pusillus*) Seed. J. Nutrition *40*:587–594, 1950.

LEVENE, C. I.: Studies on the Mode of Action of Lathyrogenic Compounds. J. Exp. Med. *116*:119–133, 1962.

LEVENE, C. I., and GROSS, J.: Alterations in State of Molecular Aggregation of Collagen Induced in Chick Embryos by β-Aminopropionitrile (Lathyrus Factor). J. Exp. Med. *110*: 771–789, 1959.

McKAY, G. F., and LALICH, J. J.: A Crystalline "Lathyrus Factor" from *Lathyrus odoratus.* Arch. Biochem. *52*:313–322, 1954.

MENNIN, S., and THOMAS, D. W.: Comparative Effects of an Osteolathyrogen and a Neurolathyrogen on Brain and Connective Tissues. Proc. Soc. Exp. Biol. Med. *134*:489–491, 1970.

PETRI, E.: *Pathologische Anatomie und Histologie der Vergiftungen*, in Lubarsch, O., and Henke, F.: Handbuch der speziellen pathologischen Anatomie und Histologie, 1930. Berlin, J. Springer, vol. 10.

PONSETI, I. V., and SHEPARD, R. S.: Lesions of the Skeleton and Other Mesodermal Tissues in Rats Fed Sweet-Pea Seeds. J. Bone and Joint Surg. *36-A*:1031–1058, 1954.

SEYLE, H.: Lathyrism. Rev. Canad. Biol. *16*:1–82, 1957.

YEAGER, V. L., and TAYLOR, J. J.: Lathyrism and Aging. Proc. Soc. Exp. Biol. & Med. *129*:44–46, 1968.

ZAHOR, Z. and MACHOVA, M.: Dissecting Aneurisms of the Large Arteries of Chick Embryos Due to (Sweat Pea) Lathyrism. Nature, Lond. *192*:532–533, 1961.

LARKSPUR

Delphinium sp.

Larkspurs of several different species cause considerable poisoning of cattle and horses on the ranges of the Western United States. Symptoms appear in a short time after the plant is eaten and terminate favorably or unfavorably usually within twenty-four hours. While there are salivation, repeated swallowing and signs of nausea, the most prominent symptoms are related to extreme neuro-muscular weakness with sprawling gait, staggering and finally falling and inability to rise. Muscular quivering is followed toward the end by convulsions and death. The post-mortem lesions are acute catarrhal gastroenteritis (hyperemia chiefly) and the widespread venous congestion typical of gradual cardiac failure. Congestion is especially prominent in the kidneys, as well as in the vena cava and large veins.

Larkspur

MARSH, C. D., CLAWSON, A. B., and MARSH, H.: Larkspur Poisoning of Livestock. Bull. 365. U.S. Dept. Agr. 1916.

YELLOW STAR THISTLE

A plant which grows abundantly in dry, weedy pastures in the northern valleys of the state of California, *Centaurea solstitialis*, popularly known as the yellow star thistle, is credited, on the basis of clinical and experimental studies, with causing an equine central nervous disorder called "chewing disease" by stockmen.

Signs appear suddenly after the animal has been eating the plant for from one to three months and has consumed several hundred pounds of it. They consist essentially of hypertonicity of the muscles of the face, lips and tongue due to hyperirritability of the nervous mechanism controlling them, the whole being dependent upon loss of central control from the higher centers. Local reflexes and sensation remain intact. The horse performs involuntary chewing movements but is unable effectively to obtain food or swallow it. The lips are rigid and the skin is puckered, although the angles of the mouth are not necessarily retracted as in the risus sardonicus of some other nervous disorders. The mouth may be held half open with the tongue protruding, although the animal is able to withdraw the latter and there is no (flaccid) paralysis. A mild degree of somnolence usually prevails, and some disturbance of gait, but death eventually results from starvation or thirst in horses so severely affected that they are unable to drink.

Post mortem, the dorsum of the tongue is regularly coated with the dried salivary and other material which accumulates with cessation of swallowing, and there is often a tendency to local edema and buccal ulceration, perhaps from injury in efforts to eat. Some cases develop entero-colitis, which may or may not be due directly to the poison. The fundamental lesion was found by Cordy (1954) to consist in localized encephalomalacia (necrosis) involving the anterior portions of the globus pallidus and substantia nigra. The necrotic areas were sharply demarcated, roundly elongated and as much as 10 to 15 mm. in greatest dimension. Slightly yellowish or buff in color, the areas were gelatinous and bulging in the early stages, distinctly soft at one or two weeks of age and were cavities filled with semifluid debris at three weeks. The lesions were usually bilaterally symmetrical; when they were unilateral the peripheral disturbances were contralateral. Microscopically, the early lesions (two to five days) showed pyknosis and karyolysis of neuroglial nuclei and gradual disappearance of neurons, with a very limited glial proliferation and slight accumulation of scavenger cells (gitterzellen). With time, the proliferated neuroglia increased (gliosis), as well as the number of scavenger cells until, at three to six weeks, a definite glial capsule had formed and some of the scavenger cells had developed into bizarre forms and giant cells. While there were minute hemorrhages in the dead areas, hyperemia was not a feature. Cordy summarized the changes under the name of nigropallidal encephalomalacia.

A very similar disease with essentially the same lesions has been produced in horses by feeding dried Russian knapweed (*Centaurea repens*) (Young, Brown, and Klinger, 1970).

Yellow Star Thistle

CORDY, D. R.: Nigropallidal Encephalomalacia in Horses, Associated with Ingestion of Yellow Star Thistle. J. Neuropath. and Exper. Neurol. *13*:330–342, 1954.
FOWLER, M. E.: Nigropallidal Encephalomalacia in the Horse. J. Am. Vet. Med. Assn. *147*:607–616, 1965.
METTLER, F. A. and STERN, G. M.: Observations on the Toxic Effects of Yellow Star Thistle. J. Neuropath. *22*:164–169, 1963.
YOUNG, S., BROWN, W. W., and KLINGER, B.: Nigropallidal Encephalomalacia in Horses Fed Russian Knapweed Centaurea repens, L.: Am. J. Vet. Res. *31*:1393–1404, 1970.

BOTULISM

Botulism, or poisoning by the toxin of *Clostridium botulinum*, figures prominently in veterinary diagnoses; especially those made in the earlier decades of this century. The existence of the condition in chickens is well established, the complete flaccid paralysis being graphically described by the popular name of "limberneck." Wild ducks die of a similar condition caused by toxins developed in vegetation decaying in the anaerobic conditions of stagnant pools. The condition was formerly known as **"alkali disease"** (Quortrup, 1941). Cattle die from a paralytic toxemia known as **"loin disease"** which Schmidt has shown to result indirectly from phosphorus deficiency. The cattle, lacking adequate dietary phosphorus, chew the bones of their deceased herd-mates. Bits of decomposed flesh still adhering to the bones frequently harbor soil-borne *Clostridia* and their toxins. **"Lamsiekte"** in South Africa is a similar disorder. Symptoms of botulism in horses, as in other species, are those of a gradually increasing paralysis, the functions of swallowing and of vision being among the first to suffer. Paralytic prostration follows and ends after a total course of twenty-four hours, more or less, in death from failure of the respiratory muscles. However, most of the cases of equine "botulism," as of "forage poisoning" (p. 887), have become equine encephalomyelitis (p. 356) with advancing knowledge, so that serious doubts may be entertained as to any appreciable frequency of botulinus poisoning in horses. In dogs and cats, as well as sheep and swine, the disease probably does not occur although a certain experimental susceptibility can be demonstrated. Gastroenteritis has been given as a prominent post-mortem lesion, but commonly the true diagnosis has been open to question in the cases showing this lesion. It is doubtful that there are any gross lesions of botulism beyond the petechiae and congestion characteristic of terminal anoxia. Except in typical cases of "limberneck," it is unsafe to render a diagnosis of botulism unless symptoms are produced by oral administration of the suspected material to a guinea pig, while a control previously immunized by antitoxin remains healthy. (See page 576.)

Botulism

ALLEN, T : Botulism in Cattle. J. Am. Vet. Med. Assn. *106*:163–164, 1945.
QUORTRUP, E. R., and HOLT, A. L.: Botulism Type C in Minks. J. Am. Vet. Med. Assn. *97*:167–168, 1940.
——————: Botulinus-Toxin-Producing Areas in Western Duck Marshes. J. Bact. *41*:363–372, 1941.

ANGUINA

Anguina agrostis is one of the many species of minute nematodes which infest plants. In the case of this species, microscopic larvae invade the seeds of certain grasses causing the seed to become an enlarged reactive mass known as a gall. The multitudinous larvae remain dormant in the gall until it is softened by moisture, when they escape and reproduce. Among the species of grass liable to be infested by this parasite are Chewings fescue, creeping red fescue, various kinds of bent grass, orchard grass, buffalo grass, red top, creeping timothy, sweet vernal grass, velvet grass, annual blue grass and Kentucky blue grass.

As has been shown by Galloway, working on the irrigated grass fields of arid Central Oregon (U.S.A.), horses and cattle, as well as experimental rats and chickens, are poisoned when they consume sufficient amounts of infested grass seeds, either mixed with the hay or in "screenings," the discarded imperfect seeds separated from harvested grass seed. The grass in which this occurred in Galloway's experience was Chewings fescue grass (*Festuca rubra* v. *commutata*).

Formerly viewed as manifestations of forage poisoning, the signs indicate that the toxic substance, which can be extracted with boiling alcohol, is a nerve poison. Prominent among these symptoms are staggering, knuckling of the feet, tucking the head between the forelegs, falling and clonic spasms. The illness may arise when the toxic material has been consumed for two weeks, more or less. Death may follow in a matter of hours or the nervous symptoms may continue for a week or more. Gross lesions are not discernible; microscopic changes apparently have not been studied. Diagnosis is made by soaking the suspected seeds and galls and demonstrating the microscopic larvae, which are very numerous.

Anguina

GALLOWAY, J. H.: Grass Seed Nematode Poisoning in Livestock. J. Am. Vet. Med. Assn. *139*:1212–1214, 1961.
HAAG, J. R.: Toxicity of Nematode Infested Chewings Fescue Seed. Science. *102*:406–407, 1945.
SHAW, J. N. and MUTH, O. H.: Some Types of Forage Poisoning in Oregon Cattle and Sheep. J. Am. Vet. Med. Assn. *114*:315–317, 1949.

CARBON DISULFIDE

This highly volatile liquid has a number of industrial and laboratory uses, but domestic animals come in contact with it when it is administered as a treatment against gastric or intestinal parasites, chiefly in horses and swine. Serious excesses in dosage have been rare, but a more frequent accident has been the breaking of a capsule in the patient's pharynx. Violent spasm of the regional musculature is the result, and fatal arrest of respiration is a possibility. Signs of poisoning include transient local pain and inflammation but are largely related to its nerve-depressant action, dullness and lethargy being followed by lower-neuron paralysis (p. 1376) and coma. Lesions, other than localized gastritis and enteritis in areas of contact, are neurological. Nerve cells are destroyed here and there in the brain and cord, and fiber tracts and peripheral nerves suffer demyelinization.

ORTHO-TRICRESYL PHOSPHATE

This substance, contained in a type of synthetic rubber used for shoe soles, scraps of which were eaten by chickens, was shown clinically and experimentally to be highly fatal. Signs in chickens were inappetence, fetid diarrhea and progressive paralysis of the legs. Sensation, at least of pain, was not lost. The poisoning was invariably fatal in three or four weeks. Lesions consisted principally of enteritis with atrophy of the unused gastrointestinal tract and a full gallbladder. There was wallerian degeneration of the myelin sheaths of peripheral nerves, principally the sciatic and lumbosacrals, which resembled histologically the lesion of thiamine deficiency (p. 985).

Ortho-tricresyl Phosphate

HARTWIGK, H.: Lähmungen bei Hühnern durch Weichigelit. Monatsh. f. Veternirm. 5:53–55, 1950.

LEAD

Animals are sometimes poisoned by lead salts through the licking of painted surfaces, which is a habit of calves especially, or through the ingestion of paint or putty left in cans or otherwise discarded. Puppies are most often poisoned by chewing or eating objects painted with lead-base paints, old paint chipped from surfaces to be repainted, linoleum containing lead and less frequently broken wet cell batteries, plumber's lead compounds or lead-containing roofing material (Zook, Carpenter and Leeds, 1969). Children may be poisoned from these same sources or possibly from lead-glazed cooking ware. Water-fowl have been poisoned by metallic lead shot ingested from the sludge of lake-bottoms, in which the discharges from the guns of many hunters had accumulated (Coburn, Metzler, and Treichler, 1951; Trainer and Hunt, 1965). Fumes from burning storage batteries, cutaneous absorption from gasoline containing tetra-ethyl lead and other mechanisms have been rarely incriminated. Habitual exposure to fumes from lead smelters has poisoned horses working in or near them. Wind-borne contamination of pastures in the vicinity of such smelters may reach 130 mg. of lead per kg. of dry forage and accumulations of lead in the soil to levels reaching 1000 p.p.m. have been associated with poisoning of cattle and horses. Orchard sprays frequently contain lead arsenate, but the arsenical ion is the one of princi-

Lesions at necropsy include petechiae and ecchymoses on and in the heart and in many other places. These occur especially in association with convulsions and are explainable on the basis of dyspneic anoxia. Pulmonary congestion and edema, diffuse or localized, are the rule. The heart usually stops in systole. In spite of the startling symptoms of central nervous disorder, there are few changes in the central nervous cells and tissues. This, of course, is in conformity with the rapid and complete recovery that may follow some of the most violent symptoms. Some have reported Nissl's degeneration and necrosis of neurones, especially in the ganglia of the medulla, cerebellum and brain stem; others have found no central nervous lesions beyond congestion and increased cerebrospinal fluid. In the few cases in which symptoms have been prolonged for a day or two, the usual changes of acute toxic hepatitis and acute toxic tubular nephrosis have been noted, centrilobular necrosis being especially prominent. Focal necroses have been noticed in the skeletal muscles. Enteritis is noticeable only if the poison has been eaten. Dehydration and rapid depletion of depot fat are usual in these cases. The biochemist can demonstrate accumulation of chlorinated compounds in the body tissues, chiefly the stored fat.

Chlorinated Hydrocarbons

ANONYMOUS: Pesticide, Chemicals, Established Tolerance Levels in Meat, and Acceptability for Use in Slaughter Animals and on Agricultural Premises. J. Am. Vet. Med. Assn. *147*: 616, 1965.

BAXTER, J. T.: Some Observations on the Histopathology of Aldrin Poisoning in Lambs. J. Comp. Path. *69*:185–191, 1959.

DALGAARD-MIKKELSEN, S., RASMUSSEN, F., and SIMONSEN, I. M.: Toxicity for Cattle of the Weed-Killer 2-methyl-4 chlorophenoxy acetate. Nord Vet. Med. *11*:469–474, 1959. Engl. summary. Abstr. Vet. Bull. No. 536, 1959.

DAVIS, K. J. and FITZHUGH, O. G.: Tumorigenic Potential of Aldrin and Dieldrin for Mice. Toxicol. appl. Pharm. *4*:187–189, 1962.

ELY, R. E. *et al.*: Lindane Poisoning in Dairy Animals. J. Am. Vet. Med. Assn. *123*:448–449, 1953.

HABER, W. G. and LINK, R. P.: Toxic Effects of Hexachloronaphthalene on Swine. Toxicol. appl. Pharm. *4*:257–262, 1962.

HAMILTON, D. G.: Gammexane (Benzene Hexachloride) Poisoning in Horses. J. Roy. Army Vet. Corps. *26*:92–94, 1955.

HARRISON, D. L. *et al.*: Dieldrin Poisoning of Dogs. II. Experimental Studies. N.Z. vet. J. *11*:23–31, 1963.

HAYMAKER, W., GINZLER, A. M., and FERGUSON, R. L.: The Toxic Effects of Prolonged Ingestion of DDT on Dogs with Special Reference to Lesions in the Brain. Am. J. Med. Sci. *212*:423–431, 1946.

HAYES, W. J., JR.: Review of the Metabolism of Chlorinated Hydrocarbon Insecticides Especially in Mammals. A. Rev. Pharmac. *5*:27–52, 1965.

JUDAH, J. D.: Metabolism and Mode of Action of DDT. Brit. J. Pharmacol. *4*:120–131, 1949.

KITSELMAN, C. H.: Long-term Studies on Dogs Fed Aldrin and Dieldrin in Sublethal Dosages, with Reference to the Histopathological Findings and Reproduction. J. Am. Vet. Med. Assn. *123*:28–30, 1953.

LILLIE, R. D., and SMITH, M. I.: Pathology of Experimental Poisoning in Cats, Rabbits and Rats with 2,2 bis-parachlorphenyl-1,1,1 trichloroethane. Pub. Health Rep. *59*:979–984, 1944.

LINK, R. P., BRUCE, W. N., and DECKER, G. C.: The Effects of Chlorinated Hydrocarbon Insecticides on Dairy Cattle. Ann. New York Acad. Sci. *111*:788–792, 1964.

LÖLIGER, H.-CH.: Beitrag zur Histologie der Vergiftung mit aldrin-und dieldrinhaltigen getreidebeizen bei Huhnern. Monatsheft f. Veterinärmed *11*:685–688, 1956.

MCENERNEY, P. J.: Accidental Poisoning of Dairy Calves by Benzene Hexachloride. Cornell Vet. *41*:292–295, 1951.

NELSON, A. A. *et al.*: Histopathological Changes Following Administration of DDT to Several Species of Animals. Pub. Health Rep. *59*:1009–1020, 1944.

PEARSON, J. K. L., *et al.*: An Outbreak of Aldrin Poisoning in Suckling Lambs. Vet. Rec. *70*:783–785, 1958.

RADELEFF, R. D., *et al.*: The Acute Toxicity of Chlorinated Hydrocarbon and Organic Phosphorus Insecticides to Livestock. U. S. Dept. Agr. Tech. Bull. No. 1122, 1955.

RADELEFF, R. D.: Chlordane Poisoning: Symptomatology and Pathology. Vet. Med. *43*:343–347, 1948.

————: Toxaphene Poisoning, Symptomatology and Pathology. Vet. Med. *44*:436–442, 1949.

RESSANG, A. A., *et al.*: Aldrin, Dieldrin and Endrin Intoxication in Cats. Commun. Vet., Bogor. *2*:71–88, 1959. (In Engl.) Abstr. Vet. Bull. No. 3266, 1959.

VIRGILI, R., and MARCHIAFAVA, G.: Quadri anatomo-pathologici nell' intossicazione acuta sperimentale da DDT con particolare riferimento al sistema nervoso. Riv. di malariol. *28*: 107–124, 1949. (Abstr. Vet. Bull. No. 1474, 1951.)

ORGANIC PHOSPHATES

Under the group name of *organic phosphates* are included certain "nerve gases" devised for use in warfare and a number of valuable insecticides. Tetra-ethyl pyrophosphate (TEPP) is one belonging to both categories. The insecticides are usually best known by specific trade names, the more important of which are currently Parathion, o,o-diethyl p-nitrophenyl thiophosphate, and Malathion, o,o-diethyl dithiophosphate. Others in this group are: Carbyl (Sevin), Carbophenothion (Trithion), Ciodrin, Coumaphos (Co-Rad), Demetron, Diazinon, Dichlorvos (DDVP), Dioxathion, Di Syston, Endosulfan, ENP, Ethion, Guthion, Methyl Parathion, Mevinphos (Phosdrin), Naled (Dibrom), Phorate (Thiomet), Ronnel and Trichlorophon (Dipterex). Known as anticholinesterases, these organic phosphates have essentially similar effects, which are dependent upon an ability to prevent or inhibit the action of cholinesterase. This leaves the acetylcholine of the sympathetic and parasympathetic nerve endings free to act continuously and without release of the effectors at the end of each stimulus. The oral lethal dose of parathion for dogs is estimated by Tsaggare, 1967, as 25 to 35 mg./kg. body weight; for cats, 15 mg./kg.; for rabbits, 40 mg./kg. body weight.

Signs include excessive salivation, the saliva being copious but watery. There is respiratory difficulty with labored and exaggerated respiratory movements, the mouth often being held partially open. Before death, there are loud pulmonary rales and soft grunts. Twitching and fasciculation of muscles occur but only exceptionally convulsions. Asphyxia is the main cause of death. Signs commonly arise within an hour or two after a single contact with the poison, which may well be by inhalation or cutaneous absorption, more often than by ingestion. Somewhat exceptionally, death has come within five minutes after tetra-ethyl pyrophosphate was sprayed on the skin of cattle (Radeleff, 1954). Non-fatal cases recover within forty-eight hours, as a rule. Susceptibility varies greatly among individuals of any species and can be increased by frequently repeated mild exposure. The greater susceptibility appears to be due to exhaustion of the body's store of cholinesterase.

Post-mortem lesions are decidedly minor. Hemorrhages appear in various locations, especially the heart, lungs and gastrointestinal tube. Pulmonary congestion and edema is a prominent, but not necessarily constant, lesion. Parenchymatous degeneration (p. 42) of the liver and kidneys has been reported, Fontanelli, 1955, but is probably exceptional. Denz, 1951, reported a characteristic shrinking and vacuolation of the epithelial cells lining submaxillary (but not sublingual) and parotid salivary and the lacrimal glands (in rats). Eosinophilic granules were found in the cells lining the tubular parts of the submaxillary gland, also. The thymus and spleen (but not the lymph nodes) were depleted of lymphocytes.

Holmstedt, Krook and Rooney, 1957, reported generalized vascular congestion and pulmonary edema to be the most conspicuous lesion in experimental poisoning of dogs and guinea pigs.

Berger and Bayliss, 1952, have described a promising histochemical method for the detection of cholinesterase at motor end plates in teased preparations of skeletal muscles which should be useful to help detect fatal accumulations of anticholinesterase.

Decrease in the level of cholinesterase in circulating red blood cells is considered to be good evidence of toxicity by organic phosphates (Anderson, Machin and Hebert, 1969).

Organic Phosphates

ANDERSON, P. H., MACHIN, A. F., and HEBERT, C. N.: Blood Cholinesterase Activity as an Index of Acute Toxicity of Organophosphorus Pesticides in Sheep and Cattle. Res. Vet. Sci. 10:29–33, 1969.

ASHDOWN, D., DAHMS, R. G., RIDGWAY, W. O., and STILES, C. F.: Hazards in Use of Parathion for Green-bug Control. J. Econ. Entomol. 45:82–84, 1952.

BELL, R. R., PRICE, M. A., and TURK, R. D.: Toxicity of Malathion and Chlorthion to Dogs and Cats. J. Am. Vet. Med. Assn. 126:302–303, 1955.

BERGNER, A. D., and BAYLISS, M. W.: Histochemical Detection of Fatal Anticholinesterase Poisoning. U.S. Armed Forces Med. J. 3:1637–1644, 1952.

COX, D. H., and BAKER, B. R.: A Diagnostic Test for Organic Phosphate Insecticide Poisoning in Cattle. J. Am. Vet. Med. Assn. 132:485–387, 1958. (Also swine, Ibid. 133:329–330, 1958.)

DENZ, F. A.: Poisoning by P-Nitrophenyl Diethyl Thiophosphate (E605): A Study of Anticholinesterase Compounds. J. Path. and Bact. 63:81–91, 1951.

DZHUROV, A.: Pathology of Acute Parathion Poisoning in Cattle. Nauchni. Trud. vissh. Vet. Med. Inst. 16:59–66, 1966. V.B. 37:1398, 1967.

ERNE, KURT: The Detection of Parathione in Biological Material. Nord. Vet. Med. 9:450–454, 1957.

FONTANELLI, E.: Su due casi di avvelenamento nel bovino da estere dell'acido tiofosforico. (Parathion.) Zooprofilassi. 10:486–492, 1955.

GALATI, P.: (Lesions in Cattle and Buffaloes Dying of Acute Parathion Poisoning). Acta Med. Vet. Napoli 7:387–411, 1966. V.B. 37:3354, 1967.

HOLMSTEDT, B.: Pharmacology of Organophosphorus Cholinesterase Inhibitors. Pharmacol. Rev. 2:567–688, 1959.

HOLMSTEDT, B., KROOK, L. and ROONEY, J. R.: The Pathology of Experimental Cholinesterase-inhibitor Poisoning. Acta pharmacol. et toxicol. 13:337–344, 1957.

McCOY, J. W.: A Case of Parathion Poisoning. Southwest. Vet. 16:196, 1963.

MUKULA, A. L.: Detection of Parathion Poisoning. In Engl. Acta Pharm. Tox. Kbh. 17:304–314, 1960.

PETTY, C. S.: Histochemical Proof of Organic Phosphate Poisoning. Arch. Path. 66:458–463, 1958.

RADELEFF, R. D.: TEPP (Tetra-ethyl Pyrophosphate) Poisoning of Cattle. Vet. Med. 49:15–16, 1954.

TSAGGARE, TH.A.: (Pathological Changes in Animals Poisoned with Parathion.) Epistem. epet. kteniatrik. Skhol. (Ann. Rep. Vet. Fac. Thessaloniki) 6:245–315, 1967. V.B. 37:5311, 1967.

YOUNGER, R. L.: Toxicity Studies of Certain Organic Phosphorus Compounds in Horses. Am. J. Vet. Res. 26:776–779, 1965.

CYCADA

Plants of the order cycadales, particularly *Zamia integrifolia, Z. portoricoensis, Z. latafoleatus, Cycas circinalis, Bowenia serrulata,* and *Macrozamia lucida,* are coarse, woody, fern-like and grow in Australia, New Guinea, Puerto Rico, Dominican Republic, and Florida. Poisoning of cattle, associated with these plants, may result in nervous signs which have prompted such colloquial names as: "wobbles," "zamia paralysis," cycad ataxia, *derriengue* (Dominican Republic) and *ranilla* (Puerto Rico). Although the plants grow in Florida, no poisonings of this type have been reported from the United States.

The clinical signs are chiefly neurologic, with ataxia involving the hindquarters initially. A peculiar involvement of the hind legs results in swaying, flexion of the hock and fetlock joints, wobbling and malpositioning of the legs. The lesions are concentrated in the spinal cord: Degeneration of myelin is evident in nerve fibers of all funiculi of the cord throughout its length. The Marchi and Guillery silver staining methods are particularly useful in demonstrating these lesions (Hall and McGavin, 1968).

Cycada

HALL, W. T. K., and McGAVIN, M. D.: Clinical and Neuropathological Changes in Cattle Eating the Leaves of *Macrozamia lucida* or *Bowenia serrulata* (Family *Zamiaceae*). Path. Vet. 5:26–34, 1968.

MASON, M. M., and WHITING, M. G.: Caudal Motor Weakness and Ataxia in Cattle in the Caribbean Area Following Ingestion of Cycads. Cornell Vet. 58:541–554, 1968.

Group Q: Poisons causing degeneration of cardiac and skeletal muscles

Coffee Senna   Coyotillo   Hairy vetch (p. 885)

COFFEE SENNA

Coffee senna (*Cassia occidentalis*, L.) received its common name because of the use of the bean as a substitute for coffee. The plant is an annual shrub which grows natively in the Southeastern United States as well as in many other parts of the world. The plant has drab green leaves and bright golden yellow flowers. The seed pods are green with brown transverse bars when immature and become brown when mature. Other sennas are known to have cathartic properties and some may be toxic to animals (Kingsbury, 1964). Among these plants are: *Cassia fistula* (Senna of commerce), *C. lindheimeriana*, *C. fasciculata* (partridge pea) and *C. tora* (sicklepod). Reported as poisonous to livestock first in 1911 (O'Hara, Pierce, and Read, 1969), episodes of toxicity in horses, cattle, and sheep have been recorded over the years. Experimental poisoning has also been recorded in cattle, rabbits, sheep and goats.

Calves given daily oral doses of ground beans of *Cassia occidentalis* at the dose rate of 0.05 per cent, or more, of their body weight survive at a rate inversely proportional to the dosage (O'Hara, Pierce, and Read, 1969). Signs of poisoning are anorexia and diarrhea, followed by hyperpnea, tachycardia and progressive muscular incapacitation with stumbling and ataxic gait. Elevated levels of serum glutamic oxaloacetic transaminase and phosphocreatine kinase are constant and hemoglobin appears in the urine of about half of these cases. Death follows prostration and recumbency by a few hours.

The gross lesions consist of focal or diffuse pallor of skeletal muscles generally distinguishable from the chalky whiteness and granular consistency observed in white-muscle disease (p. 1049). Stippling of pale muscles may be seen in calves. The myocardium is usually mottled or streaked with pale or yellow zones. These areas are sometimes concentrated adjacent to the endocardium, in others more diffusely distributed. Subepicardial hemorrhages may be seen, particularly along

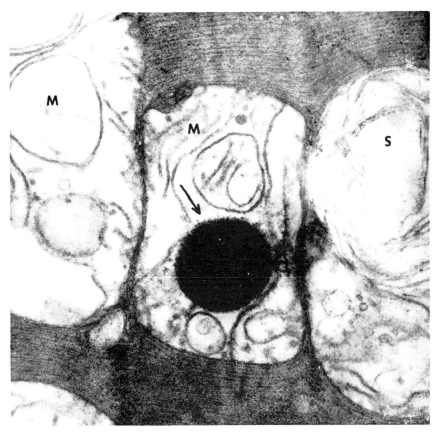

FIG. 17–32.—Poisoning due to coffee senna. Electron micrograph of myocardium of a calf poisoned with *Cassia occidentalis* ($\times$ 43,200). Note electron dense spherule (arrow) in swollen mitochondrion of myocardial muscle cell. Note disorganized cristae and spheromembranous structure(s) in mitochondrion. (Courtesy of Dr. W. Kay Read and *Laboratory Investigation*.)

the course of the coronary arteries. Effusion into the pericardial sac sometimes occurs. The lungs are usually diffusely dark red, partially airless and heavy. The interlobular septums are thickened by edema. Trachea and bronchi are filled with serous fluid which is white and frothy in part. Blood flows freely from the cut surface of the lung.

The earliest lesions seen with the light microscope in cardiac muscle (Read, Pierce and O'Hara, 1968) consist of numerous small indistinct vacuoles among the myofibrils, in some cases giving them a distinctly fenestrated appearance. These vacuoles are demonstrated with electron microscopy to be due to swelling of the mitochondria with loss of their matrix and fragmentation and disorganization of cristae. Electron-dense spherical inclusions sometimes appear in these dilated mitochondria (Fig. 17–32). Depletion of glycogen and spheromembranous degeneration of the sarcotubular system accompany the changes in mitochondria.

The lesions of skeletal muscles seen by light microscopy (Henson, *et al.*, 1965) are compatible with classic Zenker's necrosis of muscle (p. 22). The affected muscle fibers are swollen, eosinophilic (amorphous) and sometimes fragmented. Occasional nuclei are necrotic and some proliferation of sarcolemmal nuclei is evident. Calcification is not reported.

Coffee Senna

BROCQ-ROUSSEAU, and BRUERE, P.: Accidents Mortels sur des cheveaux due a la graine de *Cassia occidentalis*, L. Compt. rend Soc. biol. *92*:55–557, 1925.

DOLLAHITE, J. W., and HENSON, J. B.: Toxic Plants as the Etiologic Agent of Myopathies in Animals. Am. J. Vet. Res. *26*:749–752, 1965.

HENSON, J. B., *et al.*: Myodegeneration in Cattle Grazing *Cassia* Species. J. Am. Vet. Med. Assn. *147*:142–145, 1965.

MERCER, H. D., *et al.*: *Cassia occidentalis* Toxicosis in Cattle. J. Am. Vet. Med. Assn. *151*: 735–741, 1967.

MOUSSU, R.: L'Intoxication par les graines de *Cassia occidentalis* L., est due à une Tox-albumine. Compt. rend. Soc. biol. *92*:862–863, 1925.

O'HARA, P. J., PIERCE, K. R., and READ, W. K.: Degenerative Myopathy Associated with Ingestion of *Cassia occidentalis* L.: Clinical and Pathologic Features of the Experimentally Induced Disease. Am. J. Vet. Res. *30*:2173–2180, 1969.

READ, W. K., PIERCE, K. R., and O'HARA, P. J.: Ultrastructural Lesions of an Acute Toxic Cardiomyopathy of Cattle. Lab. Invest. *18*:227–231, 1968.

COYOTILLO

The coyotillo plant (*arwinskia humboldtiana*) is a spineless shrub with pinnately veined leaves, small greenish flowers and ovoid, brown-black fruit (Dewan, *et al.*, 1965). The fruit has been shown to cause, in sheep and goats, a toxicosis called "limberleg" which is manifest by progressive weakness of legs, muscular incoordination, recumbency and death (Marsh, Clawson and Roe, 1928). In 1789, Indian children reportedly lost the use of their limbs. and some died after eating the fruit of the coyotillo. (Clavergo, cited by Marsh, Clawson and Roe, 1928.)

This shrub is native to Southwest Texas and Mexico and in some regions grows profusely (Sperry, *et al.*, 1955).

The **lesions** in this toxicosis are found in cardiac and skeletal muscle, peripheral nerves and liver. In the myocardium disseminated focal lesions of coagulation necrosis involve a few muscle fibers in each location. A few fibers lose their sarcoplasma. In skeletal muscle, any or all muscles may be involved and the microscopic lesions are typical Zenker's necrosis (p. 22). The isolated muscle fibers are swollen, eosinophilic, often fragmented and occasionally associated with infiltration of lymphocytes and macrophages and proliferation of sarcolemmal cells (Dewan, *et al.*, 1965). Toxic hepatitis is also a feature with focal necroses of small numbers of hepatic cells, usually at the center of the lobules plus some mild fatty change. Peripheral neuropathy with segmental demyelination has been found in goats (Charlton and Pierce, 1969).

Associated with these lesions are severe increases in the serum concentration of glutamic oxaloacetic transaminase and moderate increases in glutamic pyruvic transaminase. The serum alkaline phosphatase may be slightly decreased.

Coyotillo

CHARLTON, K. M., and PIERCE, K. R.: Peripheral Neuropathy in Experimental Coyotillo Poisoning in Goats. Texas Rpts. Biol. and Med. *27*:389–399, 1969.

CHARLTON, K. M., and PIERCE, K. R.: A Neuropathy in Goats Caused by Experimental Coyotillo (*Karwinskia humboldtiana*) Poisoning. II. Lesions in the Peripheral Nervous System—Teased Fiber and Acid Phosphatase Studies. Path. Vet. *7*:385–407, 1970.

————: A Neuropathy in Goats Caused by Experimental Coyotillo (*Karwinskia humboldtiana*) Poisoning. III. Distribution of Lesions in Peripheral Nerves. Path. Vet. *7*:408–419, 1970.

—————: A Neuropathy in Goats Caused by Experimental Coyotillo (*Karwinskia humboldtiana*) Poisoning. IV. Light and Electron Microscopic Lesions in Peripheral Nerves. Path. Vet. 7:420–434, 1970.

CHARLTON, K. M., *et al.*: A Neuropathy in Goats Caused by Experimental Coyotillo (*Karwinskia humboldtiana*) Poisoning. V. Lesions in the Central Nervous System. Path. Vet. 7:435–447, 1970.

DEWAN, M. L., *et al.*: Toxic Myodegeneration in Goats Produced by Feeding Mature Fruits from Coyotillo Plant (*Karwinskia humboldtiana*). Amer. J. Path. 46:215–226, 1965.

DOLLAHITE, J. W., and HENSON, J. B.: Toxic Plants as the Etiologic Agent of Myopathies in Animals. Amer. J. Vet. Res. 26:749–752, 1965.

MARSH, C. D., CLAWSON, A. B., and ROE, G. C.: Coyotillo (*Karwinskia humboldtiana*) as a Poisonous Plant. U.S.D.A. Tech. Bull. 29, 1928.

SPERRY, O. E., *et al.*: Texas Range Plants Poisonous to Animals. Texas Agric. Exp. Sta. Bull. 796:23–24, 1955.

Group R: Poisons causing teratogenic or other effects on the embryo or fetus.

Veratrum californicum	Lupin (p. 882)
Thalidomide	Selenium (p. 901)
	Loco (p. 951)

VERATRUM CALIFORNICUM

This impressive perennial plant grows profusely in eleven Western states, reaching 3 to 8 feet in height. Its common names include: skunk cabbage, western helibore, false helibore and wild corn. It is included in the lily family (Lileacea) in which are classified seven other species in this genus which are indigenous to North America. *Veratrum veride*, which grows in the Eastern United States, and *V. album*, a European species, are the source of several alkaloids, some of which are used medicinally. Among these specific alkaloids are: veratridine, protoveratrine, veratrine, cevadine and jirvine.

A striking and grotesque congenital malformation of lambs was first described by Binns, *et al.*, 1959, as occurring in sheep pastured on mountain ranges in Southern Idaho, located at altitudes up to 10,000 feet (Fig. 17–33). The deformed lambs were usually born alive, singly or with a living or dead twin which may or may not have been affected. The malformations are limited to the head and represent several defects, the commonest being partial or complete cyclopia. A single eye or two fused eyes usually occupy a single orbit. The two fused eyes give the startling appearance which caused the sheepmen to call them "monkey-faced lambs." The upper jaw may be slightly distorted with a cleft palate or almost totally absent. The nose is distorted in varying degrees and the lower jaw usually protrudes drastically. A large median cutaneous protuberance often occurs over the single eye. The cerebral hemispheres are often fused and hydrocephalus involves the lateral ventricles. The optic nerves may be fused.

In many cases the pituitary of the fetus is absent and this is associated with **prolonged gestation** (p. 1372) and a very large fetus which is not delivered except by hysterotomy.

In a series of carefully conducted experiments, Binns and co-workers have clearly established that this congenital malformation results from the consumption of the fresh or dried plant *Veratrum californicum*, or extracts thereof, by the ewe during her thirteenth to fifteenth days of pregnancy. The active principle has not been precisely identified at this writing but one of the alkaloids of *Veratrum californicum*, veratramine, has been shown (Keeler and Binns, 1966) to have some

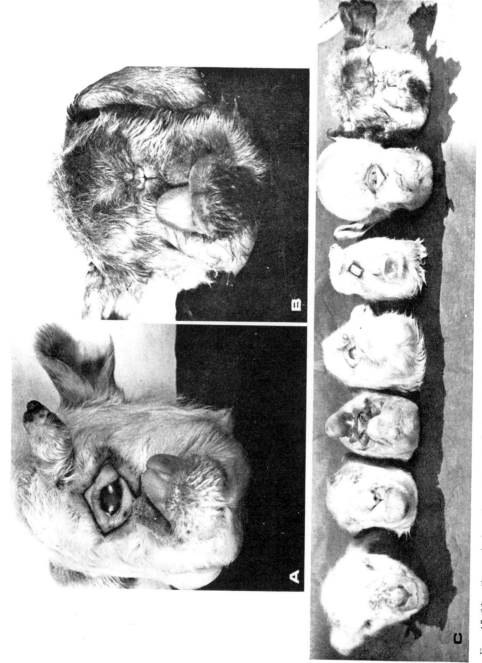

Fig. 17–33.—Congenital malformations in newborn lambs resulting from feeding their mothers a plant, *Veratrum californicum* (false helibore) on the fourteenth day of gestation. *A*, A lamb's head with cyclopia and other anomalies. *B*, A lamb with anophthalmia and other defects. *C*, Several lambs' heads with varying congenital deformities. Normal lamb at left. (Photographs courtesy of Dr. Wayne Binns, United States Department of Agriculture.)

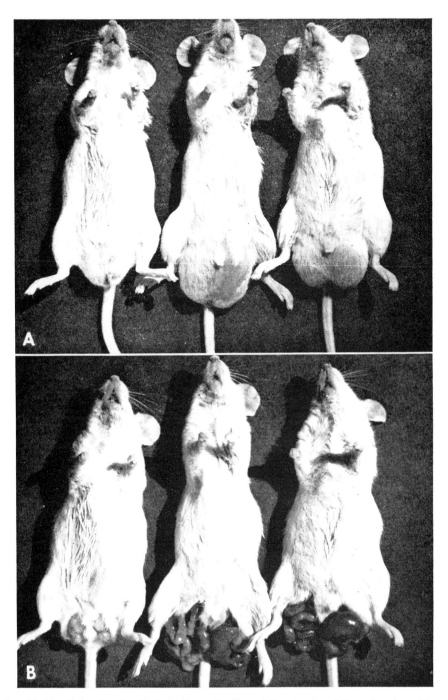

FIG. 17–34.—Poisoning by diethylstilbestrol. Scrotal hernias in adult male mice. Normal mouse on the left. *A*, Intact mice. *B*, Scrotum incised to reveal intestinal content in two affected mice. (Courtesy of Dr. W. J. Hadlow and Proceedings of *The Animal Care Panel.*)

teratogenic effects. Ewes given veratramine orally on the thirteenth and fourteenth days of pregnancy often aborted, or gave birth to abnormal lambs. These lambs did not have the cyclopian type malformations of the head but did have varying degrees of lack of control of skeletal muscles, slight lateral bowing of the front legs, slight to severe flexure of the knees or looseness of the hock joints.

Veratrum californicum

BINNS, W., *et al.*: A Congenital Cyclopian-type Malformation in Lambs. J. Am. Vet. Med. Assn. *134*:180–183, 1969.
BINNS, W., *et al.*: Cyclopian-type Malformation in Lambs. Arch. Environ. Health *5*:106–108, 1962.
BINNS, W., *et al.*: A Congenital Cyclopian-type Malformation in Lambs Induced by Maternal Ingestion of a Range Plant, *Veratrum californicum*. Am. J. Vet. Res. *24*:1164–1175, 1963.
BINNS, W., *et al.*: Toxicosis of *Veratrum californicum* in Ewes and Its Relationship to Congenital Deformity in Lambs. Ann. New York Acad. Sci. *111*:571–576, 1964.
KEELER, R. F., and BINNS, W.: Chemical Compounds of *Veratrum californicum* Related to Congenital Ovine Cyclopian Malformations: Extraction of Active Material. Proc. Soc. Exp. Biol. Med. *116*:123–127, 1964.
————: Possible Teratogenic Effects of Veratramine. Proc. Soc. Exp. Biol. Med. *123*: 921–923, 1966.

THALIDOMIDE

This tranquilizing drug, introduced in Germany in the late 1950's, was eventually associated with a large number of congenitally malformed babies whose mothers had taken the drug during pregnancy. The most striking malformations in these infants were absence of limbs (amelia) or shortening of the arms or legs to the point at which they resembled a seal's flippers (Phocomelia, *phoke* = seal, *melos* = extremity). Other anomalies have also been described in these children (Toms, 1962).

Although not a naturally-occurring teratogen for animals, thalidomide has been shown to produce congenital anomalies comparable to those seen in children in several species. Administration of 50 or 200 mg. thalidomide daily to female rhesus monkeys (*Macaca mulatta*) started after mating, appeared to kill the embryo, or prevent implantation since no young were born (Lucey and Behrman, 1963). Administration of the drug to rabbits (150 mg./kg. body weight daily) from day eight to day sixteen of pregnancy resulted in stillborn and deformed offspring. Rats apparently reabsorbed fetuses *in utero*, but produced no deformed offspring when placed on a similar regimen (Somers, 1962, Vickers, 1967). Congenital abnormalities in tail vertebrae, sternebrae and extremities also occur in puppies whose mothers are given thalidomide during pregnancy (Weidman, Young and Zollman, 1963).

Baboons respond in much the same way as human patients do (Hendrickx, Axelrod, and Clayborn, 1966), minimal doses to the mother produce teratogenic effects. Thalidomide also may produce phocomelia in the armadillo (*Dasypus novemcinctus mexicanus*) and a choriocarcinoma of the uterus with metastases has been associated with its administration (Marin-Padilla and Benirschke, 1963). Injury to the myocardium of armadillo embryos has also been demonstrated (Marin-Padilla and Benirschke, 1965).

Thalidomide

HENDRICKX, A. G., AXELROD, L. R., and CLAYBORN, L. D.: "Thalidomide" Syndrome in Baboons. Nature (Lond.) *210*:958–959, 1966.

LUCEY, J. F., and BEHRMAN, R. E.: Thalidomide: Effect on Pregnancy in the Rhesus Monkey. Science *139*:1295–1296, 1963.

MARIN-PADILLA, M., and BENIRSCHKE, K.: Thalidomide-induced Alterations in the Blasto-cyst and Placenta of the Armadillo, *Dasypus novemcinctus mexicanus,* Including a Chorio-carcinoma. Amer. J. Path. *43*:999–1016, 1963.

————: Thalidomide Injury to the Myocardium of Armadillo Embryos. J. Embryol. Exp. Morph. *13*:235–241, 1965.

SOMERS, G. F.: Thalidomide and Congenital Malformations. Lancet *1*:912–913, 1962.

TOMS, D. A.: Thalidomide and Congenital Malformations. Lancet *2*:400, 1962.

VICKERS, T. H.: The Thalidomide Embryopathy in Hybrid Rabbits. Brit. J. Exp. Path. *48*:107–117, 1967.

WEIDMAN, W. H., YOUNG, H. H., and ZOLLMAN, P. E.: The Effect of Thalidomide on the Unborn Puppy. Staff Meeting Mayo Clinic *38*:518–522, 1963.

Group S: Miscellaneous or unclassified poisons.

Smallhead sneezeweed	Yew	Nitrogen dioxide
Box	Phalaris grass	Cobalt
Grasstree	Sorghum	Hexachlorophene
Stinkwood	Sesbania	Chloroquine
Pokeweed	Estrogen	Zinc
		Gidyea tree

Brief mention will be made of several poisons which are infrequent in animals or have been inadequately studied. The original descriptions will be found in the references.

Smallhead sneezeweed (*Helenium microcephalum*).—This plant with such intriguing and descriptive common and scientific names, grows in Texas and Mexico. Many losses of cattle, sheep and goats have been attributed to eating this plant. Dollahite, Hardy and Henson (1964) have demonstrated this toxicity by feeding studies with calves, goats, rabbits and sheep. The flowering plants were more toxic than those in earlier stages of growth. Experimentally poisoned animals exhibited signs of excess salivation, nasal discharge, bloating and severe abdominal pain within an hour and died within twenty-four hours after eating these plants. Accelerated pulse and respiratory rates, vomiting and diarrhea were often exhibited. The gross lesions consisted of pulmonary edema, hydro-thorax and ascites, hyperemia and edema in the submucosa of the rumen and reticulum. Microscopically, edema of nervous tissue and lung, submucosa of rumen and reticulum were conspicuous. Mild toxic tubular nephritis was seen occasionally plus some fatty change in cardiac muscle.

Box (*Buxus sempervirens*).—The common box, boxwood or boxtree is native to Europe and Asia and is widely grown in the warmer climates of the United States as an ornamental or hedge. Losses of sheep, horses, pigs, cattle and camels have been reported as a result of eating the leaves and stems of this plant. Severe gastroenteritis, sometimes with bloody diarrhea are reported with death in a very short time. Several alkaloids have been extracted from the plant, including boxine—a severe emetic or purgative. (Couch, 1937, Kingbury, 1964, van Soest, Gotink and v.d. Vooren, 1965 and Reynard and Norton, 1942.)

Grasstree (*Xanthorrhoea resinosa, X. hastile*).—This plant has been reported to cause poisoning of cattle in Australia. These animals apparently only eat this plant when other feed is not available. The principal signs are "lurching to one side" and dribbling urine. In some animals, signs appear or are exacerbated two to three weeks after they have stopped eating the plant (Hall, 1965).

Stinkwood (*Zieria arborescens*).—This is another Australian poisonous shrub which may cause death of cattle. The principal signs and lesions are related to massive pulmonary edema (Munday, 1968).

Pokeweed (*Phytolacca americana*).—Although boiled young shoots of this plant have been recommended for human consumption, poisoning has resulted in swine from eating the roots and in cattle from the tops of the plant (Kingsbury and Hillman, 1965). Signs of poisoning have appeared overnight after feeding green plants cut with corn silage. The signs were severe diarrhea and purgation, subnormal temperature and severe drop in milk flow. Death has not been reported.

Yew (*Taxus cuspidata, T. baccata, T. canadensis*).—These ornamental shrubs are rarely eaten by animals but severe toxicity has been ascribed to them. The European variety, *T. baccata*, is a more frequently reported cause of poisoning on that continent, principally affecting cattle. The Japanese yew, *T. cuspidata*, a popular ornamental shrub in the United States has been incriminated in deaths of horses, deer, reindeer, and burros. Cattle have been reported to die after eating *T. canadensis* but the toxicity of *T. brevifolia* has been imputed but not confirmed.

Signs of poisoning may be missed, the animals may simply be found with the offending plant in mouth and stomach. Nervous manifestations such as trembling, dyspnea, and collapse may be evident during a very short course. Lesions have not been recognized (Lowe, 1970, Kingsbury, 1964).

Phalaris grass (*Phalaris tuberosa*).—This pasture plant, introduced into Australia from South Africa, has been occasionally incriminated as the cause of an acute death or chronic "phalaris staggers" in sheep. Sheep may die suddenly a few hours after grazing on a pasture of Phalaris, with no signs or lesions evident. Others may exhibit convulsive movements, staggering, hyperexcitability, tremors or convulsions before death. The toxic principles are believed to be tryptamine alkaloids. Green pigment, chemically related to tryptamine, is deposited in the kidneys and in neurones (Gallagher, Koch and Hoffman, 1966).

Sorghum (*Sorghum sudanese*, sudan grass).—Horses, grazing in pastures rich in sudan grass have been observed to develop chronic cystitis and occasionally ataxia. The urinary bladder in prolonged cases becomes thick-walled due to fibrosis, the epithelium is ulcerated and abscesses may occur in the wall. The vagina may also be ulcerated and presumably infected and abortion may occur. The urine may contain deposits of calcium carbonate (a common finding in equine urine) and in one case *Streptococcus zooepidemicus* was recovered. The basis for the ataxia described in some cases has not been explained (Knight, 1968, Romane, 1966).

Sesbania (*Sesbania punicea*, purple sesbane, purple rattlebox).—This South African shrub or small tree has been reported to be toxic to most domestic animals and poultry. The whole plant is poisonous; the seeds, flowers and leaves, in order, each contain the toxic element. The poisoning is manifest by irritation of the gastrointestinal tract and cardiac failure. Terminal renal failure has been noted in some cases (Terblanche, *et al.*, 1966). Several North American species are also known to be poisonous (Kingsbury, 1964). These are known under various scientific and common names. *Sesbania vesicaria*, bagpod, bladderpod, or coffeebean, is a vigorous annual which grows especially in damp soils in the Coastal Plain from North Carolina and Florida to Texas.

Sesbania drummondii, coffeebean, rattlebush or rattlebox, is a perennial shrub or small tree with a distribution similar to *S. vesicaria*. Sheep and goats have been poisoned under natural conditions, cattle experimentally. *S. punicea* has been described as growing in Florida to Louisiana after its introduction as an ornamental from Mexico. The toxic principle in these plants is suspected to be a saponin, but has not been clearly identified.

Estrogens. — These hormones have been known to cause poisoning under two generally different conditions. Synthetic estrogen, *diethylstilbestrol*, is used in feed for cattle to stimulate economical growth and usually causes no overt ill effects in these animals. On occasion however, the "premix" containing the synthetic estrogen has been erroneously mixed with feed under preparation for laboratory mice (Hadlow, 1955, 1957). Certain inbred strains of mice are very sensitive to estrogens and the effect upon a breeding colony is dramatic. In one incident in such a breeding colony of white mice, the number of pregnancies declined rapidly from 1000 a week to 20 per week. Litter size was reduced and many young were stillborn. About 90 per cent of the adult males suddenly exhibited scrotal hernias and sections of testes revealed complete azospermia. After removal of the offending adulterated feed, reproduction gradually resumed in the mouse colony (Fig. 17-34).

A second source of estrogens is in natural plants such as subterranean clover. This clover poisoning is a major problem to sheep in certain parts of Australia. Different strains of clover vary in estrogen content and toxicity. The effects include stillbirths, neonatal deaths, dystocia, prolapse of uterus and infertility in ewes. Virgin ewes may undergo precocious mammary development and lactation. Castrated males (wethers) may also lactate.

Nitrogen Dioxide. — This gas has been incriminated as a cause of "silo-fillers disease" in man (Lowry and Schuman, 1956) and pulmonary adenomatosis in cattle (Seaton, 1958, Cutlip, 1966). Intratracheal instillation of nitrogen dioxide gas in controlled doses into cattle results in severe respiratory distress, methemoglobinemia and death. Animals which survive for eleven to fourteen days following this exposure, exhibit severe pulmonary consolidation and emphysema of the lungs. The respiratory epithelium undergoes squamous metaplasia in the trachea and proliferation in the rest of the bronchial tree. The alveolar epithelium proliferates and fills alveoli in some lobules; in others, fibrin precipitates in alveoli to form a hyaline membrane. The bronchiolar epithelium becomes redundant and subepithelial fibrosis is conspicuous. Invasion by leukocytes into affected lungs may be extensive.

Cobalt. — Cobalt has been shown to be necessary for bacterial synthesis of vitamin B_{12} in the rumen and some soils have been demonstrated to be deficient in this element. This has led to application of cobalt sulfate to the soil and sometimes to injudicious dosing of ruminants with this salt (MacLaren, Johnston and Voss, 1964). Overdoses have led to death of cattle within a few hours. The principal findings at necropsy indicate severe congestion of the abomasal mucosa and microscopic evidence of toxic nephrosis (p. 1266). Cobalt may be demonstrated by spectrographic analysis to be present in liver and kidney.

Hexachlorophene (2,2 methylene bis [3,5,6-trichlorophenol]). — This drug is used to treat sheep infected with **Fasciola hepatica** (p. 796). Thorpe, 1969, has demonstrated that single doses of hexachlorophene (25 or 50 mg./kg. body weight) administered to sheep cause a significant effect upon spermatogenesis. Similar effects have been found in male rats (Thorpe, 1967). Following a single oral dose, spermatozoa and spermatids disappear from the testis, leaving only spermatogonia and spermatocytes. This effect may be transitory but could cause significant decrease in conceptions if it occurred during the breeding season. Hexachlorophene has also been shown to inhibit activity of certain enzymes in the liver, namely adenosine triphosphatase, succinic dehydrogenase, and glutamic dehydrogenase. Fatty change may also occur in the liver.

Chloroquine.—Chloroquine has been used for the suppression or treatment of malaria in man as well as for treatment of systemic or discoid lupus erythematosus and rheumatoid arthritis. Tests of this drug in swine have revealed some interesting toxicologic effects (Gleiser, *et al.*, 1968). Daily doses of 25 mg./kg. body weight per orum were not lethal but pigs were killed by doses of 50 to 100 mg./kg. per day. The significant pathologic lesions included a diffuse myopathy of skeletal muscles; degenerative changes in neurons of central nervous system and retina, necrosis of lymphocytes, and edema of the retina. The changes in skeletal muscles resembles Zenker's necrosis (p. 22). By light microscopy the changes in neurons appeared as swollen, foamy cytoplasm with displacement of nuclei. Electron micrographs disclosed this foamy cytoplasm to contain numerous lamellated, membranous bodies.

Zinc.—Deficiency of this element associated with parakeratosis of swine and its necessity in metabolism are discussed elsewhere (p. 1015). It seems inevitable that poisoning with zinc will occur as a result of over-zealous administration of zinc compounds. Experimentally, toxicity has been demonstrated in sheep and cattle (Ott, *et al.*, 1966). Depressed or depraved appetites result in cattle fed zinc oxide in the diet at the rate of 0.9 gm. or more per kg. of feed. Zinc accumulates in the blood, liver, pancreas, kidney and bone and in lesser amounts in hair, spleen, lung and heart. After prolonged periods, hemoglobin and packed cell volumes in the blood are decreased. Lesions have not been described.

Gidyea Tree.—The leaves and pods of this tree (*Acacia georginae*) have been shown to contain a poisonous principle which may be lethal to sheep and cattle (Whittem and Murray, 1963). This poisoning is reported from the Georgina River basin in eastern Northern Territory and western Queensland of Australia, where it is known as **Georgina River poisoning.** Of particular interest is the finding that the active poison is the fluoroacetate ion. It is possible that this tree may concentrate fluoroacetate in its leaves and pods, under specific conditions, from soils rich in fluorine. Monofluoroacetic acid in significant quantities has been isolated from the "gifblaar" plant (*Dichapetalum cymosum*) in South Africa where severe losses of livestock have been associated with eating this plant. See also sodium monofluoroacetate poisoning, page 853.

The most significant lesion is reported (Whittem and Murray, 1963) to occur in the myocardium. Focal necroses of myocardial fibers, usually followed by leukocytic infiltration and in some cases fibrosis, are seen microscopically. These are associated with gross petechiae and ecchymoses under the endocardium and epicardium and occasional focal scars in the myocardium.

BECK, A. B., and GARDINER, M. R.:   Clover Disease of Sheep in Western Australia. J. Dept. Agric. West. Aust. 6:390–392 and 395–400, 1965. V.B. 36:3330, 1966.

COUCH, J. F.:   The Chemistry of Stock-poisoning Plants.   J. Chem. Educ. 14:16–24, 1937.

CUTLIP, R. C.:   Experimental Nitrogen Dioxide Poisoning in Cattle.   Path. Vet. 3:474–485, 1966.

DOLLAHITE, J. W., HARDY, W. T., and HENSON, J. B.:   Toxicity of *Helenium microcephalum* (Smallhead Sneezeweed).   J. Am. Vet. Med. Assn. 145:694–696, 1964.

GALLAGHER, C. H., KOCH, J. H., and HOFFMAN, H.:   Disease of Sheep Due to Ingestion of *Phalaris tuberosa*.   Aust. Vet. J. 42:279–284, 1966.

——————:   Poisoning by Grass.   New Scientist.   25 Aug. 1966:412–414, 1966.

GLEISER, C. A., et al.:   Study of Chloroquine Toxicity and a Drug-induced Cerebrospinal Lipodystrophy in Swine.   Amer. J. Path. 53:27–45, 1968.

HADLOW, W. J., GRIMES, E. F., and JAY, G. E., JR.:   Stilbestrol Contaminated Feed and Reproductive Disturbances in Mice.   Science 122:643–644, 1955.

HADLOW, W. J., and GRIMES, E. F.:   Influence of Stilbestrol-contaminated Feed on Reproduction in a Colony of Mice.   Proc. Anim. Care Panel 6:19–25, 1955.

HADLOW, W. J.:   Stilbestrol Poisoning in Mice.   J. Am. Vet. Med. Assn. 130:300–303, 1957.

HALL, W. T. K.:   Grasstree Poisoning of Cattle.   Qd. Agric. J. 91:504–506, 1965.

KINGSBURY, J. M.:   *Poisonous Plants of the United States and Canada*.   Englewood Cliffs, N. J., Prentice-Hall, 1964.

KINGSBURY, J. M., and HILLMAN, R. B.:   Pokeweed (*Phytolacca*) Poisoning in a Dairy Herd. Cornell Vet. 55:534–538, 1965.

KNIGHT, P. R.:   Equine Cystitis and Ataxia Associated with Grazing of Pastures Dominated by Sorghum Species.   Austral. Vet. J. 44:257, 1968.

LOWE, J. E., et al.:   *Taxus cuspidata* (Japanese Yew) Poisoning in Horses.   Cornell Vet. 60: 36–39, 1970.

LOWRY, T., and SCHUMAN, L. M.:   Silo-filler's Disease—A Syndrome Caused by Nitrogen Dioxide.   J. Amer. Med. Assn. 162:153–160, 1956.

MACLAREN, A. P. C., JOHNSTON, W. G., and VOSS, R. C.:   Cobalt Poisoning in Cattle. Vet. Rec. 76:1148–1149, 1964.

MUNDAY, B. L.:   *Zieria arborescens* (Stinkwood) Intoxication in Cattle.   Aust. Vet. J. 44: 501–502, 1968.

OTT, E. A., et al.:   Zinc Toxicity in Ruminants.   IV. Physiological Changes in Tissues of Beef Cattle.   J. Anim. Sci. 25:432–438, 1966.

OTT, E. A., et al.:   Zinc Toxicity in Ruminants.   III. Physiological Changes in Tissues and Alterations in Rumen Metabolism in Lambs.   J. Anim. Sci. 25:424–431, 1966.

OTT, E. A., et al.:   Zinc Toxicity in Ruminants.   II. Effect of High Levels of Dietary Zinc on Grains, Feed Consumption and Field Efficiency of Beef Cattle.   J. Anim. Sci. 25:419–423, 1966.

OTT, E. A., et al.:   Zinc Toxicity in Ruminants.   I. Effect of High Levels of Dietary Zinc on Grains, Feed Consumption, and Feed Efficiency of Lambs.   J. Anim. Sci. 25:414–418, 1966.

REYNARD, G. B., and NORTON, J. B. S.:   Poisonous Plants of Maryland in Relation to Livestock.   Univ. of Maryland, Agric. Exper. Station.   Tech. Bull. A10, 1942.

ROMANE, W. M., et al.:   Equine Cystitis Associated with Grazing of Sudan Grass.   J. Am. Vet. Med. Assn. 149:1171, 1966.

SEATON, V. A.:   Pulmonary Adenomatosis in Iowa Cattle.   Am. J. Vet. Res. 19:600–609, 1958.

TERBLANCHE, M., et al.:   A Toxicological Study of the Plant *Sesbania punicea*, Benth. J. S. Afr. Vet. Med. Assn. 37:191–197, 1966.   V.B. 37:1817, 1967.

THORPE, E.:   Some Pathological Effects of Hexachlorophene in the Rat.   J. Comp. Path. 77:137–142, 1967.

——————:   Some Toxic Effects of Hexachlorophene in Sheep.   J. Comp. Path. 79:167–171, 1969.

VAN SOEST, H., GOTINK, W. M., and v.d. VOOREN, L. J.:   Poisoning in Pigs and Cows by Boxtree Leaves (*Buxus sempervirens*).   Tijdschr. Diergeneesk. 90:387–389, 1965.   V.B. 35: 2732, 1965.

WHITTEM, J. H., and MURRAY, L. R.:   The Chemistry and Pathology of Georgina River Poisoning.   Aust. Vet. J. 39:168–173, 1963.

18

Diseases and Disorders of Metabolism: Deficiency Diseases

It is possible to demonstrate the indispensability of a large number of dietary substances by depriving experimental animals of them. While the usefulness of fundamental research is not questioned, a casual perusal of the long list of abnormalities which can be shown experimentally to follow withholding of various vitamins, minerals or amino acids tends to confuse more than to enlighten and accords to deficiencies a prominence which they do not possess in actual diagnosis and therapy. Therefore, only those deficiencies which are known to occur under conditions of veterinary medical practice will be discussed here. Most of these deficiencies arise as the result of the restricted diets often imposed upon domestic animals by their caretakers through either ignorance or greed on the part of husbandmen. The current tendency to feed livestock various artificially manufactured products and by-products, as well as certain unnatural substances (hormones, antibiotics, synthetics) designed to cause abnormal gains in weight or excessive production of milk or eggs, serves to introduce a continuous succession of new diseases, the diagnosis of which is often far from simple.

Deficiency of a single nutrient is rare as a natural disease, although some examples can be cited: iodine deficiency leading to goiter; iron deficiency leading to anemia; ingestion of thiaminase leading to thiamine deficiency; molybdenum toxicosis leading to copper deficiency. But in general nutritional diseases in both man and lower animals are multiple deficiencies. This creates a more complex disease state which is often difficult to analyze, and also makes it difficult to make comparisons with the single nutrient deficiencies produced in the laboratory. The bulk of nutritional research has concerned single nutrient deficiency.

Obviously lack of a specific nutrient(s) in the diet is the simplest and most easily understood cause of nutritional disease. But other and more usual causes include: (1) The diet may be of generally poor quality (*e.g.* predominantly roughage) or volume may be inadequate (simple starvation). (2) *Interference with intake* arising from anorexia, mechanical obstruction, dental disease and so forth, have the same net effect as inadequate supply. (3) Other conditions can lead to deficiency states by *interfering with absorption of nutrients.* Lack of digestive secretions from hepatic or pancreatic disease, hypermotility of the intestinal tract, and formation of insoluble complexes such as between calcium and phytate are examples. (4) *Interference with storage or utilization* of a nutrient may have the same effect as a simple dietary deficiency. As example, in thyroiditis, insufficient normal tissue may be available for the proper utilization of iodine. (5) *Increased*

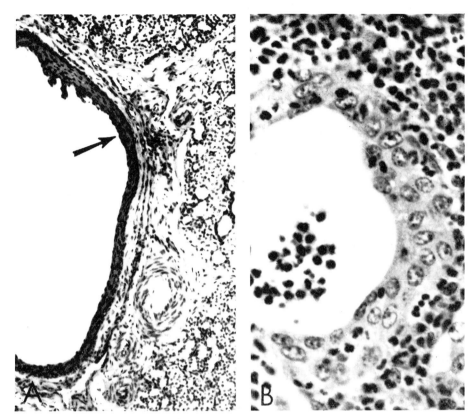

Fig. 18–1.—Vitamin A deficiency. *A*, Squamous metaplasia of a major duct in the salivary gland of a calf. *B*, Squamous metaplasia of a collecting tubule in the kidney of a mink. Also note purulent exudate in the lumen of the tubule and interstitium.

excretion represents another mechanism leading to deficiency disease. Loss of potassium associated with diarrhea, or calcium loss in hyperparathyroidism are examples. (6) *Increased requirements* associated with pregnancy, lactation or hyperthyroidism can lead to deficiency states if the diet is not adjusted. (7) *Inhibition of nutrients* by specific inhibitors or analogs also results in deficiency. Analogs are known for several of the B vitamins.

General Reference

Follis, R. H.: *Deficiency Disease*. Springfield, Charles C Thomas, 1958.

HYPOVITAMINOSIS A

Herbivorous animals obtain their vitamin A (retinol) in the form of carotene, a yellow pigment (or group of pigments) which occurs with chlorophyll in all green plants. By a slight chemical change, one molecule of carotene is converted into two molecules of vitamin A, the change taking place in the intestinal mucosa. Vitamin A is then transported via the lymph to the general circulation and ultimately to the liver where it is stored. Carnivorous animals usually depend upon animal tissues of their food, the liver obviously being especially desirable in this respect. The vitamin is fat-soluble and, since certain fishes store large amounts of it, cod-liver oil and shark-liver oil constitute concentrated sources of this vitamin. Certain species such as man and bovines can also absorb carotenoids directly and subsequently convert them to vitamin A in the liver. In all species, bile salts and pancreatic juice are necessary for the absorption of vitamin A and carotenoids.

The biochemical events of absorption, transport and storage of vitamin A and its precursors have recently been reviewed by Olson (1969).

The earliest sign of deficiency of vitamin A is **night blindness** (nyctalopia). The animal is unable to see as well as it should in partial darkness, as can be determined by placing obstructions in front of it under nocturnal conditions. Changes in cellular morphology consist in retinal degenerations not easily detected, but it has been determined that night vision is dependent upon a continuous chemical interchange involving the light-induced bleaching of a pigment in the rods of the retina, known as rhodopsin or visual purple, and its restoration. Rhodopsin is composed of vitamin A aldehyde (retinene) and the protein opsin. Descriptions of morphologic alterations in the retina have varied from the absence of lesions to accumulation of eosinophilic debris and macrophages between the rods and pigmented epithelium with thinning of the outer nuclear layer in rabbits, to degeneration of rods and the outer nuclear, outer molecular and inner nuclear layers in rats.

While nyctalopia is not likely to be noticed unless sought, the classical early symptom is xerophthalmia, which means dryness of the eye. The deficiency of lacrimal secretion responsible for this dryness is due to interference with the glands and partial obstruction of their ducts by squamous metaplasia and thickened linings. Apparently because of the lack of the protective tears, animals, especially horses and cattle, when suffering from this deficiency, are subject to recurrent episodes of conjunctivitis and keratitis. The latter are doubtless precipitated by dust, foreign particles and infection. The keratitis may or may not be of such severity as to lead to ulceration and opacity, but healing is the rule, subsequent attacks being not improbable.

The epithelial changes in the lacrimal glands are an index to the fundamental disorder of vitamin A deficiency, which is squamous metaplasia and pronounced cornification of many columnar and cuboidal epithelial surfaces. A demonstrable quantitative atrophy or even necrosis often precedes the metaplasia. These changes involve the digestive tract and especially the glands which open into it, the respiratory mucous membranes, where the protective cilia are lost, and practically all genitourinary surfaces and glands. Partially or wholly as the result of impairment of epithelial protection, respiratory infections are unusually frequent. Mastitis of unusual frequency and severity has been observed in deficient dairy herds.

In birds, the mucous glands which open into the esophagus and pharynx become distended with inspissated secretion because their ducts are occluded by the increased thickness of their epithelial linings, which have undergone squamous metaplasia and hyperkeratosis. The spherical nodules, 1 to 2 mm. in diameter, spaced at rather wide but regular intervals over the mucosa are pathognomonic of hypovitaminosis A. Accompanied by coryza and other upper respiratory inflammations, doubtless infectious, and by general malaise and inanition, this condition goes by the name of **nutritional roup.**

Probably the most important effect of this epithelial dysplasia is to be found in the urinary tract. Practically all male cattle, sheep and goats subjected to prolonged severe deficiency of vitamin A die of urinary obstruction caused by urinary calculi lodged at the sigmoid flexure. Desquamated clumps of epithelial cells from the renal pelves or other urinary surfaces are considered to form nuclear granules upon which mineral salts precipitate. Females escape the effects of this **urolithiasis** because of the less constricted urethra.

Also of importance is interference with maternal reproduction. Excessive cornification is at least sufficient to upset the cycle of epithelial changes as shown by the vaginal smear (p. 1302), cornified epithelium being constantly present. It is known that in experimentally deficient rats the embryo undergoes implantation but is resorbed a short time later. While difficult to prove, strong clinical evidence supports the view that the same happens in other species including cattle and that this defect, based upon imperfect endometrial function, is an important cause of infertility in the bovine. Atrophy of seminiferous epithelium is demonstrable in deficient rats but it is doubtful that testicular function deteriorates in domestic animals, however, more thorough studies are needed on this point.

Severe deficiency of this vitamin also alters normal bone growth and remodeling, especially of cranial bones, resulting in a disparity between growth of the nervous system and its bony enclosure. This apparently results from a replacement of subperiosteal resorption by osteoblastic activity. Probably the only noticeable effects of this, as far as domestic animals are concerned, are to be seen in occasional fetal malformations and, as found in certain experimental work, in a failure of the optic foramina to grow to sufficient diameter. This is believed by some to be the cause, through constriction of the optic nerve, of the frequent blindness in newborn calves from experimentally deficient mothers. However, these troubles appear to be extremely rare with the degree of deficiency encountered under natural conditions.

Increased cerebrospinal fluid pressure regularly follows vitamin A deficiency. In part, reduction in size of the cranial vault may explain the increased pressure, however, in that pressure returns to normal levels when adequate dietary vitamin A is provided, other mechanisms undoubtedly participate. Present evidence suggests that absorption of cerebrospinal fluid via arachnoid villi is impeded. In experimentally deficient calves, the dura mater is thickened over the anterior cerebellum and tentorium cerebelli where arachnoid villi are abundant.

Comparable to differentiation of periosteal cells, odontogenic epithelium also fails to differentiate in experimentally deficient animals, resulting in a reduction in the deposition of enamel. Although similar lesions may occur spontaneously the role of vitamin A deficiency and dental disease has not been assessed in domestic animals.

Lastly, fetal malformations must be mentioned. In addition to blindness at birth, the exact pathogenesis of which is often obscure, calves have been born with an island of hairy skin in the middle of the cornea (dermoid, p. 1418), with jaws that did not fit each other and with other deformities. Litters of pigs have been born without eyes. These and similar developmental anomalies have occurred among animals experimentally deprived of vitamin A with a frequency altogether too great to be explained by the laws of chance. Surprisingly, developmental anomalies have also been reported to result from great excesses of the vitamin. Prolonged gestation (p. 1372) has also been reported in hypovitaminosis A in cattle. This may be related to fetal anomalies.

Except through the secondary development of some fatal disorder such as urinary obstruction, deficiency of vitamin A does not cause death. Deficient animals fatten as well as any and have been maintained in a condition of marketable obesity for indefinite periods. The tissue changes are reversible, and complete return to normal can be expected if the deficiency is corrected. In any species, the liver stores an amount ample for a considerable period, during which complete experimental deprivation produces no symptoms. This period is usually five or six months in cattle and probably horses, two or three months in sheep and goats. Dogs and cats are susceptible to this deficiency but suffer from it only when kept under very unusual conditions. In cats squamous metaplasia of the respiratory tract, conjunctiva, salivary glands and endometrium have been reported. These animals appear to be unable to convert carotene to vitamin A.

Hypovitaminosis A

DUTT, B., and VASUDEVAN, B.: Clinical Syndromes and Histopathological Changes in Vitamin "A" Deficiency in Cow Calves. Indian Vet. J. *39*:584–587, 1962.
DUTT, B.: Effect of Vitamin A Deficiency on the Testes of Rams. Brit. Vet. J. *115*:236–238, 1959.
EATON, H. D.: Chronic Bovine Hypo- and Hypervitaminosis A and Cerebrospinal Fluid Pressure. Amer. J. Clin. Nutr. *22*:1070–1080, 1969.
GALLINA, A. M., *et al.*: Bone Growth in the Hypovitaminotic A Calf. J. Nutr. *100*:129–142, 1970.
HAYES, K. C., MCCOMBS, H. L., and FAHERTY, T. P.: The Fine Structure of Vitamin A Deficiency. I. Parotid Duct Metaplasia. Lav. Inv. *22*:81–89, 1970.
HAYES, K. C., NIELSEN, S. W., and EATON, H. D.: Pathogenesis of the Optic Nerve Lesion in Vitamin A-Deficient Calves. Arch. Ophthal. *80*:777–787, 1968.
MARSH, H., and SWINGLE, K. F.: The Calcium, Phosphorus, Magnesium, Carotene and Vitamin A Content of the Blood of Range Cattle in Eastern Montana. Am. J. Vet. Res. *21*:212–221, 1960.
MILLS, J. H. L., *et al.*: Experimental Pathology of Dairy Calves Ingesting One-Third the Daily Requirement of Carotene. Acta Vet. Scand. *8*:324–346, 1967.
NIELSEN, S. W., *et al.*: Parotid Duct Metaplasia in Marginal Bovine Vitamin A Deficiency. Am. J. Vet. Res. *27*:223–233, 1966.
OLSON, J. A.: Metabolism and Function of Vitamin A. Fed. Proc. *28*:1670–1677, 1969.
PALLUDAN, B.: The Teratogenic Effect of Vitamin A Deficiency in Pigs. Acta Vet. Scand. *2*:32–59, 1961.
SCHMIDT, H.: Vitamin A Deficiencies in Ruminants. Am. J. Vet. Res. *2*:373–389, 1941.
SORSBY, A., READING, H. W., and BUNYAN, J.: Effect of Vitamin A Deficiency on the Retina of the Experimental Rabbit. Nature (London) *210*:1011–1015, 1966.
SPRATLING, F. R., *et al.*: Experimental Hypovitaminosis-A in Calves. Clinical and Gross Post-Mortem Findings. Vet. Rec. *77*:1532–1542, 1965.

HYPOVITAMINOSIS B

The original vitamin B is now known to include a number of specific chemical compounds, thiamine (vitamin B_1), riboflavin (B_2), nicotinic acid ("Niacin"), pantothenic acid, pyridoxine (B_6) and cyanocobalamin (B_{12}). A number of other factors such as folic acid, biotin, and para-amino-benzoic acid are also usually included in the vitamin B group. Since these substances have largely the same source (yeast, grains and seeds) and since the lesions resulting from their deficiency tend to overlap, all can be considered together, the term B-complex being in common use for the group. The long used descriptive name of "the antineuritic vitamin" gives an insight into many aspects of the B-group.

The disease entities in veterinary medicine which have been recognized as depending on lack of one or more components of the group are (1) polyneuritis of birds including "curly-toe paralysis," (2) Chastek paralysis of foxes, (3) canine pellagra (blacktongue), (4) a chronic enteritis of pigs.

The **polyneuritis** of birds is largely or entirely an experimental disease, although it afforded the first experimental demonstration of the existence of these vitamins. There is myelin degeneration of the peripheral nerve fibers with weakness of the limbs or ascending paralysis. This condition is due entirely or principally to deficiency of thiamine. Small chicks have developed, under ill-advised but not necessarily experimental feeding conditions, a spastic paralysis which causes the toes to be continually curled in volar flexion, even when bearing weight (curly-toe paralysis, p. 1376). This has been traced to a deficiency of riboflavin.

Chastek paralysis of foxes, named from the fur farm where the disease was first studied, is a fatal ascending paralysis preceded by anorexia, weakness and diarrhea. Study has shown it to be caused by a diet of fish (several species). The bodies of these fish contain an enzyme which neutralizes or destroys thiamine, so that the disease becomes a severe deficiency of the latter substance. The fundamental lesions appear to be degenerations and necrosis of certain nerve cell bodies near the ventricles of the brain.

A similar deficiency occurs in cats as the result of a diet (usually canned) containing whole fish without adequate supplementation. Within three or four days after indisposition first makes its appearance, incoordination of movement, ataxia, postural abnormalities, and dilation of pupils pass into convulsions and terminate in coma and death. The lesions include focal hemorrhages in the periventricular gray matter which are bilaterally symmetrical and often visible to the unaided eye. Microscopically, edema, gliosis and gitter cells can also be seen. Thiamine administered parenterally prevents the disease and cures it in its early stages. At least two poisonous plants, Bracken fern (p. 907) and equisetum (p. 949) owe much (but not all) of their toxicity to their ability to destroy or neutralize thiamine.

Thiamine deficiency is also recognized to play a role in the Wernicke encephalopathy of man.

The striking feature of thiamine deficiency in all species of animals is the constant localization and bilateral symmetry of the lesions in the central nervous system. Although in advanced lesions there is almost complete destruction of all tissue elements, recent evidence suggests that the primary lesions develop in glia.

Blacktongue, or canine pellagra, is a supposed entity characterized by severe cyanosis of the distal portion of the tongue which, in severe cases, makes it practically black. In milder forms, which include those usually produced experimentally, the tongue shows only superficial ulceration along its borders. Regularly there are petechial or ecchymotic hemorrhages throughout the digestive canal with patches of hemorrhagic enteritis or gastritis. The symptomatologic entity resulting includes precipitous anorexia, salivation, foul-smelling ulceration of the buccal mucosa, vomiting and bloody diarrhea with their resultant dehydration and emaciation. Death is usually stated to be accompanied by fever, presumably from terminal bacterial infection.

Rather extensive experimental studies have seemed to show that this syndrome, like human pellagra, results from a diet consisting largely of Indian corn (maize) and foods made from it and it has been called canine pellagra. Experimentally the same syndrome has been produced by various diets lacking nicotinic acid and the amino acid, tryptophane, both of which are almost non-existent in corn. The experimental disorder is considered to have been prevented by feeding yeast or meat, but in one experiment (Follis, 1958) cod-liver oil had to be given in addition. The interpretation is current that both canine and human pellagra result from a deficiency of nicotinic acid of the B complex coupled with a low level of tryptophane, but the possibility of an "antivitamin" or direct toxic action from corn has not been excluded. Somewhat at variance with the experimental interpretations is the fact that it is practically impossible to find any veterinary practitioner today who has experienced a case combining the above symptoms and lesions with pathogenetic circumstances similar to those used in the experiments. The clinical syndrome and the post-mortem lesions correspond to those that are today recognized as characteristic of leptospirosis. Indeed it seems to be a single syndrome that has been carried down through the years of the last half-century successively as Stuttgart disease (first seen at Stuttgart, Germany), then as canine typhus, canine pellagra and now as leptospirosis. The possibility may well be entertained that the accidental presence of this latter infection may have beclouded experimental results. Without the systematic clinical examinations and diagnostic tests which practical veterinary medicine demands it seems plausible that leptospirosis and uremia, known instigators of such a clinical picture, would not have been recognized. The widespread skepticism as to the existence of a naturally occurring deficiency disease with the manifestations above described appears to be not unjustified.

The porcine enteritis, attributed to a similar deficiency and the feeding of unsupplemented corn, occurs in pigs not long after weaning and is characterized by chronic diarrhea, anorexia and stunted growth. The principal lesion is a very severe patchy mucous colitis with necrosis of the worst areas followed by secondary infection with the necrophorus organism. It was originally suggested by experimenters that a deficiency of the type described for corn (above) might be the primary cause of the well-known necrophorus enteritis ("necro"), but this was incompatible with the fact that pigs on any diet may have "necro." It must also be assumed that many pigs escape the effects of deficiency, for millions of pigs have been raised with reasonable success on the unbalanced diet afforded by corn alone.

There are a number of other poorly defined syndromes, including some forms of dermatitis, which have been ascribed to deficiencies of various members of the B-complex but these are at present in a position of uncertainty.

Human pellagra, as has been implied above, occurs in persons who subsist mainly on corn products, usually combined with fat pork. The lesions include severe chronic exfoliative dermatitis of hands and exposed areas, and glossitis with severe atrophy of the epithelium and flattening of the papillae. Various nervous degenerations are also present. There is thus a considerable similarity to the canine pellagra described above.

Human beriberi, on the basis of experimental causation by a diet of polished rice, is comparable to the polyneuritis of fowls. Clinically three features are salient; (1) neuromuscular weakness, ataxias and paresthesias with degenerative changes in the nervous system; (2) bradycardia, cardiac weakness and insufficiency with minimal degenerative changes in the myocardium; and (3) edema. The disease is considered to be due to a complicated deficiency of thiamine, other units of the B complex and general dietary inadequacy.

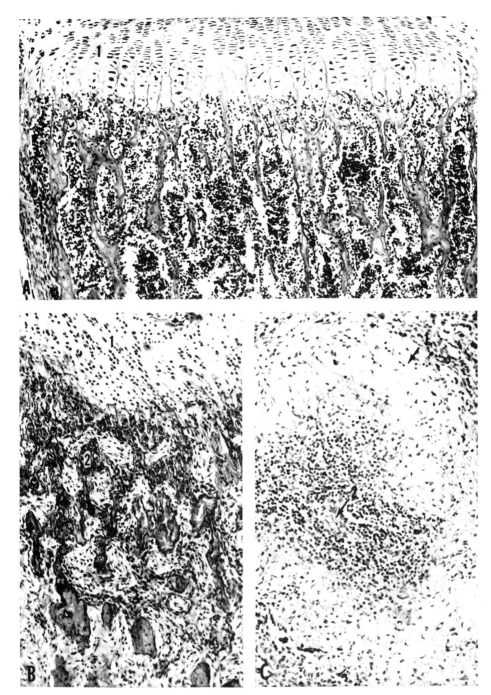

FIG. 18–2.—Scurvy in the guinea pig. *A*, Femur of normal guinea pig (× 90). Epiphyseal cartilage (*1*), new-formed bone (*2*) and hematopoietic marrow (*3*). *B*, Femur of scorbutic guinea pig (× 100). Distorted epiphyseal cartilage (*1*), disrupted spicules of new bone (*2*) and fibrous marrow (*3*). *C*, Amyloidosis of spleen of scorbutic guinea pig (× 150). Amyloid (*1*) surrounds and displaces lymphocytes of the splenic corpuscle. Central artery (*2*). (Courtesy of Armed Forces Institute of Pathology.) Contributor: Army Medical Nutrition Laboratory.

It should be noted that necrotic cardiac fibers and microscopic scars have been found in pigs in experimental thiamine deficiency, the existence of a clinical parallel being a justifiable presumption. It is possible that this deficiency should be considered in the diagnosis of unexplained sudden death in these animals.

Bovine animals synthesize abundant amounts of B complex through the growth of the ruminal bacteria. Hence they are not subject to deficiency of this vitamin except as young animals before the rumen is functioning. A potential exception is the suggestion that thiamine deficiency may play a role in polioencephalomalacia in ruminants (p. 1409). Although thiamine has been demonstrated to have therapeutic benefit in this disorder, whether thiamine deficiency is the cause remains to be established.

In horses, abundant amounts of riboflavin appear to be important in the avoidance of periodic ophthalmia. Other than this, no equine deficiencies of the B complex are known, except as part of equisetum and Bracken fern poisoning (p. 907, 949).

Experimentally produced deficiency of **pantothenic acid** in swine causes areas of mucous, hemorrhagic and necrotizing colitis with consequent diarrhea. There are also necrosis of neurones of the dorsal spinal ganglia, and myelin and axonal degenerations in the brachial and sciatic nerves, which result in an ataxic and

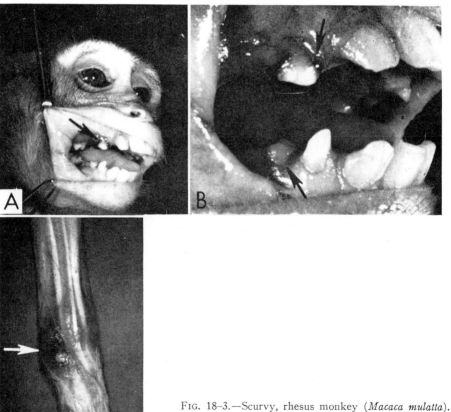

Fig. 18–3.—Scurvy, rhesus monkey (*Macaca mulatta*). *A* and *B*, Loosening of teeth and gingival hemorrhage (arrows). *C*, Subperiosteal hemorrhage at distal tibia (arrow). (Courtesy of New England Regional Primate Research Center, Harvard Medical School.)

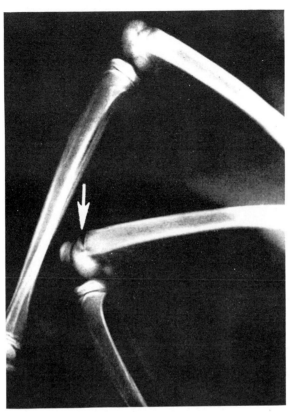

Fig. 18–4.—Scurvy, rhesus monkey (*Macaca mulatta*). Epiphyseal fracture (arrow) of the distal femur. (Courtesy of New England Regional Primate Research Center, Harvard Medical School.)

jerky gait and terminal recumbency. Deficiency of pantothenic acid can also be produced in dogs (as well as in monkeys, rats, etc.). In chicks, it causes a dermatitis. However, deficiency of this substance does not enter into clinical practice because of the wide availability of the vitamin.

Experimental deficiency of pyridoxine (B_6) has been produced in dogs, pigs, monkeys and rodents, and is characterized by cutaneous hyperkeratosis and acanthosis, by anemia and by nervous disturbances. However, since its production involves removal of the natural ingredients of foods by alcoholic extraction, the advent of this deficiency among our clinical diseases does not appear imminent!

Hypovitaminosis B

CHITTENDEN, R. H., and UNDERHILL, F. P.: The Production in Dogs of a Pathological Condition Which Closely Resembles Human Pellagra. Amer. J. Physiol. *44*:13–17, 1917.

DENTON, J.: A Study of the Tissue Changes in Experimental Blacktongue of Dogs Compared with Similar Changes in Pellagra. Amer. J. Path. *4*:341–347, 1928.

GOLDBERGER, J., and WHEELER, G. A.: Experimental Blacktongue of Dogs and Its Relation to Pellagra. Publ. Health Rep. *43*:172–177, 1928.

JUBB, K. V., SAUNDERS, L. Z., and COATES, H. V.: Thiamine Deficiency Encephalopathy in Cats. J. Comp. Path. *66*:217–227, 1956.

MADHAVAN, T. V., BELAVADY, B., and GOPLAN, C.: Pathology of Canine Black Tongue. J. Path. Bact. *95*:259–263, 1968.

MARKSON, L. M., and TERLECKI, S.: The Aetiology of Cerebrocortical Necrosis. Brit. Vet. J. *124*:309–315, 1968.

ROBERTSON, D. M., WASAN, S. M., and SKINNER, D. B.:   Ultrastructural Feature of Early Brain Stem Lesions of Thiamine-Deficient Rats. Amer. J. Path. *52*:1081–1097, 1968.
SAUNDERS, L. Z.:   Thiamine Deficiency Encephalopathy in Cats, in *Comparative Neuropathology*, Innes, J. R. M. and Saunders, L. Z., New York, Academic Press, 1962.
SMITH, D. T., PERSONS, E. L., and HARVEY, H. I.:   On the Identity of the Goldberger and Underhill Types of Canine Blacktongue. Secondary Spirochetial Infection in Each. J. Nutrition *14*:373–377, 1937.

HYPOVITAMINOSIS C

The history of vitamin C, now chemically identified as **ascorbic acid,** a derivative of hexose, goes back to the "lime-juicers" of the 18th century. This nickname was given to the British ships-of-war, since their sailors were required to consume the juice of limes, which had been found to prevent in some unknown way that scourge of long voyages, the disease known as **scurvy** or **scorbutus.**

The lesions of human scurvy consist chiefly in subperiosteal hemorrhages and failure of proper ossification of long bones, failure of wounds to heal and occasionally a hyperkeratotic papular dermatitis. In guinea pigs, defective formation of dentine is a part of the picture. Focal necroses of the myocardium sometimes occur and may be a cause of sudden death. The bony changes, of course, are painful, explaining much of the symptomatology. The classical gingivitis and bleeding gums have not been found in experimental avitaminosis C and probably represented a mixed deficiency. The fundamental disturbance is inability of fibroblastic cells to form either collagen fibers or osteoid tissue. This accounts for non-healing of wounds and the bony disorder, which is a widened zone of calcified but unossified cartilage at the sites of endochondral bone formation. The cartilaginous side of the epiphyseal junction, therefore, presents a convexity which bulges into the retarded, weakened and disordered osseous side.

Scurvy does not occur in the ordinary domestic species for the reason that they either synthesize their own ascorbic acid or live on green plants, which always contain this vitamin. The veterinarian, however, may well encounter it in guinea pigs, which are extremely susceptible and die after three or four weeks without green plants or some other source of ascorbic acid. Both New- and Old-World monkeys have the same susceptibility as humans.

Hypovitaminosis C

LEHNER, N. D. M., BULLOCK, B. C., and CLARKSON, T. B.:   Ascorbic Acid Deficiency in the Squirrel Monkey. Proc. Soc. Exp. Biol. Med. *128*:512–514, 1968.

HYPOVITAMINOSIS D

Vitamin D is formed from steroid precursors or provitamins of which two have been found in nature; ergosterol (provitamin D_2) is found in plants and 7-dehydrocholesterol (provitamin D_3) is found in animal tissues. To be effective, these steroids, either in the skin of the animal or its food, must be exposed to the radiant action of violet and ultraviolet light, ordinarily of sunlight, which converts ergosterol to vitamin D_2 (ergocalciferol) and 7-dehydrocholesterol to vitamin D_3 (cholecalciferol). In case the vitamin is not available in the food, a comparatively short exposure to direct sunlight (two minutes per day for chickens in midsummer) is adequate for normal health.

The principal role of vitamin D is to maintain serum calcium at optimal levels

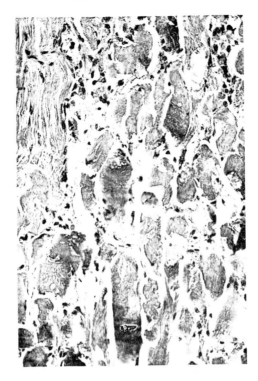

FIG. 18–5.—Nutritional myopathy, white-muscle disease, skeletal muscle of a cow ($\times$ 195). Fragmentation of muscle fibers with swelling and early calcification. (Courtesy of Armed Forces Institute of Pathology.) Contributor: Dr. J. F. Ryff.

for its numerous physiological functions (p. 1001). Two vitamin D dependent processes serve to elevate serum calcium; (1) calcium transport across the intestine and (2) mobilization of calcium from bone. The latter function is dependent upon parathyroid hormone. Great progress has recently been made which explains in part how vitamin D mediates these functions. It is now known that following ingestion or formation in the skin, vitamin D is transported to the liver by means of an α_2-globulin where it is converted to 25-hydroxycholecalciferol (25-HCC). The 25-HCC is then carried by an α_2 globulin to the kidney where it is oxygenated. The resultant product, "1- oxygenated 25-HCC," then circulates, and at the level of bone and intestine, acts on DNA to make messenger RNA which is coded for the production of specific proteins or enzymes responsible for calcium transport. The recent demonstration of the role played by the kidney in producing the active vitamin D metabolite may explain, in part, certain metabolic bone diseases associated with chronic renal failure (p. 1064).

Young chickens provide means for very precise studies of this deficiency; they are hatched with enough vitamin for the first two weeks of life; if more is not received from the food, chicks kept in darkness die between the eighteenth and twenty-first days of life (so-called leg-weakness). Although other metabolic disorders may also cause it, the disease resulting from deficiency of vitamin D is rickets, which will be described with the other diseases of bone (p. 1058). There is also retarded and abnormal dentition.

Hypovitaminosis D

DeLuca, H. F.: Recent Advances in the Metabolism and Function of Vitamin D. Fed. Proc. *28*:1678–1689, 1969.
Fraser, D. R., and Kodicek, E.: Unique Biosynthesis by Kidney of a Biologically Active Vitamin D Metabolite. Nature *228*:764–766, 1970.

HYPOVITAMINOSIS E

Vitamin E has been found to consist chemically of an alcohol, or a group of closely related alcohols, named tocopherols (Gr. *tokus*—child-birth; *phero*—·to carry). Four naturally occurring tocopherols have been discovered, alpha-, beta-, delta-, and eta-tocopherol. Alpha-tocopherol is the most active biologically. Alpha-tocopherol occurs especially in the germs of seeds and extracts thereof (wheat-germ oil).

Vitamin E deficiency has been held responsible for a variety of pathological processes in domestic animals. Based on experimentally induced deficiency and clinical observations, the following conditions are believed to result:

Rats:	Necrosis of the germinal cells of the seminiferous tubules and aspermatogenesis; necrosis of skeletal and cardiac muscle; retarded development, death and resorption of embryos; axonal degeneration in the central nervous system; hepatic necrosis, deposition of ceroid in adipose tissue.
Mice:	Necrosis of skeletal and cardiac muscle, hepatic necrosis, kidney necrosis.
Rabbits:	Necrosis of skeletal muscle; steatitis (yellow fat disease).
Calves and Lambs:	Necrosis of skeletal and cardiac muscle (white muscle disease).
Pigs:	Necrosis of skeletal and cardiac muscle (Herztod); hepatic necrosis (*hepatosis dietetica*); steatitis (yellow fat disease); exudative diathesis; anemia.
Cats:	Steatitis (yellow fat disease).
Dogs:	Ceroid deposition in smooth muscle; necrosis of skeletal muscle; testicular degeneration; axonal degeneration in the central nervous system.
Monkeys:	Necrosis of skeletal muscle; anemia.
Chicks:	Exudative diathesis; necrosis of skeletal, cardiac and gizzard muscle; encephalomalacia, decreased egg production, fertility and hatchability.
Mink:	Necrosis of skeletal muscle; steatitis (yellow fat disease).
Guinea Pig:	Necrosis of skeletal muscle.

The exact function of vitamin E at the molecular level is not understood, a fact which makes it exceedingly difficult to explain the diverse group of lesions attributed to its deficiency. To complicate our understanding, a complex physiological link between selenium, sulfur-containing amino acids (methionine, cysteine) and vitamin E has been demonstrated. It appears that certain of the lesions listed above are the result of vitamin E deficiency, others from selenium deficiency, and a third group due to a combined deficiency. Selenium has reportedly been used successfully to treat muscular dystrophy of sheep, calves, and chicks, *hepatosis dietetica* in pigs and exudative diathesis of poultry.

In view of these experimental findings, alpha tocopherol and selenium have been used in the treatment of a great variety of reproductive, muscular and other diseases of man and animals.

In the domestic animals, the need for the artificial addition of alpha tocopherol to the diet has at times been problematical. However, experimental deficiency studies now indicate that most species require this nutrient. Greatest attention

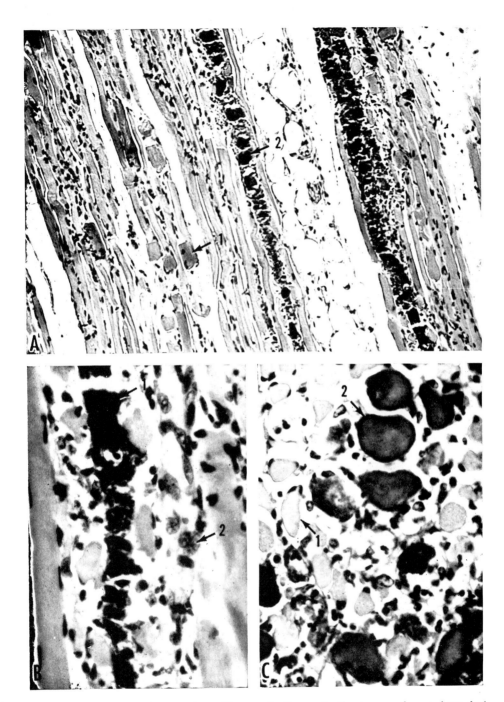

FIG. 18–6.—Nutritional myopathy, white-muscle disease, in the tongue of a newborn foal. *A*, Low power (× 150) to show fragmentation of muscle bundles (*1*) and calcification (*2*). *B*, Longitudinal section (× 500) of muscle bundles. Calcification within muscle bundles (*1*), proliferation of sarcolemmal nuclei (*2*). *C*, Cross section of muscle fibers (× 500). Note normal (*1*) and calcified (*2*) muscle bundles. (Courtesy of Armed Forces Institute of Pathology.) Contributor: Dr. W. O. Reed.

has been given to a condition known as **nutritional myopathy, white-muscle disease** (p. 1049) or muscular dystrophy (it is a degenerative process, not a disturbance of growth), some forms of which a number of investigators concur in attributing to a deficiency of vitamin E. The condition in which this muscular disease has been principally studied occurs in suckling lambs a few weeks old, and is commonly known as **stiff-lamb disease,** a term which explains its usual clinical features. Experimental evidence appears to link this disease adequately with deficiency of alpha-tocopherol, although clinical confusion with other conditions such as polyarthritis from umbilical infection (low-grade pyosepticemia neonatorum) has certainly occurred.

Also, it should be remembered that the affected muscles of horses dying from azoturia (p. 1046) and of swine poisoned by excessive gossypol (p. 873) show similar changes both grossly and microscopically. It is certainly safe to say that the degenerative changes conforming to "white muscle disease" are not all due to the same cause.

Acute myodegeneration in swine, which has been called **Herztod,** has also been attributed to vitamin E deficiency. In this condition there is acute necrosis of skeletal and cardiac muscle which results in sudden death. Acute hepatic necrosis or **hepatosis dietetica** (dietary hepatic necrosis) of swine has been more clearly related to vitamin E deficiency, although selenium and sulfur-containing amino acids afford protection. The lesions of the liver are characterized by massive necrosis of entire lobules. Dietary hepatic necrosis is frequently associated with myodegeneration, generalized edema (exudative diathesis) and yellow pigmentation of fat.

The yellow pigment to which reference was made earlier in this section occurs in what is known as **"yellow fat disease"** or **"steatitis."** The disorder has been encountered in mink and swine which were fed considerable amounts of fish meal, fish offal or other products of like origin. After a month, more or less, on such a diet, the animals come to have a body fat that is strangely yellowish or brownish in color although but little changed in other respects. Microscopic examination of such fat, subcutaneous or visceral, reveals droplets or amorphous bodies of a brown or yellow substance at the interstices of the adipose cells. The substance appears to be oily or waxy in nature and, for this reason, has received the name of **ceroid** (p. 84). It is insoluble in fat solvents, does not respond to stains for iron but does take and retain the red fuchsin when the usual stain for acid-fast bacteria is applied. With hematoxylin and eosin or similar tissue stains, the substance is relatively basophilic. The amount at any one interstice may be so large as to approach the volume of an adipose cell, but this material is outside those cells.

It may, however, be within phagocytic cells, and these macrophages occasionally develop to form foreign body giant cells. The ceroid is also found in the Kupffer cells of the liver, and sometimes small particles of it can be stained in the cytoplasm of the hepatic epithelial cells themselves. Phagocytes containing it occasionally migrate to the regional lymph nodes and even to the spleen. In the areas of adipose tissue it excites a slight infiltration of inflammatory leukocytes.

While the fishy odor that sometimes causes condemnation of meat from swine fed on fish meal may not be markedly ameliorated, the formation of ceroid and the yellow discoloration are inhibited and usually prevented by increased amounts of alpha-tocopherol in the diet. Since unsaturated fatty acids have notable

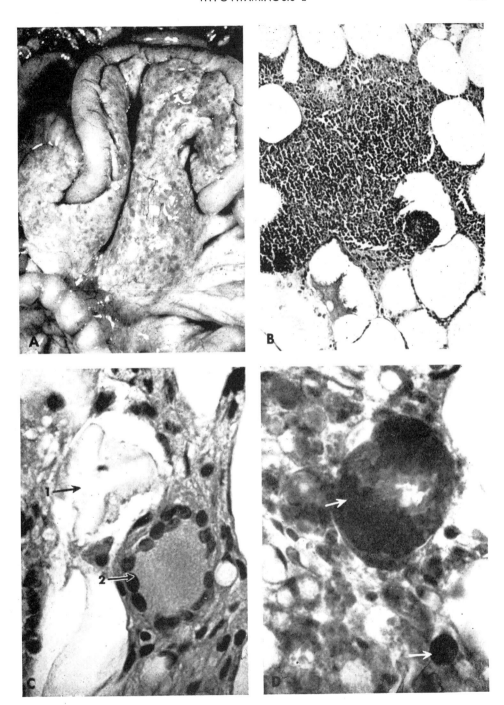

FIG. 18-7.—Steatitis in the cat. *A*, Mesenteric fat of a 1½-year-old castrated male cat. The dark spots were bright yellow color, the rest of the abundant mesenteric fat was yellowish tan. *B*, Neutrophils in adipose tissue of a young obese cat which exhibited fever and severe neutrophilic leukocytosis. H & E × 110. *C*, Adipose tissue of a cat in a late stage of the disease with altered fat (*1*) and Langhans' type giant cell (*2*). H & E × 540. *D*, A section of adipose tissue from the same cat as C, with globules of acid-fast ceroid pigment (arrows). Ziehl-Neelsen's Acid Fast Stain × 540. (Courtesy of Angell Memorial Hospital and Journal American Veterinary Medical Association.)

oxidizing properties through their attraction for H-ions, and since alpha tocopherol appears to owe its effect chiefly to its anti-oxidant powers, it is believed that the ceroid is a by-product of oxidative processes which are inhibited by a larger supply of the vitamin. Conversely it may conceivably be formed as a degradation product in the interaction of the tocopherol and the oxidant fatty acids.

A similar or identical pigment has occurred in experimental animals fed large amounts of cod-liver oil for its content of vitamin D. Apparently the oily vehicle of vitamin D exerted a similar antagonistic effect on the limited amount of vitamin E available, although signs of deficiency did not extend beyond the formation of ceroid pigment.

Steatitis in cats occurs after some weeks on certain fish diets, arising suddenly with fever and general malaise. There is severe pain when the cutaneous region is disturbed either by manipulation or by the patient's own movements and palpation reveals an abnormal denseness and lumpiness of the subcutaneous fat. These symptoms, together with a very pronounced neutrophilia, a marked "shift to the left" and often moderate eosinophilia, tend to persist for many days and may terminate fatally unless relieved by suitable treatment. By biopsy or necropsy it is seen that the fat, in addition to being markedly discolored by the yellow or brown pigment, is heavily infiltrated with neutrophils accompanied by a few leukocytes of other kinds and perhaps by Langhans giant cells. Typical deposits of acid-fast ceroid are plentiful and it has been suggested that, as irritant foreign bodies, they are the direct cause of the inflammatory reaction.

An apparently comparable steatitis, cause unknown, has been reported in the muscles of foals in New Zealand. Rarely similar fatty deposits have been found to be fluorescent, and accompanied by photosensitizational dermatitis.

Although yellow fat disease has not been reported in dogs, a histologically and histochemically identical pigment has been described in smooth muscle cells particularly of the small intestine and spleen, often imparting a grossly visible brown color to the small intestine. The condition has been called "brown dog gut" and the pigment "leiomyometoplasts," however experimental evidence indicates that the pigment is a lipofuscin similar, if not identical to, ceroid and can be induced by vitamin E deficiency.

Axonal degeneration, principally in the brain stem, which follows vitamin E deficiency in rats and dogs is not infrequently encountered in clinically normal dogs suggesting that vitamin E deficiency may be more frequent in this species than usually suspected. The degenerating axons form eosinophilic spherical bodies up to 150 microns in diameter.

Hypovitaminosis E

CHEVILLE, N. F.: The Pathology of Vitamin E Deficiency in the Chick. Path. Vet. *3*:208–225, 1966.

COUSINS, F. B., and CAIRNEY, I. M.: Some Aspects of Selenium Metabolism in Sheep. Aust. J. Agric. Res. *12*:927–943, 1961.

DAVIS, C. L., and GORHAM, J. R.: The Pathology of Experimental and Natural Cases of "Yellow Fat" Disease in Swine. Amer. J. Vet. Res. *15*:55–59, 1954.

DRAPER, H. H., and CSALLANY, A. S.: Metabolism and Function of Vitamin E. Fed. Proc. *28*:1690–1695, 1969.

DODD, D. C., *et al.*: Muscle Degeneration and Yellow-Fat Disease in Foals. N. Z. Vet. J. *8*:45–50, 1960.

DRONEMAN, J., and WENSVOORT, P.: Muscular Dystrophy and Yellow Fat Disease in Shetland Pony Foals. Neth. J. Vet. Sci. *1*:42–48, 1968.

ENDICOTT, K. M.: Similarity of the Acid-fast Pigment Ceroid and Oxidized Unsaturated Fat. Arch. Path. *37*:49–53, 1944.

GERSHOFF, S. N., and NORKIN, S. A.: Vitamin E Deficiency in Cats. J. Nutr. *77*:303–308, 1962.

GORHAM, J. R., BOE, N., and BAKER, G. A.: Experimental "Yellow-Fat" Disease in Pigs. Cornell Vet. *41*:332–338, 1951.

GRANT, C. A., THAFVELIN, B., and CHRISTELL, R.: Retention of Selenium by Pig Tissues. Acta Pharm. Tox. Kbh. *18*:285–297, 1961.

HARTLEY, W. J.: Selenium and Ewe Fertility. Proc. N.Z. Soc. Anim. Prod. *23*:20–27, 1963.

HAYES, K. C., NIELSEN, S. W., and ROUSSEAU, J. E., JR.: Vitamin E Deficiency and Fat Stress in the Dog. J. Nutr. *99*:196–209, 1969.

JONES, G. B., and GOODWIN, K. O.: Studies on the Nutritional Role of Selenium. I. The Distribution of Radioactive Selenium in Mice. Aust. J. Agric. Res. *14*:716–723, 1963.

JONES, D., HOWARD, A. N., and GRESHAM, G. A.: Aetiology of "Yellow Fat" Disease (pansteatitis) in the Wild Rabbit. J. Comp. Path. *79*:329–334, 1969.

MACHLIN, L. J., MEISKY, K. A., and GORDON, R. S.: Production of Encephalomalacia in Chickens Fed Aerated Heated Fats. Fed. Proc. *18*:535, 1959.

MICHEL, R. L., WHITEHAIR, C. K., and KEAHEY, K. K.: Dietary Hepatic Necrosis Associated with Selenium-Vitamin E Deficiency in Swine. J. Am. Vet. Med. Assn. *155*:50–59, 1969.

MONLUX, W. S., JOHNSON, D. F., and SMITH, H. A.: Muscle Degeneration in Texas Cattle. Southwestern Vet. *5*:103–107, 1952.

MUNSON, T. O., et al.: Steatitis ("Yellow Fat") in Cats Fed Canned Red Tuna. J. Am. Vet. Med. Assn. *133*:563–568, 1958.

NAFSTAD, I., and NAFSTAD, H. J.: An Electron Microscopic Study of Blood and Bone Marrow in Vitamin E-Deficient Pigs. Pathologia Vet. *5*:520–537, 1968.

NAFSTAD, I.: Studies of Hematology and Bone Marrow Morphology in Vitamin E-Deficient Pigs. Pathologia Vet. *2*:277–287, 1965.

NEWBERNE, P. M., and HARE, W. V.: Axon Dystrophy in Clinically Normal Dogs. Amer. J. Vet. Res. *23*:403–411, 1962.

PAYNE, W. J. A.: A Possible Vitamin E Deficiency Occurring in a Herd of Pigs Fed Standard Rations in the Tropics. Nature, Lond. *183*:828–829, 1959.

SCOTT, M. L., et al.: Selenium-Responsive Myopathies of Myocardium and of Smooth Muscle in the Young Poult. J. Nutr. *91*:573–583, 1967.

STOWE, H. D., and WHITEHAIR, C. K.: Gross and Microscopic Pathology of Tocopherol-deficient Mink. J. Nutr. *81*:287–300, 1963.

TRAPP, A. L., et al.: Vitamin E-Selenium Deficiency in Swine: Differential Diagnosis and Nature of Field Problem. J. Am. Vet. Med. Assn. *157*:289–300, 1970.

VAN VLEET, J. F., HALL, V., and SIMON, J.: Vitamin E Deficiency: A Sequential Study by Means of Light and Electron Microscopy of the Alterations Occurring in Regeneration of Skeletal Muscle of Affected Weanling Rabbits. Amer. J. Path. *51*:815–830, 1967.

HYPOVITAMINOSIS K

Vitamin K, a fat-soluble vitamin synthesized as 2-methyl-1, 4-naphthaquinone and very closely related compounds, is necessary for the proper formation of prothrombin, and clotting factors VII, IX, and X (p. 104). However, since the substance is widely prevalent in nature and is freely synthesized by intestinal bacteria, no clinical deficiency occurs in healthy animals. An exception to this statement may possibly arise as the result of prolonged dosing with salicylates or certain bacteriostatic drugs. In obstructive jaundice and possibly in severe and long-continued diarrhea, there may not be enough bile in the digestive canal for successful absorption of the vitamin and under such circumstances it needs to be administered to prevent hypoprothrombinemia. (See hemorrhage, p. 119.) It is at least a partial antidote for coumarin, the active substance in poisoning by sweet clover and by "Warfarin" (p. 906). In other respects, the vitamin is of experimental interest only.

Hypovitaminosis K

SUTTIE, J. W.: Control of Clotting Factor Biosynthesis by Vitamin K. Fed. Proc. *28*: 1696–1701, 1969.

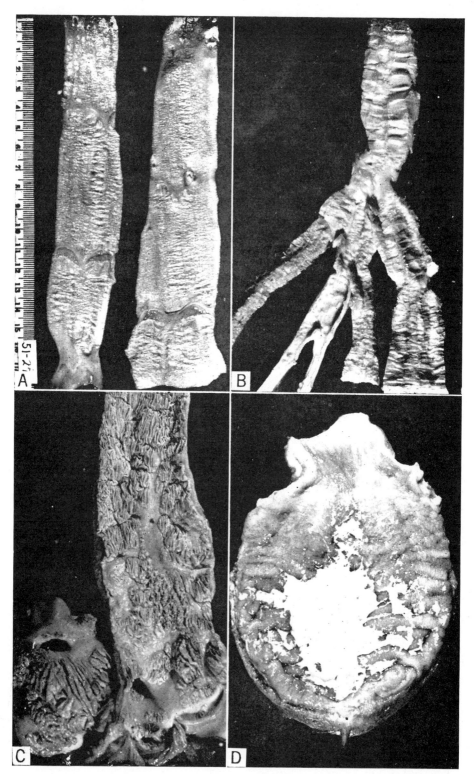

Fig. 18–8.—Hypervitaminosis D. Lesions in a pregnant Jersey cow, six years, which had been given 30 million Units of Vitamin D (viosterol) for twenty days preceding parturition, and killed one day later. *A*, Jugular vein with transverse corrugations in roughened intima. *B*, Terminal aorta and its branches with mineralization of media resulting in loss of contractility and elasticity, and irregular plaques visible from the intimal surface. *C*, Aortic valves and aortic arch. Raised, rugose plaques of calcareous material are very conspicuous from the intimal surface. *D*, Urinary bladder, containing white granular material. (Courtesy of Dr. C. R. Cole, Ohio State University.)

HYPERVITAMINOSIS

It is scarcely possible to give amounts of the vitamins so great as to be harmful except in the case of Vitamin D and Vitamin A. Even here the amount required to produce damage is far beyond ordinary therapeutic dosages.

Hypervitaminosis D.—Although several times the normal requirement is necessary to produce toxicity, hypervitaminosis D is occasionally encountered in man and animals. The deleterious effects are due to hypercalcemia resulting from increased intestinal absorption of calcium, and increased mobilization of calcium from the skeleton. The predominant tissue change is metastatic calcification (p. 56) as phosphate salts, comparable to hydroxyapatite crystals of normal bone. The mineral deposits often contain histochemically demonstrable iron and are usually PAS positive. Tissues most frequently affected are the intima and media of large arteries, where the lesions resemble Mönckeberg's arteriosclerosis (p. 1153), myocardium, gastric mucosa, lung and kidney. There is bone resorption with fibrous replacement and excessive deposition of osteoid which has been termed "hypervitaminosis D rickets." Although once considered a paradox, bone resorption is a direct effect of vitamin D in maintaining serum calcium (p. 991).

Hypervitaminosis A.—In man, acute vitamin A intoxication has been described

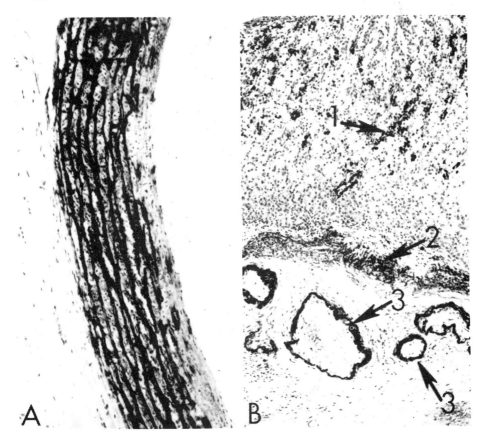

FIG. 18–9.—Hypervitaminosis D, cebus monkey. *A*, Metastatic calcification of the aorta. *B*, Metastatic calcification of the gastric mucosa (*1*), muscularis mucosa (*2*) and arteries (*3*) in the muscularis. (Courtesy of New England Regional Primate Research Center, Harvard Medical School.)

following ingestion of a single massive dose and following consumption of large quantities of polar bear liver. Chronic hypervitaminosis A has occurred in food faddists, and individuals using large daily doses of vitamin A for dermatologic conditions. In animals there are several reports of experimentally induced hypervitaminosis A, but few examples of natural poisoning. Skeletal lesions have received the greatest attention but description of the changes have been conflicting. It appears that in part, species variation is responsible for the conflicting reports. Osteoporosis and retarded bone growth due to decreased osteoblastic activity and destruction of the cartilaginous growth plate are described as the predominant changes in pigs, rats and cattle. The striking abnormality in man and cats is the development of multiple exostoses of the skeleton. Seawright and co-workers (1964, 1965, 1967) have presented evidence to indicate that hypervitaminosis A is the cause of a naturally occurring skeletal disease of cats termed **deforming cervical spondylosis**. The exostoses in this condition, which principally develop on the cervical and thoracic vertebrae, forelimbs and ribs, are histologically

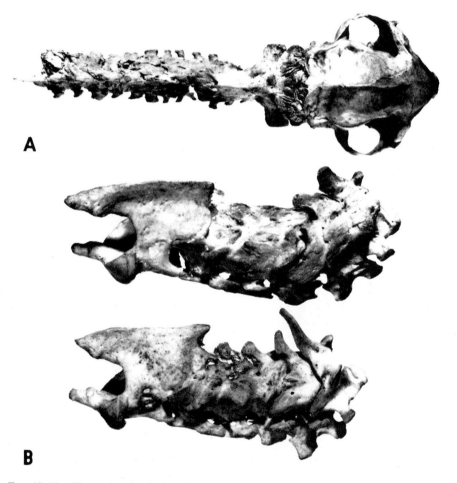

FIG. 18–10.—Hypervitaminosis A, feline. *A*, Dorsal aspect of vertebral column and cranium in a natural case of the disease. Exostoses have resulted in fusion of vertebrae and fusion of the atlas to the occipital bone. *B*, Fusion of vertebrae in an experimentally induced case. Courtesy of Dr. A. A. Seawright.

irregular masses of cartilage and new subperiosteal bone. In the experimentally induced disease, collections of large foamy macrophages occur in the liver, lungs, spleen and lymph nodes and a lipoidal material is present in renal tubular epithelium. These changes are believed to represent storage sites of excess vitamin A.

In contrast to hypovitaminosis A, excess vitamin A results in a drop in cerebrospinal fluid pressure, believed to result from a decreased formation of cerebrospinal fluid. Toxic levels of vitamin A administered by parenteral routes induce calcification of arteries, heart and kidney comparable to the changes seen in hypervitamosis D. It is of interest that the toxicity and lesions of hypervitaminosis D can be ameliorated in part by the administration of relatively large amounts of vitamin A.

Hypervitaminosis

BURGISSER, H., JACQUIER, C., and LEUENBERGER, M.: Hypervitaminosis D in Pigs Schweiz. Arch. Tierheilk. *106*:714–718, 1964.

CAPEN, C. C., COLE, C. R., and HIBBS, J. W.: The Pathology of Hypervitaminosis D in Cattle. Path. Vet. *3*:350–378, 1966.

CALHOUN, M. C., ROUSSEAU, J. E., JR., and HALL, J. J.: Cisternal Cerebrospinal Fluid Pressure During Development of Chronic Bovine Hypervitaminosis A. J. Dairy Sci. *48*:729–732, 1965.

CLARK, I., and SMITH, M. R.: Effects of Hypervitaminosis A and D on Skeletal Metabolism. J. Biol. Chem. *239*:1266–1271, 1964.

EATON, H. D.: Chronic Bovine Hypo- and Hypervitaminosis A and Cerebrospinal Fluid Pressure. Amer. J. Clin. Nutr. *22*:1070–1080, 1969.

IRWIN, C., and BASSETT, A. L.: The Amelioration of Hypervitaminosis D in Rats with Vitamin A. J. Exp. Med. *115*:147–156, 1962.

GREY, R. M., *et al.*: Pathology of Skull, Radius and Rib in Hypervitaminosis A in Young Calves. Path. Vet. *2*:446–467, 1965.

HUNT, R. D., GARCIA, F. G., and HEGSTED, D. M.: Hypervitaminosis D in New World Monkeys. Amer. J. Clin. Nutr. *22*:358–366, 1969.

LUCKE, V. M., *et al.*: Deforming Cervical Spondylosis in the Cat Associated with Hypervitaminosis A. Vet. Rec. *82*:141–142, 1968.

SEAWRIGHT, A. A., and ENGLISH, P. B.: Cervical Spondylosis—Cats. J. Path. Bact.: *88*:503–509, 1964.

SEAWRIGHT, A. A., ENGLISH, P. B., and GARTNER, R. J. W.: Hypervitaminosis A and Hyperostosis of the Cat. Nature, Lond. *206*:1171–1172, 1965.

————: Hypervitaminosis A and Deforming Cervical Spondylosis of the Cat. J. Comp. Path. *77*:29–39, 1967.

STREBEL, R. F., GIRERD, R. J., and WAGNER, B. M.: Cardiovascular Calcification in Rats with Hypervitaminosis A. Arch. Path. *87*:290–297, 1969.

WOLKE, R. E., NIELSEN, S. W., and ROUSSEAU, J. E., JR.: Bone Lesions of Hypervitaminosis A in the Pig. Am. J. Vet. Res. *29*:1009–1024, 1968.

WOLKE, R. E., *et al.*: Qualitative and Quantitative Osteoblastic Activity in Chronic Porcine Hypervitaminosis A. J. Path. *97*:677–686, 1969.

METABOLISM OF CALCIUM

In considering the disorders of calcium metabolism, two separate aspects are presented, the mobilized calcium in the blood and the organized calcium in the bones. Disorders involving the bones include rickets, osteomalacia and osteitis fibrosa cystica, which are discussed in the section on bones (p. 1058) and in connection with parathyroid disorders (p. 1365). In general, it can be said that in case the assimilation of calcium from the food is deficient for any reason, the concentration of the element in the circulating blood is maintained at or near the normal level by its withdrawal from the bones, a process which is under the control of parathyroid hormone, vitamin D and calcitonin (thyrocalcitonin). Hence, when signs of hypocalcemia (deficiency in the blood) arise we do not ordinarily expect to find the cause in a shortage of the element in the diet.

The classical signs and symptoms of **hypocalcemia** are displayed when all the parathyroids are removed experimentally, and are known as **parathyroid tetany.** Arising about two days after the removal, there are intermittent tonic spasms with tremors, paresthesias and muscular pain, the whole syndrome being referable to hyperirritability of the peripheral nervous system. However, tetany can also occur in connection with various other disorders, apparently unrelated, such as gastrointestinal disturbances, pregnancy and after thyroidectomy. (In the last instance it seems possible that the parathyroids may have been accidentally extirpated along with the thyroid lobes.) Tetany may develop whenever the amount of calcium in the blood falls below a certain critical level, which, for most species, is about 7 mg. of calcium per 100 ml., or when the calcium present is not adequately ionized. Theoretically, such tetany can result from excessive phosphorus in the blood, alkalosis or failure of a sufficient supply of calcium in the diet. Actually, however, the normally functioning parathyroid supplies deficits of this kind from the bones.

Interference with the normal flow of bile, coupled with a diet rich in fats, may produce steatorrhea and the formation of calcium soaps in the intestine to the point that hypocalcemia results and leads to **coeliac rickets.** Likewise, there are kidney disorders (nephrosis, nephritis) sufficiently severe that, due to inability to excrete phosphates in the urine, hyperphosphatemia develops which causes hypocalcemia. Cases are known in the human where tetany has resulted from severe loss of calcium (below 7 mg. per 100 ml.) in connection with these disorders. Persistence of such renal drain upon the calcium reserves leads to **renal rickets** and also to a certain degree of compensatory hyperplasia of the parathyroids. The so-called "rubber jaw" of dogs is one way in which this disturbance is manifested (p. 1064). Nephrosis may also lead to hypocalcemia by causing marked loss of protein which leads to a lowering of total serum protein and the protein bound or nondiffusible fraction of serum calcium.

Hypocalcemia often occurs in acute pancreatitis (p. 1239). Presumably calcium is rapidly depleted in extracellular fluids by its fixation as insoluble calcium soaps with fatty acids released during fat necrosis accompanying acute pancreatitis.

Hypocalcemic tetany may also accompany alkalosis which causes a reduction in serum ionized calcium.

Contrary to what occurs in parathyroid tetany, there are instances where hypocalcemia appears to depress nervous and general body activity. This is regularly seen in milk fever (see below).

In veterinary practice, hypocalcemia is a principal or subordinate factor in milk fever of cows, probably in the so-called eclampsia of lactating bitches, and, with hypomagnesemia, in grass tetany (p. 1004).

Hypercalcemia occurs in severe hypervitaminosis D, as mentioned in the preceding section. It also occurs in hyperparathyroidism (p. 1366) from parathyroid tumors or in hyperparathyroidism compensatory to nephritis, and even to rickets and similar disorders when the cause is not an actual deficiency of elemental calcium. Hypercalcemia tends to cause metastatic calcification and urolithiasis as the excess of calcium is eliminated in the urine.

MILK FEVER

Milk fever—"no milk and no fever," a saying attributed to the late Dean George H. Glover of Colorado State—is the prevalent designation of a frequently encountered, sudden, acute hypocalcemia of parturient dairy cows and less often, of ewes, nanny goats, sows and even bitches. Synonyms designed to circumvent the paradoxical appellation above include parturient paresis and parturient apoplexy, but such terms are not without objection.

With or without premonitory irritability, excitement and muscular incoordination, the recently parous cow usually becomes recumbent and somnolent, if not, indeed, comatose. Prior to the advent of modern treatments, most cases were fatal after a number of hours, but in 1897 Schmidt began achieving a high percentage of cures by the intramammary injection of a solution of potassium iodide, theorizing that some toxin was elaborated in the udder. Later this was changed to the injection of oxygen into each teat orifice until the udder was rather tensely inflated, and then it was found that inflation with air would suffice just as well. Recovery in a few hours was the rule.

Little and Wright, in 1925, Dryerre and Greig, in 1928, as well as many others showed that milk fever is characterized by a level of blood calcium equal to about half the normal (mean 5.13, minimum 3.00 mg. per 100 ml.), and that the severity of the symptoms was proportional to the degree of hypocalcemia. In most cases there is also hypophosphatemia and slight hypermagnesemia. The present-day treatment consists in the intravenous injection of perhaps 50 grams of calcium borogluconate (other salts of calcium have been used) in appropriate solution, and disappearance of the symptoms is sometimes only a matter of minutes. Treatment with high levels of vitamin D_3 has also been used satisfactorily.

The nature of this malady seems apparent from the blood analyses, the spectacular success of treatment and also from the historical fact that the disease first began to be recognized contemporaneously with the development of the modern, heavily producing dairy breeds, the earliest references to it, according to Hutyra and Marek (1938), being those of Eberhardt in 1793, Price in 1806, Jorg in 1808, and Fabe in 1837. However, the reason for the disturbed calcium homeostasis has not been answered satisfactorily. Comparative studies between cows with parturient paresis and healthy post-partum cows have not elucidated the basic disturbance. Calcium loss in milk or urine is not greater in cows with paresis. Disturbed endocrine function has been a tempting conclusion, but to date investigations have not revealed a clearly defined abnormality in parathormone, thyroxin, estrogen or adrenal cortical steroid metabolism.

Most emphasis has been directed to parathormone. It has been hypothesized that the basic defect lies in the parathyroid gland which fails to cause mobilization of sufficient calcium to meet demands of lactation. This hypothesis has not been proved. Recent studies by Capen and Young (1967) offer a new approach which includes the hypothesis that the basic defect in milk fever is a sudden release of thyrocalcitonin at parturition. Although the stimulus for the apparent release is unknown, their data demonstrated degranulation of parafollicular cells (origin of thyrocalcitonin) and reduced thyrocalcitonin activity in the thyroid glands of cows with parturient paresis. Their data and that of Sherwood and co-workers (1966) suggest hyperactivity of parathormone synthesis rather than hypoactivity.

The susceptibility to milk fever is inherent in the individual. We know of one cow which, before she went to market at twelve years of age, had had 9 calves and had been afflicted with milk fever following 7 of the 9 calvings. The owner became so adept in predicting the time of parturition and the parturient paresis that he was accustomed to arrange for treatment in advance!

Although the majority of cows with milk fever respond rapidly to therapy, some individuals do not rise after calcium treatment. These cases may represent a complication of milk fever or other poorly understood maladies associated with parturition and grouped under the term "downer cow syndrome."

Gross lesions, in those which die, are practically nil, and the same is presumably true microscopically, as well, but extensive microscopic studies have not been reported.

Calcium and Milk Fever

BJORSELL, K. A., HOLTENIUS, P., and JACOBSSON, S. O.: Studies on Parturient Paresis With Special Reference to the Downer Cow Syndrome. Acta Vet. Scand. *10*:36–43, 1969.

CAPEN, C. C., and YOUNG, D. M.: The Ultrastructure of the Parathyroid Glands and Thyroid Parafollicular Cells of Cows with Parturient Paresis and Hypocalcemia. Lab. Invest. *17*:717–737, 1967.

COMAR, C. L., SINGER, L., and DAVIS, G. K.: Molybdenum Metabolism and Interrelationships with Copper and Phosphorus. J. Biol. Chem. *180*:913–922, 1949.

DRYERRE, H., and GREIG, R.: Further Studies on Etiology of Milk Fever. Vet. Rec. 8: 721–728, 1928.

FISH, P. A.: Physiology of Milk Fever; Blood Phosphates and Calcium. Cornell Vet. *19*: 147–160, 1929.

GREIG, J. R.: Calcium Gluconate as a Specific in Milk Fever. Vet. Rec. *10*:115–120, and 301–305, 1930.

HUTYRA, F., MAREK, J., and MANNINGER, R.: *Special Pathology and Therapeutics of the Diseases of Domestic Animals.* Engl. translation. Chicago, Alex Eger. Vol. III, 1938, p. 454.

LITTLE, W. L., and WRIGHT, N. C.: The Aetiology of Milk Fever in Cattle. Brit. J. Exper. Path. *6*:129–134, 1925–26. Vet. Rec. *5*:631–633, 1925.

MARSH. H., and SWINGLE, K. F.: The Calcium, Phosphorus, Magnesium, Carotene and Vitamin A Content of the Blood of Range Cattle in Eastern Montana. Am. J. Vet. Res. *21*:212–221, 1960.

NURMIO, P.: On Plasma Calcium Regulation in Paresis Puerperalis Hypocalcemia in Cattle. Acta Vet. Scand. Suppl. 26, 1–100, 1968.

PAYNE, J. M.: Recent Advances in Our Knowledge of Milk Fever. Vet. Rec. *76*:1275–1279, 1964.

SEIDEL, H., SCHROTER, J., and KOLB, E.: Determination of Sodium, Potassium, Calcium, and Magnesium in the Serum of Cows with Puerperal Paresis. Mh. Veterinaermed. *19*: 926–932, 1964.

METABOLISM OF MAGNESIUM

Our understanding of the role of magnesium in the animal body is not on a firm footing. Magnesium is present in most tissues of the animal body. The blood serum normally contains 2 to 3 mg. of magnesium per 100 ml. in the human and about 2 mg. in the bovine. For unknown reasons large numbers of apparently normal cattle have half the latter figure in cold weather. Approximately 70 per cent of the total body magnesium is in the skeleton. There is some evidence indicating that biochemically the essential role of magnesium is in the transmission of impulses at the neuromuscular junction, a low concentration of magnesium and a low ratio of magnesium to calcium in the surrounding tissue fluids facilitating, perhaps unduly, the formation of acetyl choline, which is a presumably essential feature of the transmission of impulses. At any rate, it can be said that a deficiency resulting in a blood level below 0.7 mg. per 100 ml.

causes nervous hyperirritability, and a great excess causes nervous depression, unconsciousness and death (as in euthanasia by magnesium sulfate intravenously). Experimentally, several weeks on a deficient diet are required to produce symptoms and the blood-level of 0.7 mg.

Two clinical syndromes are associated with hypomagnesemia; grass tetany of adult cattle and hypomagnesemia of calves. Clinically the two syndromes are similar and both are characterized by hypomagnesemia. However, their pathogenesis differs.

HYPOMAGNESEMIA IN CALVES

Hypomagnesemia in calves occurs in animals raised on a low magnesium diet, usually milk, the disease representing a nutritional deficiency. Serum magnesium falls to 0.5 to 0.7 mg. per 100 ml. and bone ash magnesium is reduced to about one-third of normal. Serum calcium and phosphorus remain within normal limits. Clinical signs focus on hyperirritability and tetany. Early signs include opisthotonus, very frequent movement or fixed depression of the ears, greatly exaggerated scratching, kicking at the belly, or twitching of the skin in response to slight stimuli, spastic extreme flexion of the carpus in walking, salivation, exophthalmos and apprehensiveness. These signs are intermittent and initiated by excitement or exercise. After days or weeks, terminal tonic-clonic convulsions, lasting one or two hours, are fatal at the first or second attack.

Post-mortem lesions in the experimental cases of Blaxter and co-workers (1954) were largely limited to agonal hemorrhages (heart, intestinal and mesenteric serosae) and congestion of viscera. Contraction of segments of stomach (abomasum) and intestines persisted after death. Microscopically, thrombosis of venules of the heart, surrounded by necrosis and inflammatory reaction, was seen. Beyond this and the hemorrhages and congestion, there were no microscopic lesions of note. Neither the central nervous tissue nor muscles contained lesions of significance.

On the other hand, Moore and co-workers (1938) performed autopsies on 38 calves which had died from experimentally produced hypomagnesemia and found rather extensive lesions, the most prominent of which was calcification of the intimal layer of the heart and large blood vessels. This calcification was apparently an example of metastatic calcification (p. 56) rather than that due to previous necrosis. The lesions took the form of slightly raised, light-colored plaques, a few millimeters in diameter, on the intimal surfaces, in which there was an increase of fibrous and elastic elements. These animals also showed toxic degeneration of the renal tubules and early cirrhotic tendencies. The amount of calcium in the diet of these calves was reported as low or normal, but it would appear that the conditions of metastatic calcification were somehow met. Similar calcification of the endocardium and blood vessels, as well as of muscle and kidney, has since been reproduced by other investigators in calves, rats and dogs. However, evidence from experimental studies indicates that necrosis of myofibers precedes calcification.

GRASS TETANY

Although also characterized by low serum magnesium, hypomagnesemia in adult cattle is not analogous to the deficiency disease described above in calves.

When cattle, sheep and rarely horses, have been pastured for some time exclusively on very lush and succulent grasses of various kinds, they are likely to undergo sudden tetanic convulsive seizures. Premonitory hyperirritability, apprehensiveness or incoordination are often overlooked. Such an attack is commonly fatal, perhaps after a period of terminal recumbency in a state of partial coma or paresis. **Grass staggers** is a colloquial synonym based on the incoordination of the limbs. If the grass in question happens to be young and vigorously growing wheat which is being used for pasturage, a common practice in wheat-growing areas, the condition is often called **wheat poisoning.** The terminal convulsive attack may be initiated by excitement and exercise. If these are incident to the animal's being transported by rail or truck the term "railroad sickness" or "lorry disease" may be heard. (Lorry, motor truck.)

The symptoms are obviously similar to those of experimental hypomagnesemia. Post-mortem lesions may be non-existent or there may be, as in experimental hypomagnesemia, agonal hemorrhages associated with a convulsive death (really an asphyxiative death due to immobilization of the respiratory muscles; see Hemorrhage, p. 119). A similarity to milk fever is also obvious in the more comatose cases. The blood shows a hypocalcemia and a much more severe hypomagnesemia. Bone ash magnesium is not reduced. Disturbance of the potassium level may also be noted. Grass tetany is usually considered to be primarily due to the low magnesium but with the hypocalcemia playing a prominent secondary part. Calcium gluconate intravenously often cures the acute attack. There is no clear explanation of why the lush grass brings on these blood disorders; the grass is not deficient in either magnesium or calcium. It has been suggested that the high crude protein content of such a diet may be the underlying factor. It is known that as the dietary level of protein is increased, the dietary requirement of magnesium is increased. The exact relationship between magnesium and protein is not understood but in ruminants increased levels of ammonium in the rumen may interfere with the utilization of magnesium. Also, diets with high potassium or calcium content may depress magnesium absorption.

Another tetanic condition is the **winter tetany** occurring in cows. As has been stated, many cows in apparently normal health have only half the normal blood magnesium when wintered on fresh blue-grass. Some of these do sicken with typical tetanic symptoms, which are fatal in many instances. Pronounced hypocalcemia accompanies the hypomagnesemia, and calcium gluconate is more often curative than are magnesium compounds. Coupled with the fact that a majority of the cows are recently post-parturient, these features suggest a confusing similarity to milk fever. Indeed it may be questioned whether there is any fundamental difference. Both the abrupt onset of lactation and disorders of dietary metabolism seem capable of causing serious depletion of the blood's supply of calcium or magnesium or of both. However, in contrast to grass tetany the hypomagnesemia of winter tetany appears to be the result of prolonged nutritional deficiency.

Hypomagnesemia also occurs in sheep. Both the winter tetany type due to magnesium deficient diets and the acute grass tetany type have been described.

Magnesium

BLAXTER, K. L., and ROOK, J. A. F.: The Magnesium Requirements of Calves. J. Comp. Path. and Therap. *64*:176–186, 1954.

duction of erythrocytes in compensation for hemorrhagic or hemolytic anemia from some other cause, such as ancylostomiasis, the amount of iron required for rapid regeneration of blood cells is correspondingly increased, so that without a fully adequate supply iron-deficiency anemia may develop. The post-mortem lesions of anemia have been given (p. 125).

Tremendously excessive amounts of iron are stored in various tissues in hemochromatosis (p. 73), a disease in which control and limitation of absorption appear to have been lost. Whether it be the excessive storage that accompanies hemochromatosis or the limited and transient splenic storage which occurs in hemolytic anemia or other blood destruction, stored iron appears in the form of hemosiderin (p. 71).

Like sulfur, iron is able to enter the calcium phosphate compound of the bone and cause rickets (osteomalacia). The compound thus formed is $Fe_3(PO_4)_2$. The disorder has occurred in poultry. A similar displacement is also theoretically possible when aluminum, magnesium or beryllium are in excess.

As will be seen, minute amounts of copper and cobalt are necessary for the successful utilization of iron in hematopoiesis.

A recent practice of injecting medicinals containing iron, usually iron-dextran intramuscularly in growing swine has resulted in brown-stained areas at the site of injection (usually the ham) which have damaged the meat when the hog was slaughtered as much as three months later.

Iron

CANTRILL, S., *et al.*: Iron Absorption from the Gastro-Intestinal Tract. Aust. J. Exp. Biol. Med. Sci. *40*:17–36, 1962.
D'ARCY, P. F., and HOWARD, E. M.: The Acute Toxicity of Ferrous Salts Administered to Dogs by Mouth. J. Path. Bact. *83*:65–72, 1962.
MANIS, J. G., and SCHACHTER, D.: Active Transport of Iron by Intestine: Features of the Two-Step Mechanism: Effects of Oral Iron and Pregnancy. Amer. J. Physiol. *203*:73–86, 1962.
MOLLER, F.: Investigations on Iron Metabolism in Pigs. Abst. Vet. Bull. No. 2075, 1963.
MOORE, R. W., REDMOND, H. E., and LIVINGSTON, C. W., JR.: Iron Deficiency Anemia as a Cause of Stillbirths in Swine. J. Am. Vet. Med. Assn. *147*:746–748, 1965.

METABOLISM OF COPPER

Copper occurs in most tissues of the animal body, including the central nervous system, which contains some 20 to 30 mg. per kilogram of dry matter. Minute amounts are essential to the utilization of iron in hematopoiesis, its precise function not having been ascertained. Thus in copper deficiency anemia is a usual development. In most species this occurs as a microcytic hypochromic anemia (p. 124).

Herbivorous animals raised in a few localities where the soil is almost devoid of this element have been found to suffer from disorders of the blood-forming tissue, of the hair or of the central nervous system. The anemia which occurs is often of subclinical degree. In Florida, a disease characterized by anemia and unthriftiness and colloquially called "salt sick" is cured by giving copper plus iron.

Copper is also an essential component of the enzyme tyrosinase which is required for the normal production of melanin (p. 65). Therefore achromotrichia represents another feature of deficiency. The condition is not related to the graying of human hair A disorder expressively described as "steely wool" is considered to be due to copper deficiency. Changes in the physical nature of hair and wool also develop. Wool loses its crimp and becomes more hair-like.

As indicated, disorders of the central nervous system also follow copper deficiency. In England and Australia, sheep and sometimes goats have a disease called **"enzoötic ataxia"** or "swayback" which occurs on copper-deficient soils and is considered to be due to a shortage of that element in the animal's metabolism. **As** the names imply the symptoms are chiefly incoordination and weakness of the posterior limbs. Spastic paralysis and sometimes blindness occur. The lesions are most pronounced in new-born lambs and consist in demyelinization, and even extensive softening, necrosis and disappearance of much of the white matter in the central portions of the cerebral hemispheres and spinal cord. In the severest cases, there is little left of the hemispheres but the cortical shell of gray matter. Such a lesion is distinguished from internal hydrocephalus by the irregular and obviously necrotic lining of the cavity and the absence of histological structures there. Milder forms involve only areas of demyelinization, symmetrically located, with "gitter" cells (p. 1387) and necrotic nerve cells. There is no inflammatory reaction. Innes and Shearer (1940) have suspected a relationship between this condition and Schilder's disease of humans. The condition is further discussed on page 1402.

A disease considered to be due also to deficiency of copper occurs in adult cattle in Australia and the United States, known as "falling disease" because the cows commonly fall and die very suddenly. Anemia and loss of weight occur, but there are usually no definite premonitory symptoms. Lesions include marked hemosiderosis of the spleen, liver and kidneys, presumably as the result of the anemia, and diffuse fibrous scarring of the heart muscle. The latter, no doubt, accounts for the sudden death. The details of the pathogenesis of this condition have not been fully elucidated, but copper has been shown to be essential for the maintenance of the structural elements of the myocardium and arteries. In swine, rabbits and chicks fed low copper diets, there is defective elastogenesis resulting in fragmentation, disruption and elimination of elastic fibers in the cardiovascular system. The disorder has been shown to result from a decrease in intramolecular crosslinkage of elastin.

Copper deficiency also results in extensive skeletal changes. Although reference is made to "rickets," fractures and impaired gaits the nature of the lesions has not been studied under conditions of natural deficiency. In experimental animals, a form of osteoporosis develops which is remarkably similar to the osseous lesions of scurvy (p. 990). The epiphyseal cartilage is normal or thicker than normal and it calcifies normally but it does not degenerate. There is cessation of, or reduced, osteoblastic activity with reduced formation of osteoid. Bone resorption is apparently not impaired. These features are in direct opposition to the changes of rickets (p. 1058).

An excessive amount of molybdenum in the pasturage or forage necessitates much larger amounts of copper in the diet. This situation arises on some soils.

An excess of copper is treated under the heading of Copper Poisoning (p. 866).

Wilson's disease (hepatolenticular degeneration) in man is caused by deranged copper metabolism, presumably a defect in ceruloplasmin (an α-globulin transport system) synthesis. It is characterized by low ceruloplasmin levels, high non-bound plasma copper, increased tissue copper concentration, hepatic necrosis and cirrhosis, and progressive cerebral damage, particularly of the basal ganglia.

Lesions in the central nervous system have been described in copper poisoning in sheep. Copper poisoning is discussed in Chapter 17 (p. 866).

Copper

BULL, L. B., *et al.*: Ataxia in Young Lambs. Bull. Council Sci. Indust. Research, Australia *113*:72, 1938.

COULSON, W. F., *et al.*: Cardiovascular System in Naturally Occurring Copper Deficiency and Swayback in Sheep. Am. J. Vet. Res. *27*:815–818, 1967.

DOHERTY, P. C., BARLOW, R. M., and ANGUS, K. W.: Spongy Changes in the Brains of Sheep Poisoned by Excess Dietary Copper. Res. Vet. Sci. *10*:303–304, 1969.

EVERSON, G. J., HYAN-CHANG CHOW TSAI, and TONG-IN WANG: Copper Deficiency in the Guinea Pig. J. Nutr. *93*:533–540, 1967.

GOODRICH, R. D., and TILMAN, A. D.: Copper, Sulfate and Molybdenum Interrelationships in Sheep. J. Nutr. *90*:76–80, 1966.

HOWELL, J., DAVISON, A. N., and OXBERRY, J.: Observations on the Lesions in the White Matter of the Spinal Cord of Swayback Sheep. Acta Neuropath. *12*:33–41, 1969.

INNES, J. R. M., and SHEARER, G. D.: "Swayback" A Demyelinating Disease of Lambs with Affinities to Schilder's Encephalitis in Man. J. Comp. Path. & Therap. *53*:1–41, 1940.

LEWIS, B., TERLECKI, S., and ALLCROFT, R.: The Occurrence of Swayback in the Lambs of Ewes Fed a Semi-purified Diet of Low Copper Content. Vet. Rec. *81*:415–416, 1967.

McGAVIN, M. D., RANBY, P. D., and TAMMEMAGI, L.: Demyelination Associated with Low Liver Copper Levels in Pigs. Austr. Vet. J. *38*:8–14, 1962.

OWEN, E. C., *et al.*: Pathological and Biochemical Studies of an Outbreak of Swayback in Goats. J. Comp. Path. *75*:241–251, 1965.

PRYER, W. J.: The Liver Copper Levels of Foetal and Maternal Pigs. Aust. J. Sci. *25*: 498, 1963.

RUCKER, R. B., PARKER, H. E., and ROGLER, J. C.: Effect of Copper Deficiency on Chick Bone Collagen and Selected Bone Enzymes. J. Nutr. *98*:57–63, 1969.

SAVAGE, J. E., *et al.*: Comparison of Copper Deficiency and Lathyrism in Turkey Poults. J. Nutr. *88*:15–25, 1966.

SHIELDS, G. S., *et al.*: Copper Metabolism. XXXII. Cardiovascular Lesions in Copper Deficient Swine. Amer. J. Path. *41*:603–622, 1962.

SIMPSON, C. F., and HARMS, R. H.: Pathology of the Aorta of Chicks Fed a Copper-Deficient Diet. Exp. Molec. Path. *3*:390–400, 1964.

WAISMAN, J., CARNES, W. H., and WEISSMAN, N.: Some Properties of the Microfibrils of Vascular Elastic Membranes in Normal and Copper-Deficient Swine. Amer. J. Path. *54*: 107–119, 1969.

WAISMAN, J., and CARNES, W. H.: Cardiovascular Studies on Copper-Deficient Swine. X. The Fine Structure of the Defective Elastic Membranes. Amer. J. Path. *51*:117–135, 1967.

METABOLISM OF COBALT

Small amounts of cobalt, usually provided by the soil and the herbage which grows upon it, are necessary in ruminants only. Without sufficient cobalt, the numbers of bacteria in the rumen decline and the prevailing species change unfavorably. Since vitamin B_{12} is synthesized by ruminal bacteria and since cobalt is an essential constituent (4 per cent) of that substance, it appears that the lack of adequate cobalt is deleterious to the bacteria, preventing their growth, and to the host animal through absence of vitamin B_{12}. The latter is essential in erythropoiesis, in growth and probably in other ways. As stated, disease due to deficiency of cobalt appears to be limited to ruminants. Attempts to produce it in experimental animals have failed, although the element does stimulate erythropoiesis, even to the extent of producing polycythemia.

"Grand Traverse disease" of the American Great Lakes region, "pine" in England (so-called because they pine away and die), "hill sickness" in New Zealand and "coast disease" and **enzoötic marasmus** in Australia are examples of a cachectic syndrome in which cattle or sheep, after grazing on a certain pasturage for several months, lose their appetites, waste away and die while still in the midst of ample amounts of the same food plants. Since affected animals were anemic, attempts were naturally made to cure them by giving iron. It was found that certain impure iron salts would do this, but that the curative properties of such salts ("limonite" in Australia) were not proportional to their iron content. Further study showed that cobalt, existing as an impurity, was the effective ingredient. Iron, indeed, is stored in excess in the tissues of the sick animals. In the "coast disease" of Australian sheep, both cobalt and copper have been found to be lacking, the symptoms and lesions combining those characteristic of enzoötic marasmus with demyelinization and destruction of certain tracts in the spinal cord.

The lesions of enzoötic marasmus are anemia and marked hemosiderosis of the liver, spleen, kidneys and other organs. The hemosiderin, or material indistinguishable from it, probably represents a storage of iron which should be, but cannot be, utilized. Fatty change of the liver is also prominent.

Excessive amounts of cobalt have been shown experimentally to cause polycythemia.

Cobalt

ANDRES, E. D., HART, L. I., and STEPHENSON, B. J.: Vitamin B_{12} and Cobalt Concentrations in Livers from Healthy and Cobalt-Deficient Lambs. Nature, Lond. *182*:869–870, 1958.
DECKER, D. E., and SMITH, L. E.: The Metabolism of Cobalt in Lambs. J. Nutr. *43*: 87–100, 1951.
FILMER, J. F.: Enzootic Marasmus of Cattle and Sheep. Aust. Vet. J. *9*:163–179, 1933.
FILMER, J. F., and UNDERWOOD, E. J.: Enzootic Marasmus; Treatment with Limonite Fractions. Aust. Vet. J. *10*:83–87, 1934.
KEENER, H. A., PERCIVAL, G. P. and MORROW, K. S.: Cobalt Deficiency in New Hampshire with Sheep. J. Anim. Sci. *7*:16–25, 1948.
O'MOORE, L. B., and SMYTH, P. J.: The Control of Cobalt Deficiency in Sheep by Means of a Heavy Pellet (containing cobaltic oxide). Vet. Rec. *70*:773–774, 1958.
TOKARNIA, C. H., *et al.*: Cobalt Deficiency in Cattle in the State of Ceara, Brazil (TT). Arq. Inst. Biol. Anim. Rio de J. *4*:195–202, 1963.
UNDERWOOD, E. J., and FILMER, J. F.: The Determination of the Biologically Potent Element Cobalt in Limonite. Aust. Vet. J. *11*:84–92, 1935.
WESSELS, C. C.: Cobalt in Relation to Ruminant Nutrition in South Africa. J. S. Afr. Vet. Med. Assn. *32*:289–312, 1961.

METABOLISM OF MANGANESE

Small amounts of manganese are essential for several mechanisms of the body. Experimental deficiency in rats on artificially concocted diets results in aspermatogenesis, weak and defective offspring and retarded growth. In rats, rabbits, swine, and cattle and avians there is suppression of epiphyseal cartilage cell proliferation and reduced osteoblastic activity resulting in decreased growth, rarefaction of bone, bowing and fractures, joint deformities and tendon slippage. However, deficiency of this element does not occur clinically except in birds although it has been suggested as a cause of spontaneous lameness and joint deformity in swine. In chickens and turkeys, a deformity of the hock joint known as **perosis** or "slipped tendon" is frequent at an age of several weeks. In this condition, the epiphyseal cartilage fails to ossify, as it normally should at twelve weeks in chickens; the epiphysis loosens and the tendon of the gastrocnemius slips medially. Deficiency of choline has also been blamed for this disorder. Many deformed chicks, having short, thick legs and wings and globular heads, are hatched from eggs of manganese-deficient hens, an interesting example of a developmental defect due to malnutrition.

Manganese

AMDUR, M. O., NORRIS, L. C., and HEUSER, G. F.: The Need for Manganese in Bone Development by the Rat. Proc. Soc. Exp. Biol. Med. *59*:254–255, 1945.

BARNES, L. L., SPERLING, G., and MAYNARD, L. A.: Bone Development in the Albino Rat on a Low Manganese Diet. Proc. Soc. Exp. Biol. Med. *46*:562–565, 1941.

MILLER, R. C., *et al.*: Manganese as a Possible Factor Influencing the Occurrence of Lameness in Pigs. Proc. Soc. Exp. Biol. Med. *45*:50–51, 1940.

NEHER, G. M., *et al.*: Radiographic and Histopathological Findings in the Bones of Swine Deficient in Manganese. Am. J. Vet. Res. *17*:121–218, 1956.

METABOLISM OF ZINC

Zinc was recognized as a dietary essential to the animal economy in very small amounts over three decades ago, but clinical deficiency has only recently been described. **Parakeratosis** of swine, first described by Kernkamp and Ferrin (1953), is now accepted to be the result of zinc deficiency. Although the exact circumstances which bring about zinc deficiency in swine are not entirely understood, it has been established that excess dietary calcium interferes with zinc absorption. Addition of zinc to the ration and adjusting calcium intake dramatically cures or prevents parakeratosis. Available evidence suggests that calcium in conjunction with either phytate or phosphate forms a complex with zinc, making it unavailable for absorption.

Parakeratosis usually appears in young swine ten to twenty weeks of age and is manifested by circumscribed erythematous areas, 3 to 5 cm. in diameter, particularly in the skin of the abdomen and medial surfaces of the thighs. An elevated, scaly character is soon assumed by these affected areas, and the lesions become widespread with a symmetrical distribution. The surface layer of keratin becomes increasingly thick, rough, horny and fissured. The hairs are not lost but are often entangled and matted in the superficial horny material. The appetite may be impaired and the rate of gain somewhat reduced, but often signs are inconstant and probably not specific.

The microscopic appearance of the affected skin is dominated by parakeratosis and acanthosis with elongation and congestion of dermal papillae and disappearance of the stratum granulosum. In the thick, horny parakeratotic layer, retained nuclei are usually seen in undulating, irregular rows and sometimes are mixed with cellular debris. In some areas, the stratum germinativum is thinner than normal, but acanthosis appears to be the rule.

Experimental zinc deficiency was first induced in rats and mice, but has also been described in lambs, calves, dogs and monkeys. In each of these species the ensuing disease is dominated by loss of hair or wool and acanthosis and parakeratosis of the skin, esophagus and oral mucosa. Lesions have also been reported in the testicle and bone, but it has not clearly been shown whether they result from zinc deficiency or inanition.

Syndromes attributed to zinc deficiency have been reported in cattle and sheep, however, other than in swine, the status of naturally occurring deficiency of zinc in domestic animals is presently unknown.

Zinc

BARNEY, G. H., *et al.*: Parakeratosis of the Tongue—A Unique Histopathologic Lesion in the Zinc-Deficient Squirrel Monkey. J. Nutr. *93*:511–517, 1967.

OTT, E. A., *et al.*: Zinc Deficiency Syndrome in the Young Calf. J. Anim. Sci. *24*:735–741, 1965.

KERNKAMP, H. C. H., and FERRIN, E. F.:   Parakeratosis in Swine.   J. Am. Vet. Med. Assn. *123*:217–220, 1953.

KIENHOLZ, E. W., *et al.*:   Effects of Zinc Deficiency in the Diets of Hens.   J. Nutr. *75*:211–221, 1961.

MACAPINLAF, M. P., *et al.*:   Production of Zinc Deficiency in the Squirrel Monkey (*Saimiri sciureus*).   J. Nutr. *93*:499–510, 1967.

MILLS, C. F., *et al.*:   The Production and Signs of Zinc Deficiency in the Sheep.   Proc. Nutr. Soc. *24*:21–22, 1965.

OBERLEAS, D., MUHRER, M. E., and O'DELL, B. L.:   Effects of Phytic Acid on Zinc Availability and Parakeratosis in Swine.   J. Anim. Sci. *21*:57–61, 1962.

PIERSON, R. E.:   Zinc Deficiency in Young Lambs.   J. Am. Vet. Med. Assn. *149*:1279–1282, 1966.

PRASAD, A. S. (Ed.):   *Zinc Metabolism.*   Springfield, Charles C Thomas, 1966.

ROBERTSON, B. T., and BURNS, M. J.:   Zinc Metabolism and the Zinc-Deficiency Syndrome in the Dog.   Am. J. Vet. Res. *24*:997–1002, 1963.

VALLEE, B. L.:   Biochemistry, Physiology and Pathology of Zinc.   Physiol. Rev. *39*:443–490, 1959.   (359 references.)

VAN PREENEN, H. J., and PATEL, A.:   Tissue Zinc and Calcium in Chronic Disease.   Arch. Path. *77*:53–56, 1964.

METABOLISM OF IODINE

Iodine received into the circulation is, even within minutes, stored in the thyroid gland, where it is gradually converted into the active principle of the thyroid hormone, thyroxin.

Deficiency of iodine causes **goiter** (p. 1360). The usual type of goiter seen in animals makes its appearance with birth and is the hyperplastic type characteristic of cretinism in the human.   As has been seen in the case of a number of other elements, the amount of iodine available to the animal is dependent on the amount in the soil.   Certain areas (the Great Lakes region and the Pacific Northwest in the United States, the Swiss Alps, etc.) are known as endemic, goiter-producing regions because of their iodine-deficient soils and water.

The goiters in new-born colts, calves, lambs and pigs are often of very conspicuous size.   In swine, there is a strong tendency for the pigs to be born with little or no hair—"**hairless pigs.**"   Untreated, such animals either develop very poorly or die.   The condition is easily avoided by administration of minute amounts of iodine to the pregnant mother.   After birth, the same treatment applied to the offspring is only moderately successful.

A great excess of absorbed iodine produces the condition known as **iodism.** This occurs when iodine or its compounds are administered internally or externally in maximum dosages over a period of time.   It is characterized by lacrimation and exfoliation of dandruff-like epidermal scales and possibly cutaneous eruptions and pharyngitis.

Iodine

ANDREWS, F. N., *et al.*:   Iodine Deficiency in New-born Sheep and Swine.   J. Anim. Sci. *7*:298–310, 1948.

EVVARD, J. M.:   Iodine Deficiency Symptoms and their Significance in Animal Nutrition and Pathology.   Endocrinology *12*:539–590, 1928.

KALKUS, J. W.:   A Study of Goiter and Associated Conditions in Domestic Animals.   Exper. Sta. Bull. No. 156, Washington State College, Pullman, 1920.

WELCH, H.:   Hairlessness and Goiter in New-Born Domestic Animals.   Exper. Sta. Bull. No. 119, Montana State College, Bozeman, 1917.

METABOLISM OF PROTEINS AND AMINO ACIDS

The usual difficulty here is simply a lack of total protein, which results in slow growth and poor reproductive and other functions.   One of the writers (Smith) has seen lambs experimentally deprived of all protein. The condition was fatal in about two months, with mucoid degeneration (p. 52) at the coronary groove of the heart and elsewhere and other signs of general malnutrition.

About ten of the amino acids are known to be indispensable and a variety of symptoms and lesions have been produced by experimental exclusion of various ones. However, such deprivations do not occur except experimentally.

Several common farm feeds are moderately deficient in certain essential amino acids and may cause difficulty if fed alone. Indian corn (maize) is especially deficient in lysine and tryptophan; other grains, linseed meal and cotton-seed meal are less so in descending order. Peanuts are deficient in methionine and soybeans are less markedly so. The principal signs of deficiency of amino acids in general are hypoproteinemia, anemia, poor growth and delayed healing of wounds. Any of these disorders have other more frequent causes.

Even in experimentally induced protein deficiency the lesions are not specific. The major pathological changes include: cessation of cell proliferation of epiphyseal cartilages; reduced osteoblastic activity; failure of collagen formation; atrophy of endocrine glands including testicle and ovary; atrophy of thymus and lymphoid tissues; anemia; hypoproteinemia and edema. These lesions develop in animals following protracted periods of inanition which accompanies many diseases including nutritional deficiencies. The pathologist must exert extreme caution in assigning these changes to a specific nutrient deficiency or other cause.

Specific effects have been attributed to certain amino acid deficiencies. Experimental deficiency of tryptophan, a precursor of niacin (p. 984), results in alopecia, cataracts, corneal vascularization, necrosis of skeletal muscle and fatty change in the liver. Methionine deficiency also results in fatty change of the liver presumably owing to its role in choline synthesis. Lysine deficiency in rats causes achromatrichia.

LIPID METABOLISM

Fat is an important dietary component because it supplies essential fatty acids, serves as a carrier for fat-soluble vitamins, has high caloric value and adds palatability to food. Deficiency of fat *per se* probably does not exist in domestic animals. Deficiency of essential fatty acids (linolenic, arachidonic and linoleic) has been produced and studied in experimental animals and is often suggested as a cause of ill-defined dermatoses in animals. Dietary supplementation with fats occasionally results in improvement of certain skin disorders, but virtually no sound study has demonstrated fatty acids to be specific for the "cure." For changes to take place in the skin of dogs, experimental fatty acid deficiency requires months to years. The earliest change is dryness followed by alopecia and scaling. Microscopically the epidermis is thickened due to increase in cells and hyperkeratosis. Hair follicles become hypercellular and plugged with keratin, and sebaceous glands increase in size. The dermis becomes edematous and infiltrated with mononuclear cells.

Lipid

HANSEN, A. E., and WIESE, H. F.: Fat in the Diet in Relation to Nutrition of the Dog. I. Characteristic Appearance and Gross Changes of Animals Fed Diets With and Without Fats. Texas Rep. Biol. & Med. *9*:491–515, 1951.

HANSEN, A. E., HOLMES, S. G., and WIESE, H. F.:   Fat in the Diet in Relation to Nutrition of the Dog.   IV. Histologic Features of Skin From Animals Fed Diets With or Without Fat. Texas Rep. Biol. & Med. 9:555–570, 1951.
HANSEN, A. E., SINCLAIR, J. G., and WIESE, H. F.:   Sequence of Histologic Changes in Skin of Dogs in Relation to Dietary Fat.   J. Nutr. 52:541–554, 1954.
HOILUND, L. J., et al.:   Essential Fatty Acid Deficiency in the Rat.   I. Clinical Syndrome, Histopathology, and Hematopathology.   Lab. Invest. 23:58–70, 1970.

DIABETES MELLITUS

This disease is seen frequently in humans, not too uncommonly in dogs and cats and is reported rarely in horses, cattle and swine.   Spontaneous diabetes in Chinese hamsters, sand rats and certain strains of mice has provided valuable laboratory models for the disease.

Diabetes means a flowing; mellitus refers to honey.   The name thus gives a reasonably good introduction to the nature of this disease: An increased flow of urine (polyuria) which is so sweet that it is attractive to bees.   The polyuria is doubtless due to the inability of the renal epithelium to concentrate the urine against the osmotic attraction and possibly other effects of the sugar contained therein.   Polydipsia follows as a result of the polyuria.   The sugar, which is the glucose absorbed from the digested food, reaches an abnormally high concentration in the blood, **hyperglycemia**.   The amount of glucose in the blood is normally about 80 to 100 mg. per 100 ml.   When this amount rises above a "renal threshold" of about 150 to 170 mg. the kidneys begin to excrete the excess and there is sugar (glucose) in the urine, glycosuria.   Glucose in the blood is normally the animal's principal source of energy, but in this disease there are two fundamental defects of metabolism: (1) the liver cannot convert glucose to glycogen for storage, and (2) the tissues cannot oxidize it or use it for energy.   It is for these reasons that the glucose continues to circulate in the blood until it can be excreted by the kidneys.

Insulin, a hormone produced by the pancreatic islets, is able to correct these defects so that glucose is utilized in the normal way or is stored against future needs in the form of glycogen.   This fact was demonstrated by the famous work of Banting and Best of Toronto in 1921, who succeeded in making an effective pancreatic extract.   Proof of the relationship of the islets is derived from the following facts.   (1) Experimental removal of the pancreas in dogs produces diabetes. (2) Injection of alloxan, a substance structurally related to urea, concurrently produces diabetes and destroys the pancreatic islets.   (3) A similar concurrent production of diabetes and destruction of the islets results from repeated injections of anterior pituitary extract, the phenomenon possibly being one of initial stimulation and subsequent exhaustion.   (4) In many naturally occurring cases of diabetes, destructive lesions of the pancreatic islets can be demonstrated post mortem.   The **cause** of diabetes mellitus can therefore be said ordinarily to be an inadequacy of the hormone secreted by the pancreatic islets.   This may be an absolute deficiency of insulin, or a relative or absolute unavailability due to binding or other mechanisms or an abnormality in the target cells preventing the action of insulin.   In addition to insulin, hormones from the anterior pituitary, the adrenal and possibly from the thyroid have a part in the regulation of glucose metabolism and rare cases of diabetes appear to have an origin in derangements of these hormones, the islets functioning normally.

The **symptoms** of diabetes mellitus are briefly hyperglycemia, glycosuria, poly-**uria, polydipsia,** and voracious appetite, often leading to obesity in spite of the urinary loss of much or all of the carbohydrate portion of the ration. Later there is emaciation. Acidosis and ketosis with ketonuria are frequent findings. The lesions of the disease are those found in the islets. These may include hydropic degeneration of the beta cells, fibrosis, hyalinization or even complete disappearance of the islets, but the most common lesion is the disappearance of granules from the beta cells. This change requires special staining technique (Gomori's); by hematoxylin and eosin the islets appear normal. Owing to the accompanying ketosis there is fatty change in the liver and kidney. In dogs, diabetes is often associated with acute or chronic pancreatitis. In these cases, damage to the islets is part of the destructive processes in the pancreas as a whole and not a primary degenerative lesion of the beta cells. Cataracts develop in the majority of dogs with diabetes of long duration.

The presence of diabetes brings on certain secondary effects which may be more harmful than the diabetes. The more important of these include ketosis which, as would be expected, arises because the body fat is being consumed in lieu of the unassimilable carbohydrate. With the ketosis there is commonly hyperlipemia and hypercholesterolemia. In humans, there is often arteriosclerosis, which, in accord with present theories, is possibly traceable to the hypercholesterolemia. The arteriosclerosis may be responsible for hypertension, which is frequent, as well as for certain vascular changes in the retina and kidneys. Vascular lesions as seen in diabetes mellitus in man have received little attention in diabetic animals. However, changes develop in dogs which, though of much lesser degree, bear resemblance to the vascular lesions of the retina and glomerulus in human diabetes. The afferent glomerular arterioles are thickened at their junction with the glomeruli due to a thickening of the media which stains weakly with PAS and eosin. The glomerular mesangium also becomes thickened, resulting from the deposition of a PAS-positive substance which appears continuous with the afferent arteriole. Only rarely are thickenings encountered in the peripheral part of the glomerular capillaries which resemble the diffuse or focal nodular glomerulosclerosis (Kimmelstiel-Wilson nodules) of human diabetes. Lesions in retinal capillaries comparable to those seen in man occur in dogs and cats but are usually less advanced and the frequency is decidedly lower. These changes cannot be studied in tissue section; they are observed to best advantage in whole mounts of retina digested with trypsin following the method of Kuwabara and Cogan (1960). The typical changes include degeneration of capillary pericytes which appear as mural ghost cells, and the presence of microaneurysms.

Diabetes Mellitus

DIXON, J. B., and SANFORD, J.: Pathological Features of Spontaneous Canine Diabetes Mellitus. J. Comp. Path. *72*:153–164, 1962.

GEPTS, W., and TOUSSAINT, D.: Spontaneous Diabetes in Dogs and Cats. A Pathological Study. Diabetologia *3*:249–265, 1967.

GROEN, J. J., FRENKEL, H. S., and OFFERHAUS, L.: Observations on a Case of Spontaneous Diabetes Mellitus in a Dog. Diabetes *13*:492–499, 1964.

KANEKO, J. J., and RHODE, E. A.: Diabetes Mellitus in a Cow. J. Am. Vet. Med. Assn. *144*:367–373, 1964.

KEEN, H.: Spontaneous Diabetes in Man and Animals. Vet. Rec. *72*:555–557, 1960.

KING, J. M., KAVANAUGH, J. R., and BENTINCK-SMITH, J.: Diabetes Mellitus with Pituitary Neoplasms in a Horse and a Dog. Cornell Vet. *52*:133–145, 1962.

KUWABARA, T., and COGAN, D. G.: Retinal Vascular Patterns. I. Normal Architecture. Arch. Ophthal. *64*:904–911, 1960.

MEIER, H.: Diabetes Mellitus in Animals. A Review. Diabetes *9*:485–489, 1960.

PATZ, A., *et al.*: Studies on Diabetic Retinopathy. II. Retinopathy and Nephropathy in Spontaneous Canine Diabetes. Diabetes *14*:700–708, 1965.
RICKETTS, H. T., *et al.*: Spontaneous Diabetes Mellitus in the Dog. An Account of 8 Cases. Diabetes *4*:288–294, 1953.
WILKINSON, J. S.: Spontaneous Diabetes Mellitus. Vet. Rec. *72*:548–555, 1960.

DIABETES INSIPIDUS

This disease is a specific and extreme form of polyuria with consequent polydipsia and has no relation to diabetes mellitus. It is characterized by a remarkably voluminous excretion of urine, which is very dilute and free from glucose. The cause is deficiency of antidiuretic hormone, which has the effect of inhibiting diuresis in the kidney, and is usually associated with a tumor or other lesion involving the pituitary stalk or the supra-optic nuclei in the hypothalamus. Secretion of this hormone by the posterior pituitary is believed to be under nervous control of the hypothalamus. Pituitrin, an extract from the posterior pituitary, tends to relieve the condition.

Diabetes Insipidus
CAPEN, C. C., MARTIN, S. L., and KOESTNER, A.: Neoplasms in the Adenohypophysis of Dogs. Path. Vet. *4*:301–325, 1967.
FRAZER, T. W.: Diabetes Insipidus in the Dog. Vet. Rec. *76*:543, 1964.
VOLTIN, H., and SCHROEDER, H. A.: Familial Diabetes Insipidus in Rats. Amer. J. Physiol. *206*:425–426, 1964.

DEHYDRATION

Unfortunately many veterinary patients, ill with various diseases, actually die because of excessive loss and inadequate replacement of water. Clinicians learn to detect this situation partly by a slight wrinkling of the skin, which seems just a bit too big for the body it covers, and, of course, by a gauntness of the flanks and abdomen. Frequently, the patient is too weak or apathetic to get water in the usual way and injections of water or physiological saline solution are necessitated. A blood-cell count made on such a patient gives an abnormally high count of both white and red cells, relative polycythemia. Conditions tending to cause dehydration are (1) fever, (2) diseases accompanied by vomiting or diarrhea, (3) severe hemorrhage, (4) polyuria as in diabetes. Dehydration resulting from renal disease, protracted diarrhea or vomiting and metabolic disturbances such as diabetes mellitus are obviously complicated by other deficiencies such as sodium loss, potassium loss and by altered acid-base balance. Pathologic findings in dehydration are minimal. Little or no fluid will be evident in the pericardial, pleural and thoracic cavities and the serosal membranes are dry and appear to have lost their usual glistening character.

Dehydration
SINHA, R. P., and GANAPATHY, M. S.: Studies on Experimental Dehydration in Canines with Particular Reference to Clinical Picture, Haemoglobin Concentration, Hematocrit, Specific Gravity of the Plasma Sodium Concentration. Indian Vet. J. *44*:127–136, 1967.

KETOSIS

Ketosis, also known as **acetonemia,** is a condition in which "ketone bodies," or "acetone bodies," appear in the blood and thence in the urine. The ketone substances are the three chemical compounds, beta-hydroxybutyric acid, acetoacetic acid and acetone. Numerous theories have been advanced to explain the biochemical events leading to ketosis, but the pathogenesis of ketosis, especially the "specific disease" termed bovine ketosis, remains in a state of confusion. No attempt will be made here to discuss the various hypotheses and experimental data available, our intention being to concentrate on the salient features of the disease; however certain biochemical events deserve brief comment. In all species, ketosis develops in response to a decrease in the availability of blood glucose, whether from hypoglycemia or inability to utilize glucose as in diabetes mellitus. To compensate for the "lack" of glucose, oxidation of fatty acids provides an alternate source of energy. This is accompanied by production of ketone bodies, which serve as a source of cellular energy. If the serum levels of ketone bodies do not reach a "pathological" level, the process is considered a normal physiological process of supplying tissues with a readily utilizable fuel when glucose is not available. However, in the face of a high rate of gluconeogenesis which accompanies clinical ketosis, oxaloacetate becomes unavailable to allow the incorporation of fatty acids into the tricarboxylic acid cycle which results in continual production of ketone bodies which eventually reach harmful levels.

The symptoms of ketosis include anorexia, depression and terminal coma. The animal often has a sickly sweet smell derived from ketone bodies. **Lesions** are primarily chemical. The **ketone substances** are detected in the blood serum by appropriate tests, but the usual diagnostic procedure is a test for acetone in the urine. If this is strongly positive, it can be assumed that the acetoacetic and beta-hydroxybutyric acids are also present. In cows, it may be more convenient to test the milk for acetone than the urine. The concentration of acetone in the milk is comparable to that in the blood; in the urine, it is several times greater. A noticeable degree of **hyperlipemia** accompanies the mobilization of stored body fat. This may be considered as explaining the deposition of fat in the cells of the liver and kidneys which accompanies ketosis; or the fat may be considered an ordinary **fatty change** attributable to toxic characteristics of the ketone substances. **Acidosis,** a depletion of the body's reserve of alkaline ions, chiefly those in $Na\,H\,CO_3$, results from the neutralization of the two ketone acids. It is thought to be this loss of alkali which is mainly responsible for the symptoms manifested. **Hypoglycemia** and a reduction in hepatic glycogen are also consistent findings in bovine ketosis.

Causes.—The usual cause of ketosis in animals is **starvation.** The animal then derives its necessary energy by oxidation of its stored fats, later of proteins of the muscles. The usual clinical case of ketosis in bovines results from loss of appetite and failure to eat. It is thus dependent upon the presence of some other disorder, most often ruminal indigestion, atony, etc. Some of the coarser roughages, such as straw, contain but little digestible carbohydrate, so that the development of ketosis becomes very easy. Coarse dry roughages contain carbohydrate mostly in the form of cellulose. This is to some extent digestible with the aid of the lytic activities of bacteria normally growing in the rumen. Rather minor functional disturbances of the rumen often cause an environment unfavorable for bacterial growth with an abrupt shortage of carbohydrate and development of ketosis. Digestive disorders which prevent assimilation cause it in any species. These forms of ketosis, whether in the bovine or monogastric animals have been termed **primary nutritional ketosis** (simple starvation) and **secondary ketosis** (starvation on account of some other disease).

Primary spontaneous ketosis is a phrase applied to bovine ketosis which develops in cattle under a good plane of nutrition and in the absence of another recognizable disorder which interferes with appetite or nutrient utilization. A hereditary predisposition has been presumed but adequate proof is lacking. This form of bovine ketosis is most frequent in cows during the first few weeks after parturition.

Ketosis is also caused by diabetes mellitus (p. 1018) and by severe toxic damage to the liver, as from phosphorus or carbon tetrachloride, which prevents the metabolism and storage of glycogen (p. 40). It is possible to produce ketosis in carnivora and omnivora by a **ketogenic diet,** that is, one containing much fat and little carbohydrate. This is sometimes done with a view to producing acidosis and a more acid urine, which is unfavorable to the formation of certain kinds of urinary calculi or the growth of certain pathogenic bacteria. Temporary deficiency of adrenal glucocorticoids has also been advocated as a cause.

PREGNANCY DISEASE OF EWES

Known also as "pregnant-ewe paralysis" and toxemia of pregnancy, this disease is at once an outstanding example of ketosis and of a toxemia of pregnancy. The symptoms are depression, somnolence and coma but not true paralysis. These are characteristic of ketosis and hypoglycemia, and verification is furnished by chemical examination of the blood. However, the disease, which is frequently seen and usually fatal in a few days, occurs only in the last weeks of pregnancy and usually in ewes carrying twins or triplets. Birth or abortion is likely to be curative if not postponed too long. The **lesions** are severe fatty change of the liver, kidneys and heart (ketosis) with terminal subepicardial petechiae and ecchymoses (toxemia).

The **causes** are a combination of the toxic waste products of mother and fetuses, plus dietary difficulties of the kind which cause ketosis. Sometimes these are plain starvation, but more often there is semi-starvation on a very non-nutritious ration such as corn stalks or wheat straw. If the ewe was previously well supplied with stored fat, ketosis is even more likely to arise. An abrupt diminution in the accustomed amount of exercise is also contributory. Some believe this is because ketone substances are consumed in the muscles, a physiological concept which is not altogether proved. Since the disease rarely occurs in non-pregnant sheep, it is evident that either set of causes without the other can usually be endured.

Ketosis and Pregnancy Disease

AMBO, K., *et al.*: Studies on Ketosis in Ruminants. II. Principal Site of Ketone Body Formation (TT). Jap. J. Vet. Sci. *23*:265–273, 1961.
JASPER, D. E.: Acute and Prolonged Insulin Hypoglycemia in Cows. Am. J. Vet. Res. *14*:184–191, 1953.
————: Prolonged Insulin Hypoglycemia in Sheep. Am. J. Vet. Res. *14*:209–213, 1953.
KREBS, H. A.: Bovine Ketosis. Vet. Rec. *78*:187–192, 1966.
KRONFELD, D. S.: The Hypoglycemia of Bovine Ketosis: Its Metabolic Origin and Clinical Effects. Proc. 17th World Vet. Congr., Hanover *2*:1315–1317, 1963.
PEHRSON, B.: Studies on Ketosis in Dairy Cows. Acta Vet. Scand. Suppl. *15*:1–59, 1966.
PROCOS, J.: Ovine Ketosis. I. The Normal Ketone Body Values. Onder. J. Vet. Res. *28*: 557–567, 1961.
RODERICK, L. M., HARSHFIELD, G. S., and HAWN, M. C.: The Pathogenesis of Ketosis: Pregnancy Disease of Sheep. J. Am. Vet. Med. Assn. *90*:41–50, 1937.

Saba, N., *et al.*: Some Biochemical and Hormonal Aspects of Experimental Ovine Pregnancy Toxaemia. J. Agric. Sci. Camb. *67*:129–138, 1966.

Sampson, J.: The Significance of Hypoglycemia. J. Am. Vet. Med. Assn. *112*:350–352, 1948.

Van Den Hende, C., Oyaert, W., and Bouckaert, J. H.: I. Fermentation of Glutamic Acid by Rumen Bacteria. II. Metabolism of Glycine Valine, Leucine, and Isoleucine by Rumen Bacteria. Res. Vet. Sci. *4*:367–381 and 382–389, 1963.

19
The Skin and Its Appendages

Consideration is to be given in this chapter to those diseases of the skin and adnexa which are of unknown or uncertain etiology; diseases of known causation are described elsewhere in this book. Especial attention is invited to Chapter 7 (neoplasms), Chapter 9 (inherited diseases), Chapter 10 (pox, vesicular exanthema, aphthous fever, vesicular stomatitis, contagious ecthyma, papillomatosis), Chapter 12 (staphylococcal infections), Chapter 13 (dermatomycoses, epizoötic lymphangitis, blastomycosis, maduromycosis), Chapter 14 (dourine), Chapter 15 (helminth and arthropod parasites), Chapter 16 (ionizing radiation) and Chapter 17 (photosensitization, hyperkeratosis) and Chapter 18 (parakeratosis or zinc deficiency). The mammary glands are anatomically part of the integument but are considered with the reproductive system of which they are a functional part.

ANATOMY AND HISTOLOGY

The skin of animals presents particular problems to the pathologist, not only because of the complexity of its components in various parts of the body, but also because of the many differences between species. Knowledge of normal histology is therefore particularly important to the interpretation of lesions of the skin.

The skin has three principal layers: the epidermis, dermis (or derma) and subcutis (or hypodermis) each of which has definite structure and function and is subject to specific pathologic changes. The **epidermis,** the most superficial layer, is made up of stratified squamous epithelium in which the following layers can be distinguished in those parts of the body in which the skin is thickest:

Stratum corneum, or horny layer, is the most superficial and consists of flattened cells which have lost their nuclei and consist principally of keratin.

Stratum lucidum, or clear layer, lies just under the stratum corneum, is present only in some regions of the skin and consists of a layer two or three cells thick which appears as a clear wavy stripe in histologic sections. It contains eleidin which comes from the dissolution of keratohyalin granules found in the deeper adjoining layer.

Stratum granulosum, or granular layer, is made up of rows 2 to 5 epithelial cells in depth in which the cells are rhomboid-shaped and whose cytoplasm is filled with dark-staining basophilic keratohyalin granules. The origin of these granules is unknown.

Stratum germinativum, Malpighian layer, or stratum spinosum, is made up of polyhedral cells which are cylindrical in the deeper portions and flattened toward the surface. The deepest row of cells in this stratum, the **basal layer,**

consists of distinctive cuboidal cells with hyperchromatic nuclei. The bulk of this Malpighian layer contains cells which are joined by spines, which suggested the name spiny, spinose, or prickle-cell layer. Melanin pigment may be present in the basal layer or in cells superficial to it, and mitotic figures are seen here. In some parts of the skin, the stratum germinativum is widened at regularly spaced intervals, forming the **rete ridges** which extend into the dermis.

The **dermis,** which lies just beneath the epidermis, is made up of connective tissue rich in collagen and elastic fibers. It provides strength and elasticity to the skin and brings nutrients to the epidermis through its vasculature. It may be divided into two indistinctly separable papillary and reticular layers. The **papillary layer** is most clearly distinguishable in the dermal papillae which lie between the rete pegs. This most superficial part of the dermis is made up of a fine meshwork of connective tissue fibrils among which are found elastic fibrils, capillaries and lymphatics. The deeper **reticular layer** of the dermis makes up its bulk and consists principally of dense collagenous connective tissue in which are distributed elastic fibers, blood and lymphatic vessels and the adnexa of the epidermis. Large individual cells (melanophores) laden with granules of melanin pigment may be found in any part of the dermis, particularly in dark-skinned animals. Other individual cells may also be normally present, such as mast cells, histiocytes, plasma cells and occasionally eosinophils.

The **adnexa** include the specialized structures which arise from the epidermis. They are for the most part contained in the dermis but may extend into the subcutis in some situations. The adnexa include:

Sudoriferous or sweat glands ("merocrine" glands)
Apocrine glands
Specialized tubular glands: as lacrimal, mammary glands
Sebaceous glands and modified sebaceous glands; *e.g.*, perianal glands
Hair follicles of two types, those of common or "guard" hairs and tactile hairs
Tactile follicles are distinguished in tissue sections by the large surrounding
vascular spaces and the sensory nerve which can usually be seen.

The **subcutis** or hypodermis is not always sharply demarcated from the dermis but is usually distinguished by its loose areolar connective tissue, large nerves and blood vessels, fat (panniculus adiposus) and its muscular layer (panniculus muscularis). It contains some elastic fibers but is generally poor in collagen.

The nails, claws, hoofs and horns develop from the epidermis in particular, although the dermis may contribute supporting elements for some of the larger structures (horns, hoofs).

The pathologist must be fully aware of normal variations in the components of the skin in different body regions in order to interpret accurately any deviations from the normal. The skin is generally thinnest in the axillae and over the abdomen and thickest over the back and loins. The dermis contributes most to the difference in thickness, whether it involves different anatomic sites or different species. The elephant's skin, for example, has a very heavy dermal layer; the epidermis is not much thicker than that of other species. Most animals are fully covered with hair, but hairless areas do occur, particularly inside the flanks and on the abdomen. The long tactile hairs which are found around the lips and nostrils of many animals are distinguished by a specialized hair follicle which has large blood sinuses in its wall and especially prominent nerve fibers. The guard or common hairs always emerge from the skin at an angle and in carnivores several hair shafts emerge through the mouth of one follicle although each has its separate root. The fine wool hairs of sheep emerge vertically from the skin and the follicles are richly supplied with plump sebaceous glands.

Apocrine glands, which are found only in certain regions of the human skin, are the predominant tubular gland in many animals and may be found in any skin region. The ducts of these apocrine glands empty into the hair follicles in contrast to the sudoriferous glands whose ducts emerge through the epidermis between hair follicles. The deep secretory portion of the apocrine glands of the dog, cow and goat have a serpentine arrangement whereas in the horse, sheep, pig and cat this portion is wound up into a bail (glomiform). In the dog, sac-like diverticula may normally occur.

These differences, here very briefly outlined, emphasize the particular importance of the normal anatomy in the exact skin region which is being studied. It is highly advisable to have "control" sections available for comparison whenever possible.

Anatomy and Histology of Skin

ARCHAMBEAU, J. O.: Histologic Parameters and Elemental Composition of Skin of Swine. J. Invest. Derm. *52*:399, 1969.

BLOOM, W., and FAWCETT, D. W.: *A Textbook of Histology*, 8th Ed. Philadelphia, W. B. Saunders Co., 1966.

CREED, R. F. S.: Histology of Mammalian Skin, with Special Reference to the Dog and Cat. Vet. Rec. *70*:1–7, 1958.

GOLDSBERRY, S., and CALHOUN, M. L.: The Comparative Histology of the Skin of Hereford and Aberdeen-Angus Cattle. Am. J. Vet. Res. *20*:61–68, 1959.

KOZLOWSKI, G. P., and CALHOUN, M. L.: Microscopic Anatomy of the Integument of Sheep. Am. J. Vet. Res. *30*:1267–1279, 1969.

LOVELL, J. E., and GETTY, R.: The Hair Follicles, Epidermis, Dermis and Skin Glands of the Dog. Am. J. Vet. Res. *18*:873–885, 1957.

LYNE, A. G., and HOLLIS, D. E.: The Skin of the Sheep: A Comparison of Body Regions. Aust. J. Biol. Sci. *21*:499–527, 1968.

MONTAGNA, W., and YUN, J. S.: The Skin of the Domestic Pig. J. Invest. Derm. *43*:11–21, 1964.

NIELSEN, S. W.: Glands of the Canine Skin. Am. J. Vet. Res. *14*:448–454, 1953.

SEARLE, A. G.: *Comparative Genetics of Coat Colour in Mammals.* London, Logos Press, 1968.

SPEED, J. G.: Sweat Glands of the Dog. Vet. J. *97*:252–256, 1941.

STRICKLAND, J. H., and CALHOUN, M. L.: The Integumentary System of the Cat. Am. J. Vet. Res. *24*:1018–1029, 1963.

TRAUTMAN, A., and FIEBIGER, J.: *Fundamentals of the Histology of Domestic Animals.* Translated and Revised by Habel, R. E., and Biberstein, E. L., Ithaca, N. Y., Comstock Publishing Co., 1952.

WEBB, A. J., and CALHOUN, M. L.: The Microscopic Anatomy of the Skin of Mongrel Dogs. Am. J. Vet. Res. *15*:274–280, 1954.

DEFINITIONS

Certain terms are used by the pathologist in consideration of lesions of the skin which are not necessarily applicable to the rest of the human or animal body. Definitions of some commonly used terms in gross or histologic description follow:

Acanthosis—thickening of the epidermis as a result of hyperplasia of the Malpighian layer. This may occur with or without hyperkeratosis.

Ballooning degeneration—isolation of the cells of the epidermis from one another, particularly in the deeper layers, following intracytoplasmic edema and vacuolization; leading to vesiculation. Often seen in viral diseases.

Bulla (bleb)—cavitation in the epidermis, similar to but generally larger than a vesicle.

Dyskeratosis—an abnormality of development with distinctive alterations in epidermal cells. Two types are distinguished: **benign**—disorganization of epidermal cells especially in the granular layer, with swollen, eosinophilic cytoplasm, sometimes containing elementary viral particles (pox, contagious ecthyema); **malignant**—anaplastic changes in the epidermis manifest by hyperchromatism, changes in polarity, increase in mitotic activity and enlargement of nuclei. This is generally considered a step toward carcinoma.

Erosion (excoriation)—superficial loss of epithelium, usually produced mechanically.

Fissure—a linear defect in the epidermis, which may be crusted and tender. Most often occurs at points of cutaneous mobility and at mucocutaneous junctions.

Hyperkeratosis—thickening of the keratin layer (stratum corneum) usually but not invariably associated with thickening of the granular layer (stratum granulosum).

Liquefactive degeneration—obliteration of the dermal-epidermal junction by edema and leukocytic infiltration in the basal layer of epidermis and the adjacent dermis.

Parakeratosis—The retention of nuclei in the keratin layer (stratum corneum), usually with diminution or absence of the granular layer (stratum granulosum). This change is more frequent on moist surfaces and is characterized grossly by scaling of flaky, loosely adherent material (dandruff).

Pseudoepitheliomatous hyperplasia—severe acanthosis with downward growth of the epidermis. This occurs at the margins of indolent ulcers, burns, and might be mistaken for carcinoma.

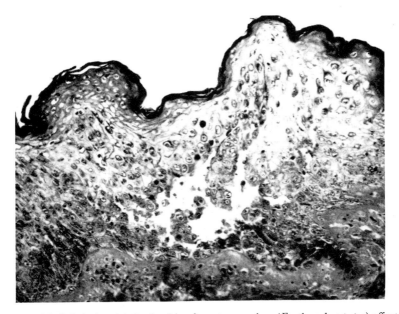

FIG. 19–1.—Epithelial viral vesicle in the skin of a patas monkey (*Erythrocebus patas*) affected with herpesvirus. (Courtesy Dr. H. R. Seibold.)

Pustule—a vesicle filled with pus.

Reticular colliquation—a change in the epidermis in which nuclei become pyknotic or karyorrhectic and the cytoplasm of several cells becomes granular, coalescent, partially disintegrated and edematous with the remaining cytoplasm forming reticulated septa separating lobules of fluid. This lesion occurs in viral diseases in which vesicles are a feature.

Spongiosis—intercellular edema of the epidermis. Severe spongiosis leads to vesiculation, as in eczema.

Ulcer—a break in the continuity of the epidermis with exposure of the underlying dermis.

Urticaria—a circumscribed area of edema and swelling involving principally the papillary layer of the dermis. In *urticaria pigmentosa*, a rare disease of man, aggregation of mast cells gives the lesions some resemblance to mast cell tumors of dogs.

Vesicle—a circumscribed cavity in the epidermis filled with serum, plasma or blood and covered by a thin layer of epidermis which is greatly elevated above the surface. Vesicles may be single or multiple and may coalesce to form larger bullae.

Definitions and General Texts

ALLEN, A. C.: *The Skin*, a *Clinicopathologic Treatise*, St. Louis, C. V. Mosby Co., 1954.
ANDERSON, W. D.: *Pathology*, 5th Ed., St. Louis, C. V. Mosby Co., 1966.

NEOPLASMS

Neoplasms of the skin are of particular interest in veterinary medicine for they are not only common, but are usually quite accessible for surgical excision or other means of treatment. The general and identifying features of neoplasms are discussed in Chapter 7, p. 190; only a few points need to be added in connection with those which are peculiar to the skin. The site of origin of particular neoplastic entities is of interest because its determination can be of value in helping to identify a particular new growth and may influence the prognosis and effectiveness of treatment. Table 19–1 will help recall some common cutaneous neoplasms of animals.

Table 19–1.—Sites of Origin of Cutaneous Neoplasms

Epidermis:
  Squamous cell carcinoma
  Papillomatosis
  Melanoma, malignant and benign
Dermis:
  Mast cell tumor
  Myelocytoma
  "Venereal" tumor
  Equine sarcoid and bovine fibro-
    papillomas
Adnexa: (*in dermis and subcutis*)
  Basal cell carcinoma
  Hair matrix tumor (benign calcifying
    epithelioma)
  Adenoma and adenocarcinoma of
    ceruminous glands

Adnexa (continued):
  Adenoma and adenocarcinoma of perianal
    glands
  "Mixed tumor" of sweat glands
  Adenoma and adenocarcinoma of
    sweat and apocrine glands
Subcutis:
  Hemangioendothelioma
  Hemangioma
  Hemangiopericytoma
  Neurofibroma and neurofibrosarcoma
  Lipoma
  Lymphangioma

Neoplasms of Skin

CHRISTIE, G. S., and JABARA, A. G.: Canine Sweat Gland Tumors. Res. Vet. Sci. *5*:237–244, 1964.

FEZER, G.: Histologische Klassifizierung der Hautdrüsentumoren bei Hund und Katze. Inaug. Diss. Tierarztl. Fak., Munchen, 1968. V.B. *39*:262, 1969.

FRESE, K.: Statistical Studies on Skin Tumours in Domestic Animals. Zentbl. Vet. Med. *15A*:448–459, 1968. V.B. *39*:745, 1969.

HEAD, K. W.: Skin Diseases. Neoplastic Diseases. Vet. Rec. *65*:926–929, 1953.

MILLS, J. H. L., and NIELSEN, S. W.: Canine Haemangiopericytomas—A Survey of 200 Tumours. J. Small Anim. Pract. *8*:599–604, 1967.

NIELSEN, S. W., and COLE, C. R.: Cutaneous Epithelial Neoplasms of the Dog—A Report of 153 Cases. Am. J. Vet. Res. *21*:931–948, 1960.

SCHÄFFER, E.: Histologische Klassifizierung epithelialer Hauttumoren bei Hund und Katze. Inaug. Diss. tierarztl Fak. Munchen pp. 139, 1967. V.B. *38*:242, 1968.

TESTI, F.: Epithelial Tumours of the Skin in Domestic Animals. Acta Med. Vet. Napoli. *9*:479–517, 1963.

WEISS, E., and FEZER, G.: Histological Classification of Sweat Gland Tumours in Dogs and Cats. Berl. Munch. tierarztl. Wschr. *81*:249–254, 1968. V.B. *39*:263, 1969.

NON-NEOPLASTIC CYSTS

Epidermal Inclusion Cyst.—Epidermal inclusion cysts are most frequently encountered in the dog. They usually are firmly attached within the dermis and appear as small nodules which slowly increase in size. The overlying skin usually remains covered with hair until the nodule attains a large size. Incision of the nodules reveals one or more spherical cysts with a thin wall and a gray, grumous, somewhat desiccated content. These cysts usually are cured by surgical excision; occasionally they may become ulcerated and infected. (See Figure 19–2.)

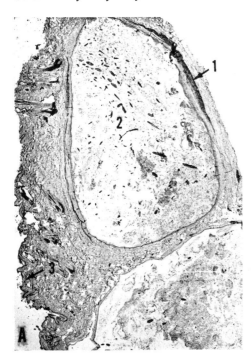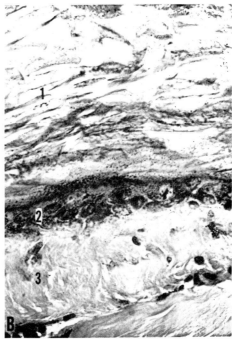

FIG. 19–2.—Epidermal inclusion cysts in the skin of a dog. *A*, Cyst (× 9) in dermis, with squamous wall (*1*), keratinous contents (*2*). Epidermis (*3*). *B*, Same lesion as *A* (× 490). Flakes of keratin (*1*) in the center of the cyst, stratified squamous epithelium (*2*) and dense collagen (*3*) in the cyst wall. (Courtesy of Armed Forces Institute of Pathology.) Contributor: Dr. Edward Baker.

Microscopic examination discloses the cyst wall to be made up of flattened squamous epithelium surrounded by a dense collagenous capsule. Skin adnexa are not present in association with the cyst wall. The cyst contains concentrically and irregularly laminated masses of keratin, occasionally mixed with amorphous tissue debris. Sometimes the epithelial wall of the cyst ruptures, stimulating an intense foreign body reaction around the extruded cyst contents.

The origin of these epidermal inclusion cysts is not entirely explained, but in the dog at least they appear to result from the occlusion of the mouth of hair follicles and subsequent isolation of the involved epithelium. The continuous desquamation of keratin by the stratified squamous epithelium which makes up the cyst wall soon fills the internal space and forces the cyst to expand.

Epidermoid or Dermoid Cyst.—The epidermoid cyst is grossly similar to the epidermal inclusion cyst but is differentiated by the character of the cyst wall which is made up of epidermis supplied with skin adnexa. Sebaceous glands, hair follicles and sweat glands may be present singly or in combination. In some instances, in addition to the keratinaceous and oily debris found in the cyst, fragments of hairs may be present. Epidermoid and epidermal inclusion cysts have essentially the same biologic significance. The epidermoid cyst has no connection with the teratomatous "dermoid" of the ovary (Chapter 26, 1308) nor with congenital "dermoid" of the eye (Chapter 29, p. 1418).

Complex epidermoid cysts occur quite often in the midline of the back of one breed of dog—the Rhodesian ridgeback. These are elongated sacs lined by stratified squamous epithelium with adnexa (hair, sebaceous and apocrine glands) and extend deep into the tissues, often reaching to the bodies of the vertebrae (Fig. 19-4). These have been compared to **trichostasis spinulosa** (Hare, 1932, Stratton, 1964) and may have some relationship to spina bifida (p. 1392).

Epidermoid cysts must be distinguished from the **hair matrix tumor** (benign calcifying epithelioma, epithelioma of Malherbe) which is somewhat similar in

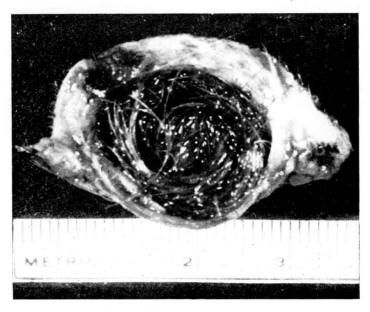

Fig. 19–3.—Epidermoid cyst in the skin of the tail of a seven-year-old castrated male bloodhound. Note hair in cyst. (Courtesy of Angell Memorial Animal Hospital.)

appearance but has a different significance. This lesion can be distinguished microscopically by its content, which has a definite pattern of multiple whorls, suggesting hair follicles, even though nuclei and all details are lost. It is apparent that the contents develop from the outer rim of viable cells by loss of nuclei and differential staining, but have a much more definite structure than the concen-

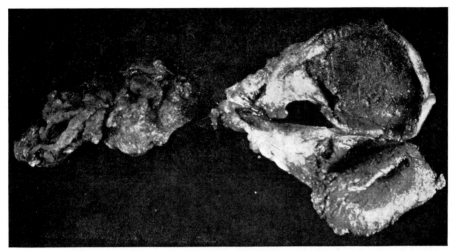

Fig. 19–4.—Epidermoid cyst removed surgically from the midline of the back of a male Rhodesian ridgeback dog, age one year. The opened sac at the right was near the skin, the tissue at the left extended down to the vertebra. (Courtesy of Angell Memorial Animal Hospital.)

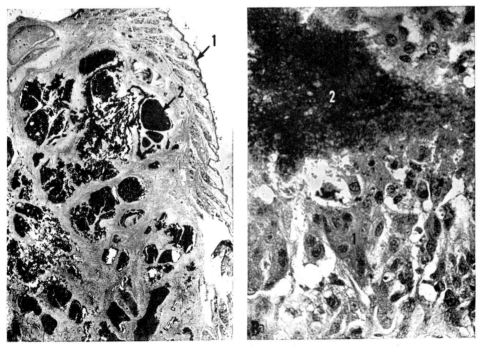

Fig. 19–5.—Calcinosis circumscripta, skin of a dog. A, Low magnification (× 7). Epidermis (1) circumscribed deposits (2) of calcium salts in the dermis. B, Same specimen as A (× 440). Epithelioid cells (1) surrounding calcium salts (2). (Courtesy of Armed Forces Institute of Pathology.) Contributor: Dr. S. W. Stiles.

trically laminated pattern in the epidermal inclusion or cyst which results from extrusion of keratin from its wall. The wall of the hair matrix tumor is also more complex, consisting mostly of basal cells which often form abortive hair follicles. Calcification is apt to occur in the contents of the hair matrix tumor (p. 230).

Sebaceous Cyst.—A sebaceous cyst arises from dilatation of a sebaceous gland or its duct and is essentially similar to an epidermoid cyst except that the contents are even more rich in sebaceous material and may contain cholesterol clefts.

Sudoriferous Cyst.—Cysts of sweat glands arise on the basis of occlusion of their ducts, usually as the result of changes in the epidermis. They may be single or multiple, are filled with watery fluid and lined by a single layer of simple columnar or cuboidal epithelium. They usually do not become very large.

Calcinosis Circumscripta.—Circumscribed masses of calcium salts are sometimes recognized in the dermis of the dog. Similar deposits which occur in human skin have been designated as "calcinosis circumscripta," a term which is descriptive of the animal lesion to which the name may be applied, at least until more is known about its cause and significance. The lesion appears as a mass 1 to 10 cm. in diameter containing a cluster of chalky-white granular foci separated by thin strands of connective tissue. The entire nodule thickens the dermis and elevates the epidermis. The cut surface reveals its chalky appearance and gritty consistency. (See Figs. 19–5 and 6.)

Microscopically, the lesion is seen to be composed of multiple spherical loculi sharply demarcated from the adjacent stroma and from one another. In early stages these loculi contain amorphous material which is basophilic in H & E

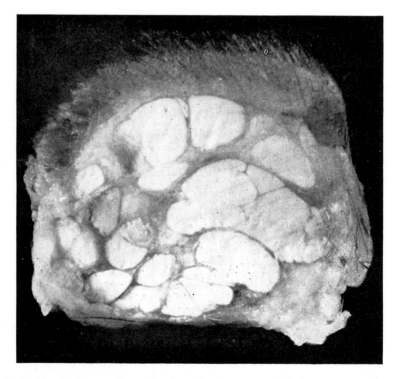

FIG. 19–6.—Calcinosis circumscripta, skin of a male, three-year-old dachshund. Freshly cut specimen somewhat enlarged. (Courtesy of Angell Memorial Animal Hospital.)

stained sections, PAS positive, stains deeply with alcian blue and is occasionally metachromatic. Calcification in the form of fine granules extends inward from the outer borders of these loculi. The border first consists of stroma but eventually is made up of epithelioid and multinucleated giant cells.

Christie and Jabara (1964) propose that the lesion of calcinosis circumscripta arises from cystic apocrine sweat glands and therefore should be called "cystic apocrine calcinosis." This appears plausible and may eventually prove to be correct but does not explain the identical lesions which we have observed in the tongue. Further, in early lesions studied by one of us (Jones) it was not possible to demonstrate a morphologic relation to apocrine glands. We consider that the question of the pathogenesis of this lesion is not yet settled.

Non-neoplastic Cysts

CHRISTIE, G. S., and JABARA, A. G.: Apocrine Cystic Calcinosis: The Sweat Gland Origin of Calcinosis Circumscripta in the Dog. Res. Vet. Sci. 5:317–322, 1964.
CORDY, D. R.: Apocrine Cystic Calcinosis in Dogs and Its Relationship to Chronic Renal Disease. Cornell Vet. 57:107–118, 1967.
HARE, T.: A Congenital Abnormality of Hair Follicles in Dogs Resembling Trichostasis Spinulosa. J. Path. Bact. 35:569–572, 1932.
HOWELL, J. McC. and ISHMAEL, J.: Calcinosis Circumscripta in the Dog with Particular Reference to Lingual Lesions. Path. Vet. 5:75–80, 1968.
KUNGE, A.: Über multiple Kolkeinlogerung in der Unterhaut der Extremitäten des Hundes. Arch wiss. prakt. Thierheilk. 54:462–478, 1926.
STRATTON, J.: Dermoid Sinus in the Rhodesian Ridgeback. Vet. Rec. 76:846–848, 1964.
THOMPSON, S. W., II., SULLIVAN, D. J., and PEDERSEN, R. A.: Calcinosis Circumscripta. A Histochemical Study of the Lesions in Man, Dogs and Monkey. Cornell Vet. 49:265–285, 1959.

HELMINTH AND ARTHROPOD DISEASES OF SKIN

Helminths and arthropods very frequently parasitize the integument of animals, producing a variety of pathologic manifestations. These parasites and the diseases which they cause are described in Chapter 15, but because of their importance, Table 19–2 was prepared to permit the student to visualize the variety of such parasites which affect domestic animals, and to provide a convenient reference to other information on the subject elsewhere in this book.

Table 19–2.—*Parasitic Diseases of the Skin*

Hosts	Parasite	Location of Lesion	Page Ref.
Cattle, sheep, dog, man, swine, horse	*Sarcoptes scabiei*, var. *bovis, ovis, canis, suis*, etc.	Epidermis generally (scabies or sarcoptic mange)	821
Dog, cat, man, swine, sheep, cattle	*Demodex folliculorum*	Fair follicles, sebaceous glands, dermis, lymph nodes, (demodectic mange)	821
Sheep, cattle, horses, rabbits	*Psoroptes communis*, var. *ovis, bovis, equi*, and *cunuliculi*	Epidermis of ears and elsewhere	821
Cattle, sheep, horses, and goats	*Chorioptes bovis*	Epidermis of feet and base of tail	821
Swine	*Demodex phylloides*	Hair follicles and sebaceous glands	816

Table 19–2.—*Parasitic Diseases of the Skin (Continued)*

Hosts	Parasite	Location of Lesion	Page Ref.
Dogs, cats, sheep, deer, and rarely man	*Thelazia californiensis*	Conjunctiva, membrana nictitans	782
Dogs, cattle	larvae of *Rhabditis strongyloides*	Dermis and hair follicles	780
Cat	*Notoedres cati*	Epidermis, esp. of neck (notoedric mange)	821
Cattle	larvae of *Hypoderma bovis* and *lineatum* (ox warble)	Subcutis and dermis of back	811
Cattle	*Thelazia rhodesi*	Conjunctiva, membrana nictitans	782
Cattle	*Onchocerca gutturosa*	Dermis and subcutis	778
Cattle	*Onchocerca gibsoni*	Subcutis	778
Cattle (U. S.)	*Stephanofilaria stilesi*	Hair follicles and dermis, usually of abdomen	781
Cattle (Indonesia)	*Stephanofilaria dedoesi*	Hair follicles and dermis of shoulders, eyelids, neck, withers, dewlap	781
Cattle (India)	*Stephanofilaria assamensis*	Dermis of shoulders and elsewhere	782
Cattle (Malaya)	*Stephanofilaria haeli*	Dermis and epidermis of lower parts of legs	782
Sheep and deer	microfilaria of *Elaeophora schneideri*	Dermis of head, face, poll	779
Sheep	*Psorergates ovis*	Epidermis generally	814
Horses	microfilaria of *Onchocerca cervicalis*	Dermis of abdomen and pectoral region	778
Horses	larvae of *Habronema majus*	Dermis, pectoral region	772
Horses	larvae of *Drachia megastoma*	Dermis, pectoral region	772
Horses	larvae of *Habronema muscae*	Dermis, pectoral region	772
Horses, asses, mules	*Parafilaria multipapillosa*	Nodules, subcutis	778
Horses, asses, mules	*Onchocerca reticulata*	Subcutis, dermis	778
Man	larvae of *Schistosomes* of birds and mammals	Dermis ("swimmer's itch")	805
Man	larvae of *Ancylostoma*	Dermis ("creeping eruption")	738
Mice	*Psorergates simplex*	Epidermis generally	819
Poultry	*Dermanyssus gallinæ*	Epidermis generally	814
Chicken	*Cnemidocoptes mutans*	Scales of legs	814
Chicken	*Cnemidocoptes gallinæ*	Feather follicles	814
Dog, rabbit, cat	*Cheyletiella parasitivorax*	Epidermis generally	814
Dog, mink, otter, raccoon	*Dracunculus insignis*	Subcutis of limbs	751

DERMATOSES OF UNKNOWN ETIOLOGY

Any disease of the skin may be considered a dermatosis, but those to be discussed in this chapter include only those of unknown or uncertain etiology or which are not discussed elsewhere in this book.

Acanthosis Nigricans.—A dermatosis of obscure etiology, acanthosis nigricans is recognized in man and in the dog. Its principal clinical features in the dog are the presence of symmetrical patches of heavily pigmented, rough, thick skin, particularly in the flanks, axillae, inguinal, circumanal and abdominal regions. These changes are persistent, gradually spread to other parts of the body and may produce a disagreeable odor. The lesions are usually poorly circumscribed, vary in diameter from 1 to 8 cm., but surprisingly result in little epilation in most cases, although in some instances this becomes a prominent feature. The cutaneous lesions are in some instances associated in man and in animals with adenocarcinomas, particularly involving the liver, but any causal relationship to such neoplasia is not established. A causal relation to pituitary thyroid stimulating hormone is indicated by the work of Bornfors (1959).

The microscopic appearance of the involved skin is dominated by acanthosis and hyperkeratosis of the epidermis. The dermal papillae are elongated in relation to the overlying acanthotic epidermis and may be congested, but the dermis is otherwise not affected. Hair follicles and adnexa may be slightly decreased in number or unchanged. Cystic dilatation of apocrine or sweat glands may occur. Increased amount of melanin, suspected from the gross appearance, is not always easily measured in histologic sections. This is especially difficult to assess in animals which normally have a deeply pigmented skin. However, careful comparison with adjoining unaffected skin will usually disclose excessive amounts of melanin in the epidermis and dermis of the involved areas.

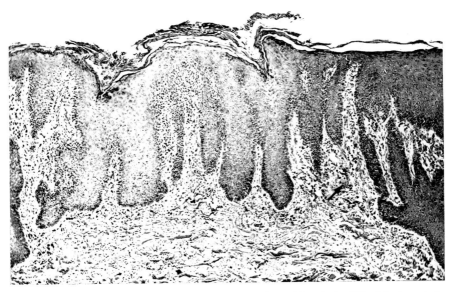

FIG. 19–7.—Ancanthosis nigricans, skin of a dog. Thick epidermis ($\times$ 50) with elongated rete pegs. Melanin is increased in the epidermis and dermis (arrows). (Courtesy of Armed Forces Institute of Pathology.) Contributor: Dr. M. A. Troy.

Dermatoses of Unknown Etiology

BORNFORS, S.: Acanthosis Nigricans in Dogs. Acta Endocr. Copenhagen. Suppl No. 37, 63, 1959.

CURTH, H. O., and SLANETZ, C. A.: Acanthosis Nigricans and Cancer of the Liver in a Dog. Amer. J. Cancer *37*:216–223, 1939.

MONTGOMERY, H. *Dermatopathology.* New York, Harper & Row, 1967.

Eczema.—Eczema is a term commonly applied in a rather broad and somewhat loose sense to the clinical differentiation of cutaneous lesions in animals. It is unfortunately true that such lesions are not often submitted for microscopic study. Eczema is generally thought to occur in response to exposure to an allergen to which the skin has been sensitized.

In histologic features, the eczematous skin is thought to pass through many phases of development from early erythema through papular, vesicular, pustular and exfoliative stages. The lesions observed microscopically will depend upon the stage at which the specimens are taken. In the experience of one of us (Jones), the earliest lesions start with varying degrees of acanthosis with edema and congestion in the underlying papillary layer. The vesicles begin as areas of spongiosis or intercellular edema in the stratum germinativum. This intercellular edema eventually coalesces to form vesicles which in turn enlarge in the severest lesions to produce bullae. Pustules may supervene in the involved epithelium and exfoliation of the superficial layers usually follows as healing occurs. The underlying dermis exhibits inflammatory changes of varying degrees of intensity.

Parakeratosis of Swine.—An afebrile dermatosis of young swine has been described by Kernkamp *et al.* (1953), and named parakeratosis from one outstanding feature. This is described as a deficiency of zinc on page 1015.

Keloid.—A keloid is a hypertrophic scar of the dermis which results from certain types of injury, particularly burns. It occurs more frequently in certain races of people such as the Japanese and Negro, and sometimes is seen in animals. The hypertrophic scar tissue elevates the epidermis, which frequently becomes ulcerated. Histologically, the keloid is made up of heavy bands of eosinophilic collagen in which thinner collagen fibers and fibroblasts are rather haphazardly mixed. The skin adnexa are usually absent and the epidermis may be atrophied or excoriated. Elastic fibers are usually sparse.

Feline Intradermal Granulomas.—Granulomatous inflammation associated with necrosis of dermal collagen has been described by Bucci (1966) and one of us (Jones) has seen numerous similar lesions among biopsy specimens from cats. These lesions appear on the skin of any site, elevating it with nodular or linear configurations. Ulceration may occur and some lesions appear to be self limiting. Ulcerative lesions in the lips, oral and pharyngeal mucosa are often associated with cutaneous lesions, particularly on the feet or legs. The lesions on the lips are often referred to as "rodent ulcer"; "eosinophilic granuloma" is also applied to the oral lesions, more frequently to those of the dermis. The term "linear granuloma" is used to describe the elongated lesions in the dermis which are often bilaterally symmetrical, involving lateral or medial surfaces of both legs or both axillae. More than one disease entity may be involved, but the histologic features in biopsy specimens are similar, justifying consideration of this to be one entity until more can be learned. The cause is at present undetermined although allergy is suspected to be a component. Microorganisms have not been demonstrated.

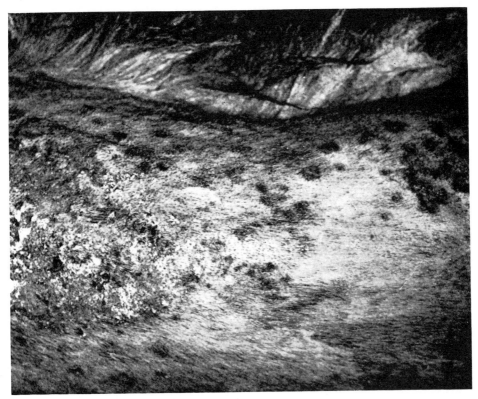

Fig. 19–8.—Eczematous dermatitis, skin of the abdomen of a female collie, age five years. (Courtesy of Angell Memorial Animal Hospital.)

The lesions are limited for the most part to the dermis. In early lesions, foci of necrosis of collagen may be found and the inflammatory reaction is evidently the result of this necrosis. Epithelioid cells, giant cells, and leukocytes (eosinophils often in great numbers) make up this cellular reaction. The necrotic collagen often forms discrete masses surrounded by epithelioid and foreign-body giant cells.

Feline Intradermal Granuloma

Bucci, T. J.: Intradermal Granuloma Associated with Collagen Degeneration in Three Cats. J. Am. Vet. Med. Assn. *148*:794–800, 1966.
Conroy, J. D.: Diseases of the Skin, pp. 346–347 in *Feline Medicine and Surgery*. E. J. Catcott (ed.). Wheaton, Ill., Amer. Vet. Public, 1964.

Equine Cutaneous Granulomas.—The horse especially is prone to develop chronic, ulcerated and bloody granulomas, chiefly on the limbs. Commonly they are known to have originated as wire-cuts or similar cutaneous injuries. The granulation tissue in many instances grows unceasingly and results in large, raw masses which are cured only by radical surgery, if at all. Clinically they have to be differentiated from equine sarcoids (pp. 196, 512) and other tumors.

It has long been accepted that the reasons for such untractable wound-healing are an unusual susceptibility of the equine species coupled with the continued irritation of uncontrolled movement and unavoidable contamination of the raw surfaces with bacteria and dirt. For some of these cases this concept is still retained but in the warmer parts of the world, where these granulomas are often known as *summer sores, bursatti* or colloquially as "leeches," other causes have been discovered.

In the latter group of cases complete gross examination of the granulation tissue should reveal here and there a limited number of yellowish-white specks, mostly visible to the naked eye, which prove to consist of a denser and more or less separable material. The presence of these bodies appears to be diagnostic.

Microscopically the granulomas of this group are composed of rather loosely arranged, newly formed fibrous tissue with large numbers of hyperemic capillaries and an active inflammatory process in which eosinophils tend to be predominant among the other leukocytes. The characteristic bodies mentioned above prove to be sharply bounded, necrotic masses which with hematoxylin and eosin take a startlingly conspicuous deep red color, although interspersed with necrotic nuclei. Cellular remnants suggest that many may have been eosinophils; peripherally the other cells, fibroblastic in nature, with much red cytoplasm, are often radially oriented, forming a minutely spinous fringe.

In the case of some patients, distorted sections of helminths are readily seen within some of these necrotic masses and the lesion is accepted as cutaneous habronemiasis (p. 772). In other individuals no evidence of helminths is discoverable but careful observation reveals coarse, septate hyphae of a fungus. Pale and practically unstained by hematoxylin-eosin, they are faintly visible in the red-staining mass of necrotic cells. Stains such as the Gridley-fungus stain show that the mycelial fragments are numerous, especially around the periphery of the necrotic bodies. Bridges and Emmons, 1961 and 1962, have identified two organisms from such lesions: *Hyphomyces destruens* and *Entomorphthora coronata*, the former from the leg and the latter from the skin of the nostril.

It would appear then that these troublesome lesions of the horse may signify any one of three entities, a non-specific granulation tissue, cutaneous habronemiasis or a "phycomycosis." To date, the two etiologic agents have never been found in the same individual. Differentiation should be readily possible by histopathologic methods. It may be that similar lesions with similar fungal pathogenesis occur occasionally in other species but habronemiasis is limited to the horse.

Equine Cutaneous Granulomas

BRIDGES, C. H., and EMMONS, C. W.: A Phycomycosis of Horses Caused by *Hyphomyces destruens*. J. Am. Vet. Med. Assn. *138*:579–589, 1961.
BRIDGES, C. H., ROMANE, W. M., and EMMONS, C. W.: Phycomycosis of Horses Caused by *Entomophthora coronata*. J. Am. Vet. Med. Assn. *140*:673–677, 1962.

Exudative Epidermitis of Swine.—A specific pustular dermatitis was described and reproduced experimentally by Hjärre (1948) who named it **contagious pyoderma** or **impetigo contagiosa suis.** The currently favored name in the United States, **exudative epidermitis,** was first used by Jones (1956). Other names are apparently synonyms: "seborrhea oleosa" (Kernkamp, 1948), "greasy pig disease" and "acute or chronic generalized dermatitis" (Mebus, Underdahl and Twiehaus, 1968).

Staphylococcus hyos, described by Underdahl, Grace and Twiehaus (1965), has been isolated repeatedly from natural cases and has been used to reproduce the disease experimentally. It is possible that natural outbreaks are made more severe by presence of other organisms, particularly viruses. An antecedent viral infection has been postulated but no evidence produced for it.

The disease usually affects only young swine during their first month of life. It has been reported from most places where swine are raised on a large scale, including Germany, Holland, Ireland, Norway, Sweden, United States, Canada and Australia (Obel, 1968). The cutaneous manifestations usually appear suddenly around the eyes and ears, and soon spread to the trunk and other parts of the body. The lesions appear first as sharply delineated patches, red or yellow tinged which soon become covered by a greasy exudate which may be removed easily, revealing hyperemic skin underneath. In chronic cases the exudate eventually sloughs, leaving congested, healing skin underneath.

Microscopically, in the early lesion, the epidermis becomes acanthotic with severe spongiosus in the upper layers of the stratum spinosum. A superficial parakeratotic layer is soon formed and covers a vesicle. Granules are lost in the stratum granulosum and the papillary layer of the dermis is hyperemic. Acanthosis and intercellular edema tend to persist in the epidermis and vesicles become pustules. Coccoid organisms are usually demonstrable in these pustules. Periodic acid Schiff (PAS)—positive material appears in epithelial cells and intercellular spaces. Some microabscesses may extend into hair follicles. The dermis in late stages becomes intensely infiltrated by leukocytes as the overlying epidermis contains abscesses or becomes excoriated.

One reported complication in spontaneous and experimentally induced cases is a severe ureteritis with edema of the ureter sufficient to produce occlusion. Hydronephrosis is reported to follow and pyelonephritis might be an expected result.

Exudative Epidermitis of Swine

HJÄRRE, A.: Kontagious pyodermi hos svin (Impetigo contagiosa). Skand. Vet. Tidskr. *38*:662–682, 1948.
JONES, L. D.: Exudative Epidermitis of Pigs. Am. J. Vet. Res. *17*:178–193, 1956.
KERNKAMP, H. C. H.: Seborrhea Oleosa in Pigs. North Amer. Vet. *29*:438–441, 1948.
L'ECUYER, C.: Exudative Epidermitis in Pigs. Clinical Studies and Preliminary Transmission Trials. Canad. J. Comp. Med. *30*:9–16, 1966.
MEBUS, C. A., UNDERDAHL, N. R., and TWIEHAUS, M. J.: Exudative Epidermitis. Pathogenesis and Pathology. Path. Vet. *5*:146–163, 1968.
OBEL, A. L.: Epithelial Changes in Porcine Exudative Epidermitis. The Light-Microscopical Picture. Path. Vet. *5*:253–269, 1968.
UNDERDAHL, N. R., GRACE, O. D., and TWIEHAUS, M. J.: Porcine Exudative Epidermitis: Characterization of Bacterial Agent. Am. J. Vet. Res. *26*:617–624, 1965.

Folliculitis.—Inflammation of the hair follicles (folliculitis) is quite common, especially in the dog. Aside from the parasitic and mycotic infections described in Chapters 15 and 13, respectively, folliculitis of unknown etiology is encountered with moderate frequency by the veterinary pathologist. The lesions are usually localized in irregular areas and the skin appears grossly thickened, indurated and hairless. Ulceration of the overlying epidermis is frequent, usually as a result of prolonged gnawing or scratching of the part by the animal. Surgical specimens are usually submitted because of a suspected neoplasm.

Histologically, the lesions are seen to be related to inflammatory and necrotizing changes in the deep parts of the hair follicles. Necrosis of the epithelium results in the isolation of bits of hairs or contents of sebaceous glands; either of

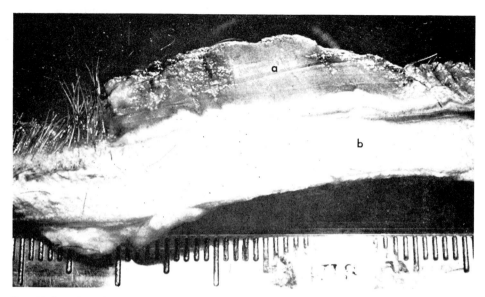

FIG. 19–9.—"Brand papilloma" in the skin of a six-year-old male Hereford. Note the thick keratin layer (a) at the site of the scar caused by a hot-iron brand; dermis (b).

these evoke an intense local foreign body reaction. The dermis adjacent to these items of debris may contain microabscesses, or, more frequently, aggregates of epithelioid cells and foreign-body type giant cells. The surrounding dermis becomes quite thick as the result of proliferation of collagenous connective tissue. The overlying epidermis may be unchanged, acanthotic, or ulcerated.

In **acne,** a type of folliculitis, the sealed-off hair follicles or sebaceous glands become enlarged, filled with pus and surrounded by intense inflammation. In **furunculosis,** abscesses in the dermis, hair follicles or sebaceous glands may reach rather large size then rupture through the epidermis. This leaves a rounded hole in the epidermis and a pit or canal leading down into the dermis.

"Brand Papillomas."—Exuberant growth of epidermis with a thick overlying layer of keratin is sometimes observed in the skin of cattle adjacent to the site of a brand. Squamous cell carcinomas rarely arise at these injured sites (see Brand Cancer, p. 275). These lesions (Fig. 19–9) have some resemblance to those seen in the bovine skin several years after injury by beta radiation following radioactive "fall out" (Fig. 16–5).

Cutaneous Amyloidosis.—Amyloid (see Chapter 2, p. 47) has been described by Hjärre and Nordlund (1942) in the skin of the horse. It appears as multiple, hard, elevated spherical nodules 5 to 25 mm. in diameter, located particularly in the skin of the head, neck and pectoral regions. The amyloid is seen microscopically in masses in the dermal papillae and in collars surrounding the sweat and sebaceous glands as well as around blood vessels. This type of amyloidosis is not associated with deposition of amyloid in the visceral organs. Its cause is unknown.

Cutaneous Amyloidosis

HJÄRRE, A., and NORDLUND, I.: Om atypisk amyloidos hos djuren. Skand. Vet.-Tidskr. *32*:385–441, 1942.

Xanthomatosis.—Collections of histiocytic cells laden with lipoid substances are occasionally encountered in the dermis and subcutis of animals. It is presumed that this finding is associated with some defect in lipoid metabolism, but studies have been so limited that its significance is not understood. The lesions are recognized in microscopic sections only. Diffuse or nodular accumulations of large cells with abundant "foamy" appearing cytoplasm are most frequent. In some cases, the presence of cholesterol is indicated by characteristic clefts (p. 25) in the tissue. Multinucleated giant cells are occasionally seen. Special stains of frozen sections reveal the lipid content of the cells.

The occurrence of familial diseases characterized by defects in lipid metabolism, as are known in man, has not yet been reported in animals. However, a disease of chickens has been described in which cutaneous xanthomatosis was a prominent feature (1958). (See page 216.)

Xanthomatosis

Peckham, M. C.: Xanthomatosis in Chickens. Am. J. Vet. Res. *16*:580–583, 1955.
Thoonen, J., Hoorens, J., and Van Mierhaeghe, E.: Xanthomatosis beim Huhn. Arch. Gelflügelk *23*:314–318, 1959.

Laminitis.—This inflammatory disease of the foot of solipeds usually has an acute onset following some event such as parturition or digestive upset. The affected horse has a fever and may be slightly lame in mild cases or may refuse to walk if severely affected. Most reports indicate that the significant lesion is due to hyperemia in the corium of the sensitive laminae (the laminated structure of the epithelium and its underlying dermis which gives rise to and supports the hoof) but careful studies by Obel (1948) indicate that the epithelium is the essential structure affected.

Laminitis is known to occur in association with (1) sudden acute indigestion resulting from overeating of a concentrated grain ration. Diarrhea and presumably a severe acute enteritis are present in these cases. (2) It occurs following the use of irritant purgatives, especially aloes. It also occurs (3) following a sudden drink of cold water, or even exposure to a sudden cold rain, when the horse is hot from strenuous exercise in hot weather. Particularly when related to these gastrointestinal disturbances the disease is often called **founder**. (4) It occurs in connection with septicemic infections such as post-parturient metritis (parturient laminitis), infected castration wounds and possibly valvular endocarditis. (5) Laminitis develops from local causes including the effects of an unusually hard drive on paved roads or standing still too long while being transported on board ship. Standing with the pressure continually on one foot because of lameness in the other causes a unilateral laminitis in the foot subjected to this continuous pressure. Cattle also occasionally have laminitis from these local stresses.

The highly specialized epidermal and dermal structures of the hoof form layers of epithelium, corium, and keratin which have orderly and intimate relationships to one another. Primary layers of epithelium are arranged in elongated, parallel fronds separated by thin bands of vascular stroma. The keratinized layer is specialized in that it forms primary and secondary onychogenic fibrils which are bound together to form the horny part of the hoof. According to Obel (1948), the primary lesion in laminitis involves the epithelium, particularly the keratogenic zones. The keratohyalin granules disappear and the onychogenic fibers are disorganized and lost. Eventually necrosis occurs in the epithelium and this is presumed to lead to the severe hyperemia and occasionally to eventual separation of the hoof from the laminae. Thus it appears that this dramatic disease results from a disturbance in the metabolism involved in production and maintenance of the cornified horny structure of the hoof. The biochemical basis for this phenomenon remains to be discovered.

If the congestion and inflammation subside within three or four days, laminitis may leave no permanent injury. If the condition persists longer, permanent deformity is likely to be the result, evidenced by the separated and downward pointing os pedis and the convex "dropped sole." Also the normally straight anterior contour of the hoof becomes concave from the coronet to the toe, which is unduly prolonged, and the unevenly growing hoof forms a series of bulging rings parallel to its coronary origin, each representing a different phase of growth.

Laminitis

Obel, N.: *Studies on the Histopathology of Acute Laminitis.* Uppsala, Sweden, Almqvist and Wiksells, 1948.
Reeks, H. C.: *Diseases of the Horses' Foot.* Chicago, Alex Eger, 1925.

Foreign Bodies in Skin.—Foreign bodies usually reach the skin through some type of wound and may consist of any material or substance. Tissue reactions vary, depending on the anatomic site and the nature of the foreign body. Keratin and hair in the dermis or subcutis may stimulate intense inflammation. This is

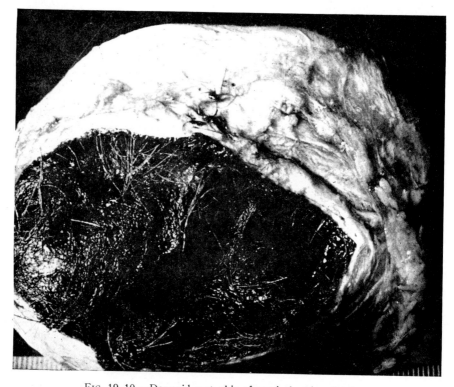

Fig. 19–10.—Dermoid cyst, skin of cervical region, bovine.

often observed when an inclusion cyst, hair matrix tumor or keratoacanthoma ruptures, exposing its keratinaceous contents directly to the dermis or subcutis. This is the usual reason for sudden increase in size, ulceration and inflammation associated with these lesions.

Other foreign bodies are found in the skin of animals upon occasion. Nettles and thorns of plants are among these. Schumacher and Majno (1967) reported thorns, believed to be from the palm (*Bactris minor*), in the skin and joints of a new world monkey, *Cebus albifrons*. These thorns, recognized in microscopic sections, produced little inflammation in the dermis but provoked an intense granulomatous response in the synovial membrane of these animals. These have been compared to blackthorn (*Prunus spinus*) described in human skin and joints by Kelly (1966).

Foreign Bodies

KELLY, J. J.: Blackthorn Inflammation. J. Bone Joint Surg. *48*:474–477, 1966.
SCHUMACHER, R. H., and MAJNO, G.: Thorns in the Skin and Joints of the Monkey. Arch. Path. *84*:536–538, 1967.

Endocrine Alopecia.—Certain changes in the skin characterized by bilateral symmetry, loss of hair and atrophy of epidermis have for many years been ascribed to "endocrine dysbalance" or "deficiency" with scant knowledge as to the causative factors involved. This view, while not wholly incorrect, is not accurate nor specific enough to permit understanding of the etiologic or therapeutic aspects of the disease. Much still needs to be learned but at least three specific endocrine disturbances are now known to cause "endocrine alopecia."

The first of these is hyperestrogenism, resulting from the prolonged administration of estrogens, such as diethylstilbesterol, or from the presence of an estrogen-secreting **Sertoli cell tumor** of the testicle (p. 260). The estrogen elaborated by this tumor not only produces changes in the skin, but causes redistribution of body fat, gynecomastia, squamous metaplasia of prostate and other evidence of feminization. This tumor is most common in cryptorchid testes of dogs. The skin in this condition loses its hair over broad, bilaterally symmetrical areas of the legs, neck, buttocks, flanks and occasionally the entire body. The hairs become brittle and are easily pulled or rubbed out and are not replaced. Depletion of hair follicles and sebaceous glands are evident in microscopic sections as is moderate atrophy of the epidermis.

The second condition in which endocrine alopecia is a prominent feature is **hypothyroidism** (p. 1357). In this disease, hair loss is gradual but has the usual bilateral symmetry. The skin in involved areas is thin, smooth and sometimes irregularly pigmented. Hair that remains over the rest of the body is usually fine and sparse. Administration of thyroxin results in improvement in vigor and return of the normal hair coat. The microscopic changes in the skin are essentially similar to those seen in hyperestrogenism.

A third syndrome in which endocrine alopecia occurs has been described by Coffin and Munson (1953) and named by them a **pituitary-adrenal state** or **canine Cushing's syndrome** (p. 1353). This disease is recognized in dogs, particularly Boston terriers, and is manifest by gradual onset of abdominal enlargement, roughness of the hair coat and symmetrical alopecia. The legs develop bare areas which extend to involve the flanks, buttocks and thighs. The hair becomes rough,

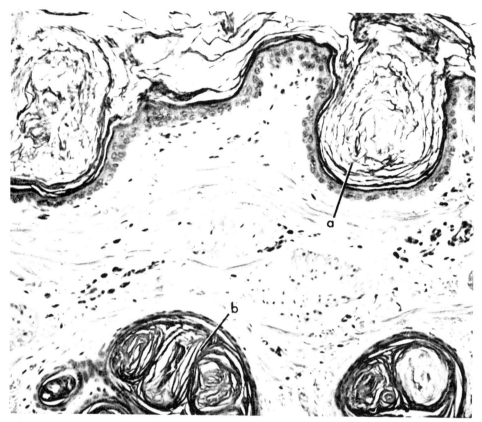

FIG. 19–11.—The skin in canine hypothyroidism. A seven-year-old female Chihuahua with characteristic clinical signs, serum cholesterol of 500 mg. per cent; protein bound iodine 1.0 mg. per cent and total serum iodide 2.6 mg. per cent. Note hyperkeratosis involving epidermis (a) and hair follicles (b). (Courtesy of Angell Memorial Animal Hospital.)

dry, and is easily broken or pulled out. The skin may be rough and scaly and bear small pustules which appear sporadically. These pustules rupture, leaving a scaly margin and a dark pigmented center. The skin is often cool to the touch. Muscular relaxation and weakness may appear, resulting in trembling and assumption of a straight-legged posture. Diabetes insipidus occurs in some cases, evidenced by polydipsia, polyuria and low specific gravity of the urine. Lymphopenia and eosinopenia are also characteristic features.

The lesions in the skin are described as atrophy of the hair follicles, sebaceous glands and epidermis with loss of dermal fat, condensation of collagen and elastic fibers and hyperkeratosis. In some severely affected animals, the dermis becomes calcified, replaced by new bone over rather large areas of the body. The pathologic findings in the rest of the body consist of enlargement of the pituitary with hyperplasia of basophil cells and formation of multiple cysts, and symmetrical hyperplasia of the adrenal cortices, which causes enlargement of the adrenals to four to eight times their normal size.

Endocrine Alopecia

AMOROSO, E. C., and EBLING, F. J.: Allergic and Endocrine Dermatoses in the Dog and Cat—II. Hormones and Skin. J. Small Anim. Pract. 7:755–775, 1966.

COFFIN, D. L., and MUNSON, T. O.:   Endocrine Diseases of the Dog Associated with Hair Loss.   J. Am. Vet. Med. Assn. *123*:402–408, 1953.

GARDNER, W. U., and DeVITA, J.:   Inhibition of Hair Growth in Dogs Receiving Estrogen. Yale J. Biol. & Med. *13*:312–315, 1940.

MONTGOMERY, H.:   *Dermatopathology*, Vol. 1 and 2, New York, Harper & Row, 1967.

THOMSETT, L. R.:   Allergic and Endocrine Dermatoses in the Dog and Cat.   III. Endocrine Disorders and Hair Loss in the Dog.   J. Small Anim. Pract. *7*:777–780, 1966.

WALTON, G. S.:   Symposium on Allergic and Endocrine Dermatoses in the Dog and Cat. I. Allergic Dermatoses of the Dog and Cat.   J. Small Anim. Pract. *7*:749–754, 1966.

20

The Musculoskeletal System

AZOTURIA

WHILE its etymological significance of "nitrogen in the urine" is no longer in accord with current concepts, the name azoturia remains well established as the designation of an important disease of horses. Other names such as paralytic hemoglobinuria are also in use.

In a typical case of azoturia, the horse begins his morning's work in fine spirits following a holiday period of one or several days on a full diet and no exercise. (Hence the name, Monday-morning disease.) It may well be a colder morning than usual, and the patient is likely to be an animal hardened and conditioned by previous hard work. Suddenly, in the course of a few steps the horse becomes practically unable to move and stands transfixed, trembling and sweating in extreme pain. Examination shows certain muscles or groups of muscles, usually but not necessarily one of the large muscles of the femoral or gluteal groups, to be slightly swollen and as hard as wood. These muscles are in a state of extreme cramp or tonic spasm. Anyone who has experienced transient cramping of the muscles of the calf of the leg (systremma) has no difficulty in understanding the animal's inability to move. Azoturia may result also from abnormal and strained positions of muscles while the horse is restrained in a casting harness: a normally ambulatory animal is thrown to the ground; a seriously crippled one arises or perhaps he does not rise. Very rarely, humans are afflicted with what appears to be an identical disease.

The **lesions** in the muscle consist of necrosis of large or small groups of fibers. Such areas, seen one to several days after the onset, are white, usually with some increase of tissue fluid. Microscopically, the change may at first qualify as what many call hyaline degeneration, but shortly all the changes of Zenker's necrosis (p. 22) are present and eventually the complete picture of necrosis is attained with absence of all but the sarcolemma and stromal elements. Thus, if the patient survives, severe disease results in atrophy of the affected muscles, which is very slowly resolved with regeneration of the sarcoplasm. Except that they are larger, the degenerated and necrotic areas are not particularly different from those seen in the so-called white-muscle disease of supposedly nutritional origin.

The urine is usually darkened to a shade of brown with excreted myoglobin. This myoglobinuria must be distinguished from hemoglobinuria. (See p. 1176.) The kidneys suffer considerable injury which becomes increasingly apparent as the patient survives a few or several days. The epithelium of the proximal convoluted tubules passes through a stage of cloudy swelling and becomes necrotic. That of the distal convoluted tubules is more prone to desquamate as it dies and

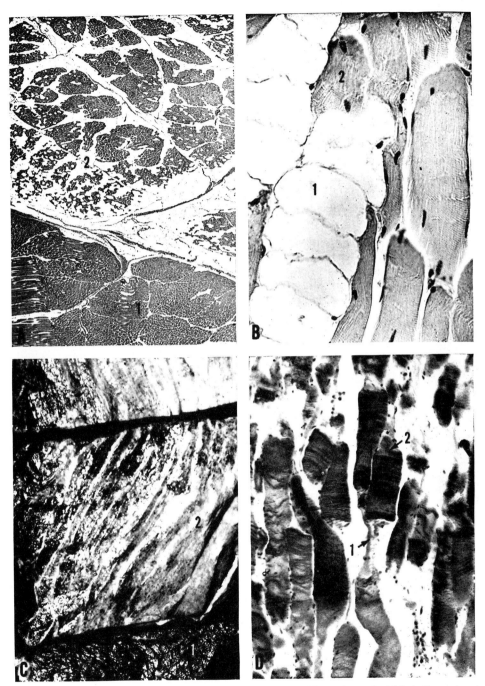

FIG. 20–1.—*A*, Steatosis, psoas muscle (× 10) of a steer.   Normal muscle (*1*) is infiltrated and replaced by fat (*2*).   *B*, The same muscle as *A* (× 330).   Note fat cells (*1*) replacing muscle bundles (*2*).   (Courtesy of Armed Forces Institute of Pathology.)   Contributor: Colonel Russell McNellis, V.C.   *C*, Azoturia, muscle of a year-old colt tangled in halter rope (lived 3 days). Normal dark red muscle (*1*) can be compared with white muscle (*2*) white and degenerating. (Courtesy College of Vet. Med. Iowa State University.)   *D*, Azoturia, muscle (× 180).   Note atrophy (*1*) and distention (*2*) of muscle fibers.   The latter appeared dark red and shiny in the section stained with hematoxylin and eosin.   (Courtesy College of Vet. Med. Iowa State University.)

the same is true of the straight tubules. Some tubules fill with a brownish pigmented material which resembles hemoglobin but is actually the closely related myoglobin. This does not appear to form the solidified casts which are characteristic of the hemoglobin of the human "crush syndrome." In other respects the lesions are very similar.

The **cause** of azoturia is in doubt. The renal damage results from myoglobin in the urine following extensive destruction of muscular tissue, although it is not known whether the myoglobin is the direct cause of that damage. The renal changes may clearly be attributed to the muscular necrosis, whatever may be the exact mechanism of their production. Biochemically, the effect on the kidneys appears entirely comparable to what occurs when muscles are extensively injured, as is seen in the well-known "crush syndrome" of human medicine.

But the original injury to the muscle is not easily explained. Ordinary muscular cramps, such as occur in man, are commonly attributed to an insufficient blood supply to the muscle, but the basic chemical difficulty is not greatly clarified by this information. From the clinical circumstances which usually precede an attack of azoturia it is easy to believe that something accumulates in the muscles during the antecedent period of abnormal inactivity. This something can scarcely be anything but glycogen, which all muscles normally store. As a muscle performs work, lactic acid ($CH_3CHOHCOOH$) is known to accumulate in it. The accepted concept is that the stored glycogen is changed by a series of intermediate steps into pyruvic acid ($CH_3COCOOH$), approximately one-fifth of which is oxidized to $CO_2 + H_2O$ with the production of energy. When the amount of oxygen immediately available is limited, the remaining four-fifths is converted to lactic acid, which may be oxidized later. Pursuant to the above conception it may well be that the amount of lactic acid formed is especially large when the supply of stored glycogen is large, not being directly proportional to the amount of work done. Confirmation of this view is found in the work of Paris (1958), who showed more than 1 per cent of lactic acid in the urine of horses after a strenuous race. Lactic acid artificially injected into the tissues in sufficient concentration is both painful and irritant in other ways. The amount of lactic acid accumulating in the muscles of a fresh, vigorously exercising horse must be very considerable. This is in accord with data and beliefs concerning azoturia which have been prevalent for a long time. Likewise, if the blood supply to a muscle is inadequate, as in cramps, there must be a deficiency of oxygen and an accumulation of lactic acid. So, shall we conclude that accumulating lactic acid irritates or stimulates the muscle to extreme contraction in equine azoturia and perhaps in human systremma and other forms of cramps? The severe contraction of the cramped muscle (hard and board-like, as already stated) certainly does not favor the free flow of blood through it which is essential for increasing the oxygen supply and oxidation of the lactic acid. If this theory be correct, a "vicious cycle" is obviously instituted: less oxygen causes more accumulation of lactic acid, which causes more severe spasmodic contraction of the muscle, which excludes the blood even more and causes a still greater shortage of oxygen. And, let us remember, the cramped, or spasmodically contracted muscle is continuing to do work, which still further augments the shortage of oxygen and the accumulation of lactic acid. The lack of blood supply and lack of oxygen are, as we well know, among the most prominent causes of necrosis (p. 17), which is the end result. As a further explanation of the severe pain, we should recall that insufficient blood supply and insufficient oxygenation were seen to be the cause of an extremely painful condition in another equine disease, thrombosis of the iliac arteries (p. 110).

There is other work suggesting that a shortage of insulin prevents catabolism of the glycogen even as far as lactic acid and that "the muscles are deprived of their energy potential." It is difficult to see how muscles deprived of energy could remain in a spasmodically contracted state, at least reasonably difficult to conceive of a general or local shortage of insulin arising so suddenly or failing to cause the usual diabetes and also difficult to ignore the demonstrated fact that lactic acid does increase.

The effect of all this upon the patient is to cause necrosis of the cramped musculature, or much of it. Clinically the board-like hardness of the muscles gradually recedes in the course of some hours or a day or two, aided, let us hope, by antispasmodic medication. The necrotic muscle, of course, relaxes; the blood supply can be presumed to be restored, except for possibly ruptured vessels; and if the horse has not died of the immediate pain and shock, it may recover but still has to run the gauntlet set up in the damaged kidneys. If the outcome here is favorable, eventual regeneration of muscle fibers is possible.

"WHITE-MUSCLE" DISEASE

At first assumed to be a single entity, "white-muscle disease" must now be considered to be an alteration which voluntary or cardiac muscle displays in a variety of injurious situations. Although the term white-muscle disease has usually been restricted to myodegenerative disorders of calves and lambs, diseases pathologically similar occur in horses, dogs and swine. The lesions of white-muscle disease or diseases consist of areas of skeletal or cardiac muscle which are pale or practically white in color and which are found microscopically to be progressing from hyaline degeneration (p. 44) to coagulative necrosis (p. 19) with fragmentation and disappearance of many muscle fibers. In some forms there is a conspicuous but poorly understood calcification of individual fibers. The condition is more properly designated a degenerative myopathy than a dystrophy, for it is scarcely a failure to develop, nutritional or otherwise, and is not comparable to the pseudohypertrophic muscular dystrophy of humans. The change may involve only a fiber here and another there, or only a certain segment of a fiber's length. Areas where many or all fibers have suffered this change are white or distinctly pale. The white area seldom involves a whole muscle but rather a certain segment of it, having straight borders parallel to the direction of the fibers. The heavy weight-bearing muscles of the croup and thigh are most likely to be involved. Indeed there is evidence that the degenerative changes and the symptoms remain latent until the muscle is subjected to considerable exertion. White areas in the heart muscle are less regularly and less sharply outlined because of the anatomical arrangement of the fibers. The process is accompanied by the presence of macrophages and lymphocytes as well as by attempts at regeneration which seldom succeed in more than the formation of highly bizarre syncytial nuclei. Persisting endomysial connective tissue may be augmented by mild fibrous proliferation where muscle fibers have disappeared. The effect, if skeletal muscles are involved, is to cause stiffness or pseudoparalysis and recumbency, soon followed by death. If the lesions are in the heart, sudden death without premonitory signs is the rule. Such hearts show fairly distinct pale or white areas in the ventricular walls or septum or in the musculi papillares. Unexplained sudden death in any animal necessitates careful examination of the heart for these lesions and microscopic confirmation if suspicious areas are found.

Causes.—The first white-muscle disease to receive careful elucidation was one that occurs with some frequency in young calves, lambs and chicks and which appears to be caused by a deficiency of alpha tocopherol. Its relation to that substance is discussed under the heading of vitamin E (p. 992). Since lambs that are affected have considerable pain and difficulty in moving the limbs, the term "stiff-lamb disease" has been used in connection with this species. Investigators have produced the condition by withholding vitamin E and cured it by supplying the same.

What may be an entirely different "white-muscle disease" is common in lambs and calves of Oregon and other parts of the western United States and has been extensively investigated by Muth (1959). In this disease the mothers have typically been maintained during pregnancy on alfalfa or clover hay grown on certain areas known consistently to produce white-muscle disease year after year. With this kind of hay alpha tocopherol had no preventive effect whatever but selenium amounting to 0.1 part per million of the total ration, given in the form of sodium selenite, was an almost perfect preventive. Muth's findings appear to be incontrovertible and have received confirmation from others. The amount of selenium in the muscles and liver of lambs affected with white-muscle disease (muscular dystrophy) has been shown to be about one-third of the normal, which is still minute, around 1 part per million. The same is true of hay which causes the disorder when fed to pregnant ewes. Experimental injection of selenium into ewes so fed brings their selenium and that of their lambs to normal and prevents the disease.

Skeletal and myocardial myodegeneration are the principal features of a disease of swine in Europe known as "Herztod," "fatal syncope," and "enzootic apoplexy." The cause is unknown, but experimentally vitamin E deficiency produces myodegeneration in swine (p. 992). Vitamin E deficiency has been suggested as the cause of two forms of myodegeneration in horses, which are apparently unrelated to azoturia (p. 1046): maxillary myositis, in which the lesions are principally restricted to muscles of mastication, and polymyositis, in which lesions occur in skeletal muscle of the limbs (principally hindquarters), jaws and heart. It remains to be established whether vitamin E deficiency is related to these conditions.

Dollahite and Henson (1965) have shown that at least two plant poisonings are characterized by whiteness of muscle grossly, necrosis with hyalinization or fragmentation of muscle fibers microscopically and marked increase (up to 18-fold) of serum glutamic oxaloacetic transaminase (SGOT, p. 25). These plants are coyotillo (*Karwinskia humboldtiana*) (p. 970) and coffee senna (*Cassia occidentalis*) (p. 968), both natives of the southwestern United States.

The presence of this type of muscular lesions in azoturia has been mentioned. They have also been noted in tetanus and at times in the musculature of swine suffering from excessive amounts of gossypol. Deficiencies of other vitamins, of phosphorus, and the presence of hypothyroidism have been blamed for white muscles, although perhaps without extensive confirmation. Hove (1954) produced an apparently identical disease in rabbits by withholding choline. Kuttler

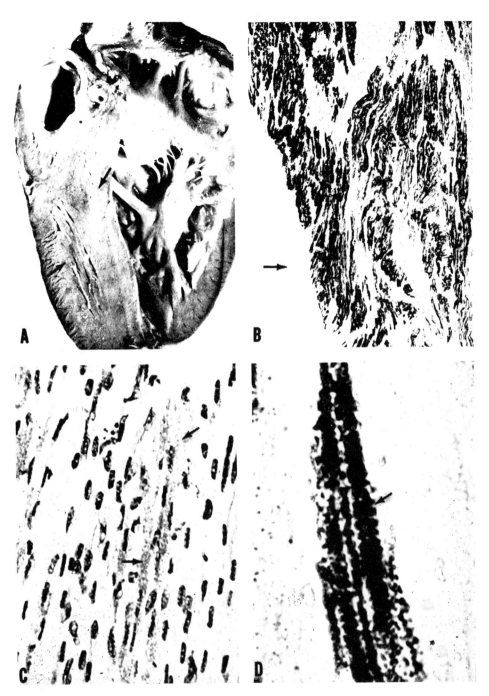

FIG. 20–2.—Myopathy (white-muscle disease) in the heart of a newborn lamb. *A*, Gray areas in the myocardium (arrows). *B*, Section of myocardium ($\times$ 45) stained with von Kossa's method to demonstrate salts of calcium (black). Arrow indicates the endocardium. *C*, Another section ($\times$ 515) stained with hematoxylin and eosin. Note dark granules (arrows) in fibers of cardiac muscle. *D*, Another section ($\times$ 600) stained with von Kossa's method. Note calcium salts (arrows) which outline the cross sections. (Courtesy of Armed Forces Institute of Pathology.) Contributor: Dr. O. H. Muth.

(1958), dealing apparently with the tocopherol form of white-muscle disease, found that the glutamic oxaloacetic transaminase of the blood serum was greatly increased. Muscles can be made "white" and more or less bloodless as the result of severe spastic contraction in nervous disorders.

In slaughtered swine a similar muscular discoloration, but without the usual dryness of typical white-muscle disease, has been pronounced and has caused numerous condemnations when the animals were raised on corn (maize) that had been stored over a period of several years. The disorder was attributed to a loss of vitamin A in the stored grain. There were no antemortem symptoms. On the whole it must be concluded that "white muscles" occur in a variety of disorders, especially if the muscles have been subjected to vigorous exercise but that the exact pathogenetic processes are as yet unknown.

EOSINOPHILIC MYOSITIS

Under the name of eosinophilic myositis, a rare disease involving the masseter, temporalis and pterygoid muscles of the dog has been recognized since about 1940. A number of cases have been reported in Northern Europe and a few in the Northern United States, usually but not invariably in the German Shepherd breed. The muscles named show prominent acute swelling, which is painful and prevents mastication. In most cases, tonsillitis and inflammation and erosion of the mu-

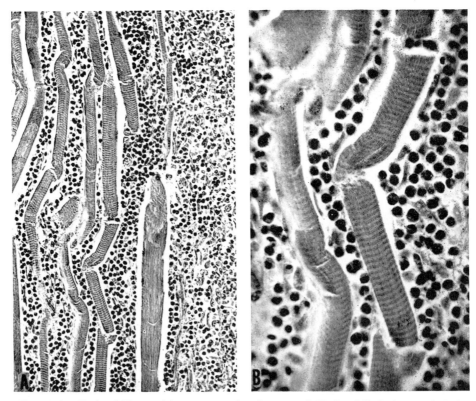

FIG. 20–3.—Eosinophilic myositis, psoas muscles of a cow. *A*, Eosinophilic leukocytes isolating and replacing muscle bundles (× 195). *B*, Detail of *A* (× 460). Distention and rupture of muscle bundles and replacement by eosinophils. (Courtesy of Armed Forces Institute of Pathology.) Contributor: Dr. C. L. Davis.

In bone diseases characterized by malacia or increased resorption of bone there is often an associated increased osteoblastic activity with osteoid formation. The stimulus to the osteoblast under these circumstances is poorly understood, but it probably represents a skeletal response to stress. Parathyroid hormone, which stimulates bone resorption, is believed to inhibit bone formation, but this is either counteracted by mechanical stress or it may be that prolonged parathormone action actually stimulates bone formation.

From this discussion it should be obvious that a diversity of endogenous and exogenous factors is necessary to maintain bone formation, growth and remodeling in homeostatic balance. These include *nutrients* such as calcium, phosphorus, magnesium, copper, vitamins D, A and C (see Chapter 18); *hormones* such as parathyroid hormone, thyrocalcitonin, thyroxin, growth hormone, adrenal cortical steroids, estrogens and androgens (see Chapter 27); *mechanical forces*; and a diversity of other influencing factors such as acid-base balance, citrate, numerous enzymes and so forth.

Before we consider specific disorders of bone a few introductory comments on **metabolic bone diseases** may help the student's understanding of a group of diseases which are often baffling. To be certain these disorders are complicated but the frequent and continued unnecessary misuse of such terms are rickets, osteomalacia and osteoporosis has led to as much confusion as has the complexity of the diseases. Metabolic bone diseases can be conveniently divided into three general types: (1) those principally characterized by porosis, (2) those principally characterized by malacia and (3) those principally characterized by petrosis. **Osteoporosis** is simply a generalized atrophy of bone, *i.e.* there is too little bone present, but what bone remains is properly calcified. Although osteoporosis is the most important metabolic bone disease in man, it is not frequent in domestic animals. The cause is usually not known, but may follow defects in bone formation or excessive resorption.

Osteomalacia (softening of bones) is characterized by failure to mineralize (calcify) osteoid into true bone. In most disorders resulting in osteomalacia there is a disturbance in calcium and phosphorus balance. The mechanism of calcification of osteoid still remains to be elucidated but the process is under control of osteoblasts which for reasons poorly understood are defective when serum calcium and/or phosphorus levels are lowered. Osteomalacia is the predominant feature of rickets (p. 1058) and osteomalacia (p. 1060). In both of these conditions there is no defect in forming osteoid, in fact excess osteoid formation is the rule. Fibrous osteodystrophy (p. 1063) represents a third disorder characterized by osteomalacia but this condition differs from rickets or osteomalacia in that a marked increase of bone resorption is a constant feature. Fibrous osteodystrophy results from a prolonged and excessive stimulation of bone by parathyroid hormone. This may result from primary hyperparathyroidism which is rare in animals, or secondary hyperparathyroidism in response to hypocalcemia. Secondary hyperparathyroidism is not infrequent in animals with chronic renal disease (p. 1064) or chronic nutritional imbalance (p. 1065), such as vitamin D deficiency, calcium deficiency or excess dietary phosphorus. Thus, fibrous osteodystrophy obviously begins as a simple osteomalacia which is subsequently altered due to increased bone resorption stimulated by parathyroid hormone. It should be clear that both rickets and osteomalacia may progress to fibrous osteodystrophy.

Osteopetrosis (p. 1070) is characterized by an excess of calcified bone (not to be confused with an excess of osteoid). Although it occurs in animals, it is infrequent. The following classification should aid the student's understanding:

1. Too little bone, *e.g.* osteoporosis.
2. Defective calcification of matrix, *e.g.* rickets, osteomalacia.
3. Increased resorption of bone (usually associated with defective mineralization), *e.g.* fibrous osteodystrophy.
4. Too much calcified bone, *e.g.* osteopetrosis.

Although the classification is helpful, the student will be quick to realize that in most metabolic disorders of bone he may find features of more than one process within a particular case. For example, with increased resorption of bone the first feature will be too little bone, *i.e.* osteoporosis; but as osteoblasts respond and produce new osteoid which fails to mineralize the disease becomes osteomalacia.

RICKETS

Rickets, sometimes called **rachitis,** is a disease characterized by failure of adequate deposition of calcium (chiefly calcium phosphate) in the bones of growing animals and children. As **adult rickets** the term is often used to include the essentially similar osteomalacia in older animals.

Gross Appearance.—Outstanding are enlargement of the ends of the long bones and of the costo-chondral articulations. The former are observable during life and in severe cases the bones of the limbs become permanently bent under the weight of the animal's body producing "bow legs" and other skeletal deformities. Due to weakening of the muscles and tendons the abdomen is pendulous, "potbellied." At autopsy the same changes are seen; the enlarged costo-chondral articulations, viewed collectively from the inner side, have been likened to a string of beads, the "rachitic rosary." This condition persists even after healing, the enlarged articulations becoming permanently calcified without regressing. Even the intestine may appear relaxed and dilated. When a long bone is sawed longitudinally the epiphyseal cartilage is seen to be abnormally wide, the result of unimpaired proliferation of the cartilage. The bones are abnormally soft and can often be cut with a knife. Routine necropsy procedure should include determination of this point by an attempt to slice a rib with a knife. In birds a crooked sternum with deviation to one side or the other is of frequent occurrence and exhibits a mild degree of rickets in early life.

Microscopic Appearance.—The principal microscopic changes are (1) an increase in the depth of the zone of proliferating cartilage adjacent to the area of ossification (zone of the metaphysis); and (2) disorderly arrangement of this cartilage, as well as a crookedness and irregularity of this zone or line as it stretches from one side of the bone to the other. Normally the cartilage cells form regular rows running lengthwise of the bone; in rickets no such rows exist. Since the whole bone is widened at this point, the area of cartilage is correspondingly increased in the transverse direction also. (3) Disorderly penetration of the cartilage by blood vessels. (4) Defective calcification and failure of normal degeneration of the cartilage. (5) A great excess of uncalcified osteoid in the metaphysis. (6) The marrow areas tend to be fibrosed with a corresponding reduction of myeloid cells. Evidence of increased resorption is usually not a feature of rickets, in fact osteoclasts are fewer in number than one might expect. If, however, secondary hyperparathyroidism in response to hypocalcemia is of sufficient degree, bone resorption and fibrous replacement become features of rickets and the microscopic appearance, especially in the diaphysis, resembles fibrous osteodystrophy. In that vitamin D is necessary for this action of parathyroid hormone, an absolute deficiency of vitamin D would preclude the development of these changes. The absence of active resorption in the usual case of rickets might well be explained by this dependency of parathyroid hormone on vitamin D. As indicated earlier, osteoid itself is resistant to the action of osteoclasts, therefore, active osteoclastic resorption, if present in rickets, is limited to mineralized bone.

Cause of Rickets and Osteomalacia.—(1) Vitamin D deficiency is the classical cause of rickets in children or young animals. In fact many pathologists restrict the use of the term rickets to vitamin D deficiency. However, the microscopic lesions described above, which develop as a result of an inadequate availability of calcium, are duplicated by any disorder favoring hypocalcemia. Thus, other causes of rickets include the following. (2) Dietary lack of calcium is a fundamental cause but in actual practice this seldom occurs, the daily requirement of new calcium being very small. (3) Since calcium is less soluble in an alkaline solution than at an acid pH, a continued excessive alkalinity of the intestinal contents is a cause, but is seldom of more than theoretical importance. The same may be said of (4) continued escape of calcium in combination with fatty acids from unassimilated fat, which has been known to occur in humans and is called coeliac rickets and (5) formation of other insoluble complexes between calcium and oxalate or phytate which prevents calcium absorption. (6) Deficiency of phosphorus obviously is able to cause rickets, since this element is essential in forming calcium phosphate. Phosphorus deficiency occurs in herbivorous animals in certain parts of the world (Gulf Coast of the United States and in South Africa) where the soil, and consequently the plants, are deficient in this element. As a rule, however, other sysmptoms, such as chewing bones or clostridial intoxication therefrom, usually direct attention to the deficiency before the impaired condition of the bones becomes apparent (p. 1009). In addition to simple dietary lack, phosphorus deficiency can arise from steatorrhea, formation of insoluble complexes and changes in the pH of intestinal contents. (7) A severely unbalanced calcium-phosphorus ratio in the diet is entirely capable of causing rickets, and such cases are encountered, especially where inexperienced persons supply mineral mixtures to livestock. If the diet contains an excessive amount of phosphorus, as when animals are fed wheat bran as a large part of their ration, or too much bone meal, such an imbalance develops for the reason that either the Ca ion or PO_4 ion tends to be excreted with the feces in combination with its counterpart, as $Ca_3(PO_4)_2$.

Significance and Effect.—Supporting weight on the poorly calcified bones is painful, and results in lameness or disinclination to move. Pathological fractures, even of the vertebral column, are not infrequent. Normal chicks, experimentally raised without sunlight or vitamin D, regularly go down with rickets, called leg weakness by poultrymen, on the eighteenth or nineteenth day after hatching and shortly die.

When the cause is corrected, normal ossification promptly begins. The strength and hardness of the bone become normal, although the deformities tend to persist for life. The roentgenologist readily detects the lack of calcification in the diseased bone, as well as the restoration which occurs during healing.

While there may be a slight (10 per cent) lowering of the serum calcium level

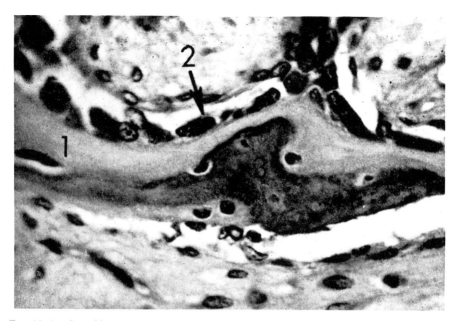

FIG. 20–4.—Osteoid seam in osteodystrophia fibrosa in a monkey. The light staining osteoid (*1*) immediately beneath a layer of osteoblasts (*2*) overlays a mature spicule of bone (*3*). Osteoid seams are the hallmark of osteomalacia.

of the blood in rickets, symptomatically and functionally speaking the action of the parathyroids maintains the blood calcium at the proper level, even at the expense of the bones. Only rarely is there severe hypocalcemia in rickets. In these cases tetany may occur. Serum alkaline phosphatase levels are elevated. As indicated earlier, in long-standing rickets, the parathyroids undergo hypertrophy, perhaps to twice or thrice their normal size. This may be looked upon as a compensatory hypertrophy (p. 92). In cases of hyperparathyroidism, as from a parathyroid tumor, the bones lose calcium but the picture is somewhat different from that of rickets, the condition being known as fibrous osteodystrophy (p. 1063).

The changes in bone which are characteristic of avitaminosis C need to be distinguished in some species from those of rickets. They are mentioned in the section dealing with that vitamin (p. 990).

OSTEOMALACIA

Osteomalacia occurs in the bones of adults through the same mechanisms as rickets in the young and is often called **adult rickets**. Since normal bone is continually being made over through the formative action of the osteoblasts, and at the same time is being destroyed by the osteoclasts, the failure of calcification and accumulation of osteoid is chiefly just beneath the periosteum and, to a lesser degree, the endosteum. As in rickets of the young, there is too much pink-staining osteoid, usually in the form of wide borders around a blue-staining calcified central portion in each bony trabecula. These osteoid borders which are lined by prominent osteoblasts are the so-called "osteoid seams" upon which the histopathological diagnosis of osteomalacia is based. As in rickets osteoid is

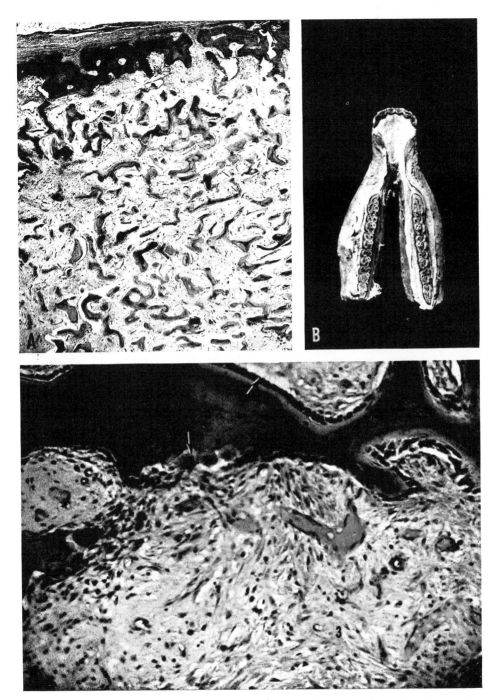

FIG. 20–5.—Equine fibrous osteodystrophy. *A*, Section of mandible (× 50) showing replacement of marrow and cortex with irregular spicules of poorly calcified bone supported by a fibrous stroma. *B*, Mandible of an affected horse. Note great thickness of mandible which was soft and easily cut with a knife. *C*, Higher magnification of *A* (× 200). Note active osteoblasts (*1*), osteoclasts (*2*) and fibrous replacement of the marrow (*3*). (Courtesy of Armed Forces Institute of Pathology.) Contributors: Colonels John H. Kintner and Rufus L. Holt.

resistant to osteoclastic resorption which allows its continual build up. Osteoclasis of calcified bone may be apparent but it is seldom a striking finding unless secondary hyperparathyroidism ensues. In the latter event resorption and fibrous replacement of bone become paramount and the pathological picture progresses to that of fibrous osteodystrophy.

Irregular diffuse thickening of the bones occurs all along the diaphysis but the

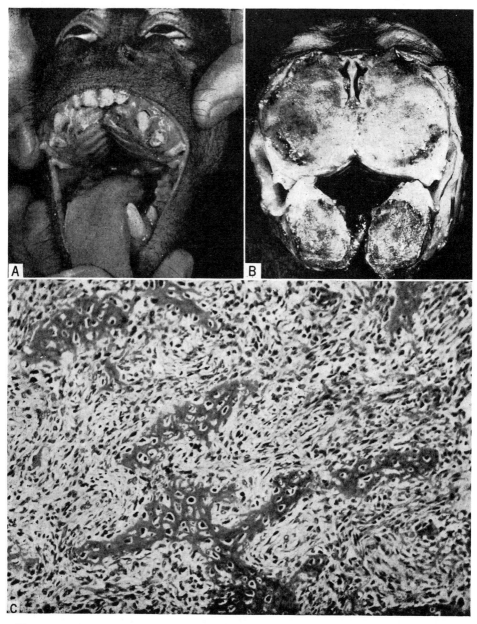

FIG. 20–6.—Fibrous osteodystrophy in a male spider monkey, 1½ years old. *A*, Thickened maxilla and deeply-embedded teeth in the living animal. *B*, Mandibles and maxillae, softened and thickened and encroaching on the nasal cavity. *C*, Section of the maxilla with zones of osteoid interspersed in fibrous marrow. H & E × 150. (Courtesy of Angell Memorial Animal Hospital.)

bone is soft, easily cut or sawed, and may become permanently deformed. As growth is no longer in progress the epiphyseal changes are absent or minimal. Enlargement at the carpal and tarsal regions occurs, nevertheless, at least in the horse. The flat bones of the head and pelvis share prominently in the thickening and distortion. Due to the stresses of weight-bearing, marked deformity of the pelvis often develops.

Causes have been given under Rickets. Significance and effect are also much the same.

FIBROUS OSTEODYSTROPHY

Also known by its Latin name **osteitis fibrosa cystica** and **osteodystrophia fibrosa,** fibrous osteodystrophy is characterized by marked bone resorption, fibrous replacement, accelerated osteoid formation which does not become mineralized (osteomalacia) and the formation of cysts. It is the direct result of the continuous and excessive action of parathyroid hormone on bone. In man the disease has also been called *von Recklinghausen's* disease. The bones in general and especially the larger ones gradually soften and become flexible and deformed. At the same time they are easily fractured and are painful when bearing weight. Roentgenological examination shows widespread areas of rarefaction, sometimes with cystic spaces in them.

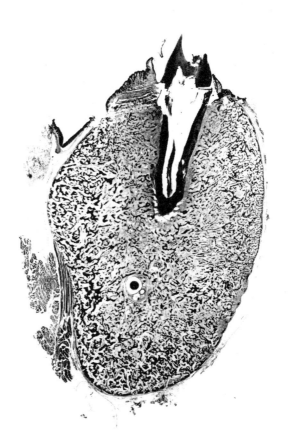

FIG. 20-7.—Fibrous osteodystrophy, wooly monkey. The cortex, lamina dura and medullary cavity of the mandible have been entirely replaced with trabecular bone in a loose fibrous stroma. (Courtesy New England Regional Primate Research Center, Harvard Medical School.)

Gross and microscopic examination of affected bones shows a marked disappearance of bone tissue which begins at the greatly enlarged Haversian canals and spreads outward from each one. The space formerly occupied by calcified bone is filled by fibrous connective tissue, with osteoclasts and osteoclastic giant cells lining receding bone in some places and the smaller osteoblasts attempting to replace the lost bone in others. The fibrous tissue may undergo cystic degeneration in places, probably because of insufficient blood supply. The bones, in addition to being deformed, may be so soft that they can be cut with a knife.

As indicated the **cause** of this startling disorder is hyperparathyroidism. The marked osteoclastic and osteolytic resorption of bone is a direct effect of parathyroid hormone. The stimulus for increased osteoblastic activity and fibrosis is less well understood though it would appear that it is a compensatory mechanism. Mechanical stress is believed to be of primary importance in initiating these attempts at healing. Parathyroid hormone itself may play a role in this stimulus but this hormone is also known to depress osteoblastic activity. Parathyroid hormone also inhibits the mineralization of osteoid even in the presence of hypercalcemia which is the usual finding in primary hyperparathyroidism. A separate function of parathyroid hormone is to increase renal loss of phosphate.

Hyperparathyroidism may be primary or secondary, but in either event the pathologic picture in bone is identical.

Primary hyperparathyroidism is usually the result of a functioning parathyroid adenoma which is rare in animals. Parathyroid adenomas have been reported in horses, cattle and dogs. In primary hyperparathyroidism there is hypercalcemia, hypophosphatemia (renal loss) and marked elevation of serum alkaline phosphatase. Metastatic calcification (p. 56) of soft tissues is a consistent finding.

Secondary hyperparathyroidism is without question the most common cause of fibrous osteodystrophy in animals. Hypocalcemia regardless of cause is the stimulus for the increased activity of the parathyroid glands. In animals secondary hyperparathyroidism occurs in nutritional deficiencies (nutritional secondary hyperparathyroidism) and in chronic renal disease.

Renal secondary hyperparathyroidism is most common in the dog in which the disorder has been termed **renal rickets** or **rubber-jaw**. Inability to excrete phosphates causes these ions to accumulate in the blood which causes a lowering of the serum calcium concentration when the serum becomes saturated with regard to calcium and phosphorus. Hyperparathyroidism in response to hypocalcemia induces resorption of bone but owing to primary renal disease the hormone does not increase urinary loss of phosphate, which continues to rise in the serum. Hyperphosphatemia is present throughout the course of the disease; serum alkaline phosphatase is also elevated. Serum calcium is usually low, but is partially compensated for by the continued release of calcium from bone. In the dog the bones of the head show pronounced softening, enlargement and roentgenologically detectable rarefaction, the jaws becoming "rubbery." Microscopically the lesions are those of fibrous osteodystrophy with osteoclastic and osteolytic resorption, fibrous replacement and active osteoblasts producing osteoid which fails to mineralize. All bones are affected to varying degrees but the lesions are most striking in the facial bones and the mandible. Metastatic calcification (p. 56) of soft tissues is a regular feature. The parathyroids are grossly enlarged. Tests for renal function are indicative of severe renal insufficiency. The role of the kidney in producing the active metabolite of vitamin D (p. 991) may be of importance to the pathogenesis of renal rickets but as yet has not been investigated.

Nutritional secondary hyperparathyroidism has been described in most domestic animals as well as many exotic species. The usual nutritional imbalances associated with the development of fibrous osteodystrophy are dietary deficiency of calcium and/or dietary excess of phosphorus, and vitamin D deficiency. As indicated under rickets (p. 1058) and osteomalacia (p. 1060), secondary parathyroid hyperplasia may develop causing these diseases to progress to fibrous osteodystrophy.

Fibrous osteodystrophy, described under the name **Bran disease,** has occurred when horses, owned by flour-millers, to whom bran was a cheap by-product, were fed almost exclusively on that substance. Changes in the head and facial outlines are commonly the first signs of the disease; it has therefore been described under the expressive designation of **big head.** The sharp features of the head, especially in the region of the zygomatic arch, and upper and lower jaws, become rounded and indefinite, giving the appearance of more swelling than really exists. Dissection shows a rather uniform thickening and rounding due to diffuse proliferation of imperfect bone in the subperiosteal region. The teeth may loosen and fall out. There is also lameness and a general tenderness of the joints. Microscopically, classical lesions of fibrous osteodystrophy are most obvious in facial bones and the mandible but the lesions are generalized throughout the skeleton. The disorder is the result of feeding diets low in calcium and high in phosphorus. Clinicopathologic findings may reveal hyperphosphatemia and hypocalcemia, but compensation may occur through the action of parathyroid hormone on bone and the kidneys. Serum alkaline phosphatase is elevated.

In young cats a diet consisting almost exclusively of beef hearts (low in calcium, high in phosphorus) has been found to cause fibrous osteodystrophy. The lesions in cats are often distinct from those seen in other species especially with respect to the amount of new bone (osteoid) formation by osteoblasts and fibrous replacement which has accounted for the disorder to be termed *osteogenesis imperfecta* and *juvenile osteoporosis.* To be certain there is often less bone, but the disorder in no way resembles osteogenesis imperfecta as seen in man which is a hereditary disease (it was once thought to be hereditary in cats). The disease is caused by a nutritional imbalance of calcium and phosphorus which results in hypocalcemia and secondary hyperparathyroidism. Unless compensated there is hypocalcemia, hyperphosphatemia and elevated serum alkaline phosphatase. The signs of the disease are nervousness and hyperirritability (hypocalcemia?), reluctance to move, abnormal stance and gait and spontaneous fractures. Microscopically in the usual case the lesions are characteristic of fibrous osteodystrophy, but rarely is there a significant production of new osteoid. Osteoblasts are present, however, and they do form osteoid but there is not the marked osteoid production leading to an increase in the overall dimensions of the bones except in rare examples. Krook (1963) refers to this expression of the disease as hypostotic type fibrous osteodystrophy in contrast to the hyperostotic type seen in horses (big head). Jowsey and co-workers (1964, 1968) have fed adult cats beef heart for thirteen months and described the resultant bone disease as osteoporosis without any evidence of fibrous osteodystrophy. They clearly showed that parathyroid activity was necessary for the development of the skeletal abnormality but suggested that the absence of fibrous osteodystrophy indicated that severe hyper-parathyroidism had not developed. These findings and similar results in mice (Ulmansky, 1965) suggest that the level of hyperparathyroidism and the age of the animal may influence the pattern of the disease, which emphasizes caution in interpreting pathogenesis of bone disease based on morphological features alone. Osteoporosis presumably of similar pathogenesis has also been described as a spontaneous disease in young cats and dogs on meat diets.

Fibrous osteodystrophy is a frequent disorder of the pet and laboratory monkey. The disease is almost exclusively encountered in New-World monkeys (*i.e.* those from Central and South America) and has been the recipient of numerous inappropriate and misleading terms such as goundou, Paget's disease, simian bone disease and cage paralysis. In monkeys the disease is characterized by facial deformity, reluctance to move, bending of long bones and multiple fractures leading to distortion of the limbs. Microscopically the lesions are classical of fibrous osteodystrophy with marked production of new bone causing gross enlargement of the skeleton, especially of the skull bones. The cause is not clear in each example but in most cases it is the result of vitamin D deficiency. Hunt, Garcia and Hegsted (1967, 1968) have clearly demonstrated that in New-World monkeys vitamin D_2 is relatively ineffective in promoting intestinal absorption of calcium and that these species require vitamin D_3 in their diet or access to ultraviolet radiation or sunshine. The substitution of vitamin D_3 for vitamin D_2 in commercial primate diets has greatly reduced the incidence of fibrous osteodystrophy in laboratory monkeys, but it still remains a frequent disorder of the pet monkey. No doubt lack of vitamin D is important to the development of the disease in the pet monkey, but the condition is also aggravated by unusual dietary programs which often contain foods high in phosphorus and low in calcium such as cereal grains (baby foods) and bananas.

Brown, Krook and Pond (1966) have proposed that atrophic rhinitis of swine (p. 1094) is an expression of generalized fibrous osteodystrophy. Atrophic rhinitis is discussed further on page 1094.

In addition to the specific examples cited, fibrous osteodystrophy of nutritional origin has been described in cattle, goats, dogs and birds and one of us (Hunt) has observed both nutritional and renal osteodystrophy in rats and hamsters.

As a rule, in all species with nutritional or renal fibrous osteodystrophy the parathyroid glands are grossly enlarged. Microscopically the enlargement is the result of an increase in size and number of light chief cells. Many chief cells become vacuolated and the number of water clear cells increases.

We have stated several times in this chapter that rickets and osteomalacia may progress to fibrous osteodystrophy if severe hyperparathyroidism develops in the course of the disease. There is little difficulty in understanding this progression, but what often appears as a dilemma is the presence of fibrous osteodystrophy in a young animal in the absence of rickets which in some species is a frequent finding. Apparently rickets only develops if the ion product of calcium and phosphorus is low and in many cases of fibrous osteodystrophy the ion product is maintained at a normal level due to the action of parathyroid hormone or is actually elevated due to hyperphosphatemia. Calcification of cartilage (which fails in rickets) is directly dependent on calcium availability; rachitic cartilage will calcify *in vitro*. Calcification of osteoid, however, requires maturation under control of osteoblasts and is not directly related to calcium availability; osteoid from animals

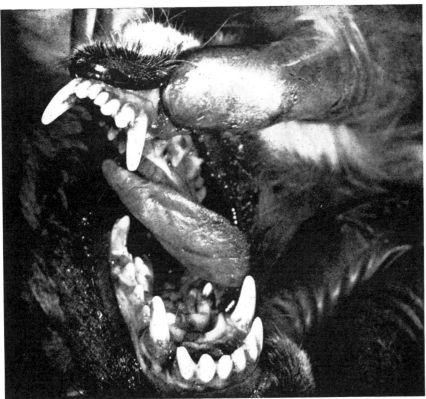

FIG. 20–8.—The flexible "rubber jaws" of a five and one-half-year-old male terrier with chronic interstitial nephritis. Normal jaws cannot be distorted in this manner. (Courtesy of Angell Memorial Animal Hospital.)

with osteomalacia or fibrous osteodystrophy does not calcify *in vitro*. However, it seems likely that other physiological factors and possibly other dietary deficiencies or excesses which may be present in certain diets (such as a 100 per cent beef heart diet) influence the course of both rickets and fibrous osteodystrophy in young animals.

OSTEOPOROSIS

Osteoporosis, properly speaking, is an atrophic disorder in which the bones are less resistant to cutting and sawing but at the same time brittle and porous. The porosity is due to widening of the Haversian canals, possibly in connection with an increased blood supply, and the fragility is augmented by a diminution in the thickness of the bony trabeculae and the whole zona compacta. There is no failure of, or deficiency in, calcification in what remains of the trabeculae and no increase of osteoid, as there is in osteomalacia. Normally throughout life there is continual rearrangement of the trabeculae, osteoblasts forming new bone, osteoclasts dissolving it (apparently through the action of an enzyme, acid phosphatase). In osteoporosis, the destructive phase of this process exceeds production. The levels of serum calcium and serum phosphorus are usually normal.

Causes are not fully understood. The disorder occurs in senility, disuse atrophy, as when surgical fixation of a limb is necessitated in the treatment of some injury of bone or joint, in a variety of obscure hormonal imbalances involving the adrenals, thyroid or pituitary, and in some other conditions. Causative mechanisms are thought to include absence of the stimulation coming from the stresses and strains of movement, malnutrition, especially with respect to proteins, and possibly deficiency of estrogen (human post-menopausal), excessive adrenal cortical hormone, hyperpituitarism, and hyperthyroidism (p. 1358). Vitamin C deficiency (p. 990) and copper deficiency (p. 1011) also result in osteoporosis. Considerable attention is presently being directed toward calcium deficiency as a cause of osteoporosis. We have already indicated the role of calcium deficiency in rickets, osteomalacia and fibrous osteodystrophy. The role of calcium deficiency in osteoporosis is yet to be defined but osteoporosis has been produced experimentally in cats (Jowsey, 1968) and mice (Ulmansky, 1965) by feeding meat diets which are low in calcium. Also, osteoporosis is seen spontaneously in cats subsisting on such a diet, however as previously indicated, in many cats rather than leading to osteoporosis, meat diets lead to fibrous osteodystrophy.

Osteoporosis, as here defined, is rare but not unknown in animals. The cases that have been designated by that name have usually proved to depend on inadequate calcium deposition and, hence, come under the heading of osteomalacia. In contrast to diseases characterized by malacia (*i.e.*, rickets, osteomalacia and fibrous osteodystrophy) in most examples of osteoporosis there is no obvious increase in resorption, no increase in osteoblastic activity, no fibrous replacement and no excess of osteoid. To the contrary the bone appears quiescent.

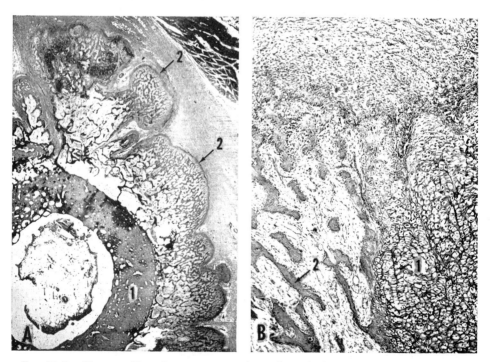

FIG. 20–9.—Hypertrophic pulmonary osteoarthropathy. *A*, Cross section of tibia of a dog (× 3¾). Note cortex of bone (*1*) and bulbous new bone (*2*) on its exterior surface. *B*, Higher magnification (× 40). Note cartilaginous (1) and osseous (2) components. (Courtesy of Armed Forces Institute of Pathology.) Contributor: Dr. H. R. Seibold.

PULMONARY OSTEOARTHROPATHY

Also known as Marie's disease for its discoverer (in man, 1890), this rather rare disease occurs in the dog and in man, and has been reported in sheep, deer, horse and lion. Often preceded a few months earlier by a cough, dyspnea or other

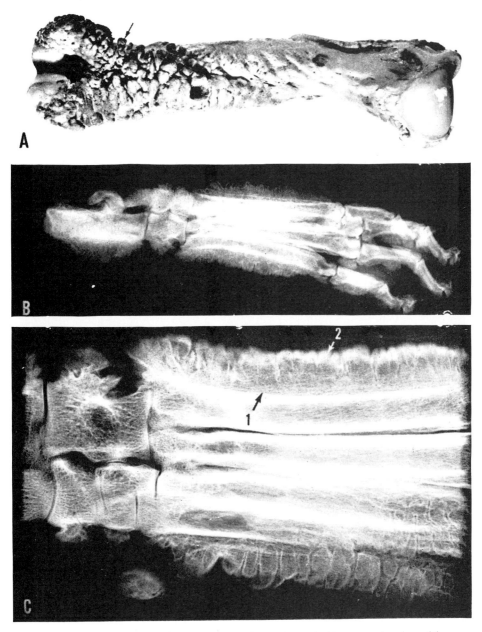

FIG. 20–10.—Hypertrophic pulmonary osteoarthropathy. *A*, Humerus of a dog with severe exostosis. Note knob-like projections of bone from the cortex. Contributor: Dr. H. R. Seibold. *B*, Roentgenograph of the forelimb of a dog. Note severe exostosis on external surfaces of metacarpal bones, phalanges and carpus. *C*, Roentgenograph of the specimen collected at necropsy from *B*. The cortex of the bone is sharply demarcated at (*1*) and the new bone growth (*2*) is all external to the cortex. (*A* and *C*, Courtesy of Armed Forces Institute of Pathology.) Contributor: Dr. H. R. Seibold.

pulmonary disturbances, the characteristic lesions are chronic proliferation of new bone producing marked thickening and deformity of the limbs. The new bone is formed just beneath the periosteum, which is pushed outward, but the osteophytic growths are very irregular so that the bone is made very rough. The bones usually affected are those of all four limbs from the femoro-tibial and shoulder joints to the phalanges. The joint surfaces are not involved, although there is much periarticular proliferation and enlargement. Occasionally a bone may attain twice its normal diameter. There is considerable pain on movement and ultimately on palpation. Terminal effects of the osseous and pulmonary lesions together are fatal.

There are ordinarily important and extensive lesions in the lungs, most often either a bronchogenic carcinoma or other primary neoplasm. In some countries, advanced pulmonary tuberculosis is frequently present; chronic bronchiectatic, purulent processes are occasionally found. The writer (Smith) has seen one case occasioned (presumably) by a large esophageal sarcoma which compressed and incapacitated a considerable portion of one lung. In humans, chronic heart diseases and insufficiencies have been concomitant with osteoarthropathy. In one canine case, there were several heartworms (*Dirofilaria immitis*) impeding the circulation. In a few human cases, there have been lesions outside the thorax which apparently obstructed circulation to the limbs.

In view of the above circumstance, the **cause** has been postulated as a long-standing anoxia although some have suspected the presence of an obscure toxemia. Accordingly an experimental anastomosis shunting a part of the blood past the lungs is stated to have produced the osteoarthropathy. It has also been theorized that increased pulmonary circulation without a corresponding demand for blood in the systemic circulation has resulted in excessive flow of blood in the extremities and consequent proliferation. Very recently it has been demonstrated that severing the vagus nerve has quickly cured the disorder, the fundamental mechanism being under study. Vagotomy results in a prompt fall in blood flow in the limbs which supports the hypothesis that increased peripheral blood flow is responsible for the bony growths. Presumably the intrathoracic lesions induce a neural reflex involving the vagus and resulting in abnormal peripheral blood flow. There is agreement that the bony growth is in no way neoplastic, neither do metastatic neoplasms in the lungs appear to be associated invariably with pulmonary osteoarthropathy.

OSTEOPETROSIS

In humans, a frequently used synonym for osteopetrosis is marble-bone disease. In this rare disease, those bones which are of endochondral origin are enlarged to the point of deformity, heavy and dense with calcium but surprisingly brittle. Not only are their outside dimensions increased but the marrow cavity is reduced or all but obliterated. Microscopically, it is seen that the cartilage does not disappear, as it must do in normal bone development, but persists, is calcified and is surrounded by osteoid which becomes heavily calcified. Owing to the virtual absence of marrow space, there is severe myelophthisic anemia (p. 129) with extra-medullary hematopoiesis.

In addition to its rare occurrence in humans, in whom it is considered hereditary, it has been reported in rabbits, mice and rats in which it is also hereditary and a single report by Thomson (1966) describes a similar disease in an Aberdeen Angus calf. The condition is of principal interest in veterinary medicine as it occurs in chickens. On the basis of transmission experiments, as well as the concomitant presence of typical lesions in the soft tissues, it is considered to be one form of leukosis. Another form of osteopetrosis is a feature of fluorosis (p. 928).

EXOSTOSES

Whenever injured, bone, like other connective tissues, may react with a chronic proliferative inflammation. This results in a bony growth, in reality a granulation tissue composed of bone instead of the usual fibrous tissue which is seen in other locations. Such proliferations are usually rather strictly localized and are called exostoses, or osteophytes. The horse is especially subject to exostoses on the limbs, just as he is to excessive fibrous granulation tissue arising in the soft tissues. An exostosis or group of exostoses arising on the second or, less commonly, on the first phalanx is a ringbone. It causes serious and painful periarthritis. Small exostoses at the ends of the second and fourth metacarpal (rarely metatarsal) bones are called splints. Because of their less sensitive surroundings, they usually do not cause lameness. Exostoses frequently form on the medial portions of the distal bones of the tarsus. Such a lesion is called a (bone) spavin. It is a serious and stubborn cause of lameness even though small.

Microscopically, an exostosis is seen to consist of compact bone of the usual appearance except there is no arrangement into Haversian systems. The outer limit of the original normal bone is usually visible as a slender line; the new bone appears as an added layer. In some cases, the extreme tip of an exostosis is formed of hyaline cartilage. Adjacent soft tissues may show inflammatory changes. The mature and orderly microscopic structure of an exostosis serves to distinguish it from a bony neoplasm.

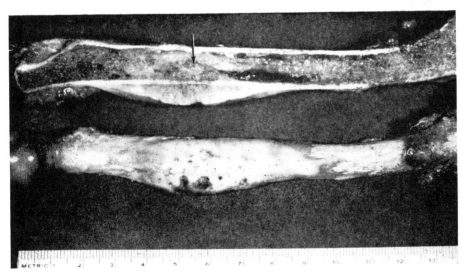

Fig. 20–11.—Secondary, metastatic tumor in femur of a twelve-year-old spayed female Kerry Blue Terrier. The primary was a bronchiolar-alveolar cell carcinoma of the lung. (Courtesy of Angell Memorial Animal Hospital.)

The **cause** of an isolated exostosis is usually a single local trauma. The exostoses on the horse's legs are causally related to the continued strains and stresses of the horse's strenuous physical exertions. Some equine families are considered to be more susceptible to these disorders than others, but to a considerable extent, at least, this situation is based upon mechanically disadvantageous con-

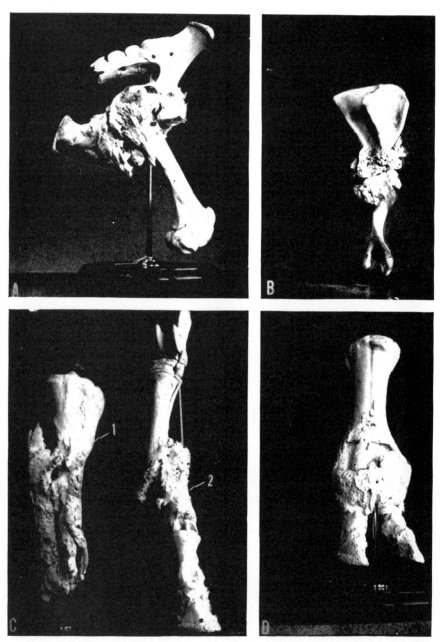

Fig. 20–12.—*A*, Periarthritis and long-standing luxation of the coxofemoral joint of a cow. *B*, Exostosis following arthritis of the scapulo-humeral joint in a pig. *C*, Attempted healing of two unreduced fractures in the tibia (*1*) and metatarsus (*2*) of two different horses. *D*, Exostosis involving the metacarpophalangeal joint in a cow. Mark Francis Collection. Texas School **Veterinary** Medicine.

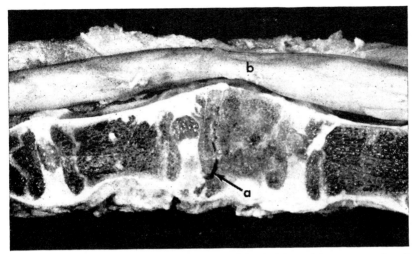

Fig. 20–13.—Fracture of a vertebra through the epiphysis (*a*) resulting compression of spinal cord (*b*). A nine-month-old female German Shepherd which had been hit by a car. (Photograph courtesy of Angell Memorial Animal Hospital.)

dimensions and restoration of the marrow cavity. Until the latter is accomplished the bone formed in this or other healing processes, which are essentially reactions to injury and, therefore akin to proliferative inflammation (p. 165), has the structure of cancellous (spongy) bone, the bony trabeculae being numerous but very irregular, the marrow initially fibrous. In the external layers of the bony callus this cancellous bone is seen attached to the outside of the layer of compact bone which formed the original shaft. In those rather frequent cases where the healing segments are not fixed in absolute rigidity during the healing process a cartilaginous union often precedes the formation of bone. The more lateral ends of the line of union, where a tilting movement would be most pronounced, may thus show areas of hyaline cartilage in contrast to the proliferating bone which constitutes normal healing.

EPIPHYSEAL NECROSIS

Epiphyseal necrosis, most often of the head of the femur or humerus, is occasionally encountered in domestic animals and laboratory rats and mice. It regularly follows fracture of the femoral neck which interferes with the vascular supply to the epiphysis, but it is also encountered without a clearly defined pathogenesis; although vascular interference is most likely the underlying cause in all examples.

Aseptic necrosis of the femoral head of the latter type is most frequent in dogs where, like its human counterpart, it has often gone by the eponym *Legg-Perthes* disease and *Calvé-Perthes* disease. Osteochondritis of the hip, juvenile osteochondrosis of the hip and coxa-plana have also been applied to this condition, which as indicated is not associated with fractures or obvious interference with the vascular supply to the femoral head. The disease is restricted to miniature breeds such as the miniature pinscher, Lakeland Terrier, toy and miniature poodle, fox terrier, pug and griffin. The disease has been reviewed in detail by Ljunggren (1967) who examined 238 spontaneous cases. His observations revealed that the disease develops in adolescent dogs with initial symptoms of lameness appearing between four and eleven months of age. The affected leg is painful, especially upon abduction and there may be crepitation of the hip joint, shortening of the affected leg and muscle atrophy. In radiographs the earliest changes are a widening of the joint space and the presence of single or multiple foci of decreased density of the femoral head which, as the disease progresses, become more numerous and larger giving a "moth-eaten" appearance to the head of the femur. The head of the femur eventually develops an irregular contour and fragments. Gross lesions, which are best observed after midsagittal sectioning, vary from subtle changes in shape of femoral head to fragmentation; the articular cartilage is often brownish and roughened. Ljunggren (1966) described the microscopic changes as commencing with excessive production of endosteal bone followed by osteonecrosis and necrosis of marrow. Subsequent to necrosis, there is obviously fibroplasia, osteoclasis and additional new bone formation. Ljunggren theorized that the development of *Legg-Perthes* disease was related to premature closure of cartilaginous growth plates and that miniature breeds were predisposed to the disease due to earlier sexual maturity.

INFECTIOUS DISEASES OF BONE

The infections which occasionally localize in bone include brucellosis, tuberculosis, actinomycosis and coccidioidomycosis. Brucellosis ordinarily forms an intra-osseous abscess, or sometimes a focus of caseation necrosis encapsulated by fibrous tissue with a mixture of leukocytes including many eosinophils. In swine and calves, a fairly frequent location is within one or two adjoining vertebrae, the condition being called **spondylitis.** Each of the other three diseases produces its typical granulomatous lesion, which is able to grow and proliferate by destroying the bony tissue around it. The bone tissue reacts with a reparative proliferation at the same time that adjoining areas are being dissolved. The result is a pronounced local enlargement which proves to be very much honeycombed when the soft tissues are removed by maceration. This type of lesion is especially conspicuous in actinomycosis as it involves the jaw bones of cattle. In the case of tuberculosis, the bone lesion is usually part of a generalized process; in the few reported cases of coccidioidomycosis, the same may be true; in actinomycosis and brucellosis, the bone lesion is usually the only manifestation. The marrow may or may not be invaded in any of these conditions.

Echinococcosis.—Very rarely the "hydatid cysts" representing the cystic stage of the canine tapeworm, *Echinococcus granulosus*, are found in bone, at least in man. Presumably the same is possible in the farm animals which can serve as intermediate hosts to this parasite.

Neoplasms.—The primary tumors of bone are the fibroma, fibrosarcoma and the osteogenic sarcoma. The adamantinoma and epulis form in or upon bone. All are discussed in the section on Neoplasms (pp. 201 and 239).

Diseases of the bone marrow are considered with the Hemic and Lymphatic System.

PROTRUSION OF INTERVERTEBRAL DISCS

Except in the aged, where they become fibrocartilaginous, the intervertebral discs consist of a central semi-solid mucoid connective tissue, the nucleus pulposus, enclosed in a thick fibrous zone, the annulus fibrosus. In response to sudden strains and, it is thought, following a certain degree of degeneration

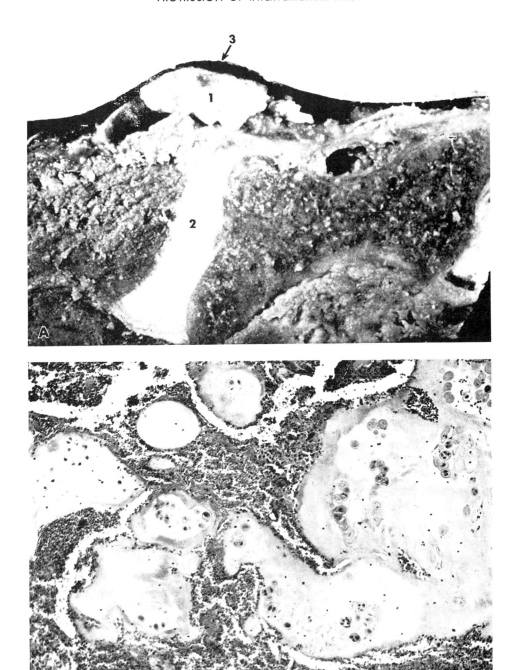

FIG. 20–14.—*A*, Protrusion of intervertebral disc in a five-year-old male dachshund. The protruded material (*1*) from cervical disc 5–6 (*2*) has compressed the spinal cord at (*3*). The vertebral column and spinal cord were fixed in formalin, then cut sagittally. *B*, Chondroid material, hemorrhage, and debris from the nucleus pulposus which has undergone "chondroid" degeneration and has been expelled into the vertebral canal through a diseased annulus fibrosus. H & E × 150. (Courtesy of Angell Memorial Animal Hospital.)

which is possibly of hereditary origin, the annulus fibrosus may be partially ruptured so that a bulging mass protrudes into the spinal canal. The lumbar or last thoracic discs are most likely to suffer this accident, although the cervical discs are not immune. In many instances no symptoms are produced, but in other cases severe and rather sudden pain and reflex immobility result from pressure upon nervous elements. In humans, there is ordinarily impingement upon one of the spinal nerves as it passes through the intervertebral foramen, and the symptoms are severe pain referred to the area of distribution of the nerve involved. Since this is usually one of those making up the sciatic nerve, the condition is often called sciatica. In the dog, the spinal canal is less spacious and the protruding mass usually presses directly upon the spinal cord. Symptoms then are those of partial or complete paralysis of the innervated regions, often the whole of the hind quarters. In severe cases, there may be local hemorrhage and necrosis of the area under pressure, with eventual wallerian degeneration of fibers coming from the destroyed nerve cells. Fortunately many cases, even of complete posterior paralysis, are not quite so severe and, with adequate nursing, slowly recover as the protruding nucleus pulposus is resorbed. Although the protrusions usually occur dorsally, ventral protrusion of degenerated discs is also encountered, but obviously protrusion in this direction is of less importance. With healing the ventral protrusion causes the development of osteophytes which may progress to ankylosing spondylitis (spondylosis deformans) (p. 1081).

The pathologist needs to realize that a very careful examination of the floor of the spinal canal is necessary to establish with certainty the presence or absence of this lesion. It is claimed that some ruptures merely cause bulging of the dorsal longitudinal ligament, which overlies them, and this subsides during the manipulations of the autopsy. On the other hand, roentgenologists frequently demonstrate a mild calcification of a degenerated disc even when no protrusion or any acute symptoms are attributable to it.

As far as known this condition is rare in domestic animals other than the dog and is less frequent in the cat. As indicated in the dog, protrusion of intervertebral discs is preceded by degenerative changes in the annulus fibrosus and nucleus pulposus. Two morphologically distinct degenerative processes are apparent in dogs. One in dogs of chondrodystrophoid breeds (dachshunds, Pekinese, French Bulldogs) develops at an early age and the other occurs in aged dogs of all breeds. In the former type, the changes are characterized by chondroid metaplasia of the nucleus pulposus followed by calcification. Granular amorphous material accumulates between the fibers of the annulus fibrosus which leads to disruptions of its normal lamellated structure. The lamellae themselves undergo hyalin degeneration and fragmentation. In nonchondrodystrophoid breeds the changes in the annulus fibrosus are similar to those seen in chondrodystrophoid breeds, however in the nucleus pulposus the degenerative change is characterized by a collagenization, described as fibroid degeneration, rather than chondroid metaplasia and calcification is rare.

In cats the condition is analogous to that seen in nonchondrodystrophoid dogs.

ARTHRITIS AND PERIARTHRITIS

Acute inflammation of a joint is commonly serous, fibrinous or purulent. The serous form is equivalent to an excessive formation of synovia, which distends the joint capsule and forms a "puffy" swelling. The articular and synovial surfaces show nothing more than a slight hyperemic redness. This type of arthritis is usually due to mild, and often to repeated trauma; when infection is present the intracapsular exudate is fibrinous or, in the presence of pyogenic organisms, purulent. In such cases, the articular surfaces are likely to be eroded and there is extreme pain. The surrounding tissues are edematous.

In chronic arthritis, which is also known as osteoarthritis and degenerative joint disease, there tends to be proliferation of the mesothelium and soft tissues lining the non-articular surfaces of the joint capsule. The proliferated tissue takes very irregular forms, often projecting into the joint cavity as bizarre but smooth, mesothelial-covered "synovial fringes." Such a projecting "tag" may be caught between the articulating surfaces and produce sudden severe pain, which slowly subsides after the projecting tissue escapes from the compression. Not too infrequently some of the more pedunculated projections may be broken off, or may become detached because of atrophy of the narrow neck. These bits of tissue remain alive by absorption of nutrients from the joint fluid and are slowly kneaded into rounded or elliptical bodies of tissue, to which are given such names as **corpora libra,** free bodies, melon-seed bodies or joint-mice. Being subject to impingement between the articulating surfaces they also may at any moment be responsible for sharp pain by placing undue pressure upon an area of joint surface. Rarely such free bodies may be formed of compressed, unorganized fibrin or of fragments of cartilage.

If the inflammatory process has destroyed much of the smooth articular surface of a joint (eburnation), fibrous and osseous adhesions between the apposed surfaces tend to form and marginal osteophytes (exostoses) develop. After some time, for instance several months, the two bones will be completely joined together by a union of solid bone. This process of bony fusion is called **ankylosis** and the obliterated joint is said to be ankylosed. It is interesting to note that after a few years (in the human) two ankylosed bones are united as a single bone, the marrow cavity passing completely through what was formerly the epiphyses and the joint cavity.

Chronic proliferative or ankylosing arthritis, like the mild serous type, is usually due to trauma, often to repeated strains and the concussion of severe work on hard surfaces in the case of horses. Chronic arthritis may also follow infectious processes such as swine erysipelas and may develop from an acute arthritis. However, chronic arthritis is more frequently seen without an association with trauma or infection, in which case it has been termed primary chronic arthritis or primary osteoarthritis. The cause is not usually known, but structural defects, congenital or acquired, predispose to osteoarthritis. For example, osteoarthritis is a feature of hip dysplasia in dogs (p. 1083), "wobbles" in horses (p. 1397), necrosis of the femoral head in dogs (p. 1075), and canine elbow dysplasia. The latter disorder, which is believed to be of hereditary origin, is most frequent in German Shepherd dogs and is associated with an ununited anconeal process.

Acute suppurative or acute fibrinous arthritides (which may progress to chronic arthritis) may be due to wounds which open the joint cavity to infective microorganisms, but they are more frequent as articular localizations of generalized septicemic or pyemic infections. The most common of these is the pyosepticemia of the new-born (pyosepticemia neonatorum, "joint-ill") resulting from infection of the umbilicus at birth. A variety of microorganisms may be

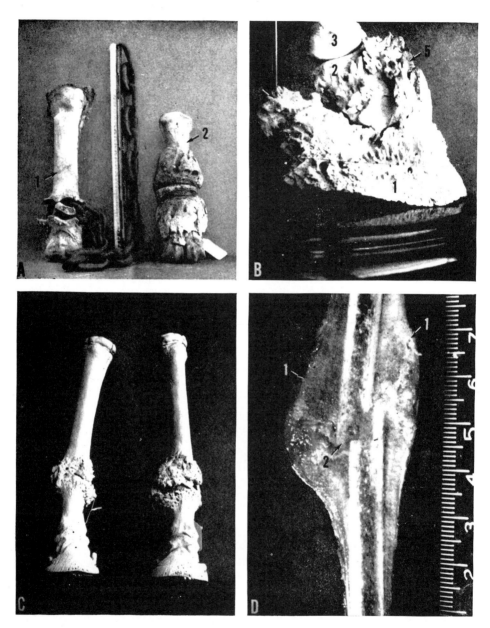

FIG. 20–15.—A, Chronic proliferative osteitis resulting from forgotten hobbles used in pioneer days. A chain around an equine (1) and two wires around a bovine metatarsus (2). B, Ossification of lateral cartilage (sidebone) and low ringbone in a horse. Third phalanx (1), second phalanx (2), first phalanx (3), ossified lateral cartilage (4) and exostosis of second phalanx (5). C, Exostosis around fetlock joint (high ringbone) in both legs of a saddle horse. A, B and C from: Mark Francis Collection, Texas School Veterinary Medicine. D, Fracture of rib of a year-old Guernsey calf. Note bony callus (1) surrounding the fracture (2). (Courtesy of College of Veterinary Medicine, Iowa State University.)

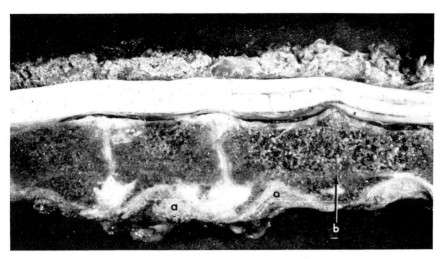

FIG. 20–16.—Ankylosing spondylitis (a) fusing lumbar vertebrae of a fifteen-year-old crossbreed terrier. Note loss of intervertebral disc (b). (Courtesy of Angell Memorial Animal Hospital.)

associated with infectious arthritis in both new-born and adult animals. In foals *Shigella equirulus* (p. 606) is the most common organism recovered but other organisms such as *Streptococcus spp.*, *Salmonella spp.* and *Escherichia coli* are also recovered with frequency. *Erysipelas rhusiopathiae* (p. 585) is notable for causing a chronic low grade arthritis and periarthritis in swine, lambs and turkeys. *Corynebacterium ovis*, *Escherichia coli* and *Streptococcus spp.* are also frequent causes of arthritis in sheep. *Mycoplasma spp.* are important causes of arthritis in swine (p. 532), sheep (p. 531), goats (p. 531), and cattle (p. 526). A member of the psittacosis-lymphogranuloma group of agents is a cause of arthritis in sheep (p. 552). *Hemophilus suis* (p. 589) produces polyserositis with arthritis in swine. *Brucella spp.* and *Streptococcus spp.* also not infrequently cause a suppurative arthritis in swine. Tuberculous arthritis which may develop in any species and which often localizes in the vertebral column is characterized by the usual granulomatous reaction, which in a joint is of very limited extent. In rats mycoplasma, *Streptobacillis moniliformis*, *Diplococcus pneumoniae* and *Corynebacterium kutscheri* are frequent causes of arthritis. It should be clear from this list that arthritis is an important manifestation of many infectious diseases, but noticeably absent are generalized infections of dogs and cats. Aside from occasional joint involvement in infections such as cryptococcosis, there is little information about infectious joint disease in these species. Most examples of infectious arthritis in dogs and cats are the result of penetrating wounds in which case the ordinary pyogenic bacteria are responsible.

Ankylosing spondylitis also known as spondylosis deformans is most frequent in dogs, cats, cattle and swine and relatively rare in other domestic animals. It results from the formation and ultimate fusion of osteophytes (exostoses) on the ventral aspect of adjacent vertebral bodies. In dogs and possibly other species ventral prolapse of intervertebral discs is believed to be the cause. Infectious spondylitis can also lead to ankylosis of vertebrae. It has been described as an occupational hazard of stud bulls but the cause has not been established.

Hemophilic arthropathy is not common owing to the fact that most animals

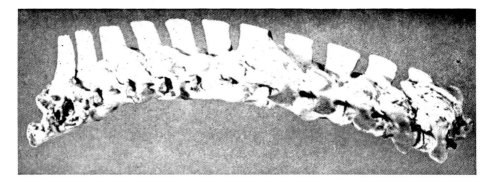

A

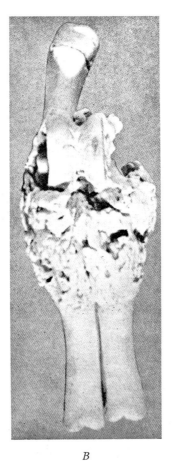

B

FIG. 20–17.—*A*, Thoracic and lumbar spondylitis in a swine which, at the age of three months, was inoculated with a pure culture of *Erysipelothrix rhusiopathiae*. Most of the joints developed a proliferative and ankylosing inflammation which was continuously progressive until euthanasia at three years of age. (Courtesy of Dr. Dennis Sikes, Georgia Sch. Vet. Med.)

B, Tarso-metatarsal arthritis in a pig inoculated with *Erysipelothrix rhusiopathiae* at three months of age; euthanasia at three years of age. Same animal as *A*. (Courtesy of Dr. Dennis Sikes.)

with hemophilia (p. 1175) die at an early age. However, hemophilic joint disease has been reported in dogs, and the lesions include hemarthrosis and hemosiderosis, fibrosis and proliferation of synovial tissues. In advanced cases degeneration of articular cartilage and osteoarthritis are present.

"Rheumatism" is occasionally diagnosed in old dogs and old cows, its exact manifestations being variable and obscure. The problem of **rheumatoid arthritis** certainly does not exist in veterinary medicine as it does in the human family.

Navicular disease is a bursitis and terminal arthritis involving the equine distal sesamoid, or navicular bone, usually in a foreleg. The earlier changes are hyperemia and inflammation of the lining surfaces of the bursa podotrochlearis; these are soon followed by erosion and ulceration of the cartilage which serves as a bearing surface for the deep flexor tendon; the latter becomes frayed and will eventually rupture. The bone itself becomes rarefied and inflamed and has been known to disintegrate.

DYSPLASIA OF THE ACETABULUM IN DOGS

Under the name of "hip dysplasia" a disorder has been described in growing dogs most notably German Shepherds which usually first manifests itself as an unexplained luxation of the coxo-femoral articulation. At autopsy it is found that the acetabular cavity is extremely and abnormally shallow, its lips being flattened and atrophic. It has been logically assumed that the luxation resulted because of the shallowness of the cavity so that the head of the femur was inadequately supported. There is evidence that this dysplasia (the shallowness) is

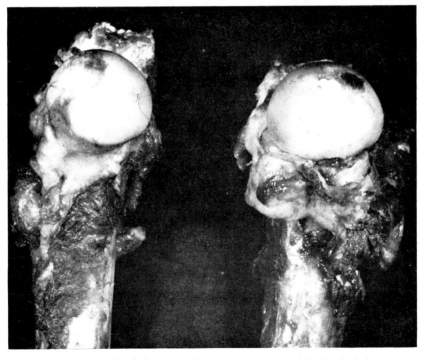

Fig. 20–18.—Osteoarthritis of the femoral heads subsequent to hip dysplasia in a ten-year-old male German Shepherd. The femoral heads are flattened and the articular surfaces eroded. (Courtesy of Angell Memorial Animal Hospital.)

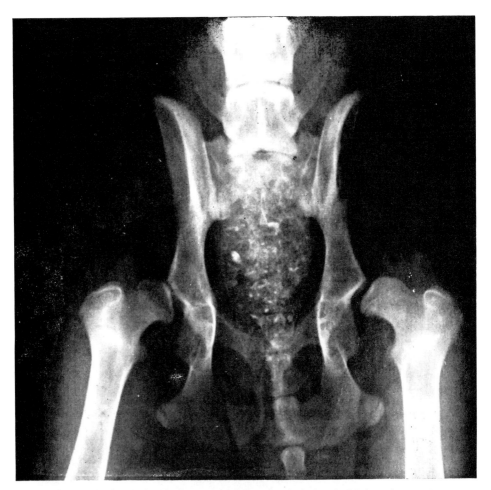

FIG. 20–19.—Hip dysplasia. Radiograph of severe dysplasia (grade IV) in a six-month-old male German Shepherd. Note that the acetabula are shallow, the femoral heads are not within the acetabulum on either side. The articular surface of the femoral head on the right is flattened. (Radiograph courtesy of Dr. G. B. Schnelle, Angell Memorial Animal Hospital.)

inherited. On the other hand, most of the necropsies have been performed after the dislocation has been in existence for some weeks and it has been shown experimentally that dislocation, uncorrected for as little as four weeks, can, in growing pups, produce dysplasia even to the extent that the acetabular cavity is amost obliterated (disuse atrophy). It has been noted that in the dogs subject to the dysplasia the several muscles concerned with pressing the head of the femur into the cavity and holding it there are much smaller, lighter in weight, and therefore weaker, than in normal dogs. This again leads to a concept of disuse atrophy as far as the bony tissues are concerned. May it be that it is the degree of development of these muscles that is the inherited characteristic?

Rupture of the Round Ligament of the Hip Joint.—This disorder has been reported by Rainey (1958) in Australia as occurring with some frequency in cattle in an area of copper and cobalt deficiency in the soil and herbage.

Imperfections of the Fibula.—The fibula of the horse often shows very rudimentary development. It has two centers of ossification but quite commonly bony union of the two never occurs. This leaves an irregular line between the two which has been mistaken roentgenographically for a fracture. Such imperfections are not unusual and do not cause interference with function.

SELECTED REFERENCES

Muscular Diseases

ADAMS, O. R.: Fibrotic Myopathy and Ossifying Myopathy in the Hindlegs of Horses. J. Am. Vet. Med. Assn. *139*:1089–1092, 1961.

ANDERSON, P.: Nutritional Muscular Dystrophy in Cattle, with Special Reference to the Functional State of the Thyroid. Acta Path. et Microbiol. Scand. Supp. *134, 48*:7–91, 1960.

ASHMORE, C. R., and ROBINSON, D. W.: Hereditary Muscular Hypertrophy in the Bovine. I. Histological and Biochemical Characterization. Proc. Sec. Exp. Biol. Med. *132*:548–554, 1969.

AZZONE, G. F. and ALOISI, M.: Changes Induced by E-Avitaminosis on the Proteins of Rabbit Muscle Extracts. Biochem. J. *69*:161–170, 1958.

BLAXTER, K. L.: Muscular Dystrophy in Farm Animals: Its Cause and Prevention. Proc. Nutr. Soc. *21*:211–216, 1962.

BLAXTER, K. L. and SHARMAN, G. A. M.: Prevention and Cure of Enzoötic Muscular Dystrophy in Beef Cattle. Nature, London *172*:1006–1007, 1953.

BLAXTER, K. L., WATTS, P. S., WOOD, W. A., and MACDONALD, A. M.: Histopathology of Muscular Dystrophy and Its Relation to Muscle Chemistry. Brit. J. Nutrition *6*:164–169, 1952.

BLAXTER, K. L., and MCGILL, R. F.: Muscular Dystrophy. Vet. Rev. & Annotations. *1* Pt. 2:91–114, 1955.

BLINCO, C. and MARBLE, D. W.: Blood Enzyme Relationships in White Muscle Disease. Am. J. Vet. Res. *21*:866–869, 1960.

BURTON, V. *et al.*: Nutritional Muscular Dystrophy in Lambs—Selenium Analysis of Maternal, Fetal and Juvenile Tissues. Am. J. Vet. Res. *23*:962–965, 1962.

BYWATERS, E. G. L. and DIBLE, J. H.: Acute Paralytic Myohaemoglobinuria in Man. J. Path. and Bact. *55*:7–15, 1943.

CAPOCASA, O.: Mallattie neonatali de carenza da Vitamina "C" ed "E." Atti. Soc. ital. sci. vet. Cortina d'Ampezzo *7*:874–877, 1953.

CHEVILLE, N. F.: The Pathology of Vitamin E Deficiency in the Chick. Path. Vet. *3*:208–225, 1966.

COTCHIN, E.: Muscular Dystrophy in Lambs ("Stiff-Lamb Disease") in a Flock in Berkshire. Vet. J. *104*:102–108, 1948.

DAM, H., PRANGE, I., and SØNDERGAARD, E.: Muscular Degeneration (White Striation of Muscles) in Chicks Reared on Vitamin-E Deficient, Low-fat Diets. Acta path. et microbiol. Scandinav. *31*:172–184, 1953.

DOBSON, K. J.: Congenital Splayleg of Piglets. Aust. Vet. J. *44*:26–28, 1968.

DODD, D. C. *et al.*: Muscle Degeneration and Yellow Fat Disease in Foals. N. Z. Vet. J. *8*:45–50, 1960.

DOLLAHITE, J. W., and HENSON, J. B.: Toxic Plants as the Etiologic Agents of Myopathies in Animals. Am. J. Vet. Res. *26*:749–752, 1965.

EKMAN, L., ORSTADIUS, K., and ABERG, B.: Distribution of Se[75]-tagged Sodium Selenite in Pigs with Nutritional Muscular Dystrophy. Acta Vet. Scand. *4*:92–96, 1963.

GARDINER, M. R.: White Muscle Disease (Nutritional Muscular Dystrophy) of Sheep in Western Australia. Austr. Vet. J. *38*:387–391, 1962.

GOTO, M.: Studies on the Waxy Degeneration of Muscles in Domestic Animals. II. On the Changes of the Myocardium and Skeletal Muscles in Tetanus. Jap. J. Vet. Sci. *12*:231–237, 1950. English summary. Abstr. Vet. Bull. No. 1271, 1952.

GZHITSKI, S. Z.: Pathogenesis and Treatment of Equine Myohaemoglobinaemia. (Translated Title) Veterinariya, Moscow *30*:40–43, 1953. Abstr. Vet. Bull. No. 1119, 1955.

HADLOW, W. J.: Myopathies of Livestock. Lab. Investig. *8*:1478–1498, 1959.

HAMILTON, J. M., and MCCANCE, C. McB.: Eosinophilic Myositis in Cattle. Vet. Rec. *83*:471–472, 1968.

HARTLEY, W. J.: White Muscle Disease and Muscular Dystrophy. Aust. Vet. J. *39*:338–339, 1963.

HAWK, P. B., OSER, B. L., and SUMMERSON, W. H.: *Practical Physiological Chemistry.* 13th ed., 1954. New York. Blakiston Division, McGraw-Hill Book Co., Inc.

HICKEY, F.: Muscular Dystrophy in Calves and Lambs (White Muscle Disease). Review of Causative Theories and Treatment. N. Z. Agriculturist *11*(No. 1):3–5, 1958.

HJÄRRE, A. and LILLEENGEN, K.: Wachsartige Muskeldegeneration im Anschluss an C-Avitaminose bei Kalbern. Ein Beitrag zur Aetiologie und Pathogenese des sog. "Welssen Fleisches" beim Kalbe. Virchow's Archiv. f. path. Anat. *297*:565–593, 1936.

HOGUE, D. E.: Selenium and Muscular Dystrophy. J. Am. Vet. Med. Assn. *133*:568, 1958.

HOVE, E. L. and COPELAND, D. H.: Muscular Dystrophy in Rabbits as a Result of Chronic Choline Deficiency. Fed. Proc. *13*:461, 1954. Abstr. Vet. Bull. No. 3242, 1954.

HUCHET, J.: La myosite éosinophilique des bovidés. Thesis, Alfort. 1945. Abstr. Vet. Bull. No. 1734, 1950.

KASPAR, L. V. and LOMBARD, L. S.: Nutritional Myodegeneration in a Litter of Beagles. J. Am. Vet. Med. Assn. *143*:284–288, 1963.

KEELER, R. F. and YOUNG, S.: Electrophoretic and Histological Evidence for Muscle Regeneration in Ovine Muscular Dystrophy. Nature, Lond. *193*:338–340, 1962.

KENNEDY, P. C.: Experimental Bovine Trichinosis: An Attempt to Produce Eosinophilic Myositis. Cornell Vet. *45*:127–152, 1955.

KUSCHER, A.: Eosinophile Muskelentzündung beim Hund. Wein, tierärztl. Monatschr. *27*:177–186, 1940. Abstr. Vet. Bull. p. 623, 1941.

KUTTLER, K. L. and MARBLE, D. W.: Relationship of Serum Transaminase to Naturally Occurring and Artificially Induced White Muscle Disease in Calves and Lambs. Am. J. Vet. Res. *19*:632–636, 1958.

LILLEENGEN, K.: Vaxartad Muskeldegeneration (s. k. fiskkott) hos Kalv. [Waxy Muscular. Degeneration (So-Called "Fish Flesh") in Calves.] Svensk Vet. Tidskr. *49*:231–289, 1944. (English summary.)

LOMBARDO, B. and MALOSSI, E.: Un Caso di Miosite Cronica Eosinofilica in un Bovino da Macello. Vet. Ital. *12*:808–811, 1961.

LUDVIGSEN, J.: "Muscular Degeneration" in Hogs (Preliminary Report). Proc. XVth Internat. Vet. Congr. Stockholm *1*:602–606, 1953.

MAKLETOW, B. W.: Myopathy of Dogs Resembling White Muscle Disease of Sheep. N. Z. Vet. J. *11*:52–55, 1963.

MARIN, O. S. M. and DENNY-BROWN, B. E.: Changes in Skeletal Muscle Associated with Cachexia. Am. J. Path. *41*:23–40, 1962.

MARSH, H.: Diseases of Young Lambs. J. Am. Vet. Med. Assn. *81*:187–194, 1932.

————: Treatment of Stiff Lambs with Wheat Germ Oil. J. Am. Vet. Med. Assn. *108*:256, 1946.

McLOUGHLIN, J. V. and GOLDSPINK, G.: Post-mortem Changes in the Colour of Pig Longissimus Dorsi Muscle. Nature, Lond. *198*:584–585, 1963.

METZER, H. J. and HAGAN, W. A.: The So-called Stiff Lambs. Cornell Vet. *17*:35–44, 1927.

MIGAKI, G. and BRANDLY, P. G.: Eosinophilic Myositis in Cattle. Proc. 65th Ann. Meet. U.S.L.S.A., Minneapolis pp. 190–193, 1962.

MOON, C. and WOOD, A. C.: Eosinophilic Myositis in a Dog. J. Am. Vet. Med. Assn. *125*:312–313, 1954.

MUTH, O. H.: White Muscle Disease (Myopathy) in Lambs and Calves. J. Am. Vet. Med. Assn. *126*:355–361, 1955.

MUTH, O. H. *et al.*: White Muscle Disease (Myopathy) in Lambs and Calves. VI. Effects of Selenium and Vitamin E on Lambs. Am. J. Vet. Res. *20*:231–234, 1959.

MUTH, O. H. and ALLAWAY, W. H.: The Relationship of White Muscle Disease to the Distribution of Naturally Occurring Selenium. J. Am. Vet. Med. Assn. *142*:1379–1384, 1963.

PARIS, R.: Lactic Acid in the Urine of Thoroughbred Racehorses after Exercise. Austr. Vet. J. *34*:111–115, 1958.

PROCTOR, J. F. *et al.*: Relation of Selenium, Vitamin E and Other Factors to Muscular Dystrophy in the Rabbit. Proc. Soc. Exp. Biol. New York *108*:77–79, 1961.

RIBELIN, W. E.: Azoturia and the Crush Syndrome. J. Am. Vet. Med. Assn. *119*:284–288, 1951.

RIGDON, R. H.: Perosis Secondary to Naturally Occurring Muscle Necrosis in the Duck. Am. J. Vet. Res. *24*:1030–1037, 1963.

SALISBURY, R. M. *et al.*: Exudate Diathesis and White Muscle Disease of Poultry in New Zealand. Abstr. Vet. Bull. No. 1662, 1962.

SCHOFIELD, F. W.: The Etiology of Muscular Dystrophy in Calves and Lambs. Proc. XVth Internat. Vet. Congr. Stockholm *1*:597–601, 1953.

SEIBOLD, H. R., and DAVIS, C. L.: Generalized Myositis Ossificans (Familial) in Pigs. Path. Vet. *4*:79–88, 1967.

SOVA, Z. and BLAZEK, K.: [Biochemistry and Histopathology in Eosinophilic Myositis of. Dogs.] Sborn. čes. Akad. Zemědělsk. Věd. *3*(31)835–844, 1958. Abstr. Vet. Bull. No. 1897, 1959.

SOVA, Z. and JICHA, J.: "Determination of Serum Glutamic Oxalacetic Acid and Serum Glutamic Pyruvic Acid Transaminase in Horses with Myoglobinaemia (TT)". Berl. Munch. tierarztl. Wschr. 76:385–387, 1963.

THURLEY, D. C., GILBERT, F. R., and DONE, J. T.: Congenital Splayleg of Piglets: Myofibrillar Hypoplasia. Vet. Rec. 80:302–304, 1967.

VAN VLEET, J. F., HALL, B. V., and SIMON, J.: Vitamin E Deficiency. A Sequential Light and Electron Microscopic Study of Skeletal Muscle Degeneration in Weanling Rabbits. Amer. J. Path. 52:1067–1079, 1968.

VAWTER, L. R. and RECORDS, E.: Muscular Dystrophy (White Muscle Disease) in Young Calves. J. Am. Vet. Med. Assn. 110:152–157, 1947.

WEST, W. T. and MASON, K. E.: Histopathology of Muscular Dystrophy in the Vitamin E-Deficient Hamster. Am. J. Anat. 102:323–349, 1958.

WHITNEY, J. C.: Atrophic Myositis in a Dog: The Differentiation of This Disease from Eosinophilic Myositis. Vet. Rec. 69:130–131, 1957.

————: Progressive Muscular Dystrophy in the Dog. Vet. Rec. 70:611–613, 1958.

WINTOR, H. and STEPHENSON, H. C.: Eosinophilic Myositis in a Dog. Cornell Vet. 42:531–537, 1952.

YONEMURA, T. and SHIGA, K.: Studies on Multiple Myo-degeneration of Sheep in Hokkaido. 21st Rep. Govt. Exper. Sta. Animal Hyg. Tokyo, 1949, pp. 1–10. Abstr. Vet. Bull. No. 3778, 1952.

YOUNG, S. et al.: Nutritional Muscular Dystrophy in Lambs—Morphologic and Electrophoretic Studies on Preparations of Fetal and Juvenile Muscle; Selenium Analysis of Maternal, Fetal, and Juvenile Tissue; The Effect of Muscular Activity on the Symmetrical Distribution of Lesions. Am. J. Vet. Res. 23:955–971, 1962.

Skeletal Diseases

BALL, V. H.: L'ostéo-arthropathie hypertrophiante pneumonique chez les fauves en captivité Rev. gén. de méd. vét. 35:417–432, 1926.

BANE, A. and HANSEN, H.-J.: Spinal Changes in the Bull and Their Significance in Serving Ability. Cornell Vet. 52:362–384, 1962.

BELANGER, L. F.: Osteolysis in Pathological Material. Cornell Vet. 58:Supplement 115–135, 1968.

BIENFET, V., et al.: A Primary Parathyroid Disorder. Osteofibrosis Caused by Parathyroid Adenoma in a Shetland Pony. Recovery After Surgical Removal. Ann. Med. Vet. 108: 252–265, 1964.

BOYD, W.: *Textbook of Pathology.* 6th ed., 1953, Philadelphia, Lea & Febiger, p. 911.

BRION, A. J. and FONTAINE, M.: A Hemorrhagic and Rachitic-like Syndrome in Chickens Due to Nitrofural-Medicated Feed. Poultry Sci. 37:1071–1074, 1958.

BRODY, R. S.: Renal Osteitis Fibrosa Cystica in a Wire-Haired Fox Terrier. J. Am. Vet. Med. Assn. 124:275–278, 1954.

BROWN, W. R., KROOK, L., and POND, W. G.: Atrophic Rhinitis in Swine. Etiology, Pathogenesis, and Prophylaxis. Cornell Vet. 56:Suppl. No. 1, 1–108, 1966.

BUTLER, W. F., and SMITH, R. N.: Age Changes in the Annulus Fibrosus of the Non-Ruptured Intervertebral Disc of the Cat. Res. Vet. Sci. 6:280–289, 1965.

CALKINS, E. et al.: Idiopathic Familial Osteoporosis in Dogs ("Osteogenesis Imperfecta"). Ann. N. Y. Acad. Sci. 64:410–423, 1956.

CAMPBELL, J. R.: Bone Dystrophy in Puppies. Vet. Rec. 74:1340–1347 and 1348, 1962.

CARLTON, W. W. and HENDERSON, W.: Histopathological Lesions Observed in the Long Bones of Chickens Fed a Copper-Deficient Diet. Poult. Sci. 41:1634, 1962.

CARRÉ, H. J.: Une enzöotie d'ostéite hypertrophiante chez le mouton. Compt. rend. Soc. de biol. 123:557–558, 1936.

COHRS, P. and SCHULZ, L. C.: Sur Pathogenese der spontanen und Experimentellen Rotlaufarthritis des Schweines. Mh. Vet. Med. 15:608–614, 1960.

CORDY, D. R.: Osteodystrophia Fibrosa Accompanied by Visceral Accumulation of Lead. Cornell Vet. 47:480–490, 1957.

CORLEY, E. A., SOUTHERLAND, T. M., and CARLSON, W. E.: Genetic Aspects of Canine Elbow Dysplasia. J. Am. Vet. Med. Assn. 153:543–547, 1968.

COTCHIN, E.: Marie's Disease Associated with Tuberculosis in a Horse. Brit. Vet. J. 100: 261–267, 1944.

COTTER, S. M., GRIFFITHS, R. C., and LEAV, I.: Enostosis of Young Dogs. J. Am. Vet. Med. Assn. 153:401–410, 1968.

DÄMMRICH, K.: Pathologisch-anatomische un histologische Untersuchungen an Knochen Nieren und Epithelkörperchen von Hunden mit Nierenerkrankungen. Zbl. Vet. Med. 5:742–568, 1958. Abstracted Vet. Bull., No. 1541, 1959.

DELEHANTY, D. D.: Defects—Not Fractures—of the Fibulae in the Horse. J. Am. Vet. Med. Assn. *133*:258–260, 1958.

DÉVÉ, F.: L'echinococcose osseuse. A Monteverde y Cia. Montevideo, 1948. Abstr. Vet. Bull. No. 3084, 1949.

DIPLOCK, P. T.: Legg-Perthes Disease (Coxa Plana) in Cattle. J. Am. Vet. Med. Assn. *141*:462–463, 1962.

DUBOULAY, G. H., and CRAWFORD, M. A.: Nutritional Bone Disease in Captive Primates. Symp. Zool. Soc. Lond. *21*:223–236, 1968.

DUCKWORTH, J. et al.: Dental Mal-Occlusion and Rickets in Sheep. Research Vet. Sci. *2*:375–380, 1961.

DURAND, M. and KCHOUK, M.: Le "Krafft," une osteopathie dystrophique du dromadaire. Arch. Inst. Pasteur, Tunis. *35*:107–152, 1958. Abstr. Vet. Bull., No. 489, 1959.

ESPERSEN, G.: Multiple Maxillary and Mandibular Cysts in Horses. Thesis, Copenhagen, pp. 110, 1962.

FELDMAN, W. H. and OLSON, C.: Spondylitis of Swine Associated with Bacteria of the Brucella Group. Arch. Path. *16*:195–210, 1933.

FETTER, A. W., and CAPEN, C. C.: Ultrastructural Evaluation of the Parathyroid Glands of Pigs with Naturally Occurring Atrophic Rhinitis. Path. Vet. *5*:481–503, 1968.

FUJIMOTO, Y., et al.: Electron Microscopic Observations of the Equine Parathyroid Glands with Particular Reference to Those of Equine Osteodystrophia Fibrosa. Jap. J. Vet. Res. *15*:37–51, 1967.

GOODBARY, R. F. and HAGE, T. J.: Hypertrophic Pulmonary Osteothropathy in a Horse. J. Am. Vet. Med. Assn. *137*:602–605, 1960.

GROENEWALD, J. W.: Osteofibrosis in Equines. Onderstepoort, J. Vet. Sci. & An. Indust. *9*:601–621, 1937.

GROTH, A. H., JR.: The Comparative Histopathology of Rickets and an Osteodystrophy in Immature Iowa Swine. Am. J. Vet. Res. *19*:409–416, 1958.

HAGE, T. J. and MOULTON, J. E. Skeletal Coccidioidomycosis in Dogs. Cornell Vet. *44*: 489–500, 1954.

HANSEN, H.-J.: Comparative Views on the Pathology of Disc Degeneration in Animals. Lab. Investig. *8*:1242–1265, 1959.

HARRIS, M. S. et al.: Cortisone Therapy in Hamman-Rich Syndrome. Am. Rev. Tuberc. *76*:123–131, 1957.

HENRICSON, B. and OLSSON, S.: Hereditary Acetabular Dysplasia in German Shepherd Dogs. J. Am. Vet. Med. Assn. *135*:207–210, 1959.

HOERLEIN, B. F.: Intervertebral-disc Protrusion in the Dog. Am. J. Vet. Research *14*: 260–283, 1953.

HOGG, A. H.: Osteodystrophic Disease in the Dog, with Special Reference to Rubber Jaw (Renal Osteodystrophy) and its Comparison with Renal Rickets in the Human. Vet. Rec. *60*:117–122, 1948. Abstr. Vet. Bull. No. 3335, 1950.

HOLLING, H. E., BRODEY, R. S., and BOLAND, H. C.: Pulmonary Hypertrophic Osteoarthropathy. Lancet. Dec. 9th, 1269–1274, 1961.

HOLMES, J. R.: Experimental Transmission of Avian Osteopetrosis. J. Comp. Path. & Therap. *68*:439–448, 1958.

HUNT, R. D., GARCIA, F. G., and HEGSTED, D. M.: A Comparison of Vitamin D_2 and D_3 in New World Primates. I. Production and Regression of Osteodystrophia Fibrosa. Lab. Anim. Care *17*:222–234, 1967.

INNES, J. R. M.: "Inherited Dysplasia" of the Hip-Joint in Dogs and Rabbits. Lab. Investig. *8*:1170–1177, 1959.

JAFFE, H. L. and BODANSKY, A.: Experimental Fibrous Osteodystrophy in Hyperparathyroid Dogs. J. Exper. Med. *52*:669–694, 1932.

JOHNSON, L. C.: Kinetics of Osteoarthritis. Lab. Investig. *8*:1223–1231, 1959.

JONES, T. C. and SCHNELLE, G. B.: Pulmonary Hypertrophic Osteoarthropathy in Dogs. Lab. Investig. *8*:1287–1303, 1959.

JOWSEY, J., and GERSHON-COHEN, J.: Effect of Dietary Calcium Levels on Production and Reversal of Experimental Osteoporosis in Cats. Proc. Soc. Exp. Biol. Med. *116*:437–441, 1964.

JOWSEY, J., and RAISZ, L. G.: Experimental Osteoporosis and Parathyroid Activity. Endocrinology *82*:384–396, 1968.

KAYE, M. M.: Hyperostosis in Newborn Pigs. Canad. J. Comp. Med. *26*:218–221, 1962.

KERSJES, A. W., VAN DE WATERING, C. C., and KALSBEEK, H. C.: Hypertrophic Pulmonary Osteoarthropathy (Marie-Bamberger Disease). Neth. J. Vet. Sci. *1*:55–68, 1968.

KINTNER, J. H. and HOLT, R. L.: Equine Osteomalacia. Philippine J. Sci. *49*:1–89. 1932.

KROOK, L., et al.: Nutritional Secondary Hyperparathyroidism in the Cat. Cornell Vet. *53*:224–240, 1963.

KROOK, L., and LOWE, J. E.: Nutritional Secondary Hyperparathyroidism in the Horse, With a Description of the Normal Equine Parathyroid Gland. Pathologia Vet. *1*:Suppl. 1–98, 1964.

KROOK, L., and BARRETT, R. B.: Simian Bone Disease—A Secondary Hyperparathyroidism. Cornell Vet. *52*:459–492, 1962.

KROOK, L.: Dietary Calcium-Phosphorus and Lameness in the Horse. Cornell Vet. *58*: Suppl. 59–73, 1968.

LAWRENCE, W. C., NICHOLS, W. W., and ALTERA, K. P.: A Simple Method of Bone Marrow Aspiration in the Cow. Cornell Vet. *52*:297–305, 1962.

LIÉGEOIS, F. and DÉRIVAUX, J.: Hyperphosphorose alimentaire et ostéogénèse chez le porc. Ann. méd. vét. *95*:201–218, 1951.

LJUNGGREN, G.: Legg-Perthes Disease in the Dog. Acta Orthop. Scand. Suppl. No. 95, 1–79, 1967.

LORD, G. H.: Hypertrophic Osteoarthropathy in a Dog.—A Clinico-Pathological Report. J. Am. Vet. Med. Assn. *134*:13–17, 1959.

LOWBEER, L.: Skeletal and Articular Involvement of Brucellosis in Animals. Lab. Investig. *8*:1448–1460, 1959.

MALHERBE, W. D.: Some Observations on Rickets and Allied Bone Diseases in South African Domestic Animals. Ann. N. Y. Acad. Sci. *64*:128–146, 1956.

MANSSON, J. and NORBERG, I.: Dysplasia of the Hip in Dogs. Hormonally Induced Flaccidity of the Ligaments Followed by Dysplasia of the Acetabulum in Puppies. Medlemsbl. Sverig. Vet Forb. *13*:330–332, 335–339, 1961.

MARTIN, J. E., COLE, W. C., and WHITNEY, R. A.: Tuberculosis of the Spine (Pott's Disease) in a Rhesus Monkey (*Macaca mulatta*). J. Am. Vet. Med. Assn. *153*:914–917, 1968.

McROBERTS, M. R.: A Dental Malocclusion Associated with Rickets in Growing Lambs. Proc. Nutr. Soc. 20(No. 2):pp xxxvii-xxxviii of abstracts, 1961.

MATHER, G. and LOW, D.: Chronic Pulmonary Osteoarthropathy in the Dog. J. Am. Vet. Med. Assn. *122*:167–171, 1953.

MORGAN, J. P., CARLSON, W. D., and ADAMS, O. R.: Hereditary Multiple Exostosis in the Horse. J. Am. Vet. Med. Assn. *140*:1320–1322, 1962.

MURPHY, H. M.: A Review of Inherited Osteopetrosis in the Mouse: Man and Other Mammals Also Considered. Clin. Orthop. July-Aug.:97–109, 1969.

NIELSEN, S. W. and McSHERRY, B. J.: Renal Hyperparathyroidism (Rubbre Jaw Syndrome) in a Dog. J. Am. Vet. Med. Assn. *124*:270–274, 1954.

NILSSON, S. A.: Clinical, Morphological and Experimental Studies of Laminitis in Cattle. Acta vet. Scand. 4(Suppl. #1):304, 1963.

NISBET, D. I. *et al.*: Osteodystrophic Diseases of Sheep. I. An Osteodystrophic Condition of Hoggs Known as Double Scalp or Cappi. J. Comp. Path. *72*:270–280, 1962.

NISBET, D. I., BUTLER, E. J., and SMITH, B. S.: Osteodystropic Diseases of Sheep. J. Comp. Path. *76*:159–169, 1966.

NORDIN, B. E. C.: The Pathogenesis of Osteoporosis. Lancet. May 13, 1961. pp. 1011–1014, 1015.

OMAR, A. R.: Osteogenesis Imperfecta in Cats. J. Path. Bact. *82*:303–314, 1961.

PALMER, N. C.: Osteodystrophia Fibrosa in Cats. Aust. Vet. J. *44*:151–155, 1968.

PANISSET, L. A.: L'ostéo-arthropathie hypertrophiante d'origine tuberculeuse chez le chien. Rev. gén. de méd. Vét. *33*:165–184, 1924.

PAPP, E. and SIKES, D.: Electrophoretic Distribution of Protein in the Serum of Swine with Rheumatoid-like Arthritis. Am. J. Vet. Res. *25*:1112–1119, 1964.

PEARCE, L.: Hereditary Osteopetrosis of the Rabbit. J. Exper. Med. *92*:601–624, 1950.

PLATT, H.: Canine Chronic Nephritis. III. The Skeletal System in Rubber Jaw. J. Comp Path. & Therap. *61*:197–204, 1951.

PLATT, B. S. and STEWART, R. C. J.: Transverse Trabeculae and Osteoporosis in Bones in Experimental Protein-Calorie Deficiency. Brit. J. Nutr. *16*:483–495, 1962.

POLEY, P. P. and TAYLOR, J. S.: Hypertrophic Pulmonary Osteoarthropathy Associated with Bronchogenic Giant-cell Tumor in the Left Lung of a Dog. J. Am. Vet. Med. Assn. *100*:346–352, 1942.

PUNTONI, P.: Su due casi di osteoartropatia ipertrofizzante pneumica osservati nel cane in esito a bronco-polmonite da corpo estraneo. Ann. Fac. Med. Vet., Pisa. *10*:168–191, 1958.

RAINEY, J. W.: Rupture of the Round Ligament of the Hip Joint in Cattle. Austr. Vet. J. *34*:160, 1958.

RAISZ, L. G.: Physiologic and Pharmacologic Regulation of Bone Resorption. New Eng. J. Med. *282*:909–916, 1970.

RAY, J. D.: Arthritis in Lambs and *Erysipelothrix rhusiopathiæ*. J. Am. Vet. Med. Assn. *77*:107–108, 1930.

REIFENSTEIN, E. C. and ALBRIGHT, F.: Paget's Disease. New Eng. J. Med. *231*:343–355 1944.

—————: Juvenile Osteoporosis (Osteogenesia Imperfecta)—A Calcium Deficiency. J. Am. Vet. Med. Assn. *139*:117–119, 1961.

—————: An Analysis of the Present Status of Hip Dysplasia in the Dog. J. Am. Vet. Med. Assn. *144*:709–721, 1964.

RISER, W. H., PARKER, L. J., and SHIRER, J. F.: Canine Craniomandibular Osteopathy. J. Am. Vet. Rad. Soc. *8*:23–31, 1967.

RISER, W. H.: Hypertrophic Osteopathy of the Mandibles and Cranium in West Highland Terriers. J. Am. Vet. Med. Assn. *148*:1543–1547, 1966.

ROBERTS, E. D., *et al.*: Pathologic Changes of Porcine Suppurative Arthritis Produced by Streptococcus equisimilis. Am. J. Vet. Res. *29*:253–262, 1968.

ROBERTS, E. D., SWITZER, W. P., and RAMSEY, F. K.: Pathology of the Visceral Organs of Swine Inoculated with *Mycoplasma hyorhinis*. Am. J. Vet. Res. *24*:9–18, 19–31, 1963.

ROONEY, J. R.: Epiphyseal Compression in Young Horses. Cornell Vet. *53*:567–574, 1963.

ROSSI, L.: L'osteo-artropatia ipertro-fizzante d'origine tubercolare del cane. Clinica vet. *49*:67–77 and 133–147, 1926.

ROWLAND, G. N., CAPEN, C. C., and NAGODE, L. A.: Experimental Hyperparathyroidism in Young Cats. Path. Vet. *5*:504–519, 1968.

SALGUES, M. R.: Lesions anatomiques et modifications tissulaires et humorales au cours de l'ostéomalacie des animaux domestiques. Rec. méd. vét. exot. *13*:22–38, 1940.

SCHALES, O.: Hereditary Patterns in Dysplasia of the Hip. No. Am. Vet. *38*:152–155, 1957.

SCHLUMBERGER, H. G.: Polyostotic Hyperkeratosis in the Female Parakeet. Am. J. Path. *35*:1–24, 1959.

SCHMIDT, W.: "The Ligamentum Teres and the Joint Capsule of Healthy and Arthritic Hip Joints in Dogs, and a Study of Sub-Chrondal Cysts (TT)." Berl. Munch. tierarztl. Wschr. *76*:245–250, 1963.

SCHNELLE, G. B.: Congenital Dysplasia of the Hip (Canine) and Sequelæ. Proc. Am. Vet. Med. Assn. 1954, pp. 253–258.

—————: Canine Hip Dysplasia. Lab. Investig. *8*:1178–1189, 1959.

SCHRYVER, H. F.: Symposium on Equine Bone and Joint Diseases. New York State Veterinary College, Cornell University, Ithaca, N. Y. 2–3 June 1967. Cornell Vet. *58*: Suppl. 1968.

SCOTT, P. P., McKUSECK, V. A., and McKUSECK, A. B.: The Nature of Osteogenesis Imperfecta in Cats. Evidence That the Disorder is Primarily Nutritional, Not Genetic, and Therefore Not Analogous to the Disease in Man. J. Bone Joint Surg. (Amer.) *45-A*:125–134, 1963.

SCOTT, P.: Osteodystrophies. Vet. Rec. *84*:333–335, 1969.

SHUPE, J. L.: Degenerative Arthritis in the Bovine. Lab. Investig. *8*:1190–1196, 1959.

SHUPE, J. L. and STORZ, J.: Pathologic Study of Psittacosis-Lymphogranuloma Polyarthritis of Lambs. Am. J. Vet. Res. *25*:943–951, 1964.

SIKES, D.: A Rheumatoid-like Arthritis in Swine. Lab. Investig. *8*:1406–1413, 1959.

SIKES, D., NEHER, G. M., and DOYLE, L. P.: Studies on Arthritis in Swine. Experimental Erysipelas and Chronic Arthritis in Swine. Am. J. Vet. Res. *16*:349–366, 1955.

SIKES, D., *et al.*: Ankylosing Spondylitis and Polyarthritis of the Dog: Physiopathologic Changes of Tissues. Am. J. Vet. Res. *31*:703–712, 1970.

SIKES, D.: Experimental Production of Rheumatoid Arthritis of Swine: Physiopathologic Changes of Tissues. Am. J. Vet. Res. *29*:1719–1731, 1968.

SMITH, W. S., IRETON, R. J., and COLEMAN, C. R.: Sequelæ of Experimental Dislocation of a Weight-Bearing Ball-and-Socket Joint in a Young Growing Animal. J. Bone & Joint. Surg. *40A*:1121–1127, 1957.

SMYTHE, A. R.: Some Clinical Aspects of Tuberculosis in the Dog (Osteoarthropathy). Vet. Rec. *9*:421–433, 1929.

SNAVELY, J. G.: The Genetic Aspects of Hip Dysplasia in Dogs. J. Am. Vet. Med. Assn. *135*:201–207, 1959.

SOKOLOFF, L.: Osteoarthritis in Laboratory Animals. Lab. Investig. *8*:1209–1217, 1959.

STORTS, R. W., and KOESTNER, A.: Skeletal Lesions Associated with a Dietary Calcium and Phosphorus Imbalance in the Pig. Am. J. Vet. Res. *26*:280–294, 1965.

SWANTON, M. C.: Hemophilic Arthropathy in Dogs. Lab. Investig. *8*:1269–1277, 1959.

THEILER, SIR ARNOLD: Osteodystrophic Diseases of Animals. Vet. J. *90*:183–206, 1934.

THOMSON, R. G.: Failure of Bone Resorption in a Calf. Path. Vet. *3*:234–246, 1966.

TREVINO, G. S.: Renal Osteitis Fibrosa Cystica in a Cocker Spaniel, the "Rubber-jaw" Syndrome. Southwestern Vet. *8*:338–340, 1955.

TRUM, B. F.: Pathogenesis of Osteoarthritis in the Horse (Particularly as Related to Nutritional Aspects). Lab. Investig. *8*:1197–1208, 1959.

ULMANSKY, M.: The Effect of "Meat Diet" on Long Bones of Mice. Amer. J. Path. *47*: 435–445, 1965.

VAN PELT, R. W., and LANGHAM, R. F.: Degenerative Joint Disease in Cattle. J. Am. Vet. Med. Assn. *148*:535–542, 1966.

VAUGHAN, L. C.: Studies on Intervertebral Disc Protrusion in the Dog. III. Pathological Features. Brit. Vet. J. *114*:350–355, 1958.

VERGE, J.: Les ostéopathies hypertrophiantes: Étude de deux cas chez le lion. Rev. gén. de méd. Vét. *43*:1–22, 1934.

WALLACH, J. D., and FLIEG, G. M.: Nutritional Secondary Hyperparathyroidism in Captive Psittacine Birds. J. Am. Vet. Med. Assn. *151*:880–883, 1967.

WILKINSON, G. T.: The Pathology of Navicular Disease; the Macroscopical Pathological Features of the Disease. Brit. Vet. J. *109*:38–42, 1953.

WILLIAMSON, W. M., LOMBARD, L. S., and FIRFER, H. S.: Fibrous Dysplasia in a Monkey and a Kudu. J. Am. Vet. Med. Assn. *147*:1049–1052, 1965.

WOOLDRIGE, G. H. and HOLMES, J. W. H.: Pulmonary Tuberculosis in the Dog with Complications Involving Bones of the Limbs. Vet. Rec. *49*:508–509, 1937.

WU, K., and FROST, H. M.: Bone Formation in Osteoporosis. Arch. Path. *88*:508–510, 1969.

ZESKOV, V.: Prelog Eosinofilnom Panesititisu U. Njemackih Ovcara. Doctoral Thesis, Veterinarski Arhiv, Zagreb, knijiga XXXII/1962, svezak 5–6. 1961. 146–149.

21

The Respiratory System

THE AIR PASSAGES

The mucous membrane of the nares, paranasal sinuses, pharynx, larynx, trachea and bronchi is subject to injury by chemical and infectious agents brought to it in the inspired air. Chemical injury is infrequent, being due to accidental inhalation of such gases as ammonia and chlorine, as well as war gases; injury by infectious microorganisms, including viruses, is frequent and often severe. As might be expected, the more external of the respiratory passages are more accessible to such injurious agents; the deeper structures, such as the bronchi, are less often attacked but the effects of infections here are most severe and more ominous than in the upper part of the respiratory tract. It is entirely possible, however, for these mucous membranes to be attacked via the hematogenous route by infections which have an affinity for them. For instance, when material containing the virus of bovine malignant catarrhal fever is injected subcutaneously, the respiratory mucous membranes become the principal seat of disease just as if the infection had gained primary access to them.

Rhinitis (inflammation of the nasal mucosa), **sinusitis, pharyngitis, laryngitis, tracheitis** and **bronchitis** usually commence as acute mucous (catarrhal) inflammations of the respective mucous membranes. They tend somewhat later to become purulent or fibrinous, depending on the nature of the infectious agent, and fulfill the descriptions already given in the general study of inflammation. In most cases the infectious process, like the human "cold," starts as a rhinitis, and the extent to which it spreads into the lower air passages depends upon its virulence and the susceptibility of the patient. Some of them reach the lung parenchyma itself, causing pneumonia. Among the acute infections localizing in the upper air passages are strangles (*Streptococcus equi*), equine rhinopneumonitis and influenza in the horse, pasteurellosis, malignant catarrhal fever, infectious bovine rhinotracheitis and calf diphtheria in cattle, pasteurellosis, influenza and inclusion body rhinitis in swine, the distemper virus and probably the bronchisepticus organism (*Alcaligenes* or *Brucella bronchiseptica*) in the dog, feline viral rhinotracheitis and probably other viruses in cats, and the various coryza-producing viruses and bacteria in poultry. Several of the chronic granulomatous infections may be localized in these structures, particularly glanders, bovine nasal granuloma, rhinosporidiosis and tuberculosis. The lesions are those characteristic of each specific disease. *Cryptococcus neoformans* is occasionally encountered as a cause of rhinitis in animals, especially cats.

In sheep, the larvae of the **bot-fly**, *Oestrus ovis* (p. 811), some 2 cm. long when fully grown, migrate up the nares, usually into the frontal sinus, sometimes into

taneous examples of the disease and correlated with the many organisms that have been claimed as causes, nutritional deficiency as the sole offender must be approached with care. Perhaps a synergistic combination of nutritional deficiency and infection is essential or synergism between organisms, or it may be likely that atrophic rhinitis has more than a single cause.

Atrophic Rhinitis

BAUSTAD, B., TEIGE, J., JR., and TOLLERSRUD, S.: The Effect of Various Levels of Calcium, Phosphorus and Vitamin D in the Feed for Growing Pigs with Special Reference to Atrophic Rhinitis. Acta Vet. Scand. *8*:369–389, 1967.

BRION, A. J., and FONTAINE, M. P.: Étude sur la rhinite atrophique du porc. Les lésions nerveuses. Essai d'interprétation étiologique et pathogénique. Canad. J. Comp. Med. *22*: 88–95, 1958.

BROWN, W. R., KROOK, L., and POND, W. G.: Atrophic Rhinitis in Swine, Etiology, Pathogenesis, Prophylaxis. Cornell Vet. *56*:Suppl. 1, 1–108, 1966.

DUNCAN, J. R., RAMSEY, F. K., and SWITZER, W. P.: Pathology of Experimental *Bordetella bronchiseptica* Infection in Swine: Pneumonia. Am. J. Vet. Res. *27*:467–472, 1966.

DUNCAN, J. R., *et al.*: Pathology of Experimental *Bordetella bronchiseptica* Infection in Swine: Atrophic Rhinitis. Am. J. Vet. Res. *27*:457–466, 1966.

MAEDA, M., INUI, S., and KONNO, S.: Lesions of Nasal Turbinates in Swine Atrophic Rhinitis. Nat. Inst. Anim. Health Quart. (Tokyo) *9*:193–202, 1969.

SCHOFIELD, F. W., and JONES, T. L.: The Pathology and Bacteriology of Infectious Atrophic Rhinitis in Swine. J. Am. Vet. Med. Assn. *116*:120–123, 1950.

SWITZER, W. P.: Studies on Infectious Atrophic Rhinitis of Swine. J. Am. Vet. Med. Assn. *123*:45–47, 1953; Vet. Med. *46*:478–481, 1951; *48*:392–394, 1953; Am. J. Vet. Res. *16*:540–544, 1955; *17*:478–484, 1956.

PORCINE RHINOHYPERPLASIA

This condition, called *bull-nose* by farmers, and also known as necrotic rhinitis, is characterized by irregular and asymmetrical proliferation of fibrous and sometimes bony tissue over the region of the snout. The skin is usually intact but may show old ulcerated areas. Within the proliferated tissue there are old, inspissated abscesses and foci of caseous necrosis. The proliferation is thus to be explained as a process of encapsulation and chronic inflammatory reaction. In severe cases, the nasal and maxillary bones and the paranasal sinuses may be involved in the process and considerably distorted, with resulting dyspnea. The cause is infectious although probably not specific. A variety of microorganisms have been demonstrated, including the necrophorus bacillus and a spirochetal organism which may have special significance. They enter the tissues through slight and often unseen wounds in the skin or adjoining mucosae of the region, including those made by the bites of other little pigs. Poor sanitation is predisposing, probably through increasing the numbers of soil-borne organisms.

EPISTAXIS

Epistaxis, or **nosebleed,** occurs infrequently in the domestic animals. If not caused by some trauma such as a heavy blow or the passing of the stomach tube, it is likely to be an indication of an ulcerative infection or neoplasm, an hemangioma (rare) or possibly a fractured bone which has lacerated a blood vessel in the region.

LARYNGEAL HEMIPLEGIA

Normally at each inspiration the arytenoid cartilages of the larynx are drawn outward by their muscles, as two double doors might be swung open to admit air.

In this disease of the horse there is a paralysis, usually partial, of one of the arytenoid cartilages which leaves it vapid in the rushing air currents. Commonly the muscles have enough strength to hold it open during ordinary breathing but not during the more violent respiration which goes with vigorous exercise, when the air current draws the flap of tissue into mid-stream. The result is that at each inspiration this fluttering obstruction not only limits the amount of air which can reach the lungs, but also sets up a considerable sound, which is responsible for the disease being called **roaring.**

The affected crico-arytenoideus muscle shows atrophy of many of its fibers, which progresses until they disappear completely, with replacement by fibrous tissue. This latter often shows considerable mucoid degeneration (p. 52), so that grossly the degenerated muscle is said to look like fish flesh. The recurrent laryngeal nerve supplying the muscle shows the successive stages of demyelinization and wallerian degeneration (p. 1381).

It is almost always the left arytenoid cartilage, crico-arytenoideus muscle and recurrent laryngeal nerve which are involved in this disorder. This is believed to be because of the unique course of the left nerve around the arch of the aorta and along the deep face of that vessel, where it is subjected to the strong aortic pulsations and apparently injured thereby. Causes of certain infrequent cases which may be on either side include pressure by enlarged granulomatous lymph nodes, tumors, abscesses, aneurysms and esophageal swelling. Congenital defects have been suspected. Many cases are post-pneumonic.

PHARYNGEAL DIVERTICULITIS

In the pig, the diverticulum pharyngeum lies just dorsal to the origin of the esophagus. It is rather frequently the site of lodgement of capsules incorrectly administered for the treatment of intestinal helminthiasis or other diseases. Depending on the nature of the contained medicaments, severe inflammation or fatal gangrene may result from release of the drug in the diverticulum. Prosectors must not overlook a lesion of this kind.

Air Passages

ADAMS, O. R., *et al.*: Comparison of Infectious Bovine Rhinotracheitis, Shipping Fever and Calf Diphtheria of Cattle. J. Am. Vet. Med. Assn. *134*:58–89, 1959.

ALLEN, A. M.: Occurrence of the Nematode *Anatrichosoma cutaneum* in the Nasal Mucosa of *Macaca mulatta* Monkeys. Am. J. Vet. Res. *21*:389–392, 1960.

BINN, L. N., *et al.*: Viral Antibody Patterns in Laboratory Dogs with Respiratory Disease. Am. J. Vet. Res. *31*:697–702, 1970.

BINN, L. N., *et al.*: Upper Respiratory Disease in Military Dogs: Bacterial, Mycoplasma, and Viral Studies. Am. J. Vet. Res. *29*:1809–1815, 1968.

CAMPBELL, R. S. F., *et al.*: Respiratory Adenovirus Infection in the Dog. Vet. Rec. *83*: 202–203, 1968.

CRANDELL, R. A., CHEATHAM, W. J., and MAURER, F. D.: Infectious Bovine Rhinotracheitis —The Occurrence of Intranuclear Inclusion Bodies in Experimentally Infected Animals. Am. J. Vet. Res. *20*:505–509, 1959.

DITCHFIELD, J., MACPHERSON, L. W., and ZBITNEW, A.: Association of a Canine Adenovirus (Toronto A21–61) With an Outbreak of Laryngotracheitis (Kennel Cough). Canad Vet. J. *3*:238–247, 1962.

DOYLE, L. P., DONHAM, C. R., and HUTCHINGS, L. M.: Report on a Type of Rhinitis in Swine. J. Am. Vet. Med. Assn. *105*:132–133, 1944.

FAIRCHILD, G. A., MEDWAY, W., and COHEN, D.: A Study of the Pathogenicity of a Canine Adenovirus (Toronto A26/61) for Dogs. Am. J. Vet. Res. *30*:1187–1193, 1969.

GUSSMAN, H. J.: Endemic Infectious Adenopapillomatosis of the Nasal Mucosa in Sheep. Mh. Veterinaermed. *17*:529–532, 1962.

HARDING, J. D. J.: Inclusion Body Rhinitis of Swine in Maryland. Am. J. Vet. Res. *19*: 907–912, 1958.

KELLY, D. F.: Canine Proliferative and Necrotizing Tracheobronchitis, With Intranuclear Inclusion-Body and Hyaline Membrane Formation. Path. Vet. (Basel) *6*:227–234, 1969.

LOMBARD, C.: A New Disease in the Goat: Adenopapilloma of the Nasal Mucosa. C. R. Acad-Agric. (Fr.) *52*:536–537, 1966.

RUBAJ, B., and WOLOSZYN, S.: Enzootic Adenopapilloma of the Nasal Cavity in Sheep. Medycyna Wet. *23*:226–229, 1967.

SMITH, J. E.: The Aerobic Bacteria of the Nose and Tonsils of Healthy Dogs. J. Comp. Path. *71*:428–433, 1961.

SWANGO, L. J., WOODING, W. L., JR., and BINN, L. N.: A Comparison of the Pathogenesis of Infectious Canine Hepatitis Virus and the A26/61 Virus Strain (Toronto). J. Am. Vet. Med. Assn. *156*:1687–1696, 1970.

WHEAT, J. D.: Typanites of the Guttural Pouch of the Horse. J. Am. Vet. Med. Assn. *140*:453–454, 1962.

THE TRACHEA AND BRONCHI

The **tracheal rings** occasionally suffer permanent deformity, usually by upward compression. This condition is often asymptomatic and discovered only at autopsy. **Ossification** of the laryngeal and tracheal cartilages has been mentioned (p. 58).

Bronchiectasis is a dilatation of one or more bronchi. During violent or forced respiration, the bronchi and bronchioles dilate to full capacity and become round in cross section, but at other times all but the largest bronchi are contracted by their encircling musculature so that the mucosa is thrown into folds. In cross sections, these folds give the smaller and medium bronchi a star-like appearance. In bronchiectasis, they are dilated and the folds stretched out to a full circle, a position which persists after death. This inelasticity and failure to return to the normal contracted state are due to small amounts of fibrous tissue in and around the bronchial wall which has proliferated as the result of chronic inflammation. Commonly a number of leukocytes and reticulo-endothelial cells are still visible in the peribronchial zone. The scar tissue also acts to keep the lumen distended by tying the wall to surrounding structures. Bronchiectasis is thus an indication of a present or previous inflammation. The peribronchial tissue commonly shares in the inelasticity, so that the ability of the lung to collapse is impaired and its functional efficiency diminished. Continued irritation results from these structural derangements, as is generally evidenced by catarrhal exudation and cough. This exudative state may be enhanced by continuing or recurrent infections of low virulence. Owing to chronic irritation, squamous metaplasia of the bronchial epithelium is a frequent finding. A striking example of bronchiectasis is a consistent feature of chronic murine pneumonia (p. 432).

Bronchitis has been mentioned in common with the upper respiratory diseases. It is most often an extension of one of these infections, but may rarely represent an extension of a pneumonic process which originated in the pulmonary parenchyma. The mild or early forms are characterized by catarrhal inflammation; later the exudate usually become fibrinous or purulent. The virulence and the importance of an upper respiratory infection can usually be gauged by how far it extends from the nares toward the lungs, bronchitis being the most formidable of the subpneumonic infections.

Canine tracheobronchitis or *"kennel cough"* is a clinical designation for a disease

SV-5
CAV-II

characterized by intermittent coughing. Although clinically the disease may appear as a single entity, there is little reason to consider it a specific disease with a single cause, anymore so than the human cold. Various viruses, including adenoviruses, influenza viruses and herpesviruses have been reported to induce tracheobronchitis in dogs but their respective roles in the natural disease is not established. There are very few reports describing the gross or histopathologic features as the disease is not fatal. Inclusion bodies in tracheal and bronchial epithelium, similar to those produced by adenoviruses and herpesviruses, are occasionally encountered in dogs with a history of coughing.

Bronchial Asthma.—This disease is characterized by attacks lasting from one to many hours of very difficult, wheezing respiration, especially expiration, due to spasmodic contraction of the encircling musculature of the bronchioles and smaller bronchi, as well as to the production of large amounts of viscid mucous exudate which is strongly inclined to adhere to the bronchial walls. While some cases are secondary to a bronchial infection, the majority are allergic reactions to a great variety of inhaled organic substances to which the individual has become hypersensitive. That contraction of smooth muscle is an outstanding manifestation of the anaphylactic state has been demonstrated many times by suitable laboratory experiments.

The principal lesions in fatal cases include extensive infiltration of the bronchial and bronchiolar walls with lymphocytes, mononuclears and usually large numbers of eosinophils, accumulation of dense mucous exudate in the lumens, as well as in the epithelial cells which produce it, and frequently an astonishing hyaline thickening of the bronchial basement membranes. The mucus sometimes condenses in peculiar spiral strings called Curschmann's spirals. There is marked secondary emphysema.

Asthma is chiefly a human disease, but it has possibly occurred in cattle and certainly, though rarely, in cats and dogs. In the latter, it has been produced artificially in experimental work. Attacks are relieved by epinephrine and similar drugs in dogs and cats, as in humans, a fact which affords further evidence of the similarity of the disease in the different species. The sensitizing allergens have not been adequately studied in veterinary medicine.

PNEUMONITIS, PNEUMONIA

Pneumonitis can properly refer to any inflammatory disease of the lungs but with many persons it carries the special implication of a more or less chronic reaction in which a prominent part is taken by fibroblasts of the interstitial tissue and the lining cells of the alveoli (reticulo-endothelial cells, epithelioid cells, septal cells). The term pneumonia is usually reserved to apply to one of the acute infectious inflammations with copious exudate filling the alveoli.

Acute inflammation of the lung, which is **pneumonia, occurs** in all species but from a variety of causes. In practically all instances the **gross** and **microscopic lesions** are (to the diagnostician) disconcertingly similar regardless of what particular bacterium or virus was the cause.

It is traditional and somewhat advantageous to consider the disease in four successive stages, congestion, red hepatization, gray hepatization and resolution, although there certainly are no clear demarcations between any of these stages. The classical **stage of congestion** involves what we have defined as active hyper-

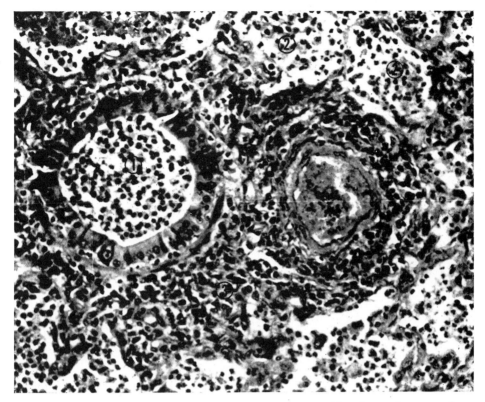

FIG. 21–3.—Pneumonia associated with equine rhinopneumonitis. Lung of a young horse (× 280). Mononuclear and polymorphonuclear cells fill the bronchioles (*1*), alveoli (*2*), and interstitial stroma (*3*). (Courtesy of Armed Forces Institute of Pathology.) Contributor: Army Veterinary Research Laboratory.

emia (p. 130) plus inflammatory edema (p. 136). The capillaries are distended with blood, and the alveoli are filled with serous fluid (recognized microscopically by a pink-staining, homogeneous precipitate). The fluid is really a serous inflammatory exudate (p. 153), as has been previously stated, but custom decrees the term edema. When the cause is a chemical irritant, this stage is attained in less than two minutes after its application. (See injection of chloroform under Serous Inflammation, p. 154.) When the cause is an infectious agent, its development requires a very few hours.

In the **stage of red hepatization,** the affected area of lung is consolidated or hepatized so that it has about the same degree of firmness as liver tissue (*hepar*, liver). Completely hepatized lung tissue sinks in water. It is still red because of a certain amount of hemorrhage by diapedesis (p. 119) into the alveoli. While a considerable quantity of serous fluid may still remain in the alveoli, the hepatization results from the filling of the alveoli with a cellular exudate, mixed, in some cases, with fibrin. With the erythrocytes there are neutrophils, lymphocytes and large mononuclear cells, the proportions depending upon the type and virulence of the causative agent. This stage of pneumonia is reached in about two days.

The **stage of gray hepatization** follows. The lung tissue is still hepatized. Perhaps, instead of really gray we should consider it merely less red than it was

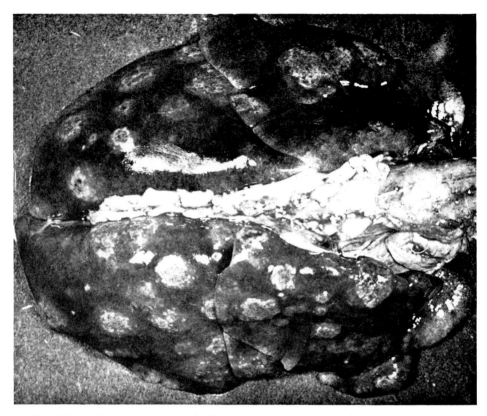

FIG. 21–4.—Purulent pneumonia in the lungs of a one-year-old female tortoiseshell cat.
(Courtesy of Angell Memorial Animal Hospital.)

earlier. Microscopically, the hyperemia is somewhat less in evidence and the erythrocytes have disappeared from the alveolar contents, giving way to white cells and fibrin. The proportions of the different components of the exudate vary, chiefly with the causative organisms. If pyogenic bacteria are prominent invaders, the exudate consists largely of polymorphonuclear neutrophils, and we speak of a purulent pneumonia. In human lobar pneumonia, the causative organism is *Diplococcus pneumoniae* and the exudate is almost exclusively fibrinous. A predominantly fibrinous pneumonia is seen once in a great while in animals, but we are not prepared to generalize as to the causative infection. In a considerable proportion of animal pneumonias, the predominant reactive cell is a large cell with a rounded central nucleus and a rather extensive cytoplasm. Some of these must be monocytes from the blood, others doubtless come from the reticulo-endothelial system and there is considerable evidence that many, perhaps a majority, are descendants of proliferating cells of the lining of the alveolus, which most histologists consider to be simple squamous epithelium. Partly because of this presumed origin and partly because they often bear a startling resemblance to individualized epithelial cells, they often go by the name of **epithelioid cells.** Avoiding the issue of histological origin, the name "septal cells" has been used by some. Regardless of their origin, these cells serve as macrophages and probably have other functions characteristic of reticulo-endothelial cells. A goodly number of lymphocytes are usually mixed with any of the other types.

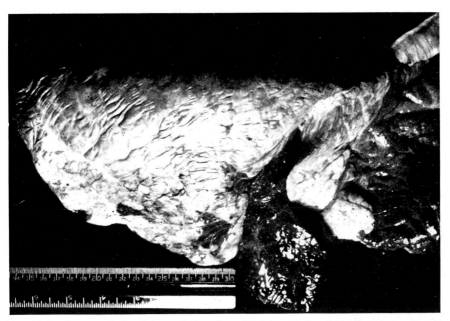

FIG. 21–5.—Pneumonia involving apical and cardial lobes of the right lung of a male calf, four months of age. *Pasteurella spp.* was isolated from the affected lobes.

In favorable cases, the **stage of resolution** supervenes in about a week after the onset of pneumonia. The invading pathogens having been overcome and destroyed, and, the hyperemia having subsided, the cells and fibrin which filled the alveoli are gradually but rather rapidly liquefied, it is believed, by lytic substances produced by neutrophils. In a matter of a very few days, the material which filled the alveoli is coughed up as a semi-solid material or drained away by the veins and lymphatics in a completely liquefied state. The lining cells of the alveoli, most of which perished during the inflammatory period, are regenerated within a few days and the lung returns to morphological, and soon thereafter, functional normality.

As a general concept, it is well to think of any pneumonia, or any given pneumonic area of lung, as passing through these successive stages. It must be recognized, however, that some pneumonias, especially those caused by viruses, show little tendency toward suppuration and tend to terminate, either by recovery or by death, from toxicity without advancing beyond a stage of sero-fibrinous exudate ("edema") accompanied by a limited number of septal or epithelioid cells.

Along with these fundamental exudative changes several other features require attention. While pneumonia itself is a reaction taking place in the alveoli and their walls, the interlobular septa and other connective tissue structures are also distended with exudate, especially with the serous fluid. There is usually, but not always a discernible bronchitis in the pneumonic area. This is recognized by desquamation and disappearance of the epithelial lining cells, by an infiltration of lymphocytes and other leukocytes in the wall of the bronchus or bronchiole and an accumulation of exudate, usually polymorphonuclear, in the lumen. However, if a bronchial lumen contains pus or other exudate while the epithelium and wall still appear normal, it may be concluded that the exudate came from some other area, the bronchus merely serving as a drainage way.

The pleura over the pneumonic area may or may not share in the inflammatory process. If pleuritis (see below) is present the exudate is usually fibrinous or fibrino-purulent on its surface and the causative organism or secondary invaders can be isolated there.

In some pneumonias, it is only in the immediate vicinity of the bronchi and bronchioles that the inflammatory changes and consolidation are in evidence, the infection having entered by the bronchial route. Such a form is known as **peribronchial** pneumonia, or even as **peribronchitis** and peribronchiolitis. This can scarcely be because of the mildness of the case, for many of them come to autopsy. It seems more logical that they be considered cases in which death from a bronchogenous infection came at an early stage.

In the vicinity of the pneumonic changes, there are almost sure to be areas of atelectasis and areas of emphysema (see below). The former are due to plugging by masses of exudate of the bronchioles which served them. The emphysema involves alveoli which expand unduly because of decreased space occupied by neighboring alveoli which are either atelectatic or consolidated.

Unfortunately the prompt and complete resolution described above does not always occur and **complications** develop. One of these is the spreading of the pneumonic process to new areas of lung tissue. These must then proceed through the same series of stages, recovery of the patient being delayed by the time required for these stages. This is characteristic of lobular pneumonia (see below) in debilitated individuals. Of considerable import also is the fact that areas of lung adjoining the pneumonic parts usually suffer from marked inflammatory edema, which may represent spread of the pneumonia but which, at any rate, interferes seriously with pulmonary function.

With delayed resolution in a given area, certain **chronic changes** may develop. The alveolar lining cells, normally flat and inconspicuous, may undergo hyperplasia and resemble cuboidal epithelium. Their nuclei are very dark and the cells are conspicuous, sometimes being known as **cells of Tripier**. The condition has also been called **fetalization** of the lining cells, since they resemble those of the fetal lung. In Marsh's ovine chronic progressive pneumonia (p. 1112) this change becomes extreme, so that the area of lung may strikingly resemble an adenoma.

If a fibrinous or partially fibrinous exudate remains long (two or three weeks) in the alveoli the same thing happens that occurs when fibrin persists in a thrombus or in a fibrinous exudate (p. 156) elsewhere: The fibrin is organized by fibroblasts which build into it from surrounding tissues. Such an area is then converted permanently into fibrous tissue, a process known as **carnification** (*carno, carnis*, flesh).

The **distribution** and **extent of lesions** deserve attention. From statements in the preceding description, it will be inferred that the areas of pneumonic consolidation do not necessarily involve a major portion of the pulmonary tissue, and this is true. It is unusual for more than a third of the total of the two lungs to be hepatized and frequently the process is much more limited. In the great majority of pneumonias, which are bronchogenous in origin, the anterior and ventral portions of the lungs are first and most extensively affected. These are the apical and cardiac lobes in those species whose lungs are divided into lobes. Evidence indicates that this is because infective particles, when inhaled, fall most readily into the bronchial system of these lobes. The pneumonic process commonly progresses centrally in these lobes and may eventually involve the anterior part of the diaphragmatic lobes, not to mention the intermediate lobe in species which have it. The disease may be localized in one lung but more frequently it attacks both.

There are two routes by which pathogenic organisms may enter the lungs, via the bronchi, the **bronchogenous** route, and via the blood stream, the **hematogenous** route. The former is the more frequent. Coming down the arborization of the bronchial system, it is obvious that infected particles may drop into certain bronchioles and not into others. Around each infected bronchiole, a pneumonic area forms and extends to the limits of the histological lobule supplied by the bronchiole in question. Other lobules become infected in the same way, with the result that the affected portion of the lung is spotted with hepatized and relatively normal lobules in an irregular pattern. This form constitutes **lobular pneumonia.** Since its origin is by way of the bronchial passages, it is also known as **bronchial pneumonia** or bronchopneumonia. While in some instances, infected particles fall or are sucked through a normal bronchial passage way, in other cases the infection and the inflammation spread along the lining of the bronchus, infecting it bit by bit. In this case, the bronchopneumonia is accompanied by bronchitis and bronchiolitis.

Hematogenous pneumonia arises when the blood carries pathogenic organisms to produce, at least temporarily, a condition of septicemia. This happens in the case of certain viral infections, like psittacosis. It also occurs with bacterial septicemias. Pasteurellosis, while often bronchogenous, may reach the lungs in this way as is proven by the fact that the causative organisms often invade the pericardial space, which can be reached in no other way than by the blood. Pneumonia of hematogenous origin may be lobular or it may be **lobar,** meaning that it involves not a lobule here and a lobule there, but that it affects all lobules in a considerable area, even a whole lobe. The term **fibrinous pneumonia** is often used synonymously with lobar pneumonia, but fibrinous describes the character of the exudate rather than the anatomical distribution, and should not be considered as a substitute for the term lobar. The virulence of the invading pathogen is of greater importance than the route by which the pathogen reaches the lung in determining if the resultant pneumonia is lobular or lobar. Many pneumonias arising by the bronchogenous route are lobar in distribution, if the offending organism is highly virulent or the host lacks resistance; in fact many examples of lobar pneumonia in animals are aerogenous in origin.

The distinction between lobar and lobular pneumonia is less important in veterinary than in human medicine, where lobar pneumonia is a specific disease with a specific cause, the *Diplococcus pneumoniae*, a fibrinous reaction and a specific course and treatment. Most pneumonias in animals are lobular.

The **causes** of pneumonia are infections; bacterial, viral and exceptionally fungal. **Chemical irritants,** such as gases like chlorine, sulfur dioxide, mustard gas, and ether vapor used as an anesthetic and various irritating medicinal substances accidentally introduced via the trachea when intended for the esophagus, should be added to the list of causes conditionally. They are frequent inciting causes, but usually they merely produce an area of injury or necrosis with a distinctly limited inflammatory reaction. Inhaled bacteria, finding a fertile field of growth in the injured and debilitated area, then continue the irritation and are responsible for most of the pneumonic process. Chemicals do not reproduce themselves; bacteria multiply indefinitely. Likewise **metazoan parasites** produce an initial injury, the injured area then becoming infected with inhaled bacteria which would not be able to colonize the healthy tissue.

The microorganisms most frequently demonstrated in pneumonic tissues include the following: *Pasteurella multocida*, staphylococci, streptococci, *Corynebacterium pyogenes*, *Pseudomonas aeruginosa* (also known as *Bacillus pyocyaneus*), which affect most mammalian species; *Corynebacterium equi* and *Streptococcus equi* in horses. *Pasteurella multocida* and *Corynebacterium pyogenes* are most prominent in the bovine, ovine, caprine and porcine species. *Hemophilus suis* may be added to the extent that pneumonia develops in some cases of swine influenza. In canines we find streptococci, staphylococci, *Klebsiella sp.* and *Brucella* (*Alcaligenes*) *bronchisepticus*, pneumonias most often being a sequel to the virus of canine distemper. In felines Pasteurella is the usual bacterium, again usually preceded by one of the viruses to which cats are subject. In non-human primates *Pasteurella multocida*, *Diplococcus pneumoniae*, *Salmonella spp.*, *Klebsiella pneumoniae* and staphylococci are frequent causes of pneumonia.

It would be a matter of great diagnostic convenience if a characteristic type of pneumonic reaction could be attributed to each individual causative agent but only a few generalities are possible. In foals a distinctly suppurative exudate with neutrophil polymorphs filling the alveoli is likely to be due to *Corynebacterium equi*. In other hosts a strongly suppurative reaction may be seen at times but can hardly be used to identify the offending pathogen. A reaction that is strongly fibrinous is suggestive of *Pasteurella sp.* although not all *Pasteurella* pneumonias are fibrinous by any means. Streptococcal pneumonias are likely to be fibrinous.

It is possible to make the general statement that pneumonia having a virus as its cause is usually characterized by a serous and mononuclear reaction, whereas most pneumonias of bacterial causation produce an exudate in which the smaller leukocytes and fibrin predominate. A number of viruses, mycoplasma and members of the psittacosis-lymphogranuloma group of agents, either cause pneumonia independently or predispose to one or more of the bacterial invaders so that pneumonia becomes a feature of the typical syndrome produced by them. These include the agents of equine rhinopneumonitis, bovine contagious pleuropneumonia, canine distemper, feline pneumonitis, a contagious mycoplasma pleuropneumonia of pigs and contagious pleuropneumonia of goats. For the most part pneumonias produced by these agents, in the absence of secondary bacterial invaders (and excluding bovine and caprine pleuropneumonia), are not comparable to the exudative lobular and lobar pneumonias described above. Instead the inflammatory reaction is predominantly interstitial and appropriately the lesion is termed **interstitial pneumonia.** Sometimes referred to as **viral pneumonia,** interstitial pneumonia is characterized by exudation within the interalveolar septa. The septa become greatly thickened by infiltrating lymphocytes, macrophages, and plasma cells, the accumulation of serum or fibrin, and by an increase in connective tissue fibers. Hyperplasia of alveolar lining cells (p. 1104) is a frequent finding. Exudation of neutrophils into the alveoli is not a usual feature, however free lining cells and macrophages may occupy the alveoli. In some infections, such as canine distemper, measles and parainfluenza-3 in calves, multinucleated giants cells are a component of the exudate in the septa and the alveolar lumens. Focal accumulation of lymphocytes often producing distinct nodules with germinal centers is a feature of many interstitial pneumonias such as in swine, calves, sheep and rats caused by mycoplasmas and chlamydiae.

Chilling of the body or a part of it lowers resistance and predisposes to pneumonia as it does to other respiratory infections. Extreme fatigue and severe hunger lower resistance to most infections, respiratory as well as others. How chilling and fatigue lower resistance is somewhat of a mystery; but how often have most of us associated our own "colds" (or other afflictions) with wet feet, a chill, or being tired?

Effects.—Many cases of pneumonia are fatal. The pneumonia may be accompanied by morbid changes in other organs, as, for instance, in pasteurellosis (p. 608). When the pulmonary disease alone is responsible for death, it may occur because too many of the alveoli are filled and unable to do their part in aerating the blood. This happens especially if non-hepatized areas are in a state of congestion and edema, conditions which also prevent the erythrocytes from getting and purveying oxygen. However, pneumonia is often fatal with very considerable portions of the lung tissue still functional. In such cases, death is attributed to toxic effects from the microorganisms and their products.

Bronchiectasis and carnification have been mentioned as unfavorable sequelae. In a few cases in which the invading organisms belong to the pyogenic group and are of high virulence, **abscesses** may form in the hepatized tissue. More frequently, however, pulmonary abscesses are of embolic origin in an otherwise healthy lung. In a few other pneumonias from non-pyogenic pathogens of high virulence, areas of tissue are killed by the toxins produced and gangrene results, but pulmonary gangrene usually has other causes.

Special Types of Pneumonia.—A number of types of pneumonia commonly receive special recognition because of peculiar characteristics.

Embolic pneumonia is characterized by numerous pneumonic foci which are rather evenly scattered through all lobes of both lungs, the greatest number of foci being near the pleural surface until they become confluent and their site of origin becomes obscured. The sub-pleural location is attributable to the fact that this area contains the largest proportion of small arteries and arterioles in which an embolus may be lodged. In contrast, the hematogenous pneumonia which accompanies septicemic diseases is diffuse. However, it is more frequent that lodged emboli produce individualized abscesses (rarely other types of reaction, such as specific granulomas) rather than areas of hepatization. Microscopically, embolic pneumonia can be seen in its earlier stages to differ from bronchopneumonia in that the foci spread out from blood vessels and not from bronchi.

Verminous pneumonia is another form in which there is departure from the usual antero-ventral distribution of lesions. In verminous pneumonia, the diaphragmatic lobes have their full share of pneumonic areas because these depend upon the localization of the worms. The larvae of ascarid worms pass through the lungs, especially in swine, but may leave only negligible lesions (p. 734). The inflamed areas in verminous pneumonia are usually small, scattered and in different chronological stages, a fact of diagnostic value. The adult nematodes are usually found in the bronchi and bronchioles where they incite a mucopurulent bronchitis. However, the exact site of localization of the adult nematodes varies between lungworms. The more common lungworms and site of localization are listed on page 766. Their embryonated ova or larvae are conspicuous in the bronchial exudate, with which they leave the lungs for the extraneous part of their existence. True pneumonic lesions develop when the tissue which the worms have injured is attacked by inspired pathogens from the throat region. Each individual inflammatory focus, small, large or perhaps confluent, thus has the usual characteristics of bronchopneumonia, some of the usual organisms being demonstrable. However, there is considerable tendency to chronicity, not only through the consecutive development of different foci, but also within the individual lesions. These heal with difficulty or not at all until the worm lives its life-span and disappears (several weeks), and there is often considerable reaction of the foreign-body type (p. 177) and fibrous encapsulation. In the meantime, an extensive and fatal bacterial pneumonia may or may not develop.

Gangrenous pneumonia is in veterinary medicine almost synonymous with what is variously called **aspiration pneumonia, foreign-body pneumonia, medication pneumonia, lipid pneumonia** and others of similar import. As previously stated it is possible for some pneumonia-producing pathogens of high virulence to kill tissue outright, which then becomes subject to invasion by putrefactive saprophytes thus fulfilling the specifications of gangrene, but such cases are rare. Pulmonary embolism and infarction with saprophytic invasion of the dead infarct are also possible but rare.

The usual cause of gangrenous pneumonia is the introduction into the lungs of medicines intended for the esophagus. Henceforth, what happens is largely dependent on the nature and quantity of the material introduced. Many drugs are highly irritant and entirely capable of producing necrosis of the pulmonary tissue, which is much less resistant than the mucus-protected lining of the stomach. Oily drugs are especially harmful, not because of their immediately irritating properties but because the oil, especially mineral oil, is not capable of being absorbed and cannot be eliminated. In any case, these medicines are not sterile, nor is the pharyngeal mucosa over which they pass. We thus have an irritant chemical substance and a rather massive concentration of various kinds of bacteria in the same place. The result is very often, but not invariably, necrosis of the area followed by gangrene (p. 26). In animals whose cough reflexes are impaired by anesthesia, paralysis or coma, there is always the possibility of aspiration of drops of exudate, particles of food or vomitus. Indeed whole grains, heads of wheat or parts of ears of corn are occasionally found in the lungs of the herbivorous animals. These usually carry high concentrations of bacteria of many kinds. Gangrene of the area involved is a common result, preceded by a very intense inflammation.

The definitive lesion of gangrenous pneumonia is death of tissue. It is accompanied by intense hyperemia and exudative and even hemorrhagic inflammation in the surrounding living tissue. The dead tissue soon liquefies (liquefaction necrosis) so that it can almost be said that the characteristic lesion is cavitation. Like other necrotic tissue, the remaining dead tissue may be white or black depending on the amount of blood in it. As putrefying bacteria multiply, foul odors appear. The liquefied material may be of pasty consistency at one stage but ultimately becomes entirely fluid. These changes are commonly well established in a course of two or three days, although death may come earlier. Very few victims recover.

Hypostatic Pneumonia.—Hypostatic congestion has been described (p. 132). The porous nature of pulmonary tissue is especially conducive to hypostatic congestion, as a result of which edema (p. 134) of the area is likely to develop.

Tissue devitalized by these two circulatory disorders may well fall prey to inhaled upper respiratory pathogens which would be promptly destroyed in a healthy lung. Pneumonia thus develops, in recumbent patients, in the lower parts of the lower lung as a feature, all too frequently terminal, of many diseases.

Pneumonitis.—There is considerable diversity in the use of this term, which literally means an inflammation of the lungs. In general, it has been used for inflammatory conditions of the lung to which one hesitates to apply the term pneumonia. The latter, we have already described in the classical way as an acute exudative filling of the lung alveoli, clinically with a rather typical febrile course. Many consider the term pneumonitis synonymous with interstitial pneumonia (p. 1106). While this is quite acceptable, we find that due to the inconsistencies in the use of the term, it is best avoided.

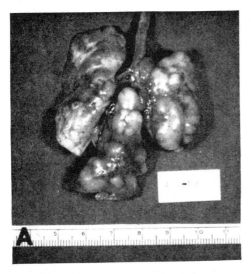

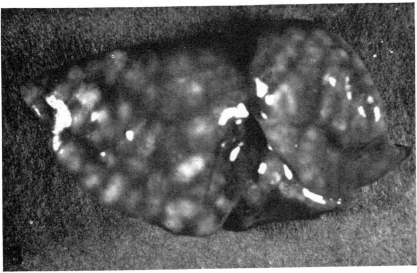

Fig. 21–6.—Chronic murine pneumonia, rat. *A*, Bronchiectatic nodules. *B*, Focal consolidation. (Courtesy of Animal Research Center, Harvard Medical School.)

Granulomatous Pneumonia.—There are a group of infectious organisms which often localize in the lung which do not induce pneumonia comparable to the acute exudative pneumonias nor interstitial pneumonias already described. These include many of the higher bacteria and fungi. Although tuberculous pneumonia occurs rarely as an acute febrile pulmonary inflammation which is clinically and pathologically much like the pneumonia already described, the usual tuberculous involvement of the lung is a very different matter; having a much slower course and being characterized by granulomatous rather than exudative lesions. This latter is well termed tuberculous pneumonia.

In the same group are the other granulomatous infections as they involve the lungs, actinomycosis, actinobacillosis, coccidioidomycosis, histoplasmosis, glanders, chronic aspergillosis, the usual chronic form of blastomycosis and rarely mucormycosis and others. *Blastomyces dermatitidis* occasionally causes diffuse pneumonia in the dog, although granulomatous lesions are more usual.

Known collectively as the **pneumoconioses** (p. 62) (*konis*, dust), chronic inflammatory reactions to several inhaled mineral contaminants constitute forms of granulomatous pneumonia. Such substances include various dusts from mines, quarries, grinding, sand-blasting and other industries, the most formidable being silica (SiO_2), beryllium and asbestos. Bauxite (impure Al_2O_3), graphite and carbon are less important. Considerable quantities inhaled over a period of time are necessary to cause important disease, but eventual fatalities are not uncommon. The reaction to silicon dioxide is typically in the form of dense fibrous nodules, the condition being known as **silicosis. Asbestosis** is characterized by a more cellular and a more diffuse reaction and by "asbestos bodies" which can be found microscopically in the lesions. These are brownish, club-shaped filaments bearing some resemblance in size and shape to the broken mycelial filaments seen in mucormycosis (p. 666). The "beryllium granuloma" resembles a non-caseating tubercle, even showing Langhans' giant cells. Asteroid inclusion bodies of unique appearance are occasionally seen in the giant cells. The pneumoconioses are largely limited to humans and experimental animals for the reason that the domestic animals are seldom exposed to the dusts which cause them. Horses and mules used in quarries and mines are subject to the same atmospheric contamination as the men and develop the same lesions, but such use of draft animals is largely past. The dust pneumonia of pigs belongs with the acute pneumonias. Anthracosis is frequent in dogs required to sleep in coal bins.

Trachea, Bronchi, Lungs

ANDRADE DOS SANTOS, J., and MILANEZ, F. R.: Broncopneumonia por Tecido Vegetal em Bovino. Arq. Inst. Biol. Animal. 2:3–13, 1959, Ministerio da Agricultura, Brasil.
BETTS, A. O.: *Ascaris lumbricoides* as a Cause of Pneumonia in Pigs. Vet. Rec. 66:749–751, 1954.
DUNCAN, J. R., RAMSEY, F. K., and SWITZER, W. P.: Pathology of Experimental *Bordetella bronchiseptica* Infection in Swine: Pneumonia. Am. J. Vet. Res. 27:467–472, 1966.
EGGERT, M. J., and ROMBERG, P. F.: Pulmonary Aspergillosis in a Calf. J. Am. Vet. Med. Assn. 137:595–596, 1960.
FARRELL, R. K., LEADER, R. W., and GORHAM, J. R.: An Outbreak of Hemorrhagic Pneumonia in Mink. Cornell Vet. 48:378–384, 1958.
FORD, T. M.: An Outbreak of Pneumonia in Laboratory Rats Associated with *Diplococcus pneumoniae* Type 8. Lab. Anim. Care 15:448–451, 1965.
FULTON, J. S., BURTON, A. N., and MILLAR, J. L.: Virus Pneumonia in Swine. J. Am. Vet. Med. Assn. 123:221–224, 1953.

GOTO, M.: Pathological Studies on So-Called Bovine Influenza. Jap. J. Vet. Sci. *21*: 123–130, 153–160, 1959. (Engl. summary.) Abstr. Vet. Bull., No. 1419, 1960.

HAGEN, K. W.: Enzootic Pasteurellosis in Domestic Rabbits. I. Pathology and Bacteriology. J. Am. Vet. Med. Assn. *133*:77–80, 1958.

HAMDY, A. H., and POUNDEN, W. D.: Experimental Production of Pneumonia in Lambs. Am. J. Vet. Res. *20*:78–83, 1959.

HOERLEIN, A. B., and MARSH, C. L.: Studies on the Epizootology of Shipping Fever in Calves. J. Am. Vet. Med. Assn. *131*:123–127, 1957.

JOSHI, N. N., BOACKWOOD, A. C., and DALE, D. G.: Chronic Murine Pneumonia: A Review. Canad. J. Comp. Med. *25*:267–273, 1961.

MACKENZIE, A.: Pathological Changes in Lungworm Infestation in Two Cats with Special Reference to Changes in Pulmonary Arterial Branches. Res. Vet. Sci. *1*:255–259, 1960.

McKERCHER, D. G.: Feline Pneumonitis. Am. J. Vet. Res. *13*:557–561, 1952.

NIELSEN, S. W.: Comparative Pathology of Pulmonary Diseases *in The Lung*, Chapter 15, pp. 226–244, Int. Acad. Path. Monograph No. 8, Baltimore, The Williams & Wilkins Co. 1967.

NEWBERNE, P. M., SALMON, W. D., and HARE, W. V.: Chronic Murine Pneumonia in an Experimental Laboratory. Arch. Path. *72*:224–233, 1961.

OMAR, A. R.: The Aetiology and Pathology of Pneumonia in Calves. Vet. Bull. *36*: 259–273, 1966.

ROBERTS, E. D., SWITZER, W. P., and L'ECUYER, C.: Influence of Pasteurella multocida and Mycoplasma hyorhinis (PPLO) on the Histopathology of Field Cases of Swine Pneumonia. Cornell Vet. *52*:306–326, 1962.

TRAUTWEIN, G., HEMBOLDT, C. F., and NIELSEN, S. W.: Pathology of Pseudomonas Pneumonia in Mink. J. Am. Vet. Med. Assn. *140*:701–704, 1962.

WAYT, L. K.: Experimental Stenosis of the Pulmonary Artery in Calves. Am. J. Vet. Res. *20*:265–269, 1959.

PULMONARY ADENOMATOSIS

There has long been uncertainty as to the correct histological classification of the cells that line the alveoli of the lungs. According to the comprehensive review by Omar (1964), electron microscopy assists us to the conclusion that the alveoli have a continuous lining of epithelial cells and that scattered below these there are smaller "septal" cells from which reactive proliferation causes the development of the large round cells of reticulo-endothelial appearance so frequently seen in many inflammatory states. At any rate, these lining cells may be released into the alveolar lumen or remain to form a very hyperplastic lining which, in extreme cases, has the appearance of simple cuboidal or even columnar epithelium, often forming papillary projections. (See also, "fetalization," p. 1104.) The histological resemblance of such extreme areas to an adenoma tempts one to place a neoplastic interpretation upon them, hence the term, pulmonary adenomatosis. Adenomatous metastases in the regional lymph nodes have been reported. This adenomatous change is pronounced in many (but not all) cases of jaagsiekte and to a lesser degree in Marsh's ovine progressive pneumonia. Similar changes are seen in various chronic inflammations of the lung, including verminous pneumonia and toxoplasmosis (p. 684); they have even been found in sheep pox and in guinea pigs inoculated with non-specific pneumonia-producing organisms. They may accompany pulmonary emphysema of cattle (p. 1124). A case of "pulmonary adenomatosis" has also been reported in a horse (Mahaffey, 1962) and the late C. L. Davis contributed a case to the Army Institute of Pathology (now Armed Forces Institute of Pathology) in which lesions comparable to jaagsiekte were present in a goat. Pulmonary adenomatosis has also been described in mice (Horn, *et al.*, 1952), opossums (Sherwood, *et al.*, 1969), and chinchillas (Helmboldt, *et al.*, 1958).

Thus adenomatosis is encountered in a variety of species and under varied circumstances. On one extreme, in jaagsiekte, adenomatosis represents the principal lesion of the disease, it may metastasize and is best considered neoplastic, while at the other end of the scale in diseases such as toxoplasmosis or chronic exudative pneumonias, it is only one aspect of the pulmonary disease and is best considered a proliferative inflammatory reaction.

Pulmonary Adenomatosis—General

BELL, E. T.: Hyperplasia of the Pulmonary Alveolar Epithelium in Disease. Amer. J. Path. *19*:901–907, 1943.

BENSLEY, R. D., and BENSLEY, S. H.: Studies of the Lining of the Pulmonary Alveolus of Normal Lungs of Adult Animals. Anat. Rec. *64*:41–49, 1935–36.

COWDRY, E. V., and MARSH, H.: Comparative Pathology of South African Jaagziekte and Montana Progressive Pneumonia of Sheep. J. Exper. Med. *45*:571–586, 1927.

DURAN-REYNALS, F., *et al.*: The Pulmonary Adenomatosis Complex in Sheep. Ann. New York Acad. Sci. *70*:726–742, 1958. (A Review.)

GEEVER, E. F., NEUBUERGER, K. T., and DAVIS, C. L.: The Pulmonary Alveolar Lining under Various Pathologic Conditions in Man and Animals. Amer. J. Path. *19*:913–937, 1943.

HELMBOLDT, C. F., JUNGHERR, E. L., and CAPARO, A. C.: Pulmonary Adenomatosis in the Chinchilla. Am. J. Vet. Res. *19*:270–276, 1958.

HORN, H., CONGDON, C., and STEWART, H. L.: Pulmonary Adenomatosis in Mice. J. Nat. Cancer Inst. *12*:1297–1315, 1952.

DE KOCK, G.: The Transformation of the Lining of the Pulmonary Alveoli with Special Reference to Adenomatosis in the Lungs (Jaagziekte) of Sheep. Am. J. Vet. Res. *19*:261–269, 1958.

MAHAFFEY, L. W.: Respiratory Conditions in Horses. Vet. Rec. *74*:(No. 47):1295–1314, 1962.

NORRIS, R. F.: Pulmonary Adenomatosis Resembling Jaagziekte in the Guinea Pig. Arch. Path. *43*:553–558, 1947.

OMAR, A. R.: The Characteristic Cells of the Lung and their Reaction to Injury. Vet. Bull. *34*:371–382, 431–443, 1964.

PEGREFFI, G., MURA, D., and CONTINI, A.: La pleuropulmonite contagiosa degli ovini da microorganismi del gruppo pleuropulmonite contagiosa (P.P.L.O.). Atti Soc. Ital. Sci. Vet., (Rimini-Ravenna. 1957.) *11*:829–833, 1958. Abstr. Vet. Bull. No. 3905, 1958.

PIEROTTI, P.: Adenomatosi Polmonare del Cavallo. Atti. Soc. Ital. Sci. Vet. *14*:356–358, 1960.

SHERWOOD, B. F., ROWLANDS, D. T., JR., and HACKEL, D. B.: Pulmonary Adenomatosis in Opossums (*Didelphis virginiana*). J. Am. Vet. Med. Assn. *155*:1102–1107, 1969.

SIMON, M. A.: So-Called Pulmonary Adenomatosis and "Alveolar Cell Tumors." Amer. J. Path. *23*:413–427, 1947.

STEWART, H. L.: Pulmonary Cancer and Adenomatosis in Captive Wild Mammals and Birds from the Philadelphia Zoo. J. Nat. Cancer Inst. *36*:117–138, 1966.

SWAN, L. L.: Pulmonary Adenomatosis of Man. Arch. Path. *47*:517–544, 1949.

MARSH'S OVINE PROGRESSIVE PNEUMONIA

This slowly progressing and eventually fatal pulmonary disease is characterized by little or sometimes no exudate in the alveoli. Instead, the interalveolar septa are rather uniformly thickened with a limited amount of fibrous tissue and infiltrated with many lymphocytes and somewhat larger mononuclear cells belonging to the reticulo-endothelial group. In the peribronchial zones, there are heavy concentrations of these cells. Even more conspicuous are areas of young lymphocytes which represent hyperplastic proliferation (see Hyperplastic Inflammation, p. 169) of the lymph nodules which normally are inconspicuous in this location, although they are somewhat more prominent in sheep than in other species. The peribronchiolar smooth muscle is also markedly increased. In many cases, the lining cells of the alveoli are hypertrophic, resembling cuboidal epithelium, the

Maedi

RESSANG, A. A., STAM, F. C., and DEBOER, G. F.:   A Meningo-Leucoencephalomyelitis
Resembling Visna in Dutch Zwoeger Sheep. Path. Vet. *3*:401–411, 1966.
SIGURDSSON, B.:   Maedi, a Slow Progressive Pneumonia of Sheep; an Epizoological and
Pathological Study. Brit. Vet. J. *110*:255–270, 1954.
————————:   Adenomatosis of Sheep's Lungs. Experimental Transmission. Arch. Ges.
Virusforsch. *8*:51–58, 1958. Abstr. Vet. Bull., No. 2923, 1958.
SIGURDSSON, B., GRIMSSON, H., and PALSSON, P. A.:   Maedi, a Chronic Progressive Infection
of Sheep's Lungs. J. Infect. Dis. *90*:233–241, 1952.

PLEURITIS

Inflammation of the pleura is known as pleuritis or by the older name of
pleurisy. The ordinary forms of pleuritis belong to the acute exudative inflammations, usually being either serous, fibrinous or purulent. If the pleuritis accompanies pneumonia, the pleuritic area overlies the hepatized portions of lung
parenchyma, the condition being called **pleuropneumonia.** But there are many
cases of pneumonia without pleuritis, and it is entirely possible for pleuritis to
exist without pneumonia. The pulmonary pleura is first involved, as a rule,
but the infection and the inflammatory reaction promptly spread to the contiguous areas of parietal pleura.

The usual attack of pleurisy begins with acute hyperemia and swelling of the
thin covering membrane. During this stage, the friction of the visceral and
parietal surfaces at each respiratory movement is very painful, causing a typical
type of breathing. After about two days a serous exudate appears, which lubri-
cates and separates the two surfaces, and the pain is assuaged. The exudate
may remain serous, filling the pleural cavity and compressing the lungs, or it
may become fibrinous or purulent. Often all forms co-exist resulting in a sero-
fibrino-purulent pleuritis. Microscopically, the pleural layer is infiltrated with
lymphocytes and other inflammatory cells. Its thickness is increased several
fold by edema fluid which fills the intercellular spaces and distends the numerous
but previously unseen lymph vessels. Capillaries are numerous and greatly
dilated. The surface layer of mesothelial cells is largely destroyed and the surface
is covered with a thin or thick layer of fibrin or with adherent dead neutrophils
and other elements characteristic of a purulent exudate.

With the lapse of a few days the amount of sero-purulent exudate collecting
in the pleural cavity may become so great as to interfere seriously with expansion
of the lungs, requiring drainage by thoracocentesis. In such cases, the exudate
is very likely to become fibrinous, depending largely on the kind of organism
which is causing it. The layers of fibrin on each of the two apposing surfaces
tend to become organized by immigrating fibroblasts and the two surfaces often
become tied together by strands of fibrous connective tissue. These are known
as **adhesions**; the inflammatory process is then called **adhesive pleuritis.** It is
not unusual to find large areas of lung surface inseparably joined to the chest wall.
Most animals so affected die while the process is still active. Some survive the
causative infection with adhesions of limited extent. These adhesions cause
pain with respiratory movement, but this diminishes as the anatomical structures
adjust themselves. There is no permanent disability in most cases.

The **causes** of pleuritis are always infectious and, in general, they are the same
kinds of organisms which cause pneumonia. Infection of the pleura may result
by direct extension from the lung, but many cases of pleuritis arise by the hema-

togenous route without involvement of the lungs, especially in septicemic diseases of young animals. An important variant is seen in those bovines in which a swallowed metallic foreign body penetrates from the reticulum into the pleural cavity, carrying infection with it. A majority of these, however, penetrate the pericardium and produce "traumatic pericarditis" rather than pleuritis. **Tuberculous pleuritis** is a fairly common accompaniment of tuberculosis of other parts. It manifests itself as "**pearly disease,**" in which pleural surfaces, especially those of the thoracic wall, become studded with protruding, irregularly spherical tubercles, dense, white and shiny and thus reminiscent of pearls. They commonly approximate a diameter of 3 to 10 mm. Tuberculous infection may be hematogenous or it may be a direct extension from a tuberculous lung or possibly from a thoracic lymph node. In swine pleuritis is part of a generalized serositis in two infections, Glasser's disease (p. 590) caused by *Hemophilus suis* and a serositis (p. 522), caused by mycoplasma.

A considerable accumulation of purulent exudate (pus) in the pleural cavity is known as **empyema. Hydrothorax** denotes accumulation of (non-inflammatory) edema fluid in the pleural cavity. The watery fluid has the low specific gravity (1.017 or less) and the low protein content (4 per cent or less) characteristic of a transudate (p. 137). Hydrothorax is one of the manifestations of generalized edema, usually cardiac or renal (p. 138). **Chylothorax** denotes the presence of chyle in the pleural cavity. This rare condition results from rupture or erosion of the thoracic duct. The chyle has a milky appearance. However, it is possible for edema fluid or serous exudate to appear milky from a high content of emulsified fat or albumin. Exudates may also accompany intrathoracic neoplasms. **Pneumothorax** is a rare condition in which air gains access to the pleural cavity. This may occur through a rupture of the chest wall, or through rupture of an emphysematous "bulla" or of some other air-containing lesion of the lung. There are pain and dyspnea, and if the entrance of air is considerable, the lung on the affected side is collapsed and unable to function, since it is only a surrounding negative pressure in the thoracic cavity that causes the lung to expand at inspiration. In the horse, such an accident is likely to be fatal, for the right and left pleural cavities usually communicate and the pneumothorax becomes bilateral. Cases are on record, nevertheless, where penetrating thoracic wounds have been followed by recovery.

Among the non-inflammatory disorders which may involve the lung, congestion, edema, infarction, thrombosis and embolism have been treated at the appropriate places in the section on General Pathology.

Hemorrhages, usually recent, but sometimes old, with clotted fibrin occur in the lungs not only from septicemias and the other causes listed in the discussion of hemorrhage (p. 119), but also as a result of uremia, presumably because of toxic injury to capillary walls. This may be an important explanation of the hemorrhages of leptospirosis.

While the lungs share in any generalized **passive congestion,** usually acute and terminal, due to a failing heart muscle, it will be remembered that the usual chronic passive congestion is a result of interference with the prompt passage of blood through the left side of the heart. The resulting brown induration (p. 72) with its "heart-failure cells" due to phagocytized hemosiderin has been described. The possibility of hypostatic pneumonia supervening was mentioned under that heading. Besides the local effects, there is generalized anoxia over the body,

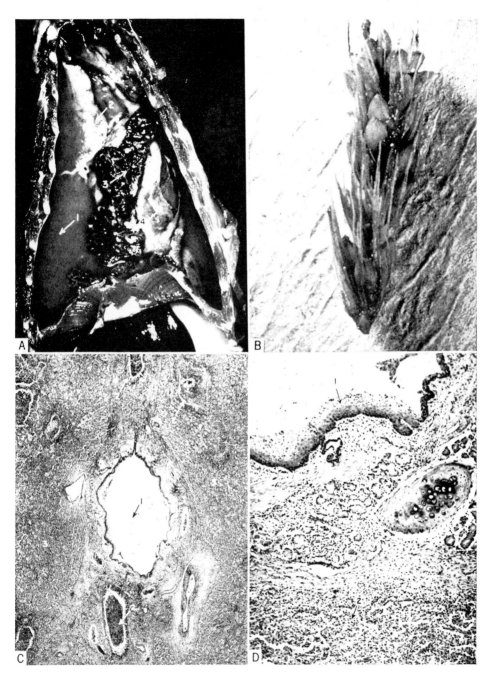

FIG. 21–8.—Pyothorax and pneumonia secondary to aspiration of a grass awn by a male cat, age one and one half years. *A*, The thorax at necropsy, containing purulent fluid (*1*), fibrinous exudate in mediastinum (*3*) and fibrinous exudate on pericardium (*4*). *B*, Grass awn found in major bronchus at necropsy. *C*, Bronchus (*1*) in which the grass awn was found, secondary bronchi (*2*) and alveoli (*3*) are filled with purulent exudate. *D*, Higher magnification of *C*. Squamous metaplasia of bronchial epithelium (*1*) and consolidation (*2*) of alveoli. H & E × 125. (Courtesy of Angell Memorial Animal Hospital.)

which, if severe, leads to lipidosis and related changes in the liver and kidney especially.

In either acute or chronic passive congestion of the lungs, **edema** of those organs develops in accordance with principles elucidated in the study of that subject (p. 134). In those numerous cases in which recent and relatively acute pulmonary congestion and edema are prominent at autopsy, there is always the question whether one is dealing with active hyperemia and inflammatory edema which would have developed into full-fledged pneumonia if the patient had lived a few hours longer. The relative scarcity of pathogenic organisms when such lungs are submitted to bacterial culture suggests that most of these cases are the result of a failing heart rather than pneumonia. The tendency for the accumulation of fluid to be greatest in the more dependent portions of the lungs and the presence of congested vessels elsewhere in the body tend to confirm this interpretation. Acute hypersensitivity reactions may account for pulmonary edema, but in these examples there is diffuse involvement of all lobes. Anaphylaxis is a classic example, but hypersensitivity may also play a role in the pulmonary emphysema-adenomatosis syndrome of cattle (p. 1124).

The gross differentiation of the lung that is congested and edematous from one that is pneumonic may confuse the inexperienced. The former is voluminous with little or no tendency to collapse, well rounded and grayish pink, especially in the dorsal parts of the diaphragmatic lobes. It is doughy and "pits on pressure" but it does yield to pressure of the finger, while the hepatized lung is incompressible save for a slight "give" which lets the finger descend just a bit before it comes to an abrupt standstill. From the cut surface, a watery fluid, clear or blood stained, runs out either freely or upon the application of pressure, depending on the degree of severity. The microscopic differentiation is obvious from the nature of the processes involved.

Fibrin **emboli** lodge in the lungs if they are released into the circulation elsewhere but, on the whole, this is a rare accident in veterinary medicine. Fatty emboli are even more rarely recognized. Thrombi form in the vessels of the lungs during the course of severe pneumonias.

As has already been explained (p. 28), **infarction** of the lung is unlikely to occur when the pulmonary and bronchial circulations are of normal force. Large infarcted areas tend to become gangrenous upon the advent of saprophytic bacteria, which are sure to be inhaled from time to time.

ATELECTASIS

This term means failure of the alveoli to open or to remain open; in other words, the empty alveoli are collapsed and do not contain air. The usual atelectasis involves one or more relatively small areas of lung. Such an area is slightly depressed and shrunken as compared to the surrounding tissue, and is sharply demarcated from it. The atelectatic area is dull red in color and has the feeling and consistency which one would expect, for instance, in liver. However, the hepatized tissue of pneumonia is swollen and not shrunken. Atelectatic, as well as hepatized, tissue sinks in water, or almost sinks if it still contains a bit of air. No fluid can be squeezed from its cut surface. Microscopically, the alveoli are compressed into scarcely recognizable slits, all lying parallel in a direction deter-

described as pulmonary adenomatosis (p. 1111). Hyperplasia of bronchiolar epithelium and musculature may also be evident.

Further inquiry is needed to explain the pathogenesis and to determine the causes of the syndrome. Schofield (1948) and others have related the syndrome to the consumption of rape (p. 925), turnip tops and possibly other plants in the *brassica* group. Monlux (1953) reported on a supposed poisoning by spoiled sweet potatoes. Consumption of a number of other plants, especially when growth was unusually lush (Tucker 1962) has been suggested, under apparently well-founded suspicion, as a causative factor. Moldy hays have also been held responsible. The bovine disorder is morphologically similar to silo-filler's disease in man which is recognized as resulting from inhaled nitrogen dioxide. Seaton (1957, 1958) has experimentally caused such lesions by forcing cattle to inhale NO_2 or other oxides of plants, artificially produced. Infestation with the lung-worm *Dictyocaulus viviparous* has also been suggested as a cause. Dickinson and co-workers (1967) have reproduced a similar pathologic picture by injecting large doses of DL-tryptophan. The morphologic similarity to the human malady "farmer's lung" has prompted the concept that the disease in cattle may have an allergic basis. Farmer's lung in man is caused by a hypersensitivity reaction to inhaled spores of *Thermopolyspora polyspora* and possibly other actinomycetes from moldy hays. This similarity lends credence to the incrimination of moldy hays in the bovine disease, and is further supported by the finding of Jenkins and Pepys (1965) that in many cattle which develop respiratory disease after exposure to musty hay, there are antibodies to *T. polyspora*. It may be that of the various theories or causes advanced, all act through a single mechanism based on hyper-sensitivity. Further investigations should answer this hypothesis.

An essentially identical pulmonary disease has been described in sheep by Pascoe and McGavin (1969) in Australia.

Pulmonary Emphysema-Adenomatosis Syndrome

Anon. "Fog Fever" and Farmer's Lung. Lancet, July 31, 1965. p. 224.

DICKINSON, E. O., SPENCER, G. R., and GORHAM, J. R.: Experimental Induction of an Acute Respiratory Syndrome in Cattle Resembling Bovine Pulmonary Emphysema. Vet. Rec. *80*:487–489, 1967.

JENKINS, P. A., and PEPYS, J.: Fog-Fever. Precipitin (FLH) Reactions to Mouldy Hay. Vet. Rec. 77:464–466, 1965.

KOBAYASHI, M., *et al.*: Antigens in Moldy Hay as the Cause of Farmer's Lung. Proc. Soc. Exp. Biol. N. Y. *113*:472–476, 1963.

LOWRY, T., and SCHUMAN, L. M.: Silo-Filler's Disease.—A Syndrome Caused by Nitrogen Dioxide. J. Amer. Med. Assn. *162*:153–160, 1956.

MONLUX, W., FITTE, J., KENDRICK, G., and DUBUISSON, H.: Progressive Pulmonary Adenomatosis in Cattle. Southwestern Vet. 6:267–269 (Spring), 1953.

MOULTON, J. E., HARROLD, J. B., and HORNING, M. A.: Pulmonary Emphysema in Cattle. J. Am. Vet. Med. Assn. *139*:669–677, 1961.

OMAR, A. R., and KINCH, D. A.: Atypical Interstitial Pneumonia, A Condition Resembling Fog Fever in Young Calves. Vet. Rec. *78*:766–768, 1966.

PASCOE, R. R.: Atypical Interstitial Pneumonia. Vet. Rec. *85*:376–377, 1969.

PEPYS, J., and JENKINS, P. A.: Precipitin (F.L.H.) Test in Farmer's Lung. Thorax *20*: 21–35, 1965.

SCHOFIELD, F. W.: Acute Pulmonary Emphysema of Cattle. J. Am. Vet. Med. Assn. *112*: 254–259, 1948.

SEATON, V. A.: Pulmonary Adenomatosis in Iowa Cattle. Am. J. Vet. Res. *19*:600–609, 1958.

———: Pulmonary Adenomatosis in Cattle Produced by Nitrogen Dioxide Poisoning. No. Amer. Vet. *33*:109–111, 1957.

TUCKER, J. O., and MAKI, L. R.: Acute Pulmonary Emphysema of Cattle. Experimental Production, Etiology. Am. J. Vet. Res. 23:821–826, 1962.

HEAT EXHAUSTION

(Heat Prostration, Heat Stroke)

Under certain conditions, animals are unable to eliminate sufficient heat to maintain body temperature at a level compatible with life. In the absence of adequate clinical study or a satisfactory history, the pathologist may have difficulty recognizing this syndrome and be at a loss for an adequate explanation of the animal's death. In those instances in which an adequate history is available it will be evident that the animal has been exposed to unusually high heat and humidity, a confined space and some psychological stress (fear, excitement). Often a dog will be bathed at a kennel, placed in a drying cage (or small cage) on a hot, humid day, then found dead an hour or two later. A common story is that the dog was left for a "short time" (usually actually two or more hours) in the back of a station wagon while the mistress (or master) is shopping and the dog is very ill or dead when the shopping is finished. Other cases may involve shipping in a small, poorly-ventilated crate or confinement in a truck, airplane or railroad car in which the temperature and humidity become excessive. Swine may be affected when shipped in hot humid weather or during or after parturition under these conditions. Poorly conditioned horses may also succumb under these conditions. Any animal confined out in hot sun may be affected. Pet monkeys and cats are susceptible to this condition. Failure of a ventilating or cooling system may also be responsible for this syndrome.

The essential signs are very high fever (106° to 110° F.) which may be lowered by cold water or other cooling methods, severe hyperpnea and respiratory distress (dog), severe discomfort, congested mucosae, tachycardia, excitement, collapse and sudden death. Fetuses in pregnant animals (swine) may die *in utero* and be delivered or remain to produce severe metritis.

The **gross lesions** are dominated by severe, generalized hyperemia which is most severe in the respiratory tract, especially in the lungs, tracheal and bronchial mucosae. Lungs may also be edematous and occasionally contain focal consolidations of bronchopneumonia. Other organs, such as heart, kidneys, meninges, lymph nodes and muscles may also be severely congested.

Preexisting heart (dirofilariasis for example) or pulmonary disease (focal pneumonia) may accentuate the effect of heat and may contribute to death of the animal. Unexpectedly extensive autolysis is often evident, particularly in dogs and swine.

The **microscopic lesions** are compatible with those seen grossly. The vasculature of the lungs is severely engorged and edema is evident in alveoli. Centrilobular necrosis, disassociation of hepatocytes and congestion are often found in the liver. Subendocardial and subepicardial hemorrhages are found in the heart. Capillary congestion is evident in kidneys, meninges, lymph nodes and other structures.

The **diagnosis** of heat exhaustion depends upon consideration of several factors. The persistent high fever, distress and sudden death of an animal which could have been exposed to high temperature and humidity should arouse suspicion. The gross hyperemia, especially of the respiratory system, unusually rapid autolysis and absence of lesions of other specific infectious disease are helpful factors in arriving at a diagnosis.

OSSIFICATION IN THE LUNGS

In cows and in old dogs, there occur from time to time cases in which considerable areas of lung are found with spicules or tiny plates of bone extensively distributed in the alveolar walls. These may reach a length of a millimeter or more. They lie entirely within the alveolar septum, which is thickened to accommodate them. Blood vessels are not involved. The bony formations never appear in the pleura nor in the peribronchial areas.

The older German writers regarded the ossification as inflammatory in nature.

Pires (1942) found the spicules of bone to be closely related to the alveolar epithelium and points out that, if we adopt the recently held view that this lining "epithelium" is of mesenchymal origin, the ossification can be explained as metaplasia of the lining cells. There appear to be no objective data on accompanying disorders or circumstances which would cast light on the underlying cause, but this may well be chronic irritation of some sort or a metabolic deficiency. The condition, of course, is not to be confused with simple calcification of tissue. This shows no bone cells and no lacunae.

Equine habronemiasis sometimes results in small, hard, yellowish-gray nodules with a caseous or calcified center. These hard centers are only lightly joined to the surrounding thin layer granulation tissue and are easily separated from it. Eosinophils are usually numerous in the granulation tissue. A microscopic larva is sometimes demonstrable in them, identified as belonging to one of the *Habronema* stomach worms.

Ossification

CREECH, G. T.: Arteriosclerosis in Cattle Associated with Pulmonary Ossification. Am. J. Vet. Rec. 2:400–406, 1941.

PIRES, R. E.: Ossificação em pulmao de bovino. Rev. Fac. méd. vét., Univ. São Paulo 2: (Fasc. 2):77–84, 1942.

TUMORS

Most tumors encountered in the lungs are metastatic growths, for reasons explained in the section on Neoplasms (p. 190). Wm. S. Monlux (1952) has ably reviewed the primary neoplasms of the lung as far back as 1851, when the first recorded primary neoplasm was reported in a donkey. In the literature or in his own collection, Monlux found the following primary pulmonary tumors (types and nomenclature slightly condensed):

In canines: adenocarcinomas (bronchiolar-alveolar cell carcinomas), 34; other carcinomas, chiefly squamous-cell, 28; chondroma, 1; lipoma, 1; total, 64.

In felines: adenocarcinomas, 2; other carcinomas, 4; cholesteatoma, 1; spindle-cell sarcoma, 1; total, 8.

In equines: adenocarcinomas, 13; other carcinomas, 14; chondro-adenomas, 2; fibroma, 1; fibro- and myxosarcoma, 1 each; total, 32.

In bovines: adenocarcinomas, 9; other carcinomas, 19; chondromas, 4; total, 32.

In ovines: adenomas, 4; adenocarcinomas, 4; other carcinomas, 2; embryonal nephroma (?) 1; teratoma, 1; total, 12.

Musky lorrikeet, 1 adenocarcinoma; Malayan civet, 1 carcinoma; rabbit-eared bandicoot, 1 carcinoma; jaguar, 1 adenocarcinoma; tiger, 1 squamous-cell carcinoma; donkey, 1 chondroma; guinea pigs, rabbits, mice and birds, numerous reports, not compiled.

Monlux found no reason to believe from the available data that recent years have brought any increase in pulmonary neoplasms in animals.

Futher discussion of neoplasms and further references are found in Chapter 7.

Neoplasms

MONLUX, W. S.:   Primary Pulmonary Neoplasms in Domestic Animals.   Southwestern Vet. (College Station, Texas) 6:131–133, and Special Ed., October, 1952.

22

The Cardiovascular System

THE HEART

A common lesion for which the aspiring prosector must be constantly watchful is **dilatation of the heart.** As the name implies, this is a pathological enlargement of one or more of the cardiac chambers, most frequently of the right ventricle. The left ventricle, because of its thicker wall, offers more resistance to the dilative force; the auricles expand less noticeably and less extensively because the absence of an "intake" valve prevents the development of any great internal pressure. Cardiac dilatation, then, is recognized by a rounded bulging of one or both ventricles; the line from the atrio-ventricular level to the apex, which normally is almost straight, assumes an outward curvature that is often very noticeable. Palpation reveals the muscular wall to be yielding and flexible, a condition to which the adjective flabby is conventionally applied. Rarely a weakened, sac-like **aneurysm** develops.

Acute dilatation arises suddenly and leads to death in a few hours or a few days. It is usually the terminal breakdown which brings the end in some one of the acute febrile diseases. The cause in such cases is presumed to be the cumulative effect of toxic products upon the heart muscle. The condition is thus akin to the myocardial exhaustion to be discussed presently, although there are many cases of fatal myocardial exhaustion in which appreciable dilatation does not occur. It is believed also that sudden extreme exertion can cause acute dilatation, recovery being possible.

Chronic dilatation of the heart develops over a period of one or many months and is readily distinguished from the acute disorder by the hypertrophy which almost always accompanies it, both changes being of a compensatory nature. As will be seen from a perusal of the causes, which are the same as those of hypertrophy, this form of dilatation is most likely to involve the left ventricle.

Hypertrophy develops in either ventricle when conditions arise requiring the accomplishment of more work in the form of a greater output of blood per unit of time or the development of a greater pressure in order to force the blood along its normal channels. The hypertrophic cardiac wall is thicker, often much thicker, than normal; if there has been dilatation of the ventricle, it is also larger both in external and internal dimensions. The weight of such a heart is abnormally great. However, in veterinary practice, where patients of different breeds and species vary tremendously with respect to what is normal, the increased thickness and a rubbery firmness are the best gross indices of cardiac hypertrophy. Microscopically, the individual myocardial fibers are increased in thickness; their nuclei are numerous, enlarged and tend to be especially plump and square-ended.

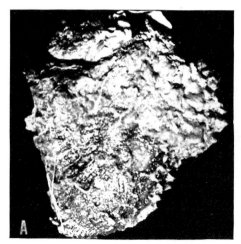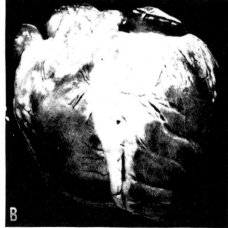

FIG. 22–1.—*A*, Chronic organizing fibrinous pericarditis in a sow. *B*, Acute dilatation of the right heart of a young Guernsey cow which died with circulatory collapse following cesarean operation. Note rounded outline of the heart, viewed from its anterior aspect. (Courtesy College Veterinary Medicine, Iowa State University.)

The cause of cardiac hypertrophy may lie within the heart itself in the form of stenosis or insufficiency (leaking) of the valve through which the ejected blood must pass (p. 131), or it may be found in leakage of the valve through which the blood enters. In the valvular insufficiencies, when functionally compensated, there is also dilatation of the ventricle in question. In this way, it may hold a volume large enough to permit a certain portion to leak backward and still to propel the normal amount forward. Such a cardiac disorder is said to be "fully compensated." Extra-cardiac causes of ventricular hypertrophy are those disorders which oblige the ventricle to pump against abnormally high resistance. The right ventricle, therefore, undergoes hypertrophy when there are obstructive processes in the lungs, such as the diffuse increase of fibrous tissue that thickens the alveolar walls in some chronic inflammatory processes (including "heaves," p. 1123), in chronic passive congestion (brown induration, p. 72), pneumoconiosis (p. 1110) or pulmonary stenosis. Hypertrophy of the left ventricle results from aortic stenosis, arterial hypertension in general and especially from nephrosclerotic (p. 1278) changes of whatever nature. An adherent pericardium (p. 1135) tends to cause hypertrophy of the part involved as an aid in overcoming the immobilizing effect of the adhesions. The exact mechanism by which compensatory hypertrophy and dilatation are induced in the unintelligent and unthinking myocardial tissues remains a mystery. It is customary to speak of such compensatory or adaptive changes (p. 93) as "designed" to remedy the functional defect, which they often accomplish with considerable success.

Myocardial Exhaustion.—We use this term to refer to a condition which is often called **toxic myocarditis,** toxic myocardium, or myocardial failure. However the condition is named, it occurs with great frequency and is the usual immediate cause of death in many acute infectious diseases, as well as in many poisonings. The action of toxic substances, probably abetted by anoxia, is its cause and, if time permits, fatty change and necrosis tend to appear and to be followed by lymphocytic infiltrations. However, in a majority of cases the animal dies with a clinically failing heart, dyspnea and widespread venous congestion, while little can be found in the heart grossly but flabbiness (see Dilatation) and even less is discernible microscopically. Another factor in deaths of this kind may be a loss of tone in the peripheral and splanchnic vessels, which leaves the cardiac chambers only partly filled, the cardiac action thereby impaired and the coronary vessels ischemic.

Advanced and well-marked inflammatory reactions to be found in exceptional cases in this group may be comparable to the cardiac lesions seen in deficiency of potassium (p. 1007), thiamine (p. 984) or tocopherol (p. 992), but usually the visible changes are much less conspicuous than those which can be seen in fatal deficiencies of any of those substances.

High-Altitude Disease.—Since it is essentially a condition of slow cardiac failure, we may consider a disease which arises in cattle, less frequently in sheep and horses, which are pastured on mountainous ranges at an elevation above 2500 meters (7600 feet). A corresponding condition known as "miners' disease" occurs in men laboring in the high Andes. Dyspnea and weakness occur, as in any cardiac insufficiency, but frequently the first sign of illness noticed by the stockman is subcutaneous and more deeply placed edema of the ventral body wall. This is usually most prominent in the sternal region, or brisket; hence, the disease is often called **"brisket disease."** Animals may be gradually acclimatized to the low oxygen-content of the rarefied atmosphere at these altitudes, their erythrocyte count reaching a level well above the usual normal and the oxygen-carrying capacity is increased so that normal health is maintained. With careful nursing and removal to a lower altitude, recovery may ensue in those which do become ill but, under common husbandry conditions, the disease is usually eventually fatal.

Lesions in fatal cases include acute dilatation generally of both ventricles and chronic passive congestion. The latter is notable in the large veins, the spleen and especially in the liver, where the typical "nutmeg liver" (p. 1235) usually develops. Cardiac edema (p. 134) develops, as mentioned. Polycythemia is often found. Blood pressure in the pulmonary artery and its branches is increased (pulmonary arterial hypertension) with a corresponding enlargement of the heart. Replacing the inhaled air with oxygen causes the hypertension to subside. In appropriate geographical areas the lesions are practically diagnostic.

Degenerative Changes.—Several of the degenerations described in Chapter 2 occur in the heart, but the details given there need not be repeated. Cloudy swelling, or albuminous degeneration, is described by some but is not easily recognized either grossly or microscopically. Mucoid degeneration (p. 52) is not rare in the subepicardial fat of the coronary border, resulting from cachexia and malnutrition. Hyaline degeneration of muscle fibers occurs as a prenecrotic change and a part of the picture of the "toxic myocarditis" of myocardial exhaustion and in company with the lesions of the deficiencies mentioned in that section. Fatty infiltration, it will be recalled, is excessive extension of the coronary adipose tissue among the cardiac muscle fibers. Fatty change leads to the appearance of minute droplets of lipid within the muscle fibers. It is detected with certainty only by fat stains. The pigment of brown atrophy (p. 83) has the myocardial fibers as a favorite site of localization. Melanosis (p. 66) rarely involves epicardial or endocardial surfaces, especially those on or near the heart valves.

Infarcts (p. 28) of the myocardium are all too common in humans, sudden infarction constituting the usual "heart attack." The cause ordinarily is arterio-sclerotic or atherosclerotic obstruction of a coronary artery, or thrombosis of one of those vessels. The extent of the infarct depends on the location of the obstruction; many of them slowly heal with replacement of the necrotic area of muscle by a fibrous scar. Lesions of this kind are quite uncommon in veterinary patients, although it has been found possible to produce them experimentally.

Congestion and hyperemia follow the usual laws. Edema fluid tends to drain into the pericardial cavity, so that edema of the heart muscle itself is rare. Both the external and internal surfaces of the heart are common sites for the hemorrhages of anoxia, toxemias and septicemias. The subepicardial hemorrhages tend to be of petechial size; the subendocardial are usually ecchymoses. They conform to the general statements already made on the subject of hemorrhages (p. 119).

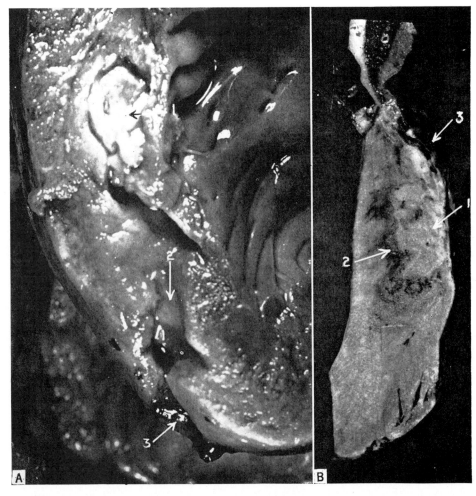

Fig. 22–2.—Infarction of the heart. A, Infarction of left ventricle of a twelve-year-old male mongrel terrier. Necrosis of myocardium (1) has led to formation of a channel in the left ventricle and rupture (3). Death followed this cardiac tamponade and hemopericardium. B, Infarction of the intraventricular septum of a four-year-old spayed female poodle. The gray-colored necrotic myocardium (1) is separated from the normal myocardium by a zone of hemorrhage. Subendocardial hemorrhage is seen at (3). (Courtesy of Angell Memorial Animal Hospital.)

MYOCARDIUM

Myocarditis, as a diffuse exudative inflammation of the heart muscle, is an uncommon disease in animals. Infections, which are the usual inciters of such inflammations, usually localize in the outer or inner coverings of the myocardium, rather than in the muscle itself, or take the form of abscesses or similarly circumscribed foci. This may well be attributable to the dense and solid character of the myocardium which renders it less favorable for the growth and spread of microorganisms than the adjacent surfaces and spaces.

Degenerative and infiltrative changes have already been considered under the titles of Myocardial Exhaustion and Acute Dilatation. Occasionally a heart is seen in which there is an appreciable degree of proliferation of the interstitial reticulum in the form of cells of reticulo-endothelial type, with large, pale vesicular nuclei. A few lymphocytes are also present in most cases. The cause of this mild subacute inflammation is seldom readily identifiable but is probably toxic, coupled perhaps with a mild allergic state. Foci of such cells sometimes bear a superficial resemblance to the Aschoff nodule of human rheumatic fever, but no clearly comparable rheumatic heart disease exists in animals.

A special type of reactive cell peculiar to the heart is known as the **Anitschow cell** (sometimes called the myocardial reticulocyte or the Aschoff cell, but never to be confused with the Aschoff body). With inconspicuous cytoplasm, this cell is characterized by an elongated, ellipsoidal nucleus, along the center of which lies a longitudinally placed rod of deeply staining chromatin. The diameter of this rod is very close to one-third of that of the whole nucleus; on each side of it is another third which remains clear and unstained. The periphery of the rod bears minute projections from some of which fine lines of chromatin, barely visible, extend across the clear zone to tie the rod to the nuclear membrane, which, though thin, is also distinctly stained.

Unless seen in longitudinal section, the Anitschow cell may be confused with other kinds of cells, but the true Anitschow cell is held to be of histiocytic (reticulocytic) origin and is restricted to the heart. In spite of the fact that it may be seen in the cellular aggregate known as the Aschoff body of (human) rheumatic heart disease, it occurs in many forms of injury to the myocardium and many (presumably all) mammalian species. It is occasionally seen congregated into syncytial giant cells and can be shown to have phagocytic properties.

Along with the cells characteristic of inflammation in general the earlier stages of inflammatory reactions in cardiac and striated muscle also include the presence of "myogenic" or "sarcolemma cells" whose nuclei have a prominent central nucleolus with a resultant similarity to the appearance of the Anitschow cell in cross section. These often form syncytial giant cells but the nuclear characteristics serve to differentiate such giant cells from the foreign-body giant cells that may be present but which have dense, homogeneous nuclei.

Certain of the infectious granulomatous diseases (p. 615), especially tuberculosis and caseous lymphadenitis, rarely localize in the heart and initiate their characteristic lesions, which may be single or multiple, the intervening areas being free of abnormalities. Such lesions are the result of hematogenous spread of the infection in question from a focus somewhere else. Similar hematogenous spread occurs in the case of infections by the pyogenic cocci, although invasion of the heart is exceptional. The lesions resulting are **abscesses;** they may be large or small, many or few, thickly or thinly encapsulated. The site of origin may be in any infected region of the body, the uterus, a joint or an infected umbilicus in the newborn being especially likely locations. Similar metastasis of the necrophorus organism (p. 623) leads to a circumscribed area of coagulative necrosis, more or less completely encapsulated as in the case of abscesses and granulomas. This also is rare in the heart. Toxoplasmosis is a specific myocardial infection (p. 684).

Scars of white fibrous tissue are occasionally seen in the myocardium. While such a scar might well represent a healed myocardial infarct in the human, in animals a healed abscess or parasitic lesion is a more likely explanation. The size, shape and location should afford a clue to previous events.

Neoplasms.—The tumor derived from the myocardium is the rhabdomyosarcoma. Such neoplasms occur rarely in various species. The most frequently encountered neoplasm in the heart is the malignant lymphoma. A very considerable proportion of these growths involve the heart in cattle. Some result in the formation of one or more discrete masses but many infiltrate among the muscle bundles. An area of rather faint white streaks parallel to the course of the muscle fibers should be considered malignant lymphoma until shown to be otherwise. These, as well as the aortic body tumor, are treated in Chapter 7, page 208.

Malignant hemangioendothelioma (p. 204) occasionally is found in the right auricle of the canine heart either as a primary tumor or as a metastasis from the spleen or other site. A type of myxoma and rhabdomyomatosis in the guinea pig is sometimes observed. Some consider this a type of congenital anomaly.

Parasites.—Heartworms (*Dirofilaria immitis*, p. 745) occupy the right ventricle and pulmonary artery, sometimes filling the available space with astonishing completeness. It is remarkable how long life may continue despite the obvious interference with function. *Cysticercus cellulosae* (p. 790), the intermediate stage of the pork tapeworm of man, forms cystic cavities about 3 or 4 by 10 mm., elongated in the direction of the muscular fibers. The cysts may be few or so numerous as to riddle the myocardium. *Cysticercus bovis* is much less prone to involve the heart but may do so. Sarcosporidial (p. 694) cysts are common in the heart muscle.

PERICARDIUM

Pericarditis includes inflammation of both the parietal and visceral surfaces of the pericardial cavity, in other words, the inner surface of the sac and the outer surface of the heart, the epicardium. The exudate formed naturally accumulates in the lumen of the pericardial sac. While, for reasons not clearly understood, moderate amounts of serum and fibrin sometimes tend to accumulate in the sac as a result of **uremia**, true pericarditis is always infectious and nearly always exudative. The source of infection may be regarded as always hematogenous except when it enters by direct extension, the latter form constituting the common "traumatic pericarditis" of bovines. It is doubtful that extension from an infected pleural cavity or surface ever occurs, for the membrane of the pericardial sac, covered with pleural mesothelium on the outside and pericardial on the inside, the whole scarcely thicker than a sheet of paper, forms an effective barrier between the two cavities. Similarly, infection involving the epicardial surface seldom shows any appreciable spread into the underlying myocardium.

Hematogenous Pericarditis.—The pericardial surfaces are commonly involved, with the pleura and lungs, in pasteurellosis (p. 608), (including fowl cholera) and less commonly in certain viral diseases, among which are hog cholera, equine viral pneumonitis and psittacosis. Just how often the pericarditis itself is due to a virus and how often to a secondary bacterial invader has not been adequately investigated. As is usual on serous membranes, the inflammation tends to be of the fibrinous or sero-fibrinous type. The amount of serous fluid accumulating in the pericardial cavity may be very considerable, but it can usually be distinguished from hydropericardium (p. 1136) both grossly and microscopically by the presence of fibrin, leukocytes or even erythrocytes. In other instances, the exudate is chiefly fibrinous, appearing at the very first as a cloudiness of the epicardial surface and shortly as a thin mesh-work of fine fibrin. This conforms to the usual course for fibrinous inflammations (p. 156), but in these cardiac diseases it is more common for either death or recovery to supervene before the exudate advances to organization or adhesions.

Traumatic Pericarditis.—This form is ordinarily a disease of bovine animals, and in cows kept in frequent and close proximity to stables and the usual activities of the farmstead it is all too frequent. In such places, there are almost sure to be old nails, bits of wire and similar hardware which cattle swallow as a result of their not-too-discriminatory feeding habits. Many of these sharp metallic objects penetrate the wall of the reticulum (p. 1200) and slowly move, encompassed in reactive granulation tissue, through the diaphragm and into the pericardial sac (a distance of only a few centimeters). Carrying cocci or other common bacteria with them, they initiate acute infectious pericarditis. The exudate is most often fibrinous or fibrino-purulent in nature and copious in amount. Cattle usually live for a number of days or weeks after the start of the process, so that the exudate has time to become extensive, organized in its deeper zones and adherent to the formative surface. A common picture at time of death is the **cor rugosum,** or "shaggy heart." Such a heart is covered with a layer of white or blood-stained fibrin several millimeters thick, of which the deeper part is being organized into vascular fibrous tissue. The more superficial unorganized portion is of indefinite depth with irregular shreds and strings of fibrin hanging from it. More or less sero-purulent fluid may distend the pericardial space, or the cavity may be empty and collapsed. In the latter case, the organizing fibrin reaches from the epicardial to the outer pericardial surface, joining the two inseparably over a large part of their area—adhesive pericarditis. Obviously such an exudate exerts pressure, and if adhesive, it tends to immobilize the heart muscle more or less rigidly. In spite of attempts at compensatory hypertrophy, the mechanical interferences, coupled with the toxic effect of the pathogenic organisms and their products, eventually bring the master pump to a standstill and death ensues. Accompanying lesions are those of chronic venous congestion or of toxemia (pp. 119, 130) depending upon the rapidity or slowness of the developing process. The granulation tissue with its fistulous tract reaching from the diaphragm and reticulum may be extensive or slender. The wire or similar object is commonly still present, reaching into or through the wall of the sac and not infrequently penetrating into the myocardium itself at time of death. On the other hand, iron rusts and dissolves rather quickly in the body fluids and may have completely disintegrated before death occurs, only the narrow sinus tract, its lining blackened by iron sulfide, remaining as evidence of the fatal accident.

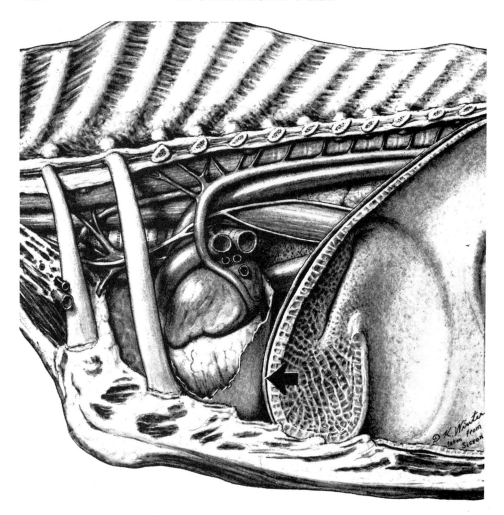

FIG. 22–3.—The anatomic relationships in traumatic pericarditis. Foreign bodies penetrate the wall of the reticulum, diaphragm and pericardium in the direction indicated by the arrow. (Modified after Sisson.)

Hydropericardium is the accumulation of fluid (lymph) in the pericardial sac. It can be distinguished from inflammatory edema, which is a serous exudate, by the absence of other aspects of an inflammatory process, for hydropericardium is true non-inflammatory (p. 134) edema of the pericardium and heart. The amount of fluid encountered naturally varies greatly; in a general way, it might be stated that a quantity equal to about one-half the capacity of a ventricle of the same heart would represent a pronounced case of hydropericardium. The causes are any of the usual causes of edema (p. 137), cardiac and nutritional edema probably being somewhat more important in this respect than renal edema. The effect is to interfere with the flow of venous blood returning to the heart, but this is commonly overshadowed by other effects of the basic disease.

In **hemopericardium,** hemorrhage fills the sac with blood. The sudden escape of blood into the pericardial sac, perhaps through rupture of an atrial or myocardial wall, is sometimes referred to as **cardiac tamponade.** Its effect is similar, although more dramatic, to hydropericardium because it also interferes with venous return to the heart.

ENDOCARDIUM

Another infectious disease of the heart is **endocarditis,** inflammation of the endocardial lining. Endocarditis may be **mural** (*murus,* wall), when the lesions are located on the lining of an auricle or ventricle, but it is much more frequently **valvular,** the lesions being located on the valves. Doubtless because of the greater pressure and mechanical strains to which the structures are subjected, valvular endocarditis is much more frequent on the left side of the heart than on the right, and also more frequent and more extensive on the atrioventricular than on the semilunar valves. Bovines are an exception to this statement, according to the statistics of Winqvist (1945) and of Evans (1957), the reasons being obscure. Species and age affect the incidence only in accordance with the various susceptibilities to the several infections of which endocarditis is a manifestation.

The lesion of endocarditis involves death and disappearance of the endothelium, although this may be preceded by hyperemia and infiltration of inflammatory cells and fluid in the affected area. Upon the raw surface left by the destroyed endothelium, a clot forms. Like other clots, it is initiated by the lodgment of platelets and the deposition of fibrin. As the days pass, the clot grows continually in size and, like other clots (p. 108), its deeper parts are organized by fibrous tissue. Thus the mass becomes essentially inflammatory granulation tissue (p. 165), which, under a covering zone of still unorganized exudate, may attain consider-

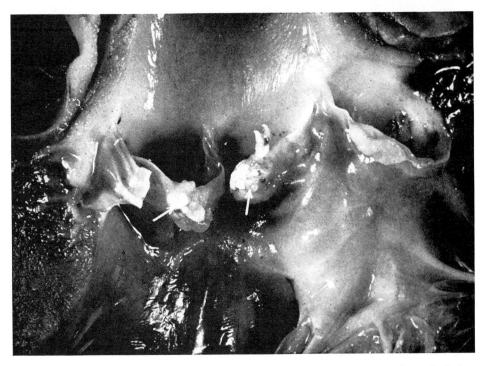

Fig. 22–4.—Endocarditis of aortic semilunar valves of an eight-year-old spayed female dachshund. Nodular lesions (arrows) on margin and surface of valves. (Courtesy of Angell Memorial Animal Hospital.)

able size (one to several centimeters) and a totally irregular and bizarre shape. Such growths are often called "vegetations," presumably because of their similarity in shape to the head of a cauliflower, or, if small and wart-like, they are called verrucae, the corresponding **"vegetative endocarditis"** and **"verrucous endocarditis"** being in use. In the case of some species and infections, healing is possible, the uneven surface being covered by regenerated endothelium. Thereupon the vascular, fibrous structure, like other granulation tissue, slowly matures into a denser, non-vascular, scar-like mass. In mural locations, lesions which are not too protuberant may subside into a flat, shiny white scar of fibrous tissue.

As can be readily imagined, the effect of one or more nodules of new tissue, when located on the wall of a ventricle or an auricle, might not be too serious but when on a valve, as they almost always are, there is important and often disastrous interference with function. The "vegetations" or verrucae tend to form at points of contact of the valve cusps with each other, hence there is every probability that their location will be such as, not only to obstruct the lumen, but also to prevent perfect closure of the valve. They may also induce contraction of the cusp or occasionally tie it down to the heart wall or to the chordae tendineae. Mere inflammatory thickening of the cusps lessens their flexibility and ability to close properly. Valvular stenoses or insufficiencies are the result to be expected from any of these changes.

In dogs, even though they have died of some other disease, it is not unusual

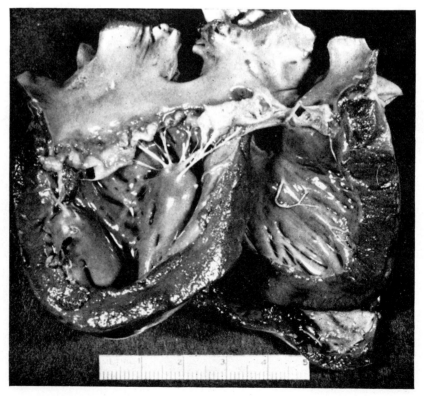

Fig. 22–5.—Thickened, nodular left atrioventricular valve. The valve and the left ventricle were also dilated. From a ten-year-old female crossbreed "spitz" dog. (Courtesy of Angell Memorial Animal Hospital.)

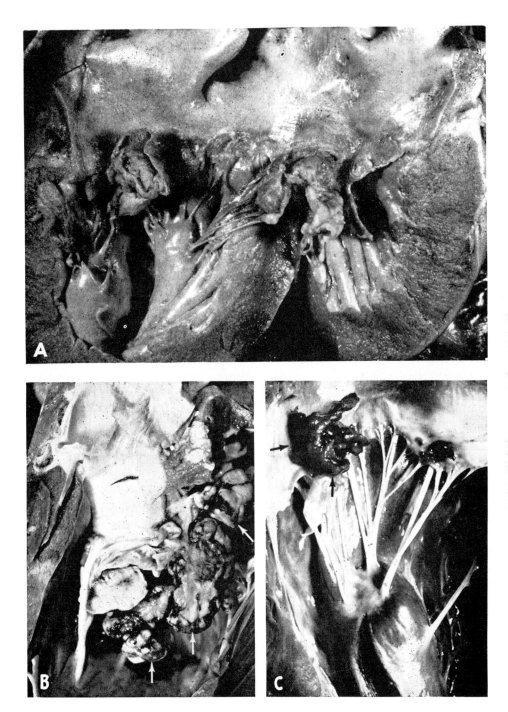

FIG. 22–6.—*A*, Acute bacterial endocarditis involving the left atrioventricular valves of a fifteen-year-old male crossbreed terrier dog. (Courtesy of Angell Memorial Animal Hospital.) *B*, Valvular endocarditis in a cow. Note thick, irregular masses firmly attached to the bicuspid valve (arrows). (*B*, Courtesy of Armed Forces Institute of Pathology.) Contributor: Dr. C. L. Davis. *C*, Smaller lesions in the bicuspid valve of a cow, *Corynebacterium pyogenes* was isolated from the lesions.

to encounter valves, usually the tricuspid, with cusps rather evenly reduced in height, white and glistening and with their outer margins smoothly but markedly thickened. These are indicative of an old, healed lesion. Without accurate statistics, it is the impression of one of the writers (Smith) that these cases are more prevalent in cold climates and that they frequently accompany the granular, contracted kidneys of chronic nephritis (p. 1263). Any statement regarding the cause would be entirely speculative.

As to the causes of endocarditis in animals generally, it may be said that the disease is a feature of certain specific infections, mostly septicemias. In horses, streptococci, chiefly *Strep. equi*, the cause of strangles, *Shigella equirulis* (*Bacterium viscosum equi*, *B. nephritidis equi*) and possibly other organisms found in umbilical infections (pyosepticemia neonatorum) of foals, have been held responsible for endocarditis. The meningococcus (*Neisseria meningitidis*) has had this effect in horses used for the production of antiserum for meningitis. In cattle, streptococci of undetermined species, *Staphylococcus aureus*, *Corynebacterium pyogenes* and paracoliform organisms causing diarrhea ("white scours") of calves have been incriminated. Endocarditis is rare in sheep but *Streptococcus fecalis* has been found in the blood and hearts of affected lambs. A rather frequent disease in swine, endocarditis is due to the organism of swine erysipelas or to streptococci with about equal frequency. *Corynebacterium pyogenes* is a much less important cause in swine.

An important form of endocarditis in humans is that which accompanies rheumatic fever and rheumatic heart disease. The valvular lesions typically consist of small verrucae and are accompanied by a myocarditis characterized by focal reticulo-endothelial proliferations, just visible to the naked eye, which are known as Aschoff bodies. This disease appears to have no natural counterpart in animals, although similar lesions have resulted in dogs experimentally infected under suitable conditions with the streptococcus derived from the human disease. Naturally occurring endocarditides in animals show no evidence of an allergic origin, nor are they accompanied ordinarily by arthritis, both of which are features of the human disease (The swine erysipelas organism [p. 586] is capable of causing both endocarditis and non-exudative periarthritic proliferations, but these are very seldom found together.) The proliferative (vegetative) valvular lesions of some size usually seen in animals have much more in common with human "subacute bacterial endocarditis" than with rheumatic heart disease.

Mulberry heart disease designates a poorly understood syndrome which brings death to young, thrifty pigs in a matter of hours. The whole heart at death is in a state of firm contraction and spotted with hemorrhages, thus suggesting the appearance of a mulberry. Edema is the most impressive lesion, however, with hydropericardium, limited hydroperitoneum and pronounced pulmonary edema. The edema fluid may clot owing to its high protein content. The gastrointestinal tract is inactive, its contents dry, although there may be marked hyperemia of the fundic portion of the stomach. If death is delayed for perhaps a day, softening of the white matter in the cerebral gyri may be detected. The cause is not know but may well be an unknown toxic substance in the food, although a limited amount of experimental work has failed to reveal it. A relationship to enterotoxemia (p. 1211), with or without hypersensitivity, has been suspected. This disease has also been called "dietetic microangiopathy" (Mowen, 1965).

Table 22–1.—Cardiovascular Malformations in 290 Dogs (Patterson, 1968)

Malformation	Number	Percentage of Total
Patent ductus arteriosus	82	25.3
Pulmonic stenosis	57	17.5
Subaortic stenosis	40	12.3
Persistent right aortic arch	23	7.1
Ventricular septal defect	20	6.2
Tetralogy of Fallot	11	3.4
Atrial septal defect (ostium secundum inc. patent foramen ovale)	12	3.7
Persistent left cranial vena cava	13	4.0
Mitral insufficiency.	9	2.8
Pericardial anomalies:		
Pericardio-diaphragmatic hernia	3	.9
Absent pericardium	1	.3
Incomplete pericardium	1	.3
Arterial anomalies:		
Retro-esophageal right subclavian artery . .	1	.3
Separate origin of right subclavian artery from ascending aorta	2	.6
Ebstein's anomaly of tricuspid valve	1	.3
Tricuspid insufficiency	1	.3
Double outlet, right ventricle	1	.3
Anomalous pulmonary venous drainage	1	.3
Conduction disturbance—without gross malformations:		
Right bundle branch block	2	.6
Wolff-Parkinson-White syndrome	1	.3
Arteriovenous fistula	1	.3
Incompletely diagnosed	42	12.9
TOTAL	325	100

Note: In 32 dogs, more than one malformation was found.

esophageal right subclavian artery, arteriovenous fistulae, and anomalous origin of the right subclavian artery from the ascending aorta. The significance and frequency of these anomalies are yet to be established.

Frequency and Etiology of Cardiovascular Anomalies.—The studies of Detweiler, Hubben and Patterson (1968) contribute to the understanding of these anomalies in dogs. According to these authors, the prevalence rate of cardiovascular malformations among dogs studied in a large university veterinary clinic was 6.8 per 1000 admissions. Purebred dogs have higher, breed-specific prevalence rates than mongrels and patent ductus arteriosus in the dog (as in man) is more prevalent in females than males. These workers present evidence that genetic factors have a bearing on the occurrence of several such cardiovascular anomalies. The frequency of many can be increased by selective matings in certain families of dogs.

Patterson (1968) has reported cardiovascular anomalies in 290 dogs, studied over a 13-year period. His data are summarized in Table 22–1.

Congenital Cardiovascular Anomalies

BELLING, T. H., JR.: Ventricular Septal Defect in the Bovine Heart—Report of Three Cases. J. Am. Vet. Med. Assn. *138*:595–598, 1961.

BURT, J. H.: Anomalous Posterior Vena Cava of a Dog. J. Am. Vet. Med. Assn. *108*:152, 1946.

CORDY, D. R., and RIBELIN, W. E.: Six Congenital Cardiac Anomalies in Animals. Cornell Vet. *40*:249–256, 1950.

DAWES, G. S., et al.: Patent Ductus Arteriosus in Newborn Lambs. J. Physiol. 128: 344–361, and 361–383, 1955.

DENNIS, S. M., and LEIPOLD, H. W.: Congenital Cardiac Defect in Lambs. Am. J. Vet. Res. 29:2337–2340, 1968.

DETWEILER, D. K.: Genetic Aspects of Cardiovascular Diseases in Animals. Circulation 30:114–127, 1964.

DETWEILER, D. K., HUBBEN, K., and PATTERSON, D. F.: Survey of Cardiovascular Disease in Dogs. Am. J. Vet. Res. 21:329–359, 1960.

ELIOT, T. S., et al.: First Report of the Occurrence of Neonatal Endocardial Fibroelastosis in Cats and Dogs. J. Am. Vet. Med. Assn. 133:271–274, 1958.

FLICKINGER, G. L., and PATTERSON, D. F.: Coronary Lesions Associated with Congenital Subaortic Stenosis in the Dog. J. Path. Bact. 93:133–140, 1967.

FREIGANG, B., and KNOBIL, E.: Patent Ductus Arteriosus with Pulmonary Hypertension and Arteritis in a Rhesus Monkey. Yale J. Biol. Med. 40:239–242, 1967.

HACKEL, D. B., et al.: Interatrial Septal Defect in a Chimpanzee. Lab. Invest. 2:154–163, 1952.

HAMLIN, R. L., SMETZER, D. L., and SMITH, R. C.: Interventricular Septal Defect (Roger's Disease) in the Dog. J. Am. Vet. Med. Assn. 145:331–340, 1964.

HARE, T.: Patent Interventricular Septum of a Dog's Heart. Vet. Rec. 55:103–107, 1943.

HARE, T., and ORR, A. B.: Patent Ductus Arteriosus with Patent Interventricular Foramen of a Dog's Heart. J. Path. Bact. 34:799–800, 1931.

HUEPER, W. C.: Aortic Abnormalities in Dogs Used for Experimental Purposes. Arch. Path. 39:375–380, 1945.

KITCHELL, R. L., STEVENS, C. E., TURBES, C. C.: Cardiac and Aortic Arch Anomalies, Hydrocephalus and Other Abnormalities in Newborn Pigs. J. Am. Vet. Med. Assn. 130: 453–457, 1957.

LEV, M., NEUWELT, F., and NECHELES, H.: Congenital Defect of the Interventricular Septum, Aortic Regurgitation and Probable Heart Block in a Dog. Am. J. Vet. Res. 2:91–94, 1941.

LINTON, G. A.: Anomalies of the Aortic Arches Causing Strangulation of the Esophagus and Trachea. J. Am. Vet. Med. Assn. 129:1–5, 1956.

LJUNGGREN, G., et al.: Four Cases of Congenital Malformation of the Heart in a Litter of Eleven Dogs. J. Small Anim. Pract. 7:611–623, 1966.

McLEOD, W. M.: Unusual Bovine Left Coronary Artery. J. Am. Vet. Med. Assn. 128:39, 1956.

MEYEROWITZ, B.: Defectus Interventricularis Septi in Heart of Pig. Am. J. Vet. Res. 3: 368–372, 1942.

MONTI, F.: Le cardiopatie congenite in pathologia comparata. Nuova Vet. 27:33–43, 65–79, 107–111, and 146–150, 1951.

NAYLOR, J. R.: Regurgitation in Pups. I. Persistent Aortic Arches. J. Am. Vet. Med. Assn. 130:283–284, 1957.

OLAFSON, P.: Congenital Cardiac Anomalies in Animals, J. Tech. Meth. & Bull. Inter. Assn. Med. Mus. 19:129–134, 1939.

PATTERSON, D. F.: Epidemiologic and Genetic Studies of Congenital Heart Disease in the Dog. Circulation Res. 23:171–202, 1968.

PRIOR, J. T., and WYATT, T. C.: Endocardial Fibro-elastosis. Amer. J. Path. 26:969–987, 1950.

ROBERTS, S. J., et al.: Persistent Right Aortic Arch in a Guernsey Bull. Cornell Vet. 43: 537–543, 1953.

ROONEY, J. R., and FRANKS, W. C.: Congenital Cardiac Anomalies in Horses. Path. Vet. 1:454–464, 1964.

ROONEY, J. R., II, and WATSON, D. F.: Persistent Right Aortic Arch in a Calf. J. Am. Vet. Med. Assn. 129:5–7, 1956.

SASS, B., and ALBERT, T. F.: A Case of Eisenmenger's Complex in a Calf. Cornell Vet. 60:61–65, 1970.

SEIBOLD, H. R., and EVANS, L. E.: A Complex Cardiac Anomaly in a Calf. J. Am. Vet. Med. Assn. 130:99–101, 1957.

STOWENS, D.: Pediatric Pathology, 2nd Ed., Baltimore, The Williams & Wilkins Co., 1966.

VAN NIE, C. J.: Congenital Malformations of the Heart in Cattle and Swine. A Survey of a Collection. Acta Morph. Neerl. Scand. 6:387–393, 1966.

————: Anomalous Origin of the Coronary Arteries in Animals. Path. Vet. 5:313–326, 1968.

WEGELIUS, O., and VON ESSEN, R.: Endocardial Fibroelastosis in Dogs. Acta Path. Microbiol. Scand. 77:66–72, 1969.

THE ARTERIES

Arteriosclerosis.—In considering disease of the arteries, the disorder or group of disorders recognized as arteriosclerosis confronts us with universal preeminence. This disease is of infinitely more importance in man than it is in animals and has been studied principally in relation to the human species. Let us summarize, then, as briefly as possible what is known or believed about arteriosclerosis in man before proceeding to consider its various aspects in animals.

Under the general term arteriosclerosis, which literally means hardening of the arteries, are included three different lesions, which probably are distinct etiological entities. The first is **atherosclerosis,** the first half of the word being derived from a Greek word *athere,* which means a mushy substance. The name is appropriate, for in this condition a mushy substance of nondescript nature forms in the intimal layer. It is chiefly the large, elastic arteries such as the aorta and its immediate branches which are affected, although the coronary and cerebral vessels are also involved. The mushy substance consists largely of fatty material, lipoids and cholesterol mixed with the remains of necrotic cells. The cholesterol frequently takes crystalline form as shown by cholesterol clefts (p. 26). Some

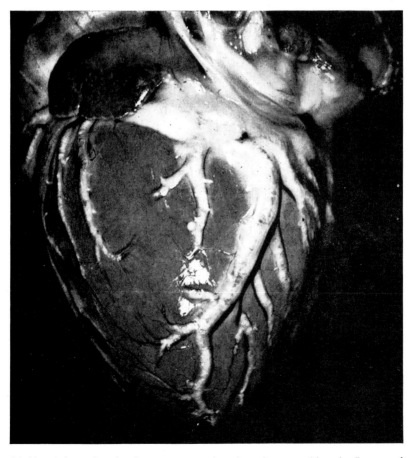

Fig. 22–10.—Atherosclerosis of coronary arteries of a nine-year-old male German shepherd. The major branches of these arteries are yellowish and thickened due to lipid in the media. See Figure 22–11 for microscopic appearance. (Courtesy of Angell Memorial Animal Hospital.)

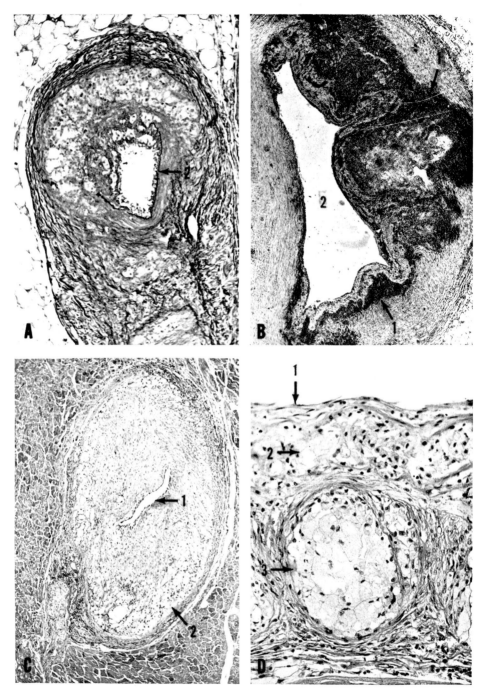

Fig. 22–11.—Xanthomatosis or atherosclerosis in the coronary arteries of a dog. *A*, Cross section of a coronary artery (× 80). Elastica stain. Lipid-laden cells in media (*1*) and intima. Note rupture of internal elastic membrane (*2*). *B*, A section (× 35) of another segment of the same coronary artery, stained for lipid by Sudan III. Note sudanophilic material (*1*) particularly in the media. The lumen is indicated by (*2*). *C*, A branch of the coronary artery. Hematoxylin and eosin stain (× 55). Endothelium at (*1*). Lipid-laden foam cells in media (*2*). *D*, Higher magnification (× 175) of a wall of a coronary artery. Endothelium (*1*), lipid-laden macrophages in subintima (*2*), and in media (*3*). (Courtesy of Armed Forces Institute of Pathology.) Contributor: Dr. Wayne H. Riser.

lipoid-filled "foam cells" of xanthomatous (Fig. 22–11D) type may be seen. Calcification often supervenes in the more necrotic areas. The foreign material is covered by a gradually thickening subendothelial layer of fibrous tissue, which tends to undergo hyaline degeneration (p. 44). Studies using the electron microscope and direct immunohistochemical techniques have demonstrated in man and animals that smooth muscle cells migrate into the intima and contribute to the development of the atheromatous plaque. It has also been shown in cattle (Knieriem, 1967) that smooth muscle cells migrate into the intima in the absence of lipid accumulation, to play a predominant role in the development of the arteriosclerotic plaque. It is not evenly distributed but forms localized gray or yellow areas in the arterial lining called atheromatous plaques. They may reach a height of several millimeters and obviously offer considerable obstruction to the flow of blood. In small vessels like the coronaries, the obstruction often terminates fatally through myocardial infarction.

Extensive studies have given rise to several theories on the causation of atherosclerosis. It appears that the formation of atheromatous plaques is affirmatively related to a high level of cholesterol and of total lipids in the blood and also to a high ratio of cholesterol to phospholipids. The formation of such plaques is also favored by hypertension (high blood pressure). On the basis of these facts and considerable experimentation in rabbits, monkeys and dogs, not to mention pertinent clinical evidence, the theory that diets too high in fats and cholesterol are causative has many adherents, although some incongruities have yet to be explained. Certain other theories deserve attention in a complete presentation of the matter but will be omitted here.

The second of the arteriosclerotic entities is known as the **medial sclerosis** of Mönckeberg, also as **medial calcification.** Instead of affecting the large, elastic arteries of the body, it involves the medium-sized, muscular arteries. There are hyaline and fatty degenerative changes in the muscular tissue of the media, leading to necrosis. The process is gradual and, as a typical sequence (p. 24) to necrosis, calcification regularly supervenes. Rarely ossification (p. 58) occurs in the vessel wall. This form of arteriosclerosis goes with advancing age but not necessarily with hypertension. It is thought to be related causally to prolonged or habitual over-stimulation of the medial musculature by the vasomotor (sympathetic) nerves. Experimentally, a similar calcification has been produced in dogs and rabbits by excessive administration of epinephrine (adrenalin). Nicotine is said to have a similar effect. The well-known tendency of excesses of vitamin D (p. 999) to produce medial calcification of arteries is considered to be on the same basis. Extensive calcification of the aorta and large thoracic arteries (media only) has been seen in young cattle, otherwise normal, when slaughtered for beef (Gailiunas, 1958).

The third entity of arteriosclerotic disease is **diffuse arteriolar sclerosis,** or **arteriolosclerosis.** The term hyperplastic sclerosis has been used and is suggestive of some of the changes that occur in the small peripheral arteries called arterioles, located especially in the kidney, spleen and pancreas. The hyperplasia consists in proliferation of the cells of the intima, producing concentric lamellations which nearly or completely fill the lumen. The intima may be replaced with connective-tissue hyalin or there may be swelling and necrosis of the medial layers with marked compression of the lumen. The latter change occurs when the disease is of rapid development and may be considered related to

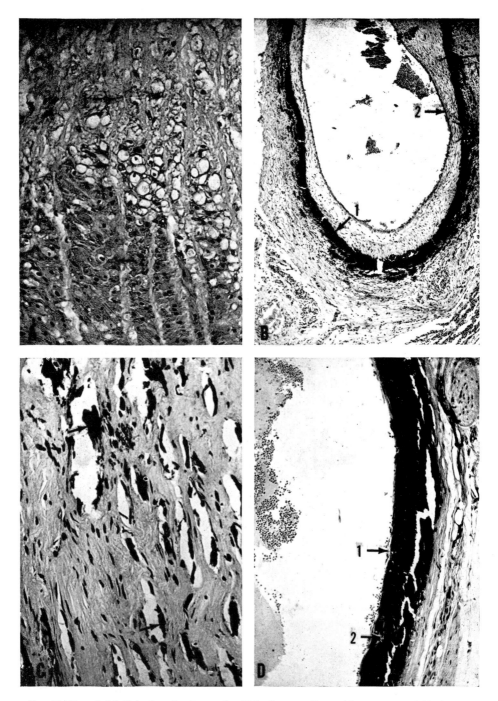

FIG. 22–12.—*A*, Medial sclerosis of aorta (× 300) of a cow. Scarred but not yet calcified area (*1*) is distinguishable from the normal media (*2*). Contributor: Dr. E. L. Stubbs. *B*, Medial calcification (*1*) in a bovine pulmonary artery (× 45) Intima (*2*). Contributor: Dr. J. F. Ryff. *C*, Calcification (arrows) of the media of a bovine aorta (× 300). Contributor: Dr. E. L. Stubbs. *D*, Calcification (*2*) in an artery (× 130) of a cat which died of uremia. Intima (*1*). (*A*, *B*, *C* and *D*, Courtesy of Armed Forces Institute of Pathology.) Contributor: Dr. Edward Baker.

"malignant hypertension," a rapidly developing increase of blood pressure. Hyperplastic reduplication of the lamina elastica interna is also a frequent finding.

All of the above changes are counted, not only as lesions of arteriosclerosis, but of hypertension, which is one of the commoner disorders with which the human race contends. The two conditions are not always coexistent but are inextricably interrelated, just how, no one knows with certainty, in spite of intensive research. Neither can we claim, in spite of wide acceptance, that agreement is entirely universal on the classification of the lesions as we have described them or on the propriety of considering them all as manifestations of a single disease.

In attempting to evaluate the features and even the existence of arteriosclerotic disease in the domestic animals, it is necessary to remember that the thickening of arterial walls, especially through proliferation of the intimal tissue (endarteritis) occurs frequently in the vicinity of many chronic inflammatory processes, whatever their cause. Such localized arterial lesions should not be interpreted as signs of arteriosclerosis without confirmation in other areas. Similarly, calcification of the walls of arteries may well have local or metabolic causes not concerned with true arteriosclerotic disease. It is not safe to speculate, in the absence of much precise data on blood pressures in our animal patients, that hypertension is not a feature of either of these conditions.

Irregular thickenings of the intima of the aorta and other large arteries are seen occasionally in cattle, dogs, swine and other species and these have been compared with human arteriosclerotic changes. Lindsay, Chaikoff and Gilmore (1952, 1955) have made an especially thorough study of such lesions in 14 old dogs ranging in age from eight to seventeen years, 5 of them ill with cardiac symptoms. Twelve younger dogs in apparently normal health were also studied and formed a sort of control group. These investigators were able to find fibrous thickening or intimal plaques in the aortas in a majority of the dogs of both groups, although in some cases the plaques were as small as $\frac{1}{2}$-mm. in diameter. Changes in the media were also found in most cases. In one dog twelve years of age, a myocardial infarct 4 cm. in greatest diameter was found. The investigators quoted drew the conclusion that spontaneous arteriosclerosis is high in dogs, while making the interesting observation that neither lipoidosis nor deposition of cholesterol was involved. It is to be noted, however, that none of their dogs died of the disease, all being given euthanasia by means of pentobarbital, and many were in normal clinical health. Moorehead and Little (1945) found localized intimal plaques with splitting and reduplication of internal elastic membranes in most dogs, even in ten-day-old puppies. Gottlieb and Lalich (1954) found rather similar plaques, up to 10 mm. in diameter, in the aortas of healthy swine slaughtered for food. The incidence rose with increasing age, attaining 25 per cent in young adults. A number of experimenters have produced arteriosclerotic, or rather, atherosclerotic changes in dogs, rabbits and also chickens through the medium of an artificially produced lipemia and cholesterolemia. This has been accomplished by means of a highly abnormal diet, by large doses of diethyl stilbesterol, by removal of the thyroid or by inactivating it with thiouracil.

The importance of considering animals of all ages, particularly those toward the end of the life span, is emphasized by the finding of advanced lesions in aged animals (Fankhauser, Luginbuhl and McGrath, 1965, Jones and Zook, 1965,

Marcus and Ross, 1967). Too often, experimental samples do not include the appropriate older age groups.

Extensive studies of atherosclerosis in animals and man over the past few years have been reported in a recent book edited by Roberts and Straus (1965).

Bovine Arteriosclerosis.—A severe generalized arteriosclerotic disease of cattle has been reported from certain tropical areas, particularly Jamaica, British West Indies, Argentina and Hawaii. Its colloquial names in these places are, respectively, "Manchester Wasting Disease," "enteque seco" and "Naalehu Disease." This latter term comes from the name of the district in Hawaii meaning "covered with gray ashes" (Lynd, *et al.*, 1965). The disease is manifest by progressive emaciation, stiffness of joints, and weakness due to impaired circulation. The lesions occur in the major and minor vasculature, as severe calcification and sclerosis of media and intima. Calcification is particularly evident in elastic tissues, especially in the lung. This calcification in the lung is accompanied by emphysema, and ossification with formation of bone (Fig. 3–3).

The disease in Hawaii is associated with a specific region and mildly affected cattle may recover after removal to areas where the disease does not occur (Willers, *et al.*, 1965). The report of Worker and Carrillo (1967) indicates that the disease is associated with the consumption of leaves and stems of a plant identified as *Solanum malacoxylon* (syn: *S. glaucum* Dun.). Ingestion of this plant, or its administration into the rumen via a rumen fistula reportedly elevates the blood levels of inorganic phosphorus and calcium of cattle.

Arteritis is characterized by the presence of inflammatory exudate, usually neutrophilic or other leukocytes, within the layers of the vessel wall. Chronic fibrosis is also to be included provided it is within the wall and not merely perivascular. This inflammatory state may arise in an artery which passes through inflamed and infected surroundings or which contains an infected thrombus or embolus, but it is remarkable how well the vessel walls usually resist infection under such circumstances. A more frequent form of arteritis is that which arises in the anterior mesenteric artery of the horse, or rarely elsewhere, as the result of invasion by larvae of *Strongylus vulgaris*. The acute exudation and subsequent or concomitant fibrous thickening of this verminous arteritis have been described (p. 752).

A specific arteritis of medium-sized muscular arteries is known in the horse infected with the agent of equine viral arteritis (p. 498). Another inflammatory disease of arteries occurs in rats of some strains. The mesenteric artery and its branches are particularly involved. This is often referred to as **polyarteritis nodosa** (Young, 1965, Cutts, 1966). A similar lesion has been described in mice (Conklin, *et al.*, 1967).

Lesions similar to those described in man as **periarteritis nodosa** have been described in several species (Figs. 22–14 and 22–15) although their etiology is not known nor is any relationship to the human disease established.

An **aneurysm** is a pathological dilatation of an artery (or a cardiac chamber), usually, but not invariably, saccular in shape and definitely circumscribed. The vessel wall is stretched beyond its capacity to resist, and certain layers, ordinarily the intima and media, will be found to have been wholly or partly ruptured. If the development has been gradual, replacement of the damaged tissues by an excess of fibrous tissue is the rule. A number of kinds of aneurysms are described on the basis of form or etiology. One requiring attention is the **dis-**

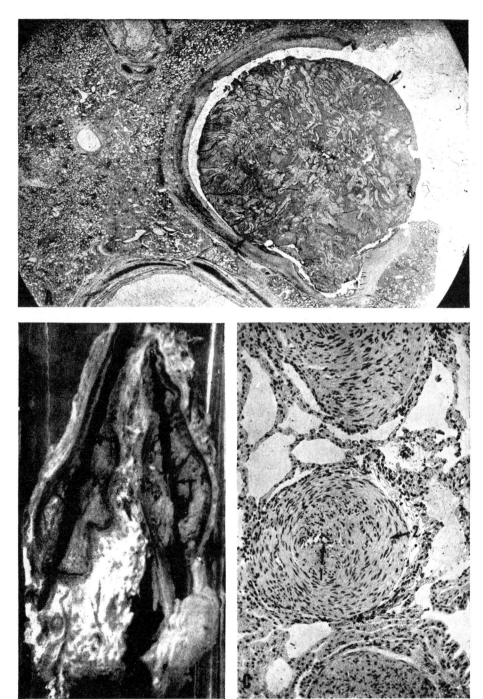

Fig. 22–13.—*A*, Thrombosis of the pulmonary artery (× 5) of a horse. Contributor: Dr. J. R. M. Innes. *B*, Verminous arteritis, anterior mesenteric artery of a horse. A single larva of *Strongylus vulgaris* is seen at (*1*) and although the wall is necrotic and thickened by inflammation, the lumen (*2*) appears reasonably patent. Specimen in Mark Francis Collection, Texas Sch. Vet. Med. *C*, Medial hypertrophy, branches of the pulmonary artery (× 130) of a cat. Intima (*1*) is surrounded by some sclerosis but the greatest increase in diameter is due to the thickened media (*2*), probably the result of infection with *Aleurostrongylus abstrusus* or *Toxocara cati*. (*A* and *C*, Courtesy of Armed Forces Institute of Pathology.) Contributor: Dr. Leo L. Lieberman.

secting aneurysm. This is due to fracture or necrosis in the medial layer of the aorta or some other large artery. Through an interruption of the inner coat or sometimes apparently through the vasa vasorum, the blood current gains access to the medial defect. Under the considerable arterial pressure, the blood then splits the inner cylindrical layer from the outer, much as the intact cylinder of bark can sometimes be separated from the inner wood of a twig. The blood thus flows in two tubes, one inside the other. Once started, this arrangement may extend for a considerable distance or even for the length of the aorta, the blood returning to its normal channel when one of the main arterial branches is encountered.

The causes of aneurysms are damage done by inflammatory or arteriosclerotic and degenerative disease. Syphilitic aortitis is a classical, but by no means the unique, cause in humans. However, there are evidences of nutritional causes for dissecting aneurysm in rats, where it accompanies poisoning by the sweet pea (*Lathyrus odoratus*, p. 951), (Bachhuber and Lalich, 1954) and in turkeys where a diet containing aflatoxin has appeared to have a causative relationship (Carnaghan, 1955, McSherry, *et al.*, 1954, Pritchard, Henderson and Beall, 1958). The injurious effects of aneurysms lie chiefly in the danger of rupture of the vessel or in the formation of a thrombus on the damaged and roughened intimal wall.

Atrophy of arteries and arterioles occurs in ergotism (p. 927) and the similar poisoning by fescue grass (p. 928). Continuously contracted, the bloodless arteries grow smaller and accompany the surrounding tissues to their gangrenous destruction.

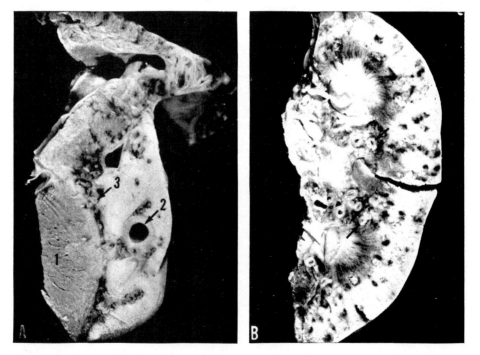

Fig. 22–14.—Periarteritis nodosa or generalized arteritis in a bovine. *A*, Myocardium (*1*), large unaffected coronary artery (*2*) and many thick-walled arteries (*3*) in epicardium. *B*, The kidney with many redundant, thick-walled arteries (arrows). (Courtesy of Armed Forces Institute of Pathology.) Contributor: Dr. C. L. Davis.

The natural atrophy that occurs in those vessels which normally change into ligaments with the advent of post-natal life is a more gradual process than might be expected. For instance, the closing of the umbilical arteries begins when they are severed at birth but may require as much as two months for completion (in the calf). The lumen is contracted but remains filled with hemolyzed and eventually with clotted blood; its slow recession can be followed inch by inch from the umbilicus to the bladder, as a central core of fibrous tissue progresses upward. This may be viewed as disuse atrophy (p. 91), similar to the change which occurs when a vessel is ligated.

Medial hypertrophy of branches of the pulmonary artery is frequently recognized in the domestic cat. The affected arteries have thick, hyperplastic muscular walls and often intimal fibrosis which effectively narrows the lumen (Fig. 22–13C). Present evidence indicates that this lesion is related to prior infection with *Aleurostrongylus abstrusus* (p. 768) or *Toxocara cati* (p. 734) (Stunzi, *et al.*, 1966, Hamilton, 1966.)

Equine Intimal Bodies.—Mineralized hyaline bodies have been noted from time to time in the intima of arterioles of horses (Marcus and Ross, 1967). In ordinary paraffin-embedded sections these bodies appear as pleomorphic, densely stained bodies in the vascular endothelium. The exact pathologic significance of these structures is unknown but they have been characterized morphologically at light and electron microscopic levels by Montali, Strandberg and Squire (1970). This work indicates that these bodies are "mineralized, degenerate cellular and intercellular elements that arise from subendothelial cells and intercellular material of the vascular wall" (Figs. 22–16, 22–17, 22–18, 22–19).

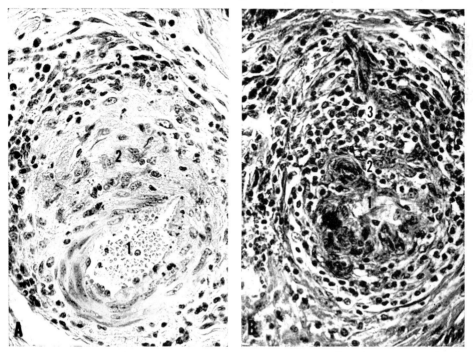

FIG. 22–15.—Periarteritis nodosa in bovine arteries. *A*, A mildly affected artery (× 330). The arterial lumen (*1*), media (*2*) and adventitia (*3*). *B*, A severely affected artery. Lumen (*1*), media (*2*) and adventitia (*3*). (Courtesy of Armed Forces Institute of Pathology.) Contributor: Dr. C. L. Davis.

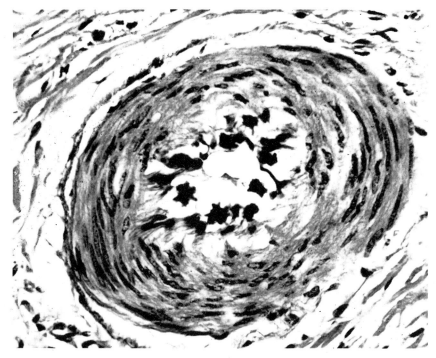

FIG. 22–16.—Equine intimal bodies. Irregularly shaped dense bodies in intima of an arteriole. (Courtesy of Dr. Richard J. Montali and *Laboratory Investigation*.)

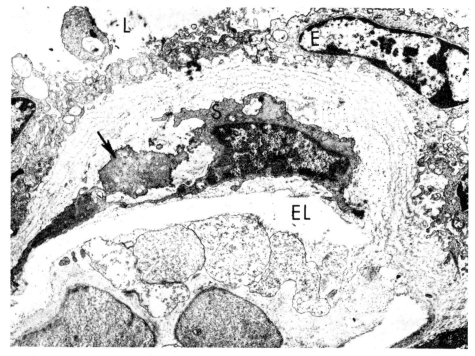

FIG. 22–17.—Equine intimal body. Electron micrograph (× 8,200). L = lumen of arteriole; E = nucleus of endothelial cell; EL = internal elastic lamina; S = subendothelial cell; arrow = irregular dense mass associated with cytoplasm of subendothelial cell. (Courtesy of Dr. Richard J. Montali and *Laboratory Investigation*.)

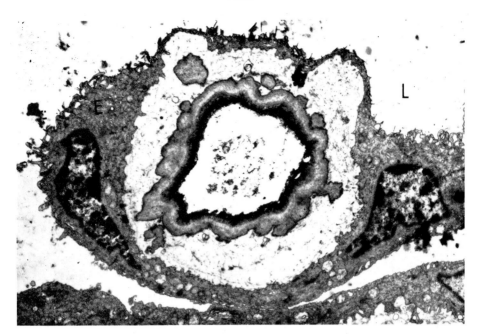

FIG. 22–18.—Equine intimal body with a hollow core (× 8,000). E = endothelial cell, surrounding central mass; L = lumen of arteriole. (Courtesy of Dr. Richard J. Montali and *Laboratory Investigation*.)

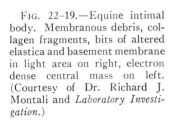

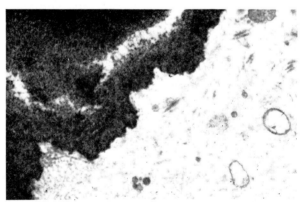

FIG. 22–19.—Equine intimal body. Membranous debris, collagen fragments, bits of altered elastica and basement membrane in light area on right, electron dense central mass on left. (Courtesy of Dr. Richard J. Montali and *Laboratory Investigation*.)

VEINS

Phlebitis is inflammation of a vein. It is characterized by the presence of any of the usual inflammatory exudates (p. 152). Most frequently neutrophilic leukocytes predominate; in chronic forms inflammatory fibrous tissue surrounds the vein. These can hardly be expected to be confined within the thin wall of a vein but phlebitis occurs usually within a more extensive inflamed and infected area through which the vein passes. Or, it may represent spread of the inflammatory process to the wall when an infected embolus lodges in the lumen or a thrombus forms there. Commonly the term phlebitis is employed, with its emphasis on the venous lesion, when there is especial concern for the spread of the infectious inflammation along the venous passageway, or perhaps when the process starts by virtue of injury incurred by the vein itself, as in the case of repeated, unsterile and unskillfully made therapeutic venipunctures. Phlebitis involving the smaller veins is a regular feature of extensively infected wounds, of septic metritis or of similar processes. The principal dangers from such inflamed (and usually infected) veins are two: necrosis resulting in local hemorrhage, and formation of thrombi, parts of which may become detached as emboli (p. 113).

Varicose veins are those that are markedly dilated and, at the same time, elongated so that, in order to find a place for the excess length, they follow an irregular, tortuous course. They thus hold an abnormal amount of blood, which tends to become static. Local anoxia and malnutrition result, together with a certain amount of pain. The condition also favors thrombosis within the vein, although this is not a frequent complication unless there is operative or other intervention. In animals, they occur chiefly in the hind legs, the saphenous and other superficial veins being involved. The usual cause is trauma or traumatic hindrance of return flow at some point in advance of the varicose area.

Telangiectasis is a marked dilatation of each of an abnormal cluster of blood vessels. The structure of their walls usually characterizes them as capillaries, although occasionally the more complicated structure of veins may be present. A type occurring beneath the skin or mucous membrane and elsewhere in humans is considered to be hereditary. The usual telangiectasis in veterinary parlance is a similar dilatation of a group of sinusoidal capillaries in one or more lobules of the bovine liver. The gross appearance is that of a small (one to several millimeters), irregular spot which is slightly depressed and so dark with venous blood as to be almost black. The lesions are often numerous in livers of animals slaughtered for food and cause condemnation of the affected parts. They are thought to be causally related to infection of the liver with the necrophorus organism (p. 623). Extreme examples of telangiectasis may simulate hemangioma.

LYMPHATIC VESSELS

Lymphangitis is diagnosed under much the same circumstances as phlebitis, that is, when we are concerned with an infectious inflammatory process which may spread by way of lymphatic vessels. The extremely thin vascular wall is, in itself, scarcely capable of harboring any significant inflammatory exudate; the disease process belongs originally to the surrounding tissues. The specific lymphangitides, such as equine epizoötic lymphangitis (p. 664), cause the subcutaneous and other lymphatic vessels to be visibly distended and somewhat thickened, but the lesions are principally in the contiguous tissues, including the normally microscopic lymphoid aggregates which are interspersed along the vessels. Failure of drainage, of course, produces edema (p. 134) of the part in question.

Lymphatic vessels are regenerated or reinforced by the formation of collateral vessels within a few (four to ten) days following operative or traumatic destruction, their function of drainage being only very transiently interrupted.

Tumors of blood and lymph vessels, hemangiomas and lymphangiomas, respectively, are treated in Chapter 7, p. 204.

Arteries, Veins and Lymphatics

ALTERA, K. P., and BONASCH, H.: Periarteritis Nodosa in a Cat. J. Am. Vet. Med. Assn. *149*:1307–1311, 1966.
ANDREWS, E. J., and KELLY, D. F.: Naturally Occurring Aortic Medial Necrosis in a Dog. Am. J. Vet. Res. *31*:791–795, 1970.

ARNOLD, R. M., and BRAS, G.: Observations on the Morbid Anatomy and Histology of Manchester Wasting Disease of Cattle in Jamaica, and Related Conditions in Other Countries of the Americas. Am. J. Vet. Res. *17*:630–639, 1956.

ARNOLD, R. M., and FINCHAM, I. H.: Cardiovascular and Pulmonary Calcification Apparently Associated with Dietary Imbalance in Jamaica. J. Comp. Path. *60*:51–64, 1950.

BACHHUBER, T. E., and LALICH, J. J.: Production of Dissecting Aneurysms in Rats Fed *Lathyrus odoratus.* Science *120*:712–713, 1954.

BIBRACK, B.: The Pathogenesis and Etiology of Obliteration of the Phalangeal Arteries in the Horse. Zbl. Vet. Med. Ser. A. *10*:67–84, 1963.

BISHOP, S. P., COLE, C. R., and SMETZER, D. L.: Functional and Morphologic Pathology of Equine Aortic Insufficiency. Path. Vet. *3*:137–158, 1966.

BLOOM, F.: Xanthomatosis of the Arterial Media in a Dog. Amer. J. Path. *22*:519–537, 1946.

BOSTROEM, B., and SCHOEDEL, W.: Uber die Durchblutung der arteriovenosen Anastomosen in der hinteren Extremität des Hundes. Arch. f.d. ges Physiol. *256*:371–380, 1953.

CARLSTRÖM, D., et al.: Chemical Composition of Normal and Abnormal Blood Vessel Walls. Chemical Nature of Vascular Calcified Deposits. Lab. Invest. *2*:325–335, 1953.

CARNAGHAN, R. B. A.: Atheroma of the Aorta Associated with Dissecting Aneurysms in Turkeys. Vet. Rec. *67*:568–569, 1955.

CARRILLO, B. J., and WORKER, N. A.: (Enteque seco: Arteriosclerosis and Metastatic Calcification of Toxic Origin in Grazing Animals.) Revta Investnes Agropec. *4*:9–30, 1967. V.B. *38*:1090, 1968.

CLARKSON, T. B., BULLOCK, B. C., and LEHNER, N. D. M.: Pathologic Characteristics of Atherosclerosis in New World Monkeys. Prog. Biochem. Pharmac. *4*:420–428, 1968.

COLOMBO, S., and CERIOLI, A.: (Significance and Pathogenesis of Calcification of the Arteries in Cattle.) Att. Soc. Ital. Sci. Vet. *18*:426–430, 1964. V.B. *36*:290, 1966.

————: Endocardial Thickening in Cattle. Att. Soc. Ital. Sci. Vet. *19*:388–392, 1966. V.B. *37*:343, 1967.

CONKLIN, J. W., et al.: Necrotizing Polyarteritis in Aging RF Mice. Lab. Invest. *16*: 483–487, 1967.

CUTTS, J. H.: Vascular Lesions Resembling Polyarteritis Nodosa in Rats Undergoing Prolonged Stimulation with Oestrogen. Brit. J. Exp. Path. *47*:401–404, 1966.

DAHME, E. G.: Atherosclerosis and Arteriosclerosis in Domestic Animals. Ann. New York Acad. Sci. *127*:657–670, 1965.

DAS, K. M., and TASHJIAN, R. J.: Chronic Mitral Valve Disease in the Dog. (A Preliminary Report on 550 Consecutive Necropsies.) Vet. Med. Small Anim. Clin. *60*:1209–1216, 1965.

DOEGLAS, A.: Een Methode tot Klinische Bloeddrukbepaling bij Honden. (A Method for Measuring Blood Pressure in Dogs.) Tijdschr. v. diergeneesk. *77*:123–136, 1952.

EGGEN, D. A., STRONG, J. P., and NEWMAN, W. P., III.: Experimental Atherosclerosis in Primates: A Comparison of Selected Species. Ann. New York Acad. Sci. *162*:110–119, 1969.

ENGELKE, J.: Endemisches Vorkommen der Periarteritis nodosa beim Schwein. Inaug. Diss. Hanover. Path. Inst. der Tierarztl. Hochschule. pp. 16, 1949.

FANKHAUSER, R., LUGINBUHL, H., and McGRATH, J. T.: Cerebrovascular Disease in Various Animal Species. Ann. New York Acad. Sci. *127*:817–859, 1965.

FARRELLY, B. T.: Pathogenesis and Significance of Parasitic Endarteritis and Thrombosis in the Ascending Aorta of the Horse. Vet. Rec. *66*:53–61, 1954.

FINLAYSON, R., SYMONS, C., and FIENNES, R. N. T. W.: Atherosclerosis: A Comparative Study. Brit. Med. J. Feb. 24, 1962, pp. 501–507.

FRENCH, J. E., JENNINGS, M. A., and FLOREY, N. W.: Morphological Studies on Atherosclerosis in Swine. Ann. New York Acad. Sci. *127*:780–799, 1965.

FRENCH, J. E., et al.: Intimal Changes in the Arteries of Ageing Swine. Proc. Roy. Soc. Ser. B. *158*:24–42, 1963.

FRY, R. J. M., HAMILTON, K. H., and LISCO, H.: Thrombi in the Left Atrium of the Heart in Mice. Arch. Path. *80*:308–313, 1965.

GAILIUNAS, P.: Calcification of Arteries in Young Cattle. Case Report. J. Am. Vet. Med. Assn. *132*:533, 1958.

GEER, J. C., et al.: Fine Structure of the Baboon Aortic Fatty Streak. Amer. J. Path. *52*:265–286, 1968.

GEISSINGER, H. D., and ANDRESS, C. E.: A Case of Porcine Endocarditis Associated with *Staphylococcus aureus.* Canad. Vet. J. *8*:236–238, 1967. V.B. *38*:875, 1968.

GOMAN, E. M., FEIGENBAUM, A. S., and SCHENK, E. A.: Spontaneous Aortic Lesions in Rabbits. Part 3. Incidence in Genetic Factors. J. Atheroscler. Res. *7*:131–141, 1967.

GOTTLIEB, H., and LALICH, J. J.: Occurrence of Arteriosclerosis in the Aorta of Swine Amer. J. Path. *30*:851–855, 1954.

GRESHAM, G. A., et al.: Atherosclerosis in Primates. Brit. J. Exp. Pathol. 46:94–103, 1965.

GUPTA, P. P., TANDON, H. D., and RAMALINGASWAMI, V.: Spontaneous Vascular Lesions in Indian Pigs. J. Path. 99:19–28, 1969.

GYORKEY, F., and REISER, R.: Experimental Dietary Arteriosclerosis in Young Swine: A Histopathological, Histochemical and Biochemical Study. Acta Morph. Hung. 12: 415–427, 1964. V.B. 35:1017, 1965.

HAMILTON, J. M.: Pulmonary Arterial Disease of the Cat. J. Comp. Path. 76:133–145, 1966.

————: Experimental Lung-worm Disease of the Cat. Association of the Condition with Lesions of the Pulmonary Arteries. J. Comp. Path. 76:147–157, 1966.

HARDING, J. D. J.: A Cerebrospinal Angiopathy in Pigs. Path. Vet. 3:83–88, 1966.

HATCH, F. T.: Critique of Current Theories in the Pathogenesis of Arteriosclerosis. Conn. State Med. J. 16:887–894, 1952.

HELMBOLDT, C. F., JUNGHERR, E. L., and HWANG, J.: Polyarteritis in Sheep. J. Am. Vet. Med. Assn. 134:556–561, 1959.

HOLZWORTH, J., et al.: Aortic Thrombosis with Posterior Paralysis in the Cat. Cornell Vet. 45:468–487, 1955.

HOPWOOD, R. T.: Perivascular Fibrosis of Splenic Follicular Blood Vessels in Macaca mulatta. Am. J. Vet. Res. 23:1303–1306, 1962.

HUMPHREYS, E. M.: Atherosclerosis in the Coronary Arteries of Rats. J. Athero. Res. 4: 416–434, 1964.

JONES, T. C., and ZOOK, B. C.: Aging Changes in the Vascular System of Animals. Ann. New York Acad. Sci. 127:671–684, 1965.

JORDAN, G. L., DEBAKEY, M. E., and HALPERT, B.: Coronary Atheromatous Change Induced by Chronic Hypercholesterolemia in Dogs. Amer. J. Path. 35:867–875, 1959.

KELLEY, F. B., JR., TAYLOR, C. B., and HASS, G. M.: Experimental Atheroarteriosclerosis. Arch. Path. 53:419–436, 1952.

KNIERIEM, H. J.: Electron-microscopic Study of Bovine Arteriosclerotic Lesions. Amer. J. Path. 50:1035–1065, 1967.

KOHLER, H.: Endarteritis obliterans der zehenarterien beim pferde. Frankf. Ztschr. f. Path. 62:326–344, 1951.

KRAUSE, C.: Zur frage der arteriosklerose bei Rind, pfered und hund. Beitr. z. path. Anat. u.z. allg. Path. 70:121–178, 1922.

LANDI, A.: Su di un particolare caso di calcificazione nell aorta di un cane. Atti. Soc. ital. sci. vet., Sanremo 6:202–205, 1952.

LIKAR, I. N., and ROBINSON, R. W.: Bovine Arterial Disease. I. Localization of Lipids in the Abdominal Aorta in Relation to Bovine Atherosclerosis. Arch. Path. 82:555–560, 1966.

————: Lipid Distribution and Pattern in Abdominal Aorta with and Without Naturally Occurring Lesions. Arch. Path. 82:561–565, 1966.

LINDSAY, S., and CHAIKOFF, I. L.: Coronary Arteriosclerosis of Birds; Comparison of Spontaneous and Experimental Lesions. Arch. Path. 49:434–446, 1950.

LINDSAY, S., CHAIKOFF, I. L., and GILMORE, J. W.: Arteriosclerosis in the Dog, Spontaneous Lesions in the Aorta and Coronary Arteries. Arch. Path. 53:281–300, 1952. In the Cat; Arch. Path. 60:29–38, 1955.

LINDSAY, S., et al.: "Arteriosclerosis in the Dog." II. Aortic, Cardiac, and Other Vascular Lesions in Thyroidectomized-hypophysectomized Dogs. A.M.A. Arch. Path. 54:573–591, 1952.

LINDSAY, S., CHAIKOFF, I. L.: Naturally Occurring Arteriosclerosis in Nonhuman Primates. J. Atheroscler. Res. 6:36–61, 1966.

LLOYD, H. E. D.: Arteriosclerosis in Certain Wild Animals Dying in Captivity. J. Comp. Path. & Therap. 69:98–104, 1959.

LOFLAND, H. B., et al.: Atherosclerosis in Cebus albifrons Monkeys. I. Sterol Metabolism. Exp. & Molec. Path. 8:302–313, 1968.

LUCKÉ, V. M.: Renal Polyarteritis Nodosa in the Cat. Vet. Rec. 82:622–624, 1968.

LUGINBUHL, H.: Angiopathien im Zentralnervensystem bei Tieren Schw. Arch. f. Tierh. 104:694–700, 1962.

LUGINBUHL, H., RATCLIFFE, H. L., and DETWEILER, D. K.: Failure of Egg-yoke Feeding to Accelerate Progress of Atherosclerosis in Older Female Swine. Virchows. Arch. Path. Anat. 348:281–289, 1969.

LYND, F. T., et al.: Bovine Arteriosclerosis in Hawaii. Am. J. Vet. Res. 26:1344–1349, 1965.

McALLISTER, W. B., JR., and WATERS, L. L.: Vascular Lesions in the Dog Following Thyroidectomy and Viosterol Feeding. Yale J. Biol. & Med. 22:651–700, 1950.

MacNINTCH, J. E., et al.: Cholesterol Metabolism and Atherosclerosis in Cebus Monkeys in Relation to Age. Lab. Invest. 16:444–452, 1967.

MALINOW, M. R., and MARUFFO, C. A.: Aortic Atherosclerosis in Free-ranging Howler Monkeys (*Alouatta caraya*). Nature, Lond. *206*:948–949, 1965.

————: Naturally Occurring Atherosclerosis in Howler Monkeys (*Alouatta caraya*). J. Atheroscler. Res. *6*:368–380, 1965.

MALINOW, M. R., and STORVICK, C. A.: Spontaneous Coronary Lesions in Howler Monkeys (*Alouatta caraya*). J. Atheroscler. Res. *8*:421–431, 1968.

MARCUS, L. C., and ROSS, J. N.: Microscopic Lesions in the Hearts of Aged Horses. Path. Vet. *4*:162–185, 1967.

McCOMBS, H. L., ZOOK, B. C., and McGANDY, R. B.: Fine Structure of Spontaneous Atherosclerosis of the Aorta in the Squirrel Monkey. Amer. J. Path. *55*:235–252, 1969.

McCULLY, K. S.: Vascular Pathology of Homocysteinemia: Implications for the Pathogenesis of Arteriosclerosis. Amer. J. Path. *56*:111–128, 1969.

McGRATH, J. M., and STEWART, G. J.: The Effects of Endotoxin on Vascular Endothelium. J. Exp. Med. *129*:833–848, 1969.

McSHERRY, B. J., et al.: Dissecting Aneurysm in Internal Hemorrhage in Turkeys. J. Am. Vet. Med. Assn. *124*:279–283, 1954.

MIDDLETON, C. C., et al.: Naturally Occurring Atherosclerosis in the Squirrel Monkey (*Saimiri sciurea*). Circulation *28*:665–666, 1963.

MIDDLETON, C. C., et al.: Atherosclerosis in the Squirrel Monkey. Arch. Path. *78*:16–23, 1964.

MONTALI, E. J., STRANDBERG, J. D., and SQUIRE, R. A.: A Histochemical and Ultrastructural Study of Intimal Bodies in Horse Arterioles. Lab. Invest. *23*:302–306, 1970.

MOORE, L. A., HALLMAN, E. T., and SHOLL, L. B.: Cardiovascular and Other Lesions in Calves Fed Diets Low in Magnesium. Arch. Path. *26*:820–838, 1938.

MOOREHEAD, R. P., and LITTLE, J. M.: Changes in the Blood Vessels of Apparently Healthy Mongrel Dogs. Amer. J. Path. *21*:339–353, 1945.

OKA, M., BRODIE, S. S., and ANGRIST, A. A.: Sex-dependent Vascular Changes in Young, Adult, Aged and Hypertensive Rats. Amer. J. Path. *53*:127–147, 1968.

PICK, R., et al.: Production of Ulcerated Atherosclerotic Lesions in Cockerels. Circulation Res. *11*:811–819, 1962.

PRIOR, J. T., and HUTTER, R. V. P.: Intimal Repair of the Aorta of the Rabbit Following Experimental Trauma. Amer. J. Path. *31*:107–123, 1955.

PRITCHARD, W. R., HENDERSON, W., and BEALL, C. W.: Experimental Production of Dissecting Aneurysm in Turkeys. Am. J. Vet. Res. *19*:696–705, 1958.

RATCLIFFE, H. L., and SNYDER, R. L.: "Coronary Arterial Lesions in Chickens: Origin and Rates of Development in Relation to Sex and Social Factors." Cir. Res. *17*:403–413, 1965.

RINEHART, J. F., and GREENBERG, L. D.: Arteriosclerotic Lesions in Pyridoxine-deficient Monkeys. Amer. J. Path. *25*:481–491, 1949.

ROBERTS, J. C., and STRAUS, R. (ed.): *Comparative Atherosclerosis*. New York, Harper & Row, 1965.

ROONEY, J. R., PRICKETT, M. E., and CROWE, M. W.: Aortic Ring Rupture in Stallions. Path. Vet. *4*:268–274, 1967.

RUBIN, L. F., and PATTERSON, D. F.: Arteriovenous Fistula of the Orbit in a Dog. Cornell Vet. *55*:471–481, 1965.

SCHENK, E. A., GAMAN, E., and FEIGENBAUM, A. S.: Spontaneous Aortic Lesions in Rabbits. I. Morphologic Characteristics. II. Relationship to Experimental Atherosclerosis. Circulation Res. *19*:80–95, 1966.

SHERWOOD, B. F., et al.: Bacterial Endocarditis, Glomerulonephritis and Amyloidosis in the Opossum (*Didelphis virginiana*). Amer. J. Path. *53*:115–126, 1968.

SIMPSON, C. F., and HARMS, R. H.: Pathology of Aortic Atherosclerosis and Dissecting Aneurysms of Turkeys Induced by Diethylstilbestrol. Exp. & Molec. Path. *5*:183–184, 1966.

SKOLD, B. H., GETTY, R., and RAMSEY, F. K.: Spontaneous Atherosclerosis in the Arterial System of Aging Swine. Am. J. Vet. Res. *27*:257–273, 1966.

ST. CLAIR, R. W., et al.: Changes in Serum Cholesterol Levels of Squirrel Monkeys During Importation and Acclimation. Lab. Invest. *16*:828–832, 1967.

STEINER, A., and KENDALL, F. E.: Atherosclerosis and Arteriosclerosis in Dogs Following Ingestion of Cholesterol and Thiouracil. Arch. Path. *42*:433–434, 1946.

STOUT, C.: Atherosclerosis in Exotic Carnivora and Pinnipedia. Amer. J. Path. *57*:673–687, 1969.

STRAUCH, C.: Zur kenntnis der spontanen Arterienveranderungen beim Hunde mit besonderer Berucksichtigung der arteriosklerose. Beitr. z. path. Anat. u.z. allg. Path. *61*: 532–549, 1916.

STRONG, J. P., and TAPPEN, N. C.: Naturally Occurring Arterial Lesions in African Monkeys. Arch. Path., *79*:199–205, 1965.

STUNZI, H., TEUSCHER, E., and PERICIN-RAUHUR, D.: Die hyperplasia der arteria pulmonalis bei feliden. Path. Vet. *3*:461–473, 1966.

SUZUKI, M., *et al*.: "Experimental Atherosclerosis in the Dog: A Morphologic Study." Exp. Molec. Path. *3*:455–467, 1964.

WILENS, S. L., and PLAIR, C. M.: The Relationship between Cortical Hyperplasia of the Adrenals and Arteriosclerosis. Amer. J. Path. *41*:224–232, 1962.

WILLERS, E. H., *et al*.: Experimental Studies of Bovine Arteriosclerosis in Hawaii. Am. J. Vet. Res. *26*:1350–1355, 1965.

WISSLER, R. W.: Recent Progress in Studies of Experimental Primate Atherosclerosis. Prog. Biochem. Pharm. *4*:378–392, 1968.

WORKER, N. A., and CARRILLO, B. J.: "Enteque Seco," Calcification and Wasting in Grazing Animals in the Argentine. Nature *215*:72–74, 1967.

YOUNG, Y. H.: Polyarteritis Nodosa in Lab Rats. Lab. Invest. *14*:81–88, 1965.

YOUNGER, R. K., *et al*.: Rapid Production of Experimental Hypercholesterolemia and Atherosclerosis in the Rhesus Monkey: Comparison of Five Dietary Regimens. J. Surg. Res. *9*:263–271, 1969.

ZEEK, P. M.: Periarteritis Nodosa and Other Forms of Necrotizing Angitis. N.E. J. Med. *248*:764–772, 1953.

ZINSERLING, W. D.: Uber bindegewebige intimaverdickungen und spontane lipoidose der Aorta und anderer Organe bei Hunden. Beitr. path. Anat. u. allg. Path. *88*:241–314, 1932.

23
The Hemic and Lymphatic Systems

THE BONE MARROW

When one hears the term, bone marrow, it is the red marrow to which reference is made. The fatty marrow is inert with respect to hematopoiesis and merely fills space left by the functional red marrow. In early life all marrow is red; by the time of maturity this has normally been replaced by fatty marrow in the long bones, beginning at the distal ends of the limbs and leaving, perhaps, a bit of red marrow at the proximal epiphyses of the humerus and femur. Even the red marrow commonly contains some adipose cells, the functional myeloid and related cells being scattered among them, all held together by a reticulum of connective tissue, with numerous blood vessels.

The cells of the bone marrow form a series of graduations from the large, round myeloblast with its central spherical nucleus and very limited basophilic cytoplasm to the polymorphonuclear leukocytes, neutrophilic, eosinophilic or basophilic, or to the nucleated erythroblast with its acidophilic cytoplasm and its successor, the non-nucleated erythrocyte. Many intermediate types are recognized by hematologists, but they can seldom be identified in sections. Megakaryocytes, also called bone-marrow giant cells, are huge, irregularly nucleated cells scattered among the others. Mononuclear reticulo-endothelial cells form a part of the supporting framework. While the great majority of the cells are engaged in the formation of more blood cells, a process called hematopoiesis, the reticulo-endothelials have, among others, the function of converting into bilirubin the hemoglobin from red blood cells which have completed their life-span and disintegrated. In birds and lower forms, the erythrocytes retain their nucleus, as the student is aware. In these creatures, birds, reptiles and amphibians, the erythrocytes are formed within vascular sinuses and the granulocytes develop outside such spaces. Whether the same occurs in mammals has not been positively determined but this may well be true, since the erythrocytes are frequently seen to be developing in close groups.

Bone-marrow cells deteriorate rapidly after death. They are usually studied from biopsies obtained during life. A segment of the sternum is usually punctured by means of a fine canula, but in horses and cattle, puncture of a rib has been found more feasible. The iliac crest has also been used with success in most animals as well as in man. Smears obtained from biopsies are essential to cellular identification and determination of myeloid:erythroid ratios. Tissue sections prepared from autopsy material are necessary to evaluate aplasia, hypoplasia or hypertrophy and to identify focal lesions such as granulomas or metastatic neoplasms.

Hyperplasia of the bone marrow is also known as hypertrophy, since the change involves an enhanced function. It is recognized grossly in the form of an increase in the amount of red marrow and a decrease of the fatty marrow, as compared with the normal for a given age. In pronounced hyperplasias which have existed for a considerable time, the red marrow is found to have replaced the adult fatty marrow of the long bones to a very considerable extent, beginning at the proximal ends of the femur and humerus and extending distally through the extremities. The finer bony trabeculae which reach from the endosteal zone into the marrow cavity tend to disappear before the advancing hyperplastic marrow tissue. In judging the degree of hyperplasia of bone marrows an accurate knowledge of the normal is necessary. In general, at the time a normal animal is half grown there is practically no red marrow in the marrow cavity of the radius, tibia and bones distal to them. Toward the proximal end of the humerus and femur a minimal amount of marrow can be expected at this age. As the animal approaches maturity even this disappears. Red marrow, of course, fills the marrow spaces of the spongy, or cancellous, bone of the epiphysis proper at all ages, as well as that of the flat bones, namely the ribs, sternum and bones of the skull and pelvis. In case a biopsy of bone marrow is to be made the sternum or iliac crest are the customary sites although many find the tuber coxae more readily feasible in large animals. There are two principal varieties of **myeloid hyperplasia,** as the condition is synonymously designated.

Erythroblastic hyperplasia is characterized by red marrow which microscopically is found to consist principally of the precursors of erythrocytes, namely erythroblasts and normoblasts. This occurs in and is a reaction to most of the anemias (p. 123) except toxic aplastic anemia, which owes its existence to inability of the marrow to function. In human pernicious anemia, with its deficient erythrocyte-maturing factor, and in the similar anemia due to the fish tape-worm, *Diphyllobothrium latum*, megaloblasts become numerous and the terms megaloblastic anemia and megaloblastic hyperplasia are applicable.

Leukoblastic hyperplasia, on the other hand, is characterized by a predominance of the precursors of leukocytes, usually mature and immature neutrophilic granulocytes and their predecessors, the myelocytes and myeloblasts. This variety of hyperplasia occurs in consequence of those infections which are accompanied by leukocytosis and a vigorous pyogenic reaction. If, however, the pyogenic disease is prolonged for several weeks, the myeloid cells and their progeny become exhausted, leaving little but erythroblastic cells and some lymphoid cells. The leukocytosis is naturally replaced by a leukopenia (p. 172).

A leukoblastic reaction with large numbers of eosinophilic granulocytes and their predecessors is found in many human cases of ancylostomiasis and trichinosis and the same may be presumed to be true in animals. In lymphoid leukemia (malignant lymphoma, p. 208), areas of marrow may be largely replaced by lymphoid cells. In myeloid leukemia, the neoplastic myeloma cells take possession of many areas of the marrow. In these cases, as well as in leukoblastic hyperplasia, the marrow grossly tends toward a grayish color without the yellowish tinge of fat.

Hypoplasia of the bone marrow occurs in connection with toxic aplastic anemia (p. 129), being, indeed, the cause of it. The proportion of fatty marrow is greater than normal and frequently such hematopoietic tissue as remains is scattered in little islands through the fatty marrow. Microscopically, it may be principally

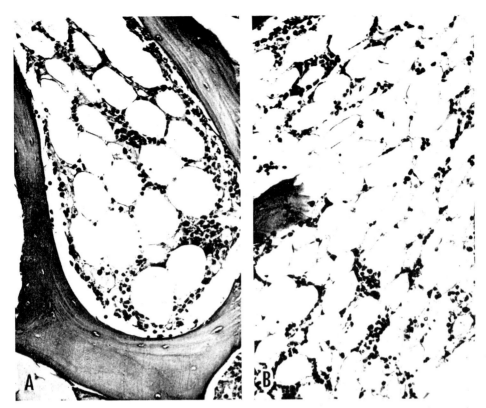

FIG. 23–1.—Hypoplasia of the bone marrow in a dog with hypochromic microcytic anemia. *A*, A rib ($\times$ 195). *B*, Sternum ($\times$ 195). Note paucity of hematopoietic cells as in rib. (*B*, Courtesy of Armed Forces Institute of Pathology.) Contributor: Dr. E. E. Ruebush.

the erythropoietic forms of developing cells that are missing or the deficiency may involve all cell types. In **leukopenia** (p. 172), which results from the marrow-depressant action of certain infections, the more mature forms of the leuko-blastic series of cells, especially the neutrophilic granulocytes and their predecessors, are largely or entirely absent.

Agranulocytosis must be mentioned here. The term refers to a more or less complete absence of granulocytes from the circulating blood. This, in turn, is due to a complete aplasia of the leukoblastic cells of the bone marrow. It is thus related to aplastic anemia (p. 129) and probably attributable to very similar toxic causes. A number of commonly used medicines are known to have a depressant action on the bone marrow and are cited under the latter type of anemia. Since the tissues are deprived of the protection of leukocytes, the condition is usually fatal in a few weeks at most as the result of some infection which would be trivial in a normal individual. Agranulocytosis is diagnosed with a fair degree of frequency in human medicine. In animals, it doubtless occurs when the same causes are operating but this is apparently rather seldom.

Summarizing, it may be said that hyperplasia of the bone marrow is a reaction tending to mend damage to the circulating cells it is charged with producing. Hypoplasia and aplasia result from injury to the marrow itself by toxins or generalized infections with deficiencies and abnormalities of the circulating blood as the result.

Osteomyelitis is an inflammatory process in the bone marrow due to infection, which gains access to the marrow through a local wound (fracture, etc.) or by hematogenous metastasis. It is thus a localized process, involving usually a single bone, in contrast to the widespread character of hyperplasia, hypoplasia and aplasia. The infection is usually pyogenic and the reaction purulent, although specific infections such as tuberculosis and coccidioidomycosis also produce their typical lesions in the bone marrow. Due to the difficulty of drainage and other anatomical considerations, osteomyelitis was much to be feared prior to the advent of modern antibiotics and is still difficult to treat. The condition is recognized grossly by a painful accumulation of pus which eventually causes softening and necrosis of the overlying bony wall and makes its way to the body surface. Microscopically, accumulation of neutrophilic polymorphonuclear leukocytes, and perhaps fibrin and other inflammatory elements at times almost to the exclusion of the myeloid cells, reveals the nature of the condition.

Fibrosis of the bone marrow, with or without **myxomatous degeneration** (p. 52), occurs as a rare accompaniment of or sequel to hypoplasia or aplasia. The cause is obscure: possibly some forms represent exhaustion of a previously active marrow. Myxomatous degeneration is prominent in starvation.

THE CIRCULATING BLOOD

Anemia, a deficiency of erythrocytes or of hemoglobin or both, has been studied on page 123.

Polycythemia is an excess of circulating erythrocytes. In the great majority of cases, an excessive number of erythrocytes noted in the blood-cell count is purely relative; the total number of cells is not increased but the total volume of plasma is decreased. This is the result, ordinarily, of **dehydration,** the bane of the clinician, the importance and frequency of which are not always realized. Dehydration may result from severe vomiting, diarrhea or hemorrhage, but usually it is due to the fact that the animal patient is too weak to get to its source of water. It is in such cases purely a nursing problem, but one of prime importance to the welfare and comfort of the patient. Death from disease may not be always preventable, but death from thirst should be avoided.

An absolute, rather than relative, polycythemia, also known as erythrocytosis, results from prolonged but mild anoxemia. This occurs as a feature of life in high altitudes and compensates for the fact that a "lung-full" of air at a high altitude is considerably less (by weight) than it is at sea-level, (see also p. 1131). A sufficient degree of anoxia to cause erythrocytosis also sometimes occurs in such diseases of the heart as patent foramen ovale and patent ductus arteriosus, as well as in severe pulmonary emphysema, fibrosis or other disorders interfering with oxygenation of the blood.

Polycythemia which is not related to anoxia nor relative to reduced plasma volume (both of which are secondary polycythemia) is known to occur in man as **polycythemia vera,** a disease of adults, and **familial polycythemia** which occurs in childhood. In both there is an absolute increase in erythrocyte count of unknown cause. Tennant and associates (1967) have described a disease in Jersey cattle which appeared to be an inherited primary polycythemia. The pattern of inheritance indicated control by an autosomal, recessive gene. Polycythemia developed during the second month of life, persisted throughout the first year and subsided

at maturity.   Clinical signs included congestion of mucous membranes, dyspnea
and retarded growth.   Hematologically there was marked elevation in erythrocyte count, hemoglobin and packed cell volume without the appearance of immature erythrocytes.   There was no change in other cellular elements.   Two reports
have described apparent primary polycythemia in cocker spaniels (Cole, 1954;
Donovan and Loeb, 1959), and a single report has described the disease in a cat
(Reed, *et al.*, 1970).

Other abnormalities of the circulating blood include excesses of leukocytes,
which are **leukocytosis** (p. 172) if inflammatory and **leukemia** (p. 213) if neoplastic.   An abnormally low number of leukocytes constitutes **leukopenia** (p. 172).
In tissues, leukocytes of one type or another participate in most inflammatory
reactions (p. 169) and are victims of certain specific infections and poisons.   Aside
from these "general" degenerative inflammatory and neoplastic reactions of
leukocytes, few specific diseases focus on the leukocyte.

Chediac-Higashi Syndrome.—Although this disorder involves many tissues
and cell types, most attention has focused on abnormal granules in peripheral
leukocytes and accordingly we will briefly consider this rare syndrome under
circulating blood.   Described in man, cattle, mink and mice, the Chediac-
Higashi syndrome is characterized by the presence of giant granules or cytoplasmic
inclusions in neutrophils, eosinophils, basophils, monocytes and lymphocytes as
well as in many other cell types, such as hepatocytes, renal tubular epithelium,
neurons, endothelial cells and melanocytes.   Ultrastructural studies indicate that
the granules are abnormal lysosomes, but their exact significance is unknown.   In
man, cattle and mink the disease is inherited by an autosomal recessive gene.
All affected individuals are partial albinos; in mink the coat color of this partial
albinism is known as Aleutian or "blue" and all Aleutian mink have the Chediak-
Higashi syndrome.   Other characteristics of the disease include photophobia
(albinism), hemorrhagic tendencies and a marked susceptibility to infections
which usually accounts for the cause of death.   In mink there is increased susceptibility to the virus of Aleutian disease (p. 501), which may, of course, affect mink
of any coat color.   No satisfactory explanation has been found to explain the
increased susceptibility to infection or the hemorrhagic tendency.

Cyclic Neutropenia.—Also known as "gray Collie syndrome," cyclic neutropenia is confined to the collie breed and only occurs in dogs with a gray (dark
pewter gray to silver) coat color.   A similar disorder is known in man.   Not all
gray collies suffer from cyclic neutropenia, a fact clearly illustrated by the studies of Ford (1969) who demonstrated that at least three types of gray or silver
collies exist which are controlled by separate genes.   Dominant gray or slate gray
is inherited as a dominant gene and only appears if observable in one parent.
Dominant gray collies are normal.   Maltese gray collie pups appear in litters of
nongray parents.   The controlling gene is recessive and the dogs are normal.
Lethal gray which is light silvery gray (almost white) is also inherited as a recessive gene which is apparently not an allele to maltese gray.   Lethal gray collies
suffer from cyclic neutropenia and generally die before maturity.   As its name
suggests, the outstanding characteristic of this disease is a periodic neutropenia
occurring at regular intervals of eight to twelve days.   Neutrophils may completely disappear from the peripheral blood only to reappear with a "rebound"
neutrophilia.   The cause of the neutropenia is apparently a failure of maturation
of stem cells.   The controlling mechanism is not known, nor do we have an expla-

nation for the periodicity of this failure. The dogs are extremely susceptible to infections, which if not controlled lead to their death. Whether other primary abnormalities are associated with the disease and contribute to death has not been determined. Cheville (1968) described fundic ectasia with incomplete pigmentation of the retina, maladsorption and diarrhea and failure of maturation of the gonads as part of the picture. It is not known whether these lesions are linked to the controlling lethal gray gene. He also reported amyloidosis which would appear to be related to chronic infection.

Reticulo-endotheliosis.—Reticulo-endotheliosis as described by Gilmore, Gilmore and Jones (1964) is a reticuloproliferative disease of cats characterized by proliferation of undifferentiated (reticulum) cells in bone marrow, spleen, liver and lymph nodes and their entrance into peripheral blood. The principal clinical signs are anorexia, listlessness, loss of weight, fever, splenomegaly, hepatomegaly and enlargement of lymph nodes. Hematologic findings include anemia and usually leukocytosis. Total leukocyte counts as reported in Gilmore's series of 10 cats ranged from 6,100 to 53,000/cmm. of blood. In each example reticulum cells accounted for up to 55 per cent of the circulating leukocytes and up to 76.8 per cent of cells in the bone marrow. The cells have large round red-purple eccentric nuclei with a fine chromatin pattern, a single pale blue nucleolus and abundant dull blue cytoplasm with azurophilic granules. There is no evidence of maturation to another cell type. The disease is rapidly progressive, leading to death in two to four weeks after clinical signs are first noted. Gross findings are dominated by marked splenomegaly and enlargement of the liver and lymph nodes. Microscopically, reticulum cells fill the vascular and lymphatic spaces in these organs, remaining individually discrete without forming solid sheets or invading connective tissues. Extramedullary hematopoiesis was found by Gilmore and associates in the liver, spleen and lymph nodes.

The cause of reticulo-endotheliosis is not known. It is distinguishable from malignant lymphoma with leukemia (p. 208) but no doubt the two have often been confused. Whether the disease is malignant is not clearly established, but is somewhat only of academic importance. The interpretation of many reticuloproliferative diseases of man and animals vacillates between neoplastic and proliferative inflammation depending on who is doing the interpretation and the prevailing fashion. No doubt, in reticuloproliferative disorders a broad gray zone exists between simple proliferation and malignancy.

Purpura Hemorrhagica.—Encountered principally in humans and horses, purpura hemorrhagica denotes a syndrome characterized by many hemorrhages, petechial or ecchymotic in size, in the skin and external and internal mucous membranes. In the horse there is usually much subcutaneous edema, perhaps localized about the head or commonly in the form of numerous subcutaneous swellings several centimeters in diameter suggestive of urticaria. The cutaneous hemorrhages frequently bleed into these plaque-like collections of edema fluid. The disease is afebrile throughout most of its stormy course, of variable severity but frequently fatal. In veterinary medicine practically all reported cases have supervened when the patient appeared to be recovering from some infectious or necrotizing disease, such as equine strangles or other respiratory infection, often with streptococcal organisms as the cause.

The Latin word, purpura, refers merely to the purple color of the hemorrhagic spot (in a white skin). Hence, in some quarters there has been a confusing tendency to designate as "purpura" any disease characterized by multiple hemorrhages into the tissues. Such confusion can at least be avoided in veterinary medicine with its frequently encountered and usually well-defined acute hemorrhagic diseases (p. 119). Classically, purpura hemorrhagica is the result of a severe deficiency of platelets in the circulating blood (thrombocytopenia). This form of purpura is appropriately termed thrombocytopenic purpura and is discussed below, but limited studies on horses with purpura hemorrhagica have usually shown no thrombocytopenia, nor defects in coagulation. Marked neutrophilia and mild icterus have been reported and in one study (King, 1949) hemorrhagic focal necroses were found in the voluntary muscles. Possibly from the resultant release of myoglobin, there were also renal lesions comparable to those seen in the "crush syndrome" of humans and experimental animals (and azoturia, p. 1046). The most striking feature of purpura in horses is edema of subcutaneous tissues.

That edema and hemorrhage by diapedesis, such as occurs in this disease, could result from injury to the capillaries seems self-evident. While the degree of permeability or impermeability of capillary walls has defied accurate elucidation, the concept of increased permeability in inflammation is well founded, if not understood (p. 147). There is no reason to discredit the possibility of a similar state of increased permeability in equine purpura hemorrhagica and in many examples of this disorder such an injurious change in capillary walls must be thought to exist for as indicated above the thrombocytopenia proves to be minor or absent.

How, then, do the non-thrombocytopenic examples of purpura hemorrhagica differ from the numerous hemorrhagic disorders attributed to infections, toxic substances or anoxia? (p. 119.) The identifying characteristic of purpura hemorrhagica is that it appears in company with, but late in the course of an infection such as those mentioned, developing when convalescence had seemed to be well established. Etiologically speaking, this fact seems to tie it to a hypersensitization or anaphylaxis developing as a reaction to, but not a primary feature of, the original infection. That the manner of pathogenesis involves injury to capillary walls seems probable but is not proven. The other feature distinguishing purpura hemorrhagica from one of the primary hemorrhagic diseases is the fact that one of the latter with hemorrhagic lesions as extensive as those typically seen in purpura hemorrhagica would prove promptly fatal, probably within hours. The course of purpura hemorrhagica, even in fatal cases, is seldom less than several days.

In domestic species other than the equine this disease is certainly rare. There are reports of purpuric lesions in swine and one of the production of such lesions in dogs by the administration of sesame oil as a vehicle for estradiol benzoate (Cruz, et al., 1945). The equine species has long shown a strong propensity for developing antibodies; just possibly the preponderance of purpura hemorrhagica in this species is a further indication for an immunologic origin for the disease.

Thrombocytopenic Purpura.—A reduction in number of circulating platelets results in purpura hemorrhagica; owing to a prolongation of bleeding time. Edema and hemorrhage of subcutaneous tissues, mucous membranes and internal organs similar to equine purpura hemorrhagica described above characterize the clinical and pathological findings. In animals, thrombocytopenia is most often associated with disorders which cause extensive destruction of bone marrow, such

as may result from lymphomatous or other neoplastic invasion, ionizing radiations (p. 824) or the various inciters of aplastic anemia (bracken fern poisoning,
p. 907; trichlorethylene-extracted soybean meal poisoning, p. 914). Not to be
overlooked as a cause of thrombocytopenia is the simple hypothesis of exhaustion
of supply in the course of repeated attempts to seal leaking capillaries. Thrombocytopenia may also develop in the course of bacterial and viral infections. For
example thrombocytopenia is a regular finding in equine infectious anemia
(p. 481), and transient thrombocytopenia has been reported (Foster and Cameron,
1968) in sheep with experimental *tick-borne fever*. Tick-borne fever is usually a
mild transient infection of sheep and cattle in Great Britain caused by *Rickettsia
phagocytophilia*. Thrombocytopenia of unknown cause (idiopathic thrombocytopenia) is encountered on occasion in animals, but reports are few. Very possibly
certain examples of idiopathic thrombocytopenia are immunologic in origin.
Immunologic thrombocytopenia has been recognized in baby pigs caused by
maternal isoimmunization and in a horse and dogs as an autoimmune disease
(p. 1174). The disorder in pigs which has been described in Norway, Sweden,
Finland, England and Canada is analogous to isoimmune hemolytic anemias
(erythroblastosis fetalis, Rh phenomenon, p. 126). Following numerous pregnancies, antibodies against platelets of the offspring are developed in the sow
during gestation, resulting from mating with a boar possessing platelet antigens
different from those of the sow. Purpura which may lead to death develops in
the pig eight to seventy-two hours after birth, apparently receiving the anti-
thrombocyte antibodies in the colostrum. In addition to the usual lesions of
purpura, megakaryocytes may be absent from the bone marrow. Autoimmune
hemolytic anemia with thrombocytopenia has been reported in dogs (Lewis, *et al.*,
1963, 1965) and limited evidence suggests its occurrence in horses (Farrelly, *et al.*,
1966).

    Immunohemolytic Anemias.—Isoimmune hemolytic anemias (erythroblastosis
fetalis) has been considered in Chapter 5 (p. 126). What remains to be discussed
here is autoimmune hemolytic anemia. A general discussion of autoimmunity
will be found in Chapter 8 (p. 312). Autoimmune hemolytic anemia which has
been documented in dogs (Lewis, *et al.*, 1963, 1965) and apparently in horses
(Farrelly, *et al.*, 1966) results from an immune response directed against the
animals own erythrocytes (and other tissues). Erythrocytes coated with the
autoantibody directed against them, become spherical in shape (spherocytes;
spherocytosis), become more fragile, may agglutinate and are actively destroyed
by the spleen, leading to anemia. The coated erythrocytes are detected by the
direct Coomb's test, which is necessary to establish the diagnosis. The Coomb's
test employs a specific anti-canine-globulin (or anti-horse, human etc.), usually
prepared in rabbits, which when mixed with washed erythrocytes coated with
autoantibody (globulin) causes agglutination. In the series of dogs with autoimmune hemolytic anemia reported by Lewis, the disorder had features remarkably similar to systemic lupus erythematosus in man, and the "L. E. cell test"
also proved of diagnostic value (Lewis, 1965). In addition to anemia and spherocytosis, peripheral blood changes consistent with active erythropoiesis (p. 124)
are evident as well as thrombocytopenia (p. 1173). Other clinical and pathological
features may include splenomegaly, lymphoadenopathy, purpura and glomerulonephritis. Lameness is seen in some affected dogs which may be the result of a
"rheumatoid arthritis" (Lewis and Hathaway, 1967). A disease resembling lupus

erythematosus also occurs in NZB/BL mice (p. 1261). The disease in mice and man has been suggested to be a viral infection. Ultrastructural studies of affected mice and men have revealed viral particles in tissue, but their etiological importance has not been established.

Hemophilia.—Once considered a single disorder, it is now recognized that hemophilia represents a number of different disorders characterized by hereditary defects in clotting mechanisms. In man, hereditary defects are known to occur for most of the numerous coagulation factors discussed in detail on page 104; whereas in animals the number of distinct disorders are fewer. However, in horses, dogs, swine, laboratory rodents and birds hereditary defects of factors VII, VIII, IX and XII have been reported.

Hemophilia A or **classic hemophilia** is the result of a deficiency of factor VIII (antihemophilic globulin, p. 104) and is the most common form of hemophilia in man and domestic animals. In man the disorder is inherited as a sex-linked recessive gene, and the affected individual which has been carelessly called a "bleeder," is in danger of bleeding to death from every trivial cut or bruise. While this is true in the case of cuts and similar injuries, in which stopping the loss of blood depends on the formation of a clot, the "bleeding time," which is the duration of bleeding from a minute puncture of the skin, remains normal. This is because these latter wounds are closed by an accumulation of platelets (thrombocytes) which remain normal in this disease. Clotting time (in a glass tube) is prolonged. Prothrombin time is normal. An identical condition, which is also inherited as a sex-linked-recessive trait, occurs in certain families of dogs. Hemophilia A has also been described in horses. Details of inheritance are not established, but all reports have concerned males. In swine hemophilia A has been reported, but is transmitted as a simple mendelian recessive, not sex linked.

Hemophilia B or **Christmas disease** results from a deficiency of factor IX (p. 104). It is known in man and dogs, and is inherited as a sex-linked characteristic in both species. Hemorrhagic problems are less pronounced than in hemophilia A. Bleeding time and prothrombin time are usually normal, whereas clotting time is prolonged.

Factor VII deficiency in both man and dogs is not characterized by a marked hemorrhagic tendency. The usual finding is increased susceptibility to bruising with extensive edema. In dogs factor VII deficiency is inherited as an autosomal characteristic. Bleeding times and clotting times are normal but prothrombin time is prolonged.

Factor XII deficiency (Hageman trait, p. 104) has been observed in horses but it is not associated with clinical manifestation of hemorrhage.

Blood Groups in Animals.—As is well known, human beings can be separated into four principal groups, A, B, AB or O, according to the presence or absence of (iso-) agglutinins in the serum and the corresponding absence or presence of (iso-) agglutinogens in the cells. Group A contains agglutinogen A and its cells are agglutinated by those sera which contain agglutinin anti-A (also known as A, alpha). These are the sera of group B and group O. Group B contains agglutinogen B and is agglutinated by the sera which contain agglutinin anti-B (also known as B, beta). These latter are the sera of group A and group O. Group C cells contain no agglutinogen, hence they are not susceptible to agglutination, although the serum of type O agglutinates the cells of all the other groups. The cells of group AB contain both agglutinogens A and B, therefore these cells are agglutinated by serum of any one of the other three groups, but serum A-B, containing no agglutinins, does not agglutinate any of the other cells.

The objective, in selecting blood for a transfusion is to see that the transfused erythrocytes are not agglutinated by the patient's (recipient's) serum, for the agglutination is an index of other more vital effects of the antigen-antibody reaction, the chief of which is hemolysis. In other words, if the donor's cells are agglutinated, they will also be hemolyzed, with the various disturbances characteristic of a transfusion reaction. These include shock and circulatory collapse, with oliguria probably due to ischemia of the renal cortex, but which, even though transient, is often accompanied by occlusion of the lower renal tubules by casts of hemoglobin-containing material, the uremia-producing "lower-nephron disease" (p. 1268).

Among the domestic animals the presence of different blood groups based upon iso-agglutination has been reported in horses, mules, donkeys, cattle, sheep, swine, dogs and cats. In most, if not all of these, however, the agglutinins are not naturally occurring and preformed, as they are in the human, but develop only after the patient has had at least one sensitizing transfusion. If the donor was of a foreign type or group, the patient then is likely to develop agglutinins against the donor's cells in the course of ten to fourteen days, much as other antibodies are developed following exposure to an antigen. In horses, Lehnert (1952) found blood types A, B, AB and O, similar to those in the human, but it appears doubtful that the agglutinins (and hemolysins) are as potent or the grouping as clear-cut as in the human. Stormont and associates (1964) have reported over a score of identifiable blood factors in horses and cattle. Mustakallio and Rislakki (1949) found no blood groups in cattle by agglutination tests but demonstrated groups A and B by indirect tests for hemolysis. Ferguson (1947) found very weak bovine antigens comparable to those of humans but clinical significance was attained only when a patient was repeatedly transfused at intervals.

Young et al. (1952) found five iso-antibodies which could be developed in dogs which were made the recipients of a previous transfusion. "Anti-A" was a potent hemolysin, while anti-B, -C, -D and -E were agglutinins of little or no clinical significance. The hemolytic anti-A was found in 63 per cent of dogs, the remainder being A-negative, and they considered the danger of serious transfusion reaction after the first transfusion to be sufficient to justify precautionary cross-matching of the donor and recipient bloods or the limitation of donors to A-negative dogs.

The various iso-agglutinins of the human behave genetically as dominant and recessive mendelian characters; hence, in certain combinations conclusions can be drawn as to the blood group of an unknown parent when the group of the offspring and of the other parent are known. While, as previously indicated, animals usually are born with only the iso-agglutinogen, these also appear to be inherited according to definite laws, and Ferguson has shown certain possibilities of utilizing them to determine parentage after producing the corresponding agglutinins by one or more transfusions into a suitable recipient.

No doubt most animal erythrocytes possess numerous antigens (there are many besides A and B in man) but their relative importance to disease is either not known or of little apparent importance.

Hemoglobinemia and Hemoglobinuria.—The presence of free hemoglobin in the blood or in the urine is a symptom but is sometimes carelessly considered as if it were a disease in itself. For instance, there was an inclination formerly to use hemoglobinuria as a longer (and more sophisticated?) name for the disease of muscles known as azoturia. Even if the pigment in the urine were hemoglobin, instead of myoglobin, the colored urine is only one symptom of the disease, as it is of various others.

Hemoglobin occurs normally in the erythrocytes, and only there. From the principles set forth in connection with anemia (p. 123), we learn its history in case it is released from disintegrating erythrocytes and that when the amount of hemoglobin in the blood plasma passes a certain level (the renal threshold), it is excreted in the urine, giving to the latter a reddish or brownish color. It follows that whenever there is hemoglobinemia of any considerable degree there is also hemolytic anemia, not to mention hemolytic icterus, which develops if the rapid destruction of erythrocytes continues.

Hemoglobinuria is diagnosed tentatively but with considerable reliability by the brownish color of the urine. A microscopic examination of the urinary sediment, separated preferably by centrifugation, otherwise by settling in a tall vessel, is necessary to eliminate hematuria, which is the presence of whole blood and blood cells in the urine. This latter is essentially hemorrhage into the urinary passages anywhere from the glomerulus to the external meatus. Its causes and significance are obviously quite unrelated to the presence in the urine of hemoglobin without blood cells. Simple chemical tests serve to eliminate other possible sources of brownish discolorization, as well as to detect minute amounts of hemoglobin which escape visual observation.

Hemoglobinemia of a degree insufficient to produce hemoglobinuria, of course, may exist and can be detected only by an appropriate test upon the blood serum.

The **causes** of hemoglobinemia and hemoglobinuria are to be sought first among the causes already given for hemolytic anemia (p. 126). Prominent among the infections are bovine bacillary hemoglobinuria (which should rarely be diagnosed without bacteriological confirmation), severe forms of leptospirosis in the bovine and piroplasmoses. Anaplasmosis, on the other hand, is said never to reach a sufficiently violent state to cause hemoglobinuria.

Hemoglobinuria is probably more often a symptom of toxic diseases than it is of infections. Some hemoglobinuric toxins probably remain unknown, but we do recognize in this category poisoning by copper, chlorates, the pasture plant, rape and, in some cases, by ricin (castor beans). Poisonous mushrooms, eaten by humans, produce marked hemoglobinuria. In humans, severe hemolysis with icterus and hemoglobinuria results from eating a bean, *Vicia flava*. Venoms of most snakes and some of the more poisonous scorpions and spiders belong in the same class. The toxemic state which results from the decomposition of large amounts of dead tissue following extensive burns or freezing causes notable hemoglobinuria as does also severe crushing trauma (the "crush syndrome") (myoglobin?). The hemolysis which follows transfusions of incompatible blood, of course, results in hemoglobinuria. The various benign **paroxysmal hemoglobinurias** seen in humans have not been recognized in animals.

The term **post-parturient hemoglobinuria** has been applied to an obscure toxic disorder which is often fatal in cattle in the western United States, Australia and other localities. It appears usually but not invariably in cows that have given birth to calves a few weeks previously. The hemoglobin in blood and urine results from severe hemolysis of circulating erythrocytes, the red-cell count often being less than 2,000,000 in spite of active hematopoiesis (nucleated red cells, etc.). Hemolytic jaundice develops except in peracute cases. Marked hypophosphatemia is an accompaniment. Acute toxic hepatitis is suggested by centrilobular necrosis and midzonal fatty change, although these changes are attributed by some merely to anoxia resulting from the severe anemia. The lesions of hemoglobinuric nephropathy may be mild to severe (p. 1268). Suspected **causes** range from a deficiency of phosphorus in the diet and in the soil to accumulation of toxic products which the parturient uterus failed to discharge. Some cases possibly have been confused with plant poisonings, including a diet excessive in the leaves of the sugar beet, which is a plentiful farm crop in some of the affected regions.

Myoglobinuria.—Although completely unrelated to disorders of the hemic and lymphatic systems, hemoglobinuria must be differentiated from myoglobinuria. The causes of myoglobinuria are discussed in Chapter 20. The molecular weight of myoglobin is approximately one fourth the weight of hemoglobin which accounts for a much lower renal clearance. Myoglobin appears in the urine when plasma levels reach approximately 20 mg. per 100 ml., whereas hemoglobin does not appear in the urine until plasma levels approach 100 mg. per 100 ml. As a result of this difference, plasma is generally not colored by myoglobin, whereas in those diseases causing hemoglobinuria the plasma is red. Obviously caution must be used to prevent mechanical hemolysis in obtaining blood specimens. Both myoglobin and hemoglobin react to the usual tests for occult blood. The two pigments can be distinguished by spectroscopic techniques.

THE SPLEEN

By far the most common problem which confronts the pathologist as he examines the spleen has to do with its size, for, as with soldiers' uniforms, there appear to be two sizes: too large and too small. While we shall presently mention some pathological enlargements, the great majority of spleens encountered at autopsy are essentially normal. It is well to remember that the spleen is a "great reticulo-endothelial sponge" (Boyd) which holds a large but varying amount of blood. From the arterioles, the blood slowly percolates through the multitudinous, ill-defined spaces of the splenic pulp, and is collected into the venous sinuses. This is by no means accidental but serves to expose the blood to the action of the reticulo-endothelial and lymphoid cells which are the principal components of the splenic parenchyma, and which perform such functions as destruction of decadent erythrocytes, conversion of hemoglobin, elaboration of antibodies and many others. There is evidence, indeed, that the flow of blood through the maze of poorly recognizable compartments among the cells of the splenic pulp is controlled by little vascular sphincters which open and close at the proper time.

Obviously the spongy organ can hold a very considerable amount of blood, varying with the state of the sphincters, if they exist, and, at any rate, with the degree of contraction or relaxation of the muscular trabeculae and capsule (muscular in animals). Furthermore, the concentration of blood cells varies, doubtless according to changing needs of the body, and the stored blood is often highly cellular.

It is entirely understandable, then, that when an animal dies of hemorrhage, the spleen is small, "dry" and "atrophic," in other words simply empty, for no living thing perishes without exhausting every resource that might counteract the attack which threatens it. The same is generally true when death comes from one of the many diseases which destroy blood cells (hemolytic anemias), although the picture in such cases is influenced by accumulation of various white cells if the cause is an infection, by the presence of hematopoietic cells in some anemias, by an increase of phagocytic reticulo-endothelial cells needed to dispose of fragmented erythrocytes or other waste particles, by the augmentation of reticulo-endothelium for the production of antibodies, by enlargement of the splenic (Malpighian) corpuscles in lymphoid hyperplasia (p. 95), by fibrosis, congestion and other changes.

Evaluation of the net results thus becomes more than a little complicated, and this situation is enhanced by the difficulty of recognizing each cell type and the total impossibility of ascertaining the functions and purposes of the cells by means of microscopic sections. While the term **splenitis** is in use by some to refer to some of the cellular accumulations to which allusion has just been made, we prefer to limit the concept of splenic inflammation to those infrequent cases where the spleen itself is the object of attack and to view its various reactions to generalized disease as functional changes designed or fitted, as they certainly are, to counteract certain disorders of the body as a whole through the medium of its circulating blood.

Splenic Enlargements, Splenomegaly.—In a broad sense, the latter term can be used to indicate any abnormal increase in size of the spleen, the following different kinds existing.

Acute Congestion of the Spleen.—The acutely congested spleen is enlarged, but not excessively so, and somewhat soft. Its cut surface is dark and bulges moderately, with blood oozing from it. Microscopically, there may be little change beyond a large number of erythrocytes in the pulp and sinuses or the lesion may be combined with others, such as a decrease or increase of splenic cells.

The most frequent example of acute splenic congestion encountered in veterinary pathology is that which results from the use of Nembutal or similar barbiturates for procuring a humane death, the usual procedure when pet animals have to be given euthanasia. One of the actions of the drug is to relax smooth muscle, including that of the spleen, with the result that the organ fills with dark, venous blood at the moment of death.

Acute congestion is also common as a part of the picture of generalized venous congestion which accompanies a failing heart. The immediate cause of death in a great variety of diseases is this congestive heart failure.

Chronic Passive Congestion.—The spleen is moderately enlarged and filled with blood but is firm or a little tough because of the increase of fibrous tissue.

The microscopic lesions, which result from long continued venous pressure, are (1) distention of the sinusoids and pulp-spaces with blood, (2) often an appreciable hyperplasia of the endothelium of the sinusoids so that the lining cells resemble cuboidal epithelium, (3) marked diffuse fibrosis throughout the pulp, the fibrous tissue being an attempt to strengthen the walls of the sinusoidal spaces, (4) even a thickening of the trabeculae with additional fibrous strands, and (5) accumulation of phagocytized hemosiderin from erythrocytes which have been entrapped in the nearly static blood and hemolyzed in excessive numbers.

Chronic passive congestion of the spleen is comparatively infrequent in animals owing to the infrequency of the causative disorders. The latter include anything which will produce increased pressure, or back pressure, in the splenic vein, such as thrombotic obstructions in, or pressure of tumors or abscesses upon, the vascular drainage system anywhere from the spleen to the heart. Cirrhosis constricts the venules through which the splenic blood must traverse the liver and causes congestion of the spleen as well as the other structures drained by the portal vein. Even right-sided valvular lesions (p. 132) of the heart and fibrosis of the lungs leave their marks upon the spleen in the form of venous back-pressure.

In humans, a poorly understood condition known as **Banti's disease** simulates chronic passive congestion with respect to its diffuse fibrosis. Banti's disease, however, produces a more startling picture with marked enlargement of the total size of the organ, peculiar "siderotic nodules" thought to result from old hemorrhages and the ultimate accompaniment of cirrhosis and gastric hemorrhages. In the opinion of many, Banti's disease is related to chronic passive congestion also in being a result of increased venous pressure in the spleen. The condition is not known in animals.

Acute Splenic Swelling.—This form of splenic enlargement is associated with infectious inflammations and by some is called acute splenitis, although the primary inflammation is not in the spleen. The increase in size is moderate. The organ is mushy in consistency and the purplish pulp bulges from the cut surface, from which the protruding surplus is easily removed by scraping. The enlargement is found **microscopically** to be due to an augmentation of the pulp, in which there are increased numbers of lymphocytes, reticulo-endothelial cells, neutrophilic granulocytes and erythrocytes in varying proportions. The accumulation of blood cells, which is less than that seen in severe congestion, has been explained on the basis of obstructive pressure on the venules and sinuses by proliferated reticulo-endothelial tissue, a postulate which is perhaps only occasionally applicable. However implemented, it is theorized that thus delaying the blood in its passage through the spleen serves a useful purpose by exposing it longer to the actions of the several kinds of leukocytes and to humoral antibodies produced there.

In a majority of cases, the most numerous of the reactive cells are lymphocytes. In a few instances, there is a proliferation of masses of reticulo-endothelial cells which develop almost an epithelioid appearance. Some cases of brucellosis furnish an example of this, although such a change is usually more prominent in the lymph nodes. In cases of septicemia from pyogenic bacteria (p. 158), areas of heavy neutrophilic infiltration occur; such a spleen is often called a **septic spleen**. In anthrax, the swelling is greater than in most other inflammatory diseases and the considerable amount of blood in the organ makes it unusually soft, the **"blackberry-jam spleen."** However, the spleen is softened rapidly as a result of post-mortem autolysis, and some very humiliating diagnostic errors have been made through overlooking this fact.

Fat-storage Diseases.—In the human spleen, great enlargement occurs in a group of rare diseases known variously as lipid-storage disease, reticulo-endothelial granulomas and by other names. Gaucher's disease is the best known member of the group. All are characterized by proliferation of reticulo-endothelial cells which phagocytize lipoid substances and swell to huge dimensions thereby.

The causes and the chemistry of these disorders are poorly understood. They have been demonstrated in animals but are exceedingly rare.

Lymphomatous Enlargement.—The various forms of malignant lymphoma and leukemia have been discussed (p. 208). In the usual experience with lymphomas in animals, whether they be leukemic or aleukemic, the spleen is moderately or greatly enlarged in one-fourth or one-third of the cases. Why some of these processes attack some lymphoid organs and spare others is not known. The picture in the affected spleen is not that of a discrete metastasis of a lymphoid neoplasm, but rather a replacement or rebuilding of the organ with amorphous lymphoid tissue lacking splenic (Malpighian) corpuscles or any other histological structure.

Splenic Enlargement in Anemia.—The spleen is usually enlarged and filled with blood in cases of hemolytic anemia. This appears to be a feature of the mechanism for the final disposal of the injured or disintegrating erythrocytes. It is possible that the hypothetical sphincters play a part in holding the blood in the spleen longer than the usual time. There is a varying degree of hyperplasia of the reticulo-endothelial tissue, whose cells perform the function of final hemolysis, and this hyperplasia contributes also to the enlargement of the organ. What causes a certain erythrocyte to be phagocytized and destroyed while its fellows escape is an intriguing but unanswered question. Presumably some cellular injury, visible as in piroplasmosis, or invisible as in some other diseases, renders the erythrocyte both vulnerable and attractive to the phagocytes. In one form of hemolytic anemia (autoimmune) the cells swell and become relatively spherical (spherocytes) before they are phagocytized, a change presumably indicative of injury to them. It has also been suspected that in hemolytic anemias the phagocytic reticulo-endothelial cells become more voracious through some change in their chemical constituents. In such spleens, there is also a marked accumulation of hemoglobinogenous pigment in the form of phagocytized hemosiderin. When the amount of hemosiderin is great, giant cells of the foreign-body type may also be numerous in the splenic pulp. These have to be distinguished from megakaryocytes, which appear in extramedullary hematopoiesis. The latter have very irregularly multilobed nuclei; the foreign-body giant cells tend to have multiple nuclei clustered together in the central portion of the cell and not infrequently piled one upon another.

Reticulo-endothelial hyperplasia leading to splenic enlargement may also accompany diseases which are not characterized by anemia. Such is the case in histoplasmosis, leishmaniasis and East Coast fever.

An entirely different basis for splenic enlargement is **splenic hematopoiesis.** The total increase in size is only moderate. Microscopically, there are clumps and areas of cells recognizable as members of the myeloid and hematopoietic groups, myelocytes, hemocytoblasts, nucleated and mature erythrocytes and megakaryocytes. Myelocytes are also scattered through the pulp in some cases but are recognized with difficulty.

These hematopoietic changes occur in connection with myelophthisic anemias, (p. 129), the bone marrow being unable to function because it is wholly or partially non-existent. Splenic hematopoiesis also occurs in other chronic forms of anemia, especially in the young, when, without any deficiency of the essential raw materials, the normal marrow is unable to meet the demands for new cells. In other forms of anemia, the size of the spleen is not directly affected. At times

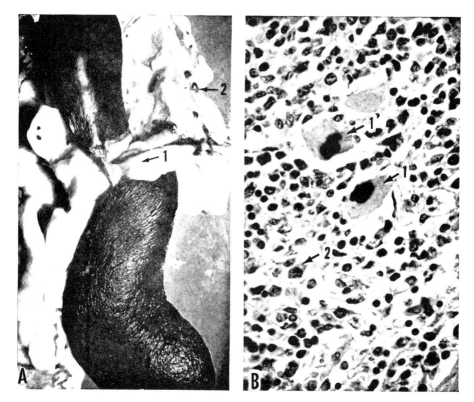

Fig. 23–2.—*A*, Rupture of the spleen (*1*) of a seven-year-old Scottish Terrier, with implants of spleen (*2*) in the mesentery. The dog was hit by a car one year prior to necropsy. *B*, Extramedullary hematopoiesis, spleen of a dog. Megakaryocytes (*1*) and myeloid cells (*2*) are evident. (*B*, Courtesy of Armed Forces Institute of Pathology.) Contributor: Dr. John Mills.

caution must be exercised in judging the significance of extramedullary hematopoiesis, as it is to be expected in most perinatal animals and persists throughout life in species such as rats and mice.

Abscesses, large or small, numerous or few, form in the spleen as the result of blood-borne pyogenic infections. Abscesses or encapsulated areas of necrosis or liquefaction occasionally result from infection brought in on penetrating foreign bodies which chance to wander into the spleen from the reticulum instead of pursuing their usual course toward the heart. In such cases, there usually are extensive fibrous adhesions along the path taken by the nail, wire or other body. Especially in the experimental animals and birds, some infections of septicemic distribution produce myriads of minute gray spots in or on the spleen. Sometimes these prove to be minute abscesses or lymphocytic foci; more often they are foci of necrosis.

Tuberculosis and other **granulomas** produce their typical lesions in the spleen when the specific organisms happen to be carried there from other regions. While tuberculosis of the bovine spleen is rare it will be noted that metastasis to the spleen is always via the systemic circulation, a consideration which is often of importance in tracing the origin of infectious or neoplastic lesions in the spleen, as in meat inspection.

Lymphoid Hyperplasia.—The general aspects of the increase of lymphoid tissues of the body which accompanies many infectious processes of some duration have been described (p. 95). In the spleen, this frequently encountered reaction takes the form of enlargement of the individual splenic corpuscles (Malpighian bodies). The increase is principally in the zone of densely packed lymphocytes but occasionally in young animals large, pale germinal centers develop within the splenic corpuscle. Grossly, the corpuscles appear as bulging, fuzzy, whitish nodules from 1 to 3 mm. in diameter scattered through the splenic pulp. The latter is usually increased in amount and dark red or purple in color (acute splenic swelling) in these same spleens, and from the same cause, which is still acutely active.

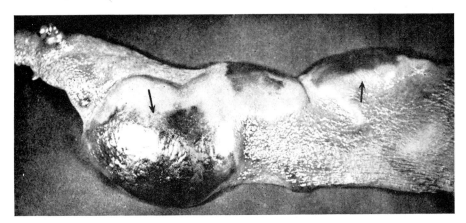

Fig. 23–3.—Infarction of the spleen of a ten-year-old female springer spaniel. The infarcts (arrows) near the apex are elevated and partially hemorrhagic. (Courtesy of Angell Memorial Animal Hospital.)

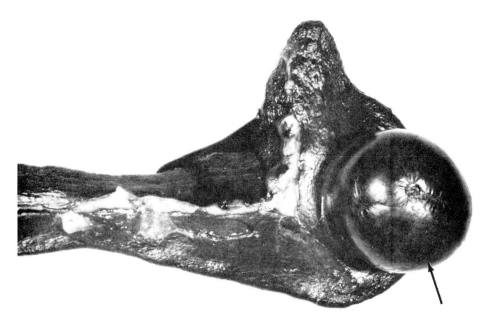

Fig. 23–4.—Nodular hyperplasia ("splenoma") of the spleen of a fourteen-year-old male collie. (Courtesy of Angell Memorial Animal Hospital.)

Upon complete recovery from the causative infection, the enlarged corpuscles gradually return to normal size. Just how great a part increased lymphoid tissue has in overcoming the infection is, of course, not susceptible of precise measurement, but to the diagnostic pathologist, the lymphoid reaction is a valuable clue to the existence of a sometimes poorly evidenced infection such as canine distemper or its sequelae. Lymphoid hyperplasia need not involve all Malpighian corpuscles. In old dogs, single or on occasion two or three distinct nodules from one to several centimeters in diameter may be found projecting above the capsule. These are composed of almost solid masses of lymphocytes, which may be present in "whorls" mimicking corpuscles but lacking the central arteriole of a normal corpuscle (Fig. 23–4).

Infarctions occur occasionally in the spleen, usually being hemorrhagic but not invariably so. They tend to be conical with the base at the capsule, as explained in the general discussion of infarcts (p. 28) but may be so large as to occupy a whole end or a considerable segment of the spleen.

A lesion consisting of a raised, subcapsular area, almost black in color and usually multiple, occurs in 50 per cent of cases of hog cholera (swine fever). These have been classed as hemorrhagic infarcts, although some have been confused with mere hemorrhages. The obstruction of blood essential to infarction is considered to be due to thickening of capillary walls and minute thrombi in them.

Amyloidosis involves the splenic corpuscles, as previously explained (p. 47). It is rare except in animals which have been used for the production of hyperimmune serums.

In old dogs **siderotic plaques** or **Gamma-Gandy bodies** are frequently found on the splenic capsule. They appear as yellow, dry encrustations. Microscopically yellow-brown, iron positive pigment in trabeculae and capsule is mixed with deep blue (with hematoxylin) fibers which react to the usual stains for calcium salts. Although usually considered a senile change, the significance is not known; it may be that they are sites of previous hemorrhages.

Cysts in the spleen may prove to contain the scolices of *Echinococcus granulosus* in the herbivorous and omnivorous species. However, this parasite is practically nonexistent in the United States.

Rupture of the spleen is a not infrequent accident in the dog for reasons which must be evident in a world of automotive transportation. A considerable number of dogs so injured survive, and the two or more healed fragments of the spleen are found at autopsy years later. There are even cases in which several small fragments of spleen are spattered over the adjoining areas and become implanted in the mesentery to live and carry on such functions as do not require anatomically normal vascular connections. Accessory spleens of varying sizes originate also as congenital malformations but these are rare.

Primary **neoplasms** of the spleen are rare with the exception of hemangiomas. Metastases from primary tumors in other locations are somewhat frequent but less so than in the lungs and liver, as would be expected from the relative blood supplies.

THE LYMPH NODES

Acute Lymphadenitis.—The alert student will recognize the error in the designation *adenitis* for inflammatory lesions involving lymph nodes which are not glands. However, the use of the term lymphadenitis is so well entrenched in the literature and vocabulary of veterinarians as well as physicians that it has become the accepted (although erroneous) way to communicate inflammatory lesions of lymph nodes.

By far the most frequent disorder of lymph nodes to concern the veterinary pathologist is the acute swelling which is characteristic of most of the acute septicemic diseases. Prominent among these are anthrax, pasteurellosis, hog cholera, swine erysipelas and others. In septicemias such as these, the infection is rather generally spread throughout the body and, accordingly, the reaction usually involves many, or perhaps nearly all of the nodes with little regard for anatomical location.

A comparable process is seen when a particular organ or region of the body is involved in an acute infectious inflammation, for the lymph nodes which drain the affected part undergo a similar acute inflammatory swelling. For instance, the bronchial lymph nodes are enlarged in the presence of pneumonia, the mandibular and pharyngeal nodes swell in the case of rhinitis or an infected tooth and the supramammary nodes respond similarly to mastitis. The reason for this is obviously that the infectious irritant is drained into the regional lymph nodes. It produces approximately the same effects in the node as it did in its original location, including pain as well as the other aspects of inflammation. The total results are frequently beneficial by virtue of the filtering capacity of the node to prevent further progress of the pathogenic organisms. If this fails, the filtering attempt is repeated at the next group of lymph nodes along the lymph-vascular route.

The **lesion** which accounts for the swelling is a combination of exudation with proliferation of the lymphoid and reticular (reticulo-endothelial) tissues of the node. The exudate most frequently is chiefly serous and the lymph nodes are described grossly as edematous (inflammatory edema). They are swollen, somewhat soft and the cut surface bulges slightly. There is always hyperemia, and in some of the septicemias the nodes are "hemorrhagic." This means that considerable amounts of blood accompany the incoming lymph so that the node is red grossly, and microscopically contains large numbers of erythrocytes in the lymph sinuses. In a minority of cases when the infecting organism is in the pyogenic group (p. 158), the exudate in the regional lymph nodes is clearly purulent, the sinuses containing large numbers of neutrophilic granulocytes. Abscesses develop rarely and will be mentioned later.

The proliferative part of the reaction is always considerable, the lymph sinuses being narrowed or filled with lymphocytes among which are mixed a certain number of reticulo-endothelial mononuclears, a few plasma cells and a scattering of blood-borne leukocytes.

In many acute generalized infections, especially those caused by viruses, necrosis of lymphocytes is a major feature of acute lymphadenitis. This in part may be due to the depressant effect of adrenal corticosteroids on lymphocytes, but many viruses specifically destroy lymphocytes; for example, rinderpest virus and most herpesviruses.

If the outcome of the infectious process is favorable, the nodes return to normal with recovery from the primary disease process.

Abscesses develop in acutely inflamed lymph nodes less frequently than would be expected even though the reaction be of the purulent type. When this change does occur, the whole node is usually transformed into a single abscess, the

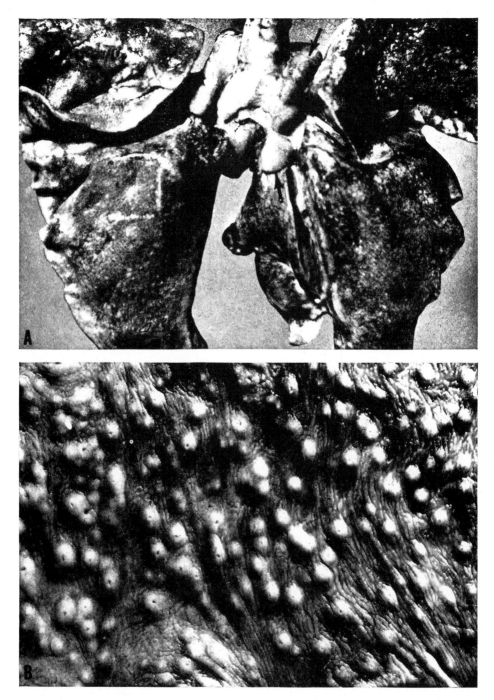

Fig. 23–5.—A, Hyperplasia of bronchial lymph nodes (arrows) in a dog with "salmon disease." B, Hyperplasia of the lymph nodules in colon of a dog with "salmon disease." Photographs courtesy of Dr. Wm. J. Hadlow.

capsule of the node becoming the capsule of the abscess. These abscesses usually rupture to the exterior, sometimes into a body cavity. This process is the rule in equine strangles, the submaxillary (mandibular) nodes regularly forming a single large abscess.

Lymphoid hyperplasia, general or regional, is the usual reaction to a number of less virulent and less rapidly progressive infections, like canine distemper, chronic pneumonitis and chronic enteritides. The affected nodes are moderately enlarged, firm and dry but neither fibrous nor calcified. **Microscopic** examination shows the increase in size to be due to lymphocytes almost exclusively. Germinal centers are numerous and surrounded by a wide zone of closely packed and darkly staining lymphocytes. In cases of generalized lymphoid hyperplasia, the lymphocyte count of the blood shows some increase from the previous level for the individual animal but does not necessarily exceed the normal maximum. A frequent picture when death comes from one of the diseases in this group is a node containing many germinal centers which are very large but with only a narrow and inconspicuous zone of mature lymphocytes around them. The germinal centers proper are large and pale because of the very active proliferation of the pale maternal lymphoblasts, even though the accumulation of mature lymphocytes is slight. This condition has the very suitable name of **lymphoid hyperplasia with lymphoid exhaustion.** The lymph nodes return to the normal state if the cause of the disease is overcome.

Chronic lymphadenitis usually represents one of the specific infectious granulomatous infections. The lesion in the lymph node is that which is typical for the disease in question regardless of location. Among the more prominent granulomatous infections of lymph nodes are tuberculosis, Johne's disease, glanders, caseous lymphadenitis and actinobacillosis.

A diffuse and extensive proliferation of solid masses of reticulo-endothelial cells is occasionally seen. The large pale cells with their expansive cytoplasm fill the lymphoid sinuses, especially in the medulla of the node. This reaction is typical of, but not limited to, **brucellosis** in swine. Rarely the reticulo-endothelial cells assume bizarre forms and develop into giant-cells with multilobed central nuclei. If they are accompanied by some fibrosis and a variable number of eosinophilic granulocytes, the proliferated tissue comes to resemble the tissue of **Hodgkin's disease** as seen in patients. The latter is usually thought to be a variant of lymphoblastic neoplasia (malignant lymphoma), although the theory that it is inflammatory has also had numerous supporters. It is questionable whether true Hodgkin's disease has even been seen in animals, although there have been reactions of striking similarity.

Other disorders found to affect lymph nodes include amyloidosis, which has been discussed (p. 47), and certain pigmentations. Anthracosis of the nodes occurs when carbon pigment is carried to them from the lungs. Hemosiderosis (p. 71), hemochromatosis (p. 73) and melanosis occur rarely. A brownish discoloration of the medullary portion, especially, seen frequently in bovine lymph nodes does not indicate ill health. It may be related to porphyrinemia (p. 84).

Aberrant parasites, including the mange mite, *Demodex folliculorum,* are seldom found in lymph nodes.

Primary neoplasms of lymph nodes are rare, but metastatic tumors, especially carcinomas and melanomas, are frequent. Malignant lymphoma, in its many varieties, usually involves a number of nodes, often remotely separated, in a diffuse replacement by structureless lymphoid tissue entirely comparable to that described for the spleen.

TONSILS

While it is common to speak of tonsils in the dog, anatomically distinct tonsils do not exist in the domestic animals, the nearest approach to these structures of the human being seen in the sheep. Diffuse inflammation in the faucial area occurs rarely and is probably best considered an aspect of pharyngitis rather than a separate entity. However, submucous lymphoid tissue is microscopically identifiable and in some species distinct crypts indent the mucous membrane. In the pig, these are prone to become infected and to form chronic abscesses a few millimeters in diameter. The most frequent neoplasms of the "tonsils" are squamous cell carcinoma and malignant lymphoma.

SELECTED REFERENCES

ARCHER, R. K.: True Hemophilia (Hemophilia A) in a Thoroughbred Foal. Vet. Rec. 73:338–340, 1961.

ARCHER, R. K., and BOWDEN, R. S. T.: A Case of True Hemophilia in a Labrador Dog. Vet. Rec. 71:560–561, 1959.

BEDOYA, V., GRIMLEY, P. M., and DUQUE, O.: Chediak-Higashi Syndrome. Arch. Path. 88: 340–349, 1969.

BIGGERS, J. D., INGRAM, P. L., and MURRAY, C. B.: Studies on Equine Purpura Hemor-rhagica. Brit. Vet. J. 105:191–200, 1949.

BLUME, R. S., et al.: Giant Neutrophil Granules in the Chediak-Higashi Syndrome of Man, Mink, Cattle and Mice. Can. J. Comp. Med. 33:271–274, 1969.

BOGART, R., and MUHRER, M. E.: The Inheritance of a Hemophilia-like Condition in Swine. J. Hered. 33:59–64, 1942.

BROCK, W. E., et al.: Canine Hemophilia. Arch. Path. 76:464–469, 1963.

BRODEY, R. S., and SCHALM, O. W.: Hemobartonellosis and Thrombocytopenic Purpura in a Dog. Am. J. Vet. Med. Assn. 143:1231–1236, 1963.

CALHOUN, M. L.: Bone Marrow of Horses and Cattle. Science 104:423, 1946.

——————: A Cytological Study of the Costal Marrow; the Adult Cow. Am. J. Vet. Research 15:395–404, 1954.

CAPEL-EDWARDS, K., and HALL, D. E.: Factor VII Deficiency in the Beagle Dog. Lab. Anim. 2:105–112, 1968.

CHEVILLE, N. F.: The Gray Collie Syndrome. J. Am. Vet. Med. Assn. 152:620–630, 1968.

——————: Amyloidosis Associated with Cyclic Neutropenia in the Dog. Blood 31:111–114, 1968.

COLE, N.: Polycythemia in a Dog. No. Amer. Vet. 35:601, 1954.

CRUZ, W. O., DA SILVA, E. M., and DE MELLO, R. P.: Manifestaçoes purpuricas na pele em caes anemiados com benzoato de estradiol. Rev. brazil. de biol. 5:367–376, 1945.

DONOVAN, E. F., and LOEB, W. F.: Polycythemia Rubra Vera in the Dog. J. Am. Vet. Med. Assn. 134:36–37, 1959.

FARQUHARSON, J., and SMITH, K. W.: Post-parturient Hemoglobinuria of Cattle. J. Am. Vet. Med. Assn. 93:37–39, 1938.

FARRELLY, B. T., COLLINS, J. D., and COLLINS, S. M.: Autoimmune Haemolytic Anaemia (AHA) in the Horse. Irish Vet. J. 20:42–45, 1966.

FERGUSON, L. C.: The Blood Groups of Cattle. J. Am. Vet. Med. Assn. 111:466–469, 1947.

FIELD, R. A., RICKARD, C. G., and HUTT, F. B.: Hemophilia in a Family of Dogs. Cornell Vet. 36:285–300, 1946.

FORD, L.: Hereditary Aspects of Human and Canine Cyclic Neutropenia. J. Hered. 60: 293–299, 1969.

FOSTER, W. N. M., and CAMERON, A. E.: Thrombocytopenia in Sheep Associated With Experimental Tick-Borne Fever Infection. J. Comp. Path. 78:251–254, 1968.

FOWLER, M. E., CORNELIUS, C. E., and BAKER, N. F.: Clinical and Erythrokinetic Studies on a Case of Bovine Polycythemia Vera. Cornell Vet. 54:153–159, 1964.

GALLEGO GARCIA, E.: El mielograma normal en la especie porcina. An. Fac. vet. Madrid 3:129–141, 1951. (Engl., Fr. and Ger. summaries.)

GILMORE, C. E., GILMORE, V. H., and JONES, T. C.: Reticuloendotheliosis, A Myeloproliferative Disorder of Cats: A Comparison with Lymphocytic Leukemia. Path. Vet. 1:161–183, 1964.

————: Bone Marrow and Peripheral Blood of Cats: Technique and Normal Values. Path. Vet. 1:18–40, 1964.

GRAUSZ, H., et al.: Diagnostic Import of Virus-Like Particles in the Glomerular Endothelium of Patients with Systemic Lupus Erythematosus. New Eng. J. Med. 283:506–511, 1970.

GRUNSELL, C. S.: Marrow Biopsy in Sheep. Brit. Vet. J. 107:16–23, 1951.

HAGAN, A. G., MUHRER, M. E., and BOGART, R.: A Hemophilia Like Disease in Swine. Proc. Soc. Exp. Biol. Med. 48:217–219, 1941.

HJÄRRE, A.: Die puerperal Hämoglobinämie des Rindes. Acta path. et microbiol. Scandinav. Supp. 7, 1930.

HOWELL, J., and LAMBERT, P. S.: A Case of Haemophilia A in the Dog. Vet. Rec. 76:1103–1105, 1964.

HUTCHINS, D. R., LEPHERD, E. E., and CROOK, I. G.: A Case of Equine Haemophilia. Aust. Vet. J. 43:83–87, 1967.

ISHMAEL, J., and HOWELL, M.: Neoplasia of the Spleen of the Dog With a Note on Nodular Hyperplasia. J. Comp. Path. 78:59–67, 1968.

JENNINGS, A. R., and HIGHET, D. R.: Some Cases of Purpura Haemorrhagica in the Horse. Vet. J. 103:369–376, 1947.

JONES, R. F., and PARIS, R.: The Greyhound Eosinophil. J. Small Anim. Pract. 4, Suppl. pp. 29–33, 1963.

KANEKO, J. J., CORDY, D. R., and CARLSON, G.: Canine Hemophilia Resembling Classic Hemophilia A. J. Am. Vet. Med. Assn. 150:15–21, 1967.

KING, A. S.: Studies on Equine Purpura Haemorrhagica; Morbid Anatomy and Histology. Brit. Vet. J. 105:35–54, 1949.

LANDING, B. H., and FREIMAN, D. G.: Histochemical Studies in the Cerebral Lipidoses and Other Cellular Metabolic Disorders. Am. J. Path. 33:1–12, 1957.

LEWIS, E. F., and HOLMAN, H. H.: Haemophilia in a Saint Bernard Dog. Vet. Rec. 63:666–667, 1951.

LEWIS, R. M., SCHWARTS, R., and HENRY, W. B.: Canine Systemic Lupus Erythematosus. Blood 25:143–160, 1965.

LEWIS, R. M.: Clinical Evaluation of the Lupus erythematosus Cell Phenomenon in Dogs. J. Am. Vet. Med. Assn. 147:939–943, 1965.

LEWIS, R. M., and HATHAWAY, J. E.: Canine Systemic Lupus erythematosus; Presenting With Symmetrical Polyarthritis. J. Small Anim. Pract. 8:273–284, 1967.

LEWIS, R. M., et al.: A Syndrome of Autoimmune Hemolytic Anemia and Thrombocytopenia in Dogs. Scientific Proc. 100th Ann. Mtg. AVMA pp. 140–163, 1963.

LIE, H.: Thrombocytopenic Purpura in Baby Pigs. Clinical Studies. Acta Vet. Scand. 9:285–301, 1968.

LITT, M.: Eosinophils in Lymph Nodes of Guinea Pigs Following Primary Antigenic Stimulation. Am. J. Path., 42:529–549, 1963.

LUND, J. E., PADGETT, G. A., and OTT, R. L.: Cyclic Neutropenia in Grey Collie Dogs. Blood 29:452–461, 1967.

LUTZNER, M. A., TIERNEY, J. H., and BENDITT, E. P.: Giant Granules and Widespread Cytoplasmic Inclusions in a Genetic Syndrome of Aleutian Mink. Lab. Invest. 14:2063–2079, 1965.

MACKENZIE, C. P.: Idiopathic (Acquired) Haemolytic Anaemia in the Dog. Vet. Rec. 85:356–361, 1969.

MADSEN, D. E. and NIELSEN, H. M.: Parturient Hemoglobinemia of Dairy Cows. J. Am. Vet. Med. Assn. 94:577–586, 1939.

————: The Production of Hemoglobinemia by Low Phosphorus Intake. J. Am. Vet. Med. Assn. 105:22–25, 1944.

MEDWAY, W., and RAPP, J. P.: A Case of Granulocytic Leukemia with Thrombocytopenic Purpura in a Dog. Cornell Vet. 52:247–260, 1962.

MEYER, R. C., RASMUSEN, B. A., and SIMON, J.: A Hemolytic Neonatal Disease in Swine Associated with Blood Group Incompatibility. J. Amer. Vet. Med. Assn. 154:531–537, 1969.

MILLER, E. R., et al.: Swine Hematology from Birth to Maturity. II. Erythrocyte Population, Size and Hemoglobin Concentration. J. Anim. Sci. 20:890–897, 1961.

MIOTTI, R.: Lymph Nodes and Lymph Vessels of the Hamster (TT). Acta Anat. 46:192–216, 1961.

MULLINS, J. C., and RAMSAY, W. R.: Hemoglobinuria and Anaemia Associated with Aphosphorosis. Austr. Vet. J. 35:140–147, 1959.

MUSTAKALLIO, E., and RISLAKKI, V.: Om blodgrupper hos nötkreatur. [Blood Groups in Cattle.] (Engl. summary.) Nord. Vet.-Med. *1*:750–758, 1949. (Abstr. Vet. Bull. No. 3346, 1951.)

MUSTARD, J. F., *et al.*: Canine Factor VII Deficiency. Brit. J. Haemat. *8*:43–47, 1962.

PADGETT, G. A.: Neutrophilic Function in Animals with the Chediak-Higashi Syndrome. Blood *29*:906–915, 1967.

————: Comparative Studies of the Chediak-Higashi Syndrome. Amer. J. Path. *51*: 553–571, 1967.

————: The Chediak-Higashi Syndrome. Advances Vet. Sci. *12*:239–284, 1968.

PADGETT, G. A., *et al.*: Comparative Studies of Susceptibility to Infection in the Chediak-Higashi Syndrome. J. Path. Bact. *95*:509–522, 1968.

PAGE, A. R., and GOOD, R. A.: Studies on Cyclic Neutropenia. Amer. J. Dis. Child. *94*: 623–661, 1957.

PARKINSON, B., and SUTHERLAND, A. K.: Post-parturient Haemoglobinuria in Dairy Cows. Austr. Vet. J. *30*:232–236, 1954.

PENNY, R. H. C.: Post-parturient Haemoglobinuria (Haemoglobineamia) in Cattle. Vet. Rec. *68*:238–241, 1956.

PHILLIPS, L. L., *et al.*: Comparative Studies on the Chediak-Higashi Syndrome. Coagulation and Fibrinolytic Mechanisms of Mink and Cattle. Amer. J. Vet. Clin. Path. *1*:1–6, 1967.

RATOFF, O. D.: Hereditary Defects in Clotting Mechanisms. Advances Intern. Med. *9*: 107–179, 1958.

REED, C., *et al.*: Polycythemia Vera in a Cat. J. Am. Vet. Med. Assn. *157*:85–91, 1970.

ROWSELL, H. C., *et al.*: A Disorder Resembling Hemophilia B (Christmas Disease) in Dogs. J. Am. Vet. Med. Assn. *137*:247–250, 1960.

ROWSELL, H. C.: The Hemostatic Mechanisms of Mammals and Birds in Health and Disease. Adv. Vet. Sci. *12*:337–410, 1968.

SANGER, V. L., MAIRS, R. E., and TRAPP, A. L.: Hemophilia in a Foal. J. Am. Vet. Med. Assn. *144*:259–264, 1964.

SAUNDERS, C. M., and KINCH, D. A.: Thrombocytopenic Purpura of Pigs. J. Comp. Path. *78*:513–523, 1968.

SAUNDERS, C. N., KINCH, D. A., and IMLAH, P.: Thrombocytopenic Purpura in Young Pigs. Vet. Rec. *79*:549–550, 1966.

SCHALM, O. W., and LING, G. V.: Hematologic Characteristics of Autoimmune Hemolytic Anemia in the Dog. Calif. Vet. *23*:19–24, 1969.

SCHRYVER, H. F.: The Bone Marrow of the Cat. Am. J. Vet. Res. *24*:1012–1017, 1963.

SQUIBB, R. L., *et al.*: Several Blood Constituents of Five Breeds of Dairy Cattle in Guatemala. Am. J. Vet. Res. *19*:112–114, 1958. [Proteins, riboflavin, ascorbic acid, carotene, vitamin A, tocopherols, alkaline phosphatase, Ca, P, Hb, R.B.C.]

STANSFELD, A. G.: The Histological Diagnosis of Toxoplasmic Lymphadenitis. J. Clin. Path. *14*:565–573, 1961.

STORMORKEN, H. R., *et al.*: Thrombocytopenic Bleedings in Young Piglets Due to Maternal Isoimmunization. Nature *198*:1116–1117, 1963.

STORMONT, C., SUZUKI, Y., and RHODE, E. A.: Serology of Horse Blood Groups. Cornell Vet. *54*:439–452, 1964.

TENNANT, B., *et al.*: Familial Polycythemia in Cattle. J. Am. Vet. Med. Assn., *150*:1493–1509, 1967.

THOMPSON, S. W., *et al.*: Perivascular Nodules of Lymphoid Cells in the Lungs of Normal Guinea Pigs. Am. J. Path. *40*:507–517, 1962.

WINQUIST, G.: Morphology of the Blood and the Hemopoietic Organs in Cattle Under Normal and Some Experimental Conditions. Acta Anatomica *22*: (Supp. 21–1), 1–157, 1954.

WRIGHT, J. N.: Blood Incompatibilities in the Dog. Cornell Vet. *52*:523–533, 1962.

————: A Study of Certain Blood Incompatibilities in the Cow and the Dog. Thesis, Cornell, pp. 49, 1961.

WURZEL, H. A., and LAWRENCE, W. C.: Canine Hemophilia. Thromb. Diath. Haemorrh. *6*:98–103, 1961.

YOUNG, L. E., O'BRIEN, W. A., SWISHER, S. N., MILLER, G., and YUILE, C. L.: Blood Groups in Dogs. Am. J. Vet. Res. *13*:207–213, 1952.

24
The Digestive System

THE MOUTH AND ADNEXA

The mucous surface of the buccal cavity, the gums, tongue and pharynx are subject to acute exudative inflammations of the usual kinds. Caustic medicines are occasionally administered and cause severe inflammation or necrosis in the mouth or pharynx. Physical trauma from sharp awns of plants may act as a inciting cause in the mouths of herbivora; sharp bones may play a similar role in dogs and cats. However, all extensive or prolonged forms of **stomatitis, as** inflammation of the buccal mucosa is called, owe their existence to the activity of pathogenic microorganisms or viruses. The buccal lesions of aphthous fever, vesicular stomatitis, vesicular exanthema, rinderpest and malignant catarrhal fever are discussed in the descriptions of those diseases. Nonspecific infections may be caused by the various pyogenic bacteria or the necrophorus organism, with inflammatory lesions characteristic of those pathogens, but only in the event that the involved area has previously suffered traumatic or chemical injury or has been otherwise devitalized.

Ulcers of variable latitude but of minimal depth are encountered with some frequency in the mouth of the dog, many of them on the less heavily epithelialized parts of the tongue. The majority of these are manifestations of uremia (p. 1294), constituting one aspect of the injury done to the whole alimentary mucosa in the course of the partial elimination of toxic urinary wastes through the mucous membrane. Buccal ulcers are a part of the syndrome of canine leptospirosis, but the pathogenetic mechanism is still that of uremia. Ulcers on the tongue have also been considered characteristic of canine pellagra, or blacktongue (p. 985). Whether the same mechanism applies in this case appears not to have been investigated. There is also a gangrenous necrosis of the whole distal end of the tongue. This commonly extends to a distance of 4 or 5 cm. from the tip of the organ, an inflammatory line of demarcation separating it sharply from the more proximal healthy tissue. Information is lacking as to the exact pathogenesis of this lesion, but it is considered diagnostic of blacktongue and responsible for the name.

Many infectious diseases result in ulceration of the oral mucosa. These include those listed above under stomatitis as well as most herpesvirus infections, blue-tongue, papular stomatitis of cattle, and the virus diarrhea : mucosal disease complex. Actinobacillosis in bovines frequently involves the tongue.

The epithelial hyperplasia and hyperkeratosis of poisoning by chlorinated napththalenes (p. 938) in bovines commonly manifest themselves on the mucosa of the tongue, lips and other buccal surfaces.

The **teeth** of animals are much less subject to caries (dental decay) than are those of humans. The comparative absence of readily fermentable carbohydrates in the diets of animals may well be credited for this fortunate difference, in the light of current doctrines on this important human disorder. Supernumerary teeth, usually rudimentary in size and development, are not rare in the horse ("wolf teeth") and occur occasionally in other species. Developmental anomalies in the form of teeth misplaced in the middle of the hard palate have been seen in the horse especially. In rickets, the development and emergence of the teeth may be greatly delayed. Rather specific changes are present in the teeth in fluoride poisoning (p. 928).

Neoplasms of various kinds arise in the several structures of the mouth and pharynx, squamous cell carcinomas being rather common in the dog and in the horse. While the lips do not exhibit the neoplastic predilection seen in man, squamous cell carcinomas of the tongue are reported with some frequency in the cat and with less in the dog. It may be supposed that these growths would show much of the local stubbornness and slow metastasis which are characteristic in the human, but extensive clinical experiences have not been reported. Fibroblastic tumors similar to the human epulis are not altogether rare in the dog. As in the human, they arise on the gums or jaws, often in proximity to diseased dental alveoli. Bizarre forms and giant cells are less in evidence than in the human epulis. True ameloblastomas are rare. In our limited experience growths arising in the horse's gingival tissues have been simply exuberant granulation tissue (p. 166). These also have usually been related to trauma or dental abnormality. Malignant melanomas may arise anywhere that the buccal or labial mucosa is pigmented, as in certain breeds of dogs. Malignant lymphoma has been known to infiltrate between the mucosa and the bone of the palate, causing extensive diffuse

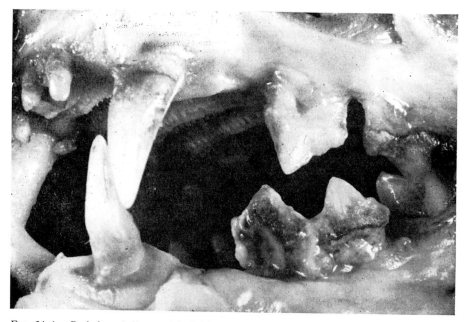

FIG. 24–1.—Periodontal disease (gingivitis) resulting in receding gums and exposure of roots of teeth of a three-year-old female tortoiseshell and white cat. (Courtesy of Angell Memorial Animal Hospital.)

swelling. Cutaneous warts involving the face and lips sometimes spread to the mucosa of the mouth, with severe effects especially in the dog. Warts occurring in the mouth only are said to result from a different virus from that which causes cutaneous warts (p. 508).

Pharyngitis (p. 1092) occurs in connection with infection of the air passages, as does tonsillitis (p. 1188). Foreign bodies in the supra-esophageal diverticulum of swine have been mentioned (p. 1098). Actinobacillosis occasionally involves the parapharyngeal lymph nodes, causing swelling which interferes with deglutition and respiration.

THE SALIVARY GLANDS

The salivary glands may participate in infectious inflammatory processes arising in their vicinity, usually from trauma. In the domestic animals there is no specific infection, comparable to mumps, which has a predilection for salivary tissue. It should be recalled, however, that the cytomegaloviruses (p. 419) have a predilection for the salivary gland, however they rarely induce sialoadenitis. In rats there are specific forms of transmissible sialoadenitis and sialodacryo-adenitis, believed to be caused by viruses. It is possible, but quite unusual, for infection to ascend the duct of a parotid or other salivary gland. Foreign bodies, such as kernels of grain or awns of plants, rarely find their way up a parotid or submaxillary duct, causing inflammation and possibly obstruction or dilatation of the duct.

Sialoliths, or salivary calculi, form in a duct or in the gland itself as a result of chronic inflammation which provides desquamated cells or consolidated exu-date as a minute nidus upon which calcum salts precipitate. Foreign bodies may also serve to start the precipitation of salts. Since the salivary secretion contains but little dissolved mineral, the process of formation of salivary calculi is possibly more akin to calcification of tissue than it is to the formation of urinary or biliary stones. At any rate sialoliths may reach astonishing dimensions, parotid calculi several centimeters in diameter and length occurring in the horse.

When its duct is occluded, a salivary gland undergoes atrophy (p. 90), but before this process is complete, a cyst may form in the obstructed duct due to the dilating effect of the imprisoned secretion. Such a cyst in the sublingual duct, lo-cated in the frenum linguae, has the special name of **ranula.** A salivary fistula occasionally forms when an injury has made an opening from the duct to the out-side of the body, proper healing being prevented by the flow of saliva through the opening.

Neoplasms arising in the parotids or other salivary glands are extremely rare in animals. Tumors in the region usually prove to be fibrosarcomas or malignant lymphomas or other forms not histogenetically related to the glandular tissue.

THE ESOPHAGUS

Inflammation of the esophagus is infrequent but, like that of the mouth, re-sults from trauma produced by foreign objects, from caustic chemicals or from infection. Because of the heavy and impervious epithelial lining, injury from elimination of toxic substances through the esophageal mucous membrane prob-ably never occurs.

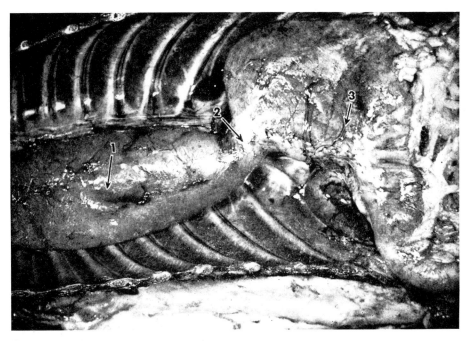

Fig. 24–2.—Dilatation of esophagus of a nine-month-old female collie, due to unknown cause, presumably congenital. The thoracic viscera and diaphragm have been removed, leaving the esophagus and stomach *in situ*. The esophagus (*1*) was not obstructed at the cardia (*2*) of the stomach (*3*). (Courtesy of Angell Memorial Animal Hospital.)

Reddened streaks of catarrhal inflammation may extend up and down the tops of the longitudinal ridges which form in the relaxed esophagus. In cattle, these suggest the presence of the poorly understood "mucosal disease" (p. 493) or of Olafson's "virus diarrhea" (p. 492).

Any considerable injury, chemical or traumatic, to the esophageal lining is much to be feared because of its tendency to produce **stenosis** of the esophageal lumen. The mechanism depends upon the production of scar tissue, which is very likely to form as such an injury heals. The scar tissue, contracting as it ages, draws the lumen into a **stricture,** or inordinate narrowing of the lumen. Injury from the swallowing of highly irritant or caustic chemicals including lye is the common cause. Surgical operations on the esophagus are formidable because of the same effect of contracting cicatricial tissue.

Choke, a complete or partial obstruction of the esophagus by foreign material, is all too common in cattle as the result of trying to swallow such things as beets, turnips, apples or small ears of corn without reducing them to small pieces. The horse practically never makes such a mistake as this, but does become choked by the gradual accumulation of ground or whole grain or tough grasses which fail to continue their passage through the whole length of the esophagus. Dogs and cats become choked by sharp pieces of bone which lodge usually in the thoracic esophagus. Contrary to popular belief, choking, as long as it is in the esophagus and not the pharynx or larynx, does not interfere seriously with respiration, although in the cow it prevents regurgitation of gas formed in the rumen with tympanites (p. 1196) of that organ which may well be fatal in some hours. Without this complication, if choke can not be relieved, death is likely in about three days because of local gangrene (from pressure and from compressed blood vessels) and resultant sapremia and toxemia.

Sometimes choking on a single foreign body results in only partial obstruction of the esophageal passageway. A common result then, especially in the dog, is that food is eaten but after some minutes is returned by vomition, only small amounts or none at all reaching the stomach. In a few weeks, the repeated stretching of the wall just above the obstruction produces a sac-like dilatation, usually asymmetrical and unilateral, known as an **esophageal diverticulum.** Perforation is another possible outcome in the case of sharp bones or similar objects.

In dogs and doubtless in related wild species, the spirurid worm *Spirocerca lupi* penetrates the mucosa and submucosa of the lower esophagus and causes a reaction in the form of subepithelial fibrous nodules as it develops there. The smoothly covered and perhaps coalescent nodules bulge into the lumen as much as 0.5 cm. Interference with esophageal function appears to be minimal (unless a sarcoma is formed, see below) and the lesions are usually found incidentally post mortem. Other parasites of the esophagus include *Gongylonema spp.* in ruminants and non-human primates and sarcoporidia in ruminants and rarely other species. A diffuse and non-localized dilation of the esophagus known as **megaesophagus** has been viewed as an entity in puppies. It is apparently paralytic in origin but the cause is rarely established. It has also been thought to result from spasm of the cardiac end of the esophagus (cardiospasm) and/or lack of reflex relaxation of the distal esophagus (achalasia). A hereditary basis has been hypothesized for the disorder in *wire-haired fox terriers* by Osborne, *et al.* (1967). Tracheo-esophageal fistula is an important but rare congenital anomaly. Obstruction of the esophagus also results from pressure from a vascular ring resulting from **persistent right aortic arch** (p. 1147).

Among **neoplasms,** carcinomas are not unknown (cat), but the only tumor of significant frequency in the esophagus of domestic animals is a fibrous and bony tumor which occurs in the lower esophagus in the dog. The histologic structure is commonly that of an osteosarcoma or osteogenic sarcoma (p. 197), the ossification doubtless representing a metaplasia from fibrous tisue. Typically the tumor not only bulges into the lumen, but also distorts and destroys considerable areas of the esophageal wall and extends into the surrounding mediastinal tissues as a highly irregular mass. Some of them reach a size sufficient to usurp a considerable portion of the thoracic cavity, and pulmonary osteo-arthropathy has developed concomitantly with certain ones, presumably through the mechanism of impaired pulmonary capacity and tissue anoxia. In many of these sarcomas, a number of the *Spirocerca lupi* worms, just mentioned, have been found, occupying indeterminate positions in the new growth. Chronic irritation from the parasites has been accused of a causative role, the hyperplastic inflammatory (p. 169) fibrous reaction having progressed to neoplasia. Indeed, the concomitant occurrence of the sarcomas and the parasites would seem too frequent to be a coincidence.

THE FORESTOMACHS OF RUMINANTS

The rumen, reticulum and omasum are called stomachs only because of their general shape and size. They store food in a manner similar to that of the crop (ingluvies) of a chicken; bacterial decomposition proceeds in them, but there is no secretory function such as characterizes a true stomach. References to the stomach, in this work, apply only to the true, secretory stomach.

The **rumen** is subject to common disorders which are functional rather than organic. **Tympanites** of the rumen, or **bloat,** consists in the accumulation of excessive quantities of gas in the organ, distending it to a dangerous degree. The gas, which can often be ignited with a match, consists largely of methane, carbon dioxide, carbon monoxide and small amounts of various others including the poisonous H_2S. These gases are the usual products of bacterial decomposition of carbohydrates and proteins and result from the action of many kinds of saprophytic bacteria upon ingested plant tissues. These fermentational processes are normal and go on continuously, but normally the gas is discharged in the form of frequent belchings or eructations through the esophagus and mouth.

Pathological bloating can obviously arise as the result of any interference with the normal eructations or from the production of gas at a rate beyond the capacity of esophageal eructations to discharge it. We do not know what mechanisms, if any, limit the amount of gas which can pass up the esophagus in a given period of time, but the escape, rather than being a passive process, requires active reverse peristaltic waves on the part of the esophagus and hence is under control of the (autonomic) nervous system. The amount of gas produced, of course, depends upon the rapidity of bacterial fermentational processes, and these are greatly favored when the food ingested is fresh, succulent, green legumes such as clovers and alfalfa. We can suspect, but cannot say with certainty, that the habitual capacity for repeated eructation may be exceeded at such times. There are various other theories on this point, however. One is that this green succulent material is very soft and that the initiation of expulsive ruminal contractions requires the mechanical irritation of rough stems and stalks upon the lining of the rumen. This explanation seems only slightly attractive when we consider that when the animal is on a diet of coarse, dry and largely indigestible straw, the rumen is well filled yet develops but little gas, with few eructations. Another theory is that the gases developed from the fresh green legumes include sufficient amounts of hydrogen disulfide to exert a toxic depressant action upon the local nervous structures. This is as yet unproved, either that important amounts of that gas are absorbed or that the H_2S would have that effect if the absorption did, indeed, occur. It is doubtful that the phenomenon of imprisoned gas in the bovine rumen is much different from that in the equine stomach or cecum (see below), where spasmodic contraction of adjacent segments of the alimentary canal are known to exert a sphincter-like action. It is common human experience that excessive fermentation in the intestine induces a certain degree of spasmodic action of the bowel. It seems not improbable that similar reflex spasms of the esophageal tube or orifice are responsible for the impounding of ruminal gases and that the increased pressure is sufficiently irritant to stimulate further spasm, a vicious circle being created. Certain it is that upon the passing of a stomach tube the excess of gas promptly escapes.

"**Frothy bloat**" constitutes an exception to the last statement and is a form of tympanites complicated by other factors than the mere excessive production of gas and its inability to escape through the tightly contracted esophagus. In this disorder, the gas is finely mixed with the fluid in the rumen in the form of very small bubbles, like the foam that one gets when he shakes an emulsion with air. The inability of the gas to escape from the foamy mixture is dependent on

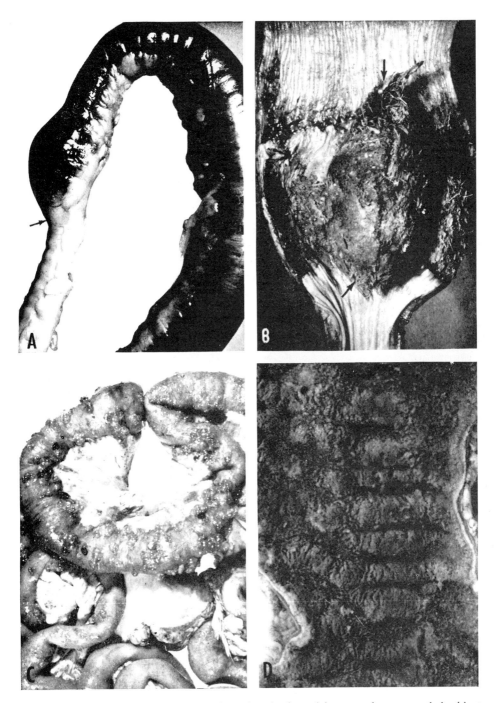

FIG. 24–3.—A, Obstruction of the small intestine of a dog. A large peach stone was lodged just above the arrow. B, Obstruction of the esophagus (choke) in a horse which died on the third day from severe toxic hepatitis and toxic tubular nephritis. The site of the large obstructing mass of ingesta is indicated by arrows. C, Intestinal emphysema, small intestine of swine. Note bubbles of air under serosa. D, Necrotizing enteritis of swine. Dark, thick, tenacious exudate consisting largely of fibrin and necrotic cells on intestinal mucosa. (Courtesy of College of Veterinary Medicine, Iowa State University.)

the surface tension of the liquid and doubtless of the colloidal state of dissolved solids. Liquids added to the mixture which reduce its surface tension tend to release the bubbles, but the chemical changes responsible for the original rise have not been satisfactorily ascertained. Possibly there is release from the ingested plant material of too much saponin, a soap-like emulsifying agent, but clinically the rapid ingestion of a large amount of succulent plants, usually leguminous, is the inciting cause.

Bloating of the preceding types is acute, arising suddenly and often causing death within an hour or two. The second form of tympanites is that which results from some physical obstruction of the esophageal or pharyngeal passageways. Choke has been mentioned earlier in this chapter as a cause of such obstruction. Strictures may have the same effect but are rare. Other causes include pressure upon the esophagus by tumors, abscesses, swollen lymph nodes and similar enlargements. Except in the case of a completely obstructing choke, these forms of bloating arise more gradually and often they are chronic or intermittent depending upon the cause.

One of the effects of severe bloating is to push the diaphragm forward, seriously limiting the respiratory capacity. Another is to compress the large veins of the abdominal cavity, seriously obstructing the general circulation. Both these mechanisms result in anoxia, which is the immediate cause of death in those cases which are fatal. If the excessive pressure is relieved by surgical or other form of intervention the above effects promptly subside.

Sheep, as well as cattle, are susceptible to bloating but, because of their more conservative eating habits, are less commonly involved.

RUMINAL ATONY AND INTOXICATION

In most cases, the weak and atonic musculature is that of a rumen which is tightly impacted with undigested roughage, although there are a few cases in which the rumen is nearly empty, except, perhaps, for an accumulation of sand or similar foreign substance. The essential feature is that the rumen stops working; there are no more contractions of sufficient force to move the contents forward along the normal digestive course nor to regurgitate them for "chewing the cud." There is little or no gas in the rumen and this fact affords a clue to what is at least an important aspect of the pathogenesis of this disorder, namely, a failure of bacterial growth. Present knowledge of just what bacterial species are involved and the pertinent aspects of their physiological processes (production of gas, acid, etc.) is not complete, nor can we always point to the exact reason why desirable species stop growing and disappear, but the absence of fermentational processes is evident in the condition of the ruminal contents. They are dull in color, soggy and solid in consistency, like unleavened bread dough. Unleavened it is, indeed, for the fermentation has stopped. Putrefactive bacteria begin, at least, to produce their characteristic odors. The wall, at autopsy, is thin and "lifeless," easily folded in any direction. Microscopically, it is difficult to describe specifically any change in the tissues other than a certain degree of quantitative atrophy.

The disease is gradual and insidious in its onset, and for a day or two after symptoms become manifest, the changes are reversible; later, it is unlikely that any known treatment will be availing. There is clinical evidence that potent toxins are absorbed from the decomposing mass, and at death toxic changes (acute toxic hepatitis, p. 1223) are discernible in the liver. However, both the clinical and pathological pictures are likely to be complicated, at the end, by ketosis (p. 1020) due to lack of assimilation of food.

RUMENITIS AND ULCERS OF THE RUMEN

The mucosa of the rumen is subject to the formation of frequent and extensive ulcers but they are seldom seen by others than meat inspectors for the reason that they occur ordinarily in young cattle fattened for market and in excellent health as far as can be determined by clinical standards. It is not unusual for a majority of a pen of animals fattened for "prime, heavy beef" on a concentrated ration such as corn and alfalfa hay to show one or more ruminal ulcers each, when slaughtered. Limited to the papillated areas, the ulcers are of entirely irregular shape but may be as large as a person's outspread hand. They are often multiple but always superficial, usually reaching no deeper than the mucosa, and have no true similarity to the human peptic ulcer. They have been found to originate in an area where the villi are somewhat swollen and loosely glued together with a slightly sticky substance. Microscopically, this substance proves to be an inflammatory exudate of sero-purulent nature and quite limited in amount. The affected villi die, become detached and disappear, leaving a smooth, raw surface. Microscopically, a rather mild leukocytic infiltration, chiefly of lymphocytes and neutrophilic granulocytes, is found in the underlying submucosa. The ulcer, now completely formed, begins to heal by proliferation of new epithelium at the outer edges. The proliferating epithelium, in a period which may be estimated as several weeks, eventually covers the largest ulcer, which meantime has shrunk greatly. At first the new epithelium is white, contrasting with the normal ruminal lining, which is black in a majority of cattle. As time goes on, nothing remains but a narrow, angular or stellate scar. This becomes a mere line and eventually disappears completely, the process probably requiring several months or a year. Bacteriological examination of the ulcer usually reveals the necrophorus organism as the principal if not the only invader.

What we believe to be a variant of the ulcerative process is the formation of a clump of little spherical white nodules attached to the mucosal surface. Diameters of 1 to 2 cm. represent the more frequent sizes. Not uncommonly they occur on the pillars, as well as in the papillated areas. The epithelium is non-pigmented, comparatively thin and always smooth, like that of the healing scars. It is underlaid by fibrous tissue which constitutes the inner bulk of the nodule. We look upon the nodules as representing an inflammatory hyperplasia rather than neoplasms, which they have been called. One reason for this view is that after examining large numbers we have seen none which reached large size; their potentialities of growth appear to be definitely limited. We have seen the nodules forming in connection with and as parts of the more usual flat scars.

The cause and pathogenesis of ulcers in the rumen are only partly clear, but they have been shown to have an important relation to a sudden shift from a diet of range grasses to the too luxurious ration of the feed-lot. Their possible connection with abscesses in the liver is discussed in the study of that organ (p. 1230).

Exceptionally, localized areas of acute rumenitis and possibly ulceration have been encountered in the vicinity of slowly dissolving capsules or boluses of such mildly stomachic drugs as tartar emetic (potassium-antimony tartrate). A more or less essential provocative factor appears to be cessation of ruminal motility so that the chemical is left concentrated in one spot.

A disorder described as **parakeratosis of the rumen** has been encountered in sheep whose diet consisted largely of "pelleted" feeds, the ground material being formed into small cylinders by a feed mill. The cornified (keratinized) layer and the underlying Malpighian layer of the epithelium are each far thicker than normal and the keratinized cells retain vestiges of their nuclei rather than losing their cellular identity in the pink-staining homogeneity which is normally expected. Whether this is wholly a retardation of a normal maturation, a failure of the aging cells to wear off and disappear, or whether there is also involved a reactive hyperplasia with more rapid production of new epithelium may well be inquired. The latter is known to occur as the result of some irritant substances in feeds (chlorinated naphthalenes, p. 938) and the existence of other irritants, presently unknown, may well be suspected.

FOREIGN BODIES IN THE RETICULUM

The bovine species is not equipped with highly sensitive prehensile organs nor a delicate sense of taste. As a consequence, cattle that are kept in farmyards, stables or in other proximity to the various mechanized activities of humans are prone to swallow metallic objects like nails, screws and bits of wire which have been carelessly allowed to get into their mangers or feed boxes. Probably some of these objects are even licked up from the surface of the ground as the cow wraps her tongue around a choice tuft of grass.

These objects almost invariably remain in the reticulum, retarded, no doubt, by the baffle-like action of the criss-crossing folds of its lining. No especial harm results from the presence of smooth foreign bodies, but the sharp ones either become entrapped in perforations they have made in one or more of the lining folds or penetrate the wall of the organ. The perforation of a fold is a relatively harmless accident as shown by the fact that many healthy cattle are slaughtered and found to have nails or wires embedded horizontally in the reticulated mucous folds with small white, scarred areas around them. Those which penetrate the wall proper are gradually pushed through it by the recurrent peristaltic movements of the organ. While migration in any direction is possible, the great majority of the objects move anteriorly. They pass through the diaphragm and into the pericardium and heart muscle, carrying infectious organisms with them, and producing the condition known as traumatic pericarditis (p. 1135). Movement is usually slow, so that a dense fibrous wall encircles the path of the wire or similar object. It is not unusual for the ordinary iron wire to become completely rusted out by the time pericardial infection reaches its usually fatal culmination. In such a case, the diagnosis can still be made by finding the dense fibrous encapsulating mass of highly variable size and shape but with a slender, blackened tract usually demonstrable along the path taken by the penetrating body. The anterior surface of the reticulum is usually adherent to the diaphragm and examination for adhesions in this region should constitute a part of every bovine necropsy. Not infrequently there are also heavily encapsulated abscesses in the vicinity. If the foreign body has chanced to take a different direction, there is localized (rarely generalized) peritonitis with abscesses anywhere among the

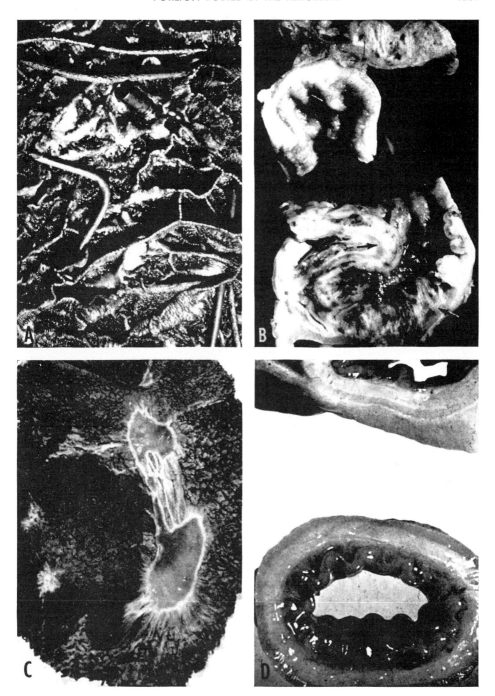

FIG. 24–4.—A, Foreign bodies in the reticulum of a cow. Note that one nail (lower right) has penetrated the wall. Objects such as these may lead to traumatic gastritis. (Courtesy College of Veterinary Medicine, Iowa State University.) B, Regional cicatrizing enterocolitis in a two-year-old dog given euthanasia because of severe diarrhea for six months. (Courtesy Texas Sch. Vet. Med.) C, Ulcers in the rumen of a fattened steer which was slaughtered in apparently normal health. The large dark area at left is undergoing necrosis and would have sloughed. (Courtesy Colorado Sch. Vet. Med.) D, Edema of the mucosa and submucosa of the ileum incarcerated in an umbilical hernia in a four-year-old mule. Death followed laparotomy and attempted relief. (Courtesy College of Veterinary Medicine, Iowa State University.)

abdominal viscera or there may be penetration of the liver or spleen. If the infection transported happens to be other than pyogenic, the lesion shows changes characteristic of the organism involved, usually caseous or liquefactive necrosis.

The **omasum** and the **esophageal groove** are seldom the seat of important pathological processes. Actinobacillosis rarely localizes in the region, producing the characteristic granulomatous reaction. Malignant lymphomas may develop neoplastic masses in any of the local tissues but are more likely to infiltrate the wall of the rumen or abomasum. A rare but curious disorder is the formation of horn-like protruding growths several millimeters in diameter and some 2 to 4 cm. in height, arising on the edges of the esophageal groove, on nearby portions of the pillars of the rumen or at the opening of the omasum. They are essentially papillomas but of no clinical importance.

THE STOMACH

Gastritis—Inflammation of the stomach is essentially an affection of its mucous lining. The symptoms, in general, are pain, anorexia and vomiting. The latter sign is invariably present in gastritis but may also be induced by reverse peristalsis initiated lower in the gastrointestinal tract, as well as by central nervous disturbances. Gastritis is usually catarrhal or hemorrhagic in type.

Acute catarrhal gastritis is recognized by an increased reddening and thickening of the entire surface or parts of it, the fundic area usually being most severely involved. There is an increase of the mucous secretion which may or may not be sufficient to be recognizable grossly. Under the microscope, one sees that the redness is due to a combination of hyperemia and desquamation of the epithelium. It is often difficult to decide whether some of the desquamation is attributable to post-mortem autolysis. In company with these changes, there is a limited amount of lymphocytic or, less commonly, neutrophilic infiltration of the mucosa and submucosa. Lymphoid hyperplasia of the normally minute lymphocytic foci in the gastric mucous membrane may result in microscopically large or even grossly recognizable nodules in the case of inflammatory processes of some days' duration.

Acute hemorrhagic gastritis is also common and is to be distinguished grossly by deeper reddening and by the presence of free blood on the surface or in the gastric contents. It should be noted that blood which has remained for any considerable time exposed to the gastric juice turns brown; commonly it is mixed with mucus as a slimy and viscid brownish substance, clinging more or less to the gastric surface. In the exact microscopic distinction as to whether an inflammation is hemorrhagic or merely catarrhal it must be recognized that the extravascular blood may be within the tissues as well as on the surface. Since these two types of gastritis differ mainly in degree, the distinction is usually academic. Of course, the presence of extravasated blood without other signs of inflammation is to be interpreted as hemorrhage.

Catarrhal or hemorrhagic gastritis is a typical effect of various locally destructive poisons but is also a characteristic lesion of certain infectious diseases including swine erysipelas. The bites or points of attachment of several kinds of parasitic helminths, especially the trichostrongyles of ruminants, leave tiny hemorrhages or inflamed spots. With large numbers of parasites, the tiny spots become more or less confluent.

Serous fluid (serous exudate, p. 153), usually termed **inflammatory edema,** may be a prominent part of the picture of gastritis, causing marked thickening of the mucosa and submucosa. The other varieties of acute inflammation are unusual in the stomach, although a fibrinous exudate may be formed in response to certain infections of a mucosa previously devitalized. Certain poisons exert specific effects upon the gastric lining when ingested in concentrated form. Mercuric chloride produces coagulative necrosis and at the same time acts as a fixative, preserving the tissue from post-mortem changes. Carbolic acid has a similar effect and turns the surface white or gray.

Hemorrhages, large and small, may occur in the gastric mucosa under any of the circumstances listed as causative in the general discussion of hemorrhage (p. 119), but localized and generalized toxic conditions occupy a prominent place among them. Uremia is among the latter, as well as canine "blacktongue" (p. 985). The principal hemorrhage-producing poisons are listed in Chapter 17, page 843. Outstanding among the hemorrhage-producing infections likely to involve the gastric mucosa are hog cholera (swine fever), anthrax and leptospirosis. Numerous small or punctate hemorrhages, some being old and faded, should lead to a search for helminth parasites, especially for the trichostrongyles of cattle and sheep. On the peritoneal surface, hemorrhages signify either hemorrhagic poisons or infections.

Chronic passive congestion, with or without (non-inflammatory) edema, represents the effect upon the stomach of the circulatory impairment which results from cirrhosis or cardiac insufficiency.

Acute dilatation of the stomach from accumulation of gas occurs in connection with spasmodic forms of indigestion with much the same results as those which follow tympanites of the bovine rumen. Spasmodic closure of the gastric openings is an essential mechanism; it is usually due to irritant substances in the stomach contents. Obstructive lesions, usually at the pylorus, result in intermittent or **chronic dilatation.** Acute dilatation is most commonly seen in horses where it may lead to rupture. Acute gastric dilation, described as "bloat," occurs in non-human primates.

Impaction of the stomach in the horse as the result of rapid ingestion of an excessive amount of ground feed or heavy grains (wheat, Indian corn) is especially dangerous. Even without gaseous fermentation, which is usual, absorption of toxic products of partial digestion, circulatory derangement and shock may be fatal in a number of hours or may cause laminitis (p. 1041).

Parasites.—A variety of parasites may infest the stomach. In horses *Gastrophilus spp.* larvae are very common. The roundworm, *Hyostrongylus rubidus*, invades the mucosa in swine. In ruminants, stomach worms are a major problem. The more common nematodes are *Hemonchus spp., Ostertagia spp.*, and *Trichostrongylus axei*.

Ulcers.—Some of the infectious or toxic inflammations are ulcerative, especially in the later stages, and some of the hemorrhages owe their origin to erosions or ulcerations, but all these ulcers are acute and superficial. Chronic, indurated ulcers comparable to the human peptic ulcer do not occur naturally in any of the domestic species.

Ulceration of the non-glandular (stratified squamous epithelium) stomach in swine is a frequent and often serious disease. The ulcers are irregular in shape and may be single or multiple, varying in size from a few millimeters to several centimeters in diameter. Histologically the ulcers extend into the submucosa but rarely beyond and are associated with edema, arteritis, infiltration of neutrophils and eosinophils and hyperplasia of submucosal lymphoid follicles. Adjacent epithelium is acanthotic and parakeratotic: changes which are believed to develop prior to erosion and ulceration. Blood in varying quantities may be admixed with the stomach contents. Healed ulcers leave contracted scars. Depending on the degree of ulceration, clinical signs may be inapparent as death may result from acute gastric hemorrhage without premonitory signs. More often the affected animals are weak, pale (anemia) and dyspneic. Vomiting may occur and the feces may be tarry. The cause of gastric ulceration in swine is not known. The most promising hypothesis suggests vitamin E deficiency, but the pathogenesis is not clear. Diets deficient in vitamin E and high in unsaturated fatty acids have been shown experimentally to be ulcerogenic. Ulcers have been seen in association with hepatosis dietetica (p. 994). Deficiencies of vitamins A, and D, zinc, and copper have also been suggested, as has hyperacidity, but all are unproved. Gelatinized corn rations have been associated with ulceration.

Stress of confinement and transportation may also play a role in the development of ulcers. No doubt ulcers may be incited by more than a single factor, but the syndrome in swine suggests that most gastric ulcers are part of a single disease process. Ulceration of the glandular stomach of swine is much less frequent and not associated with ulceration of the non-glandular stomach.

Ulceration of the non-glandular portion of the stomach is occasionally encountered in foals. Rooney (1964) believes they are related to mechanical trauma by *Gastrophilus intestinalis* larvae, stones, etc. Ulceration of the glandular mucosa also occurs in horses and is common in calves. Trauma and stress are believed to be causative factors but vitamin E deficiency has also been suggested. In calves mucormycosis commonly develops in gastric ulcers as well as in ulcers of the colon.

Ulcers of the pyloris and proximal duodenum are often associated with generalized mast cell tumors ("mast cell leukemia") in cats (p. 236).

Torsion of the stomach is occasionally encountered in dogs. The cause is unknown, but it is seen most often in large breeds. **Displacement of the abomasum** occurs in cattle, chiefly in the postpartum period.

Neoplasms.—Malignant lymphomas rather frequently involve the stomach by infiltrating extensively into the wall and the mucous folds (bovine), causing marked thickening. Leiomyomas occasionally arise from the gastric musculature. Other tumors, including carcinomas, are almost nonexistent. The latter, however, are not unknown, at least in the horse and the dog. In the dog they are usually scirrhous, presenting a contracted, scarred or distorted gastric wall which grossly may suggest a healed ulcer rather than carcinoma. Peritoneal metastases are usually present, which are also scirrhous.

Foreign bodies are occasionally encountered, for instance, a rubber ball in the stomach of a dog. Piliconcretions may be in the stomach but are more likely to be found in the intestine (p. 1214).

THE INTESTINE

Enteritis.—The term enteritis commonly refers to inflammation of any or all parts of the intestinal tract, but in some quarters its significance is limited to the small intestine. The former usage will be followed here. The outstanding sign of enteritis is diarrhea; unless the disorder is very mild, there are also pain and anorexia.

Acute enteritis may conform to any one of the five types of acute exudative inflammation (p. 153), and subacute lymphocytic and chronic proliferative forms are by no means lacking. The whole small intestine may be rather uniformly inflamed, or even the small and large intestines together, but it is more usual that the inflammation be more pronounced toward one end or the other of the small intestine or perhaps relatively localized as a colitis, cecitis (also known as typhlitis) or proctitis. The location of the reaction, of course, coincides with the site of greatest concentration of the irritant, be it chemical or infectious. Toxic substances which are ingested may be held for some time in the stomach so that their principal effect is a gastritis. Other toxic substances are of such a nature that the stomach rather quickly advances them to the intestine, where most of their effect is felt. There is also the factor of solubility; those which dissolve slowly may progress to the intestine before becoming extensively dissolved. The rather high acidity in the stomach and the relative alkalinity in the intestine are also important influences on solubility and absorption. If the irritant is of infectious nature, the time required for adequate multiplication of the organisms may be instrumental in determining where their harm is greatest. A rather common situation is for the upper small intestine to be severely inflamed with the ileum remaining relatively normal. This is ordinarily attributable to the injurious substance having been dissipated or at least diluted before it reached the lower portions of the bowel. The length of time during which the ingesta remain in a given place is also important and may be responsible for a cecitis or colitis with little or no damage in the more rapidly emptying small intestine. When inflammation is principally in the colon, the possibility of its being caused by a toxic substance in process of elimination there should be entertained. Numerous toxic substances of endogenous or exogenous origin are eliminated from the blood into the bowel, some of them principally in the large bowel (mercury, uremic products), causing injury and an inflammatory reaction in the mucous membrane through which they pass. Lastly, the peculiar affinities of a particular infecting organism have to be considered: the coccidia of most mammals confine themselves almost entirely to the last part of the large bowel although certain species localize in the small intestine; the various avian coccidia have different sites of predilection, the cecum or the upper small intestine, depending on the species of coccidium. Some microorganisms depend upon metazoan parasites to provide a mode of entry, and hence localize in the area favored by the metazoan species. Within a given area the most superficial parts of the mucosa often show more severe injury than more protected structures: the summits of the longitudinal rugae of the rectum may be reddened with catarrhal inflammation; the tips of the villi may be dying, while the fundi of the glands show no injury.

In catarrhal enteritis, acute or chronic, the changes simulate those of catarrhal gastritis: death of epithelium and perhaps the underlying stroma in the more exposed structures, moderate hyperemia and moderate lymphocytic infiltration in the deeper parts of the mucosa. Enteritis of this kind is a common accompaniment of many infectious diseases as well as the result of toxic substances. The multitudinous bites occurring in an extensive infestation of hookworms cause confluent hemorrhages and catarrhal or hemorrhagic enteritis in the small intestine of the dog. Somewhat less conspicuous injury is done to the cecum and large colon of the horse in the case of severe strongylosis (p. 752). In canine autopsies, a mild degree of catarrhal duodenitis and jejunitis is found with such frequency as to be almost routine.

Occasionally, a truly mucous exudate is encountered, of such intensity that the microscopic section reveals streams of blue-staining epithelial mucin (p. 52) stretching out from the intestinal glands (crypts). Clinically this type of reaction, occurring in the large bowel, is revealed by sheets or strings of white, inspissated mucus on the formed feces. The soft fecal discharges of the bovine are an obvious exception, but in the constipation, which often accompanies this benign and transitory enteric disturbance, formed feces flecked with visible aggregations of solidified mucus sometimes appear even in cattle.

Like its gastric counterpart, **hemorrhagic enteritis** is chiefly a violent form of the acute catarrhal. Its distribution is practically always patchy for the simple reason that an animal could scarcely remain alive until a hemorrhagic enteritis had become widespread. This form is usually the enteric manifestation of a locally destructive poison in concentrated form or of one of the highly virulent infections, such as anthrax. Salmonella species, commonly *S. enteritidis* or *S. typhimurium*, have been reported as causing acute catarrhal, and often hemorrhagic, enteritis in cattle, horses and monkeys. In swine, *Salmonella cholerae suis* is the common cause of acute enteritis, but there are numerous reports of a vibrio (*V. coli*) causing severe and fatal enteritis in young pigs. Shigellosis is an important cause of hemorrhagic enteritis in most species of non-human primates. Viruses have also been incriminated.

Purulent enteritis is infrequent but occasionally occurs where mechanical injuries from helminth parasites (*e.g.*, hookworms, nodular worms) have opened the tissues to invasion by pyogenic bacteria. Chronic muco-purulent enteritis in the dog, apparently of non-specific origin, is characterized by dense, slightly tenacious, semi-solid, whitish exudate lying to a depth of 2 or 3 mm. over the duodenal and jejunal surfaces.

Fibrinous Enteritis.—Acute fibrinous inflammation is probably of less rarity in the large intestine of cattle than elsewhere. The fibrinous exudate is often of the pseudomembranous type and as the inflammation subsides, the pesudomembrane may be loosened to pass out with the feces in the form of a long, hollow cast bearing an uncanny resemblance to the lining of a stretch of intestine.

A more diphtheritic (p. 156) form of acute fibrinous inflammation sometimes involves either the small or large intestine of the pig. Limited data indicate that it is due to the activities of the organism, *Salmonella cholerae suis (suipestifer)*.

The much more usual fibrinous enteritis in the pig is chronic, the well-known **necrophorus enteritis,** or **"necro."** The term "necrotic enteritis" has also been used, but the careful pathologist will naturally suspect that it is the tissue rather than the enteritis which undergoes necrosis! The lesions occur in the large intestine and, to some extent, in the last portion of the ileum. They consist of patches, large or small, of thick, rough, brownish or grayish diphtheritic exudate which is tightly adherent to the dead and living tissue beneath. As is usual with diphtheritic exudates (p. 156), the underlying cells undergo coagulative necrosis and the fibrils of the exudate extend into and among them, tying the whole into a crust-like layer. Fecal material becomes mixed with the superficial portions of the exudate. The exudative areas may line a considerable portion of the bowel, or they may be limited to raised patches here and there. Not infrequently they form rather perfect circular structures known as "button ulcers." Since necrophorus enteritis frequently accompanies severe outbreaks of hog cholera, the button ulcers were at one time considered diagnostic of that viral disease.

As the name implies, the necrophorus organism (presently *Spherophorus necrophorus*) plays an important part in producing the lesions of this disease, but it is generally believed to be a secondary invader, supervening upon primary injury caused by some other infection, possibly the *Salmonella* just mentioned. Whatever its precise bacteriological status may be, necrophorus enteritis is a disease which belongs to filthy or long used and contaminated pig pens; adequate sanitation and husbandry eliminate it. Deficiency of nicotinic acid in the diet may have predisposing importance but cannot be accepted as fundamental (p. 986).

Balantidiasis.—The ciliated protozoan, *Balantidium coli*, occurs in the large intestine of the pig. The rounded organism, some 50 by 75 microns in size, with an elongated, blue-staining nucleus in the central part of the pink-staining cytoplasm, is not infrequently seen in the lumens of the intestinal glands or even in the tissue of the mucosa or submucosa. When the organisms invade the tissues they must be considered in some degree pathogenic, but balantidiosis is scarcely a clinical disease, as it is in man and chimpanzees (p. 708).

Severe acute catarrhal or hemorrhagic reddening of the rectum (proctitis) and terminal colon, in cattle, is very likely to mean **coccidiosis** and necessitates search for oöcysts in the feces or for encysted forms in and beneath the epithelial cells. Both forms are numerous in coccidiosis of clinical severity (p. 679). Other protozoon parasites which are occasionally encountered as "causes" of enteritis are *Endamoeba histolytica* (dogs and monkeys), *Giardia spp.* (dogs, chinchillas), and *Globidium spp.* (horses, cattle—also localizes in other tissues, p. 698).

Chronic proliferative enteritis is seen in those granulomatous infections which involve the intestine, notably Johne's disease, tuberculosis, colibacillosis (Hjärre's disease) of fowls, histoplasmosis and others. The proliferative enteric reaction is that characteristic of each disease. Partial obstructions or other mechanical factors are occasionally responsible for localized chronic inflammations of the same general variety.

Regional cicatrizing enterocolitis, or Crohn's disease, was established as an entity in humans in 1932. An entirely comparable disease was recognized in the dog by Strande *et al.* (1954). In the general vicinity of the ileo-cecal orifice and sometimes both above and below it, the mucosa and submucosa are rather irregularly involved in asymmetrical thickening which, in the experience of one of the writers (Smith), reaches as much as 6 cm., and is strongly suggestive of mucosal neoplasia. Microscopically, the suspected neoplasm proves to consist of fibrous and reticulo-endothelial granulation tissue with many bizarre epithelioid and even multinucleated giant cells. In places, the mucous surface is ulcerated, with an acute purulent reaction. Fistulas may reach the serosal side of the bowel. Dense fibrous scarring marks attempted healing. The regional mesenteric lymph nodes may undergo a similar granulomatous enlargement. The ultimate result is partial or complete obstruction of the intestinal lumen. The cause appears to be a chronic infection, but rather extensive search has failed to identify one in either man or animal.

Muscular Hypertrophy of the Ileum in Swine.—An apparently unrelated condition of swine, characterized by marked hypertrophic thickening of the muscularis propria in the last portion of the ileum, has been confused with the above granulomatous disease under the name of **terminal ileitis**. The great thickening of the intestinal wall and stenosis of the lumen are similar although usually less abrupt. Microscopically, the thickening is not granulomatous and does not involve the mucosa and submucosa but is, rather, an extensive but orderly increase in both layers of the muscularis. This is probably to be explained, as pointed out by Neilsen (1955), on a functional basis, an adaptive hypertrophy gradually developing as the result of impaction or spasmodic contraction lower in the tract. With increasing stenosis, ingesta actually become lodged at the site of narrowing. Local pressure brings venous obstruction and edema, with bacterial and gangrenous invasion of the devitalized mucosa. Nielsen suggested the name "muscular hypertrophy of the ileum" in place of terminal ileitis.

Dodd (1968) has recently described a lesion in the ileum of a pig which he termed **"adenomatous intestinal hyperplasia"** or **proliferative ileitis,** which is apparently the same condition as described by Biester and Schwarte in 1931 as "intestinal adenoma." The lesion is characterized by multiple small mucosal nodules composed of proliferating epithelium, producing an adenomatous picture.

There is a single report of segmental hypertrophy of a $5\frac{1}{2}$ cm. length of the transverse colon of a rhesus monkey (*Macaca mulatta*) (Casey, *et al.*, 1969). In this animal the hypertrophy was principally of the muscularis.

Proliferative Ileitis in Hamsters.—What is apparently a contagious disease has been described in hamsters as proliferative ileitis (Boothe and Cheville 1967) and *enzootic intestinal adenocarcinoma* (Jonas, *et al.*, 1965). Despite the opposing interpretations (inflammatory vs. neoplastic) the diseases described in the two reports are so similar that they are considered here as a single entity which we consider inflammatory and not neoplastic. Clinically there is weight loss and diarrhea. In the report of Boothe and Cheville, the disease spread slowly, had a morbidity rate of 25 to 60 per cent and a mortality rate of 90 per cent. The lesions develop in the ileum, less often the jejunum and rarely in the colon. Grossly the ileum is dilated, thickened, studded with small white subserosal foci and often adhered to other viscera. Microscopically there is hyperplasia of the intestinal epithelium, accompanied by purulent inflammation and coagulation necrosis extending into the submucosa. The hyperplastic epithelium extends into the submucosa, muscularis and often to the serosa, forming small glands or cysts which remain after healing. Diffuse and focal collections of large histiocytes occur on the lamina propria, submucosa, muscularis and serosa as well as in mesenteric lymph nodes. Tomita and Jonas (1968) have isolated two viruses (which may be herpesviruses) from affected hamsters but their relationship in this disease is not established at present. Lussier and Pavilonis (1969) described eosinophilic intranuclear inclusion bodies in the ileal epithelium which may add support to the hypothesis of a viral etiology.

Spontaneous Ileitis in Rats.—Also described as "megaloileitis," this disease of unknown cause occurs in young rats less than two months of age. Clinically there is marked distention of the abdomen, rough hair coat and occasionally diarrhea. Approximately 50 per cent of affected rats die, the others recovering over a period of about a week. At necropsy the most striking lesion is a severe dilatation of the ileum with 7 to 10 cm. segments distended up to 1.5 cm. The distention generally terminates at or near the ileocecal junction. The contents of the ileum vary from a frothy semi-fluid to a pasty consistency. Microscopically

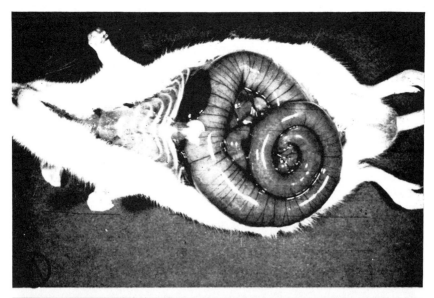

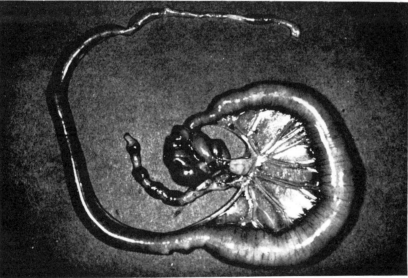

FIG. 24–5.—Regional ileitis, rat. There is marked dilation of the ileum.
(Courtesy Animal Research Center, Harvard Medical School.)

the lesions are not striking. There is hydropic degeneration and coagulation necrosis of both layers of the muscularis associated with an inflammatory cell infiltration composed of lymphocytes, macrophages, and a lesser number of neutrophils. In the mucosa a lymphocytic infiltration occurs in the lamina propria and many of the crypts of Lieberkuhn are occluded with amorphous eosinophilic material. In the healing stages of the condition, fibrovascular proliferation repairs the lesions in the muscularis. Occasionally the distended ileum becomes adhered to the abdominal wall or other viscera. In some rats with this disease there is also a necrotizing and lymphocytic myocarditis and hepatitis.

Histocytic Ulcerative Colitis of Boxer Dogs.—Confined to dogs of the boxer breed, this disorder, also termed granulomatous colitis, is similar in many respects to Whipple's disease of man. Affected dogs, which are usually less than two years of age, pass soft tan feces often mixed with blood, with great frequency (up to 15 times a day). Profuse diarrhea does not occur and throughout the course the disease is afebrile, and weight is usually maintained. Significant gross lesions are confined to the colon, cecum, and mesenteric lymph nodes. The wall of the colon and cecum is thickened and the mucosa is ulcerated often to the extent that little intact mucosa remains. Microscopically the surface of the ulcers is composed of fibrin and neutrophils, but the striking feature throughout the colonic mucosa as well as the submucosa is a marked infiltration by large macrophages, which may be accompanied by lymphocytes, plasma cells and collagen. The macrophages have pink foamy cytoplasm which is PAS positive and stains lightly with fat stains. Ultrastructural studies by Van Kruiningen (1967) have demonstrated the cells to be filled with packets of phagocytized material composed of membranes often arranged in whorls. In one dog he saw structures suggesting a psittacoid agent. Enlargement of mesenteric lymph nodes results from lymphocytic hyperplasia and aggregates of macrophages similar to those in the colon and cecum. In advanced cases peripheral lymph nodes may also be enlarged and contain similar macrophages. The cause of this disease is not known.

Winter dysentery of cattle is a comparatively mild and transient enteritis which has generally been ascribed to the bacterium *Vibrio jejuni*, however a virus has also been held as the responsible agent (Macpherson 1957). It is highly contagious in stabled herds in northern lands. The outstanding lesion is an acute mucous ileitis and jejunitis, which in exceptionally severe cases becomes hemorrhagic. Direct staining techniques, as well as cultures, demonstrate the vibrios in large numbers in the affected mucosa.

Swine Dysentery.—Also known as hemorrhagic enteritis and vibrionic dysentery, swine dysentery is an acute infection of young pigs characterized by bloody

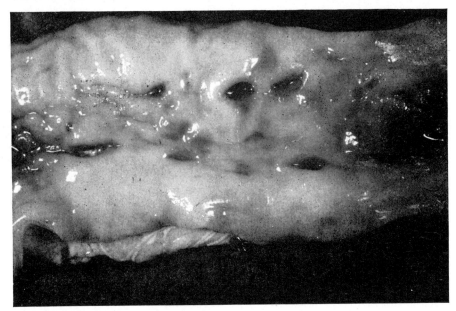

Fig. 24–6.—Ulcers in duodenum of a five-year-old spayed female cat. Neoplastic mast cells invaded the spleen. (Courtesy of Angell Memorial Animal Hospital.)

diarrhea. *Vibrio coli* is believed to be the cause, but the isolation of vibrio from normal pigs and the fact that all isolates do not regularly reproduce the disease, indicates that predisposing influences, synergism with other agents or strain variations of *Vibrio coli* may be of importance. The outstanding lesion is a hemorrhagic colitis and cecitis which often extends to the rectum. In acute cases the inflammation may be more catarrhal and less hemorrhagic and in cases of longer standing, a fibrino-necrotic membrane may overlie the colon. The small intestine is usually normal. There is regional lymphadenitis and excessive fluid in the pericardial sac. *Vibrio coli* can be demonstrated in the crypts of the mucosa and isolated to establish the diagnosis. Differential diagnosis includes salmonellosis (*Salmonella cholerae suis*) (p. 604) and necrotizing enteritis caused by *Spheropherous necropherous* (p. 623).

Staphylococcal enteritis in chinchillas.—A severe enteritis in these animals has followed long-term feeding of a mixture containing antibiotics. The normal Gram-negative bacterial flora of the intestine were found to have disappeared and to have been replaced by hemolytic *Staphylococcus aureus* in huge numbers. The animals returned to normal when the feeding was changed to more ordinary ingredients. This experience is comparable to staphylococcal infections elsewhere accompanying the indiscriminate use of antibiotics.

ENTEROTOXEMIA

Cl. perfringens Type D Enterotoxemia.—There has long been recognized in fattening lambs, and less regularly in adult sheep, a disease characterized by brief nervous symptoms and sudden death, which could be prevented by markedly decreasing the total amount of food or by changing from a high concentration of grains with little roughage to a ration consisting almost entirely of hay or similar material. While the lambs are usually found dead, if an observer is present, he may detect a period of one-half to a few hours during which opisthotonos progresses into pre-mortal coma. In a few cases, convulsions take the place of coma and death is still more prompt. Occasionally, there is the desire to push the forehead against a solid wall, which is the characteristic attitude of "blind staggers" as seen in many forms of indigestion in various species. Some investigators have found these acute symptoms to be preceded by a day or more of anorexia and diarrhea or mucus-covered feces, at least in some individuals.

Post-mortem lesions which have attracted most attention are petechial or ecchymotic hemorrhages beneath the epicardial and endocardial surfaces, the serous surfaces of the intestines, in the abdominal muscles and diaphragm and in the thymus. Hydropericardium is usually noted. In addition to distortion of certain values in the blood chemistry, there is pronounced glycosuria. Also noted by some observers are distention of the rumen and reticulum, the abomasum and the lower intestines by ingesta and gas. Mild catarrhal gastroenteritis is sometimes visible. A distended gallbladder frequently provides further evidence of digestive malfunction (p. 1236). In addition, there is often a tendency toward the development of "pulpy kidney" (p. 16). Neurologic signs are explained (at least in part) by lesions of the nervous system which consist of bilaterally symmetrical focal malacia of the basal ganglia, substantia nigra and thalamus and demyelination in the internal capsule, subcortical white matter and cerebellar peduncles.

It has been demonstrated by Bennetts (1932) and confirmed by others that the intestinal contents of these lambs contain large numbers of clostridial organisms and significant amounts of the thermo-labile toxin of *Clostridium perfringens*, type D (until recently the approved name was *Cl. welchii*, type D; another name is *Cl. ovitoxicus*). This toxin is promptly fatal to lambs and laboratory animals when injected parenterally but, under ordinary circumstances, quite harmless when given by mouth. There is nothing remarkable about the presence of the *Cl. perfringens* organisms in the digestive tract; in fact, it would be unusual if these and other soil-borne clostridia were absent. The toxin must be significant, especially since its injection appears to reproduce the characteristic disease, but it has been demonstrated in the intestine of healthy lambs, as well, and just why it is absorbed into the circulation in some individuals and not in others has never been fully explained. Experimentally, it has been made to produce the disease when introduced into the lamb's alimentary tract previously injured or at least functionally impaired by such procedures as partially paralyzing the bowel with opium and belladonna, distending it with an excessive amount of milk or irritating it with a heavy feeding of corn meal. Ligation of the jejunum has produced terminal symptomatology apparently identical with that which accompanies death from enterotoxemia.

From the evidence available, which is extensive, it would appear that this disease is initiated as the result of excessive quantities of a concentrated diet, culminating in the absorption of the fatal but normally unabsorbed toxin of *Cl. perfringens*, type D. The effectiveness of active immunizing agents against this organism is debated and difficult to determine because of the unpredictability of naturally occurring cases. It is not contended that the organism is a tissue pathogen in the ordinary sense. (But see "pulpy kidney disease," p. 16.)

Enterotoxemia caused by *Cl. perfringens* type D has also been reported in calves and goats. The clinical and pathologic findings are comparable to those in lambs.

In addition to classical *type D* enterotoxemia, *Cl. perfringens types A, B, C and E* cause enterotoxemias in animals.

Cl. perfringens Type A Enterotoxemia.—Type A enterotoxemia has been reported in lambs and calves as an acute syndrome of short course and high mortality, characterized by intense icterus and hemolytic anemia with hemoglobinuria. Lesions include icterus, anemia, excess pericardial fluid, dark kidneys, and an enlarged friable liver.

Cl. perfringens Type B Enterotoxemia.—Type B enterotoxemia, better known as "lamb dysentery," is of principal importance in lambs less than two weeks of age. Death may occur without premonitory signs but usually the lambs are found reluctant to suckle, lying down, and exhibiting signs of pain. The feces become semifluid, brownish and contain blood. The characteristic lesion is a marked hemorrhagic enteritis, often with ulceration. Petechiae and ecchymoses are common on serous membranes of the epicardium and endocardium and the pericardial cavity contains excess fluid. An essentially identical type B enterotoxemia occurs in calves, which is largely restricted to the first ten days of life and characterized by severe hemorrhagic enteritis. Type B enterotoxemia has also been reported in foals during the first two days of life. Lesions are again characterized by hemorrhagic enteritis with ulceration.

Cl. perfringens Type C Enterotoxemia.—Two distinct forms of type C enterotoxemia have been described. The first form of type C enterotoxemia to be described was "*struck,*" a disease of adult sheep in Britain. It occurs most commonly during the winter and early spring months. Clinical signs are usually not noted. The lesions are hemorrhagic enteritis with ulceration of the mucosa particularly of the jejunum and duodenum. A striking feature is peritonitis with a large volume of clear-yellow fluid in the peritoneal cavity.

In the United States a form of type C enterotoxemia known as **enterotoxic hemorrhagic enteritis** occurs in calves and lambs in the first few days of life. Clinically there is diarrhea but as with other forms of enterotoxemia, death often occurs in the absence of noted signs. The lesions as described by Griner and co-workers (1953) are similar in both species and characterized by hemorrhagic enteritis with ulceration. Hemorrhages are frequent beneath the epicardium on the thymus and elsewhere. In both species, bacteria identified as *Clostridium perfringens (welchii)*, type C, were numerous in the bowel contents. The evidence that this organism was responsible was that, in the case of the calves, the disease was reproduced by feeding a pure culture together with corn-meal and milk (a concentrated and irritant food for a newly born calf). In the case of the lambs, susceptible animals were protected by an antiserum against this organism. The condition is to be regarded as an enterotoxemia rather than as a mere enteritis for the reason that bacteria-free filtrates of the intestinal contents were promptly lethal when injected into mice, the toxic substance being inactivated by heat, as is characteristic of bacterial exotoxins. Type C enterotoxemia also occurs in suckling piglets, usually during the first week of life. Most affected pigs die within twelve to forty-eight hours after onset of clinical signs which include depression, dehydration, and diarrhea which is often bloody. The pathologic changes which have been described in detail by Hogh (1969) are dominated by a hemorrhagic or necrotizing enteritis principally affecting the jejunum. There is hemorrhagic lymphadenitis of draining lymph nodes, serosanguinous fluid in the peritoneal, pleural and pericardial cavities and hemorrhage in the epicardium, endocardium and kidneys.

Cl. perfringens Type E Enterotoxemia.—Type E *Cl. perfringens* have been found in calves and lambs but the status of the disease with respect to frequency or importance is not known. Available data do not suggest that the disease is of significance.

Veterinarians in many and probably all parts of this country see with considerable frequency sudden deaths in well-nourished calves receiving liberal amounts of milk either in buckets or from the mother. They are usually at an age (two to six months) when consumption of other feeds is beginning or well advanced. Frenzy or convulsions mark the illness but coma precedes death. Lesions are largely absent but include hemorrhages and sometimes mild catarrhal enteritis. The cases are sporadic and unpredictable, hence systematic studies have seldom been made, but it may well be that these little-understood cases belong with the enterotoxemias. Bloating is not present, nor is there any reason to suspect a deficiency of magnesium (p. 1004) or potassium (p. 1007). As stated by Schofield (1955), they are not typical of the myocardial deaths supposed to result from deficiency of vitamin E (p. 992).

EDEMA DISEASE OF SWINE

First reported by Shanks in Ireland in 1938, this disease has been encountered with some frequency in most of the swine-producing countries of the world. It attacks previously thrifty animals without warning, produces incoordination and paralyses of the limbs, pain and coma and is commonly but not invariably fatal within a number of hours or a day or two. It is not highly contagious, but herd morbidity may approach 35 per cent. Mortality may reach 100 per cent.

The edema is typically but not invariably found in the wall of the stomach, where it may involve the cardiac region or the greater curvature or the whole organ. The thickness of the gastric wall may be increased just perceptibly or it may reach 3 cm. The coiled portion of the colon, with its mesentery, is another common location of the edema, but these regions are by no means the only sites which may be involved. The body cavities usually contain small or large amounts of fluid; other parts of the intestinal tract sometimes are involved. The face and eyelids are edematous in a high proportion of cases, as can be observed during life. Less frequently, the tarsal and carpal regions and the ventral belly wall contain an excess of fluid. The parenchymatous organs of the abdomen usually appear normal, as do the brain and, usually, the lungs. Subepicardial hemorrhages sometimes occur, but inflammatory changes are typically absent from all organs. Although not noted by other investigations, Kurtz and associates (1969) have described lesions in the brain and arterioles which help to explain the clinical and pathologic features of edema disease. They noted a necrotizing arteritis in most all organs and tissues of the body. They also described focal symmetrical encephalomalacia, presumably secondary to arteritis, involving the thalamus, basal ganglia and nuclei of the brain stem. These findings are the first pathologic observations which correlate with the clinical signs of the disease.

Luke and Gordon (1950) found evidence of hypoproteinemia in cases studied by them, but, in general, metabolic and physiological studies have not been made. A number of transmission experiments indicate that the intravenous injection of supernatant fluids or bacteria-free filtrates from the edematous gastrointestinal structures or their contents will reproduce the disease. This fact, plus the erratic and unpredictable occurrence of individual cases, has led to the prevalent belief that the disease is an endogenous toxemia similar to the "enterotoxemia" of sheep possibly with hypersensitivity to the toxic substance. The findings of several investigators that beta hemolytic strains of *Escherichia coli* can be regularly isolated from pigs with edema disease, and more recently the reproduction of the disease by oral administration of these strains of *E. coli* (Smith and Halls, 1968), provides very strong evidence incriminating *E. coli* as the cause.

Gastrointestinal edema in other species has occasionally been seen. Very severe edema of the ileum has been encountered in the horse, without adequate explanation. Priouzeau (1954) has reported a chronic edematous gastritis affecting cattle which was recurrent and eventually continuous, with death from diarrhea and cachexia.

The action of some unrecognized locally destructive poison probably cannot be entirely excluded in such cases.

INTESTINAL OBSTRUCTION

The small intestine not infrequently suffers complete obstruction by **foreign bodies,** such as rubber balls, nuts or peach stones in the dog, or piliconcretions (hair-balls) in calves. **Strangulated hernias** (umbilical or scrotal, usually) cause complete obstruction in any species, being most frequent in horses and pigs. The

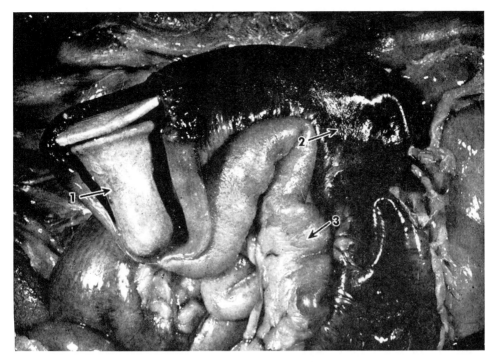

Fig. 24–7.—Obstruction of the duodenum of an eight-month-old male Doberman Pinscher puppy. The foreign body was a rubber nipple (*1*) from a nursing bottle. Note hemorrhagic wall of duodenum (*2*) proximal to the obstruction and normal-appearing intestine distal to it (*3*). (Courtesy of Angell Memorial Animal Hospital.)

long and tenuous intestine of the horse is subject to obstruction because of accidents resultant from its tortuosity and the length of the mesentery which suspends it. These are **torsion,** or twisting upon itself, or **volvulus,** in which a loop of intestine passes through a tear in the mesentery or similar abnormality. **Intussusceptions** occur in any species. In this accident, excessive peristaltic movement forces a segment of the bowel inside the segment just below it, as the smaller tube of a telescope slides into the slightly larger tube next ahead of it. In the intestine, there is actually no difference in the diameters of the outer and inner tubes. As a consequence of this fact, and of the attached mesentery, the outermost of the three layers which make up the intussusception is greatly stretched, the innermost greatly compressed. Interference with the flow of blood being greater in the thin-walled veins than it is in the less compressible arteries, venous stasis and edema promptly develop and lead, in a matter of hours, to adhesive inflammation which binds the layers together or to necrosis and gangrene. The absence of these several features serves to differentiate from true pathological intussusceptions, brought about by excessive peristalsis in diarrheic and similar conditions, others which occur rather frequently near the moment of death, even in slaughtered animals. Because of the pressure, an intussusception is usually completely obstructive to passage of the intestinal contents. **Neoplasms,** chiefly carcinomas, in the intestinal wall tend to assume an annular (ring-shaped) form and more slowly but scarcely less surely stop the movement of the ingesta.

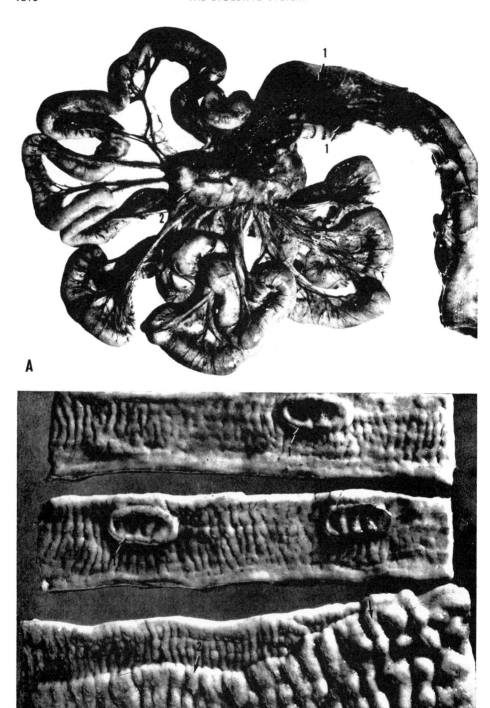

A

Fig. 24–8.—*A*, Intussusception of the ileum (*1*) into the colon of a dog with "salmon disease." Note also hyperplastic lymph node (*2*). *B*, Hyperplasia of Peyer's patches (*1*) and lymphoid tissue in terminal ileum (*2*) in a dog with rickettsiosis of "salmon disease." Photographs courtesy of **Dr. Wm. J. Hadlow.**

While the **effects** of a gradually developing obstruction may be mitigated by hypertrophy of the local muscularis (see Terminal Ileitis, above), complete blocking of the intestinal canal has definite and constant results. The lumen of the bowel for a considerable distance above the obstruction becomes greatly distended with fluid which is chiefly that of inflammatory edema (serous exudate), the accumulated ingesta constituting a minor portion. The wall is not only edematous but red with hyperemia and infiltrated with leukocytes. These changes are most marked just above (anterior to) the obstruction and gradually fade out with increasing distance from it. Below the obstruction, the bowel is empty and normal. While pathogenic and saprophytic bacteria would bring havoc to the involved section of the bowel and eventually spread to the peritoneum, usually with gangrene (and this sometimes occurs), the regular outcome of complete obstruction of the bowel is death after some hours or, in some species, a day or two unless it is surgically relieved. This is earlier than such changes would ordinarily be fatal and, on the basis of the course and symptoms, death is attributed to endotoxic shock (p. 140). If the obstruction involves the upper small intestine, vomiting is the principal sign, and loss of electrolytes constitute the greatest danger.

Intestinal impactions cause fatal obstruction in the horse. Cecal impaction is the most frequent and results when older animals are forced to subsist on coarse, dry roughage such as wheat straw. The cecum becomes progressively more atonic as it is filled with increasing amounts of undigested stalks and stems, until it is distended to unbelievable dimensions with little chance of recovery. Impaction of segments of the small colon results from one or more unusually large boluses of undigested roughage, frequently coarse alfalfa hay. The irritated intestine contracts spasmodically around the lodged bolus, tightening the obstruction.

Tympanites of the cecum is the usual form of alimentary bloating in the horse and is scarcely less formidable than its counterpart in the bovine rumen. Spasmodic or other disorders interfering with peristaltic movement through the colon and rectum appear to be causative without much relation to the kind of feed.

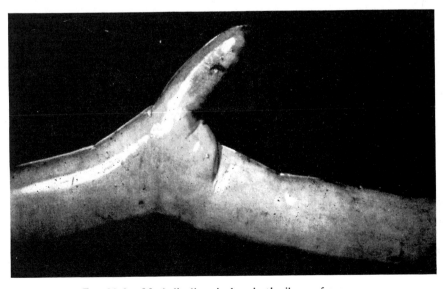

Fig. 24–9.—Meckel's diverticulum in the ileum of a pony.

Inversion of the Cecum.—Rarely in the dog, the cecum becomes inverted into the colon, projecting into the latter for a considerable distance and acting as a partial obstruction. In some cases, it protrudes from the anus during defecation. Naturally a variable degree of edema, inflammation and perhaps chronic fibrosis results locally but the disorder is not necessarily fatal.

Diverticulosis.—This disorder is very rare but not unknown, at least in calves and pigs. The diverticula, of which there are usually a series throughout a considerable portion of the bowel, consist in tiny holes in the muscular layer into which the mucous membrane is evaginated to form a lining. The whole intestinal wall at these points may thus consist of little more than mucosa plus serosa. In humans, the diverticulum is thought to mark a place of weakness in the muscularis around the point of entrance of a blood vessel. A similar nature may be presumed in animals. Due to stasis of bowel contents accumulating in these mucosal depressions, infection is likely to lead to localized inflammation, diverticulitis, which is usually purulent in type.

Meckel's diverticulum is rarely encountered as a small tube branching from the ileum and terminating after several centimeters (in the horse) in a rounded closed end. It is a congenital anomaly representing persistence of the omphalo-enteric duct of the embryo and has, in a rudimentary way, the histologic structure of the intestine. Stasis of ingesta occurs in it only exceptionally.

Prolapse of the rectum occurs probably in any species but especially in cattle and swine. The exposed portion of the bowel becomes traumatized, inflamed, as well as filled with venous blood confined there by pressure of the rectal sphincter. Here, as elsewhere, venous flow is often stopped by a degree of pressure which permits the arterial circulation to continue. Hemorrhoids, which consist, when severe, of slightly prolapsed hemorrhoidal veins and mucosa, do not occur in the domestic animals.

Atresia ani is a failure of development of the anal opening. Often there is little more than the skin and subcutis remaining imperforate, and it may be possible to establish surgically a satisfactory opening, the muscular sphincter and the rectum being adequately developed.

Neoplasms of the Intestine.—As was stated regarding the stomach, malignant lymphomas are much the commonest neoplasm in the intestine, where they infiltrate the wall or cause subserosal masses. Adenocarcinomas occur in the dog but must be considered rare; leiomyomas and leiomyosarcomas are at least as frequent. Papillomas are rare. Adenomas of the circumanal glands probably belong more with tumors of the skin than in the present group, but may be mentioned as being much more frequent than any of the preceding. In cats argentaffin cell tumors (Kultchitzky-cell tumors) similar to the carcinoid of man, are occasionally encountered.

Intestinal emphysema is occasionally seen in healthy swine at slaughter. Numerous small air-filled vesicles from 1 mm. to 2 cm. in diameter are found in the serosa, submucosa and mucosa of the small intestine and in the mesentery and mesenteric lymph nodes. Microscopically the gas bubbles occupy lymphatics. The cause is not known. Occasionally intestinal emphysema is seen in sheep with enterotoxemia (p. 1211).

Megacolon is a paralytic distension of the colon seen in pups. It results from a deficient innervation of Meissner's plexus in the wall of the bowel below the dilatation.

Pseudomelanosis coli is a somewhat misleading term applied to a darkening of the intestinal wall post mortem. It is due to a chemical combination of sulfides of the contained ingesta with iron of the hemoglobin from blood that has been hemolyzed after death. In other words, blackening of the intestine in varying degree, diffuse and widespread, is just another evidence of post-mortem autolysis (p. 15).

THE PERITONEUM

Peritonitis is nearly always infectious. Acute inflammation of the peritoneum may be localized to a given area or may be generalized over the whole peritoneal surface. This depends upon the mode of entrance of the infection and the relative resistance of the patient. The latter is largely a matter of species; dogs seldom have serious peritonitis; in horses, the introduction of any appreciable amount of infectious material into the peritoneal cavity is practically a death sentence, although antibiotics have mitigated the danger somewhat. Cattle not infrequently die of generalized peritonitis but, on the other hand, have sufficient resistance to maintain localization of many infections.

The infecting organisms are various and many cases represent invasion by more than one pathogen. Prominent among the possible causative species are the colon bacillus and its relatives and streptococci of different types and species. Corynebacteria and staphylococci may be the offenders, and occasionally the clostridium of malignant edema and other anaerobes are responsible.

The inflammatory exudate is most often sero-fibrinous or fibrinous, although suppurative peritonitis results when the invaders are exclusively pyogenic species. Certain of the granuloma-producing organisms also thrive on the peritoneal surfaces, as will be explained shortly.

The principal routes by which infections enter are (1) operative incisions through the abdominal wall, (2) rupture or perforation of the stomach, intestines or uterus, (3) direct extension through the more or less necrotic wall of one of these organs during the course of a severe infectious inflammation of its lining and (4) by the blood stream in the case of certain specific infections, such as bovine viral encephalitis. Other routes are possible, such as via the ostium abdominale of the Fallopian tube, from an infected umbilicus in the new-born, or by direct extension from an infected kidney.

The peritoneum constitutes one of the large absorptive surfaces of the body, even when compared with the gastrointestinal mucous membrane or the total of the pulmonary alveolar or renal tubular surfaces. If its thin mesothelial lining becomes coated with toxin-producing microorganisms, the consequences are sure to be of a most serious nature. The victim's best chance of survival depends upon keeping the infection localized near its portal of entry, to which end several mechanisms are well adapted. The fibrin tends to seal off infected areas and cover the invading pathogens. In those species which have a well-developed and flexible omentum, that membrane moves through some unknown attraction to cover an infected or injured area almost within minutes, becoming glued to the diseased surface. Through reflexes partly the result of pain, movements are kept to a minimum; peristalsis ceases; the abdominal wall becomes rigid; the breathing is limited to thoracic movements.

These mechanisms are not without their disadvantages. Paralytic ileus may develop in the motionless and non-digesting intestine. In this condition the bowel becomes distended with gas and the shock-like accompaniments of intestinal obstruction (see above) are likely to develop. If the patient survives, the fibrin, like fibrin elsewhere (p. 50), tends to become organized by fibroblasts and to tie the various abdominal organs to each other and to the diaphragm and abdominal wall. This process begins if the inflammation is not resolved in six to ten days. The adhesions commonly interfere considerably with peristalsis and the digestive process and may bring it almost to a standstill.

Tuberculous peritonitis is common enough that, in cattle, it has received the popular name of "pearly disease" from the large numbers of shiny gray spheres constituting individual tubercles on the diaphragmatic or other peritoneal surfaces. **Actinobacillosis** occasionally involves the peritoneal surfaces of cattle with a multitude of tiny nodular excrescences of granulation tissue, the mode of entry of the infection being obscure. Diagnosis of this condition is microscopic.

Actinobacillosis, as well as tuberculosis, has to be differentiated from **neoplastic transplantations.** Occasionally a malignant neoplasm, usually a carcinoma arising in the digestive mucosa (or the ovary in humans), gains access to the peritoneal cavity, and its cells are transplanted through movement of the surfaces and fluids to form myriads of tiny nodular growths over many peritoneal areas, both parietal and visceral. The mesothelioma occurs rarely as a primary tumor of the peritoneum.

Necrosis of abdominal fat regularly accompanies necrotizing pancreatitis (p. 1239), and is occasionally encountered in most animal species as small plaques or nodules in the abdominal cavity. The cause of the latter is not known. A peculiar form of abdominal fat necrosis of unknown cause occurs in cattle,

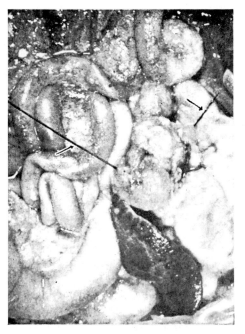

FIG. 24–10.—Chronic peritonitis in a cat following ingestion of broom straws (arrows) which penetrated the stomach.

characterized by extremely large masses of necrotic fat in the omentum, mesentery and retroperitoneal tissues. Casts of necrotic fat may encircle the intestine leading to obstruction.

HYDROPERITONEUM, ASCITES

Accumulation of watery fluid in the peritoneal cavity, in the broadest sense, is called hydroperitoneum. If, as is often the case, the fluid represents a true (non-inflammatory) edema, the term ascites is applicable. Fluid in the peritoneal cavity may, however, represent an inflammatory edema (serous peritonitis) or it may be the result, especially in male cattle and sheep, of severe acute urinary obstruction with, or even without, rupture of the bladder. With the possible exception of the inflammatory form, the amount of fluid which accumulates may be tremendous, causing great distension of the abdomen and all the symptoms that go with great abdominal pressure.

Ascites, or true edema of the peritoneal cavity, may form a part of the syndrome of generalized edema (p. 134) and be referable to any of the causes of that condition. Such cases betray themselves by the presence of edema in other places, which need not be listed here. But ascites more typically results from chronic passive congestion of the portal venous system. The special causes of that congestion are conditions which obstruct (incompletely) the flow of the portal vein, most commonly cirrhosis (p. 1225). Other causes of obstruction include pressure of neoplasms, abscesses, granulomas and enlarged lymph nodes upon the vein, as well as thrombosis within it.

Like any edema fluid, this is a true transudate, with a specific gravity less than 1.017 and with a protein content usually below 3 per cent.

Inflammatory accumulation of fluid is distinguished by the presence of other signs of inflammation and by other elements of inflammatory exudation, chiefly leukocytes and fibrin. The specific gravity and level of protein are correspondingly higher.

Urinary fluid, whether it came directly from a ruptured bladder or as a transudate concomitant with the gradual uriniferous infiltration of the tissues of the peri-urethral region, has the odor and other characteristics of urine. Evidence of urinary obstruction (p. 1283) is present in the form of calculi, cystitis, hydronephrosis or related lesions.

The effects of hydroperitoneum are those of pressure, interfering with the abdominal organs and also, through pressure upon the diaphragm, with respiration. If the fluid is surgically withdrawn, more soon accumulates. The causal disorders, of course, produce other characteristic effects, such as uremia in the case of urinary obstruction.

THE LIVER

Hepatitis

Having acquired the habit of speaking first about what is uppermost in our minds, we shall indulge that custom by giving first attention to what is at once the most important and the most intricate aspect of hepatic disease. The subject of alterative inflammation was discussed briefly in the general study of the inflammatory reaction (p. 164). Some will hesitate to consider as inflammatory certain of the degenerative changes about to be included under the heading of hepatitis, but we urge consideration of our reasons, not the least of which is the conviction that only in this way can the various hepatic phenomena common in acute and chronic toxic conditions be fitted together into an understandable and coordinated pattern.

The view that hydropic degeneration, fatty change and necrosis are the incipient stages of a process which soon becomes inflammatory is attributed to Aschoff. However we venture to quote several more recent writers. Hutyra and Marek (1926), in listing the various diseases of the liver, describe "acute parenchymatous hepatitis" as "inflammatory disease of the liver substance in which, in addition to cellular infiltration and hyperemia, there is pronounced cloudy swelling and fatty infiltration of the liver cells." Liegeois (1933) states under the heading of Acute Diffuse Hepatitis (translated): "This is also called parenchymatous, although it may be mixed, since it consists in degenerative changes in the cells and a leukocytic infiltration." Kaufmann (1929) states, "Several kinds of inflammations of the liver can be distinguished: (a) parenchymatous hepatitis marked by cloudy swelling or by fatty degeneration. . . ." Karsner (1942) begins his description of Acute Nonsuppurative Hepatitis with, "Acute hepatitis of this variety is essentially an alterative (degenerative) inflammation. The parenchymal component varies from cloudy swelling to necrosis. The interstitial or mesenchymal component is found in the form of infiltration of polymorphonuclear leukocytes or lymphoid and large mononuclear cells, or mixtures. In addition, certain authorities accept Roessle's view that the accumulation of fluid between capillaries and cord cells is an inflammatory component and represents a serous hepatitis." Boyd (1953) may be considered to summarize the matter with, "The characteristic reaction of liver cells to an injurious agent is necrosis. This may be called with equal truth either hepatic necrosis or hepatitis. . . . The term hepatitis is often used for convenience to describe all stages of the process from necrosis to healing by fibrosis."

With this introduction, and with a view to simplicity, we shall consider hepatitis under the following classifications:

1. Infectious hepatitis
2. Non-infectious or toxic hepatitis
    a. Acute toxic hepatitis, also known as acute yellow (or red) atrophy
    b. Chronic toxic hepatitis, for which the usual name is cirrhosis.

Infectious Hepatitis.—For this term to apply, the infective organisms must invade the liver and be rather diffusely distributed in it. Infections of other organs, for instance of the uterus, often cause a toxic hepatitis because of toxic substances absorbed and carried by the blood, without the metastasis of pathogens into the liver, which is essential if the hepatitis is to be classed as infectious.

The infections that may attack the liver include a few which are peculiar to the liver and several which localize elsewhere with equal or greater facility. In the former group are Rubarth's canine viral hepatitis (hepatitis contagiosa canis), a supposedly viral hepatitis of South African sheep known as Wesselbron disease (1958), histomoniasis of turkeys (entero-hepatitis), and (shared with the kidney) leptospirosis. The infectious viral hepatitis of humans holds, of course, a comparable position. In laboratory animals experimentally inoculated, a number of other infections such as brucellosis and tularemia localize in the liver as minute foci widely disseminated.

The more prominent members of the latter group are tuberculosis, syphilis (humans), coccidioidomycosis, histoplasmosis, toxoplasmosis (rarely other granulomas), herpesvirus infections (*Herpesvirus canis, Herpesvirus T*, equine rhinopneumonitis, etc.), necrobacillosis and the pyogenic infections. The features of a given case of hepatitis due to such an infection are those characteristic of the disease itself. In fact, while it is not erroneous to speak of tuberculous hepatitis, for instance, tuberculosis of the liver is more usual and possibly more meaningful. One also considers to what extent these infections are diffuse or localized in the liver. Often the granulomatous lesions are decidedly restricted and the pyogenic infections much more commonly form localized and encapsulated abscesses than diffuse infectious processes. All of the above infections are treated individually elsewhere and their characteristics need not be repeated here.

Of more importance in appreciating the general aspects of infectious hepatitis is a consideration of the routes by which infections of any sort gain access to the liver. These are, more or less in order of frequency, (1) the portal vein, (2) the hepatic artery, (3) the umbilical vein in the new-born, (4) the bile-duct system, (5) the hepatic vein, and (6) direct extension. The importance of the portal blood as a carrier of infectious material is obvious in view of its large volume and the fact that it drains the extensively exposed intestinal area. Entrance of infective material via the hepatic artery occurs when the microorganisms, as emboli or otherwise, are in the general systemic circulation. In the farm animals, infection of the umbilical structures by contact soon after birth is by no means unusual. The umbilical vein, filled with partially clotted blood, affords an excellent route of access to the liver. Coming from contaminated soil, the infections entering in this way are usually the necrophorus bacillus or the pyogenic organisms, and necrotic areas or abscesses are the usual results. Infections may ascend the biliary passages either through static secretion consequent upon obstruction or by continuous spread of the infectious inflammatory process from the duodenum and up the ductal tissues. Usually the two processes are combined. Spread of infection to the liver via the hepatic vein would appear impossible, but it occurs very rarely due to momentary reversal of the current in right-sided valvular disease, the primary source of infection usually being the diseased valve itself. A retrograde thrombus may form, reaching backward into the hepatic vein and its tributaries, the distance involved being really very short. Direct extension of infection from adjoining tissues and organs is, of course, possible. It usually depends upon a traumatic origin, such as that due to foreign bodies in the bovine reticulum.

Acute Toxic Hepatitis.—As pointed out in the introductory discussion, acute toxic hepatitis is characterized by death of hepatic cells and the changes which precede death, in other words, by hydropic degeneration, fatty change, and necrosis.

Microscopically, the necrosis is most often coagulative in type, recognized by pyknosis and acidophilic cytoplasm. Disintegration and disappearance of the cells follow.

From the standpoint of location, necrosis in the liver may take any one of five forms: (1) **Diffuse necrosis,** in which the change spreads over considerable areas without regard to lobular boundaries. This is simply a very severe manifestation of the lobular forms listed below. (2) **Focal necrosis,** in which minute necrotic areas, or foci, of sublobular size, appear here and there, occupying any part of any lobule. These are characteristic of disseminated infections, often in laboratory animals. Included here are livers of equine fetuses aborted because of rhinotracheitis (influenza abortion). (3) **Peripheral necrosis,** in which the peripheral zones of the lobules are regularly necrotic. This form is not common but results when strong toxic substances are brought to the lobule by the blood stream without any impairment in circulation of the blood and oxygenation of the cells. The peripheral cells receive the toxic blood first and suffer most from its effects. (4) **Midzonal necrosis,** in which the most pronounced necrotic changes involve the cells half way between the periphery and the center of the lobule. This form is unusual but is characteristic of human eclampsia and a few other diseases. (5) **Centrilobular necrosis,** in which the cells nearest the central vein suffer both from blood-borne toxins and from a stagnation of the circulation with consequent anoxia. This is the usual form of necrosis as seen in acute toxic hepatitis, the primary disorder being responsible for both production of toxic substances and impairment of circulation. (6) **Paracentral necrosis** is an unusual form in which the necrotic area adjoins the central vein on one side but does not surround it. Attributed to local circulatory disorder, it is a characteristic of Rift Valley fever (p. 471) and is also seen in some anemic diseases.

The typical (but not invariable) microscopic picture of acute toxic hepatitis may then be described as centrilobular necrosis with disappearance of a considerable number of the most centrally located cells, blood taking their place. More peripherally in the lobule, there are most typically hepatic cells in a state of fatty change and, peripheral to these and commonly comprising the remainder of the lobule, hydropic degeneration. When the condition is several days old, a moderate infiltration of lymphocytes into the periportal connective tissue (islands of Glisson) usually begins. The typical picture, however, is often incomplete, with the fat, or the necrosis or other elements missing.

The **gross appearance** of a liver affected by acute toxic hepatitis involves the changes already described for hydropic degeneration, fatty change and necrosis. Such a liver is usually lighter in color, even to the tan of severe fatty degeneration. It is also likely to be redder because of an increased content of blood. The majority probably are best described as showing **accentuation of the lobular markings.** In the normal liver (except that of the pig), the lobules are not discernible with the naked eye. In the livers under consideration, the lobules can usually be seen because of a difference in color between the centers and the peripheries of the lobules. If the central part of the lobule is seriously congested, it will have the redder color of blood. The more peripheral part then is relatively more yellow and often decidedly pale, because of cloudy swelling, fat or necrosis in this zone. At another stage, however, the coagulated necrotic cells of the center may be the palest part of the lobule, the more nearly normal cells of the peripheral zone retaining their natural deep brown. It is seldom possible to decide the exact status grossly, but there should be little difficulty in detecting that some of these changes are present. The size of the liver tends to be decreased as some of its parenchymal cells undergo necrosis and disappear, but the influx of blood and the accumulation of fat tend to augment its volume. Thus, no positive statement can be made as to size, although severely affected livers are usually smaller than they were during health. **Acute yellow atrophy** was formerly listed as a disease entity, usually of unknown cause. During an acute illness, the liver became yellow because of fatty degeneration and necrosis and became smaller because of

PLATE II

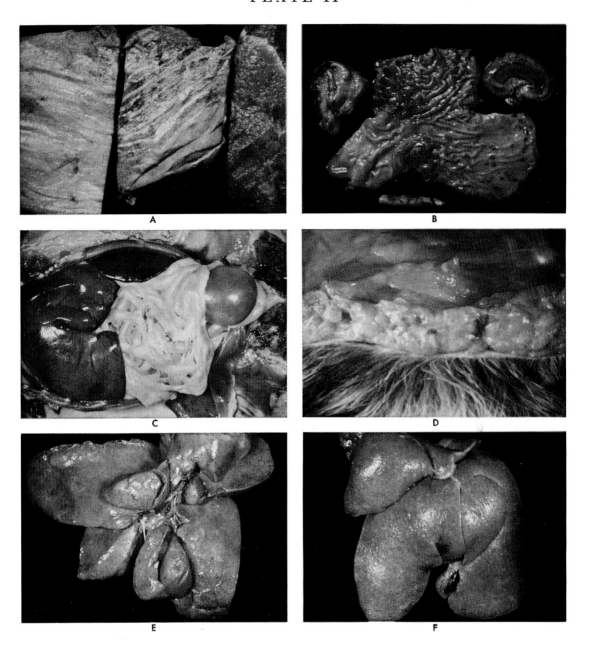

A, Azoturia in a yearling Palomino colt which became entangled in a halter robe and was unable to rise from a recumbent position. The colt was sacrified after three days. Specimens of biceps femoris and latissimus dorsi muscles are illustrated, with normal muscle for comparison. Case from Iowa School Vet. Med.

B, Icterus due to acute leptospirosis in a male springer spaniel, nine months old. The yellow color is pronounced in tissues which are naturally pale (aorta, gastric and bladder mucosa) and is discernible in darker tissues (kidney, prostate)

C, Acute hemolytic icterus and hemolytic anemia due to *Hemobartonella felis*, affecting a two-year-old male cat. Note the yellow-colored omentum contrasting with the white intestines, the pale and swollen liver and the enlarged, congested spleen. Most of this splenic enlargement is due to extramedullary hematopoiesis. The bluish object is the urinary bladder filled with hemoglobin-stained urine. (Photograph courtesy of Angell Memorial Animal Hospital)

D, Steatitis involving the subcutaneous fat of a one-year-old spayed female cat. This cat's diet consisted almost exclusively of canned red tuna. (Photograph courtesy of Angell Memorial Animal Hospital)

E, Severe fatty infiltration of the liver, secondary to diabetes mellitus in a spayed female Terrier, age 12 years. (Courtesy of Angell Memorial Animal Hospital)

F, Toxic hepatitis, following exposure to benzene, in a twelve-year-old castrated male cat. Microscopic sections revealed severe focal necrosis, fatty degeneration and bile retention. The greenish color in the gross specimen results from oxidation of bilirubin to biliverdin. (Courtesy of Angell Memorial Animal Hospital)

disappearance of many of its cells. We now know these cases to represent acute toxic hepatitis, a fact which affords at least some clue to their causes. **Acute red atrophy** was an essentially similar condition, the red of severe congestion overwhelming the yellow of the damaged cells.

The **causes** of acute toxic hepatitis are toxic substances of great variety, many of them not clearly identified. They may be divided into three groups:

(1) Chemical poisons. Included are copper, arsenic and the arsenical drugs, phosphorus (if the patient survives three days or more), mercury (unless chronic), chloroform (delayed poisoning developing two or three days after anesthesia), tannic acid (used in treatment of burns), cincophen (a proprietary drug), tetrachloroethane (industrial), trinitrotoluene (industrial), tetrachlorethylene and carbon tetrachloride. The last two are of especial interest in veterinary medicine because they are commonly used as anthelmintic drugs. Their toxicity to the patient is due to their destructive action on the liver. Coal tar pitch (p. 871) and gossypol (p. 873) cause a severe destructive type of toxic hepatitis.

(2) Plant poisons. Among those recognized at present are species of the genera *Senecio* (Nebraska, Texas, Nova Scotia, South Africa), *Amsinckia* (tar weed of Pacific Northwest), *Phyllanthus* (Texas); and, under certain circumstances of growth and preservation, the wild and cultivated lupines, vetches, velvet beans (*Macuna utilis*) and other legumes. Other forage crops are said to have similar effects when they have undergone certain types of spoilage or fermentation. Certain of the latter toxicities are not based on poisons in the plant itself but rather toxins produced by various fungi. A notable example is the hepatic injury in aflatoxin poisoning (p. 888).

(3) Metabolic poisons. Certain types of gastroenteritis are believed to generate toxic substances of this nature. Mild degrees of toxic injury accompany many of the acute infectious diseases. Toxemias of pregnancy are important in humans. The outstanding example in veterinary medicine is the so-called "pregnancy disease" of ewes, which depends upon the combined effects of pregnancy and ketosis (p. 1022).

It has been found that hepatic necrosis and icterus can be produced in experimental animals by administration of extremely high doses of follicular hormones. Also vitamin E and selenium deficiencies (p. 992) may result in acute hepatic necrosis.

Significance and Effect.—The severe acute cases are fatal within a few days, with most of the hepatic parenchymal cells necrotic and disappearing. It is such cases that constitute the classical "acute yellow atrophy." In less severe cases, the patient recovers completely, the hepatic epithelium being regenerated with considerable facility after removal of the toxic substances. All too frequently in animals the unsuspected toxic component of the feed or pasturage is continuously or repeatedly ingested in moderate amount, and the acute condition just described is superseded or accompanied by cirrhosis, the chronic form of toxic hepatitis.

CIRRHOSIS

Chronic toxic hepatitis, commonly called cirrhosis, is characterized, like most chronic inflammations, by fibrosis, the production of new fibrous tissue, hence it is to be classed as a proliferative inflammation. The formation of new tissue may be regarded as the direct response to an irritant toxic substance, comparable to the proliferation seen in tuberculosis; or it may be considered as the healing and scarring that would naturally follow death and disappearance of areas of parenchymal cells. Recent views lean toward the latter interpretation, even though no necrotic epithelial cells are seen at the moment death makes the tissue available for examination. Many definitions of cirrhosis are more complex than the parameters we have just stated, but for our purposes we shall consider any widespread fibrosis or scarring of the liver as cirrhosis.

Microscopic Appearance.—The outstanding feature of cirrhosis is proliferation of fibrous connective tissue, which begins at the islands of Glisson (portal areas) and increases to surround the lobules, which are irregularly reduced in size. The change may vary from a slight increase of the normally fibrous portal areas to a condition where the interstitial connective tissue exceeds the parenchymatous tissue of the lobules. The connective tissue may be young and cellu-

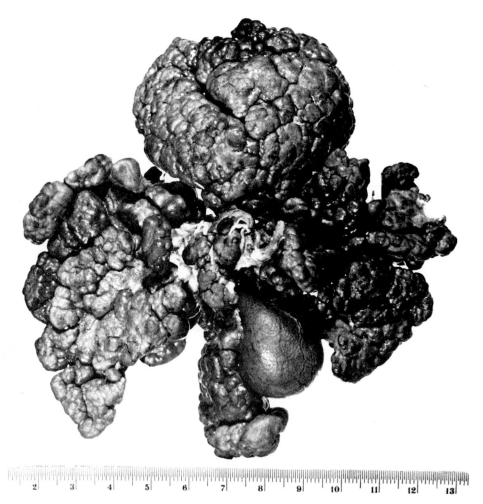

Fig. 24–11.—Cirrhosis of liver of a dog. Note extensive nodularity and atrophy. (Courtesy of Armed Forces Institute of Pathology.) Contributor: Dr. Robert Ferber.

lar, but is more often of the mature, fibrous variety. There is usually more or less infiltration with lymphocytes and mononuclear leukocytes, chiefly in the islands of Glisson. These indicate that the inflammatory process is still active. Newly formed (non-functioning) bile ducts are often seen in the connective tissue. They are recognized as tiny circles (or in longitudinal section as double lines) of small epithelial cells with darkly staining nuclei. Necrosis and the other changes described under acute toxic hepatitis may still be active within the lobules. There is often considerable regeneration of new hepatic epithelium. This usually results in marked distortion of lobular architecture. In addition, regenerative hyperplasia of individual hepatic cells may result in bizarre forms with tremendously large and hyperchromatic nuclei.

According to the exact location of the new connective tissue, different forms of cirrhosis are recognized: **portal, nodular or atrophic cirrhosis,** also known as **cirrhosis of Laennec, gin-drinker's liver, hobnail liver,** is the common type. The connective tissue tends particularly to encircle the lobule and may be very extensive. Distortion of architecture with formation of irregular nodules ("hobnails") on the surface is especially marked. The nodules consist principally of regenerated and more or less hyperplastic parenchyma. The depressions between them mark the position of contracting fibrous tissue. Proliferation of bile ducts is minimal. This is the form which follows acute toxic hepatitis.

Intralobular cirrhosis is characterized by diffuse proliferation of a rather immature type of fibrous tissue within the lobule. Whether its fundamental etiology is different from that of portal cirrhosis is uncertain. It is much less frequent than the portal form. Its appearance is comparable to that of the hypertrophic cirrhosis of Hanot, as seen in man, but it would appear to be quite dissimilar etiologically.

A form of cirrhosis distinguished by some is called **"post-necrotic cirrhosis."** As its name implies, it follows and results directly from extensive acute necrosis of hepatic parenchymal cells.

Causes.—Frequently the cause in an individual case of cirrhosis cannot be ascertained, but in general the causes of portal cirrhosis are the same as those of acute toxic hepatitis. They act more slowly, doubtless because the amount of toxic substance ingested in a given period is less. Some, perhaps many cases, represent the end result of an attack of acute toxic hepatitis. In the farm animals, chronic poisoning by plants, known and unknown, should be suspected as the most likely cause. Thus, the "walking disease" of horses described by Van Es (1929) in Nebraska proved to be cirrhosis caused by a plant of the *Senecio* genus, while walking disease of the horses in the Pacific Northwest is a cirrhosis produced by seeds of the plant *Amsinckia intermedia* (tarweed). "Hard-liver disease" of swine and cattle in that region is due to the same plant. "Hard-liver disease" of sheep in many parts of the world (Texas, South Africa), "Pictou disease" of cattle in Canada and "Winton's disease" of horses and cattle in New Zealand have been traced to other poisonous Senecios, the essential lesion being cirrhosis. It is probable that other plants, presently unrecognized, have similar toxic properties. However, cirrhosis is occasionally seen in dogs, showing that some cases in animals must be attributed to other causes than plant toxins.

Biliary Cirrhosis.—Distinguishable from portal cirrhosis only with difficulty, this form of cirrhosis has an entirely unrelated cause, namely, chronic inflammation of the intrahepatic bile ducts. With the cholangitis there is usually an ob-

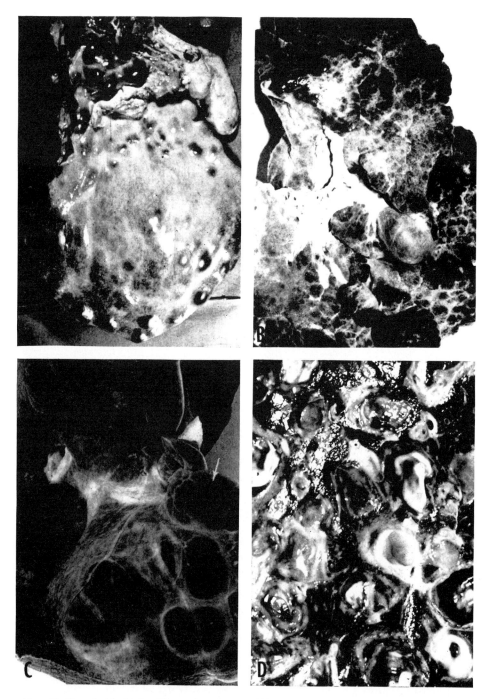

Fig. 24–12.—*A*, Cirrhosis of liver of a two-year-old steer. *B*, Cirrhosis, liver of a four-month-old pig. *C*, Large cysts in the liver of a ten-year-old female spaniel dog. *D*, Abscesses in a bovine liver. Ordinarily they are much less numerous. (Courtesy College of Veterinary Medicine, Iowa State University.)

struction somewhere in the extrahepatic ductal system (pressure of tumors, etc.) but the inflammatory process may have an infectious basis. While parasites (flukes, ascarids) are named as causes of biliary cirrhosis in humans, it is noteworthy that in animals liver flukes practically never cause more than an encircling fibrosis in the immediate vicinity of the invaded ducts, which are the relatively larger ones.

Microscopically, well-advanced biliary cirrhosis presents a perilobular fibrosis similar to that of atrophic cirrhosis, but careful observation reveals that the process is marked especially by fibrous tissue which encircles the various bile ducts. Its spread through the portal areas and around the lobules is incidental to the anatomical position of the structures. Newly formed (non-functional) bile ducts are especially numerous in this form of cirrhosis, and the infiltration of inflammatory cells (lymphocytes and mononuclears usually) is especially prominent, also. Since there is almost always some obstruction of the ductal system, from local swelling if nothing else, bile pigment (p. 73) collects in the liver and jaundice is almost always present.

Grossly, the liver in this form of cirrhosis is completely or nearly smooth. It is enlarged and is of a greenish hue because of the retained bile.

Glissonian cirrhosis presents a picture in the microscopic section quite similar to that of portal cirrhosis, but grossly the fibrous change is found to be confined to areas extending only a short distance beneath the capsule. It represents the spread of a chronic fibrosing inflammation of Glisson's capsule (the covering of the liver), hence of a regional peritonitis. It is not a true cirrhosis since the latter term applies to a condition involving the liver as a whole.

Central, or **cardiac, cirrhosis** refers to an increase of fibrous tissue around the central veins incident to chronic passive congestion. This proliferative phenomenon is characteristic of long-standing congestion in any vessel. The fibrous tissue is rarely extensive.

Pigment cirrhosis refers to the form which occurs in connection with hemochromatosis (p. 73).

Parasitic cirrhosis is occasionally seen in domestic animals, but not with the frequency that hepatic parasitism is encountered. Of greatest significance is the migration of the larvae of the swine kidney worm (*Stephanurus dentatus*) and *Ascaris lumbricoides* which if their number are great, may result in hepatic necrosis leading to cirrhosis. Infestation with liver flukes rarely leads to cirrhosis. Schistosomiasis in man may result in parasitic cirrhosis and can be anticipated to lead to cirrhosis in affected non-human primates but this has not been reported.

Effects of Cirrhosis.—Owing to the large reserve capacity of the liver, impaired hepatic function is not a common accompaniment of cirrhosis. In humans, the liver may fail in its function of inactivating estrogens with resultant atrophy of the testes and feminization. Presumably the same could occur in entire male animals. Somewhat rarely, there is inadequate formation of prothrombin and other clotting factors and interference with clotting (p. 104). Porphyrinemia and photosensitization may also result (p. 77). Decreased levels of blood protein and of vitamin A have been reported.

The principal effect of cirrhosis (ordinary portal but not biliary) is interference with the flow of the portal blood through the many hepatic ramifications on its way to the heart. The result is chronic passive congestion of the spleen (p. 1179) and of the digestive organs. Mild digestive disturbances and discomfort follow, but the chief effect of the retarded venous flow is ascites, the collection of edema fluid in the peritoneal cavity (p. 134). Jaundice is the rule in biliary cirrhosis but occurs only terminally in portal cirrhosis. On the other hand, interference with the portal circulation goes with portal but not biliary cirrhosis.

An unfortunate feature of cirrhosis is the fact that the presence of the proliferated fibrous tissue itself appears to have an irritant effect, stimulating the production of more fibrosis. Thus, the condition tends to continue to an eventually fatal termination even if the original cause be removed.

HEPATIC ABSCESSES AND RELATED CONDITIONS

Abscesses occasionally form in the liver of all species as the result of the entrance of microorganisms by any of the routes mentioned under Infectious Hepatitis. Important among these in newly born or young animals is the umbilical vein, which affords a route of metastasis or direct extension from the umbilicus. As the metastatic lesions develop in the liver, the primary site of infection at the umbilicus may even heal, without affecting the hepatic disease. Abscesses also occur in the livers of old dairy cows and others living under barnyard conditions, these being the result of extension from the wounds of penetrating foreign bodies in the reticulum (p. 1200). Abscesses under any of the above circumstances are regularly due to the entrance of pyogenic cocci or other well-recognized pus-producing species. They practically always play a central role in a generalized and fatal disease. But the much more frequent and important cause of hepatic abscesses in veterinary medicine is a disease of fattening cattle and is of a much more subtle nature. Before discussing this, it is desirable to present briefly two disorders of the bovine liver which are often concurrent and probably predisposing to the former condition.

"Sawdust Livers."—This very descriptive bit of professional slang refers to bovine livers seen frequently (and condemned) by meat inspectors. They come most often from well-fattened young cattle which appear clinically to be in perfect health. The livers contain several or many minute yellowish foci of necrosis, as if the same number of granules of sawdust had been scattered over them. The necrotic foci, 1 or 2 mm. in diameter, are scattered without grossly apparent relation to the lobular architecture. They consist of collections of hepatic epithelial cells in a state of coagulative necrosis or in the process of disappearing, mingled with or surrounded by a thin sprinkling of neutrophils and lymphocytes. They are often concomitant with telangiectasis and hepatic abscesses, and there is at least statistical evidence to link them etiologically with those conditions. It is suspected that "sawdust" foci may be the forerunners of telangiectatic spots and possibly of abscesses. It may be said with confidence, however, on purely numerical grounds that there are tremendous numbers of "sawdust" foci which never become abscesses. Vitamin E deficiency (which has been blamed for innumerable idiopathic lesions in most organs and tissues, p. 992), has been suggested as the cause of "sawdust." Todd and Krook (1966) experimentally induced lesions similar to spontaneous "sawdust" using a diet high in polyunsaturated fatty acids and poor in protein, vitamin E and selenium.

Telangiectasis.—This term denotes a dilatation of functioning blood vessels anywhere. In the liver, the lesion consists of a small group of sinusoidal capillaries within any part of a lobule which are greatly widened. The cells of the hepatic cords between the dilated sinusoids have partially or completely disappeared. Jarrett (1956) believes that the early lesion of telangiectasis consists of an accumulation of glycogen between the hepatic cell and the sinusoidal epithelium. When the glycogen penetrates the sinusoid its place is taken by blood, which erodes the column of hepatic cells. He feels there is evidence that absorption of hydrogen sulfide from the bowel may be responsible for the lesion. Grossly, the result is a dark red spot, irregular in shape, from one to several millimeters in diameter. Seen from the surface of the organ these spots tend to be slightly depressed. Appearances indicate that a telangiectatic spot may well represent a stage superseding the necrotic "sawdust" granule and, as stated above, the two often occur together in the same liver. However, telangiectasis is of some frequency not only in heavily fattened beeves, but also in old and debilitated cattle, some of which come to the autopsy room rather than the abattoir. While there is no detectable effect on the general health of the animal, telangiectatic livers are not passed for human food.

Abscesses.—Occasionally, an animal of the bovine or other species dies of abscesses of the liver, after a few days of acute but vague digestive symptoms. The liver of such an animal usually contains a dozen abscesses at least, often several times this number. Their cause is often but not necessarily apparent from other lesions revealed by the necropsy. But, as previously stated, the usual hepatic abscesses occur in heavily fattened cattle which are slaughtered in apparently perfect health. The incidence of these abscesses approximates 5 per cent of the cattle slaughtered throughout the United States, reaches 10 per cent in the Rocky Mountain area and approaches 100 per cent in some shipments from certain feed-lots. Post-mortem examination reveals no other abnormalities beyond, perhaps, the "sawdust" and telangiectasis just noted, possibly localized diaphragmatic adhesions over certain abscesses and, quite frequently, the ulcerative lesions of the rumen (p. 1199) already described as bearing a noteworthy relation to these abscesses. Bacteriological studies have incriminated the necrophorus organism (which has received with the changing times the successive appellations of *Bacillus necrophorus*, *Actinomyces necrophorus* and *Spherophorus necrophorus* and which in Europe is very logically known as *Fusiformis necrophorus*). In nearly all cases in the United States, it is found in pure culture.

The number of abscesses in the liver of one of these animals may vary from one to many but a number between 3 and 8 is typical. In size the abscesses range typically from 2 to 5 cm. in diameter. We must hasten to explain that many, probably a majority, of these "liver abscesses" are not true abscesses but circumscribed areas of coagulative necrosis. Observation has long suggested that the early lesion is one of coagulative necrosis (the usual result of infection with the necrophorus organism), and that the true abscesses consisting of encapsulated pus represent older processes. This is confirmed by the work of Jensen *et al.* (1954), who produced typical lesions by the experimental introduction of necrophorus organisms into the portal blood. They found the lesion to be entirely coagulative for the first six to eight days, with a gradual change to pus commencing beneath the fibrous capsule, the development of which began at about the same time. The central mass of coagulated necrotic tissue continued to enlarge until the thirtieth day, but by the one hundredth day it had been completely replaced by pus. By this time the capsule had grown to considerable thickness, consisting of mature fibrous tissue on the outside and immature fibrous tissue shading into

reticulo-endothelial and individual mononuclear macrophages centrally. Polymorphonuclear neutrophils were fairly numerous surrounding the central necrotic area. It is thus seen that the "abscesses" are at first necrotic areas (nodular
necroses of Hutyra and Marek, 1926) and, later, chronic abscesses with the granulomatous reticulo-endothelioid type of reaction playing an important part. The
fact that the abscesses eventually heal was also confirmed by Jensen's work, in
which fibrous scars had replaced the abscesses at stages varying from forty-five
to one hundred and eighty days after the inoculation. The scars themselves
ultimately disappear.

As we have stressed, clinical disease is rarely associated with hepatic abscesses
in cattle. Occasionally however, depressed, emaciated cattle slaughtered for
salvage are found to have hepatic abscesses, and there is little reason not to suspect that these abscesses lead to the chronic wasting condition. Erosion and
perforation of the wall of the posterior vena cava with entrance of the bacteria-
rich abscess contents into the circulation is a sporadic complication, which leads
to sudden and unexpected death in an apparently healthy animal. Rubarth
(1960) in a report of 56 cases with rupture into the posterior vena cava described
the abscesses as invariably present on the dorsal portion of the liver immediately
ventral to the vena cava. Necropsy findings in such cases include emphysema,
edema, and hemorrhages in the lungs, subendocardial and subepicardial petechiae,
congestion of the spleen and edema, hyperemia and hemorrhage of lymph nodes.
Bacterial emboli occlude capillaries in the lung, liver, kidney and myocardium.
Corynebacterium pyogenes animalis was the most frequent bacterial isolate in
Rubarth's series of Swedish cattle.

Causes.—It would be difficult indeed to explain these abscesses except as the
result of hematogenous metastasis. Jensen has demonstrated that this metastasis
is via the portal vein. While occasionally abscesses of the liver have been observed
subsequent to a necrophorus infection such as "foot-rot" (p. 623), these coinci-
dences seem to have been accidental. An infection picked up by the peripheral
venous circulation should reach the lungs and then be disseminated to all susceptible organs and tissues. While conceivably the lungs might not provide the
anaerobic environment needed by this organism, certainly other organs than the
liver should receive their share of abscesses. Thus the absence of involvement
elsewhere than in the liver is in conformity with Jensen's experimental findings.
Smith, at the suggestion of Gooch (1944), was the first to call attention to ulcers
of the rumen (p. 1199) as a probable source of infection for the portal blood, and
this theme has been further developed by Jensen and his colleagues (1954). The
latter investigators have presented evidence strongly supporting the prevalent
clinical impression that the ruminal disturbances accompany the highly concentrated grain diets of the fattening pen, and have also shown a relation to the suddenness of the change from pasturage or roughage to the ration high in concentrates. The exact mechanism by which the dietary indiscretions produce their
pathological effects has not been elucidated, but the chain of causative events
seems clear.

Hepatosis dietetica is a disorder of swine characterized by massive liver
necrosis. All evidence indicates it is caused by vitamin E:selenium deficiency
(p. 992), and is often associated with other lesions of this deficiency complex to
include: "yellow fat disease," necrosis of skeletal muscle and myocardium and
ulceration of the non-glandular stomach.

Parasitic Diseases of the Liver

Echinococcus or **hydatid cysts** occur in the livers of the farm animals (and man) in those countries where the corresponding adult tapeworm, *Echinococcus granulosus*, (*Taenia echinococcus*) is prevalent in dogs. Unilocular cysts commonly reach a diameter of 4 or 5 cm., developing over a period of months or years. During the first several months, while the cystic embryo is only a few millimeters in diameter, the surrounding tissue presents a considerable reaction with reticulo-endothelial, fibroblastic and foreign-body giant cells (p. 177) and a marked infiltration of eosinophils. The more mature cyst is tightly surrounded by a dense fibrous capsule but with little evidence of a more vigorous reaction. The cyst itself has an outer zone of hyaline, non-nucleated material approaching 1 mm. in thickness, beneath which is an inner layer of embryonal-appearing cells. From the latter, unless the cyst be sterile, which is not unusual, several minute papillary structures project into the clear fluid of the lumen. These are in the process of development into brood capsules with very thin-walled vesicles whose inner lining produces embryonal scolices some 100 microns in diameter. Typical hooklets can (with patience and good fortune) be demonstrated in the scolex, but the echinococcus cyst can be differentiated from other cysts by its general structure. If the host lives several years, the cyst dies and degenerates into a pulpy mass, of which the capsule, at least, becomes calcified. Occasionally in cattle (and man) the young cyst, for reasons which are in doubt (possibly the parasite is of a different species), pursues an abnormal form of growth, failing to attain a diameter of more than, perhaps, a centimeter, but producing a spreading mass of new subsidiary cysts. Known as an **alveolar cyst,** this formation grows indefinitely in spite of a surrounding granulomatous and fibrous reaction and parts of it may even be carried by hematogenous metastasis to establish a new growth in some other organ. A moderate eosinophilia (6 per cent) usually exists during the active phases of hydatidosis. Humoral antibodies of diagnostic value are also produced.

Liver Flukes.—These parasites of sheep, cattle and rarely horses and other species include the common *Fasciola hepatica* (*Distomum hepaticum*) and some other species of flat worms (*Trematoda*). The adult flukes live in the lumens of the intrahepatic bile ducts and reach considerable size, for example, 2 by 1 by 0.2 cm. in the case of *F. hepatica*. Before attaining their permanent domicile, the flukes, as larvae of gradually increasing size, migrate through the hepatic tissue, in many cases having penetrated the perihepatic capsule from the peritoneal cavity. In severe infestations, the local damage from the migrating larvae results in necrosis, considerable escape of blood, and abscesses or other secondary infections are possible. However, in the average case, it is not until the flukes approach their mature size in the bile ducts that clinical signs appear. These include cachexia, weakness, constipation, jaundice, anemia, and edema ("bottle-jaw," ascites). The usual lesions in the liver are those which result from the mechanical and toxic irritation of these large parasites. The lumen of the duct is necessarily dilated as the fluke grows, the wall is greatly thickened by proliferation of encircling fibrous tissue and there is a limited infiltration of lymphocytes and eosinophils. The fibrosis extends for a short distance among the liver lobules but does not constitute a true cirrhosis. Extensive calcification of the injured walls is common. The lumen of the duct becomes more or less completely closed by the body of the fluke and an accumulation of amorphous, blood-stained exudate and debris. The jaundice which develops in severe infestations is thus explainable on an obstructive basis but may be in part hemolytic, since hemolytic toxins are produced. If the patient survives, the flukes die, and pass out with the bile after about nine months. Severe infestations are fatal but, in spite of the dark picture here portrayed and various other possible complications that might be mentioned, the usual outcome is that the animal fattens sufficiently well to go to slaughter, where its liver is condemned because of a number of flukes. In many parts of the country, as many as 25 per cent of sheep's livers are condemned for this reason; in cattle, the liver condemnations vie in number with those for abscesses.

Fascioloides magna, a rather rare fluke of large size found in the livers of ruminants in northern North America and northern Europe, causes the deposition of large amounts of a deep black pigment in the liver and hepatic lymph node. The nature of the pigment appears not to have been determined (p. 70).

Dicrocoelium dendriticum in cattle produces changes similar to those induced by *Fasciola magna*, but less severe. Many other flukes infest animals but they are usually of little clinical or pathological significance.

Ascariasis.—In addition to the adults of *Capillaria hepatica* (p. 777) in monkeys, dogs, and rats, a number of parasites wander through the liver during their larval migrations, including the kidney worm of swine (*Stephanurus dentatus*) (p. 781) which leaves slight scars on the visceral surface, but the only one requiring much further attention is the ascarid of swine. It is known that these larvae pass through the liver, as well as through the lungs. It is common to see livers of pigs from three to ten months of age in which the diaphragmatic and other surfaces bear poorly outlined, diffuse white spots from 1 to 3 cm. in diameter. These spots have no definite limits nor typical shapes, appearing possibly as if they had been applied with a paint brush. Microscopic sections show that the white consists of a thin layer of excess fibrous tissue underlying the capsule and extending along the interlobular septa for a depth equal to the width of two or three lobules. These scars are commonly attributed to damage done by larval ascarids. If anyone has proved or disproved this belief, we have overlooked the fact. Tentatively, we accept this explanation of this frequent lesion (Fig. 15–2, p. 735).

Other hepatic parasites include *Eimeria stiedae, Hepatocystis kochi*, and schistosomes.

Miscellaneous Hepatic Disorders

Cysts, other than hydatid cysts, are assumed to represent a congenital malformation in which one or more primitive bile ducts lack an outlet or connection with the main biliary system. They are lined with cuboidal epithelium but contain a clear fluid having little resemblance to bile. Solitary or multiple, they are of varying sizes, even in the same liver, diameters of 2 to 5 cm. being common. They appear to be less rare in dogs, cats and swine than in other domestic species. While considered to be congenital, they are not necessarily encountered in the young. Most often they are found incidentally upon death from some other cause. The hepatic parenchyma suffers heavily from pressure atrophy and pressure necrosis when the cysts are numerous and large.

In poisoning by chlorinated naphthalenes (p. 938), the hyperplastic epithelium of the intrahepatic bile ducts occasionally becomes so irregular as to form a series of cystic spaces as much as 5 or 6 mm. in diameter along the wall of the duct.

Congestion (p. 130) of the liver is very frequent. If acute it is usually the consequence of terminal myocardial failure, which occurs in many diseases. Chronic hepatic congestion is also traceable with rare exceptions to cardiac disease, either myocardial or valvular (right-sided insufficiency or stenosis) (p. 132). A striking example of chronic hepatic congestion due to myocardial weakness is the so-called "brisket-disease" (p. 1131) which cattle have at high altitudes. Another important example exists in gossypol poisoning in swine (p. 873). Chronic pericarditis as seen in the "traumatic" pericarditis from a penetrating foreign body in bovines leads to similar congestion in the liver. Rarely, pulmonary emphysema and fibrosis cause similar impairment of the venous circulation.

Grossly, the congested liver is dark red, somewhat swollen with rounded edges, and considerable blood escapes from the severed vessels when it is incised. Microscopically, the dilated sinusoids indicate congestion whether or not they are filled with erythrocytes when examined (p. 130). Chronic passive congestion leads to the fibrous proliferation around the central veins which has been called central cirrhosis (p. 1229). It also leads to anoxic centrilobular necrosis (p. 1224), the spaces left by the destroyed cells being filled by blood. As a result the centers of the lobules are very dark. Frequently, the less severely anoxic cells in the peripheral parts of the lobule suffer from fatty degeneration, hence are lighter in color. There is thus produced a fine sprinkling of dark brown and gray reminiscent of the outside of a nutmeg. Such a liver is called, by professional tradition, a "nutmeg liver."

Infarction.—The rarity of infarcts in the liver has already been pointed out (p. 28) and attributed to the double blood supply of that organ.

Pigmentation.—Under this heading, the accumulation of dissolved (bilirubin) or precipitated (bile pigment) biliary coloring matter first comes to mind. Carotenosis must be differentiated from this discoloration as seen grossly. The liver is the most common site of the pigment of brown atrophy. It harbors large amounts of iron-containing pigment in hemochromatosis. Melanosis is occasionally seen in the liver. The blood-containing spots in telangiectasis are almost as black, when seen grossly, as if they contained melanin but are depressed and shrunken. Infestations with *Fascioloides magna* and schistosomes are associated with a peculiar black pigmentation. Arias and Cornelius (1964) have described a disorder in sheep similar to the Dubin-Johnson syndrome of man which is associated with a peculiar melanin-like pigment in hepatocytes. A similar disorder has been described in howler monkeys (Maruffo, *et al.*, 1966). All these conditions are discussed under "Pigments" (p. 60). In cadavers which have undergone considerable post-mortem autolysis, that part of the liver which has lain in contact with the gallbladder is often stained a deep green or yellow, especially in the dog.

Disorganization of Hepatic Cords.—In certain diseases which are destructive of liver tissue, including leptospirosis, one is surprised to see the hepatic cells no longer lying end-to-end in the cords or strands characteristic of its normal arrangement. Instead, each cell is separate and individualized and nearly spherical in form. The cytoplasm may also be more acidophilic than is normally the case. Rickard has studied this condition extensively and found this change to be indicative of approaching necrosis, one of the ways in which a liver cell may die.

Nuclear inclusions of a crystalline nature called *acidophilic crystalline intranuclear (ACN) inclusions* are frequently encountered in hepatocytes and renal

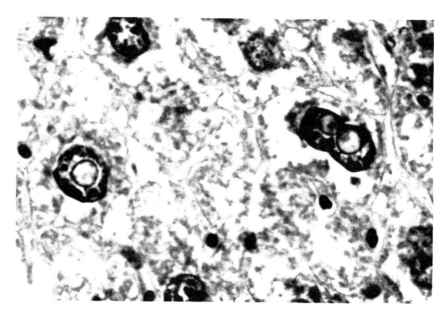

FIG. 24–13.—Cytoplasmic invaginations into hepatocyte nuclei in a mouse.
(Courtesy Animal Research Center, Harvard Medical School.)

tubular epithelium of dogs. They are usually rectangular, up to 15 microns long, and distort the nuclear membrane. Although their significance is not known, they are believed to be crystallized protein and are not related to viral infections. Invagination of cytoplasm into the nucleus produces peculiar membrane-bound intranuclear inclusions. They are encountered most frequently in the hepatocytes of aged rodents but may also be found in dogs and monkeys. In addition to the liver cytoplasmic invaginations are occasionally seen in other tissues, such as corpus luteum, interstitial cell tumors of the testes, and adenocarcinoma of the lung. Normal cytoplasmic organelles can be demonstrated within the inclusion with electron microscopy.

Neoplasms.—For obvious anatomical reasons, the liver is a frequent site of metastatic tumors, especially but not exclusively of those which are primary in the area of portal venous drainage. Primary hepatomas or hepatocellular carcinomas are not as rare in animals as formerly supposed. Adenomas and adenocarcinomas of bile duct origin are occasionally encountered in dogs and cats. Another primary neoplasm which occurs with some frequency, at least in the dog, is the hemangioma. These may reach large size, may spread to adjacent structures, and not infrequently terminate in fatal hemorrhage. The malignant lymphoma is the most frequent neoplasm in the liver. It usually forms a number of nodular metastases, often of large size, but diffuse infiltration of lymphoid cells also occurs, with gradual replacement of the normal parenchyma.

THE GALLBLADDER

Cholecystitis and cholangitis may arise from infections ascending from the duodenum and are possible as the result of blood-borne metastasis, but all these things are rare in animals. Cholecystitis also results from the chemically irritant action of the retained and concentrated bile when the escape of bile is prevented, as by pressure upon or swelling of the bile duct. Experimentally, cholecystitis is claimed to have been produced in poultry and dogs by diets high in fat and low in protein, but this has no known clinical significance. Any of the ordinary types of exudative inflammation are possible, but the usual kinds are mucous (catarrhal), characterized by excessive secretion of the mucous glands, or serous, characterized by inflammatory edema. Leukocytic infiltration is seldom extensive.

More puzzling to the student may be the proper interpretation of the degree of fullness of the organ and the character of its contents. Bile is secreted continually and stored in the gallbladder (horse and other animals lacking a gallbladder excepted), to be discharged when a full meal begins to reach the intestine (action of cholecystikinin). Throughout the period of storage, water is resorbed from the bile by the mucosa and concurrently the mucous glands scattered through the mucous membrane add a small amount of mucus, so that the organ tends slowly to become distended. At the same time fluid continues to be resorbed, leaving the solids. These, together with the slow accumulation of mucus, make the bile more and more viscous. A catarrhal cholecystitis sometimes co-exists, resulting in a markedly increased flow of mucus. With rare exceptions, such as obstruction of the common duct, these mechanisms and failure of the sick animal to eat explain the enlarged gallbladders and viscous, "inspissated bile" so often given prominence in veterinary descriptions of disease.

If the ingress of bile to the gallbladder is prevented by swelling of the cystic duct or other obstruction, the epithelium of the gallbladder secretes a clear watery fluid, filling the cavity with what has been called "white bile."

Cholelithiasis.—Biliary calculi, gallstones, or choleliths, as they may be

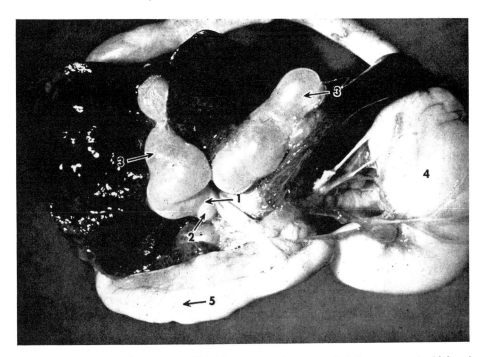

Fig. 24–14.—Obstruction of the gallbladder, presumably congenital, in a ten-week-old female Siamese kitten. The obstruction (1) was related to a small adenoma (2). The distended gallbladder was double (3) in this animal, an occasional occurrence in this species. The stomach (4) and duodenum (5) were not affected. (Courtesy of Angell Memorial Animal Hospital.)

called, occur with rarity in all of the usual domestic species, having been reported even in the chicken. They appear to be less rare in bovines than in the other farm or pet animals. They may be of minute size, like grains of sand, several hundred having been found in the bile ducts of a horse, or they may be few or single, a length of 11.5 cm. having been reported. Depending upon their composition, three types of stones are known, one being the cholesterol stone which is large, white, light in weight and contains glistening crystals of cholesterol radially arranged. The second type, called the "pigment stone," consists of dried and precipitated bilirubin as its principal ingredient. These stones are almost black in color, friable and usually small but multiple in a given patient. One of the writers (Smith) has observed gall stones of this type up to 2 cm. in diameter in cattle and swine. The third type is a heavy, pale stone consisting largely of calcium phosphate and carbonate. These are less common but the same writer has seen such a stone 2.5 cm. in diameter from a bovine animal.

The usual gallstones, however, are composites of these several ingredients, commonly being yellow to dark brown in color, light in weight, somewhat fragile, sometimes concentrically laminated and often faceted, that is, flattened on each of several sides where the stones lay side by side in the gallbladder. Commonly all the stones are of nearly identical size, presumably because they are of the same age.

The **cause** of gallstones of this, the ordinary type, is almost without question cholecystitis of infectious origin. Such infectious processes are by no means frequent in animals and have been studied only occasionally, but the pyocyaneus organism (*Pseudomonas aeruginosa*) has been isolated from cases of cholelithiasis in sheep. The mechanism of formation is doubtless similar to that responsible for urinary calculi, solid particles of dead cells or inspissated material serving as the starting point for a process of crystallization. In the case of gallstones, however, changes in the water content and colloidal state are certainly of considerable importance. It is probable that some constituents of bile are reabsorbed in the event of biliary stasis more easily than others, leaving highly abnormal residues.

Many gallstones are "silent," that is, produce no symptoms. Others, in man, cause episodes of severe pain, dyspepsia and nausea and other gastric symptoms based upon the closely related innervation of both gallbladder and stomach. The accompanying cholecystitis is doubtless more responsible for the symptoms than are the stones themselves. Presumably similar symptoms occur at times in animal patients but they have seldom been recognized clinically. Cholelithiasis has more frequently been discovered at autopsy incidental to icterus and hepatic disease of a more general nature. Obstruction of the biliary flow as the result of choleliths is possible but not usual.

Cystic Hyperplasia.—Also known as cystic mucinous hypertrophy, papillary adenomatous hypertrophy and other descriptive phrases, this lesion is frequently encountered in dogs. The mucosa of the gallbladder is thickened by numerous fronds and cysts lined by squamous to columnar epithelium. The epithelial cells and the cysts contain mucin which stains blue in hematoxylin and eosin stained tissue sections. Grossly the wall of the gallbladder is thickened and numerous multilocular, gelatinous, translucent cysts of varying size are evident. The cause and significance of the lesion are not known. Kovatch, Hildebrant and Marcus (1965) have recently described nine examples of this entity.

Neoplasms.—Primary neoplasms of the gallbladder are rare except in cattle where adenomas and occasionally adenocarcinomas are encountered. (See Fig. 7–14.)

THE PANCREAS

Disease of the pancreas is far from common in the domestic animals. Infectious, as well as neoplastic, processes can of course invade the pancreas by direct extension or metastasis, but usually they do not. Pancreatitis is the most common primary disorder encountered, which in animals is most frequent in the dog. Based on the acuteness of the disorder, the degree of necrosis, fibrosis and atrophy, pancreatitis can be conveniently classified into *acute necrotizing pancreatitis, chronic pancreatitis, chronic fibrosing pancreatitis* and *chronic pancreatitis with atrophy*. Classification is somewhat artificial, however, in that these terms in reality apply to the spectrum of variations of a single disease process; acute necrotizing pancreatitis, with recovery, will progress to chronic fibrosing pancreatitis.

Primary **acute necrotizing pancreatitis** is a tremendously painful catastrophe in human beings. It is known in dogs, cats and horses but has not been reported in ruminants. Experimentally, it has been produced in dogs by a variety of procedures. While commonly called pancreatitis, the more logical term of **acute pancreatic necrosis** is generally preferred, since the primary lesion is necrosis due directly to the local action of the pancreatic enzymes. The necrotic areas may be large or small, most often but not necessarily near the main pancreatic duct and its orifice. The tissue passes through the usual stages of necrosis (p. 17), often

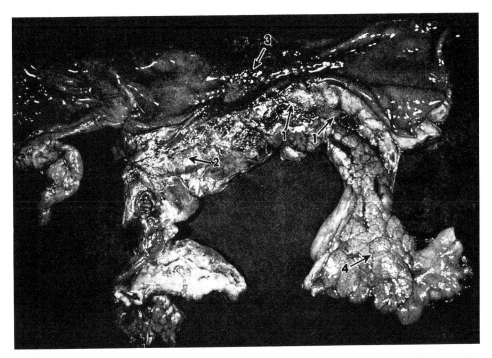

Fig. 24–15.—Necrotizing and hemorrhagic pancreatitis in a male beagle dog, age 7 years. Interstitial hemorrhage (*1*), gray necrotic areas (*2*) and congestion in duodenal mucosa (*3*). The head of the pancreas (*4*) is not affected. (Courtesy of Angell Memorial Animal Hospital.)

accompanied by hemorrhages, thrombosis and local edema, with a very limited infiltration of inflammatory cells. If the area is small and the patient survives there is usually a limited amount of fibrous encapsulation. Pancreatic necrosis of fat (p. 22) will probably have involved nearby structures as the lipolytic enzyme escapes from the damaged ducts; it can even be carried for some distance via the lymphatic channels. The lesions may be multiple at once or there may be a series of recurrent episodes. A **chronic fibrosing pancreatitis** is likely to be the termination, the organ becoming a greatly shrunken, irregularly nodular, fibrous mass. In chronic pancreatitis with atrophy, there are minimal inflammatory changes and little fibrosis. Certain of these may represent a hypoplasia. Diabetes mellitus results when most of the islets have been destroyed. The fatty feces of **steatorrhea** attest the loss of most of the exocrine glandular tissue. Diagnosis during the early, acute phase, always very difficult, is assisted by the determination of serum amylase, which is abnormally high due to interference with the normal passage of the pancreatic secretion into the intestine.

The **cause** of pancreatitis is not known, nor is the mechanism by which pancreatic enzymes become activated to cause this autodigestion. The activation of trypsinogen to trypsin has generally been blamed (and may be responsible), but there is virtually no scientific evidence to support this claim. A more recent theory focuses on the pancreatic enzyme phospholipase A (lecithinase A) which converts harmless lecithin and cephalin to their lyso-compounds. The latter have strong surface-active properties which could destroy the phospholipid layers that make up cell membranes. Although no one has demonstrated trypsin activity in pancreatitis, Creutzfeldt and Schmidt (1970) have found 10-fold increases in the lysolecithin content of the pancreas. It is postulated that pancreatitis may be initiated by the entrance of bile into the pancreatic system with subsequent conversion of lecithin (a major constituent of bile) to lysolecithin by phospholipase A. However, even with this scheme of events the activation of trypsinogen to trypsin is needed because phospholipase A requires minute amounts of trypsin for activation.

Parasites.—Small red **flukes**, *Eurytrema pancreaticum*, usually less than 1 cm. in length, may be very numerous in the pancreatic ductal system of cattle, buffalo, sheep and goats, causing chronic fibrosing pancreatitis of mild or minimal nature. They occur commonly in Brazil and Asia. (See page 808.) Rarely *Ascaris lumbricoides* may invade the pancreatic ducts, as well as the bile duct.

Pancreatic calculi are found rarely in the pancreatic ducts of cattle. They are usually hard, white and numerous, but small. They are reported to consist of carbonates and phosphates of calcium and magnesium, in company with organic substances.

Ectopic pancreatic tissue is rarely observed in dogs in the submucosa or muscularis of the gastrointestinal tract and gallbladder or in the mesentery.

Neoplasms of both acinar and islet cells are recorded in the dog. They are discussed in the section on neoplasms.

SERUM HEPATITIS OF HORSES

Known by such names as **serum hepatitis,** equine **viral hepatitis, Theiler's disease,** and possibly confused with Kimberly horse disease (*Crotalaria retusa*, p. 910) or merely acute yellow atrophy (p. 1224), a suddenly occurring and usually fatal disease of horses has been recognized since as early as 1919 (Theiler). Symptoms of acute indigestion, including those of "blind staggers" (p. 1243), develop in the course of a few hours, accompanied by marked icterus. Death in a day or two reveals a swollen, typical "nutmeg liver" (p. 1235), all parts being uniformly involved. Microscopic examination shows that the "nutmeg" appearance is due to centrilobular necrosis (p. 1224) with replacement by blood, often to the extent that only a narrow rim of hepatic cells survive around the periphery of the blood-filled lobule. The picture differs from that of the usual acute toxic hepatitis (p. 1223) in that in the portal areas (islands of Glisson) and throughout whatever hepatic parenchyma remains there is a liberal infiltration of inflammatory cells, chiefly lymphocytes and neutrophils.

The etiology is unknown and it may well be that a number of intoxications have been confused to form what has been considered a single syndrome but it is of interest that many of the afflicted horses have a history of having received a few months previously a therapeutic agent consisting of horse serum. Among such agents are immunizing sera directed against several equine infections such as African horse sickness in South Africa and equine encephalomyelitis in North America, as well as tetanus antitoxin. Also occupying a prominent place in the list is the serum of pregnant mares, which has been injected in liberal amounts in the hope of assisting placentation in brood mares. This situation has lead to a widespread suspicion that the equine species may be plagued with a virus hidden in the serum of apparently normal horses, transferable in therapeutic sera, comparable to the "serum hepatitis" of man. On the other hand, it must be noted (1) that in many instances the administration of the supposedly causative therapeutic agent occurred several months previous to the sudden development of this disease, (2) that of thousands of horses receiving therapeutic sera only a minute proportion have ever shown this disease, (3) that numerous experimental attempts to produce a hepatitis in horses by the administration of horse serum have given uniformly negative results.

The symptomatology of nervous disorder ("staggers") when the hepatitis followed the use of an anti-encephalomyelitis serum has led to a theory that the supposed virus also attacked the brain. However, convincing lesions have been uniformly lacking.

NERVOUS SYMPTOMS OF HEPATIC AND ENTERIC DISEASE

The interpretation of symptoms is a difficult art and one that we would willingly leave entirely, as we do mainly, to the clinician, were it not for the fact that in some aspects symptoms and lesions are inextricably bound together. A peculiar, poorly understood and often unrealized nervous and cerebral reaction which often accompanies hepatic malfunction in various liver diseases is something we cannot forbear to bring to the reader's attention. The late Dean Glover of the Colorado Veterinary School, teaching at a time when chronic alcoholism occupied a more central position in the etiology of cirrhosis than it does now, was wont to tell his pupils, "Boys, it will get you. Drinking will not only ruin you; it will kill you. A few small drinks a day will not make you drunk, but by the time you are fifty you will have a mild cirrhosis; you will be so chronically unhappy and ill-tempered that, in a fit of anger, you will shoot your mother-in-law. The law will hang you for that. So, see, alcohol will have taken your life." To prove that such a view is not an innovation we have only to consider the choleric individual who might commit such an act and go back to the origin of the word "choleric" and its implication of bad or disordered bile.

It is the common experience of many persons suffering from viral hepatitis, while conscious of no real pain, to feel a general revulsion against their surroundings that is second only to a disinclination to exert the effort necessary to accomplish any malevolent design that a somewhat disordered intellect might conceive. As recounted by Sherlock (1955), humans affected by various hepatic diseases are apt to suffer from changes in personality, even from amnesia or hallucinations. Children become restless and very noisy, with crying, screaming and nightmares. As the condition worsens, spells of extreme emotional instability or mental confusion may be superseded by apathy or mania. Such episodes are likely to begin in late evening, are of variable duration and may terminate in rapid recovery.

Is it any wonder, then, that horses walk incessantly until death relieves them from the hepatitis of Senecio poisoning (p. 875), or that cattle with the same disease continually force the head into a solid wall or attack their keepers? Dogs also show signs of nervous derangement ("encephalitis," probably an erroneous interpretation) in cases of interference with hepatic function (see below).

Several theories have been offered to explain this clinically obvious relationship between cerebral and hepatic malfunctions, which were the subject of comment even by Galen in the early years of the Christian era (Sherlock, 1955). At least as early as the works of Frerichs in 1860 and of Leyden in 1866, the concept of **cholemia** arose, with a connotation of the presence in the blood of harmful products of bile, quite analogous to uremia, which designates the presence of urinary poisons in the same vital fluid. The currently accepted and rather well-proven view is that the interference with cerebral function does not come directly from the bile, although bilirubinemia and jaundice are present in many cases, but, rather, that it is due to nitrogenous compounds, possibly ammonia, which are carried to the brain because of failure of the hepatic detoxifying process. As Sherlock points out, failure of the liver to free the blood of toxic nitrogenous substances can result from hepato-cellular damage of various kinds or from the presence of some vascular arrangement allowing portal blood to bypass the liver in its route into the systemic circulation. Such a collateral circulation via enlarged vessels in the abdominal wall is well known as a result of cirrhosis or it may, of course, be produced surgically. To the latter category belong experimental animals with an Eck fistula. A persistent ductus venosus is also a possibility in those species having this vessel. Among the disorders of humans in which cerebral malfunction can be attributed to failure of detoxification are not only destructive diseases of the liver, chiefly cirrhosis, but also certain transitory hepatic insufficiencies which occur in infections, severe hemorrhages and intoxications by anesthetics, barbiturates, morphine or acute alcoholism. When the detoxifying function is imperfect, the cerebral syndrome may also be traceable to an excess of nitrogenous substances in the intestine as a result of bacterial action or the presence of ammonium chloride, methionine, melena or even too large amounts of dietary proteins.

The diagnosis of hepato-cerebral disturbances in animals may be temporarily complicated by the fact that somewhat similar symptoms accompany acute gastrointestinal diseases, although such indigestions usually terminate either favorably or unfavorably after only a few hours. Toxic hepatitis (p. 1223), in any of its forms, is almost always of longer duration. The digestive symptoms to which we allude are picturesquely designated by two antiquated colloquialisms, "mad staggers" and "blind staggers." The "mad staggers," in which a horse paws, sweats, thrashes and struggles with all sorts of grotesque movements, is usually interpreted as a frenzied attempt to escape from the agony that accompanies some forms of "colic" (p. 1214). In what early writers called "blind staggers," the animal is free from violent pain, shows little inclination to move and appears to be blind. The one stance that is typical of this condition is to stand immovably with the head pressing forward against a wall or manger. Some interpret this as indicating a severe headache, which may be correct. On the other hand, animals with a trephined frontal sinus, or with intracranial abscesses or tumors may be presumed by human analogy to have a severe headache but they do not take this position. Neither is the attitude usual in animals suffering from the infectious encephalitides. That no irreversible central nervous lesion necessarily accompanies the above symptoms is proven by the fact that if recovery from the primary digestive disorder occurs, the nervous symptoms promptly disappear.

Dogs and cats (and children, we are told) react to various enteric disorders with convulsions. This is the common belief among veterinary practitioners, although, being difficult of proof, it is sometimes questioned.

The explanation of related or identical symptoms in both enteric and hepatic disorders may conceivably lie in the development of undetoxified ammonium or other nitrogenous compounds in both instances. The subject merits further study. It may be added that the rare disorder of humans known as hepatolenticular degeneration or Wilson's disease is not involved in the above-described transitory syndromes, nor is it known ever to occur in animals, although a possibly comparable condition was reported by Dobberstein (1926) under the name of Schweinberger's disease.

SELECTED REFERENCES

Andersen, A. C.: The Pathogenesis of Telangiectasis in the Bovine Liver. Am. J. Vet. Research *16*:27–34, 1955.

Anderson, W. A., Monlux, A. W., and Davis, C. L.: Epithelial Tumors of the Gall Bladder —A Report of Eighteen Cases. Am. J. Vet. Res. *19*:58–65, 1958.

Archibald, J., and Whiteford, R. D.: Canine Atrophic Pancreatitis. J. Am. Vet. Med. Assn. *122*:119–125, 1953.

Arias, I., *et al.*: Liver Disease in Corriedale Sheep: A New Mutation Affecting Hepatic Excretory Function. J. Clin. Invest. *43*:1249–1250, 1964.

Bailey, J. M., and Carbeck, R. B.: Porphyria Hepatica with Primary Psychiatric Manifestations. U. S. A. F. Med. J. *9*:1346–1350, 1958.

Barron, C. N.: Ectopic Pancreas in the Dog. Acta Anat. *36*:344–352, 1959.

Bartley, E. E. *et al.*: Bloat in Cattle. IV. The Role of Bovine Saliva, Plant Mucilaegs, and Animal Mucins. V. The Role of Rumen Mucinolytic Bacteria. J. Anim. Sci. *20*:648–658, 1961.

Belonje, C. W. A.: Field Observations on Wesselbron Disease. J. So. Afr. Vet. Med. Assn. *29*:1–12, 1958.

Benjamin, S. A., and Lang, C. M.: An Ameloblastic Odontoma in a Cebus Monkey (*Cebus albifrons*). J. Am. Vet. Med. Assn. *155*:1236–1240, 1969.

Biester, H. E., Eveleth, D. F., and Yamashiro, Y.: Intestinal Emphysema of Swine. J. Am. Vet. Med. Assn. *88*:714–731, 1936.

Biester, H. E., and Schwarte, L. H.: Intestinal Adenoma in Swine. Am. J. Path. *7*:175–185, 1931.

Birrell, J.: Infection by Vibrio As a Cause of Disease in Pigs. Vet. Rec. *69*:947–950, 1957.

Bishop, W. H.: Salmonellosis in Cattle. Australian Vet. J. *26*:253–255, 1950.

Boothe, A. D., and Cheville, N. F.: The Pathology of Proliferative Ileitis of the Golden Syrian Hamster. Path. Vet. *4*:31–44, 1967.

BOYD, W.: *Textbook of Pathology*. 6th ed., 1953. Philadelphia, Lea & Febiger, p. 496.

BRITTON, J. W., and CAMERON, H. S.: So-Called Enterotoxemia of Lambs in California. Cornell Vet. *34*:19–29, 1944.

BROBERG, G.: [Factors influencing pH and osmotic pressure in the rumen of sheep during acute overeating of foods rich in carbohydrates.] Finsk. Vet-Tidskr. *64*:450–464, 1958. Abstr. Vet. Bull., No. 483. 1959.

BULL, L. B.: Liver Diseases of Livestock from Intake of Hepato-toxic Substances. Austr. Vet. J. *37*:126–130, 1961.

BULLEN, J. J.: Enterotoxaemia of Sheep: *Clostridium welchii*, Type D, in the Alimentary Tract of Normal Animals. J. Path. and Bact. *64*:201–206, 1952.

BYRNE, M. M.: Salmonella Infection in a Foal. Irish Vet. J. *1*:94, 1947.

CAPUCCI, D. T., JR.: Porcine Gastric Ulcers in the United States: A Review. Veterinarian *4*:213–218, 1967.

CASEY, H. W., *et al.*: Segmental Hypertrophy of Colon in a Rhesus Monkey. J. Am. Vet. Med. Assn. *155*:1245–1248, 1969.

CHAPMAN, W. L., JR.: Acute Gastric Dilation in *Macaca mulatta* and *Macaca speciosa* Monkeys. Lab. Anim. Care *17*:130–136, 1967.

CREUTZFELDT, W., and SCHMIDT, H.: Aetiology and Pathogenesis of Pancreatitis (Current Concepts). Scand. J. Gastroent. *5*: Suppl. *6*:47–62, 1970.

CURTIN, T. M. *et al.*: Clinical and Pathologic Characterization of Esophagogastric Ulcers in Swine. J. Am. Vet. Med. Assn. *143*:854–860, 1963.

DEAS, D. W.: Observations on Swine Dysentery and Associated Vibrios. Vet. Rec. *72*:65–69, 1960.

DOBBERSTEIN, J.: Über einen Fall von Leberkoller des Pferdes und die dabei gefundenen Gehirnveränderungen. Deutsche tierärztliche Wchnschr. *34*:501–505, 1926.

DODD, D. C.: Adenomatous Intestinal Hyperplasia (Proliferative Ileitis) of Swine. Path. Vet. *5*:333–341, 1968.

DORN, K. *et al.*: Studies on Pigs. V. Chemical Studies on Pigs with Edema Disease. Arch. Exp. Vet. Med. *16*:1187–1203, 1962.

DOYLE, L. P.: Etiology of Swine Dysentery. Am. J. Vet. Research *9*:50–51, 1948.

————: Enteritis in Swine. Cornell Vet. *35*:103–109, 1945.

————: A Vibrio Associated with Swine Dysentery. Am. J. Vet. Res. *15*:3–5, 1944.

EGERTON, J. R., and MURELL, T. G. C.: Intestinal Emphysema in Pigs in the Western Highlands of New Guinea. J. Comp. Path. Therap. *75*:35–38, 1965.

EMSBO, P.: Terminal or Regional Ileitis in Swine. Nord. Vet. med. *3*:1–28, 1951.

FIELD, H. I., BUNTAIN, D., and JENNINGS, A. R.: Terminal or Regional Ileitis in Pigs. J. Comp. Path. and Therap. *63*:153–158, 1953.

FIELD, H. J., and GOODWIN, R. F. W.: The Experimental Reproduction of Enterotoxemia in piglets. J. Hyg., Camb. *57*:81–91, 1959. Abstr. Vet. Bull., No. 2379, 1959.

FORNEY, M. M., *et al.*: Limited Survey of Georgia Cattle for Fat Necrosis. J. Am. Vet. Med. Assn. *155*:1603–1604, 1969.

FRANDSON, R. D., and DAVIS, R. W.: Partial Strangulation of Bovine Abomasum. J. Am. Vet. Med. Assn. *124*:267, 1954.

FREDERICK, L. D.: Bovine Hepatic Disturbances. J. Am. Vet. Med. Assn. *102*:338–345, 1943.

FRERICHS, F. T.: *Clinical Treatise on Diseases of the Liver*, Translated by C. Murchison. Vol. I. New Sydenham Society, London. 1860, p. 241 (Cited by Sherlock.)

GALL, E. A., and LANDING, B. H.: Hepatic Cirrhosis and Hereditary Disorders of Metabolism. A Review. Am. J. Clin. Path. *26*:1398–1426, 1956.

GARDNER, A. F., DARKE, B. H., and KEARY, G. T.: Dental Caries in Domesticated Dogs. J. Am. Vet. Med. Assn. *140*:433–436, 1962.

GEIL, R. G., DAVIS, C. L., and THOMPSON, S. W.: Spontaneous Ileitis in Rats. Am. J. Vet. Res. *22*:932–936, 1961.

GETTY, R.: The Histopathology of a Focal Hepatitis and of its Termination ("Sawdust" and "Telang" Liver) in Cattle. Am. J. Vet. Research *7*:437–449, 1946.

GIANELLI, F.: Contributo all conoscenza delle calcolosi pancreatiche dei bovini. Atti. Soc. ital. sci. vet. *5*:218–224, 1951.

GIOVANELLI, N. E.: Estudio de una Enfermedad en Equinos con Lesion de Cirrosis Hepatica. Rev. Med. Vet. B. Aires *42*:173–180, 183–185, 1961.

GITTER, M., and LLOYD, M. K.: Haemolytic *Bact. coli* in the Bowel Edema Syndrome. II. Transmission and Protection Experiments. Brit. Vet. J. *113*:212–218, 1957.

GORLIN, R. J., *et al.*: The Oral and Pharyngeal Pathology of Domestic Animals—A Study of 487 Cases. Am. J. Vet. Res. *20*:1032–1061, 1959.

GORRIE, C. J. R.: Enteric Diseases of Swine. Swine Dysentery. Aust. Vet. J. *22*:135–137, 1946.

GREENHAM, L. W.: Some Preliminary Observations on Rabbit Mucoid Enteritis. Vet. Rec. *74*:79–85, 1962.

GRIESEMER, R. A. and KRILL, W. R.: Enterotoxemia of Beef Calves—30 Years' Observation. J. Am. Vet. Med. Assn. *140*:154–158, 1962.

GRINER, L. A. and BRACKEN, F. K.: *Clostridium perfringens* (Type C) in Acute Hemorrhagic Enteritis of Calves. J. Am. Vet. Med. Assn. *122*:99–102, 1953.

GRINER, L. A. and CARLSON, W. D.: Enterotoxemia of Sheep. I. Effects of *Clostridium perfringens* Type D Toxin on the Brains of Sheep and Mice. II. Distribution of I^{131} Radio-iodinated Serum Albumin in Brains of *Clostridium perfringens* Type D Intoxicated Lambs. III. *Clostridium perfringens* Type D Antitoxin Titers of Normal, Nonvaccinated Lambs. Am. J. Vet. Res. *22*:429–442, 443–446, 447–448, 1961.

GRINER, L. A., and JOHNSON, H. W.: *Clostrium perfringens* (Type C) in Hemorrhagic Enterotoxemia of Lambs. J. Am. Vet. Med. Assn. *125*:125–127, 1954.

GYORGY, P. *et al*.: Prevention of Experimental Dietary Hepatic Injury by Extracts of Some Tropical Plants. Proc. Soc. Exp. Biol., N. Y. *113*:203–206, 1963.

HARSHFIELD, G. S., CROSS, F., and HOERLEIN, A. B.: Further Studies on Overeating (Enterotoxemia) of Feedlot Lambs. Am. J. Vet. Research *3*:86–91, 1942.

HASTINGS, C. C.: Gastroenteritis of Swine. Cornell Vet. *37*:129–135, 1947.

HEAD, M. J.: Bloat in Cattle. Nature, Lond. *183*:757, 1959.

HEARN, E. M., and KEEP, M. E.: Torsion of the Stomach in the Dog. J. So. Afr. Vet. Med. Assn. *30*:389–391, 1959.

HEIMBERG, M. *et al*.: The Action of Carbon Tetrachloride on the Transport and Metabolism of Triglycerides and Fatty Acids by the Isolated Perfused Rat Liver and Its Relationship to the Etiology of Fatty Liver. J. Biol. Chem. *237*:3623–3627, 1962.

HOE, C. M.: Tests for Liver Dysfunction in Dogs. Nature, Lond. *192*:1045–1047, 1961.

HOGH, P.: Necrotizing Infectious Enteritis in Piglets, Caused by *Clostridium perfringens* Type C. I. Biochemical and Toxigenic Properties of the Clostridium. Acta Vet. Scand. *8*: 26–38, 1967.

————: Necrotizing Infectious Enteritis in Piglets, Caused by *Clostridium perfringens* Type C. II. Incidence and Clinical Features. Acta Vet. Scand. *8*:301–323, 1967.

————: Necrotizing Infectious Enteritis in Piglets, Caused by *Clostridium perfringens* Type C. III. Pathological Changes. Acta Vet. Scand. *10*:57–83, 1969.

HOLTENIUS, P.: On the Occurrence of Intranuclear PAS-Positive Material in Liver Cells of Cattle. Cornell Vet. *53*:322–327, 1963.

HOTTENDORF, G. H., HIRTH, R. S., and PEER, R. L.: Megaloileitis in Rats. J. Am. Vet. Med. Assn. *155*:1131–1135, 1969.

HUTYRA, F., and MAREK, J.: *Special Pathology and Therapeutics of the Diseases of Domestic Animals*. 3rd Am. Ed., 1926, translated by John R. Mohler and Adolph Eichhorn. Chicago, Alexander Eger. Vol. II, pp. 428, 430, 438, 448.

IMAI, N. *et al*.: [An infectious disease of dogs characterized by hemorrhagic enteritis.] Bull. Azabu Vet. Coll., Japan. No. *5*:11–36, 1958. Abstr. Vet. Bull., No. 2035, 1959.

IN-CHANG PAN *et al*.: Experimental Production of Edema Disease of Swine. Abstr. Vet. Bull. No. 3819, 1963.

INNES, J. R. M., and STANTON, M. F.: Acute Disease of the Submaxillary and Harderian Glands (Sialo-Dacryoadenitis) of Rats with Cytomegaly and No Inclusion Bodies. Amer. J. Path. *38*:455–468, 1961.

JARRETT, W. F. H.: Bovine Hepatic Disease. Vet. Rec. *68*:825, 1956.

JENSEN, R., CONNELL, W. E., and DEEM, A. W.: Rumenitis and its Relation to Rate of Change of Ration and the Proportion of Concentrate in the Ration of Cattle. Am. J. Vet. Research *15*:425–428, 1954.

JENSEN, R. DEANE, H. M., COOPER, L. J., MILLER, V. A., and GRAHAM, R. W.: Rumenitis-Liver Abscess Compex in Beef Cattle. Am. J. Vet. Research *15*:202–216, 1954.

JENSEN, R., FLINT, J. C., and GRINER, L. A.: Experimental Hepatic Necrobacillosis in Beef Cattle. Am. J. Vet. Research *15*:5–14, 1954.

JENSEN, R., FREY, P. R., CROSS, F., and CONNELL, W. E.: Telangiectasis, "Sawdust," and Abscesses in the Livers of Beef Cattle. J. Am. Vet. Med. Assn. *110*:256–261, 1947.

JENSEN, R., *et al*.: Parakeratosis of the Rumens of Lambs Fattened on Pelleted Feed. Am. J. Vet. Res. *19*:277–282, 1958.

JONAS, A. M., TOMITA, Y., and WYAND, D. S.: Enzootic Intestinal Adeno-Carcinoma in Hamsters. J. Am. Vet. Med. Assn. *147*:1102–1108, 1965.

JONES, J. E. T., and SMITH, H. W.: Histological Studies on Weaned Pigs Suffering from Diarrhea and Oedema Disease Produced by Oral Inoculation of Escherichia coli. J. Path. *97*:168–172, 1969.

KARSNER, H. T.: *Human Pathology*. 6th ed., 1942. Philadelphia, J. B. Lippincott Co., p. 559.

KATITCH, R. V.: Conceptions Modernes sur la Pathogénic des Enterotoxémies du Mouton. Bull. Off. Int. Epiz. *56*:929–934, 1961.

KAUFMANN, E.: *Pathology for Students and Practitioners.* 1929. Translated by Stanley P. Reimann. Philadelphia, C. Blakiston, Vol. II, p. 913.

KEAST, J. C., and McBARRON, E. J.: A Case of Bovine Enterotoxaemia. Australian Vet. J. *30*:305–306, 1954.

KENNEDY, P. C., and CELLO, R. M.: Colitis of Boxer Dogs. Gastroenterology *51*:926–929, 1966.

KERNKAMP, H. C. H., *et al.*: Epizootiology of Edema Disease in Swine. J. Am. Vet. Med. Assn. *146*:353–357, 1965.

KOCK, S. A., and SKELLEY, J. F.: Colitis in a Dog Resembling Whipple's Disease in Man. J. Am. Vet. Med. Assn. *150*:22–26, 1967.

KOVATCH, R. M., HILDEBRANT, P. K., and MARCUS, L. C.: Cystic Mucinous Hypertrophy of the Gallbladder in the Dog. Path. Vet. *2*:574–584, 1965.

KOWALCYZK, T., *et al.*: Stomach Ulcers in Farrowing Gilts. J. Am. Vet. Med. Assn. *148*: 52–62, 1966.

KURTZ, H. J., *et al.*: Pathologic Changes in Edema Disease of Swine. Am. J. Vet. Res. *30*: 791–806, 1969.

KITCHEN, R. H. *et al.*: Megaesophagus in a Dog. J. Am. Vet. Med. Assn. *143*:1106–1107, 1963.

KUTAS, F. and KARSAI, F.: The Diagnostic Value of Transaminase and Cholinesterase Determinations in Hepatic Disease of Domestic Animals. Acta Vet. Acad. Sci. Hung. *11*:277–288, 1961.

LAMBERT, R. A., and ALLISON, B. R.: Types of Lesions in Chronic Passive Congestion of the Liver. Bull. Johns Hopkins Hosp. *27*:350–356, 1916.

LAMONT, H. G.: Gut Edema in Pigs. Proc. Am. Vet. Med. Assn. 1953, pp. 186–191.

LAWSON, D. D., *et al.*: Dental Anatomy and Histology of the Dog. Res. Vet. Sci. *1*:204–210, 1960.

LEBEDEV, N. A., and ERASTOV, V. V.: Patologo-anatomicheskie izmeneniya pri paratife telyat. [Pathology and Histopathology of Calf Paratyphoid (Salmonellosis).] Trud. vsezoyuz. Inst. eksp. Vet. *14*:124–131, 1937. (French Summary.) Abstr. Vet. Bull. No. 846, 1948.

LETTOW, E.: Diagnosis of Diseases of the Liver in Dogs. Zbl. Vet. Med. *9*:75–108, 109–157, 1962.

LEYDEN, E.: *Beitrage zur Pathologie des Icterus.* 1866. Berlin, Hirschwald. (Cited by Sherlock.)

LIÉGEOIS, F.: *Traite de pathologie medicale des animaux domestiques.* Librairie Agricole, Paris. 1933. p. 158.

LOEB, W. F. and EDGE, L. I.: A Method for the Determination of Serum Amylase in the Dog. Am. J. Vet. Res. *23*:1117–1119, 1962.

LUKE, D., and GORDON, W. A. M.: Oedema of the Bowel in Pigs. Nature, London, *165*:286, 1950.

LUKES, J., and CECH, K.: Hypertrophic Cirrhosis and its Relation to Leptospiral Infection. Schweiz. Z. Path. Bakt. *13*:175–199, 1950.

LUSSIER, G., and VYTAUTAS, P.: Presence of Intranuclear Inclusion Bodies in Proliferative Ileitis of the Hamster (*Mesocricetus auratus*). A Preliminary Report. Lab. Anim. Care *19*: 387–390, 1969.

MACK, R.: Disorders of the Digestive Tract of Domesticated Rabbits. Vet. Bull. *32*:192–199, 1962.

MACPHERSON, L. W.: Bovine Virus Enteritis (Winter Dysentery). Canad. J. Comp. Med. *21*:184–192, 1957.

MARUFFO, C. A., *et al.*: Pigmentary Liver Disease in Howler Monkeys. Amer. J. Path. *49*: 445–456, 1966.

MATHEWS, F. P.: Poisoning of Cattle by a Species of Groundsel. Exper. Sta. Bull. No. 481, Texas A. & M. College, College Station. 1933.

McCULLOCH, E. C.: Hepatic Cirrhosis of Horses, Swine and Cattle Due to Seeds of the Tarweed *Amsinckia intermedia.* J. Am. Vet. Med. Assn. *96*:5–18, 1940.

MICHEL, R. L., WHITEHAIR, C. K., and KEAHEY, K. K.: Dietary Hepatic Necrosis Associated with Selenium-Vitamin E Deficiency in Swine. J. Am. Vet. Med. Assn. *155*:50–59, 1969.

MOON, H. W., and BERGELAND, M. E.: *Clostridium perfringens* Type C Enterotoxemia of the Newborn Pig. Can. Vet. J. *6*:159–161, 1965.

MOON, V.: The Origins and Effects of Anoxia. Bull. N. Y. Acad. Med. *26*:361–369, 1950.

MOON, V., and MORGAN, D. R.: Shock: The Mechanism of Death Following Intestinal Obstruction. Arch. Surg. *32*:776–788, 1936.

MORRIS, H.: Investigacion sobre la Flora Bacteriana de la Boca del Perro. Rev. Med. Vet. Parasit., Maracay *18*:85–94, 1959–60.

MUGGENBURG, B. A., McNUTT, S. H., and KOWALCZYK, T.: Pathology of Gastric Ulcers in Swine. Am. J. Vet. Res. 25:1354–1365, 1964.

MUGGENBURG, B. A., et al.: Survey of the Prevalence of Gastric Ulcers in Swine. Am. J. Vet. Res. 25:1673–1678, 1964.

MUSHIN, R., and BASSET, C. R.: Haemolytic Escherichia coli and Other Bacteria in Oedema Disease of Swine. Aust. Vet. J. 40:315–320, 1964.

NAERLAND, G. and HELLE, O.: Functional Pyloric Stenosis in Sheep. Vet. Rec. 74:85–90, 1962.

NAFSTAD, I.: Gastric Ulcers in Swine. 1. Effect of Dietary Protein Dietary Fat and Vitamin E on Ulcer Development. Path. Vet. 4:1–14, 1967.

NAFSTAD, I., and TOLLERSRUD, S.: Gastric Ulcers in Swine. 2. Effects of High Fat Diets and Vitamin E on Ulcer Development. Path. Vet. 4:15–22, 1967.

NAFSTAD, I., TOLLERSRUD, S., and BAUSTAD, B.: Gastric Ulcers in Swine. 3. Effects of Different Proteins and Fats on Their Development. Path. Vet. 4:23–30, 1967.

NEWSOM, I. E.: A Bacteriologic Study of Liver Abscesses in Cattle. J. Infect. Dis. 63:232–233, 1938.

NEWSOM, I. E., and THORP, F., JR.: The Toxicity of Intestinal Filtrates from Lambs Dead of Overeating. J. Am. Vet. Med. Assn. 93:165–167, 1938.

NICHOLS, R. E., and PENN, K. E.: Simple Methods for the Detection of Unfavorable Changes in Ruminal Ingesta. J. Am. Vet. Med. Assn. 133:275–279, 1958.

NIELSEN, N. O., et al.: Attempts to Produce Edema Disease of Swine Experimentally with Hemolytic Escherichia coli. Am. J. Vet. Res. 26:928–931, 1965.

NIELSEN, N. O., MOON, H. W., and ROE, W. E.: Enteric Colibacillosis in Swine. J. Am. Vet. Med. Assn. 153:1590–1606, 1968.

NIELSEN, S. W.: Spontaneous Hematopoietic Neoplasms of the Domestic Cat. Nat. Cancer Inst. Monogr. No. 32, Presented at Symposium on Comp. Morphology of Hematopoietic Neoplasms, A.F.I.P., Wash. D.C. March 11 and 12, 1968.

————: Muscular Hypertrophy of the Ileum in Relation to "Terminal Ileitis" in Pigs. J. Am. Vet. Med. Assn. 127:437–441, 1955.

NIELSEN, S. W., and POCOCK, E. F.: Chronic Relapsing Pancreatitis in a Dog. Cornell Vet. 43:567–572, 1953.

NIILO, L., MOFFATT, R. E., and AVERY, R. J.: Bovine "Enterotoxemia." II. Experimental Reproduction of the Disease. Canad. Vet. J. 4:288–298, 1963.

O'BRIEN, J. J.: Gastric Ulceration (of the Pars Oesophagea) in the Pig. Vet. Bull. 39:75–82, 1969.

OLAFSON, P., MacCALLUM, A. D., and FOX, F. H.: An Apparently New Transmissible Disease of Cattle. Cornell Vet. 36:205–213, 1946.

OSBORNE, C. A., CLIFFORD, D. H., and JESSEN, C.: Hereditary Esophageal Achalasia in Dogs. J. Am. Vet. Med. Assn. 151:572–581, 1967.

PAVONCELLI, R. Su di un caso di litiasi pancreatica bovina. (Engl. & Fr. summaries.) Riv. med. vet., Parma. 6:433–438, 1954 . (Abstr. Vet. Bull. No. 2506, 1955.)

PELLEGRINI, N.: Tuberculosi pancreatica del bovino. Atti. Soc. Ital. Vet. 13:420–421, 1959.

PETROV, O. V.: Changes in the Aerobic Bacterial Flora of the Small Intestine during Infectious Enterotoxaemia in Sheep (TT). Abstr. Vet. Bull. No. 379, 1962.

PHILIP, J. R. and SHONE, D. K.: Some Observations on Oedema Disease and a Possibly Related Condition of Pigs in Southern Rhodesia. J. S. Afr. Vet. Med. Assn. 31:427–434, 1960.

PICKRELL, J. A., et al.: Attempts to Produce Experimental Edema Disease in Swine by Parenterally Injecting Escherichia coli serotype 0139–K82:H1. Can. J. Comp. Med. 33:76–80, 1969.

POPPER, H. and SCHAFFNER, F.: Fine Structural Changes of the Liver. Ann. Int. Med. 59:674–691, 1963.

PRIOUZEAU, M.: Gastrite oedémateuse des bovidés. Rec. méd. vét. 130:377–380, 1954.

PRITCHARD, W. R., and WASSENAAR, P. W.: Studies on the Syndrome Called Mycotic Stomatitis of Cattle. J. Am. Vet. Med. Assn. 135:274–277, 1959.

RAMSEY, F. K., and CHIVERS, W. H.: Mucosal Disease of Cattle. North Am. Vet. 34:629–633, 1953.

REESE, N. A. et al.: Factors Influencing Gastric Ulcers in Swine. J. Anim. Sci. 22:1129, 1963.

RITCHIE, H. D., GRINDLAY, J. H., and BOLLMAN, J. L.: Flow of Lymph from the Canine Liver. Am. J. Physiol. 196:105–109, 1959.

RICHTER, W. R., et al.: Ultrastructural Studies of Intranuclear Crystalline Inclusions in the Liver of the Dog. Amer. J. Path. 47:587–599, 1965.

ROBERTS, D. S.: Studies on Vibrionic Dysentery in Swine. Aust. Vet. J. 32:114–118, 1956.

ROBERTS, S. J.: Winter Dysentery in Cattle. Cornell Vet. 47:372–388, 1957.

ROONEY, J. R.: Volvulus, Strangulation, and Intussusception in the Horse. Cornell Vet. 55:644–653, 1965.

—————: Gastric Ulceration in Foals. Path. Vet. *1*:497–503, 1964.

ROTHENBACHER, H.: Bovine Hepatitis Associated with Ruminal Protozoa. J. Am. Vet. Med. Assn. *145*:558–563, 1964.

—————: Esophagogastric Ulcer Syndrome in Young Pigs. Am. J. Vet. Res. *26*:1214–1217, 1965.

ROTHENBACHER, H. *et al.*: The Stomach Ulcer-gastrorrhagia Syndrome in Michigan Pigs. Vet. Med. *58*:806–816, 1963.

RUBARTH, S.: Hepatic and Subphrenic Abscesses in Cattle with Rupture Into Vena Cava Caudalis. Acta Vet. Scand. *1*:363–382, 1960.

SAID, A. H.: Rumenotomy and Experimental Traumatic Reticulitis in the Camel. Vet. Rec. *75*:966–969, 1963.

SANDER, C. H., and LANGHAM, R. F.: Canine Histiocytic Ulcerative Colitis. A Condition Resembling Whipple's Disease, Colonic Histiocytosis, and Malakoplakia in Man. Arch. Path. *85*:94–100, 1968.

SEIBOLD, H. R., BAILEY, W. S., HOERLEIN, B. F., JORDAN, E. M., and SCHWABE, C. W.: Possible Relation of Malignant Esophageal Tumors and *Spirocerca lupi* Lesions in the Dog. Am. J. Vet. Res. *16*:5–14, 1955.

SCHOFIELD, F. W.: Observations on the X-disease of Marsh as Seen in the Niagara Peninsula. Rep. Ontario Vet. Coll. pp. 21–25, 1939.

SCHOFIELD, F. W.: Enterotoxemia (Sudden Death) in Calves Due to *Clostridium welchii*. J. Am. Vet. Med. Assn. *126*:192–194, 1955.

SCHLOTTHAUER, C. F.: Inverted Cecum in a Dog. J. Am. Vet. Med. Assn. *125* 123–124, 1954.

SCHLOTTHAUER, C. F., and STALKER, L. K.: Cholelithiasis in Dogs. J. Am. Vet. Med. Assn. *88*:758–761, 1936.

SEIBOLD, H. R.: Pathology of Mucosal Disease in Alabama. J. Am. Vet. Med. Assn. *128*:21–26, 1956.

SELYE, H., and STONE. H. Hormonally Induced Transformation of Adrenal into Myeloid. Tissue. Am. J. Path. *26*:211–233, 1950. (Ref. p. 220).

SETCHELL, B. P. and LITTLEJOHNS, I. R.: Poisoning of Sheep with Anthelmintic Doses of Carbon Tetrachloride. III. Liver Histopathology. Aust. Vet. J. *39*:49–50, 1963.

SHANKS, P. L.: An Unusual Condition Affecting the Digestive Organs of the Pig. Vet. Rec. *50*:356–358, 1938.

SHELDON, W. G.: Fibrous Gingival Hyperplasia of a Mustache Guenon Monkey (*Cercopithicus cephus*). Lab. Anim. Care *17*:140–143, 1967.

SHERLOCK, S. *Disease of the Liver and Biliary System*. Springfield, Charles C Thomas, 1955.

SMITH, K. J. and WOODS, W.: Relationship of Calcium and Magnesium to the Occurrence of Bloat in Lambs. J. Anim. Sci. *21*:798–803, 1962.

SMITH, H. A.: Ulcerative Lesions of the Bovine Rumen and Their Possible Relation to Hepatic Abscesses. Am. J. Vet. Research *5*:234–243, 1944.

SMITH, H. W., and HALLS, S.: The Production of Oedema Disease and Diarrhoea in Weaned Pigs by the Oral Administration of E. coli: Factors that Influence the Course of the Experimental Disease. J. Med. Microbiol. *1*:45–59, 1968.

SMITH, L. D. S.: Clostridial Diseases of Animals. Adv. Vet. Sci. *3*:463–524, 1957.

SOBEL, H. J., SCHWARZ, R., and MARQUET, E.: Nonviral Nuclear Inclusions. I. Cytoplasmic Invaginations. Arch. Path. *87*:179–192, 1969.

STEVENS, C. E., *et al.*: Phlegmonous Gastritis in Cattle, Resulting from Ruminatoric Doses of Tatar Emetic. J. Am. Vet. Med. Assn. *134*:323–327, 1959.

STÖBER, M.: Die Gallenkolik des Rindes. Dtsch. tierarztl. Wschr. *68*:608–612, 647–651, 1961.

STONER, H. B.: The Mechanism of Toxic Hepatic Necrosis. Brit. J. Exper. Path. *37*:176–198. 1956.

STRANDE, A., SOMMERS, S. C., and PETRAK, M.: Regional Enterocolitis in Cocker Spaniel Dogs. Arch. Path. *57*:357–362, 1954.

SWEENEY, E. J.: The Aetiology of Dysentery of Swine. Vet. Rec. *78*:372–375, 1966.

THEILER, A.: Acute Liver Atrophy and Parenchymatous Hepatitis in Horses. Rep. Director Vet. Res., U. So. Afr. *5–6*:7–164, 1919.

THOMAS, R. M., and PRIER, J. E.: An Experimental Case of Urinary Calculus in a Steer. J. Am. Vet. Med. Assn. *120*:85–86, 1952.

THOMLINSON, J. R. and BUXTON, A.: Anaphylaxis in Pigs and its Relationship to the Pathogenesis of Oedema Disease and Gastroenteritis Associated with Escherichia coli. Immun. *6*:126–139, 1963.

TIMONEY, J. F.: Oedema Disease in Swine. Vet. Rec. *69*(No. 49, Pt. 2):1160–1171, 1957.

TOMITA, Y., and JONAS, A. M.: Two Viral Agents Isolated from Hamsters with a Form of Regional Enteritis: A Preliminary Report. Am. J. Vet. Res. *29*:445–453, 1968.

TODD, G. C., and KROOK, L.: Nutritional Hepatic Necrosis in Beef Cattle: "Sawdust Liver." Path. Vet. *3*:379–400, 1966.

UNDERDAHL, N. R., BLORE, I. C., and YOUNG, G. A.: Edema Disease of Swine. I. Preliminary Report on Experimental Transmission. J. Am. Vet. Med. Assn. *135*:615–617, 1959.

UNDERDAHL, N. R., STAIR, E. L., and YOUNG, G. A.: Transmission and Characterization of Edema Disease of Swine. J. Am. Vet. Med. Assn. *142*:27–30, 1963.

VALBERG, L. S., YOUNG, R. A., and BEVERIDGE, J. M. R.: The Effect of Unsaturation of Dietary Fat and of Antioxidants on the Development of Liver Damage. Canad. J. Biochem. Physiol. *37*:493–499, 1959.

VAN ES, L., CANTWELL, L. R., MARTIN, H. M., and KRAMER, J.: On the Nature and Cause of "Walking Disease" of Northwestern Nebraska. Exp. Sta. Bull. No. 43, Univ. of Nebraska, Lincoln. 1929.

VAN KRUININGEN, H. J. *et al.*: A Granulomatous Colitis of Dogs with Histologic Resemblance to Whipple's Disease. Path. Vet. *2*:521–544, 1965.

VAN KRUININGEN, H. J.: Granulomatous Colitis of Boxer Dogs: Comparative Aspects. Gastroenterology *53*:114–122, 1967.

VITUMS, A.: Portosystemic Communications in Animals with Hepatic Cirrhosis and Malignant Lymphoma. J. Am. Vet. Med. Assn. *138*:31–34, 1961.

WEINREB, M. M. and SHARAV, Y.: Tooth Development in Sheep. Am. J. Vet. Res. *25*: 891–908, 1964.

WILLIAMS, D. J., TYLER, D. E., and PAPP, E.: Abdominal Fat Necrosis as a Herd Problem in Georgia Cattle. J. Am. Vet. Med. Assn. *154*:1017–1021, 1969.

WOOD, J. S., BENNETT, I. L., and YARDLEY, J. H.: Staphylococcal Enterocolitis in Chinchillas. Bull. Johns Hopkins Hosp. *98*:454–463, 1956.

WRAY, C., and THOMLINSON, J. R.: Abomasal Ulceration in Calves. Vet. Rec. *83*:80–81, 1968.

WROBLEWSKI, F.: The Clinical Significance of Transaminase Activities of Serum. Am. J. Med. *27*:911–923, 1959.

WYLIE, J. A. H.: Renal and Hepatic Lesions in Experimental Leptospirosis Icterohaemorrhagica. J. Path. and Bact. *58*:351–358, 1946.

ZIMMERMAN, H. M., and HILLMAN, J. A.: Chronic Passive Congestion of the Liver. An Experimental Study. Arch. Path. *9*:1154–1163, 1930.

ZIOLECKI, A. and BRIGGS, C. A. E.: The Microflora of the Rumen of the Young Calf. II. Source, Nature and Development. J. Appl. Bact. *24*:148–163, 1961.

25

The Urinary System

THE KIDNEYS

Anatomy and Physiology

Certain features of renal structure and function are important in understanding the disorders to which the kidney is susceptible. It must be recalled that the blood entering the renal cortex is conducted first into the glomerulus by the latter's afferent arteriole. After passing through that tuft of intertwining capillaries, it is distributed by the efferent arteriole to capillaries that supply the tubules, apparently the tubular system of the same nephron to which the particular glomerulus belongs. Thus the delicate epithelial cells of the tubules, with their vital function of selective absorption, are dependent for their blood supply upon the free movement of blood through the tortuous passageways of the glomerulus. As will be explained, the glomerulus is unfortunately vulnerable to a number of lesions which interfere with this free flow of blood, and death and destruction of tubules as the result of such lesions are of frequent occurrence. Some studies indicate that the kidney may be provided with a small number of "arteriovenous shunts" which by-pass the glomeruli to carry blood directly to the tubules, but if such exist they are relatively unimportant and insufficient to obviate the effects of impeded passage through the glomeruli.

The glomeruli and their secretory function are almost equally dependent on proper conditions in the tubular regions, and there are situations in which swelling of the epithelium of the tubules raises the pressure within the non-yielding renal capsule to the point where blood is excluded from all structures of the kidney, including the glomeruli, thus stopping their function of urinary secretion.

The arteries supplying the renal cortex form no anastomoses with each other. For this reason, infarction of the renal cortex readily occurs. The infarcted areas take the form of pyramids with their bases at the capsule.

The vessels which traverse the outer medulla (arteriolae et venulae rectae) run parallel to the collecting tubules and tend to lie in groups so that when congested each group is represented by a red streak, radial in direction, which is readily visible to the naked eye.

It is computed that something like one-third of the cardiac output of blood goes to the kidney at each circuit, and that nearly 10 per cent of blood, equivalent to 16 per cent of the plasma, which passes through the glomerulus, filters freely into Bowman's capsule as the "glomerular filtrate." Only about 1 per cent of this is believed to be excreted as urine, the remaining 99 per cent being reabsorbed through the epithelium of the tubules. Electrolytes such as chlorides, carbonates, and bicarbonates, phosphates, silicates (herbivorous animals) and sulfates of ammonium, sodium, potassium and calcium, as well as various organic substances including glucose and urea, pass freely into the glomerular filtrate either to be excreted in the urine or to be reabsorbed more or less selectively by the epithelial cells.

At the same time that many are reabsorbed, a very few substances appear to be excreted by the epithelium of the tubules. These include creatinine in man but not apparently in the dog. Certain "renal clearance" tests are available for measuring the excretory power of the kidneys. The "clearance" is stated in cubic centimeters per minute and means the number of cubic centimeters of blood which, by concurrent analysis, is found to contain an amount of the substance, urea, for example, equal to that which the urine removes in the stated time.

Compounds with large molecules, especially the proteins, do not pass through the healthy glomerular filter, which is comparable to a dialyzing membrane, and do not appear in the normal urine. The presence of protein in the urine, commonly entitled simply albuminuria, is a readily determined clinical sign of injury to the glomeruli and a serious renal malfunction.

Glucose is absent from normal urine, because it is completely reabsorbed in the tubules unless its concentration in the blood is above a certain critical level called the renal threshold. The latter situation arises in diabetes mellitus, in which the glucose of the blood cannot be utilized, and at times immediately following an excessively large meal of carbohydrates.

Formation of urine can be prevented completely (anuria) or partially (oliguria) by various lesions in the glomeruli, by renal ischemia or by the excessive swelling of the tubular epithelium previously mentioned. When this occurs profound changes appear constituting the condition of uremia (p. 1294).

Glomeruli, once destroyed, do not regenerate, although those which remain may undergo some compensatory hypertrophy. Fortunately, the total number of nephrons is considerably in excess of requirements, so that many of them, or even a whole kidney, may be lost without fatal effects providing the remaining renal tissue is uninjured.

Destroyed tubular epithelium regenerates readily. The new cells have hyperchromatic nuclei but may be less columnar than their predecessors. It is not unusual to encounter tubules whose epithelium is flattened and whose lumens are large. These are variously interpreted as dilated because of obstruction, regenerated or hypertrophic with increased function compensatory to destruction of other tubules, or merely hyperplastic.

Nephron.—The essential anatomic and functional unit of the kidney is the nephron. Each kidney contains many nephrons, depending upon the species (the human kidneys are estimated to contain between one and two million). Each nephron is made up of the **glomerulus,** a spherical body which is formed by invagination of branching segments of an afferent arteriole into a terminal bud of a **renal tubule.** The renal tubule has distinct segments known as (1) the proximal convoluted tubule, (2) the loop of Henle with descending and ascending limbs and (3) the distal convoluted tubule which connects with a collecting duct which in turn empties into a duct of Bellini and then to the renal pelvis and ureter.

In the **glomerulus,** the afferent artery branches and re-anastomoses to form a capillary tuft which is intimately associated with the epithelial cells of the tubule and the visceral layer of Bowman's capsule. The glomerular space surrounds the

capillary tuft, communicates with the proximal convoluted tubule and is surrounded by an epithelial layer and a thin fibrous capsule—the parietal layer of
Bowman's capsule. At light microscopic magnification, the capillary endothelium
may be seen to be closely applied to the tubular epithelium, separated only by a
basement membrane. Under the electron microscope, much greater detail is
evident: The endothelial cell which lines the capillary lumen is stretched out
with only a thin layer of cytoplasm evident over most of its surface. This layer
may be fenestrated and is adjacent to the glomerular basement membrane which
has three layers—an electron dense layer separating two less compact layers.
The cells of the visceral layer of Bowman's capsule are in contact with the basement membrane by means of long extensions of the cytoplasm known as foot
processes, giving a name to these cells: **podocytes.** Between the foot processes,
spaces are found which form channels through which the glomerular filtrate is
believed to flow. In addition to the endothelial and epithelial cells, a third cell,
the **mesangial** or **intercapillary** cell, is found in the glomerulus. This cell is
located centrally within the capillary loops, one side of the capillary always facing
the mesangial cell. The basement membrane is thin and often incomplete in the
zone of juxtaposition with the mesangial cell (Rhodin, 1963). The cytoplasm of
the mesangial cell is similar to that of the epithelial cell but adjacent extracellular spaces contain fine reticular filaments and material similar to basement
membrane (**mesangial matrix**). The mesangium is involved in some pathologic
conditions (*e.g.* intercapillary glomerulosclerosis) which will be considered later.

The **proximal convoluted tubule** leaves the glomerulus as a short segment called
the neck piece. The tortuous tubule is lined by a single layer of cuboidal cells
which have a brush border on their luminal surface. Under the electron microscope this brush border is seen to consist of microvilli which increase the absorptive surface of the cells. Infoldings of the cell membrane also extend deep into
the cell from the base of the microvilli. Similar membranes extend into these
cells from their basal surface. Mitochondria are often found between these membranes. The **thin descending limb of** the **loop of Henle** continues the renal
tubule into the renal medulla. The epithelial cells lining this segment are flattened and contain few mitochondria. The loop is completed, usually in the
peripheral medulla, and the lining cells of this ascending limb are cuboidal and
contain numerous mitochondria. Their cytoplasm is for this reason usually
darker when viewed by light microscopy. At the point where the ascending limb
returns to the cortex, the tubule becomes the **distal convoluted tubule.** The
epithelial cells lining this segment are columnar but have clear cytoplasm and no
brush border. A few microvilli may be demonstrated with the electron microscope in these cells. Their basal surface bears deeply infolded cell membranes
which are closely aligned with many mitochondria.

At the point where the ascending limb joins the distal convoluted tubule, the
tubule lies in contact with its own afferent arteriole, near the hilus of the glomerulus. The epithelial cells at this point, called the **macula densa,** are uniformly
cuboidal and arranged in an easily recognized palisade adjacent to the afferent
arteriole. Cells in the media of the arteriole in this zone are enlarged and resemble cells of the aortic or carotid body. These cells are believed to have a
regulatory effect upon the flow of blood through the glomerulus. Together with
the **macula densa,** these cells of the arteriole form the **juxtaglomerular apparatus**
which is considered to be the source of **renin.**

In certain species, particularly the dog, rat and cat, the orifice in Bowman's capsule through which the neck piece of the proximal convoluted tubule passes may be widened under certain circumstances. This permits part of the tubule to protrude into Bowman's space and presents a puzzling feature in histologic sections. This phenomenon has been variously named "protrusions of tubular epithelium" or "infraglomerular epithelial reflux." Mullink and Feron (1967) present evidence that this histologically recognized feature is the result of postmortem change.

Anatomic differences between species are of some consequence in interpreting lesions in the kidneys. A few might be mentioned: Bovine animals have lobulated kidneys, similar to fetal lobulation in other species. Each lobule has multiple calices, a separate ureter and its blood is supplied through a single artery entering at the hilus. The kidney of the dog has a single renal ridge which extends the length of the kidney to form what amounts to a single papillus. The capsule is apt to be adherent and fat is normally present in tubular epithelium. The cat also frequently has fat in renal tubular epithelium and the kidneys are more moveable in the abdomen. The horse has many compound mucous glands in the renal pelvis.

The kidney of newborn and young animals may be recognized histologically by glomeruli which are small with hyperchromic epithelial and endothelial nuclei. The tubules are less well developed than in the adult and fewer nephrons have tubules which dip into the medulla. The young animal therefore has much less capacity to concentrate urine than does the adult.

Anatomy and Physiology

BHARADWAJ, M. B., and CALHOUN, M. L.: Histology of the Urethral Epithelium of Domestic Animals. Am. J. Vet. Res. 20:841–851, 1959.

CHRISTENSEN, G. C.: Circulation of Blood Through the Canine Kidney. Am. J. Vet. Res. 13:236–245, 1952.

CRAIGE, A. H., JR., et al.: Renal Excretion Following Intravenous Injection of Calcium Salts in the Normal Cow. Am. J. Vet. Res. 10:217–220, 1949.

EDWARDS, J. G.: The Formation of Urine. Arch. Int. Med. 65:800–824, 1940.

FISHER, E. R., COPELAND, C., and FISHER, B.: Correlation of Ultrastructure and Function Following Hypothermic Preservation of Canine Kidneys. Lab. Invest. 17:99–120, 1967.

FRIEDMAN, M., and BYERS, S. O.: Causes of the Excess Excretion of Uric Acid in the Dalmatian Dog. J. Biol. Chem. 175:727–735, 1948.

GOLDFARB, A. R., SANTAMARIA, L., and FOA, P. P.: Phosphorus Metabolism in the Dog Kidney. Proc. Soc. Exper. Bio . & Med. 84:523–526, 1953.

GRIFFITH, L. D., BULGER, R. E., and TRUMP, B. F.: The Ultrastructure of the Functioning Kidney. Lab. Invest. 16:220–246, 1967.

HUBER, G. C.: The Arteriolae Rectae of the Mammalian Kidney. Amer. J. Anat. 6:391–406, 1906–1907.

JORGENSEN, F.: Electron Microscopic Studies of Normal Glomerular Basement Membrane. Lab. Invest. 17:416–424, 1967.

LATIMER, H. B.: The Growth of the Kidneys and the Bladder in the Fetal Dog. Anat. Rec. 109:1–12, 1951.

MARSHALL, M. E., and DEUTSCH, H. F.: Clearances of Some Proteins by the Dog Kidney. Amer. J. Physiol. 163:461–467, 1950.

MAYER, E., and OTTOLENGHI, L. A.: Protrusion of Tubular Epithelium into the Space of Bowman's Capsule in Kidneys of Dogs and Cats. Anat. Rec. 99:477–510, 1947.

MOTTRAM, V. H.: Fat Infiltration of the Cat's Kidney. J. Biol. Chem. 24:11–12, 1916.

MOUSTGAARD, J.: Variation of the Renal Function in Normal and Unilaterally Nephrectomized Dogs. Am. J. Vet. Res. 8:301–306, 1947.

MULLINK, J. W. M. A., and FERON, V. J.: Infraglomerular Epithelial Reflux as a Postmortem Phenomenon in the Kidneys of Dog and Rat. Path. Vet. 4:366–377, 1967.

RHODIN, J. A. G.: An Atlas of Ultrastructure, W. B. Saunders Co., Philadelphia, 1963.

SMITH, H. A.:   *Renal Lipidosis*. Thesis. Univ. Michigan, Ann Arbor, 1949.
WOLFSON, W. Q., COHN, C., and SHORE, C.:   The Renal Mechanism for Urate Excretion in
the Dalmatian Coach-hound. J. Exper. Med. *92*:121–128, 1950.
YADAVA, R. P., and CALHOUN, M. L.:   Comparative Histology of the Kidney of Domestic
Animals. Am. J. Vet. Res. *19*:958–968, 1958.

Congenital and Hereditary Anomalies

Anomalies of the kidney have been reported in man and many other species.
Some are known to be caused by inherited factors, others are of unknown etiology.
The most frequently reported involves **aplasia** or **agenesis** of one or both kidneys.
Absence of both kidneys of course is incompatible with life and would be encountered only in the fetus, newborn or stillborn animal. On the other hand, aplasia
of one kidney results in compensatory hypertrophy of the remaining kidney and
the individual may cope with life quite well. Agenesis of kidneys has been reported in the pig, dog, cat, rat, mouse and howler monkey (*Alouatta caraya*).

Renal hypoplasia describes kidneys in newborn or young animals, which are
markedly smaller than normal with little or no function. Cordes and Dodd, 1965,
described bilateral renal hypoplasia in 19 swine, 12 of which were born dead or
died within two days of birth. Varying degrees of hypoplasia were found, from
tiny almost unrecognizable kidneys to bilobed kidneys or kidneys with distinct
fetal lobulation. All affected piglets were sired by the same boar and the evidence
indicated probable control of the defect by a single recessive autosomal gene.
This condition has also been recognized in the dog (Fig. 4–1, p. 93) and cat.

Horseshoe Kidney.—This descriptive name is applied to the appearance of
kidneys which are fused at one pole to produce a horseshoe-shaped structure
centered roughly in the midline of the abdomen. The ureters are usually intact
and the kidneys function adequately in most instances. This condition has been
reported in man and cat.

Vascular Anomalies.—Congenital variations in origin and course of renal
arteries and veins are sometimes observed, usually at time of necropsy. These
have no deleterious effects, except in those instances in which their position
partially occludes the ureter. In this instance, hydronephrosis might result.

Displacement.—The anatomic position of the kidneys is retroperitoneal in all
species, but the exact position varies between species and to some extent between
individuals. In the cat, for example, the kidneys during life may be quite moveable if the blood vessels are longer than usual. This so-called "floating kidney"
appears to have little pathologic significance.

Cysts in the Kidney.—Cysts are not infrequently seen in the kidneys of
various species but are considerably more common in swine and dogs than in the
other domestic animals. They may be solitary or very numerous, varying in
size from those just visible to the eye up to a diameter of about a centimeter in
the case of multiple cysts of the pig and dog, or of several centimeters in the case
of a single cyst. Their walls are usually thin and transparent, their contents
clear and watery, perhaps tinged with yellow. They may bulge from the surface
or lie buried in the depths of the parenchyma. Cysts may arise from gradual
distention of a nephron whose outlet has been closed, usually by the pressure of
exudates or fibrous tissue. But if the kidney contains a considerable number of
cysts, the disorder is usually that designated as the **congenital polycystic kidney.**
In man, Osathanondh and Potter (1964) have described three types of polycystic

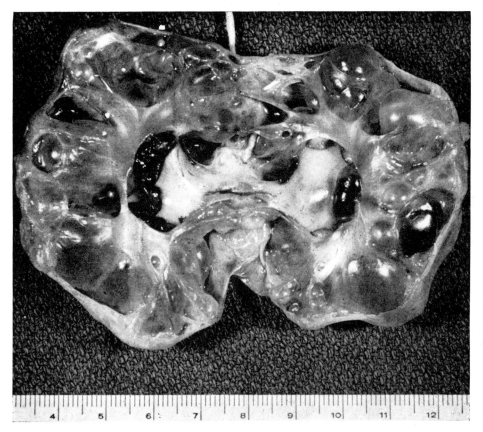

FIG. 25–1.—Polycystic kidney from an eight-year-old spayed female cat.
(Courtesy of Angell Memorial Animal Hospital.)

renal disease, each arising from abnormal fetal development, as follows: Type I, due to dilatation and hyperplasia of collecting tubules, saccular or cylindrical dilatations develop in all collecting tubules. This results in bilaterally symmetrical, sponge-like appearance in the kidneys. The dilated channels lie at right angles to the surface of the cortex, completely replacing the medulla and cortex. The cysts are lined with uniform cuboidal epithelium. This type is found only in infants because it is not compatible with prolonged survival. Cystic bile ducts are often present also and a familial, possibly hereditary, origin is postulated.

Type II congenital polycystic renal disease is considered to be due to inhibition of ureteral ampullary activity. It is believed that failure of the ureteral ampullary regions to branch results in the absence of collecting tubules and consequent failure of nephrons to develop. The cysts tend to be asymmetrical but may involve one or both kidneys. The cysts tend to be large, thick-walled and separated by dense connective tissue in which few nephrons and irregular blood vessels may be embedded. This type is compatible with life unless large parts of both kidneys are involved.

Type III polycystic kidneys, according to Osathanondh and Potter (1964) are due to multiple abnormalities of development. Normal and cystic nephrons are admixed in involved kidneys and survival is possible to adulthood, depending on the number of functional nephrons. In this type, often bilateral, masses of cysts often result in greatly enlarged kidneys. The cysts contain clear or sometimes bloody fluid (Fig. 25–1). The cysts are thought to arise from tubules or parts of nephrons. When Bowman's capsules are involved, remnants of glomeruli may be found in some cysts. This human type has been seen in cats.

Cysts, whether of the congenital type or not, tend to enlarge slowly and, by pressure atrophy, to cause progressive loss of functioning renal parenchyma, so that in early or middle life renal insufficiency develops with lethal results. This is true in dogs and cats as well as in human beings; in swine, the cystic kidney is usually revealed at slaughter. Cysts are also known in the peripelvic tissues from obstruction of the lymphatic vessels there; these are very rare.

Congenital and Hereditary Anomalies

CORDES, D. O., and DODD, D. C.: Bilateral Renal Hypoplasia of the Pig. Path. Vet. *2*: 37–48, 1965.
HUNT, H. R.: Absence of One Kidney in the Domestic Cat. Anat. Rec. *15*:221–223, 1918.
JOHNSON, C. E.: Pelvic and Horseshoe Kidneys in the Domestic Cat. Anat. Anz. *46*:69–78, 1914.
KARDEVAN, A.: Cystic Kidneys in Cattle, Originating from Bowman's Capsule. Magy. Allatorv. Lap. *19*:444–446, 1964. V.B. *35*:3967, 1965.
LEIGHTON, C.: Canine Nephrosis Associated with Absence of the Other Kidney. J. Comp. Path. and Therap. *16*:171–173, 1903.
MACK, C. O., and McGLOTHLIN, J. H.: Renal Agenesis in the Female Cat. Anat. Rec. *105*: 445–450, 1949.
MARUFFO, C. A., and CRAMER, D. L.: Congenital Renal Malformations in Monkeys. Folia Primat. *5*:305–311, 1967.
McCLURE, C. F. W.: Abnormalities in Connection with the Post-Caval Vein and Its Tributaries in the Domestic Cat. Amer. Naturalist. *34*:185–198, 1900.
McFARLAND, L. Z., and DENIZ, E.: Unilateral Renal Agenesis with Ipsilateral Cryptorchidism and Perineal Hypospadias in a Dog. J. Am. Vet. Med. Assn. *139*:1099–1100, 1969.
ROBBINS, G. R.: Unilateral Renal Agenesis in the Beagle. Vet. Rec. *77*:1345–1347, 1965.
STORY, H. E.: A Case of Horseshoe Kidney and Associated Vascular Anomalies in the Domestic Cat. Anat. Rec. *86*:307–319, 1943.
TANNREUTHER, G. W.: Abnormal Urogenital System in the Domestic Cat. Anat. Rec. *25*: 59–62, 1923.
VYMETAL, F.: Renal Aplasia in Beagles. Vet. Rec. *77*:1344–1345, 1965.

Diseases of Glomeruli

Acute Proliferative Glomerulonephritis.—A clinical syndrome associated with characteristic renal lesions has been known in children for many years and more recently has been identified as a spontaneous and experimentally-induced disease entity in animals. The human disease, which characteristically affects young children but may appear in adults, typically follows by two weeks or more an acute upper respiratory infection by streptococci. The onset of the renal disease is sudden with fever, nausea, weakness, subcutaneous edema and excretion of brown or bloody urine in scant amounts. The fever may abate in about a week but abnormalities in the urine may persist and some cases may continue as a chronic disease. Subacute or chronic glomerulonephritis (p. 1263) may eventually result.

The **lesion** in glomeruli is quite characteristic under the light microscope. Although not recognizable definitively in the gross, the kidney may be enlarged and pale with petechiae outlining the glomeruli. The glomeruli are initially congested or edematous and conspicuous at low magnification. The glomerular tufts are increased in size, with increased numbers of endothelial ("fixed tissue cells") filling Bowman's space. In this early stage, leukocytes, particularly neutrophils, appear in the glomerulus. This influx and proliferation of cells result in compression of the capillaries and the absence of red blood cells. As the disease progresses, epithelial cells also proliferate and some may adhere to the parietal layer of Bowman's capsule. These eventually form the epithelial "crescents" seen in subacute or chronic forms. Thrombosis and necrosis of glomerular capillaries may occur, with subsequent hemorrhage into the glomerulus. No obvious thickening of the basement membrane or alteration in the foot processes of epithelial cells are found by examination with the electron microscope.

Leukocytic infiltration may occur adjacent to glomeruli or in nearby interstitial tissues. Proximal convoluted tubules may contain red cell casts or red blood cells. Fatty changes may occur in the epithelium of convoluted tubules, presumably due to interference with the flow of blood through the glomeruli.

Etiology and Pathogenesis.—The causes and mechanisms involved in this so-called poststreptococcal glomerulonephritis have been under investigation for many years but not all facets are understood even yet. Direct action by the streptococci is not considered to occur because organisms are not found in the affected kidneys nor in the urine. The immunologic nature of the disease is indicated by (1) the appearance of elevated titres of antibodies to streptococci (antistreptokinase, antistreptolysin, antihyaluronidase and antideoxyribonuclease) in the plasma of patients, (2) the demonstration of gamma globulins localized in the

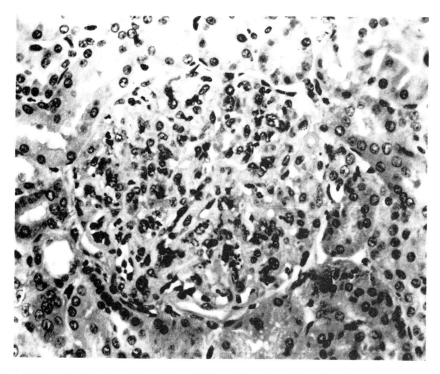

Fig. 25–2.—Proliferative glomerulonephritis. Nine-year-old male dog. Glomerulus fills Bowman's space and contains numerous nuclei, including leukocytes. The basement membrane may also be thickened. (Courtesy of Armed Forces Institute of Pathology.)

glomerular basement membranes by fluorescence antibody techniques and (3) the production of similar lesions in experimental animals with immunologic methods.

Masugi (1934) first produced an experimental model of glomerulonephritis by injecting rats with an antiserum prepared by immunizing rabbits with preparations of rat kidney. This antibody localized in the glomerular basement membranes and resulted in a glomerulonephritis sometimes referred to as "nephrotoxic nephritis." It has been found subsequently that the antigen in this system is glomerular basement membrane and that its antigenicity is not species specific. In the natural disease it is possible that some autoimmune mechanism (p. 312) may make the animal's basement membrane antigenic to its own immune mechanisms, or more likely, that bacteria or viruses may contain common antigens which are selectively deposited with antibody on basement membranes. It appears that immunologic mechanisms are involved in this disease even though not all the details are established.

Naturally occurring lesions suggestive of proliferative glomerulonephritis have been reported in sheep, cattle and goats (Lerner and Dixon, 1966; Lerner, Dixon and Lee, 1968). These workers described hypercellular glomeruli with deposition of immunoglobulin along the basement membranes of glomerular capillaries with proteinuria in some cases. The antibody deposited on the basement membranes were assumed to be antigen-antibody complexes because antibodies to glomerular basement membrane were not demonstrable. This interesting observation deserves further study to answer several questions, among them would be: why should so many apparently healthy sheep be affected?; why is the "disease" rarely progressive or accompanied by proteinuria, azotemia, or eventual uremia?; could the "hypercellular" glomeruli and mild proteinuria be within normal limits for this species?

Proliferative Glomerulonephritis

BURKHOLDER, P. M.: Ultrastructural Demonstration of Injury and Perforation of Glomerular Capillary Basement Membrane in Acute Proliferative Glomerulonephritis. Amer. J. Path. *56*:251–266, 1969.
FISHER, E. R., and FISHER, B.: Glomerular Lipoidosis in the Dog. Am. J. Vet. Res. *15*: 285–286, 1954.
FRENCH, J.: Glomerulonephrosis. A Morphologic Manifestation of Renal Cortical Ischemia in Toxic Oliguria and Lower Nephron Nephrosis. Arch. Path. *49*:43–54, 1950.
LERNER, R. A., and DIXON, F. J.: Spontaneous Glomerulonephritis in Sheep. Lab. Invest. *15*:1279–1289, 1966.
LERNER, R. A., DIXON, F. J., and LEE, S.: Spontaneous Glomerulonephritis in Sheep. II. Studies on Natural History, Occurrence in Other Species, and Pathogenesis. Amer. J. Path. *53*:501–512, 1968.
MARGOLIS, G., *et al.*: Glomerulonephritis Occurring in Experimental Brucellosis in Dogs. Amer. J. Path. *23*:983–993, 1947.
MASUGI, M.: Uber die experimentelle glomerulonephritis durch das specifische antinierenserum. Bietr. Path. Anat. *92*:429–440, 1934.
McFADYEAN, J.: Nephritis in Animals. J. Comp. Path. and Therap. *42*:58–71, 141–162, 231–241, 1929.

Membranous Glomerulonephritis.—Rather clearly distinguishable from proliferative glomerulonephritis in man, membranous glomerulonephritis also occurs naturally as a distinct entity in other animals. In individual cases, however, differentiation is not always simple and it is possible for both forms to occur simultaneously. Membranous glomerulonephritis is distinguished in the final analysis by certain features detected by study of sections with light and electron microscopy, and also by some distinguishing clinical characteristics. It is believed to be the most frequent cause of the nephrotic syndrome (p. 1266) in man and usually has an insidious onset and prolonged course in man or animals. Early studies in children associated the clinical disease with deposits of lipid in epithelial cells of proximal convoluted tubules, but changes in glomeruli were overlooked, hence the now obsolete name "lipoid nephrosis" was applied.

The morphologic changes which identify membranous glomerulonephritis are: (1) thickening, splitting and reduplication of the glomerular basement membrane, and (2) loss of the foot processes of the podocytes (epithelial cells) of the glomerulus. With the electron microscope, the earliest detectable lesions appear to be the loss of the foot processes and spaces between glomerular basement membrane and epithelial cells by the application of broad segments of the epithelium to the external surface of the basement membrane. Later in the course of the disease, the glomerular basement membrane becomes irregularly thickened with scalloped portions along its external (epithelial) border. This thickening of the basement membrane becomes severe enough to be recognized by light microscopy and is particularly evident in sections stained by periodic acid Schiff (PAS) methods. Sometimes, proteinaceous materials deposited on the external surface of the basement membrane make it appear even more thick. The thickened basement membrane is sometimes described as resembling a "wire loop" in microscopic section. The epithelial cells in the glomerulus may become swollen, and laden with fat, giving the glomerulus a hypercellular appearance. Similar lipid vacuoles in the cells of the proximal convoluted tubules may be expected.

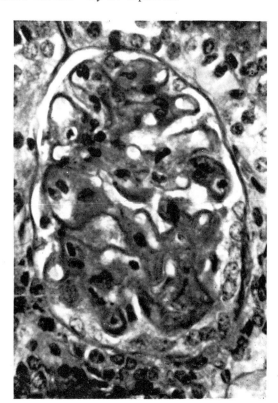

FIG. 25–3.—Diffuse membranous glomerulonephritis in mouse with chronic allogeneic disease. Note thickened basement membranes and mesangium. (Courtesy of Dr. Robert M. Lewis and *The Journal of Experimental Medicine*.)

After a prolonged course, the glomerulus may become enlarged, hypercellular and distend Bowman's capsule. The glomerular space is rarely obliterated, however, and epithelial crescents and adhesions are not usual. The glomerulus is not only dense and cellular but is essentially bloodless at this stage.

Grossly, the kidney affected with membranous glomerulonephritis is usually enlarged and pallid ("large pale kidney"), presumably due to the fatty changes and increase in interstitial fluid caused by generalized edema. In some stages, the kidney may become contracted and fibrous as an end stage. The possibility of chronic glomerulonephritis resulting from this entity must also be considered.

The etiologic factors in membranous glomerulonephritis are in general believed to involve immunologic processes which result in deposition of immunoglobulins, or immune complexes, on the glomerular basement membrane. The deposition of immunoglobulins on the basement membrane has been clearly shown by immunofluorescence techniques applied to microscopic tissue sections. In some situations, as in experimental "nephrotoxic nephritis," the antigen for this antibody is glomerular basement membrane (GBM) in others bacterial or viral antigens may be involved. Nephritogenic streptococcal antigens are not usually incriminated, as they are in proliferative ("poststreptococcal") glomerulonephritis.

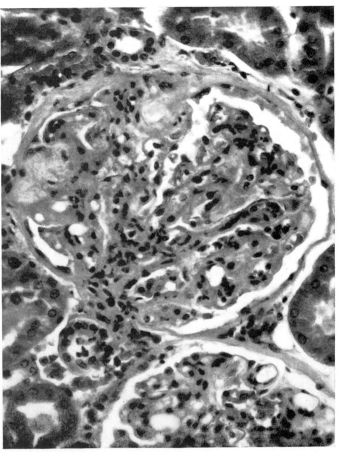

Fig. 25–4.   Membranous glomerulonephritis in an aged dog. Basement membranes thickened and adhesions to Bowman's capsule. (Courtesy of Armed Forces Institue of Pathology.)

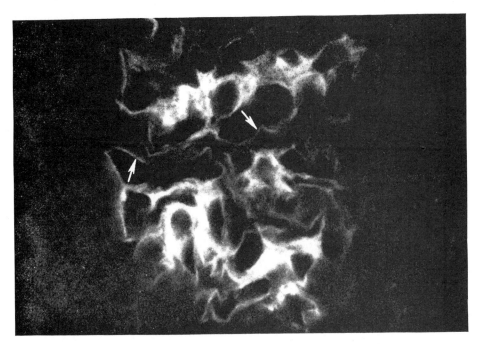

Fig. 25–5.—Fluorescent labeling of basement membranes (arrows) and mesangium (diffuse areas) of allogeneic mouse. Anti-basement membrane antiglobulin is deposited in the basement membrane and the mesangium. (Courtesy of Dr. Robert M. Lewis.)

One such antigen has been demonstrated in mice to be the lymphocytic chorio-meningitis virus. This virus produces choriomeningitis (p. 391) in mice under certain circumstances and may be transmitted congenitally to unborn mice even though they are delivered by cesarean section and raised under "germfree" conditions (Kajima and Pollard, 1970). Such congenitally infected mice even-tually develop hypergammaglobulinemia and membranous glomerulonephritis. Viral particles have been demonstrated in glomerular epithelium and are believed to be the antigen which stimulates the antibody deposited in the glomeruli. Electron micrographs reveal changes in and on both sides of the glomerular base-ment membrane. In endothelial cells, microvilli are increased and granular material is present in plasma spaces. Prolonged cytoplasmic projections of mesangial cells occur into the capillary loops. The mesangium is enlarged by fibrinoid deposits and mesangial cells proliferate. Fibrinoid material is also deposited in subendothelial spaces. Large amounts of similar material in endo-thelial cells occlude the capillary lumen. The basement membrane is thickened by fibrinoid deposits, intramembranous dense deposits, true thickening and focal irregularities. Loss of foot processes of epithelial cells is also evident.

Another naturally occurring membranous glomerulonephritis has been de-scribed in certain inbred mice, originating in New Zealand. These mice, the NZB/BL strain, were noted occasionally to die spontaneously with hemolytic anemia. Hybrids with a "normal" strain (NZW) were found to have a spontane-ous disease in which weight loss, progressive anemia, hepatosplenomegaly, alopecia, positive lupus erythematosus (LE) preparations (p. 1174) and circulating autoantibody, free and on red blood cells, were conspicuous features. Death occurred at eight to ten months of age from renal failure. Anti-mouse globulins were demonstrable in glomerular basement membranes by suitable immunofluorescence techniques and lesions of membranous glomerulonephritis were evident by light microscopy. Ultrastructural studies (Comerford, Cohen and Desai, 1968) demonstrated the earliest changes to be nodular deposits of material on the epithelial aspects of glomerular basement membrane plus small dense deposits in the mesangium. Subepithelial and subendothelial dense deposits on the basement membrane occurred subsequently. The mesangial deposits then increased in size. This glomerular lesion resembles systemic lupus erythematosus of man but differs in some minute details. A virus is also suspected in this murine disease.

Canine lupus erythematosus, described by Lewis, *et al.* (1963, 1965), is another animal disease complex which closely simulates the human syndrome. The canine disease is manifest by recurring episodes of hemolytic anemia and thrombocytopenia (p. 1174) demonstrable by the Coombs test and LE (lupus erythematosus) preparations to have an autoimmune basis, the antigen being nuclear deoxyribonucleic acid (DNA). Some canine patients are affected with a type of arthritis typical of the rheumatoid type and most eventually die from membranous glomerulonephritis. The renal lesions are typical of those described previously in this chapter.

Membranous Glomerulonephritis

BEN-ISHAY, Z., *et al.*:   Fine Structure Alterations in the Canine Kidney During Hemorrhagic Hypotension. Effects of Osmotic Diuresis. Lab. Invest. *17*:190–210, 1967.
COMERFORD, F. R., COHEN, A. S., and DESAI, R. G.:   The Evolution of the Glomerular Lesion in NZB Mice. A Light- and Electron-Microscopic Study. Lab. Invest. *19*:643–651, 1968.
FOLEY, W. A., *et al.*:   A Renal Lesion Associated with Diuresis in the Aging Sprague-Dawley Rat. Lab. Invest. *13*:439–450, 1964.
GRISHMAN, E., *et al.*:   Lupus Nephritis with Organized Deposits in the Kidneys. Lab. Invest. *16*:717–725, 1967.
GUDE, W. D., and UPTON, A. C.:   A Histologic Study of Spontaneous Glomerular Lesions in Aging RF Mice. Amer. J. Path. *40*:699–709, 1962.
GUTTMAN, P. H., and KOHN, H. I.:   Progressive Intercapillary Glomerulosclerosis in the Mouse, Rat and Chinese Hamster, Associated with Aging and X-ray Exposure. Amer. J. Path. *37*:293–307, 1960.
HELYER, B. J., and HOWIE, J. B.:   Renal Disease Associated with Positive Lupus Erythematosus Tests in a Cross-bred Strain of Mice. Nature (Lond.) *197*:197, 1963.
HENSON, J. B., GORHAM, J. R., and TANAKA, Y.:   Renal Glomerular Ultrastructure in Mink Affected by Aleutian Disease. Lab. Invest. *17*:123–139, 1967.
KAJIMA, M., and POLLARD, M.:   Ultrastructural Pathology of Glomerular Lesions in Gnotobiotic Mice with Congenital Lymphocytic Choriomeningitis (LCM) Virus Infection. Amer. J. Path. *61*:117–140, 1970.
KINDIG, D., SPARGO, B., and KIRSTEN, W. H.:   Glomerular Response in Aleutian Disease of Mink. Lab. Invest. *16*:436–443, 1967.
LAMBERT, P. H., and DIXON, F. J.:   Pathogenesis of the Glomerulonephritis of the NZB/W Mice. J. Exper. Med. *127*:507–521, 1968.
LERNER, R. A., and DIXON, F. J.:   Induced and Spontaneous Glomerulonephritis in Sheep. Fed. Proc. *25*:660, 1966.
LEWIS, R. M., *et al.*:   A Syndrome of Autoimmune Hemolytic Anemia and Thrombocytopenia in Dogs. Sci. Proc. AVMA 140–163, 1963.
LEWIS, R. M.:   Clinical Evaluation of the Lupus Erythematosus Cell Phenomenon in Dogs. J. Am. Vet. Med. Assn. *147*:939–943, 1965.
LEWIS, R. M., SCHWARTZ, R. S., and GILMORE, C. E.:   Autoimmune Diseases in Domestic Animals. Ann. New York Acad. Sci. *124*:178–200, 1965.
LEWIS, R. M., SCHWARTZ, R. S., and HENRY, W. B.:   Canine Systemic Lupus Erythematosus. Blood *25*:143–160, 1965.
LEWIS, R. M., *et al.*:   Chronic Allogeneic Disease. I. Development of Glomerulonephritis. J. Exper. Med. *128*:653–679, 1968.

Porter, D. D., Dixon, F. J., and Larsen, A. E.: Metabolism and Function of Gamma Globulin in Aleutian Disease of Mink. J. Exper. Med. *121*:889–900, 1965.

Recher, L., *et al.*: Further Studies on the Biological Relationship of Murine Leukemia Viruses and on Kidney Lesions of Mice. With Leukemia Induced by These Viruses. Nat'l. Cancer Inst. Monogr. *22*:459–479, 1966.

Sun, S.-C., *et al.*: Coxsackie B₄ Viral Nephritis in Mice and Its Autoimmune-like Phenomena. Proc. Soc. Exper. Biol. Med. *126*:882–885, 1967.

Chronic Glomerulonephritis.—This lesion currently appears to be the late stage of one or more of the various forms of glomerulonephritis. At this writing it is not known which forms of glomerular disease are most often responsible for this lesion. This end stage of glomerular disease may be encountered at necropsy and is often the lesion which results in terminal uremia. The clinical manifestations are variable and depend upon the number of glomeruli affected as well as the degree of malfunction in involved glomeruli.

Microscopically, the lesions in glomeruli include increased numbers of cells (endothelial, mesangial and epithelial) in the glomerulus with disorganization and occlusion of the lumens of glomerular capillaries. The proliferating epithelial cells may accumulate along the parietal layer of Bowman's capsule to form the so-called "epithelial crescents." Adhesions of the glomerulus to Bowman's capsule may occur and Bowman's space is often obliterated. Electron micrographs confirm the proliferation of epithelial and endothelial cells and disclose reduplication, thickening and disorganization of the glomerular basement membrane. The lumen of capillaries is usually occluded. In advanced stages, the entire glomerulus is replaced by hyaline connective tissue.

Interference with the circulation through the glomerulus obviously decreases

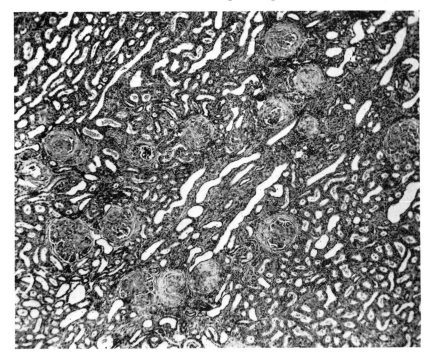

Fig. 25–6.—Chronic glomerulonephritis in a one-year-old male dog. Thick, fibrotic Bowman's capsules, fibrosis of glomerular tufts, adhesions to Bowman's capsule. (Courtesy of Armed Forces Institute of Pathology.)

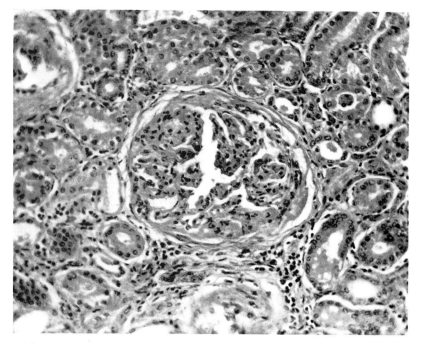

FIG. 25–7.—Chronic glomerulonephritis in a two-year-old female dog. Fibrosis of glomerular tuft, obliteration of Bowman's space, adhesions of glomerulus to Bowman's capsule. (Courtesy of Armed Forces Institute of Pathology.)

the blood supply to the tubular parts of the nephron and leads to their degeneration. Severe fibrosis of the interstitium results from this ischemia and many tubules atrophy.

As the fibrous connective tissue contracts, the kidney tends to decrease in size and increase in density. At this end stage it is difficult to reconstruct the events in glomeruli, tubules or interstitium which may have led to this combination of lesions. Such kidneys are usually smaller than normal, rough or pitted on the surface and tough to cut, often with a coarse, granular or cystic cut surface.

It is evident that chronic glomerulonephritis from the pathologist's viewpoint, represents a definite combination of lesions which obviously seriously interfered with renal function during life but whose etiology and pathogenesis cannot be discerned in each individual case. This lesion has been reported in many mammalian and reptilian species (Zwart, 1964). Presumably, it would be found in all mammals by adequate study of these species.

Chronic Glomerulonephritis

BURKHOLDER, P. M., MARCHAND, A., and KRUEGER, R. P.: Mixed Membranous and Proliferative Glomerulonephritis. Lab. Invest. 23:459–479, 1970.

DIDOMIZIO, G., and MINOCCHERI, F.: (Ultrastructural Aspects of Diffuse Glomerulosclerosis in the Dog: Pathogenesis and Lesions). Archo. Vet. Ital. 18:29–48, 1967. V.B. 37:4880, 1967.

HAMILTON, J. M.: Nephritis in the Cat. J. Small Anim. Pract. 7:445–449, 1966.

HOE, C. M., and O'SHEA, J. D.: The Correlation of Biochemistry and Histopathology in Kidney Disease in the Dog. Vet. Rec. 77:210–217 and 218, 1965.

LUCKE, V. M.: Renal Disease in the Domestic Cat. J. Path. Bact. 95:67–91, 1968.

RICHARDS, M. A., and HOE, C. M.: A Long-term Study of Renal Disease in the Dog. Vet. Rec. 80:640–646, 1967.

ZWART, P.: Studies on Renal Pathology in Reptiles. Path. Vet. 1:542–556, 1964.

Focal Glomerulitis.—In the course of many bacteremias and toxemias, changes may occur in scattered glomeruli which do not represent diffuse glomerulonephritis but are recognized in histologic sections. These glomeruli do not contain identifiable bacterial emboli but in some respects resemble focal embolic glomerulonephritis (below). The lesion of focal glomerulitis consists of swelling and proliferation of endothelial and epithelial cells in one or more lobules of the glomerulus, accompanied by focal infiltrations of neutrophil leukocytes. Involved glomeruli may be scattered throughout the kidney but do not occur in significant numbers.

Focal Embolic Glomerulonephritis.—This lesion is most often a sequel to a localized bacterial infection elsewhere in the body. In man, acute bacterial endocarditis is the most common antecedent—a situation which also occurs in other species, particularly the cow and dog. Other sources of infection may also be possible, such as bacterial pneumonia, reticulitis and other localized infections. Emboli of infected necrotic tissue are presumed to reach the glomeruli to initiate the lesion although the presence of organisms is not always demonstrable.

In some instances, however, colonies of bacteria may be demonstrable in glomeruli (Fig. 25–8) and some of these may lead to frank abscesses (Fig. 25–11C).

The lesion is recognized by light microscopy as a focal zone of necrosis, usually involving part of the glomerulus, with neutrophil infiltration and occasionally hemorrhage. Affected glomeruli are patchily scattered throughout the kidneys. In some, proliferation of epithelial cells and formation of "crescents" may occur, making the lesion difficult to distinguish from proliferative glomerulonephritis. In this latter situation, necrosis is not as conspicuous and larger numbers of glomeruli are involved nearly simultaneously.

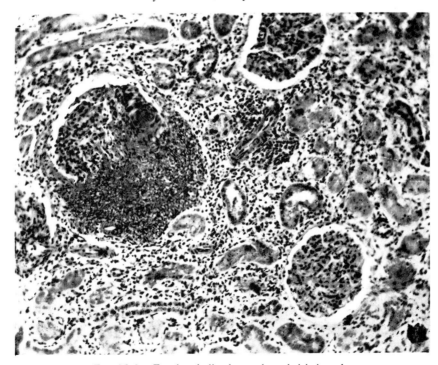

FIG. 25–8.—Focal embolic glomerulonephritis in a dog.
(Courtesy of Armed Forces Institute of Pathology.)

Affected kidneys may bear scattered petechiae and occasionally multiple tiny abscesses. In the bovine, one or more renal lobules may be affected with most of the kidney free of gross involvement. Although frank embolism is not demonstrable in each case, it seems expedient to consider this lesion in animals to be most often the result of bacterial embolism.

Amyloid in the Kidney.—Originating in close association with the walls of blood vessels, as explained in the general discussion of amyloidosis (p. 47), amyloid usually reaches conspicuous proportions in the glomeruli, dogs and horses being the most frequent sufferers. Microscopically, the amount is seen to be small in the early stages, but eventually many renal corpuscles are almost completely replaced by amyloid. The amyloid usually remains more or less lobulated, however, which facilitates distinguishing amyloidosis from hyaline scarring of glomeruli. Grossly, the change is not easily detected, but the application of an iodine solution such as Lugol's to a slice of fresh kidney which has previously been exposed to a weak acid brings out affected glomeruli as conspicuous brown spots visible to the naked eye.

As amyloid formation advances, the substance is found also among the tubules, first in the medullary tissue but eventually in all parts. When involvement is widespread (which is not often), the kidney is irregularly firm and pale. In advanced cases, oliguria, renal insufficiency and azotemia slowly develop.

Nephrotic Syndrome.—This is a clinical syndrome, best known in human patients but also occurring occasionally in animals. It should not be confused with **nephrosis,** a term used to refer to specific pathologic entities. The nephrotic syndrome is manifest by (1) proteinuria, principally albuminuria, (2) hypoproteinemia (3) generalized edema (anasarca), (4) hyperlipemia (especially hypercholesterolemia) and (5) lipiduria. The syndrome may result from any of the disseminated diseases of glomeruli (membranous glomerulonephritis, proliferative glomerulonephritis, amyloidosis, nodular glomerulosclerosis), thrombosis of renal veins, or rarely toxic tubular nephrosis.

The syndrome is believed to result from increased permeability of the glomeruli to protein, permitting it to be lost with the urine. The exact mechanism is unknown but present theories include the concepts that (1) the glomerular basement membrane is chiefly responsible for the filtration or (2) the podocytes are responsible for this function. Lesions in one or the other of these structures could account for increased permeability, resulting in the loss of protein.

Other Glomerular Lesions

ARAKAWA, M.: A Scanning Electron Microscopy of the Glomerulus of Normal and Nephrotic Rats. Lab. Invest. *23*:489–496, 1970.
PLATT, H.: A Case of Generalized Amyloidosis in the Dog. J. Comp. Path. and Therap. *59*: 91–96, 1949.

Diseases of Renal Tubules

Toxic Tubular Nephrosis.—In this condition various irritant toxic substances act directly and without any previous hypersensitization to produce fatty change and necrosis of the delicate epithelial cells lining the tubules, a sequence of degenerative changes which have already been seen to result from the actions of similar toxins on the epithelium of the liver. There are also hyperemia and, somewhat later, very limited infiltrations of lymphocytes and proliferation of fibrous tissue.

These minor evidences of inflammation have caused many to use the term nephritis to designate this lesion. We now consider the term nephrosis to be more appropriate. This pathologic entity should not be confused with the clinical "nephrotic syndrome" (p. 1266).

The proximal convoluted tubules, with their large and doubtless highly specialized epithelial cells, suffer most, especially with respect to necrosis, which may in some toxemias (as poisoning from the budding leaves of certain oaks, p. 859) leave these tubules as solid, dense-appearing masses of coagulated protoplasm. The lipidosis may be most extensive in these tubules or it may appear chiefly or exclusively in the epithelium of the ascending loops of Henle, especially in the medullary rays. This difference may well have diagnostic significance, but the exact distinctions have not been elucidated. Another change occasionally seen in the proximal convoluted tubules is a sort of albuminous degeneration in which the cytoplasm of dying cells is converted into round, pink-staining hyaline droplets of a size somewhat greater than a nucleus. This is the "hyaline-droplet degeneration" described by some authors. Calcification, usually in the form of granules no larger than one or two cells, is not unusual in tubules which persist after a limited amount of necrosis. The gross appearance of toxic tubular nephrosis is that of the large pale kidney.

If degeneration and necrosis have not become too extensive, regeneration of the epithelial lining cells is possible upon removal of the cause. Hence, a most important aspect of treatment in the case of acute nephrotoxic poisonings is the adoption of measures (the "artificial kidney") designed to avoid a fatal uremia before regeneration and restoration of tubular function can occur, a period of ten days or more. In fatal cases, the proximal tubules, at least, suffer complete destruction; the other parts of the nephron follow the same course less rapidly. In case the patient survives, the place of the lost tubules is partly taken by the fibrous tissue of chronic inflammation, producing the "small, white, granular contracted kidney." The glomeruli may survive and, with the loss of most of the intervening tubular structures, they come to lie very close together, giving the erroneous impression that their number has been increased. All of the above changes may advance rapidly in one segment of the kidney but leave an adjacent part untouched. This is probably because of a physiological tendency of one group of nephrons to function while another rests, the nonfunctioning group often escaping a transient severe concentration of the blood-borne poison. It is this mechanism which sometimes permits survival of the patient, although with permanent loss of segments of his renal parenchyma. In such a case, the remaining tubules tend to undergo a compensatory hypertrophy characterized by increase in size, with or without increase in height of their epithelial linings. Such patients secrete large volumes of poorly concentrated urine of low specific gravity.

The **causes** of toxic tubular nephrosis are toxic irritant substances brought to the kidney by the circulating blood, the previously stated facts being borne in mind by the reader that the tubules commonly suffer a limited amount of toxic injury from locally elaborated toxins in the vicinity of lesions of infectious nephritis and, also, that ischemia from occlusion of the glomerular capillaries can cause the same types of degenerative tubular injury. The blood-borne toxic substances can conveniently be divided into three classes, as follows:

1. "Chemical" poisons. In general, the same poisons which cause toxic effects on the liver (p. 1223) produce toxic nephrosis to some degree. More or less in order

of declining importance are the soluble salts of mercury (mercuric chloride, excessive doses of calomel, mercurial fungicides used to disinfect seed, such as Ceresan), of chromium (potassium bichromate), uranium (uranium nitrate), copper (copper sulfate used as a parasiticide, fungicide, molluscicide), bismuth (excessive "BIPP", bismuth-iodoform-petrolatum paste used in the treatment of wounds), cadmium, arsenic and phosphorus. Organic nephrotoxic chemicals, also somewhat in order of declining importance of the renal lesions include carbon tetrachloride (solvent, anthelmintic), tetrachloroethylene (anthelmintic), various chlorinated-hydrocarbon insecticides such as "Toxaphene," sulfonamide allergy, oxalic acid and oxalates, usually of plant origin, turpentine, cantharides, iodoform, phenol, pyrogallic acid, alpha-naphthyl thiourea (ANTU rat-poison) and others. Sodium monofluoroacetate (the rodenticide "1080") and other fluorine compounds probably belong in this group. In the case of many of these substances, the direct toxic effect is reinforced by the anoxia of renal congestion and failing circulation.

A startling picture of **hydropic degeneration** of practically 100 per cent of the epithelial cells of the kidney is produced in poisoning by dioxane, by ethylene glycol (used as "antifreeze" in automobiles), and by diethylene glycol (formerly used as a vehicle for sulfonamide drugs). The cytoplasm is distended with fluid, so that in ordinary microscopic sections the enlarged and crowded cells are strikingly clear and empty. The change is sometimes called **vacuolar degeneration.** It leads to necrosis and the patient is likely to die but the change is promptly reversible if the cause is removed. A similar picture can result from the experimental injection intravenously of concentrated solutions of sucrose, although this is transitory. A vacuolar change in the epithelium of the proximal tubules is stated to be characteristic of potassium deficiency.

2. Plant poisons, many of which undoubtedly have not been identified in accurate relation to renal pathology. Included are poisoning by the young buds of certain species of oaks, young plants of cockle-burs, which are eaten by pigs, sacahuiste, broomweed of the Southwestern United States, called snakeweed in the Great Plains (*Gutierrezia microcephala*), *Baileya multiradiata*, *Drymaria pachyphylla*, lupines, aspidium (male fern), used as a teniacide, senecios, mushrooms and moldy feeds. Oxalate-containing plants injure the kidney by deposition of crystals in the tubules (p. 859).

3. Endogenous toxemias, usually produced in the course of other diseases. Here belongs the necrosis characteristic of most of the acute infections. In the ketosis of "pregnant-ewe toxemia," severe lipidosis of the renal tubules, as well as of the liver, is a prominent lesion.

The term **hepatorenal syndrome** has been applied to the simultaneous occurrence of hepatic and renal dysfunction in the human or animal patient. The assumption that the lesions in the kidney were caused by those in the liver has not been supported by satisfactory evidence. For this reason the term has little meaning in the field of pathology.

Hypoxic (hemoglobinuric, shock, lower nephron) Nephrosis.—A syndrome differing both in tissue changes and in etiology from the ordinary toxic disorders just described exists in the form of the rather poorly understood condition which Lucké, 1946, has called "lower nephron nephrosis." While this condition has some aspects in common with the toxic tubular nephrosis just discussed, particularly the ultimate necrosis of tubular epithelium, there are two essential characteristics which mark "lower nephron nephrosis" as a different entity. These are (1) the fact that the epithelial damage is primarily in the "lower nephron," that is, the last part of Henle's loop and the distal convoluted tubule, rather than in the usually vulnerable proximal tubule and (2) the presence of dense and conspicuous casts in many of these lower nephrons. The casts stain a dirty, almost brownish red when submitted to hematoxylin and eosin, a shade quite different from the bright pink of the ordinary hyaline casts of albuminuria. While the exact chemical changes have not been elucidated, the different appearance is due to derivatives of hemoglobin (or myoglobin) and the casts are called **hemoglobin casts.** Lesions which accompany these two pathognomonic changes, at least in the late stages, include cytoplasmic disintegration and necrosis of epithelium in other than the lower parts of the nephron and localized infiltrations of lymphocytes and other inflammatory cells in the interstitial tissue. The proximal tubules are often markedly dilated, as if from obstruction lower down in the nephron.

Symptomatically, the syndrome presents itself with oliguria, anuria and uremia. Shock (p. 140) or a shock-like condition is a preceding or accompanying derangement contributing to the seriousness of the situation. Obstruction of the lower parts of the nephron by the hemoglobin casts is one postulated cause of the cessation of urinary secretion, but the number of casts is scarcely sufficient to account entirely, or even principally, for the loss of function. Excessive reabsorption of fluid through the damaged epithelial linings is thought to be an important cause of the anuria, as is also the drop in blood pressure which goes with the state of shock, an adequate "hydrostatic" pressure in the glomerular capillaries being essential to secretion.

The extra-renal disorders leading to "lower nephron nephrosis" are numerous and diverse, although the inexact boundaries assigned to this syndrome cause some variations in the list of acceptable causes. The large crushing and bruising injuries, azoturia and the extensive hemolysis which follows a transfusion with incompatible blood (p. 1176) are the most important causes in animals. They all result directly in the accumulation of free hemoglobin or myoglobin in the blood and therefore in the kidneys (see Hemoglobin, p. 69). Similar renal changes are said to occur in certain rare myoglobinurias resembling azoturia (p. 1046) but affecting other species than the equine. A practically identical syndrome, either histopathologically or clinically, also follows extensive burns and perhaps some other forms of tissue destruction. Many believe that sudden ischemia of the renal cortex resulting from a state of shock is the basis of the causative mechanism, but the fact remains that the typical cases are those in which large amounts of hemoglobin or myoglobin (almost identical chemically) are released into the blood and urine.

The urine in humans suffering this affliction is highly acid, and the suggestion has been made that this acidity is important in precipitating the hemoglobin. Whether the same acidity is present in similar cases in the herbivorous animals, whose urine is normally alkaline, we are not able to say. Lower nephron nephrosis has followed experimental transfusions in dogs, but only when the urine was made highly acid and the blood was hemolyzed in considerable amounts previous to introduction into the animal's circulation. The disorder was, however, more easily produced in dogs whose renal circulation was already impaired by pre-existing chronic nephritis or by the low hydrostatic pressure incident to a state of shock. It may well be that in most naturally occurring cases in man or animal, both hemoglobinemia and renal ischemia operate synergistically to produce the renal damage and insufficiency (De Gowin, Warner and Randall, 1938; Yuile, *et al.*, 1949).

Vacuolar (Osmotic) Nephrosis.—This term has been applied (Robbins, 1967) to a lesion in tubular epithelium in which large vacuoles displace much of the cytoplasm. The vacuoles contain fluid but not fat, glycogen, mucus or other foreign substances. The presence of this fluid is believed related to disturbances in the osmotic relationships within these cells. It is associated with disturbances in fluid balance, such as gastrointestinal and other disorders which result in severe vomiting or diarrhea. Most characteristically, this lesion is associated with severe hypokalemia. Potassium deficiency is believed to be a most significant cause, but the exact mechanism involved is not clear at this writing. The lesion does not appear to have a prolonged effect upon renal function, provided that the potassium stores are restored promptly.

Glycogen Nephrosis.—Glycogen may accumulate in the epithelium of proximal convoluted tubules and the loops of Henle in diabetes mellitus and glycogen-storage disease such as von Gierke's disease in human patients. The former disease of course is not infrequent in animals. The presence of glycogen in the renal tubular epithelium gives the cytoplasm a uniformly vacuolated appearance. These changes are reversible and apparently do not cause significant functional impairment of the kidneys.

Cholemic Nephrosis.—Bile pigments may be found in the epithelium of proximal convoluted tubules or loop of Henle in animals with obstructive icterus or severe liver disease. The bile is seen in these tubular cells as yellow granules of irregular size. Formalin-fixed gross specimens of kidney are green in color due to the change of bilirubin to biliverdin (Plate II). The fresh specimen may be yellow (icteric). Moderate degeneration of tubular epithelium may occur but severe interference with renal function is not usual. The pathogenesis of this lesion is not clearly understood although it appears that toxic products released by the liver or not detoxified by the liver may be the cause. Unconjugated bile at elevated levels may be toxic but bilirubin glucuronide (conjugated bilirubin) does not appear to be injurious to renal cells. Hepatic injury may result in excretion of large amounts of amino acids, such as cystine, arginine, histidine and tryptophan, which experimentally have been shown to damage renal tubular epithelium.

Uric Acid Precipitates.—Extensive deposits of urate crystals may sometimes impart a yellowish color to the renal pyramids. The presence of these crystals in collecting tubules may give a radial pattern to the yellowish streaks. Microscopically, the collecting tubules are seen to be filled with yellow crystals. Urates may also be found (especially in birds) in the interstitial stroma where the crystals have a radial pattern (Fig. 3-4). The urates in tubules presumably result from destruction of cells, particularly erythroblasts in newborn animals and is most likely to be seen in pigs. This change also may occur in gout (p. 58).

Cloisonné Kidney.—An interesting pigmented thickening of tubular basement membranes has been described in goats (Zahawi, 1956; Light, 1960). The pattern of these thickened basement membranes around renal tubules under low magnification suggests the inlay of metal wire in porcelain using the cloisonné technique (cloisonné — Fr. — cloison = partitioned; Latin — claudere = shut, close). The thickened basement membrane surrounds only the proximal convoluted tubules and has dark brown or grayish-brown color, even in unstained sections. The chemical nature of the material in these basement membranes has not been established although it does not appear to be either hemosiderin or melanin. Iron-positive material has been demonstrated in some places but for the most part the involved basement membranes do not contain iron. Antecedent hemosiderosis has been postulated as a possible means of staining these basement membranes. The lesion appears to be limited to goats and does not interfere with renal function.

The gross appearance of this change is striking. The renal cortex in both kidneys, in severe cases, is dark brown, almost black. This color extends through the entire cortex but is abruptly interrupted at the corticomedullary junction.

The lesion has been identified in living goats by histologic examination of specimens of kidney obtained by percutaneous biopsy (Altman, Grossman and Jernigan, 1970). These authors confirmed the absence of significant change in renal function and speculated that low levels of erythrocytic glucose-6-phosphate dehydrogenase and glutathione in normal and affected goats, plus elevated serum-iron-binding saturation, predispose to fragility of erythrocytes. The presence of ferritin deposits in affected basement membranes and hemosiderin in tubular epithelial cells in electron micrographs (Altman, Grossman and Jernigan, 1968) is also presented as evidence for intravascular hemolysis as the antecedent lesion. Further studies are needed to firmly establish the pathogenesis of this lesion.

Sulfonamides in the Kidney.—Sulfonamide medication, especially if accompanied by a limited intake of water and an acid condition of the urine, may damage the kidney in various ways, often with lethal results (p. 893). The lesions include toxic tubular degeneration and necrosis, commonly with marked inflammatory infiltrations around the tubules which are involved. As previously stated, the degeneration of tubular epithelium may be of the hydropic type; the changes may also resemble those just described for "lower nephron nephrosis." Other changes apparently based on hypersensitivity may occur, such as glomerulonephritis, periarteritis nodosa (p. 1156) and necrosis of areas of peripelvic tissue. Some of these changes have been produced experimentally in dogs. The more usual lesion, however, has been, in dogs and cattle, a plugging of the lower collecting tubules with masses of fine crystals (Fig. 17–11, p. 894), a fatal anuria resulting. The crystals of most of the sulfonamides now in use are elongated, acicular, anisotropic and yellowish in color. Since they are soluble in water, many or perhaps all of them may be dissolved out in the routine preparation of microscopic sections.

Fat in the Kidney.—Lipids or lipoids stainable by ordinary techniques can be demonstrated in the epithelium of the several parts of the tubules, the glomerular tufts, the walls of Bowman's capsules, the interstitial tissue, the walls of blood vessels, the epithelium of the pelvic lining and the tubular lumens of the kidneys of the various species of domestic animals and man (Smith, 1949). However, deposits of fat in places other than the tubular epithelium are more in the nature of curiosities than lesions of practical significance. The gross appearance of renal lipidosis is pathognomonic only in canine cases of severe fatty degeneration of the ascending arms of Henle's loops. In these instances, the medullary rays stand out as prominent white streaks, radially directed, evenly spaced and reaching from the corticomedullary junction nearly, but not quite, to the capsule. In other species and in other localizations of the fat, little more can be detected grossly than a certain degree of paleness of the cortex and a hazy distinction between the alternating cortical labyrinths and medullary rays, as one views a cut surface traversing the cortex. In many kidneys with the latter appearance, the paler band represents not the medullary ray but the labyrinth, in which the proximal tubules especially have undergone cloudy swelling with or without fatty degeneration and necrosis, the picture of toxic tubular nephrosis in general. Microscopically, the fat is in the form of clear cytoplasmic droplets as explained under the general heading of Fatty Change (p. 34).

There are experimental indications that a sudden increase in the lipids of the circulating blood may cause the deposition of small amounts of visible lipid in various structures of the kidney and in the urine. Fat apparently may be absorbed (or phagocytized) by various cells in the immediate vicinity of locally destructive lesions where it has been released from an invisible combined form in the cells that have perished. Interpretations by a number of biologists that visible fat-droplets are normal in the tubular epithelium of cats is not in accord with fairly extensive veterinary experience. At any rate, fat of practical importance in the kidney appears in the epithelium of the tubules, principally the proximal convoluted tubules and the ascending loops, and represents toxic or anoxic degeneration comparable to that in the liver. Thus the condition is an aspect of toxic tubular nephrosis (p. 1266). As in the liver, fat is also deposited in epithelial cells in the ketotic state which characterizes ovine toxemia of pregnancy (p. 1022) and similar conditions.

Very rarely in the dog, a portion of the glomerular area has been taken over by large reticulo-endothelial cells filled with fat. Other parts of the glomerulus appear normal. The condition has been called glomerular xanthomatosis in some quarters (Fisher and Fisher, 1954).

Dilated Renal Tubules.—The interpretation of this common abnormality deserves a moment of consideration. First of all, the investigator must make sure that the tubules are really dilated. It is possible to mistake enlargement of the tubular lumens resulting from atrophy or flattening of the epithelial lining cells for true enlargement of the whole tubule. Dilatation usually involves a group of tubules, or in some cases the same nephron is seen several times in cross section, in the same area. They may be either convoluted tubules, the loops of Henle or collecting tubules or a combination of these. The degree of dilatation may be slight or the tubule may be enlarged to two or three times its normal diameter. An epithelial-lined space, seen in a single cross section, may give rise to the question whether it is a greatly dilated tubule or a cyst. The lining cells are most frequently, but not always, flattened; this depends on the cause of the dilatation. In may instances, the condition is due to back pressure caused by closure, from external pressure or otherwise, of the nephron at some lower point in its course. The increased internal pressure naturally tends to compress and flatten the epithelial lining. Such internal pressure must be mild, slowly developed and long continued, for sudden and marked increase of intratubular pressure merely stops the filtration process by counterbalancing the "hydrostatic" pressure of the blood within the glomerular capillaries. It appears from careful study, however, that not infrequently nephrons become dilated through a process of hypertrophy. In such a case, the lining cells may be stretched and flattened or they may be of normal height. If they have recently proliferated or regenerated, the cells tend to be hyperchromatic, like other young cells, even though they have not yet developed to normal height. Such hypertrophy appears to be common in certain nephrons that survive when their neighbors have been destroyed through some pathological process. It is compensatory hypertrophy, the nephron adding to its own some of the load formerly carried by its departed brethren. Obviously, hypertrophic nephrons of this kind are likely to be located in or near areas of fibrosis.

Diseases of Renal Tubules

ALTMAN, N. H., GROSSMAN, I. W., and JERNIGAN, N. B.: Electron Microscopy of Caprine Cloisonne Renal Proximal Tubular Basement Membranes. Proc. 26th Ann. Mtg. Electron. Micro. Soc. Amer. Claitors, Baton Rouge, La. 192–193, 1968.
————: Caprine Cloisonne Renal Lesions. Clinicopathological Observations. Cornell Vet. *60*:83–90, 1970.
BATTIFORA, H. A., and MARKOWITZ, A. S.: Nephrotoxic Nephritis in Monkeys. Amer. J. Path. *55*:267–281, 1969.
BULGER, R. E., *et al.*: Human Renal Ultrastructure. II. The Thin Limb of Henle's Loop and the Interstitium in Healthy Individuals. Lab. Invest. *16*:124–141, 1967.
DEGOWIN, E. L., WARNER, E. D., and RANDALL, W. L.: Renal Insufficiency from Blood Transfusion; Anatomic Changes in Man Compared with Those in Dogs with Experimental Hemoglobinuria. Arch. Int. Med. *61*:609–630, 1938.
ERICSSON, J. L. E., MOSTOFI, F. K., and LUNDGREN, G.: Experimental Hemoglobinuric Nephropathy. I. Comparative Light Microscopic, Histochemical and Pathophysiologic Studies. Virchows Arch. Abt. B. Zellpath. *3*:181–200, 1969.
FOOTE, J. J., and GRAFFLIN, A. L.: Quantitative Measurements of the Fat-laden and Fat-free Segments of the Proximal Tubule in the Nephron of the Cat and Dog. Anat. Rec. *72*:169–179, 1938.
FULLER, R. H.: Lipoids in the Kidney. Arch. Path. *32*:556–568, 1941.
HELPER, O. E., and SIMONDS, J. P.: Experimental Nephropathies, III: Calcification and Phosphatase in the Kidneys of Dogs Poisoned with Mercury Bichloride, Potassium Dichromate and Uranyl Nitrate. Arch. Path. *40*:37–43, 1945.
JAENIKE, J. R.: The Renal Lesion Associated with Hemoglobinemia. J. Exper. Med. *123*:523–535, 1966.
LIGHT, F. W., JR.: Pigmented Thickening of the Basement Membranes of the Renal Tubules of the Goat ("Cloisonne Kidney"). Lab. Invest. *9*:228–238, 1960.
LUCKE, B. C.: Lower Nephron Nephrosis. Mil. Surgeon *99*:371–396, 1946.
MAISEL, B., McSWAIN, B., and GLENN, F.: Effects of Administration of Sodium Sulfadiazine to Dogs. Arch. Surg. *46*:326–335, 1943.
MODELL, W.: Observations on the Lipoids in the Renal Tubule of the Cat. Anat. Rec. *57*:13–28, 1933.
MODELL, W., and TRAVELL, J.: The Role of the Lipoid in the Renal Tubule of the Cat in Uranium Nephritis. Anat. Rec. *59*:253–263, 1934.
OTTOSEN, H. E.: A Case of Renal Sulfathiazole Concretion and Nephrosis in a Calf. Nord. Vet.-Med. *1*:410–415, 1949.
RIBELIN, W. E.: Azoturia and the Crush Syndrome. J. Am. Vet. Med. Assn. *119*:284–288, 1951.
SZEKY, A., and MIKLOVICH, N.: Histopathological Changes in the Rat Kidney Following Administration of Sulphamethylthiazole, Acta Sci. Hung. *12*:351–371, 1962.
YUILE, C. L., *et al.*: Hemolytic Reactions Produced in Dogs by Transfusion of Incompatible Dog Blood and Plasma. II. Renal Aspects Following Whole Blood Transfusions. Blood *4*:1232–1239, 1949.
ZAHAWI, S.: Symmetrical Cortical Siderosis of the Kidneys in Goats. Am. J. Vet. Res. *18*:861–867, 1957.

Diseases of the Interstitium

Interstitial Nephritis.—This term, disputed by some, is used to designate diffuse inflammation of the kidney with the exudate confined almost exclusively to the interstitial tissues. The causes are infections by various organisms, among them are leptospira (p. 560). These organisms are found in renal tubular epithelium but the inflammatory reaction to their presence is confined to the interstitium. Red blood cells, plasma and neutrophils make up the exudate in

41

early stages but are gradually replaced by plasma cells, lymphocytes and epithelioid cells as the disease progresses. Interstitial fibrosis and thickening of Bowman's capsule (periglomerular fibrosis) are also believed to be long-term effects (Fig. 25–11A). The lesions of leptospirosis are described in detail on page 560.

Pyelonephritis.—A second, and probably most frequent, involvement of the interstitium is pyelonephritis. The word signifies inflammation of the renal pelvis and parenchyma of the kidney. It usually starts with purulent infection in the renal parenchyma and soon spreads to the renal pelvis and rest of the urinary tract. Infection is believed to reach the kidney by ascending through the urinary tract or by dissemination through the vasculature. This latter is the so-called descending route of infection. Although the route of entry of infection is rarely demonstrable in individual cases, experimental evidence points toward circulatory dissemination of the organisms as the most likely means of infection. On the other hand, urinary obstruction (due to calculi, etc.) and ureteral reflux may well permit ascending infection. Pyogenic organisms generally become involved in pyelonephritis. *Escherichia coli* and *Staphylococcus aureus* have been incriminated experimentally in dogs and *Corynebacterium renale* is a well-known pathogen in bovine animals. In man, *E. coli* is the commonest pathogen; others include: *Aerobacter aerogens*, *Proteus vulgaris*, alpha hemolytic streptococci, hemolytic staphylococci, *Pseudomonas aeruginosa* and *Klebsiella pneumoniae*.

The **lesions** in the acute form of pyelonephritis consist of purulent inflammation and necrosis which involve renal parenchyma and extend into collecting ducts, calyces and renal pelvis. Classically, glomeruli and nephrons are spared, but they may become entrapped in the widespread inflammation. The lesions may be focal or diffuse, involving one or both kidneys or a single lobule (in bovines). Some lesions may be sharply circumscribed and consist essentially of abscesses. Sometimes the lesions are distributed around a single calyx, suggesting ascending infection from the renal pelvis. Extension of infection into nephrons usually results in neutrophils and granular or leukocytic casts in nephrons or collecting ducts. Purulent exudate may be found in the pelvis or just outside the pseudostratified epithelium which lines the pelvis.

Grossly, acute pyelonephritis is recognized by congestion, hemorrhages and sometimes abscesses in the renal cortex with severe congestion and pus in the pelvis—usually involving the ureters and possibly urethral and bladder mucosae.

Pyelonephritis may be accompanied by fever and malaise and often is preceded by localized or generalized infections (prostatitis, pneumonia). **Pyuria** (pus in the urine) and **bacteriuria** are constant findings and **dysuria** with frequent urination may occur. Microscopic examination of urine reveals neutrophils, granular and leukocytic casts, red blood cells and bacteria in large numbers. The acute signs may abate shortly but persistence of pus and bacteria in the urine indicates active infection which may result in active lesions characteristic of chronic pyelonephritis.

In the chronic form of pyelonephritis, usually but not always preceded by acute pyelonephritis, the kidney become grossly scarred and contracted. These scarred areas may be single, with a depressed base located adjacent to the capsule, or may be multiple, giving the kidneys a coarsely nodular appearance. In extreme cases the kidney may be small, fibrous and contracted. Microscopically, at this stage, the interstitium contains lymphocytes, plasma cells, and neutrophils; tubules **may** be atrophic and contain casts and pus (sometimes bacteria); glomerular capsules are thickened by fibrosis (periglomerular fibrosis) and blood vessels may have thickened walls with fibrinous material in the media. In the most advanced stages, fibrous connective tissue replaces the exudate in the interstitium and contraction eventually results. The tubules may be dilated and contain proteinaceous casts. Some lymphocytes and plasma cells usually persist in the interstitium. This stage usually results in death due to uremia.

Peripelvic Necrosis.—Known as **papillitis necroticans,** a necrotizing and at the same time inflammatory change affecting one or, more often, several of the renal papillae occurs in the human kidney. The distal half or two-thirds of the renal papilla is a yellowish gray and is sharply demarcated from the normal adjacent tissue by a narrow inflammatory zone and, except for its position, resembles an anemic infarct. Microscopically, the tissue is in a state of coagulative necrosis. Some of these lesions occur in connection with pyelonephritis (and concurrent diabetes in the human); others result from urinary obstruction. In the former case, the pressure of intrarenal exudates is thought to compress and close the blood vessels supplying this rather distant and isolated part of the kidney; in the case of urinary obstruction, the back pressure of the urine, acting from several directions on the protruding papilla, is supposed to produce a similar ischemia. The disorder tends to cause anuria and is likely to be fatal. A corresponding change has been seen at least in the dog, in which it involves the renal crest rather than a papilla because of anatomical differences. In one such case, amyloidosis in the basal region of the pyramids appeared to be responsible for compression of the blood vessels.

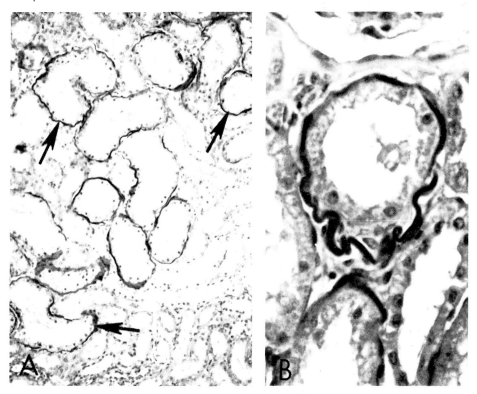

FIG. 25–9.—Cloisonné kidney, Angora goat. *A,* Deeply pigmented basement membranes (arrows) encompass renal tubules. *B,* Higher magnification of a single tubule.

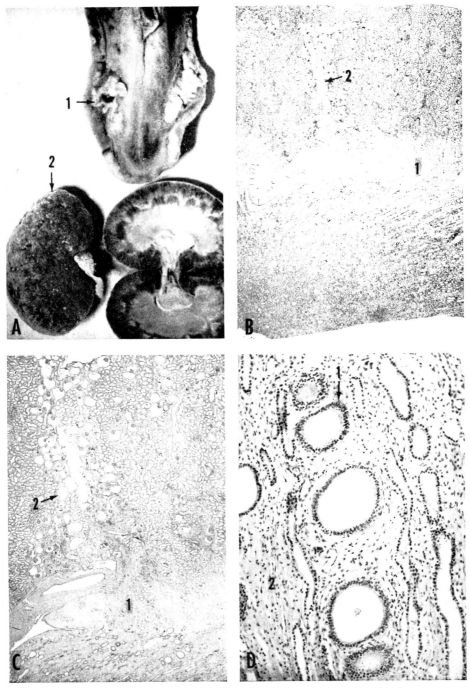

Fig. 25–10.—*A*, Nephrosclerosis, granular contracted kidney of chronic nephritis in a nine-year-old dog. Uremic ulcers of the tongue (*1*) and the pitted, contracted kidney (*2*). *B*, Nephrosclerosis, concentrated at the cortico-medullary junction (*1*) kidney of a dog ($\times$ 5). Note dilated tubules (*2*) in one nephron. *C*, The renal cortex of *B* ($\times$ 10). Scarring at cortico-medullary junction (*1*) and dilatation of Bowman's space (*2*). The renal medulla in *B* and *C* ($\times$ 100). Collecting tubules are lined with multiple rows of cells (*1*) and are spherical in outline. Note connective tissue (*2*). (*B*, *C* and *D* Courtesy of Armed Forces Institute of Pathology.) Contributor: Base Veterinarian, Barksdale AFB.

amounts pass into the urine with the exudates of acute infectious nephritis, as previously stated.

When large amounts of blood protein continually escape into the urine, edema (p. 134) results because of the deficiency of protein molecules and resulting reduction of the blood's osmotic tension. Hence, in cases of generalized edema the condition of the kidneys should always be investigated.

Hematuria is recognized and differentiated from hemoglobinuria by the microscopic demonstration of erythrocytes in a centrifuged sample of urine. If the amount of blood is large, the color of the urine becomes reddish brown. It is the result of hemorrhage anywhere from glomerulus to urethra, including hemorrhagic exudates from the kidney or bladder. Indeed, in most cases of acute exudative nephritis small numbers of erythrocytes are demonstrable in the urine.

Hemoglobinuria is the condition in which hemoglobin (p. 69), without blood cells, appears in the urine. The same brownish color as in hematuria is imparted to the urine when the condition is severe. Hemoglobinuria results from hemoglobinemia, the condition in which free hemoglobin is in solution in the blood plasma, which in turn is the result of extensive hemolysis of circulating erythrocytes by certain toxins or pathogenic microorganisms. Hemoglobin is normally eliminated through its partial decomposition by the reticulo-endothelial system and excretion of the blood pigment as bilirubin. When this mechanism becomes inadequate, the hemoglobin accumulates in the plasma to a level where it is excreted in the urinary filtrate, the reddish brown discoloration becoming more or less evident. If this situation persists for two or three days, hemolytic jaundice (p. 75) also develops.

Hemoglobinuria must be differentiated from **myoglobinuria.** Myoglobinuria, which develops from myoglobinemia (see Azoturia, p. 1046, White Muscle Diseases, p. 1049), and hemoglobinuria are disorders identical in their superficial manifestations in the blood but, whereas hemoglobin comes from perishing erythrocytes, myoglobin comes from damaged or destroyed muscle. Unfortunately there is no simple chemical means of differentiating these two similar substances, only spectrographic analysis being incontrovertible. However, these two causes of brownish pigmentation of the urine can usually be distinguished on a practical basis by examination of the blood plasma. After a sample of blood has been treated with an anticoagulant and the cells allowed to settle out (accidental hemolysis being avoided) the plasma is found to be practically unstained in the case of myoglobinemia, while in hemoglobinemia the plasma shares the discoloration of the urine. The reason is that the smaller molecules of myoglobin are easily and promptly excreted from the blood into the urine, whereas in the case of hemoglobin with its large molecules, a rather high threshold must be exceeded before the pigment is released from the plasma into the urine, a considerable amount of color being constantly retained in the plasma. The presence of hemolytic anemia (p. 126) and also of hemolytic icterus (p. 75), if present, afford indirect evidence of release of hemoglobin. Most cases of "red-water," as the stockman may call it, are hemoglobinuria or myoglobinuria; hematuria is much less frequently sufficient to cause marked discoloration of the urine.

Anuria.—This condition of complete urinary failure and the milder oliguria, in which renal excretion is pathologically reduced but not extinguished, can arise by several different mechanisms, of which the following are of principal importance (1) The changes described for glomerulonephritis prevent blood from flowing through the glomeruli, without which there can be no urinary secretion. (2) Since the renal capsule is quite inelastic, no great amount of intrarenal pressure is necessary to close the blood vessels which distribute blood within the kidney, thus again preventing glomerular filtration. Such pressure may result from tubular nephrosis. (3) Back pressure of urine already secreted but not discharged for any reason (hydronephrosis) prevents further secretion when the back pressure equals or closely approaches the effective filtration pressure ("hydrostatic" pressure with some modifications) of the blood within the glomeruli. (4) Similarly, when the general blood pressure in the arterial system falls below a certain level necessary to maintain filtration through the glomeruli, the formation of urine ceases. This is the mechanism responsible for the **extrarenal anuria** of shock and similar conditions. (5) Extreme dehydration prevents filtration until the volume of blood is sufficiently restored. (6) Destruction of the lining epithelium of the tubules in a later stage of tubular nephrosis than that mentioned in the second item of this series leaves the tubules with no control over resorption of the glomerular filtrate. The filtrate tends to diffuse back into the lymphatic and venous drainage as fast as it is formed. (7) Casts in general and especially the hemoglobin casts of "lower nephron nephrosis" (p. 1268) stop the production of urine to the extent that the nephrons are occluded. Anuria is an important feature of this disease; however, the low arterial pressure of shock (item 4, above) is probably a more important causative factor than the plugging of a certain number of nephrons.

Polyuria.—Physiologically, the amount of urine produced and its degree of concentration depend upon the amount of water ingested (as such or in the food) and not eliminated by such mechanisms as sweating, lactation and respiration. The sensation of thirst ordinarily depends upon the water balance of the body and is, therefore, secondary to the extent to which water is eliminated. Hormones (pituitary anti-diuretic, etc.) also exert their influence upon the amount of urine excreted and are the decisive factor in the disease known as diabetes insipidus (p. 1020). As far as the kidney is concerned, polyuria is an indication of moderately injured tubules. Polyuria is often marked during the regenerative stage of tubular nephrosis when the epithelial lining has developed to a place where it prevents the indiscriminate return of urinary fluid into the lymphatic and venous drainage but has not yet attained its normal state of selective permeability. Similarly when numbers of tubules have disappeared, for instance through the tubular ischemia of glomerular nephritis, those remaining commonly undergo an imperfect hypertrophy which leaves their selective permeability impaired or perhaps allows the urine to pass too rapidly through a dilated and shortened nephron without adequate concentration. Waste products are, however, successfully eliminated and there is no uremia in these cases.

Uremia.—Literally a condition of urine in the blood, uremia may be defined as a disorder in which a variety of harmful waste products normally eliminated in the urine remain in the circulating blood because of complete or partial failure of urinary excretion. The principal substances abnormally retained are urea, uric acid, creatinine and ammonia, all of which are included in the non-protein nitrogen in the ordinary laboratory examination of the blood. Also included in the list of retained substances are sulfates, chlorides and especially phosphates. The calcium content is diminished concomitantly with the rise of phosphates. As a glance at the list of retained ions would suggest, there is a strong tendency toward acidosis.

The signs cannot be attributed to any one of these hemic abnormalities. Symptoms such as headache are not easily evaluated in animals; vomiting can be explained on the basis of irritative lesions in the gastrointestinal tract; nervous hyperirritability, including convulsions in dogs, is usually ascribed to the lowering of calcium, although the status of the magnesium level would bear investigation in this regard.   In farm animals, uremia is usually due to obstructive urolithiasis; the disease develops in the course of a very few days and, because of this and the characteristics of the species, symptoms directly attributable to the changed composition of the blood are not usually observed.   In patients of any species, a urine-like odor of the breath is often present and is diagnostic.   In testing for "blood urea nitrogen," it must be kept in mind that the substance is likely to be destroyed by four or five hours of post-mortem autolysis.

The causes of uremia are either urinary obstruction, as noted above, or failure of renal function due to some one of the anuric diseases of the kidneys already described.   Outstanding among these are the small, granular contracted kidney, whatever its cause, the tubular obstructive diseases, including obstruction by sulfonamide crystals, and extensive amyloidosis.

At the necropsy, certain extrarenal lesions may be found which are more or less characteristic of uremic death, and which, if present, are of very practical significance.   In the dog and also in the cat, hemorrhagic erosions or superficial ulcers are common in the buccal or pharyngeal mucosa, as is hemorrhagic gastritis, often covering a large portion of the fundic mucosa.   Less frequently, the intestine may be similarly involved.   In cattle, the preceding lesions seldom occur, but severe catarrhal or hemorrhagic inflammation may involve the terminal part of the large intestine.   In either case, the lesions of the digestive tract are presumably due to elimination of some of the toxic substances through the affected mucous membrane.   In the case of toxic tubular nephrosis or of leptospirosis (canine), it is difficult to say how much of the injury to the digestive mucosa is attributable directly to uremic products and how much to the original injurious agent.   A uremic lesion which is common in man and occasional in dogs and cattle is an increase of pericardial fluid, often with a small amount of fibrin.   The explanation is not apparent, but the condition has not been shown to be a true inflammation (reaction to an irritant, p. 145).   The so-called uremic aortitis, rather frequently seen in dogs, consists in a proliferative roughening of the intima, usually near the heart, and sometimes extending into it (the left ventricle).   Microscopic areas of calcification are frequent in the intima of this and other blood vessels, beneath the endocardium and elsewhere.   If prolonged, uremia is often accompanied by a noticeable degree of anemia.   Toxic injury to the bone marrow (toxic aplastic anemia, p. 129) has been postulated as a cause, but the frequency of hemosiderosis in the spleen and elsewhere is suggestive of a hemolytic action.   The cerebral edema which is common in humans seldom accompanies uremia in domestic animals.

THE URETERS, URACHUS, BLADDER AND URETHRA

The Ureter.—Inflammation of the ureteral mucosa occurs as a part of inflammation of the whole urinary tract.   Because of the dense nature of the wall of this small tubular organ, the exudative or proliferative changes are less extensive and attract less attention in the ureter than in the bladder or renal pelvis. The dilatation of the ureteral lumen and the thickening of the wall which occur in ascending pyelonephritis or pyonephrosis have been mentioned. If there is partial obstruction lower in the urinary tract, the gradual dilation of the lumen of one or both ureters (depending on location of the obstruction) can be quite remarkable. Tuberculosis and possibly certain other granulomatous infections occasionally invade the wall of the ureter, producing characteristic lesions.

Strictures in the form of an irregular fold or a gradual narrowing can occur either congenitally or as the result of previous inflammation. Such damage is most likely to be due to the temporary lodgment of calculi somewhere along the tube, although a considerable proportion of strictures are located just at the ureteral inlet.

Neoplasms, usually papillomas or carcinomas, arise from the ureteral mucosa rarely. Metastatic tumors may infiltrate the wall, one of the writers (Smith) having seen the thickness of the wall of a bovine ureter increased to twenty times the normal by an infiltrating malignant lymphoma.

The Bladder. — Especially when there is interference with the normal drainage of urine, the mucosa and deeper layers of the bladder are subject to infectious inflammations of the acute fibrinous, purulent, catarrhal and hemorrhagic types. The purulent form occasionally reaches phlegmonous proportions. Chronicity leads to irregular thickening of the subepithelial connective tissue and mild corrugation of the mucous side as seen grossly. A form of cystitis occurs rarely in the dog in which numerous epithelial-lined diverticula, the nature of whose origin is uncertain, become closed at their orifices and form minute cystic spaces in the inflamed and thickened wall. Involvement by tuberculosis and possibly other infectious granulomas occurs rarely. Tubercles may be small and confined to the submucosa or may form large bulges into the lumen, with or without ulceration. Urolithiasis tends to result from long-continued cystitis of exudative type.

Hemorrhages, usually petechial, without inflammation are indicative of acute toxemias or septicemias. Petechiae in the mucosa are considered of diagnostic significance in hog cholera.

Hypertrophy of the muscular layer is recognized by raised parallel longitudinal ridges about 2 or 3 mm. in width and height (dog) visible on the serous side. It is a compensatory (or adaptive) hypertrophy designed to provide sufficient force to expel the urine against some partial obstruction, most frequently the periurethral pressure of an enlarged canine prostate.

Two helminth parasites may inhabit the urinary bladder, *Capillaria plica* in cats and *Trichosomoides crassicaudata* in rats (p. 777). These produce little or no pathologic effect.

Metastatic neoplasms, especially malignant lymphomas, may infiltrate the wall of the bladder, usually the submucosa or subserosa. The result is a series of diffuse or nodular thickenings consisting of smoothly homogeneous, white tissue. A primary tumor which is not altogether rare is a papilloma characterized by very numerous and very long, stringy papillations reminding one of the flower of a dahlia. It appears to be more frequent in cattle than in other species. The disorder known as bovine enzoötic hematuria (p. 1298) is characterized by pronounced hyperplastic proliferation of the mucosa of the bladder and almost certainly can serve as a precursor of carcinoma. Experimentally, papillomas and papillary carcinomas have been produced in the dog's bladder by very prolonged administration (over several years) of such compounds as beta-naphthylamine. This was done primarily in connection with the study of certain "aniline tumors" which have developed in people working in aniline industries. There appears, however, to be nothing in the dog's bladder comparable to the human neoplasms which develop in connection with schistosomiasis (p. 802). The precancerous squamous metaplasia called leukoplakia in the human patient has not been reported in animals, possibly because the prolonged episodes of chronic cystitis which appear to precede the disorder seldom occurs in animals. Histologically carcinomas of the bladder may be sufficiently well differentiated to resemble transitional epithelium or they may be highly anaplastic with little resemblance to the cells from which they arose. Leiomyomas are seen occasionally.

"Pervious urachus" is a congenital failure of the fetal urachus to close, which requires surgical intervention. The occasional ascent of infection from a diseased umbilicus to the kidney has been mentioned (p. 1274). Cysts rarely form in the course of a urachus which closes in some parts and not in others, leaving isolated stretches of patent lumen, or they may form in the midline of the bladder.

The Urethra.—The urethra almost never suffers from more than very transient inflammation as long as there is no interference with the drainage of urine. The passing of a catheter usually causes mild injury and inflammation which remains painful for a few days, especially in males. The principal lesion to be encountered in this organ is the lodgment of calculi. This is especially likely to occur at the sigmoid flexure in male ruminants. There is always a variable degree of hyperemia and inflammation at and above the site of lodgment, none below it. There are in animals no specific infections with a predilection for the urethra, such as gonorrheal infection in the human. The mucosa and probably its tributary glands appear to harbor such organisms as *Trichomonas fetus* in the bull, but the condition represents more a symbiosis than a pathogenesis as far as the urethra itself and its glands are concerned. A bull so infected may, however, be a source of contagion to the female, in which the infection is a cause of sterility (p. 707).

Diverticula (in the female especially) and strictures (in the male chiefly) occur rarely in the urethra, being either congenital or the result of injury by stones, catheters or compressing injuries from the outside. As in other tubular organs, a dilatation may form above a stricture as the result of pressure of accumulated fluid. The effect of obstruction in the urethra (as elsewhere) in causing hydronephrosis has been discussed (p. 1283).

Obstruction of the urethra of the male cat is a common clinical problem, especially in castrated males. Although uroliths are sometimes demonstrated, in many cases inflammation of the urethra appears to be the underlying factor in the obstruction. Some evidence indicates that a picornovirus may be involved (Rich and Fabricant, 1969).

Fistulas.—Fistulous tracts can be established between adjacent pelvic organs as a result of necrotizing processes, especially if these are preceded by adhesions between the two surfaces concerned. While all such openings are very rare in the domestic animals, it is possible for the rectum to become inflamed and adherent where it passes the bladder and for continuing destruction to lead to perforation into the bladder. Possible causes are trauma from foreign objects, usually surgical, caustic medicaments locally applied, cystic calculi, invasive neoplasms and some others, conceivably including lesions produced by nodular worms (*Œsophagostomum sp.*).

Recto-vaginal fistulas are more frequent than the recto-vesical just described. They arise from similar causes and also are at times congenital. The vesico-vaginal fistula, rather common in humans, does not occur in the domestic animals to any appreciable extent since the walls of the two organs are not contiguous as in the human female.

Bovine Enzoötic Hematuria.—Reported only from certain sharply limited regions of the world, especially the Northwestern United States, Western Canada and the Black Sea region of Turkey, Bulgaria and Yugoslavia, this is a disease of adult cattle, also water buffalo, characterized by persistent hematuria leading to (chronic hemorrhagic) anemia and death. The lesions, which arise most frequently in the bladder, but also occasionally in the ureters or renal pelvis, appear to represent a chronic but violently hyperplastic inflammation with severe hyperemia and recurrent hemorrhage. There is localized proliferation of epithelium with metaplasia either to mucin-forming columnar or to stratified squamous types or a mixture of the two. In certain cases, the hyperplastic epithelium acquires neoplastic properties, developing into a carcinoma (either squamous-cell or adenocarcinoma) which is locally invasive and may metastasize to the regional lymph nodes and the lungs. The capillaries of the inflammatory lesion also participate in the hyperplastic proliferation, sometimes to the extent of forming hemangiomas either in the stroma or projecting from the mucosal surface, and are capable, in themselves, of developing malignant qualities. The etiology appears to be well established as one long term effect of poisoning due to bracken fern (p. 908).

An **epizootic cystitis** in horses has been described in the Southwestern United States and Australia. It has been associated with grazing on Sudan or hybrid Sudan grass. (Romane, *et al.*, 1966, Hooper, 1968.)

Ureters, Urachus, Bladder and Urethra

DENNIS, S. M.: Patent Urachus in a Neonatal Lamb. Cornell Vet. *59*:581–584, 1969.
FULTON, J. D., and ARMSTRONG, J. A.: Obstruction of the Urogenital Tract in Some Rodents. J. Reprod. Fertil. *4*:309–312, 1962.
HOOPER, P. T.: Epizootic Cystitis in Horses. Aust. Vet. J. *44*:11–14, 1968.
MACHADO, A. V., RANGEL, N. M., and GIOVINE, N.: Persistent Urachus Associated with Pyelonephritis. Cornell Vet. *33*:372–376, 1943.
MARSH, H.: Urethral Occlusion in Lambs on Feed Containing Stilbesterol. J. Am. Vet. Med. Assn. *139*:1019–1023, 1961.
McCULLY, R. M., and LIEBERMAN, L. L.: Histopathology in a Case of Feline Urolithiasis. Canad. Vet. J. *2*:52–61, 1961.
ROMANE, W. M., *et al.*: Cystitis Syndrome of the Equine. Swest. Vet. *19*:95–99, 1966.

26
The Genital System

THE FEMALE REPRODUCTIVE ORGANS

The reader is, of course, familiar with the anatomy, histology and physiology of the organs under consideration, but it may be advantageous to review as briefly as possible certain features which have a special bearing on their pathology.

The Estrual Cycle.—Of unique importance in interpreting many failures of the reproductive process and lesions of the reproductive organs is a familiarity with the morphological changes which accompany the estrual cycle in normal, parous females of each species. If we consider a given cycle as starting just after an ovulation, which is convenient in those species which do not menstruate, we encounter a series of changes which are incited through the medium of chemical hormones released into the blood. The pituitary, according to extensive evidence from many investigators, secretes two reproductive hormones, the follicle-stimulating hormone, commonly abbreviated F S H, and the luteinizing hormone, L H. The ovarian (Graafian) follicle, in proportion to its size and development, liberates the hormone (or hormones), estrogen (estradiol, folliculin, theelin, etc.), which, among other actions, inhibits the production of F S H, which induced the formation of the follicle in the first place. The corpus luteum owes its existence to the L H, but as the corpus luteum grows it elaborates more and more of the hormone, progesterone. Progesterone, as it accumulates, antagonizes and diminishes the production of L H. Thus the action of these two hormones is self-limiting.

Starting at the point in the cycle where a mature follicle has just ruptured, in other words, at ovulation, we find that the production of estrogen is minimal, leaving the pituitary free to provide the high level of F S H which will cause the development and maturation of the next follicle (or follicles). But at the moment, and for approximately the first half of the cycle, the F S H remains weak and the balance with the L H is such that the latter is free to stimulate the formation of the corpus luteum. The latter, however, is soon producing considerable amounts of progesterone. This antagonizes and lowers the production of L H, which is essential for the growth and, indeed, the existence of the corpus luteum. The corpus luteum, thus, by means of the hormone which it, itself, produced, initiates its own extinction, which occurs through gradual fatty degeneration, atrophy and slow necrosis, with disappearance of the lutein cells. By the time of the next ovulation (about twenty-one days in most farm animals, twenty-eight days in humans), the corpus luteum has receded to less than half its maximum size, and in a few more weeks there remains only a scar of hyaline connective tissue, which is called the corpus albicans.

As the concentration of progesterone from the old corpus luteum recedes, the
L H of the pituitary slowly regains its ascendancy in time to build a new corpus
luteum upon rupture of the next ovulating follicle, which is accomplished by a
transformation and proliferation of the cells of the stratum granulosum and the
theca interna. Thus the life of the corpus luteum is self-limited due to repression
of the pituitary hormone which brought it into being, and, likewise, we believe,
the life of the Graafian follicle culminates in ovulation because of estrogenic repression of the pituitary's F S H.

Barring the occurrence of pregnancy, this cyclic development of follicles and
corpora lutea goes on indefinitely in some species, such as humans, monkeys,
most dairy cows and swine. In most domestic animals, it is to some extent cur-
tailed by the unfavorable environment of winter; in most wild animals, it is
entirely restricted to the invigorating spring or summer; and in some species,
such as the dog, a single cycle occurs at the long interval of six months but possibly is not dependent on seasons or environment. In some species, such as the
cat, rabbit, ferret and mink, ovulation occurs and the cycle is initiated only
with the nervous stimulation of coitus.

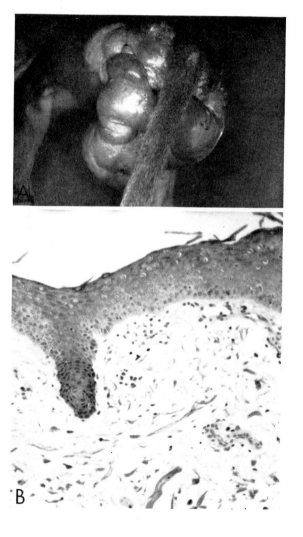

Fig. 26–1.—Sex skin in a
baboon. *A*, Marked swelling of
the perineum recurs with each
estrous cycle. *B*, Microscopically
the collagen fibers of the dermis
are separated by mucopolysaccharides. (Courtesy New England Regional Primate Research
Center, Harvard Medical School.)

While the ovarian cycle goes on as outlined, the other reproductive organs display cyclic changes, largely as a result of the alternating rise and fall of estrogen and progesterone, and these are of even greater significance in practical diagnostic pathology than those seen in the ovary (Fig. 26–1).

Endometrium.—The variable picture encountered in the endometrium is largely cyclical and needs to be understood before endometrial disorders can be properly evaluated. Unfortunately, our knowledge of the cyclic changes in animals is far from complete in various details and is based largely on what occurs in the human species. In the cow, the only domestic animal to which much study has been given, the endometrium seems to follow much the same cycle as in the human except that the variations are less pronounced and, of course, there is no menstruation. Cyclic changes may be observed in the lining epithelium, the glands, the glandular epithelium, the stroma and, to some extent, in the blood vessels.

A number of days previous to ovulation, in other words, at the beginning of the stage termed pro-estrum by physiologists, hormonal stimulation of the genital tissues may be considered at its lowest ebb. At this time, the lining epithelium of the uterus is low cuboidal and that of the glands is not much more impressive. The glands themselves are comparatively simple, straight tubular glands. The stroma consists of very closely placed, short, fibroblastic nuclei with no individual cytoplasm but lying in a rather scanty fibrillar meshwork. The blood supply is minimal. This is not unlike the post-menstrual endometrium in the human. From here onward the tendency is toward proliferation. Indeed, the ensuing stage has been given the name of the "proliferative phase." Since the proliferation is due to the influence of the follicular hormone, estrogen, from the growing follicle, the term "follicular phase" is used synonymously. The lining epithelium becomes taller. The glands become larger and more numerous; their lumens are wider and their epithelium taller. Toward the last of this stage, clear vacuoles, destined for a glandular secretion, appear underneath the nuclei of the glandular epithelium and push the latter toward the distal or superficial end of the cell. The nuclei of the stroma become larger, plumper, less deeply chromatic and develop a little individualized cytoplasm in some cases. The blood supply increases. To a slight extent similar changes can be detected in the mucosa of the oviduct: epithelial hyperplasia with increase in the number of cilia.

As ovulation occurs (stage of oestrus), the endometrium falls under the predominant influence of progesterone from the developing corpus luteum, although it is not to be supposed that estrogen is absent, for it is also produced by the corpus luteum and possibly by other, younger follicles. Under the influence of progesterone, the endometrial development continues, but in a somewhat modified manner. The epithelial cells of the glands increase in number as well as in size, which tends to make the walls of the glands tortuous with tiny folds of redundant lining. It cannot be said, however, that they reach the "saw-tooth" form which is seen in the human at this stage. These glands secrete the "uterine milk" which serves as a nutrient for the embryo. As the secretion starts, the epithelial cells lose their clear vacuoles and their nuclei subside to their usual level in the cells. To some extent, the secretion can be seen as a pale precipitate in the lumens of the glands. The cells of the stroma tend to become more rounded and less fibrous, approaching but not attaining the pre-decidual type of endometrium as it exists in the human. The capillary blood supply increases further.

This phase is known as the "secretory phase," or as the "progesterone phase." It is, as the latter name implies, a progestational endometrium adapted to the well-being and nutrition of an embryo for which the uterus has now been prepared.

If pregnancy occurs, this endometrial hypertrophy, as well as growth of the corpus luteum, continues. But if there is no conception, the hypertrophic endometrium subsides in company with the regressing corpus luteum. In the human, this would be menstruation; in the domestic animals, there is no such precipitous destruction, no sloughing, no hemorrhage. Neutrophils and other leukocytes invade the endometrium in appreciable numbers, presumably to dispose of the remains of cells that perish in the retrogressive process.

To a certain degree the other parts of the genital tract participate in this cyclic rise and fall, this proliferation and regression, but a practical use of this fact has been limited largely to the case of the vaginal epithelium. This proliferates during the endometrial proliferative phase (pro-estrum) to form a thicker layer, which tends to become cornified as the more superficial cells find themselves farther from their nutrient supply. Then regression sets in, earlier than in the endometrium (early di-estrum), numerous leukocytes infiltrating the stroma and epithelium. There is vaginal bleeding in the dog. Smears made from the vaginal surface reveal cells corresponding in type to those underlying it. It has been found possible to estimate the phase of the cycle by study of such smears, at least in the canine species. In the herbivora, the period of ovulation is characterized by a copious secretion of mucus (mucus of estrum) from the glands of the cervix.

Endometriosis.—The transplantation of a bit of endometrium by embryonic or surgical displacement, to an abnormal site, leaves viable tissue which is subject to the effects of various hormones and has no outlet for its secretions. This may result in accumulation of secretions, possibly toxemia. It is best known in women and non-human primates (Fig. 26–2).

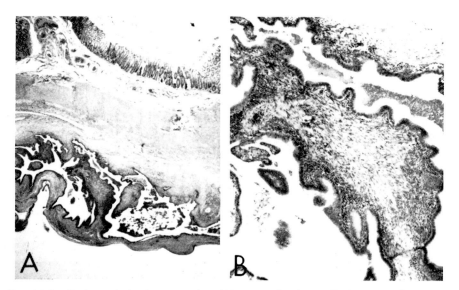

FIG. 26–2.—Endometriosis, rhesus monkey (*Macaca mulatta*). *A*, Endometrium implanted in the wall of the colon. *B*, Uterine columnar epithelium accompanied by endometrial stroma differentiates endometriosis from malignancy. Note detritus which represents evidence of menstruation. Inability of menstrual fluids to escape the body results in toxemia. (Courtesy New England Regional Primate Research Center, Harvard Medical School.)

Atretic Follicles.—Another normal phenomenon with which the pathologist needs to be familiar is the atresia (closing up) of follicles. Without trying to choose between the time-honored concept that all primordial ovarian follicles are formed before birth (400,000 in the newborn infant) and the newer contention that they are produced continually throughout reproductive life, it is certain that during each reproductive cycle a number of them progress to a stage approaching complete maturity. In most species, these can be seen in practically any ovary. But only one, in uniparous species, is able, through some unique preference which we do not understand, to attain complete maturation and send its ovum along the course designed to lead to a new life. In the case of multiple births there is, of course, one ovum for each individual born, excepting identical twins.

After each ovulation, the remaining nearly mature follicles degenerate and disappear, no doubt because they are deprived of the follicle-stimulating hormone. This process of atresia begins with simple necrosis of the cells of the stratum granulosum, perhaps preceded by fatty degeneration. Later the follicular lining is reduced to a single layer of cells of epithelial appearance or perhaps there may be no epithelial lining at all. The necrotic granulosal cells can often be seen floating uselessly in the liquor folliculi. Normally this fluid is soon resorbed, and in the bovine the follicle is replaced temporarily by a small, circumscribed spot of fibrous tissue, the corpus fibrosum. It is denser than the surrounding stroma, but not hyaline like the corpus albicans. In some species, rounded, lipoid-containing "theca-lutein cells" precede the fibrous stage. Pathologically resorption sometimes fails, fluid increases and the atretic follicle becomes a cystic follicle, or follicular cyst (p. 1307).

The Placenta.—While we shall refer the reader to other sources for most of our histological details, an accurate knowledge of the placental tissues in the several species is of such importance in the practice of pathology that it is desirable to describe them briefly here. By the placenta, we mean those tissues which are concerned in the exchange of nutrients and other substances between the blood of the mother and that of the fetus. That portion which is a part of the mother's endometrium is the maternal placenta; the part which belongs to the fetal membranes is the fetal placenta. In a general way, the fetal placenta consists of minute projections from the allanto-chorion, called chorionic villi, which penetrate with more or less intimacy into the maternal endometrium, but there are many differences among the various species. As a matter of convenience and because of their villous appearance in the single plane of a microscopic section, the narrow strips or ridges of endometrium which fill the spaces between the chorionic villi are often called maternal villi, and this somewhat erroneous term will be indulged in here. They are also called "maternal septa" of the endometrium or "endometrial septa."

Anatomically this allanto-chorion, the outermost envelope of the developing embryo, early comes to fill the uterine cavity, being pressed tightly against the endometrial lining by the fetus and fluids within. Just how much of the allanto-chorion has placental connection with the maternal tissues depends upon the species. That part of the allanto-chorion which forms villi and a placental connection is called the placental area, or the chorion frondosum (fern-like); the part which merely is held in apposition to the uterine lining is called the non-placental area, or the chorion laeve.

In the mare and sow, the whole endometrial lining and the whole allanto-chorion are placental areas. This type is known as the **diffuse placenta.** In the bitch, the placental area is in the shape of a wide band which encircles the elongated elliptical fetal sac at its middle. This is the **zonary placenta.** In the human, we have a **discoid placenta,** in which only a disc-shaped area on one side of the sac is placental.

It is of interest that in the human and similar species the chorion frondosum, which is the fetal component of this discoid placenta, is divided into 15 to 20 small sections, each derived from one primary villus, which are called cotyledons. In the bovine and ovine species, there is a fundamental similarity, but each cotyledon is separated from its neighbor by a wide non-placental area, and the total number, perhaps 100 in the bovine, are scattered over the whole of the allanto-chorion. This is the familiar **cotyledonary placenta.**

Regardless of the anatomical distribution of the placental and non-placental areas, placentas are classified histologically on the basis of the degree of closeness with which the fetal blood approaches that of the mother. One would expect to find interposed between the two the following six layers: fetal vascular endothelium, fetal connective tissue (mesenchymal), fetal chorionic epithelium, maternal endometrial epithelium, maternal connective tissue and maternal vascular endothelium. This arrangement is known as an **epitheliochorial placenta.** The fetal and maternal villi dovetail with each other or, more precisely, the fetal villi are interspersed between maternal endometrial septa in simple or complex fashion.

This type is found in the equine and porcine, as well as related, species. In the **equine,** the chorionic villi are slender, only slightly branched, in the neighborhood of 2 mm. in height, and have one layer of epithelial cells which are tall in the proximal region, but flat near the distal end of the villus. As would be expected, the maternal "villi" are covered with a single layer of low epithelial cells, a continuation of the normal simple columnar epithelium of the non-pregnant uterus.

The situation in the **porcine** species is similar although the chorionic villi are less slender and much shorter (one-half millimeter). Their single layer of columnar epithelium is readily distinguished from the apposed maternal epithelium because the latter is much flatter and stains more darkly. As gestation advances endometrial capillaries come to run exceedingly close to the maternal epithelium, and on the fetal side the chorionic capillaries even insinuate themselves between the epithelial cells, an arrangement which might be mistaken superficially for an endotheliochorial type of placenta. Especially during mid-gestation, there are numerous tiny areas (several per square centimeter), called areolae, where the fetal and maternal surfaces are separated, the space being filled by secretion of endometrial glands which converge to open at these points. This secretion is the so-called uterine milk; fetal cells in the vicinity can be observed assimilating its solid particles.

The three layers mentioned for the fetal side are regularly present in all species but, owing to an invasive power possessed by the chorionic epithelium, (the trophoblast or trophoderm according to the embryologists), certain of the maternal layers are destroyed in some species.

In the **syndesmochorial** type (syndesmo refers to connective tissue), the maternal epithelium is lacking and the chorionic villi protrude into the endometrial stroma (lamina propria). This general type is accredited to the bovine, ovine and caprine species, but some areas prove to be epitheliochorial, depending to some extent upon the stage of gestation. In these species, and especially in the bovine because of the large size of the animal, the chorionic villi are large, approaching 2 cm. in total length, and subdivide and branch repeatedly. Conforming to this complicated arborization, the maternal tissue forms deep crypts and saccules, correspondingly subdivided, into which the fetal villi fit. Not infrequently, the microscopic section is cut in such a direction that the maternal tissue forms hollow circles each enclosing a cross section of a chorionic villus, usually with a shrinkage space between them. The chorionic epithelium begins as a single layer of columnar cells, but as pregnancy advances these tend to join together, forming syncytial giant cells which lie scattered at irregular intervals along the surfaces of the chorionic villi. They are comparable to the syncytial giant cells of the human placenta but are smaller and less complicated. A majority have only two nuclei (diplokaryocytes), but cells with larger numbers are by no means nonexistent.

In the **endotheliochorial** placenta, the chorionic villi come into direct contact with the endothelium of the endometrial capillaries. This type of placenta occurs in the canine and feline species.

The chorionic villi penetrate the endometrium and destroy it to a considerable depth (down to the glandular "spongiosa"), leaving in the vicinity only the endometrial capillaries and a few stromal fibroblasts, which become large and rounded (like large mononuclears) and correspond to the specialized decidual cells of the human placenta. The chorionic villi, with their epithelium intact, thus lie in close contact with the maternal capillaries. Near the edges of the zonary placenta of these species, there is considerable accumulation of maternal blood in sinus-like spaces. This, becoming stagnant, develops grossly the greenish black color of partly hemolyzed blood in the canine.

The ultimate in chorionic invasion of the maternal tissues is found in the **hemochorial** placenta of humans and monkeys. In this type, the maternal tissues are destroyed to the extent that the blood escapes from ruptured endometrial capillaries, flows into sinus-like spaces surrounding chorionic villi, where the exchange of nutrients occurs with great ease, and then returns to the venous circulation of the mother. In rodents such as the rabbit, guinea pig and rat, the placenta is called hemo-endothelial, the maternal blood being in direct contact with the fetal capillaries.

Placentas are also classified as deciduate and non-deciduate. In the **deciduate placenta,** which happens to be also hemochorial or endotheliochorial, the penetrating chorionic villi produce practically a fusion of fetal and maternal structures so that when the fetal membranes are expelled after parturition, an outer layer of the endometrium comes loose (as a deciduous tree sheds its leaves) and is expelled with them. The deciduate placenta occurs in humans and monkeys and, to a less marked degree, in the dog and cat families. It is of interest to note that in some rather primitive wild species, the placenta is not shed or expelled, but instead, is slowly absorbed by the endometrium and leukocytes in it (contra-deciduate placenta). This is said to be true in part in the case of the sheep. In the **non-deciduate placenta** of the mare, sow, goat, cow and ewe (in spite of the statement in the preceding sentence), the fetal placenta is much less firmly adherent to the maternal and there is no shedding of maternal tissue.

42

Female Genital Tract, Histology and Physiology

ANDERSON, J. W.: Ultrastructure of the Placenta and Fetal Membranes of the Dog. Anat. Rec. *165*:15–36, 1969.

ASDELL, S. A., ALBA, J. DE, and ROBERTS, S. J.: Studies on the Estrous Cycle of Dairy Cattle; Cycle Length, Size of Corpus Luteum, and Endometrial Changes. Cornell Vet. *39*:389–402, 1949.

ASSHETON, RICHARD, VI: The Morphology of the Ungulate Placenta, Particularly the Development of the Organ in Sheep, and Some Notes on the Placenta of the Elephant and Hyrax. Phil. Tr. Roy. Soc. *198*:143–220, 1906.

BJORKMAN, N.: Ultrastructural Features of Placenta in Ungulates. Fifth Inter. Congr. Anim. Reprod. Trento, *5*:259–263, 1964.

————: Fine Structure of the Ovine Placentome. J. Anat. (Lond.) *99*:283–297, 1965.

————: On the Fine Structure of the Porcine Placental Barrier. Acta Anat. *62*:334–342, 1965.

COOPER, R. A., CONNELL, R. S., and WELLINGS, S. R.: Placenta of the Indian Elephant, *Elephas indicus*. Science *146*:410–412, 1964.

CROTTO, N. R.: Modificaciones citológicas de los epitelios vaginales en la vaca. Rev. méd. vet., Buenos Aires *34*:91–98, 1952.

DAUZIER, L., and WINTENBERGER, S.: Durée du pouvoir fécondant des spermatozoïides de bélier dans le tractus génital de la brebis et durée de la période de fécondité de l'œuf après l'ovulation. Compt. rend. Soc. de biol. *146*:660–663. 1952.

————: La remontée des spermatozoïdes dans le tractus génital de la brebis en dioestrus et anoestrus. Compt. rend. Soc. de biol., *146*:663–665, 1952.

DAVIES, J., and WIMSATT, W. A.: Observation on the Fine Structure of the Sheep Placenta. Acta Anat. *65*:182–223, 1966.

DAWSON, A. B., and KOSTERS, B. A.: Preimplantation Changes in the Uterine Mucosa of the Cat. Am. J. Anat. *75*·1–37, 1944.

DEBOIS, C. H. W., MUURLING, F., and WENSING, C. J. G.: Histological Pregnancy Diagnosis in the Sow by Means of Vaginal Biopsy. Tijdschr. Diergeneesk. *90*:1317–1326, 1965.

DRIEUX, H., and THIÉRY, G.: Placentation chez les mammifères domestiques. Rec. méd. vét. Placenta des equidés. *125*:197–214, 1949; des suidés, *125*:437–455, 1949: des bovidés, *127*:5–25, 1951; des ovidés, *128*:5–18. 1952.

EDWARDS, R. G.: Maturation in vitro of Mouse, Sheep, Cow, Pig, Rhesus Monkey and Human Ovarian Oocytes. Nature (Lond.) *208*:349–351, 1965.

FEDRIGO, G.: Aspetti della mucosa delle salpingi di pecora, bovina, Cavalla e cagna in periodo di gravidanza. Nuova vet. *28*:95–102, 1952.

GUNTHER, E.: Zur Vascularisation der Uterus-Karunkel des Schafes. Zbl. Vet. Med. *5*:171–196, 1958.

HADEK. R.: Morphological and Histochemical Study on the Ovary of the Sheep. Am. J. Vet. Res. *19*:873–881, 1958.

————: Histochemical Studies on the Uterus of the Sheep. *Ibid. 19*:882–886, 1958.

HADEK, R., and GETTY, R.: The Changing Morphology of the Uterus of the Growing Pig. Am. J. Vet. Res. *20*:573–577, 1959.

HAFEZ, E. S. E.: Techniques of Collection and Transplantation of Ova in Farm Animals. J. Am. Vet Med. Assn. *133*:506–512, 1958.

HAMILTON, W. J., and HARRISON, R. J.: Cyclical Changes in the Uterine Mucosa and Vagina of the Goat. J. Anat. *85*:316–324, 1951.

HANSEL, W., ASDELL, S. A., and ROBERTS, S. J.: The Vaginal Smear of the Cow and Causes of Its Variation. Am. J. Vet. Res. *10*:221–228, 1949.

HASHIMOTO, H.: Diagnosis of Pregnancy in the Ewe. Canad. J. Comp. Med. *25*:51–53, 1961.

HATCH, R. D.: Anatomic Changes in the Bovine Uterus During Pregnancy. Am. J. Vet. Research *2*:411–416, 1941.

HAWK, H. W., TURNER, G. D., and SYKES, J. F.: Variation in the Inflammatory Response and Bactericidal Activity of the Sheep Uterus during the Estrous Cycle. Am. J. Vet. Res. *22*:689–692, 1961.

HERRICK, J. B.: The Cytological Changes in the Cervical Mucosa of the Cow (*Bos taurus*) Throughout the Estrous Cycle. Am. J. Vet. Res. *12*:276–281, 1951.

HILTY, H.: Untersuchungen über die Evolution und Involution der Uterusmucosa vom Rind. Schweiz. Arch. f. Tierheilk. *50*:268–323, 1908.

JOHNSON, K. J. R.: Cyclic Histological Changes Occurring in the Endometrium of the Bovine. Res. Bull. Idaho Agric. Exp. Sta. No. 63, p. 20, 1965.

KINGMAN, H. E.: The Uterine Wall of the Cow. Am. J. Vet. Res. *5*:223–227, 1944.

————: The Placentome of the Cow. Am. J. Vet. Res. *9*:125–130, 1948.

KNUDSEN, O.: Endometrial Cytology as a Diagnostic Aid in Mares. Cornell Vet. *54*:415–422, 1964.

MALVEN, P. V. *et al.*: Estrogenic Activity in Bovine Luteal Cyst Fluid. J. Dairy Sci. *46*:995–996, 1963.

McCRACKEN, J. A.: Plasma Progesterone Concentration after Removal of the Corpus Luteum in the Cow. Nature, Lond. *198*:507–508, 1963.

McDONALD, L. E., and HAYS, R. L.: The Effects of Prepartum Administration of Progesterone to the Cow. Am. J. Vet. Res. *19*:97–98, 1958.

MULLIGAN, R. M.: Histological Studies on the Canine Female Genital Tract. J. Morph. *71*:431–448, 1942.

NOVAZZI, G.: Cystic Ovaries Following Estrogen Therapy in Sows. Clin. Vet. Milano *86*:1–8, 1963.

POMEROY, R. W.: Ovulation and the Passage of the Ova Through the Fallopian Tubes in the Pig. J. Agric. Sci. *45*:327–330, 1955.

RESTALL, B. J.: Histological Observations on the Reproductive Tract of the Ewe. Aust. J. Biol. Sci. *19*:673–686, 1966.

RUEBER, H. W., and EMMERSON, M. A.: Arteriography of the Internal Genitalia of the Cow. J. Am. Vet. Med. Assn. *134*:101–109, 1959.

SANGER, V. L. and BELL, D. S.: Comparative Effect of Ladino Clover and Bluegrass Pasture on Fertilization of Ova in Sheep. Cornell Vet. *51*:204–210, 1961.

SANGER, V. L., ENGLE, P. H., and BELL, D. S.: The Vaginal Cytology of the Ewe During the Estrous Cycle. Am. J. Vet. Res. *19*:283–287, 1958.

SANTAMARINA, E., and JOVEN, L. L.: Evaluation of a Diagnostic Test for Pregnancy in Mares Based on the Presence of Gonadotropic Hormones. J. Am. Vet. Med. Assn. *135*:383–387, 1959.

SCHOFiELD, B. M.: Hormonal Control of Pregnancy by the Ovary and Placenta in the Rabb t. J. Physiol. *151*:578–590, 1960.

TORPiN, R.: Placentation in Rhesus Monkey (*Macaca mulatta*). Obstet. & Gynec. *34*:410–413, 1969.

VAN NIEKERK, C. H., and GERNEKE, W. H.: Persistence and Parthenogenetic Cleavage of Tubal Ova in the Mare. Onderstepoort J. Vet. Res. *33*:195–232, 1966.

VOLLMERHAUS, B.: Untersuchungen uber die normalen Zychlischen Veranderungen der Uterusschleimhaut des Rindes. Zbl. Vet. Med. *4*:18–50, 1957. Abstr. Vet. Bull., No. 2242, 1957.

WAGNER, W. C., and HANSEL, W.: Reproductive Physiology of the Post Partum Cow. I. Clinical and Histological Findings. J. Reprod. Fert. *18*:493–500, 1969.

WAGNER, W. C., SASTMAN, R., and HANSEL, W.: Reproductive Physiology of the Post Partum Cow. II. Pituitary, Adrenal and Thyroid Function. J. Reprod. Fert. *18*:501–508, 1969.

WEBER, A. F., and MORGAN, B. B.: Cyclic Histological Changes Occurring in the Endometrium of the Virgin Heifer. J. Animal Sci. *8*:646, 1949.

WIMSATT, W. A.: New Histological Observations on the Placenta of the Sheep. Amer. J. Anat. *87*:391–457, 1950.

WYNN, R. M., and CORVETT, J. R.: Ultrastructure of the Canine Placenta and Amnion Amer. J. Obstet. & Gynec. *103*:878–879, 1969.

Diseases of the Ovary

Infections.—Tuberculosis and other granulomatous infections occasionally involve the ovary by virtue of hematogenous metastasis from lesions elsewhere. The ovary is much more resistant than most organs to the common pyogenic infections, neither does it often show lesions in the acute septicemias or toxemias. The ascent of infection via the oviduct is thought to be possible but it is extremely rare.

Endocrine Disorders.—Cystic ovaries is the common clinical term used to designate the rather frequent condition in which the ovary contains one or more clear cysts ranging in diameter from one to several centimeters.

Follicular Cysts.—The ordinary type of ovarian cyst is the follicular cyst, or cystic follicle. Such cysts have the structure of atretic follicles from which they differ in size and persistence, but they may also be regarded as follicles which approached, but did not attain, normal maturity. While ordinarily larger than the ripening normal follicle, they are not necessarily distinguishable on the basis of size alone.

The atretic follicle differs from the normal follicle in that the lining of granulosal cells, normally several layers thick, is disappearing or has disappeared. Not infrequently, the necrotic granulosal cells may be seen, singly or in bunches, floating in the liquor folliculi. There remains most frequently a single layer of cuboidal or flattened cells; at times even this last remnant of the stratum granulosum has disappeared, leaving the cavity lined only with the fibers of the theca interna. As to when the atretic follicle has become a follicular cyst, there seems to be no definite criterion. The normal course is for the follicle to grow smaller and disappear. To form a cyst this process is reversed, and the term cyst is applied when the structure becomes large enough to become conspicuous upon clinical or gross post-mortem examination. The cysts that are said to occur rarely in the human, which still retain the structures of a living ripening follicle, have not been reported in animals.

In the light of present knowledge and theories of endocrinology, it may be concluded that the **cause** of follicular cysts is a continuously excessive follicle-stimulating action, presumably F S H from the pituitary. Whether this might be due, in turn, to some abnormality in the anti-F S H effect of estrogenic substances from the corpus luteum, other follicles or adrenal is entirely speculative.

The **effect** of one or more cystic follicles may be negligible as in many human cases. However, in mares and cows, clinical experience shows that nymphomania with continual estrum is a frequent result, which is what would be expected if excessive quantities of estrogen are produced. In the canine species, Mulligan finds mammary tumors, glandular hyperplasia of the endometrium and other uterine disorders associated with follicular cysts, presumably as the result of excess of estrogens. Like other cysts, when very large they may cause pain through pressure. Occasionally, hemorrhages occur into these cysts, and an organized clot may be the end result in accordance with the same principles which govern clotting elsewhere.

Lutein Cysts.—Sometimes called ungrammatically "corpus luteum cysts," these represent an abnormal accumulation of fluid at the center of the corpus luteum, where a small fluid-containing cavity is normal. They can be distinguished from follicular cysts only by finding in their walls spherical or polyhedral, lipoid-containing cells, remnants of the atrophic and degenerating corpus luteum. Nothing definite can be said about their cause, although this could conceivably be some accidental insufficiency of blood supply.

Theca-lutein Cysts.—These are similar to ordinary lutein cysts but the polyhedral, lipid-containing cells are considered to be derived from the theca interna. These cysts occur in connection with and apparently as the result of the presence of a chorionepithelioma, a neoplasm arising from chorionic villi. While there are one or two somewhat equivocal examples of chorionepithelioma in the canine species, there appear to be no reports of this type of cyst in domestic animals.

Endometrial cysts, which in the human develop from ectopic endometrium-like tissue, have not been noted in animals.

Cysts constituting parts of a **cystadenoma** or cystadenocarcinoma of the ovary may rarely be encountered.

Dermoid cysts, which are discussed in connection with teratomas (p. 270)

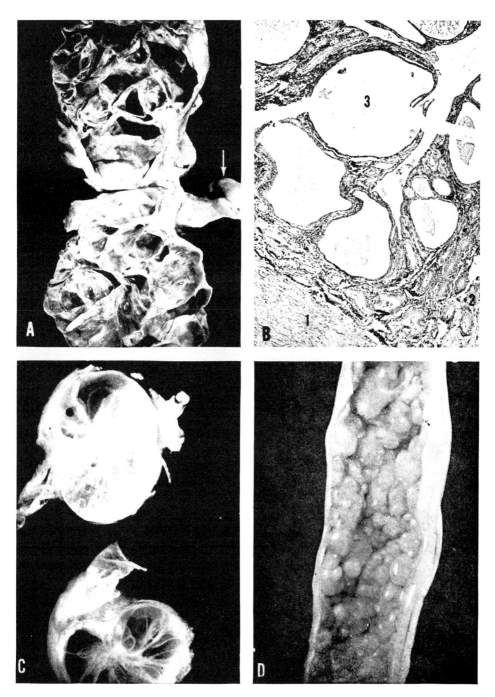

FIG. 26–3.—*A*, Multiple cysts in a canine ovary. The uterine horn is indicated by the arrow Contributor: Dr. Wayne H. Riser. *B*, Cystic glandular hyperplasia of the canine uterus ($\times$ 70), myometrium (*1*), endometrium (*2*), cyst of endometrium (*3*). (*B*, Courtesy of Armed Forces Institute of Pathology.) Contributor: Dr. C. P. Zepp, Jr. *C*, Cystic oviduct in a cow. *D*, Cystic glandular hyperplasia in the canine uterus.

occur in the ovary. They are usually readily recognizable by the hair which they almost always contain.

Parovarian cysts, one or several, are frequent, especially in the bovine. They are found attached to the mesovarium or mesosalpinx, or between their two peritoneal coverings as clear spherical cysts from one to several centimeters in diameter. They are lined with simple columnar, cuboidal or flattened epithelium. Etiologically, they arise as dilated vestigial segments of the embryonic Wolffian body. The latter consists of a main duct, known as Gärtner's duct, with a number of rudimentary branches. In accordance with their embryological origins, the cysts are sometimes referred to as cystic **hydatids of Morgagni.** In the herbivorous animals, it is possible for the cysts of *Taenia hydatigena* to be so located as to cause confusion in diagnosis, but the scolex of the tapeworm is, of course, absent from the parovarian cyst.

Retained Corpus Luteum.—Especially in the bovine, it occasionally happens that a corpus luteum spurium fails to undergo normal involution with the advance of the cycle into its di-estrual phase. Instead it continues to enlarge, reaching the proportions (2 to 4 cm.) which the corpus luteum verum normally attains in pregnancy. Presumably a disturbed hormone balance produced an excess of L H, maintaining the corpus luteum indefinitely. The latter can scarcely be

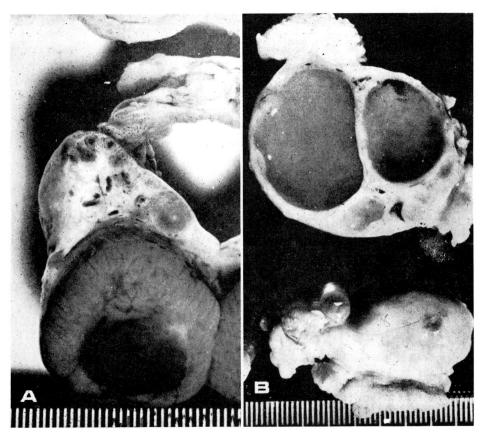

Fig. 26–4.—*A,* Cystic, "retained," corpus luteum from a sterile heifer. *B,* Follicular and parovarian cysts in a bovine ovary.

due to any shortage of the inhibitory progesterone, for the principal effect of the persistent corpus luteum is to prevent the ripening of subsequent follicles. The clinician, by digital expulsion of this corpus luteum per rectum, sets the normal cycle again in motion and the cow's breeding function is restored.

Tumors of the Ovary.—Among primary tumors of the ovary we usually think first of the cystadenoma and cystadenocarcinoma although they may not be the most frequent in all species. These neoplasms consist of large or small cavities lined with a single layer of epithelial cells. In one variety, the cells are cuboidal or low columnar and the cystic fluid is albuminous. In another variety at least in the human, the lining cells are very tall and clear and the fluid in the cavities, called pseudomucine, resembles a mucous fluid in most respects, although it is acidophilic in staining and is not precipitated by acetic acid. In many cases, complicated and reduplicated papillary projections from the lining more or less fill the cystic lumens, whereupon the tumor is called a papilliferous cystadenoma (or cystadenocarcinoma). This type tends toward malignancy. These tumors are usually thought to arise from derivatives of the germinal epithelium although Willis suggests that their origin may be similar to that of the granulosa-cell tumor.

Solid medullary carcinomas are also seen. Adenocarcinomas of the ovary are relatively frequent in domestic birds. Various tumors occasionally metastasize to the ovaries from primaries in other organs. However, there is no such entity as the Krukenberg tumor of humans, a mucoid carcinoma, often presenting its first symptoms in the ovary but proving to be metastatic from a less rapidly progressing primary in the stomach or bowel.

The **granulosa-cell tumor, arrhenoblastoma** and **dysgerminoma** are tumors exclusively of the ovary. All but the first are quite rare, although not unknown, in animals. They are described in the chapter on Neoplasms (p. 259).

Teratomas, including **dermoid cysts,** have been reported in the ovary in some of the domestic species and may prove to be more frequent than our present scanty data would indicate.

Primary supporting-tissue tumors (fibroblastomas, etc.) are extremely rare in the ovary. These organs may be the site of metastatic invasion by extra-ovarian tumors, such as malignant lymphomas, but this is not common.

The Ovary

BECK, C. C., and ELLIS, D. J.: Hormonal Treatment of Bovine Cystic Ovaries. Vet. Med. 55:79–81, 1960.

DAWSON, F. L. M.: Bovine Cystic Ovarian Disease: An Analysis of 48 Cases. Brit. Vet. J. 114:96–105, 134–142, 1958.

DONALDSON, L. E., and HANSE, W.: Cystic Corpora Lutea and Normal and Cystic Graafian Follicles in the Cow. Aust. Vet. J. 44:304–308, 1968.

DOW, C.: Ovarian Abnormalities in the Bitch. J. Comp. Path. 70:59–69, 1960.

GARM, O.: Investigations on Cystic Ovarian Degeneration in the Cow, with Special Regard to Etiology and Pathogenesis. Cornell Vet. 39:39–52, 1949.

LYNGSET, O.: Studies on Reproduction in the Goat. IV. The Functional Activity of the Uterine Horns of the Goat. V. Pathological Conditions and Malformations of the Genital Organs of the Goat. Acta Vet. Scand. 9:308–315, 364–375, 1968. V.B. 39:2739, 1969.

McENTEE, K.: Cystic Corpora Lutea in Cattle. Int. J. Fertil. 3:120–128, 1958.

MOBERG, R.: The Blood Picture in Connection with Persistency of Follicles in Cattle. Nord. Vet. Med. 17:232–236, 1965.

NELSON, L. W., TODD, G. C., and MIGAKI, G.: Ovarian Neoplasms in Swine. J. Am. Vet. Med. Assn. 151:1331–1333, 1967.

RAMAMOHANA RAO A., NARASIMHA, RAO P., and RAO, A. S. P.: Some Observations on Genital Abnormalities of Cattle. Indian Vet. J. 42:751–754, 1965.

SPRIGGS, D. N.: Cystic Ovarian Disease in Dairy Cattle. With Special Reference to Its Treatment Using a Combination of Chorionic Gonadotrophin and Progesterone. Vet. Rec. *83*:231–238, 1968.
THAIN, R. I.: Cystic Ovaries and Cystic Endometrium in Swine. Aust. Vet. J. *41*:188–189, 1965.

Diseases of the Oviducts

The Fallopian tube, or oviduct, is not readily vulnerable to many of the disorders which involve the parenchymatous organs, nor is it usually accessible to the various agents which injure the exterior of the animal body. **Salpingitis,** or inflammation of the oviduct, is the lesion of principal importance because relatively slight inflammatory changes are incompatible with successful performance of the primary function of conveying the ovum to the uterus. Conception can be rendered impossible (1) by occlusion of the tiny lumen through acute or proliferative swelling, (2) by the lethal effect of toxic inflammatory exudates upon spermatozoa, or (3) by destruction of stretches of ciliated epithelium or contractile muscle which propel the ovum to the uterus.

The signs of inflammation are the same in the oviduct as elsewhere, but the pathologist must guard against underestimating the significance of desquamated epithelium (not post mortem), dead cells and débris in the lumen, lymphocytic infiltrations, even though scanty, and proliferation of stromal elements. This is well illustrated in Gilman's (1921) series of bovine cases in which long-standing clinical sterility could not be explained until autopsy, when the oviducts, although normal grossly, showed microscopic inflammatory changes. His diagnoses of infectious salpingitis were strikingly confirmed by the presence of virulent organisms, usually *Streptococcus viridans* or *Staphylococcus aureus*. Hirth, Nielsen and Plastridge (1966) produced salpingo-oophoritis in cows by injecting semen mixed with a *Mycoplasma*.

There are occasional cases of infectious inflammations of the Fallopian tubes characterized by extensive gross lesions. These include the pyogenic infections, with abscesses and **pyosalpinx,** a condition in which the tube is distended with pus entrapped within its lumen. Included also are tuberculosis and probably other chronic infections. The gonorrheal pyosalpinx of humans does not exist in animals. A pathologically mild sero-purulent endosalpingitis may form a part of the syndrome of bovine trichomoniasis.

The cause of salpingitis is always an infection, with the more or less hypothetical exception of irritant medicines being introduced by uterine insufflation or by surgery. The principal causative microorganisms are mentioned above. They may gain entrance (1) by way of the blood stream as part of a generalized infectious process, such as tuberculosis, (2) by spread of a peritonitis through the ostium abdominale, or (3) through the ostium uterinum from a progressing endometritis. Most cases of pyogenic infection represent spread from the uterus.

Sterility has been mentioned as the chief general effect or result of salpingitis. Anatomically, there may be adhesions of the fimbria of the tube to the ovary, tubo-ovarian cysts or abscesses, or local or even generalized peritonitis. Infection and inflammation of the tubal mucosa are seldom uniform throughout the length of the tube and occlusions tend to be formed here and there rather than continuously. As a result, cysts, as well as abscesses, of microscopic or larger size, often form in the intervals of patency between occluded segments. The term

hydrosalpinx is often used in referring to a cyst of macroscopically conspicuous size.

Tumors of the oviduct are practically nonexistent although lymphoid infiltration as a localization of generalized malignant lymphoma occurs rarely.

Congenital anomalies are likewise very rare, although in bovine freemartins (p. 330) the oviduct may share in **hypoplasia** of the whole genital tract. Parovarian cysts or **hydatids of Morgagni** are occasionally seen as pedunculated, clear cysts attached to the fimbria, the tube or the mesosalpinx. As explained in connection with the ovary, they are vestiges of the Wolffian body.

Obstruction of the lumen or stagnation of the blood vessels of the oviduct may result from mechanical displacement by local tumors, abscesses or similar enlargements.

Tubal pregnancy occurs in the human oviduct when a partial obstruction from any cause permits entry of the ascending sperm but denies egress to the much larger ovum. Development of the fertilized ovum then continues in this narrow lumen until the distended tube bursts, often with fatal hemorrhage. Tubal pregnancy seems not to have been reported in animals, perhaps because of the less invasive character of their chorionic tissues.

Diseases of the Uterus and Cervix

While in a quiescent, non-gravid and non-parturient state the uterus is usually free from disease, most of its disorders being connected in one way or another with the reproductive process. Of those illnesses to which the organ is subject, inflammatory diseases require primary attention.

Metritis, Endometritis, Cervicitis

Metritis.—Inflammation of the uterus as a whole is termed *metritis*, while the milder and much more frequent inflammation which involves only the mucosa is **endometritis.** Tuberculosis and other chronic granulomatous infections may invade the uterus, the former with some frequency. In **tuberculosis** of the uterus, or tuberculous metritis, the tubercles tend to be numerous and small, being scattered through the connective tissue of the endometrium and of the intermuscular septa. They are practically always hematogenous metastases from primary infection elsewhere.

Septic metritis is a severe and often fatal inflammation of the whole uterus due ordinarily to infection introduced at or shortly after parturition. As a rule it is the hands and instruments of an operator assisting at a difficult parturition which carry the infectious organisms into the uterine cavity. The parturient uterus is an especially susceptible field for the propagation of microorganisms during this, the puerperal (*puer*- a child), period, because of decomposing (autolyzing) bits of fetal membranes and proteinaceous fluid which remain in it, a perfect culture medium maintained at body temperature and anaerobic. It also constitutes a culture flask of huge size, particularly if involution is delayed by injury of the tissues and exhaustion of the musculature suffered in the struggle of parturition.

The pathogenic organisms most likely to gain entrance and thrive in the lumen and tissues are streptococci, which are often of high virulence, staphylococci, and other pus-formers. The inflammation in such a case is suppurative in type.

Less often the organisms of tetanus, malignant edema or blackleg are carried in, each producing its characteristic local and general disease. It happens that each of these latter infections produces a minimum of exudate, but their toxins are no less deadly and the latter two are also necrotizing. Many streptococci also produce necrotizing (lytic) toxins, so that at the time of death the uterine wall, swollen and bloody, may scarcely have the strength to hold itself together. Other gross features include edematous and hyperemic swelling and the presence of more or less seropurulent exudate which, in acute cases, is likely to be stained with blood. If parturition was a recent event, shreds of fetal membranes may remain adherent to the swollen placentomes.

Microscopically, the uterine wall shows the usual constituents of acute serous and purulent exudates throughout its several layers, the serous constituent (edema) being especially prominent in acute cases. In metritis of longer standing, lymphocytes are numerous. The lining epithelium is commonly missing and the glands may contain mucus. It is interesting to note that this inflammation seldom, if ever, becomes fibrinous. The peritoneal surface of the uterus, like other peritoneal surfaces, is prone to develop a fibrinous inflammation, but this is almost always due to infection originating on the peritoneal side. The terminal period of a fatal metritis is much more likely to be accompanied by a septicemic dispersion of the infection over the body than by a direct extension through the serosa to involve the peritoneal surface. Providing there has been no mechanical perforation as the result of accident or surgery, this latter seldom occurs.

Thrombus formation in necrotic veins is a complication that should cause the veterinary pathologist to search for occluding emboli in other parts of the body when death lacks other adequate explanation.

It should not be inferred, however, that septic metritis is invariably fatal. Today's therapeutic agents present considerable hope of avoiding this outcome. In case of recovery, subsidence is gradual and a chronic purulent endometritis commonly persists for sometime.

Pyometra.—Due to the effect of gravity, exudates are not easily expelled from the uterine lumen in the quadrupeds. The constant weight and pressure of accumulating exudate sometimes produce a gradual distention of the lumen, or impede normal involution in the event that the patient has recently given birth. The result after some days or weeks is pyometra, a condition in which the uterus is greatly distended and filled with pus. The pus usually has the color and consistency of thin cream. The uterine wall may exhibit only mild inflammatory changes.

Pyometra in the farm animals is usually a sequel to parturition and imperfect involution. In the canine and feline species, it supervenes not too infrequently upon the pseudopregnancy that follows an unfruitful ovulation.

Pseudopregnancy.—Also known as **pseudocyesis,** this uterine disturbance of canines and felines represents a pathologically accentuated preparation of the endometrium for the implantation of an embryo, which, in Nature's unguided processes, would normally follow estrum and ovulation. The endometrial epithelium and its stroma proliferate as illustrated in Figure 26–5, long villous extensions proceeding from what were glands, the epithelium of the more superficial villi becoming swollen with huge amounts of clear cytoplasm. Sometimes forming histological structures suggestive of true cystic glandular hyperplasia (p. 1318), this is the same change that is normal in preparation for the development of the complex placental attachments in these species. The difference is that there are no fetal membranes. That these changes are indeed a manifestation of the hormonally stimulated processes of pregnancy, even though it be a false and mistaken one (*pseudo*—false), can, in the case of many bitches, be intriguingly demonstrated if one waits until the sixtieth or sixty-third day after estrus (the normal gestation period), when the expectant canine mother may be seen industriously arranging her nest for the instinctively anticipated accouchement which will not occur and the babies that will not be born.

These morphological and physiological characteristics of pseudocyesis would not be unhygienic or detrimental were it not for the tendency of infectious inflam-

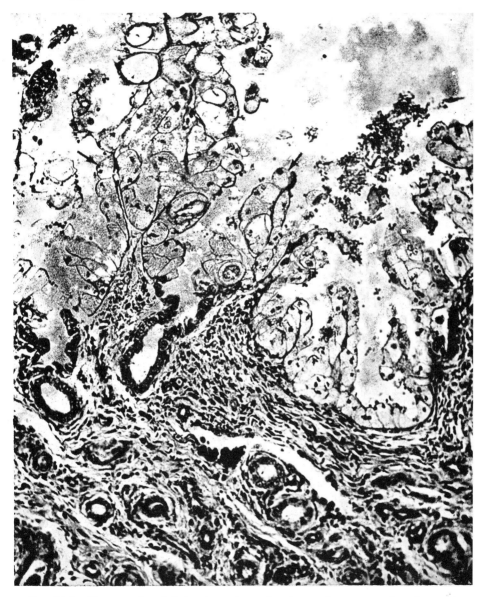

FIG. 26–5.—Hypertrophy of the canine endometrium in pseudopregnancy (pseudocyesis). Note large endometrial cells with clear cytoplasm (arrow).

matory processes to accompany them, in other words, for pyometra to supervene. There is abundant evidence to show, unfortunately, that the progesterone-influenced endometrium, whether post-parturient or psuedopregnant, affords an all too favorable field for the multiplication of pyogenic and other bacteria which may chance to arrive by hematogenous or other routes.

The tendency of the (progesterone-producing) corpora lutea to persist after each ovulation much as if pregnancy were present is characteristic of the canine species and this is doubtless the fundamental cause of pseudopregnancy. That the changes of pseudopregnancy are the result of excessive progesteronic stimulation has been shown by experimental administration of that hormone, as well as by clinical benefits derived from expressing the corpus luteum or administration of the opposing hormone, stilbestrol. On the basis of low specific gravity of the urine (characteristic of pituitary disturbance) and poor tonus of the uterine musculature (pituitrin being recognized as stimulating uterine contraction) Carlstom (see Talanti, 1959) believes that the fundamental abnormality is a low level of posterior-pituitary hormone. Talanti (1959) finds confirmatory evidence in a markedly diminished amount of stainable (by Gomori's aldehyde-fuchsin) "neurosecretory substance," which is supposed to contain the hormone. Definite endometritis developed in 50 per cent of the bitches in which Teunissen (1952) produced endometrial proliferation by means of progesterone, bacterial infection being demonstrated in nearly all.

Endometritis.—As stated previously, endometritis is an inflammation of the mucous lining of the uterus, the endometrium. It may occur as a "hang-over" from a more severe, usually post-parturient, metritis, in which case it is purulent in type, at least at first. A catarrhal endometritis occurs frequently in cows without direct connection with any previous pregnancy and even in heifers which have never been pregnant. The causative organisms appear to be some of the weaker strains of the pyogenic cocci, *Trichomonas fetus* and *Vibrio fetus*. The presence of the microorganisms may be difficult to understand but is usually traceable to previous coitus or parturition or to ill-advised therapeutic maneuvers or artificial insemination. Not a few cases have as their cause chemical irritants in the form of applied antiseptics introduced for therapeutic purposes but in a concentration too strong for the delicate mucous membrane of the uterus or cervix.

Visible changes in the endometrium are not impressive either grossly or microscopically. They include an excessive amount of mucous secretion in the lumen with or without detectable hyperemia, and microscopically a moderate or slight infiltration by lymphocytes, plasma cells, and other leukocytes; there is little more to be seen.

The principal effect of catarrhal endometritis is to prevent conception. The spermatozoa ordinarily cannot survive the toxic substances in the exudate and the ovum, even if fertilized, would perish. There is no significant detriment to the general health as long as the endometritis is no more severe than the catarrhal type. These remarks apply to all species but catarrhal endometritis is of principal importance as a chronic disease of cows.

Cervicitis and Endocervicitis.—The dense fibrous body of the cervix is resistant to inflammatory processes as well as to their causative agents, but the cervical mucosa with its extensive development of mucous glands is peculiarly prone to develop catarrhal (mucous) inflammation. In fact many of the milder cases of catarrhal endometritis should be considered chiefly catarrhal endocervicitis for the catarrhal mucus flows in both posterior and anterior directions. Microscopically, the condition is recognized by the hyperplastic cervical glands with tall, pale, mucin-containing epithelium and precipitated mucin in their lumens. The causes and the significance are essentially the same as for catarrhal endometritis.

Perimetritis.—Inflammation of the uterine serosa and subserosa as well as of the retroperitoneal fibrosa, can exist without spreading into the muscularis or mucosa. It is usually a part of a generalized peritonitis but may result from

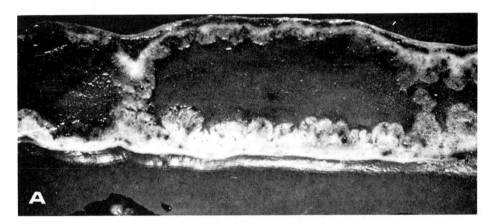

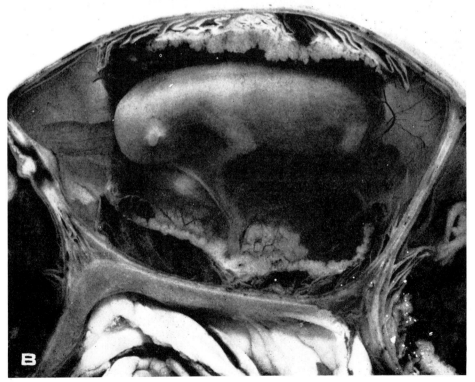

FIG. 26–6.—*A*, Pseudocyesis in a canine uterus (female cocker spaniel, age twelve years). Compare the compartmentation and thickened endometrium with the normal pregnant uterus (*B*). *B*, Normal canine fetuses *in utero* four weeks.

penetrating wounds in the area including perforations of the uterus which sometimes occur in the course of relief of dystocias. The cause is always infectious,
except that large numbers of invasive parasites, such as *Dioctophyma renale* in
the dog, may institute a foreign-body reaction without the presence of bacteria.

Cystic Glandular Hyperplasia

There is a condition seen not too rarely in the canine uterus in which the
mucosal surface of both horns is filled with a congeries of bulging cysts ranging
up to 4 or 5 mm. in diameter, most of them being much smaller and even microscopic in size. The cysts more or less fill the endometrial layer. They are lined
with a single layer of epithelium which, when not too much flattened by pressure
of the fluid within them, resembles the cells which line the normal endometrial
glands.

The cause is presumed to be hormonal, paralleling a similar disorder of the
human endometrium, which has been shown to be attributable to an excess of
estrogens. Glandular hyperplasia and even squamous metaplasia was found in
the uteri of guinea pigs accidentally receiving an excess of estrogens in their food.
There are no indications that cystic glandular hyperplasia leads to neoplasia in
our animals.

Disorders of the Gravid Uterus

Placentitis.—Infections of the placental tissues are likely to lead to early
abortions, but in some types a more or less extensive inflammatory lesion may
develop previous to, or without, expulsion of the fetus. In the human, syphilis
leaves its characteristic mark on the chorionic villi, and tuberculosis occasionally
localizes here to produce its usual granulomatous reaction. One would not be
surprised to find a tuberculous cow or other female similarly affected, although
the more rapid course of this disease in the domestic species and their lower resistance to it would favor death of the fetus before tubercles had time to develop.

Abortion, Premature Births and Still Births.—Abortion is usually defined as the
expulsion of a dead embryo or fetus previous to the end of the full term of normal
gestation. In reference to human patients, abortion is considered to be the
expulsion of an embryo or fetus prior to the stage of development which would
enable it to survive extrauterine life. Still birth is defined as the expulsion of a
dead fetus which has reached the stage of development which would ordinarily
enable it to survive outside of the uterus. It is not always possible to distinguish
these two in animals, and the legal impetus to do so is lacking. The survival of
premature infants also depends upon the quality of post-natal care available.
It is thought that there are a very considerable number of pregnancies in the
bovine that are terminated previous to full implantation (fifty to sixty days),
when the expelled embryo is so small that it is usually not observed. At the
other extreme, some abortions occur at any stage of pregnancy up to full term.
The abortion of Bang's disease occurs typically at approximately the seventh
month of gestation.

The principal infections in which abortion can be expected as a primary manifestation may be summarized as follows: In the active case of **brucellosis** (Bang's
disease) (p. 594), there occurs a placentitis which is characteristic although not
entirely pathognomonic. In the usual acute form, a rather extensive sero-purulent

exudate develops between the chorion and the endometrium in the interplacental areas (chorion laeve), tending to separate these two surfaces. The exudative reaction results in an (inflammatory) edema of the chorion with considerable infiltration of reticulo-endothelial cells, lymphocytes and plasma cells and, in some cases, neutrophils. Suitable stains show the chorionic epithelium to be loaded with the causative bacteria. Upon this exudative inflammation, necrosis supervenes to a variable depth in the allantochorion, producing a hyaline picture microscopically, and grossly a brownish color and leathery consistency.

The effect of these changes is to sever, or at least impair, the placental connection between mother and fetus, with abortion as the result. Nevertheless, some cases are milder so that the calf survives to be born alive.

A chronic proliferative form of placentitis is also described in Bang's disease in which a diffuse and sparsely arranged fibrosis, aided by thickening of the tips of the chorionic villi, ties the chorion to the endometrium. This appears to be responsible for the frequent retention of the placental membranes in those cows in which the infection is not sufficiently severe to cause abortion. It is to be borne in mind that resistance to the Brucella infection gradually develops. Many cows abort only once, a very few may have three consecutive abortions.

In swine, similar lesions occur to those in the cow, but they are likely to be more acute and more severe.

Infarction of the placenta is an important mechanism in abortion in non-human primates (Hertig and King, 1971) (Fig. 26-7).

In **vibriosis**, an abortifacient infection of sheep and cattle, a somewhat similar type of placentitis is encountered. The infection and its products kill the fetus, with abortion following about two days later, in cows between the fifth and seventh month of pregnancy, in ewes during the fifth. No permanent maternal injury results. The principal lesions include necrosis of the chorionic epithelium, serofibrinous or serous exudate (inflammatory edema) throughout the placental tissues

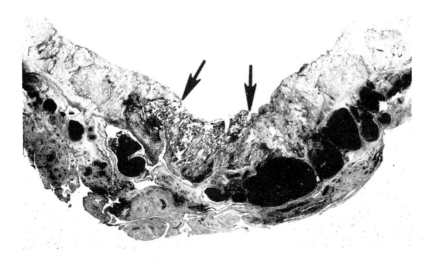

Fig. 26-7.—Infarction of the placenta in a rhesus monkey (*Macaca mulatta*). A small portion of viable tissue is evident between the arrows, the remainder is necrotic. Large thrombi fill placental vessels. Courtesy Dr. A. T. Hertig, and Dr. N. W. King, Jr., New England Regional Primate Research Center, Harvard Medical School.

and infiltration of neutrophilic and other leukocytes, especially into the chorionic villi. The fetal liver is described as containing discolored foci of necrosis a few millimeters in diameter accompanied by perivascular neutrophilic and eosinophilic infiltration. The diagnosis can often be suspected from a noticeable paleness and softness of the fluid-containing cotyledons. It is confirmed by demonstration of the usually numerous curved or even comma-shaped organisms, sometimes in spiral chains. These can be shown readily in smears or sections of the placental cotyledons, preferably stained by Giemsa's or Wright's method.

In bovine **trichomoniasis** (*Trichomonas fetus*), the infection proceeds from the vagina to the uterus, where it initiates endometritis and placentitis which range from a very mild purulent reaction to a copious pyometra. The infection tends to become chronic, with retention of the fetal membranes, usually following abortion during the first half of gestation. The retention of fetal membranes is presumably due to the same mechanism of fibrosis as is the case in brucellosis. Organisms are present in the fetal membranes and fluids but, due to the difficulty of rendering trichomonads visible in tissue, they usually have to be demonstrated by methods appropriate to wet preparations.

In **paratyphoid abortion of mares,** a purulent hemorrhagic placentitis with necrosis of the chorionic villi produces abortion between the fourth and eighth months of pregnancy.

In **equine virus abortion,** which is an infection of the fetus with the virus of equine rhinopneumonitis, the fetal membranes are said to show only edema and perhaps icterus, although a greater variety of changes are to be found in the body of the fetus (p. 429).

Epizootic bovine abortion, caused by a member of the psittacosis-lymphogranuloma group, has been recognized in restricted geographical localities (California, parts of Europe). Among the rather inconspicuous lesions reported in the fetus are minute, scarcely visible, gray foci of leukocytes in most of the parenchymatous organs.

Enzootic abortion of ewes (p. 558) also caused by a member of the psittacosis-lymphogranuloma group is associated with late abortion, and lesions similar to those of epizootic bovine abortion.

Infectious bovine rhinotracheitis (p. 436) is an important cause of abortion in cattle, usually following an outbreak of the respiratory form of the disease. Typical herpesvirus lesions are seen in the fetus (p. 438).

Listeriosis (*L. monocytogenes*) has been known to produce abortion in late pregnancy in cattle and even in sheep. When this involvement is present we are told that the usual encephalitis of listeriosis is minor or absent.

Mycotic abortion has been reported by several, fungi of the genera *Mucor*, *Aspergillus*, and others, having been isolated. Abortion occurs during the last half of gestation and lesions are often very striking, such as large plaques of thickened epidermis, swollen and necrotic placentomes and a thick, leathery chorion-allantois.

Abortion may, of course, be an incidental feature of many acute illnesses not fundamentally localized in the genital tract.

Fundamentally, the cause of most abortions is death of the fetus. The normal reaction of the uterus to a dead fetus is to expel it as a foreign body. The tissues of the placental union often are patently injured, showing inflammation, necrosis, hyalinization or other degenerative changes.   Inability of the injured placenta to transmit the supply of oxygen and nutrients is the usual reason for the death of the fetus, although in some cases, such as certain blood-borne poisonings, it may well be that the fetal body itself is fatally injured by poison that has passed through the placental barrier.   The same is true in some of the infections, including equine viral abortion.

An exception to the above statements is to be found in the case of ergot, which causes expulsion of the fetus (sometimes) through the violent and abnormal contractions which it induces in the uterine smooth muscle.   Abortions can also be produced, at least early in gestation, by anything which eliminates or neutralizes the progestational effect of the hormone of the corpus luteum verum.   This includes manual removal of the corpus luteum from its seat and the administration of large amounts of the antagonistic hormone, estrogen.

Practically speaking, then, the primary causes of abortion are as follows:

(1) Those infections which injure placental tissues, and destroy their function or, in early stages, prevent the original implantation. (See above.)

(2) Severe deficiencies which deprive the fetus, as well as the mother, of some substance essential to life.   Deprivation of oxygen is included here although we are more accustomed to think of minerals and vitamins.   If the latter deficiencies are in existence in the beginning their effect will be prevention of conception rather than abortion of an embryo or fetus already conceived.

(3) Severe acute and often septicemic infections of the mother.   In many cases, probably a majority, this type of abortion can be attributed to the anoxia mentioned under the second heading above, which supervenes because of the generalized venous congestion characteristic of these diseases.

(4) The effect of ergot, mentioned above, and similar abortifacient substances.

Abortions have been attributed to excessive nitrates in weeds growing in fertilized lowland pastures.

(5) The hormonal disturbances mentioned.   These result from artificial interference.

(6) Traumatic injury to the placental attachment, which is very rare.

Mummified Fetus.—As has been stated, a fetus which has died is ordinarily expelled, constituting an abortion.   The reason for this is that the dead fetus acts as an irritant foreign body.   This is particularly true if the fetus is invaded by pathogenic or putrefactive organisms; its continued presence then would lead to maternal infection or sapremia.   But when the cervix remains closed, the uterine contents are frequently sterile; in such a case the fetus undergoes post-mortem autolysis but not putrefaction, and may not be expelled.   The soft tissues of the fetus are gradually liquefied, and the liquid is concurrently resorbed by the maternal blood and lymph.   Months later the fetus is discovered, sometimes by accident, as a mass of bones, sometimes without, but usually with a covering of shrunken and wrinkled skin, a dried and shrivelled mummy.

Retained fetal membranes have been mentioned as a not infrequent post-partum result of placentitis.   Either acute swelling or chronic inflammatory fibrosis appears able to prevent the timely separation of the chorionic from the maternal structures.   Recent experimental evidence points to a lack of progesterone as a potent cause of the disorder, also.   The visible lesions necessary for retention are often quite slight.   Retained more than several hours the membranes undergo both post-mortem autolysis and putrefaction for they are now without a blood supply, lifeless and exposed via the open cervix to exterior contamination. This disintegration ultimately loosens their attachment to the endometrium and, as fragments, they are expelled in the course of several days.

The mother, meanwhile, suffers more or less severely from various toxic products generated by putrefactive and pathogenic bacteria which have gained access by way of the vaginal canal. Under these circumstances, the normal involution of the uterus to its pregravid condition, which should be well advanced in a few hours, is delayed indefinitely. Such a uterus is a most fertile field for the growth of bacteria including anaerobes such as the organism of tetanus, and the list mentioned in connection with septic metritis.

It happens occasionally that in the human uterus small bits of retained chorionic tissues remain attached and maintain themselves alive by absorption of nutritive material. Such chorionic villi tend to proliferate, producing an irregular mass of clear cystic structures known as an **hydatidiform mole.** From such retained fetal villi or from the hydatidiform mole, a malignant epithelial neoplasm known as a **chorionepithelioma,** or syncytioma, occasionally arises. It is recognized by its large multinucleated giant cells resembling those of the normal chorionic syncytium. Comparable proliferations of retained chorionic tissue have been reported in the dog, but they have not been duplicates of the human hydatidiform mole, nor have they fulfilled the criteria of malignancy characteristic of the true chorionepithelioma. In species having the epitheliochorial placenta, such proliferations probably never occur.

Post-partum hemorrhage is not encountered in species having the epitheliochorial or syndesmochorial placenta.

Placenta praevia, which is the formation of the placenta in such a location that it covers the internal cervical opening, and which may, in itself, lead to severe hemorrhage in the human, is limited to those species which have a discoid placenta.

Ectopic Pregnancy.—The development of an embryo elsewhere than in the uterine cavity is called ectopic pregnancy. The most frequent form of this rare accidental phenomenon is tubal pregnancy, in which the embryo, fertilized in the Fallopian tube and prevented by obstruction from reaching the uterus, continues its natural development in the tube. This applies to the human oviduct, where the chorionic villi make their way into the wall forming an hemochorial placenta. Unless relieved by operation, the eventual result is rupture and disastrous hemorrhage when the fetus reaches a certain size. In species having the less invasive epitheliochorial placenta, tubal pregnancy probably does not occur. There are, however, a number of reports of abdominal pregnancy in animals. In most of the reported cases some of which have terminated in artificial delivery of living offspring, investigation has disclosed a recent rupture of the uterine musculature that allowed the fetus to slip into the peritoneal cavity. This, of course, is not true ectopic pregnancy, but fully verified abdominal pregnancy has been reported in certain domestic species. The peritoneal surfaces are obviously not a favorable site for placentation, but the development of a full-term fetus there, later becoming mummified, has been recorded in the dog.

Hydrops Amnii.—This Latin term meaning edema of the amnion refers to a great excess of fluid in the amniotic cavity, a disorder which occurs occasionally. Frequently, the allantoic cavity shares in the excessive accumulation of fluid. The normal amniotic fluid in the mare and cow varies from 3 to 6 liters; the allantoic from 6 to 15 liters.

The causes are not always evident but include rotation of the uterus and twisting of the umbilical cord. The mechanisms here are similar to those which cause local edema elsewhere, interference with the venous drainage by compression of veins but not of the more resistant arteries. Hydrops amnii has been known to occur a second time in the same cow. The condition persists until parturition and may cause death of the fetus and abortion.

Congenital Anomalies.—The uterus and cervix may occasionally undergo anomalous development in animals. The hypoplasia and anomalies of the entire female genitalia in intersexes, and bovine freemartins are described on page 330. An interesting **segmental aplasia** of the uterus and cervix has been reported in cattle (often as "white heifer disease") and in a pony. The anomaly appears to be inherited in cattle as a single recessive gene linked to the gene determining white coat color, thus it occurs more often but not exclusively in white animals. The anatomic features of this entity usually include normal ovaries and oviducts, incompletely developed uterine horns which may distend with fluid due to lack of communication with the cervix. The cervix is hypoplastic as is the vagina. The uterus may be attached to the cervix by two cords, without lumina. These are considered to be incompletely developed remnants of the Müllerian ducts, the embryonic structures which differentiate to form the female tubular organs.

Tumors of the Uterus and Cervix.—There is no important or frequently occurring neoplasm of the uterus or cervix in the domestic animals. Rare reports of fibromas, myomas, adenocarcinomas of the corpus uteri and squamous-cell

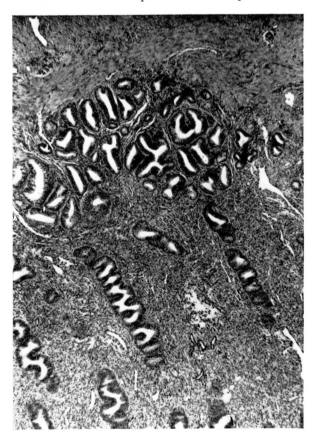

Fig. 26–8.—Carcinoma *in situ*, in the uterus of a chimpanzee. A small cluster of endometrial glands at the base of the endometrium are disorganized, have hyperchromatic nuclei, and are invading adjacent tissue. Courtesy Dr. A. T. Hertig, New England Regional Primate Research Center, Harvard Medical School.

carcinomas of the cervix are just sufficient to tell to us that they exist in domesticated and wild animals, paralleling in type the tumors seen in the human uterus. Adenocarcinomas of the bovine uterus, often with pulmonary metastases, are occasionally seen by meat inspectors. Since death from this cause is almost never reported, it may be that growth of the tumors is quite slow.

Oviduct, Uterus, Cervix and Vagina

AFSHAR, A.: Virus Disease Associated with Bovine Abortion and Infertility. Vet. Bul. *35*: 735–752, 1965.

BECK, A. M., and McENTEE, K.: Subinvolution of Placental Sites in a Post-partum Bitch. A Case Report. Cornell Vet. *56*:269–277, 1966.

BHANDARI, R. M., VELHENKAR, D. P., and SANE, C. R.: Histopathological Study of Tubercular Endometritis with Consequent Effects on Cervix. Indian J. Anim. Hlth. *6*: 281–289, 1967.

BLACK, W. G., *et al.*: Inflammatory Response of the Bovine Endometrium. Am. J. Vet. Res. *14*:179–183, 1953.

BOYD, H.: Embryonic Death in Cattle, Sheep and Pigs. Vet. Bull. *35*:251–266, 1965.

BOYD, W. L.: Some Physiologic and Pathologic Aspects of Sterility in Cattle. Cornell Vet. *24*:138–145, 1934.

BRODEY, R. S., and FIDLER, I. J.: Clinical and Pathologic Findings in Bitches Treated with Progestational Compounds. J. Am. Vet. Med. Assn. *149*:1406–1415, 1966.

BRODEY, R. S., and ROSZEL, J. F.: Neoplasms of the Canine Uterus, Vagina, and Vulva: A Clinicopathologic Survey of 90 Cases. J. Am. Vet. Med. Assn. *151*:1294–1307, 1967.

CALLAHAN, C. J., *et al.*: Prolonged Gestation in a Holstein-Friesian Cow. Clinical and Reproductive Steroid Studies. Cornell Vet. *59*:370–387, 1969.

CORDES, D. O., DODD, D. C., and O'HARA, P. J.: I. Bovine Mycotic Abortion. II. Acute Mycotic Pneumonia of Cattle. N. Z. Vet. J. *12*:95–100 and 101–104, 1964.

DAWSON, F. L. M.: Bovine Endometritis; A Review of Literature to 1947, with Special Reference to the Catarrhal Type of the Disease. Brit. Vet. J. *106*:104–116, 1950.

DENNIS, S. M., and ARMSTRONG, J. M.: Ovine Abortion due to Salmonella typhimurium in Western Australia. Aust. Vet. J. *41*:178–181, 1965.

DENNIS, S. M.: The Effect of Bacterial Endotoxin in Pregnancy. Vet. Bul. *36*:123–128, 1966.

————: Comparative Aspects of Infectious Abortion Diseases Common to Animals and Man. Int. J. Fert. *13*:191–197, 1969.

DIAZ, R., JONES, L. M., and WILSON, J. B.: Antigenic Relationship of the Gram-negative Organism Causing Canine Abortion to Smooth and Rough Brucellae. J. Bact. *95*:618–624, 1968.

DOW, C.: Experimental Reproduction of the Cystic Hyperplasia-Pyometra Complex in the Bitch. J. Path. Bact. *78*:267–278, 1959.

DOZSA, L.: Ein seltener Fall von primärer Bauchhöhlengravidität bei der Katze. Schweiz. Arch. f. Tierheilk. *92*:106–110, 1950.

DOZSA, L., OLSON, N. O., and CAMPBELL, A.: The Uterine Biopsy Technique for Following the Histologic Changes Caused by *Vibrio fetus* in the Uterine Mucosa. Amer. J. Vet. Res. *21*:878–883, 1960.

GARDNER, D. E.: Abortion Associated with Mycotic Infection in Sheep. N. Z. Vet. J. *15*: 85–86, 1967.

GIBBONS, W. J., *et al.*: The Bacteriology of the Cervical Mucus of Cattle. Cornell Vet. *49*:255–265, 1959.

GINTHER, O. J.: Segmental Aplasia of the Mullerian Ducts (White Heifer Disease) in a White Shorthorn Heifer. J. Am. Vet. Med. Assn. *146*:133–137, 1965.

GOUDSWAARD, J., and VAN KOL, N.: *Corynbacterium uteri* (*nov. spec.*) as the Probable Cause of Abortion in a Sow. Neth. J. Vet. Sci. *2*:14–18, 1969. V.B. *39*:3678, 1969.

GRIEL, L. C., JR., KRADEL, D. C., and WICKERSHAM, E. W.: Abortion in Cattle Associated with the Feeding of Poultry Litter. Cornell Vet. *59*:226–235, 1969.

HALLMAN, E. T., SHOLL, L. B., and DELEZ, A. L.: Pathology of *Bacterium abortus* Infections. Mich. State Col., Agric. Exp. Stat., Tech. Bull. 93, 1928.

HARDENBROOK, H.: The Diagnosis and Treatment of Nonspecific Infections of the Bovine Uterus and Cervix. J. Amer. Vet. Med. Assn. *132*:459–464, 1958.

HELLMANN, E., and RAETHEL, S.: (*Trichosporon capitatum* as cause of Abortion in a Cow.) Berl. Munch. Tierarztl. Wschr. *77*:380–381, 1964. V.B. *35*:541, 1965.

HILLMAN, R. B.: Bovine Mycotic Placentitis in New York State. Cornell Vet. *59*:269–288, 1969.

HILLMAN, R. B., and McENTEE, K.: Experimental Studies on Bovine Mycotic Placentitis. Cornell Vet. *59*:289–302, 1969.

HIRTH, R. S., NIELSEN, S. W., and PLASTRIDGE, W. N.: Bovine Salpingo-oophoritis Produced with Semen Containing a *Mycoplasma*. Path. Vet. *3*:616–632, 1966.

HOLLAND, L. A., and KNOX, J. H.: Vaginal Prolapse in Hereford Cows. J. Anim. Sci. *26*: 885, 1967.

JENSEN, R., MILLER, V. A., and MOLELLO, J. A.: Placental Pathology of Sheep with Vibriosis. Am. J. Vet. Res. *22*:169–185, 1961.

JONES, L. M., *et al.*: Taxonomic Position in the Genus *Brucella* of the Causative Agent of Canine Abortion. J. Bact. *95*:625–630, 1968.

KENDRICK, J. W., GILLESPIE, J. H., and McENTEE, K.: Infectious Pustular Vulvovaginitis of Cattle. Cornell Vet. *48*:458–495, 1958.

KENNEDY, P. C., OLANDER, H. J., and HOWARTH, J. A.: Pathology of Epizootic Bovine Abortion. Cornell Vet. *50*:417–429, 1960.

KENNEDY, P. C., and RICHARDS, W. P. C.: The Pathology of Abortion Caused by the Virus of Infectious Bovine Rhinotracheitis. Path. Vet. *1*:7–17, 1964.

KING, S. J., MUNDAY, B. L., and HARTLEY, W. J.: Bovine Mycotic Abortion and Pneumonia. N. Z. Vet. J. *13*:76, 1965.

KNUDSEN, O.: Partial Dilatation of the Uterus as a Cause of Sterility in the Mare. Cornell Vet. *54*:423–438, 1964.

KURTZ, H. J., *et al.*: Histologic Changes in the Genital Tracts of Swine Fed Estrogenic Mycotoxin Am. J. Vet. Res. *30*:551–556, 1969.

LANG, C. M., and BENJAMIN, S. A.: Acute Pyometra in a Rhesus Monkey (*Macaca mulatta*) J. Am. Vet. Med. Assn. *155*:1156–1157, 1969.

LINDSEY, J. R., *et al.*: Intrauterine Choriocarcinoma in a Rhesus Monkey. Path. Vet. *6*: 378–384, 1969.

LOMBARD, L., MORGAN, B. B., and McNUTT, S. H.: Some Pathologic Alterations of the Oviduct. Am. J. Vet. Res. *12*:69–74, 1951.

MAHAFFEY, L. W., and ADAM, N. M.: Abortions Associated with Mycotic Lesions of the Placenta in Mares. J. Am. Vet. Med. Assn. *144*:24–32, 1964.

McCANN, T. O., and MYERS, R. E.: Endometriosis in Rhesus Monkeys. Amer. J. Obstet. Gyn. *106*:516–523, 1970.

McDONALD, L. E., McNUTT, S. H., and NICHOLS, R. E.: Retained Placenta—Experimental Production and Prevention. Am. J. Vet. Res. *15*:22–24, 1954.

McKERCHER, D. G.: Relationship of Viruses to Reproductive Problems. J. Am. Vet. Med. Assn. *154*:1184–1191, 1969.

MERRILL, J. A.: Spontaneous Endometriosis in the Kenya Baboon (*Papio doguera*). Amer. J. Obstet. Gyn. *101*:569–570, 1968.

MILLER, F. W., and GRAVES, R. R.: Breeding History and Gross Changes Found on Autopsy in the Genital Organs of Dairy Cattle. J. Am. Vet. Med. Assn. *81*:408–410, 1932.

MIYAGI, M.: Changes in Arteria Uterina Media of Cows Caused by Pregnancy. Jap. J. Vet. Res. *13*:137–138, 1966.

MOLELLO, J. A., *et al.*: Placental Pathology. I. Placental Lesions of Sheep Experimentally Infected with *Brucella ovis*. II. With *Brucella melitensis*. III. With *Brucella abortus*. Am. J. Vet. Res. *24*:897–922, 1963.

MOLELLO, J. A., and JENSEN, R.: Placental Pathology. IV. Placental Lesions of Sheep Experimentally Infected with *Listeria monocytogenes*. Am. J. Vet. Res. *25*:441–449, 1964.

MOORE, J. A., and BENNETT, M.: A Previously Undescribed Organism Associated with Canine Abortion. Vet. Rec. *80*:604–605, 1967.

MORSE, E. V., *et al.*: Canine Abortion Apparently Due to *Brucella abortus*. J. Am. Vet. Med. Assn. *122*:18–20, 1953.

NICHOLSON, J. W. G., and CUNNINGHAM, H. M.: Retained Placenta, Abortions and Abnormal Calves from Beef Cows Fed All Barley Rations. Canad. Vet. J. *6*:275–281, 1965.

OVERGOOR, G. H. A., and VAN HAAFTEN, J. A.: (Bovine Abortion Caused by *Nocardia asteroides*). Tijdschr. Diergeneesk. *90*:150–154, 1965.

PALMER, W. M.: Macroscopic and Microscopic Changes in the Reproductive Tract of the Lactating Sow. Diss. Abstr. *26*:1262–1263, 1965.

PASCOE, R. R., SPRADBROW, P. B., and BAGUST, T. J.: Equine Coital Exanthema. Aust. Vet. J. *44*:485–490, 1968. V.B. *39*:2010, 1969.

RANBY, P. D., and RAMSAY, W. R.: A Clinical Note on the Occurrence of Oestrogen Toxicity in Pigs. Aust. Vet. J. *35*:90–92, 1959.

RASBECH, N. O.: A Review of the Causes of Reproductive Failure in Swine. Brit. Vet. J. *125*:599–616, 1969.

ROWSON, L. E. A., LAMMING, G. E., and FRY, R. M.: The Relationship Between Ovarian Hormones and Uterine Infection. Vet Rec. *65*:335–340, 1953.

SANGER, V. L., ENGLE, P. H., and BELL, D. S.: Evidence of Estrogenic Stimulation in Anestrous Ewes Pastured on Ladino Clover and Bardsfoot Trefoil, as Revealed by Vaginal Smears. Am. J. Vet. Res. *10*:288–294, 1958.

SATTAR, S. A., BOHL, E. H., and SENTURK, M.: Viral Causes of Bovine Abortion in Ohio. J. Am. Vet. Med. Assn. *147*:1207–1210, 1965.

SCHLOTTHAUER, C. F., and WAKIM, K. G.: Ectopic Pregnancy in a Dog. J. Am. Vet. Med. Assn. *127*:213, 1955.

SCHMIDT, H.: Trichomoniasis or Trichomonad Abortion in Cattle. J. Am. Vet. Med. Assn. *90*:608–617, 1937.

SCHUTTE, A. P.: Canine Vaginal Cytology. I. Technique and Cytological Morphology. II. Cyclic Changes. III. Compilation and Evaluation of Cellular Indices. J. Small Anim. Pract. *8*:301–306, 307–311, 313–317, 1967.

SIMON, J., et al.: Prevention of Non-infectious Abortion in Cattle by Weed Control and Fertilization Practices on Lowland Pastures. J. Am. Vet. Med. Assn. *135*:315–317, 1959.

SKYDSGAARD, J. M.: The Pathogenesis of Hydrallantois Bovis. I. The Concentration of Sodium, Potassium, Chloride and Creatinine in the Foetal Fluids in Cases of Hydrallantois and During Normal Pregnancy. Acta Vet. Scand. *6*:193–207, 1965.

————: II. Electrical Potential and Chemical Gradients Between the Allantoic Fluid and the Maternal Blood in Hydrallantois and Normal Pregnancy. Acta Vet. Scand. *6*: 193–207, 1965.

SOUTHCOTT, W. H., and MOULE, G. R.: Vulvitis in Merino Ewes. Austr. Vet. J. *37*:291–296, 1961.

TALANTI, S.: Observations on Pyometra in Dogs with Reference to the Hypothalamic Hypophysial Neurosecretory System. Am. J. Vet. Res. *20*:41–43, 1959.

TAUL, L. K., POWELL, H. S., and BAKER, O. E.: Canine Abortion Due to an Unclassified Gram-negative Bacterium. Vet. Med. Small Anim. Clin. *62*:543–544, 1967.

TENNANT, B., KENDRICK, J. W., and PEDDICORD, R. G.: Uterine Involution and Ovarian Function in the Postpartum Cow. A Retrospective Analysis of 2,338 Genital Organ Examinations. Cornell Vet. *57*:543–557, 1967.

TEUNISSEN, G. H. B.: The Development of Endometritis in the Dog and the Effect of Oestradiol and Progesterone on the Uterus. Acta Endocrinol. *9*:407–420, 1952.

TICER, J. W.: Canine Infertility Associated with *Pseudomonas aeruginosa* Infection. J. Am. Vet. Med. Assn. *146*:720–722, 1965.

TURNER, P. D.: *Syncephalastrum* Associated with Bovine Mycotic Abortion. Nature (Lond.) *204*:399, 1964.

TURNER, P. D.: Simultaneous Infection of a Bovine Foetus by Two Fungi. Nature (Lond.) *205*:300–301, 1965.

WEBER, A. E., MORGAN, B. B., and McNUTT, S. H.: A Histological Study of Metrorrhagia in the Virgin Heifer. Amer. J. Anat. *83*:309–327, 1948.

WEIKL, A.: (Mycotic Abortion of Cattle.) Vet. Med. Rev., Leverkusen No. 2, pp. 71–80, 1965. V.B. *36*:1744, 1966.

WESTERFIELD, C., and DIMOCK, W. W.: The Pathology of Equine Virus Abortion. J. Am. Vet. Med. Assn. *109*:101–111, 1946.

WETHERILL, C. D.: Retained Placenta in the Bovine. A Brief Review. Canad. Vet. J. *6*: 290–294, 1965.

WHITE, D. S.: A Case of Bovine Fungal Abortion. Irish Vet. J. *18*:168–172, 1964.

WHITNEY, J. C.: The Pathology of the Canine Genital Tract in False Pregnancy. J. Small Anim. Pract. *8*:247–263, 1967.

————: The Pathology of Unilateral Pyometra in the Bitch. J. Small Anim. Pract. *10*: 223–230, 1969.

WILSON, J. C., FOGGIE, A., and CARMICHAEL, M. A.: Tick-borne Fever as a Cause of Abortion and Stillbirths in Cattle. Vet. Rec. *76*:1081–1084, 1964.

WIMSATT, W. A.: New Histological Observations on the Placenta of the Sheep. Amer. J. Anat. *87*:401–459, 1950.

WINTER, A. J., et al.: Variations in Uterine Response to Experimental Infection Due to Hormonal State of the Ovaries. I. The Role of Cervical Drainage, Leukocyte Numbers, and Noncellular Factors in Uterine Bactericidal Activity. II. The Mobilization of Leukocytes and Their Importance in Uterine Bactericidal Activity. Am. J. Vet. Res. *21*:668–682, 1960.

YOUNG, S., PARKER, H., and FIREHAMMER, B. D.: Abortion in Sheep Due to Virus of the Psittacosis-Lymphogranuloma Group. J. Am. Vet. Med. Assn. *133*:374–379, 1958.

THE MAMMARY GLAND

Mastitis

Inflammation of the udder is more commonly known by the above title, derived from the Greek word *mastos*, meaning mammary gland, than it is by the corresponding Latin term, mammitis, which is derived from *mamma*, the Latin name for the same gland. The disease may occur in any mammalian species but is of the greatest frequency and importance, by far, in the dairy cow.

While localized and usually transitory inflammation can result here, as elsewhere, from trauma of various kinds, practically speaking, mastitis is always of infectious origin. Several different bacterial species cause the disease and, in general, it is scarcely possible to determine the causative organism by the type of reaction. The inflammation may partake of any of the acute exudative types except the catarrhal, there being no mucus-producing epithelium in the udder. Hemorrhagic inflammation also is exceptional. Usually acute mastitis represents a combination of the other exudative forms, serous, fibrinous and purulent. Chronic mastitis implies the additional feature of fibrous proliferation, which is common to chronic inflammations anywhere. Since the various reactions almost always overlap in a highly variable manner, there is little to be gained by attempting to classify the multitudinous cases but, in the bovine, it may be helpful to speak of different forms on a basis related as nearly as possible to their etiologies.

In studying the lesions of mastitis, it should be remembered that this is a disease of the lactating rather than of the inactive gland and histologic features must be appraised accordingly. The exudates, fluid and cellular, naturally follow the paths of least resistance, so that most of their component material finds its way into the alveolar lumens, but the intercellular spaces are also filled with leukocytes and fluids. It is thus not unusual to see an alveolus packed with dead or dying leukocytes (pus) but others may be distended chiefly with fluid, which is recognized in the microscopic section by a scanty albuminous precipitate. The epithelial lining of such alveoli is compressed, vacuolated or absent. The adjoining interalveolar stroma may or may not be infiltrated and distended with leukocytes, neutrophilic, mononuclear or lymphocytic, principally the latter. The capillaries are distended in the early acute forms but, in general, mastitis is more impressive for its exudation than for hyperemia. Clots of fibrin and leukocytes are not uncommonly seen in the smaller ducts. These are thought frequently to occlude the drainage of exudate and vitiated milk, thereby favoring the spread of the infective organisms with which they are heavily populated. The importance of drainage as a protective mechanism is well illustrated by the much greater prevalence of inflammatory change in the more dependent portions of the udder and its relative infrequency in the dorsal parts. Judging from the distribution of visible organisms, most, if not all, forms of mastitis appear to be infections fundamentally of the epithelial linings rather than of the interalveolar tissues. Pattison (1952) found the early effects of *Streptococcus agalactiae* to be hyperplastic thickening and cornification of the epithelial lining of the lactiferous duct and sinus with an infiltration of reactive cells immediately beneath. As the condition improved, the extra layers of epithelial cells were shed and the lining returned to normal. From the diseased lactiferous sinus, infection spreads up the branching ductal system to involve the alveolar epithelium and, to some extent, its supporting stroma. The rapidity and ubiquity of this spreading, which of course is dependent upon the relative virulence of the pathogen and the resistance of the host, are responsible for the principal distinctions between what may be called acute diffuse and chronic focal mastitis.

If the activity of the inflammatory process subsides, as it usually does either in a few days or when the lactational period has come to a normal or a premature termination, residual damage of various degrees is discernible. If the injury has been mild and of only a few days' duration, the mammary alveoli, like those of the lung in pneumonia, may return completely to normal. In the more severe forms and more virulent infections, unfortunately, the alveolar epithelium is often so thoroughly destroyed that regeneration is impossible. The alveolar walls then collapse against each other and fuse to form a firm mass of connective tissue, with or without a number of remaining lymphocytes. Despite a certain amount of fibrous proliferation which may have accompanied the process in chronic cases, the total volume of this non-alveolar residuum is considerably less than the space formerly occupied. This constitutes the terminal atrophy which is described in medical writings, the "shrunken quarter" of the dairyman. It is difficult to predict clinically whether any regeneration will occur at the next lactation but if the alveolar destruction has been as great as that just described, regeneration is not possible.

Gross Characteristics of Mastitis.—During life, acute inflammation of one or more of the mammary glands in any species is to be recognized by the usual cardinal signs (p. 145) of acute inflammation. Not the least obvious of these is impaired function, for secretion of milk ceases or diminishes in proportion to the severity of the case. It may be replaced by exudative fluid of abnormal appearance as described below. If the case is of longer duration or is purely inactive and residual, the shrinking and the meaty firmness upon palpation are the decisive features. The shrinking, or atrophy, is especially evident when only one or two of the bovine quarters are so affected, the others remaining of normal size. The firmness is the result of a rather diffuse fibrous proliferation which accompanies the chronic, atrophying process and augments the pre-existing fibrous tissue of the alveolar walls and interlobular septa. Occasionally, the firm tissue has a lumpy arrangement, which betrays a markedly focal form of mastitis or, possibly, old, inspissated abscesses.

Post mortem, most of the same signs are still in evidence, although heat and pain obviously no longer exist. The cut surface of normal mammary tissue in a state of active lactation is a pale pink in color. Its sharply angled and more or less rectilinear lobules are moderately conspicuous, have a diameter of several millimeters and fit together like irregularly formed bricks in a wall. A few drops of milk commonly exude and stand upon the cut surface but there is very little blood. By contrast, the cut surface of acutely inflamed mammary tissue is a darker pink or light red in color; its lobules are somewhat larger in average size (inflammatory swelling) but less distinct and the cut surface is diffusely moist. Usually a few drops of blood ooze from the larger of the severed vessels; if there is any "milk," it is yellowish and resembles pus. The degree of reddening may vary from place to place. If there is chronic fibrosis, the irregularly distributed white fibrous tissue can be seen, often rather easily. Old abscesses and similar lesions of course are obvious.

The diagnosis of mastitis may be accomplished in the living animal either by clinical signs discernible by careful examination of the udder, by demonstration of the causative organism or by **examination of the milk.** In the severe acute cases, the secretion is plainly abnormal, being a yellowish, watery fluid which is little more than blood serum, a serous inflammatory exudate (p. 153). In cases which are more chronic but still severe, the milk may be "stringy," "ropy" or "curdy." The ropy or stringy characteristic is due to the presence of long strands of coagulated fibrin, a fibrinous inflammatory exudate, in which numerous cells are usually entangled. The "curds" are small masses of coagulated casein, more or less pure, which results, in some cases at least, from the local production of acid, certain of the pathogenic organisms (streptococci) being strong acid-producers. This change, then, is chemically analogous to what happens in the souring and curdling of milk after it has been withdrawn and stored for human use. The milk may also contain macroscopically appreciable amounts of blood. These abnormal substances are best detected by directing the milk stream into a "strip cup," a black cloth serving to strain out and make visible such solidified substances.

A number of laboratory procedures can be applied to the milk for the more precise detection of mastitis. Foremost among these are the leukocyte count and the direct bacterial count. In these techniques, a measured amount of milk is spread on a slide and stained. The number and kinds of body and bacterial cells are readily ascertained. A total of 100 leukocytes per ml. is not considered abnormal, since some leukocytes of the various kinds enter the mammary tissue physiologically. The tests by brom-thymol-blue and similar indicators show an increased alkalinity. In spite of the production of acid from lactose by the streptococcal, staphylococcal and other causative organisms, if the inflammation is actively exudative, the alkalinity of the inflammatory exudate shifts the reaction in the alkaline direction. The tests for chlorides and some other substances are also tests for the presence of inflammatory exudate as an invisible contaminant of the milk. On the other hand, there are a few examples of mastitis in which little exudate is formed and the milk shows a higher acidity, detectable by measurement of the pH or by the easier coagulation of the milk upon heating or the addition of alcohol. The increased protein of an inflammatory exudate also favors coagulation by alcohol (or heating). However, the alcohol test is of minor importance in the diagnosis of mastitis.

The question naturally arises as to which of the several diagnostic methods are most accurate. Physical examination of the udder depends for its accuracy upon the skill of the examiner but obviously has its limitations in the rather numerous latent and subclinical cases. The special tests upon the milk are usually considered suitable for use in conjunction with other methods of diagnosis. Culturing alone has been said to miss a very considerable proportion of cases which were detectable by leukocyte counts upon the milk and a somewhat higher proportion of those which were diagnosed post mortem by histopathological examination. However, in making the histopathological examination, it must be remembered that the presence of considerable numbers of lymphocytes is characteristic of the process of post-lactational involution and not necessarily pathological.

Causes and Routes of Entry.—It has already been stated that the cause of mastitis is infection by pathogenic microorganisms. While there are two routes by which pathogenic organisms theoretically may gain access to the mammary tissue, all evidence indicates that hematogenous infection almost never occurs and that entrance through the lactiferous duct accounts for practically all cases of mastitis. Much of this evidence is clinical and bacteriological and will not be recounted here, but the great preponderance of cases in which one quarter of the cow's udder becomes infected independently of the others argues for accidental contamination through the orifice of the teat. There are indications that bovine udders have been infected from the mouths of calves suckling them, at least in the case of disease caused by Pasteurellae or Corynebacteria. The more usual source of infection is contamination of the milker's hands, the "cups" of the milking machine or other utensils which come in contact with the teat.

While several different pathogens are capable of causing bovine mastitis, the great majority of cases are due to *Streptococcus agalactiae* (*Strep. mastitidis*) (p. 580). This organism is the cause of the usual insidiously arising, chronic form of mastitis. *Streptococcus dysgalactiae* causes an acutely arising form, sometimes apparently originating in a traumatic injury. While the infection is eventually self-limiting, its termination may apparently depend upon the exhaustion and destruction of the susceptible acinar epithelium; in other words the affected quarter is permanently functionless. *Streptococcus uberis* also causes an acute mastitis, but the disease is typically much less severe, with early complete recovery.

Next in importance to the streptococci are staphylococci. *Staphylococcus pyogenes* causes a severe acute or fulminating infection of the gland commonly accompanied by fever and general bodily malaise. These cases are often fatal in a few days. Some go on to gangrene of the udder.

Corynebacterium pyogenes, another one of the pyogenic group of organisms, occasionally causes mastitis. The disease is usually distinctly suppurative in type with formation of large amounts of pus, often abscesses and sometimes extensive necrosis and sloughing of masses of tissue. There has sometimes been sloughing of whole quarters, followed ultimately by healing. Presumably the latter phenomenon is the result of thrombosis and infarction, although there appear to be no investigations which would eliminate direct toxic action of the bacteria. Some udders rupture, others form fistulous tracts to discharge the pus. A minority of affected cows show fever and general reaction in the early stages, with signs of pain in the joints. Occasionally, the attack is fatal, but the usual result is slow recovery with functional loss of the involved quarter or quarters. This form of mastitis attacks non-lactating or even immature glands as well as those in lactation. In Europe, it has been called summer mastitis since the non-lactating cows are often affected while in summer pasture.

Pseudomonas aeruginosa (*pyocyanea*) is a rare cause of acutely developing mastitis. Tucker (1952) reported cases which resulted from the introduction of contaminated medicaments into the teats by a dairyman. The inflammation terminated in destruction of the affected quarters.

The Pasteurella organism (*P. multocida, P. septica*) is occasionally the cause of mastitis. It is chronic and suppurative in type.

The organism of Bang's disease, *Brucella abortus*, is usually stated to remain in the udder during the quiescent inter-gestational period without producing lesions. While this is doubtless true as regards clinical mastitis, Runnells and Huddleson (1925) found well-marked inflammatory changes in the form of lymphocytic infiltrations, a purulent intra-alveolar exudate and other changes, with terminal destruction of alveoli (atrophy) in affected areas. High cell counts and other confirmatory data come from other sources. Experimental introduction of *Brucella suis* into the udders of cows produced very severe acute mastitis.

Coliform mastitis, while rare, is a rather distinct type. Acute inflammation characterized by heat, pain and soft, edematous swelling, together with discolored, fibrinous clots in the milk, arises suddenly either without previous evidence of abnormality or as an acute exacerbation of a latent infection (determined by systematic culturing at regular intervals). The causative organisms are *Escherichia coli, Aerobacter aerogenes* or their close relatives. Terminal effects are usually mild but vary; there is often return to normal in a few days; in other cases, persistent mastitis leads to involution of the quarter with restoration of normal function at the next lactation. A chronic form characterized by successive acute exacerbations may develop. There is also an acute form accompanied by fever, dehydration, severe toxic symptoms and usually death (prevented by streptomycin). Histopathological examinations of the affected glands appear not to have been made.

Aphthous fever (aftosa, foot-and-mouth disease) is accompanied by mastitis in a considerable proportion of cases. Development of this complication appears to depend upon introduction of virus into the lactiferous orifice from vesicles on nearby skin. The reaction is acute serous in type and adds considerably to the severity of the generalized disease.

A "pleuro-pneumonia-like organism" is described as causing agalactia (mastitis) in sheep and goats. The disease is not localized to the mammary gland, however.

The presence of a member of the genus *Candida* has been reported in conjunction with mastitis in cattle.

Gangrenous Mastitis.—It is not rare for a cow to develop suddenly an acute and severe inflammation, often of all four quarters of the udder which, in the course of a day or two progresses to gangrene. Starting in the distal portions and rising closer and closer to the attachment of the udder, the parts become cold and insensible; white skins show a bluish tinge. Commonly death supervenes about the third or fourth day. A similar disease occurs in sheep and is not necessarily precluded in other species. The tissue changes are those characteristic of any moist gangrene (p. 26), often with considerable amounts of fluid, a serous inflammatory exudate, or inflammatory edema. It is noteworthy that while one group of lobules is completely necrotic and gangrenous, an adjoining area may be living and only moderately altered, with just an inflammatory line of demarcation between the two.

Many of these cases appear to be infections with highly virulent staphylococci, although Mura (1950) believed the combined action of a streptococcus and *Clostridium welchii (Cl. perfringens)* to be essential in causation. It is commonly accepted that the gangrene (p. 26) supervenes upon infarction resulting from thrombosis of vessels. While this is entirely plausible on the basis of pathological principles, it is difficult to reconcile with the fact that in many cases all four quarters are synchronously affected. The possibility of a direct necrotizing action of the causative pathogen should be investigated. Numerous investigators have attributed just such an action to staphylococci.

Cryptococcal Mastitis.—Very rarely, the bovine udder is affected with cryptococcosis or torulosis (*Torula histolytica, Cryptococcus neoformans*), which leads to disastrous destruction of the mammary tissue. The mode of entry of

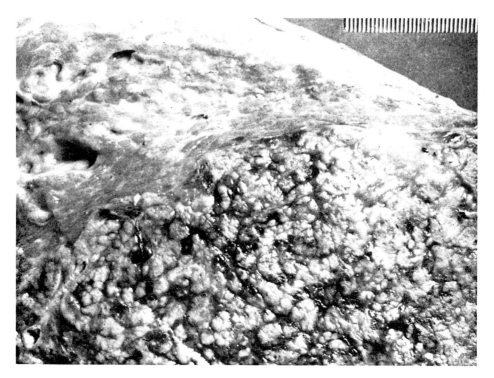

Fig. 26–9.—Gangrenous mastitis in a cow.

the infection is accepted as being via the orifice of the teat, as in other kinds of mastitis. The number of quarters involved is variable.

The affected tissue, which is often the whole quarter, is firmer than normally and grayish or almost white in color, except for occasional small hemorrhagic areas. From the cut surface exude copious amounts of a slippery, viscid fluid which resembles mucus excepting that it is less translucent. (It contains no epithelial or connective tissue mucin, p. 52.) The microscopic changes correspond to those of cryptococcosis in any location (p. 657). Briefly, in the most acutely affected areas, there is replacement of the acinar and ductal epithelium by the liquefied material just described. The yeast cells are plainly seen, but little else is visible within the relatively unchanged fibrous walls of the alveoli and ducts. In areas (or individual patients) where the infection was held to less rapid destruction, there is a limited degree of reticulo-endothelial and even fibrous reaction, with large numbers of fat-filled phagocytes or small granulomatous nodules. Diagnosis is made by demonstration of the typical yeast cells, which are described elsewhere (p. 659).

Mastitis in Sheep.—Ewes suffer from a severe acute form of mastitis often unilateral, which frequently displays considerable contagiousness. Stockmen refer to the condition as "blue bag" because of the severe venous congestion which imparts a dark bluish tinge to the exterior of the udder. Doubtless abetted by the venous stasis, the inflammatory process often is superseded by gangrene. In ewes, the gangrene is more prone than it is in bovines to limit its ravages to parts of a gland rather than the whole.

The microscopic picture, except in a few mild and almost subclinical cases, is

Infectious orchitis may result from hematogenous metastasis or from extension of infection up the genital tract and through the epididymis, as mentioned above. **Brucellosis** (Bang's disease) in the bull and in the boar commonly manifests itself as a severe orchitis, which may be both necrotizing and suppurative. In view of the well-known predilection which this infection has for reproductive tissue, it would be dangerous to offer an opinion as to whether entrance of the organism is hematogenous or by extension. Infections of other parts of the genital tube can often be demonstrated, but the vas deferens itself is seldom injured. In some cases, brucellosis of the testicle, most often unilateral, becomes chronic with much fibrous enlargement of the testicle, the functional tissue of which has been extensively or completely destroyed. The peritesticular and scrotal tissues usually share in the inflammatory proliferation, perhaps with pus between the layers of the tunica vaginalis.

An acute suppurative orchitis with or without abscesses has been described in the horse as the result of infection with the abortion-producing *Salmonella abortus-equi* (Jansen, 1947; Helmy, *et al.*, 1966). The orchitis was accompanied by fever and general bodily reaction during its acute stage.

The Brucella organism, *Brucella ovis*, causes epididymitis in rams (Simmons and Hall, 1953). Hyperplasia of the lining epithelium was a part of the microscopic picture. Brucellosis is, however, very rare in sheep.

The other abortifacient microorganisms (*Vibrio, Trichomonas*) appear not to invade the male genital system beyond its external parts. Non-specific hematogenous orchitis occurs occasionally in the course of various infections which assume a generalized form, such as equine strangles (p. 578). An organism causing a severe purulent orchitis in rams was identified as *Pasteurella pseudotuberculosis (Corynebacterium pseudotuberculosis rodentium)*, which is ordinarily a pathogen of guinea pigs (Jamieson and Soltys, 1947). The organism of blue-green pus (*Pseudomonas aeruginosa, Bacillus pyocyaneus*) has been identified in diseased male genital tracts, apparently without being responsible for marked lesions (Rempt and Zwanenburg, 1949). In a diagnostic test known as the **Strauss reaction,** male guinea pigs often develop periorchitis and a necrotizing and destructive suppurative orchitis a few days subsequent to intraperitoneal inoculation of small doses of the glanders bacillus as well as of the organisms which cause melioidosis, epizootic lymphangitis, ulcerative lymphangitis and ovine caseous lymphadenitis. In humans, mumps is a disease which often includes orchitis in its manifestations when it attacks adult males.

The **effects** of the more severe forms of orchitis are obvious: destruction of the testis, marked pain and in some cases a generalized febrile disease with fatal septicemia. The mildest forms result in at least temporary **aspermatogenesis.** This depends upon necrosis and destruction of the germinal cells lining the seminiferous tubules. The more superficial cells perish first; often the process continues until none but the sustentacular (Sertoli) cells remain to line the tubules. A high percentage of deformed and imperfect spermatozoa supervenes upon such injury to the germinal epithelium (Andreevskii, 1948), provided, of course, the disorder is slight so that some spermatogenesis still continues. Regeneration does not occur, once the germinal tissue has been completely destroyed. In evaluating these milder lesions, it should be remembered that certain areas of aspermatogenesis may be encountered in the normal testis, as if they were in a resting or dormant state.

43

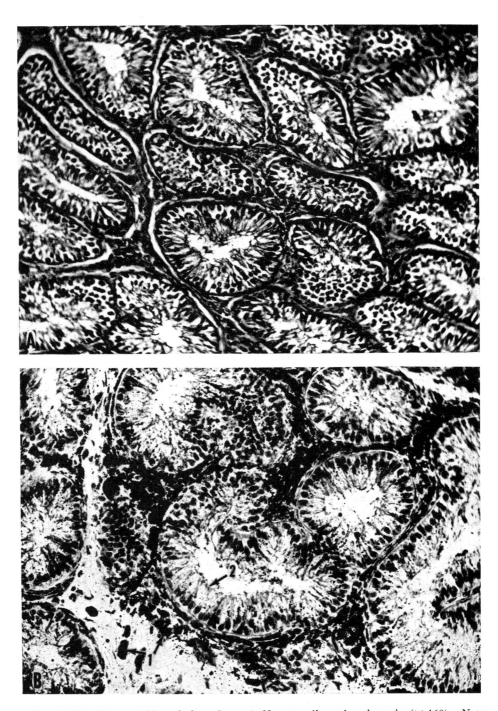

FIG. 26–10.—Cryptorchid testis in a dog. *A*, Hematoxylin and eosin stain (× 160). Note tubules are lined completely with tall columnar Sertoli cells. *B*, Section stained with Sudan III to demonstrate lipid in interstitial cells (*1*) and Sertoli cells (*2*). (*B*, Courtesy of Armed Forces Institute of Pathology.) Contributor: Dr. Leo L. Lieberman.

Semen and Spermatozoa

The study of the semen in cases of suspected masculine infertility in farm animals has become an important specialty (Weber and Morgan, 1949; Glover, 1955). For successful breeding, the number of spermatozoa must be adequate, although it can vary within wide limits, the great majority, at least, must be of normal structure, and their motility must be satisfactory. Stains have been devised which differentiate between living and dead sperms, coloring only the latter (Blom, 1950). The collection, preservation and transportation of semen for artificial insemination, chiefly of dairy cattle, have received wide attention. It is possible to maintain the viability of semen (except porcine) for many weeks by freezing it under suitable conditions at extremely low temperatures ($-79°$ C.) (Polge and Rowson, 1953).

Cryptorchidism

With a literal meaning of "hidden testicle," this relatively mild developmental disorder results from failure of one or both testes to descend, with their tunics, from their fetal position in the sublumbar region, through the inguinal canal and into the scrotal sac. While normally an event of fetal life, it is not unusual for the complete descent into the scrotum to be delayed until several months after birth. Permanent retention is most important and most frequent in the horse and dog. In cattle and sheep cryptorchidism is quite uncommon.

The cryptorchid testis fails of complete anatomical and histological development because of the disadvantages of its position, its size being small and its consistency soft. The seminiferous tubules, if formed, are rudimentary, lacking most of the layers of reproductive cells. Only quite exceptionally is there any spermatogenesis. The interstitial cells are likely to be few and buried in much fibrous tissue, but there are cases in which these cells are unduly numerous. There have been instances where the cryptorchid testis proved to be no more than a modified vas deferens, with many tributary tubules. The reason for this hypoplasia of the cryptorchid testis appears to be less a matter of the unnatural pressures upon it than it is the higher temperature of the abdominal cavity. Experimental work indicates that the cooler environment of the scrotal sac is necessary for proper development and spermatogenesis.

The anatomical cause of cryptorchidism is often discovered in the form of shortened spermatic vessels, cremaster muscle or vas deferens, but the fundamental cause is commonly suspected to be hereditary. There is limited statistical support for this theory. On the other hand, Manning (1950) induced cryptorchidism in rats previously normal by a diet of egg-whites (deficient in biotin). Of interest is the report that the testes of the elephant normally remain in the abdomen.

Indications are that testicular neoplasms arise with greater frequency in cryptorchid testes than in normal ones.

Torsion of the Testis

Especially when the spermatic cord is unusually long or relaxed, the testicle may be rotated on its axis by trauma, exercise or straining. The twisting of the blood vessels produces venous and often arterial obstruction, leading to con-

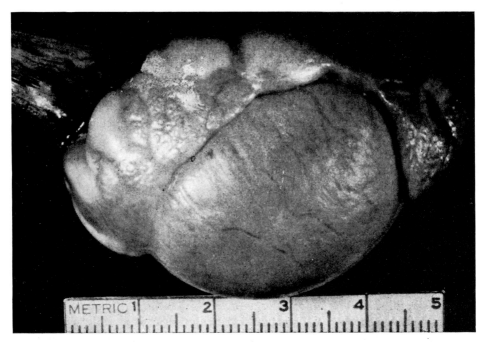

FIG. 26–11.—Sperm granulomas in epididymis of a seven-year-old male beagle. (Courtesy of Angell Memorial Animal Hospital.)

gestion and edema in mild cases. With more complete obstruction, these changes are accompanied by necrosis, at least of the delicate cells lining the seminiferous tubules. The condition is essentially that of an infarction involving the whole organ. **Infarction** of the testis or a segment of it can also occur as the result of thrombosis or embolism in the spermatic vessels, although the condition is not common.

Spermatic granuloma is a name given to small masses of granulation tissue, usually with a foreign-body reaction, which form around foci of escaped spermatozoa in the testis or epididymis. They are not altogether rare. (Fig. 6–10*B*, p. 178.)

Neoplasms of the Testicle

Primary tumors are seen most frequently in the dog, but this is probably because entire males are available for observation in far larger numbers in this than in other domestic species. The types peculiar to the testicle are the seminoma, the sustentacular-cell or Sertoli-cell tumor, the interstitial-cell or Leydig-cell tumor and the teratoma. These are discussed under their respective headings. Metastatic tumors are possible but are extremely rare.

Hermaphroditism

Since the genital tracts of both sexes develop primarily from the same embryonic primordium, it is perhaps not surprising that occasionally structures characteristic of both sexes are found in the same individual. In a true hermaphrodite, both ovarian and testicular tissue occur either in united or separate structures. A male pseudohermaphrodite has more or less normal testes, but the accessory reproductive organs resemble those of the female. In the female pseudohermaphrodite, ovaries are present but the tubular reproductive tract is rudimentary and the external genitalia bear an anatomical resemblance to those of the male. The uterus masculinus constitutes a normal persistence in the male of parts of the female genital tract. It is usually of appreciable size in the stallion and in some species, for instance, the guinea pig, it is a well-developed anatomical structure. Hermaphroditism represents a form of congenital malformation.

Various forms of intersexuality are discussed further in connection with chromosomal anomalies (p. 330). Gonadal hypoplasia is found in most species, if adequately studied, but the etiology is not known in most instances. Simple genetic inheritance is postulated in some instances (Kodagali and Kerur, 1968). A segmental aplasia of the Wolffian duct of mink, resulting in absence of the epididymis, is thought to be an inherited defect (Blom and Hermansen, 1969).

Heterotopic displacement of testicular tissue has been reported in swine (Todd, Nelson and Migaki, 1968). The testicular tissue was found embedded in or attached to the liver, spleen, mesentery, pancreas, stomach, omentum, colon, cecum and diaphragm. Grossly, these usually resembled neoplasms but histologically were seen to consist of atrophic testicular tissue resembling cryptorchic testes. The origin of these testicular implants is not known. It is postulated that they may arise from displaced germ cells or possibly from surgical procedures such as castration.

Hydrocele

Whereas hydrothorax, for example, is an accumulation of watery fluid in the thoracic cavity, hydrocele is an accumulation of watery fluid in the cavity of the scrotum. Usually the fluid lies between all adjacent layers of the tunica vaginalis and occupies all spaces between the testicle proper and the skin.

While hydrocele occurs occasionally as an accompaniment of generalized edema involving the whole ventral belly wall, it is ordinarily the result of intrascrotal disorders. These include interference with the return flow in the spermatic veins. In the majority of cases, however, hydrocele is an inflammatory edema, as shown not only by the causative circumstances, but also by the higher specific gravity and protein content of the fluid, which are such as to place it in the category of an exudate and not of a transudate (p. 137). The condition is thus a histologically mild inflammatory disease of the scrotal tissues (with or without the testis proper) and is caused most often by trauma, sometimes by local infections.

Scirrhous Cord

While elephantiasis of the scrotum comparable to that seen in humans as an effect of *Filaria (Wuchereria) bancrofti* does not occur in the domestic animals, a superficially similar gross enlargement of the scrotum and its contents occurs in scirrhous cord. The disorder is merely excessive granulation tissue (p. 166) forming on the stump of the severed spermatic cord following castration, the cause being a chronic hyperplastic proliferative inflammation resulting from untoward operative injury and infection. It is common in pigs because of their proximity to the soil, their commonly insanitary surroundings and the crude sort of surgery which is sometimes performed by stockmen. The species next most frequently involved is the equine because of the horse's notoriously poor resistance to many of the ordinary infections, chiefly pyogenic.

The mass of abnormal tissue may attain startling proportions in a very few weeks. It consists usually of dense fibrous tissue alternating irregularly with areas of more youthful and more active fibroblastic growth. Some areas contain much leukocytic infiltration. There are often thick-walled, chronic abscesses. Under the name of botryomycosis (p. 581), a form has been described in equines in which the granulation tissue assumes a reticulo-endothelial form suggestive of actinomycosis, with the formation of "rosettes." This condition is in fact attributable to a staphylococcus, but it is not meant to imply that the usual case of scirrhous cord is anything more than the ordinary type of pyogenic granulation tissue. Scirrhous cords are usually terminated by operative removal.

Accessory Structures

Epididymitis accompanies or may precede orchitis. in connection with which it has been mentioned.

Epididymitis in sheep has been ascribed to infection by *Actinobacillus seminis* by several authors (Livingston and Hardy, 1964; Simmons, Baynes and Ludford, 1966).

Inflammation of the **vas deferens** is rare because of its simple and impervious structure and excellent drainage.

The seminal vesicles and bulbo-urethral glands (in those species which have them) tend to harbor infections because of their complicated structure and poor drainage. They are thus of some importance as sites of localization of brucellosis, vibriosis and trichomoniasis, as well as for the locally less destructive *Pseudomonas aeruginosa* (*pyocyaneus*). In the bovine seminal vesicle, pronounced metaplasia of the columnar epithelial lining to a heavily cornified stratified squamous type has been noted, apparently due to avitaminosis A. Well-marked melanosis has been seen in the bulbo-urethral (Cowper's) gland of the ram.

A syndrome involving the seminal vesicles of male bovine animals has been described and given the name **seminal vesiculitis.** An organism of the psittacosis group (*Chlamydia*, p. 550) has been isolated from the semen and epididymis of affected bulls (Storz, *et al.*, 1968; Ball, Young and Carroll, 1968).

The Prostate

In cattle, sheep and swine, the prostate is little more than rudimentary in size, much of its glandular tissue being disseminated in the wall of the upper urethra. The equine prostate is also relatively small; its function, limited; its diseases, rare. The dog's prostate, however, is well developed, as if to compensate for the absence of seminal vesicles and bulbo-urethral glands in this species. The diseases of the canine prostate are of importance and appear to be entirely comparable to those seen in the human being.

Acute prostatitis occurs infrequently except in the dog. It is ordinarily suppurative, often with formation of abscesses. There may be a number of abscesses, small or microscopic in size or there may be one or two of large size, a maximum diameter of 11 cm. having been reported (Schlotthauer, 1937). With high resistance on the part of the patient, the abscess or abscesses may become heavily

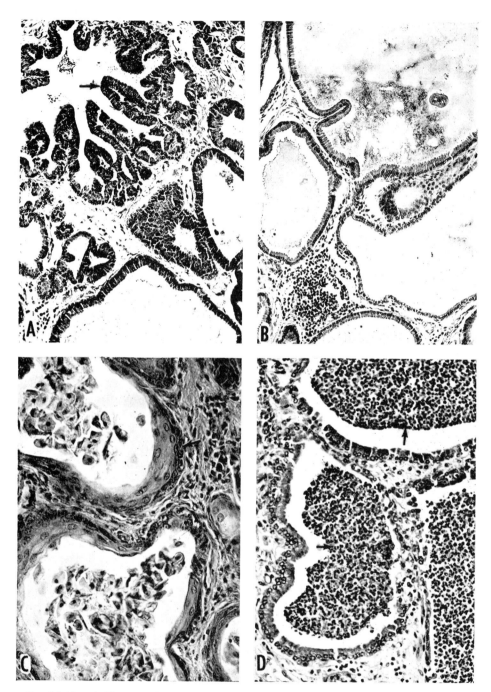

FIG. 26–12.—*A*, Hyperplasia of the canine prostate. Note tall columnar cells (arrows) in long fronds extending into the lumen of prostatic acinus. Contributor: Dr. S. Pollock. *B*, Cystic glandular hyperplasia of the canine prostate. Cysts are formed in parts of the gland. Contributor: Dr. Norman G. Simels. *C*, Squamous metaplasia (arrow) of the prostate of a dog with a Sertoli cell tumor of the testis. Contributor: Dr. Wayne H. Riser. *D*, Acute purulent prostatitis in a dog. Note acini filled with neutrophils and cellular debris. (*A–D*, Courtesy of Armed Forces Institute of Pathology.) Contributor: Dr. Albert M. Berkelhammer.

encapsulated; otherwise septicemia and a fatal outcome are entirely possible. One or another of the pyogenic cocci can usually be incriminated as the cause. Clinically, the acutely inflamed prostate is extremely painful when subjected to pressure, in contrast to the ordinary enlarged prostate, which is comparatively insensitive.

Hyperplasia of the Prostate.—Chronic prostatitis merges in an obscure fashion with what is often called clinically "benign prostatic hypertrophy." However, the condition is in reality a hyperplasia by either of the possible definitive criteria (p. 94). If we consider the matter of function, there certainly is no improvement in function; if we judge merely by the number of cells, it is immensely increased but their individual size is not greatly changed; if our criterion is a disproportionate increase of some tissue components as compared to others, this obviously exists. Hence, pathologists use the term hyperplasia.

In prostatic hyperplasia, the organ is enlarged, often immensely, because of an increase in both the size and number of glandular acini. Accompanying this glandular proliferation there is an augmentation of the fibrous tissue and smooth muscle of the septa and supporting structures. Occasionally, this increase of the supporting tissues is the predominant change, but in the great majority of cases it merely keeps pace with the epithelial hyperplasia. The epithelial cells lining the acini increase in height but they increase much more in numbers. As is the case with hyperplasia of the thyroid and other glands, the augmented cellular population is accommodated by the formation of tortuous folds in the acinar lining. These folds and ramifications may become very numerous and complicated so that the lumen of the acinus is filled with a complex maze of epithelial surfaces, each with its supporting fibrous stroma. It is only by carefully following the winding row of surface cells that the true arrangement is perceived, and it is only by the absence of anaplastic epithelium and its failure to penetrate through its basement membrane into the connective tissue stroma that the suspicion of neoplasia is eliminated. On the other hand, some acini dilate and fill with secreted fluid, thus forming cysts of microscopic or macroscopic size. The epithelial lining of these cysts is usually stretched and flattened. In some hyperplastic prostates the cystic changes are more or less predominant and the condition is known as **cystic glandular hyperplasia.** Frequently, however, the cystic changes, regarded by some as degenerative in nature, and the strictly hyperplastic increase of epithelium just described occur in the same prostate. Accompanying these hyperplastic changes, there is practically always some evidence of chronic inflammation, chiefly in the form of lymphocytic infiltrations into the interstitial tissue.

Grossly, the change is a rather uniform increase in the outside dimensions of the organ without noticeable distortion in its shape. When the urethra is opened, however, it is not unusual to see a number of smooth but roundly pointed nodules projecting into its lumen. These are commonly from 1 to 4 mm. in diameter and height and represent nodules of bulging prostatic tissue beneath the urethral mucosa. It is difficult to state what the dimensions of a normal prostate should be in a species whose individual members vary through the tremendously wide range of stature that is seen in dogs. Schlotthauer (1937, 1942) found that the weight of the normal canine prostate varies from 0.01 to 0.07 per cent of the total body weight in the case of dogs less than five years of age. Perhaps another way of expressing the same thing would be to say that the prostate of the normal young dog extends but little beyond the width of the adjoining urethra; the diameter of the former being scarcely more than one and one-half times that of the latter. The hyperplastic prostate may easily be of a width or diameter three times the normal and, when first seen at autopsy, it not infrequently approaches or surpasses the undistended bladder in size. With the exception of a slight median furrow along the dorsal aspect, the canine prostate is not divided into lobes. Neither is there any lobe or part which tends to project into the region of the sphincter of the bladder, such as develops in the human.

As the reader probably is aware, the expected clinical **effect** of prostatic hyperplasia is interference with the flow of urine through the urethra. In the human male, this not infrequently becomes serious through gradual compression or invasion of the urethral lumen. The enlargement is often pronounced just at the neck and orifice of the bladder with the formation of a "middle lobe" which actually projects into the cavity of the bladder and carries the urethral entrance with it. The "middle lobe" is said to arise as the result of hyperplasia of glandular tissue in the wall of the urethra, which must be quite comparable to the "disseminated" portions of the prostatic tissue which are normal in the several species of farm animals. There is also interference with proper closing of the sphincter, and urine may escape contrary to the patient's volition. It is now recognized that too much has been taken for granted in applying these facts of human pathology to the dog and that enlarged prostates do not cause urinary obstruction in the dog. Following the usual post-mortem routine of removing the pelvic organs as an ensemble, it is commonly possible to lift the bladder by its vertex, or anterior end, and find that, by force of gravity, the urine flows unimpeded through the urethra, whatever may be the size of the prostate or however small the unfilled urethral lumen may have appeared. Whatever obstructive effect an enlarged prostate has upon the urinary flow must be due, at least in many cases, to a filling and overcrowding the non-distensible pelvic girdle. This lack

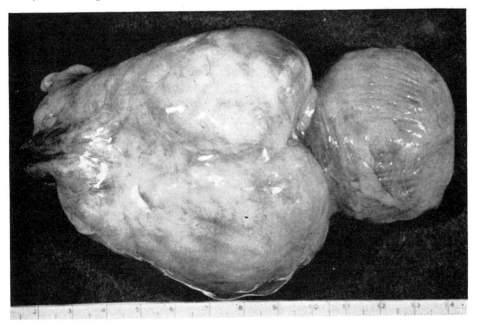

FIG. 26–13.—Benign hyperplasia of the prostate of an eight-year-old male German short-haired pointer dog. (Courtesy of Angell Memorial Animal Hospital.)

of space should be more obstructive to the passage of the rectal contents than to the flow of urine and, indeed, constipation is frequently attributed by clinicians to prostatic enlargement. This may be followed by perineal hernia when efforts at defecation are sufficiently forcible.

The **cause** of hyperplasia of the prostate is not known, either in man or dog, although a number of theoretical explanations have been proposed. In both the human and canine it is a disorder of advancing years, fifty or beyond in man, when sexual activity is supposed to be declining. But canine prostatic enlargement was found by Schlotthauer to be commencing as early as six years and there is no reason to believe that sexual activity declines at anywhere near this age. It is known that in man or animals castration prevents prostatic development in the young and causes pronounced atrophy of the organ when performed after puberty. Experimental injection of estrogenic substances into castrated rats produces hyperplasia of the prostate, but the addition of a suitable amount of testosterone prevents this. On the other hand, there are experiments indicating that an excess of the male hormone can cause prostatic enlargement. Julian (1947) divides hyperplasia into two types, one that can be produced experimentally by estrogenic stimulation and which may accompany feminizing tumors (p. 261), and a second type, "cystic hyperplasia" which he believes to be due to excessive androgenic (testosterone) stimulation.

It has also been believed that the hyperplasia was a sequel to, and result of, chronic prostatitis. The prevalent opinion at present is that the lymphocytic infiltrations, fibrosis or other evidences of chronic inflammation are the result, rather than the cause of the disturbance. On the basis of rather inconclusive statistical observations, it has been suspected that the unnatural postponement of urination required of male house-dogs was a causative factor, but our conceptions of anatomy and physiology offer little to support such a view. For the present, it seems proper to attribute hyperplasia of the prostate to imbalances in the sexual hormones, but an understanding of their precise nature awaits further elucidation. It is known that an excess of feminizing hormone will produce **squamous metaplasia** of prostatic epithelium, as in the presence of a Sertoli-cell tumor (Fig. 26–12C), or with experimental administration of estrogens.

Prostatic Calculi.—Stones occur in the prostate of the dog, but only with great rarity. They are usually small (1 to 5 mm.), hard, white and spherical. They consist chiefly of phosphates and carbonates of calcium. Usually a number of them fill a cystic cavity, of which there may be one or several. The central nucleus is practically always organic material, indicating an origin in desquamated or other dead cells. They doubtless arise in connection with chronic prostatitis and hyperplasia. Since corpora amylacea (p. 45) are extremely rare in the prostates of domestic animals, it seems doubtful that these starch-like bodies are essential predecessors of calculi. Small collections of stones are asymptomatic, others are irritant and obstructive, requiring operative removal. They can be demonstrated roentgenologically.

Prostatic neoplasms are uncommon in most domestic species but careful studies of aged dogs (Leav and Ling, 1968) have uncovered numerous adenocarcinomas of the prostate which are quite similar in histologic appearance and clinical behavior to those which occur in man. Fibromas and leiomyomas also **originate** in this organ. In the farm animals, prostatic tumors are rarely **reported.**

The Penis, Prepuce and Urethra

The external parts of these organs are subject to trauma with the usual fibrino-purulent reactions such as are seen in wounds generally. The folds of mucous membrane, especially in the prepuce, harbor various microorganisms including the trichomonad of bovine abortion, which causes a chronic, subclinical infection of the parts, whence it is transmitted to the cow. None of the other specific abortifacient organisms and viruses is transmitted in this way with any appreciable frequency and most of them probably not at all. Cultural studies of the genital mucous membranes of bulls indicate that *Pseudomonas aeruginosa* (*pyocyaneus*) (Rempt and Zwanenburg, 1949), *Corynebacterium pyogenes* and *C. renale* (Morgan, Johansson and Emerson, 1946) are rather frequently present. The first of these has rarely been incriminated in abortions. Inflammatory **phimosis** is a condition in which inflammatory swelling prevents extension of the penis from the sheath; **paraphimosis** is a similar situation, the penis being already protruded and impossible to withdraw. True congenital phimosis probably does not occur in the domestic animals because of differences in local anatomy.

Balanitis (inflammation of the glans penis or clitoris) and **posthitis** (inflammation of the prepuce) are known in most species and are considered to be caused by various pathogenic organisms. A troublesome infection in sheep, **ovine posthitis,** is reported by Southcott (1965) to be due to a gram-positive, diphtheroid bacterium which is carried by non-diseased animals but under certain conditions will cause inflammation. This organism has the ability to hydrolyze urea to produce ammonia (NH_3), and its pathogenic multiplication appears related to urine stasis. The infection may be transmitted by contact or coitus.

Balanitis and vaginitis in swine has been reported (Onstad and Saxegaard, 1967) to result from infection by the bovine virus of infectious bovine rhinotracheitis—infectious pustular vulvo-vaginitis (p. 438). The bovine infections with this agent are also described elsewhere. Bovine posthitis is also reported to resemble the ovine disease clinically but its etiology is not established. In the horse, a virus has been associated with vulvitis and balanitis (Girard, Greig, and Mitchell, 1968).

Neoplasms of the penis, usually on the glans, are of some frequency in horses and cattle. Whether the males are entire or castrated appears to make no difference, but the tumors occur almost always in older animals. In the bovine, fibromas and fibrosarcomas predominate (See Fibropapillomatosis, p. 511); in the horse, the tumor is practically always a squamous-cell carcinoma.

The **penile urethra** is subject to lodgment of uroliths (p. 1286), which occur with frequency in cattle, dogs and sheep. The stone practically always lodges at the sigmoid flexure, where the lumen is narrowest. In the dog, uroliths, especially of cystine, are apt to lodge at or near the point where the penile urethra is contained by the os penis. There are inflammation and limited distention above the stone; none below it. Strictures in the form of an irregular fold of mucous membrane have been noted at least in the bovine urethra, the cause not having been demonstrated.

Male Genital Organs

ABDEL-RAOUF, M.: The Postnatal Development of the Reproductive Organs in Bulls with Special Reference to Puberty. (Including Growth of the Hypophysis and the Adrenals). Acta endocrinol. Copenhagen. Suppl. No. 49, pp. 109, 1960.

ASHDOWN, R. R.: Persistence of the Penile Frenulum in Young Bulls. Vet. Rec. 74:1464–1468, 1962.

ASHDOWN, R. R., and FORD, C. M.: Bilateral Epididymal Spermiostasis in a Ram. Vet. Rec. 80:492–494, 1967.

ANDREEVSKII, V. Y.: Prichiny porochnosti spermy u baranov. (Reasons for Sperm Defects of Rams.) Iskusst. Osemen. sel'khoz. Zhivotn. 1:36–45, 1940. Abstr. Vet. Bull. No. 997, 1948.

BALL, L., YOUNG, S., and CARROLL, E. J.: Seminal Vesiculitis Syndrome: Lesions in Genital Organs of Young Bulls. Am. J. Vet. Res. 29:1173–1184, 1968.

BANE, A., and NICANDER, L.: Electron and Light Microscopical Studies on Spermateliosis in a Boar with Acrosome Abnormalities. J. Reprod. Fert. 11:133–148, 1966.

BARTLETT, D. E., HASSON, E. V., and TEETER, K. G.: Occurrence of Trichomonas fetus in Preputial Samples from Infected Bulls. J. Am. Vet. Med. Assn. 110:114–120, 1947.

BASSET, C. R.: Ulcerative Posthitis in Bulls. Vict. Vet. Proc. 22:38–39, 1963/64.

BENITZ, K. F., and DAMBACH, G.: The Toxicological Significance of Multinucleated Giant Cells in Dystrophic Testes of Laboratory Animals and Man. Arzneimittel Forsch. 15:391–404, 1965.

BENNETTS, H. W.: Metaplasia in the Sex Organs of Castrated Male Sheep Maintained on Early Subterranean Clover Pastures. Austr. Vet. J. 22:70–78, 1946.

BIBERSTEIN, E. L. et al.: Epididymitis in Rams. Studies on Pathogenesis. Cornell Vet. 54:27–40, 1964.

BIEBERDORF, F. W.: Actinomycosis of a Bovine Testis. J. Am. Vet. Med. Assn. 122:49–50, 1953.

BLOM. E.: En hurtig-farvningsmetode til adskillelse af levende og døde spermier ved hjaelp af Eosin-Nigrosin. (Rapid Eosin-nigrosin Staining Technique for Differentiating Living from Dead Spermatozoa.) Nord. vet. med. 2:58–61, 1950. Abstr. Vet. Bull. No. 2938, 1950.

BLOM, E., and HERMANSEN, E.: Segmental Aplasia of the Wolffian Duct (Lack of Epididymis), a Sterilizing and Hereditary Defect in the Mink. Nord. Vet. Med. 21:188–192, 1969. V.B. 39:4822, 1969.

BOUTERS, R., et al.: [Ulcerative balanoposthitis in bulls.] Vlaams diergeneesk. Tijdschr. 29:171–186, 1960. (In Flemish.) Abstr. Vet. Bull., No. 4086, 1960.

BROOK, A. H., SOUTHCOTT, W. H., and STACY, B. D.: Etiology of Ovine Posthitis: Relationship Between Urine and a Causal Organism. Aust. Vet. J. 42:9–12, 1966.

FAWCETT, D. W.: A Comparative View of Sperm Ultrastructure. Biol. Reprod. 2:90–127, 1970.

FOSTER, A. E. C.: Polyorchidism. Vet. Rec. 64:158, 1952.

FRASER, A. F., and WILSON, J. C.: Testicular Calcinosis in Domestic Ruminants. Nature (Lond.) 210:547, 1966.

GARLICK, N. L.: An Unusual Case of Monorchidism in a Stallion. J. Am. Vet. Med. Assn. 121:101–103, 1952.

GERBER, H.: Anatomie der Prostata des Hundes unter Beruchsichtigung verscheidener Altersstufen. Schweis. Arch. Tierheilk. 103, 537–567, 1961.

GILMAN, H. L.: Genital Infections in the Bull. J. Am. Vet. Med. Assn. 60:416–434, 1922.

GIRARD, A., GREIG, A. S., and MITCHELL, D.: A Virus Associated with Vulvitis and Balanitis in the Horse . . . a Preliminary Report. Canad. J. Comp. Med. 32:603–604, 1968.

GLOVER, T. D.: The Semen of the Pig. Vet. Rec. 67:36–40, 1955.

GREULICH, W. W., and BURFORD, T. H.: Testicular Tumors Associated with Mammary, Prostatic and Other Changes in Cryptorchid Dogs. Am. J. Cancer. 28:496–511, 1936.

HAFEZ, E. S. E., and JAINUDEEN, M. R.: Intersexuality in Farm Mammals. Anim. Breed, Abst. 34:1–15, 1966.

HELMY, N., et al.: Orchitis and Epididymo-orchitis in Domesticated Animals. Vet. Med. J. Giza 11:179–209, 1966. V.B. 37:4023, 1967.

ISENBERG, H. D.: Simplified Method for Staining Spermatozoa. Am. J. Clin. Path. 18:94, 1948.

JABARA, A. G.: Some Tissue Changes in the Dog Following Stilbesterol Administration. Austr. J. Exp. Biol. Med. Sci. 40:293–307, 1963.

JAMIESON, S., and SOLTYS, M. A.: Infectious Epididymo-Orchitis of Rams Associated with Pasteurella pseudotuberculosis. Vet. Rec. 59:351–353, 1947.

JANSEN, J.: Orchitis bij Hengsten, Abortus bij Merrier (Klinischbacteriologische les over Salmonella abortus-equi-infecties). (Orchitis in Stallions and Abortion in Mares due to S. abortus-equi infection.) Tijdschr. f. diergeneesk. 71:160–167, 1946. Abstr. Vet. Bull. No. 2217, 1947.

JENSEN, R., et al.: Arteriosclerosis and Phlebosclerosis in Testes of Sheep. Am. J. Vet. Res. 23:480–488, 1962.

JULIAN, L. M.: The Pathology of the Prostate Gland of Man and the Dog. Cornell Vet. 37:241–253, 1947.

KERNKAMP, H. C. H., ROEPKE, M. H., and JASPER, D. E.: Orchitis in Swine Due to *Brucella suis*. J. Am. Vet. Med. Assn. 108:215–221, 1946.

KING, N. W., and GARVIN, C. H.: Bilateral Hermaphroditism in a Dog. J. Am. Vet. Med. Assn. 145:997–1001, 1964.

KODAGALI, S. B., and KERUR, V. K.: Gonadal Hypoplasia in Gir Cattle. Indian Vet. J. 45:114–118, 1968.

————: Seminal Characters in Testes Hypoplasia. Indian J. Anim. Hlth. 7:209–212, 1969.

KONIG, H.: Genital Pathology of Bulls. Arch. Exp. Veterinaermed. 16:501–584, 1962.

————: (An Unusual Form of Orchitis in Bulls.) Schweiz. Arch. Tierheilk. 106: 529–534, 1964. V.B. 35:423, 1965.

KRAVIS, E. M. and LORBER, J. H.: Feminization Syndrome Associated with Epididymitis in a Dog. J. Am. Vet. Med. Assn. 140:803–806, 1962.

LAMBERT, G., MANTHEI, C. A., and DEYOE, B. L.: Studies on *Brucella abortus* Infection in Bull. Am. J. Vet. Res. 24:1152–1157, 1963.

LEAV, I., and LING, G. V.: Adenocarcinoma of the Canine Prostate. Cancer 22:1329–1345, 1968.

LIVINGSTON, C. W., and HARDY, W. T.: Isolation of *Actinobacillus seminis* from Ovine Epididymitis. Amer. J. Vet. Res. 25:660–663, 1964.

MANNING, W. K.: Biotin Deficiency as the Causative Agent of Induced Cryptorchidism in Albino Rats. Science 112:89, 1950.

McENTEE, K.: Pathological Conditions in Old Bulls with Impaired Fertility. J. Am. Vet. Med. Assn. 132:328–331, 1958.

MORGAN, B. B., JOHANSSON, K. R., and EMERSON, E. Z.: Some Corynebacteria Isolated from the Genital Tract of Bulls. Mich. State College Vet. 6:68–69 and 72–74, 1946.

MULLIGAN, R. M.: Feminization in Male Dogs with Carcinoma of the Testis. Am. J. Path. 20:865–873, 1944.

OETTLÉ, A. G., and HARRISON, R. G.: The Histological Changes Produced in the Rat Testis by Temporary and Permanent Occlusion of the Testicular Artery. J. Path. and Bact. 64:273–297, 1952.

ONSTAD, O., and SAXEGAARD, F.: Outbreaks of Vaginitis and Balanitis in Swine. Clinical and Pathological Findings. Nord. Vet. Med. 19:49–53, 1967.

PALLUDAN, B.: Vitamin A Deficiency and Its Effect on the Sexual Organs of the Boar. Acta Vet. Scand. 4:136–155, 1963.

————: Direct Effect of Vitamin A on Boar Testis. Nature (Lond.) 211:639–640, 1966.

PEZZOLI, G.: La torsione del testiculo. Clin. Vet. Milano. 80:353–364, 1957.

POLGE, C., and ROWSON, L. E. A.: Long-term Storage of Bull Semen Frozen at Very Low Temperatures. Rep. IInd Internat. Congr. Physiol. Animal Reproduction, Copenhagen, 3:90–98, 1952. V.B., 23:2109, 1953.

RAO, C. K., and HART, G. H.: Morphology of Bovine Spermatozoa. Am. J. Vet. Research 9:117–124, 1948.

REMPT, D., and ZWANENBURG, T. S.: *Pseudomonas Aeruginosa* (*Ps. pyocyanea, Bac. pyocyaneus*) in het Sperma van Drie Dekstieren. (Pseudomonas in Semen of Bulls.) Tijdschr. v. diergeneesk. 73:224–230, 1948. V.B. 19:356, 1949.

ROB, O.: (Degeneration of the Germinal Epithelium in Bulls: Histopathology and Spermatozoal Morphology.) Vet. Med. Praha. 11:437–444, 1966. V.B. 37:1069, 1967.

ROLLINSON, D. H. L.: Studies on the Abnormal Spermatozoa of Bull Semen. Brit. Vet. J. 107:203–214, 258–273 and 451–468, 1951.

SAXEGAARD, F., and ONSTAD, O.: Isolation and Identification of IBR-IPV Virus from Cases of Vaginitis and Balanitis in Swine and from Healthy Swine. Nord. Vet. Med. 19: 54–57, 1967. V.B. 37:3197, 1967.

SCHENKER, J.: Zur functionellen Anatomie der Prostata des Rindes. Acta Anat. 9:89–102, 1950. V.B. 21:3362, 1951.

SCHLOTTHAUER, C. F.: Diseases of the Prostate Gland in the Dog. J. Am. Vet. Med. Assn. 90:176–187, 1937.

SCHLOTTHAUER, C. F., and BOLLMAN, J. L.: The Effect of Artificial Cryptorchidism on the Prostate Gland of Dogs. Am. J. Vet. Research 3:202–206, 1942.

SIMMONS, G. C., and HALL, W. T. K.: Epididymitis of Rams. Australian Vet. J. 29:33–40, 1953.

SIMMONS, G. C., BAYNES, I. D., and LUDFORD, C. G.: Epidemiology of *Actinobacillus seminis* in a Flock of Border Leicester Sheep. Aust. Vet. J. 42:183–187, 1966.

SMITH, L. W.: Senile Changes of the Testis and Prostate in Dogs. J. Med. Research 40:31–51, 1919.

SOUTHCOTT, W. H.: Etiology of Ovine Posthitis: Description of a Causal Organism. Aust. Vet. J. *41*:193–200, 1965. V.B. *36*:45, 1966.

————: Epidemiology and Control of Ovine Posthitis and Vulvitis. Aust. Vet. J. *41*: 224–234, 1965. V.B. *36*:1286, 1966.

STORZ, J., *et al.*: Isolation of a Psittacosis Agent (*Chlamydia*) from Semen and Epididymis of Bulls with Seminal Vesiculitis Syndrome. Amer. J. Vet. Res. *29*:549–555, 1968.

SULLIVAN, D. J., and DROBECK, H. P.: True Hermaphrodism in a Rhesus Monkey. Folia primat. *4*:309–317, 1966.

TODD, G. C., NELSON, L. W., and MIGAKI, G.: Multiple Heterotopic Testicular Tissue in the Pig. A Report of Seven Cases. Cornell Vet. *58*:614–619, 1968.

WHITE, P. T., and JOHNSON, P., JR.: Strangulated Hernia of a Cryptorchid Dog. J. Am. Vet. Med. Assn. *126*:312, 1955.

ZEMJANIS, R., *et al.*: Testicular Degeneration in *Macaca nemestrina* Induced by Immobilization. Fertil. & Steril. *21*:335–340, 1970.

ZUCKERMAN, S., and GROOME, J. R.: Aetiology of Benign Enlargement of the Prostate in the Dog. J. Path. and Bact. *44*:113–124, 1937.

ZUCKERMAN, S., and McKEOWN, T.: The Canine Prostate in Relation to Normal and Abnormal Testicular Changes. J. Path. and Bact. *46*:7–19, 1938.

Chapter

27

The Endocrine System

THE ADRENAL GLANDS

The adrenal glands may share, either through direct extension or blood-borne metastases, in degenerative, inflammatory and neoplastic processes which affect other parts of the animal body. Hemorrhages, usually petechial, infarctions and similar disturbances may appear in the adrenals from the same causes as elsewhere. If one adrenal deteriorates for any one of a variety of reasons, its fellow is prone to undergo compensatory hypertrophy. Hence, except in the case of primary neoplasms, or altered control by the pituitary, functional disease is likely to develop only if involvement is bilateral.

The Adrenal Cortex.—Each adrenal gland consists of two parts, cortex and medulla, which embryologically, as well as functionally, are separate organs. As in some other structures such as the combined openings of the urinary and genital tracts, one wonders if the arrangement of the adrenal medullary tissue inside the cortical does not represent an anatomical makeshift; indeed in some lower animal species, the two tissues are anatomically separate.

The adrenal cortex arises from the urogenital ridge, in common with the several urinary and genital organs; thus it is of mesodermal origin. This tissue, under the stimulus and control of a hormone, or hormones, from the pituitary gland (adrenocorticotropic hormone, ACTH) and juxtaglomerular apparatus of the kidney (renin-angiotensin), secretes a number of hormones of its own which control a variety of body functions. Because of the essential nature of these hormones, complete loss of adrenocortical tissue is fatal. Chemically the hormones are sterols, having a steroid nucleus which relates them to cholesterol, ergosterol and other forms of vitamin D, to the sex hormones, certain carcinogenic compounds and the drug, digitalis.

In general, the hormones produced by the adrenal cortex (1) favor the retention, and inhibit renal excretion of sodium (but not potassium) and chlorides, thereby maintaining an osmotic pressure sufficient to retain appropriate amounts of water in the blood and tissues. Hormones of this group are under control of renin-angiotensin from the juxtaglomerular apparatus and are believed to come from the zona glomerulosa and are designated, on the basis of chemical structure, as mineralocorticoids. They include aldosterone (natural) and desoxycorticosterone (synthetic). (2) Certain ones favor gluconeogenesis, raising the level of blood sugar and increasing the glycogen in the liver. They also tend to reduce the numbers of eosinophils in the blood and of lymphocytes in either the blood or lymphoid tissues. These hormones are called glucocorticoids; cortisone (17-hydroxy-11-dehydroxycorticosterone) and hydrocortisone (17-hydroxycorticosterone) are the outstanding examples. They come from the zona fasciculata and are under control of ACTH. (3) The adrenal sex hormones are androgenic and masculinizing, an effect which has been mentioned in connection with adreno-cortical tumors (p. 252). These hormones are characterized by a ketone group on the 17th carbon atom and, therefore, are known as the 17-ketosteroids. They are believed to come from the zona reticularis. Some effects of some of the hormones are more or less antagonistic to those of others, a proper balance being essential to health. Many of them are concerned, along with epinephrine from the medulla, in maintaining many bodily functions in their normal state of activity (homeostasis) against the "stress" (p. 186) of unfavorable environmental situations. Other effects attributable to cortical hormones include stimulation of delivery of erythrocytes and neutrophils into the circulating blood but an inhibition of the same process as applied to lymphocytes and eosinophils. There is, in fact, a general depression of the lymphoid tissues. Deposition of body fat is favored, although it is likely to be peculiarly localized. Sweating is increased. This, probably with other factors, assists in toleration of high ambient temperatures. Production of melanin in the skin is augmented. Blood pressure tends to be raised. Excretion of calcium is somewhat increased. Proliferation of cells of the reticulo-endothelial and fibroblastic groups is inhibited. It is to this latter action that the drug cortisone (and indirectly ACTH, adrenocorticotropic hormone) owes its value; chronic proliferative inflammations are inhibited, as are also certain immunologic processes. Where these inflammations are excessive (p. 182), such inhibition is desirable, bringing symptomatic and often morphological relief. In the case of active infections (such as the granulomas), the same action is harmful and may be lethal.

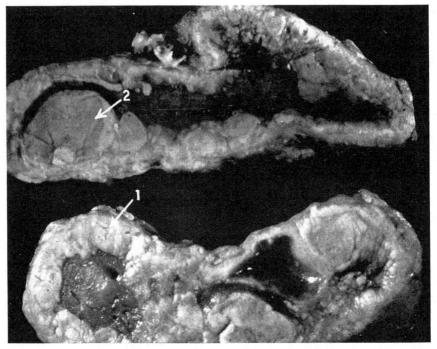

Fig. 27–1.—Hyperplasia (1) and adenoma (2) of adrenal cortex of a twelve-year-old male English Setter. (Courtesy of Angell Memorial Animal Hospital.)

The practical details of these hormonal effects are best pursued by examining the results of naturally induced hypo- and hyperadrenalism. **Adrenal insufficiency** is classically represented by Addison's disease, a fatal disorder of humans described in 1855. In this disease, there is a gradually developing weakness with feeble heart action, accompanied by very low blood pressure, decrease in blood volume (due to excessive excretion of sodium and chlorides and consequent loss of fluid), frequently hypoglycemia (due to failure of gluconeogenesis) and shock. Severe gastrointestinal malfunctions, including vomition, are the rule. A spectacular symptom regularly present is a marked increase in the pigmentation of the skin. This is believed to be due to an excess of a pituitary "melanocyte-stimulating hormone" which develops reciprocally to a fall in an inhibitory adrenocortical hormone. Lesions of Addison's disease in other organs are of interest in showing the effects of adrenal insufficiency upon other structures and functions. The pituitary gland shows a decrease of basophils and an increase of chromophobes. Both the thyroid and the heart are often small and atrophic with areas of atrophic or dying fibers in the myocardium. Lymphoid tissue is often markedly increased in the thyroid and in the lymphoid organs. These abnormalities are present in status thymico-lymphaticus (p. 187), and it may be that the latter disorder is primarily a disease of the adrenals.

The cause of Addison's disease is the destruction of both adrenal glands. Frequently, this is the result of tuberculous involvement but histoplasmosis, amyloidosis, bilateral metastatic tumors and what are believed to be the direct toxic effects of some drugs and chemicals in hypersensitive individuals are also causes of the same destructive lesions. We are not certain whether a condition identical to Addison's disease has been observed in animals. A few cases of apparently comparable nature have been reported. Atrophy of the cortex appears to be a feature of "fatal syncope" of pigs with an allergic reaction to an unaccustomed food perhaps being an inciting cause. There is, of course, no reason why extensive tuberculosis or a similar process might not destroy the adrenals unless it be that the animal patients would, in all probability, die from other lesions while the disease was at an earlier and less widespread stage.

Hyperadrenalism is frequently manifested by masculinization. In the adult female, this amounts to defeminization. In the infant female, it may even be characterized by pseudohermaphroditism. In the growing male, there is precocious maturity, sexual and somatic. The urinary excretion of 17-ketosteroids is increased, a fact which may be utilized diagnostically. As will be surmised, hyperadrenalism is not a frequent disorder. When recognized, it is usually indicative of the presence of an adrenal cortical tumor (p. 252) or adenoma of the pituitary (basophil and chromophobe adenomas) which produces ACTH resulting in bilateral hyperplasia of the adrenal cortices. It must be remembered also that masculinization can be the result of the arrhenoblastoma (p. 259) of the ovary and of the interstitial-cell tumor of the testis. Precocious sexual development may also rarely be traceable to tumors in the region of the hypophysis and hypothalamus. At the same time, in dealing with adrenal tumors, it should be pointed out that many of them are entirely inactive as far as hormones are concerned.

Hyperadrenalism in man results in a characteristic syndrome called Cushing's disease. A similar syndrome occurs in dogs with either adrenal cortical tumors or neoplasms of the pituitary which produce ACTH. Although adrenal cortical

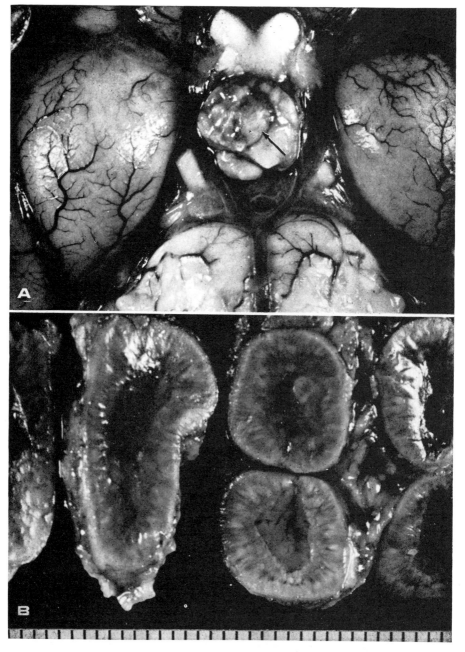

FIG. 27–2.—*A*, Adenoma of the pituitary of a ten-year-old spayed female Boston Terrier with canine "Cushing's" syndrome. *B*, Hyperplasia of adrenal cortices, same dog. (Courtesy of Angell Memorial Animal Hospital.)

tumors are not infrequent in other species (especially cattle and sheep), they apparently are rarely functional. In dogs the clinical signs are muscular weakness, bilaterally symmetrical alopecia, abdominal distension and hyperpigmentation of the skin. If hyperadrenalism is the result of a functioning pituitary tumor, which is the usual, diabetes insipidus (p. 1020) almost regularly occurs. Clinicopathologic findings include leukocytosis, neutrophilia, eosinopenia and lymphopenia. Gross findings will include either adrenal cortical neoplasia or, if secondary to a pituitary neoplasm, bilateral cortical hypertrophy. Metastatic calcification of the skin, lung, skeletal and cardiac muscle and kidney is frequent. In man Cushing's disease results in osteoporosis but few reports have described this lesion in dogs.

Bilateral nodular hyperplasia of the adrenal cortex without evidence of hyperadrenalism is a very frequent finding in older dogs. The cause is not known but its presence necessitates caution in interpreting endocrinological disorders.

The Adrenal Medulla.—The adrenal medulla produces the well-known and important hormone epinephrine, or adrenalin, as well as another closely related endocrine substance, but the medulla is not essential to life. In common with

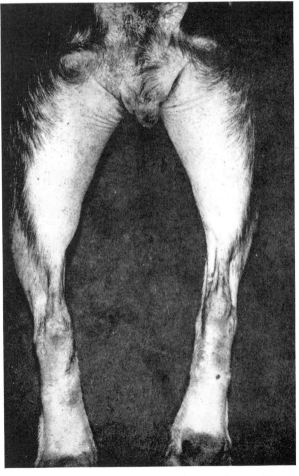

FIG. 27–3.—Symmetrical alopecia of the thighs of a ten-year-old spayed female Boston Terrier with hyperadrenalcorticism. (Courtesy of Angell Memorial Animal Hospital.)

the adrenal cortex, it bears a relation to some forms of essential hypertension in human beings.

The medulla has no noteworthy diseases of its own excepting its primary neoplasms (p. 253). Since the medullary tissue shares with the sympathetic nervous tissue an embryogenetic origin in the neural crest, the tumors arising from it are related to nervous tissue. The rapidity of post-mortem autolysis in this structure (p. 15) should not be overlooked.

Cysts are occasionally encountered in the cortex or medulla. Their cause and significance are not known. Concretions, particularly at the corticomedullary junction, are not infrequently found, especially in Old-World monkeys. They may mineralize in which case they stain blue with hematoxylin and eosin. Amyloidosis of the adrenal is occasionally seen. The adrenal cortex may be the site of extramedullary hematopoiesis.

Adrenal

BARONE, R., and BACQUES, C.: Les glandes surrénales des équidés domestiques. Bull. Soc. sci. vét. Lyon *54* and *55*:383–405, 1952–53.

BELL, J. T., and WEBER, A. F.: A Comparative Study of Lipid Accumulation in the Adrenal Glands of Cows. Am. J. Vet. Res. *20*:53–60, 1959.

BROCH, O. J., and HAUGEN, H. N.: The Effects of Adrenaline on the Number of Circulating Eosinophiles and on the Excretion of Uric Acid and Creatinine. Acta Endocrinol. *5*:143–150, 1950.

BUSH, I. E., and FERGUSON, K. A.: The Secretion of the Adrenal Cortex of Sheep. J. Endocrinol. *10*:1–8, 1953.

CHRISTIAN, J. J.: The Relation of Adrenal Weight to Body Weight in Mammals. Science *117*:78–80, 1952.

COFFIN, D. L., and MUNSON, T. O.: Endocrine Diseases of the Dog Associated with Hair Loss. Sertoli-cell Tumor of Testis, Hypothyroidism, Canine Cushing's Syndrome. J. Am. Vet. Med. Assn. *123*:403–408, 1953.

COWIE, A. T., and STEWART, J.: Adrenalectomy in the Goat and Its Effects on the Chemical Constituents of the Blood. J. Endocrinol. *6*:197–204, 1949.

DÄMMRICH, K.: Die Beeinflussung des Skeletts durch die Hormone der Nebennierenrinde under besonderer Berucksuchtigung des "Morbus Cushing" beim Hund. Berl. u. Münch. Tierarztl. Wochshaft. *75*:331–337, 1962.

ELIAS, H.: Growth of the Adrenal Cortex in Domesticated Ungulata. Am. J. Vet. Res. *9*: 173–189, 1948.

FORSIUS, P. I., and HAIKONEN, M.: Iakttagelser Rörande Farplasmats binjurebarkhormoner (Adrenal Cortical Hormones in Sheep Plasma.) Nord. vet.-med. *7*:154–156, 1955. (Engl. and Ger. summaries.)

GOBETTO, A., PELLEGRINI, S., and PELLEGRINI, N.: The Cortical Substance of the Adrenal During Pregnancy; Histological Observations on Cows, with Reference to Sudanophile Substances (TT). Ann. Fac. Med. Vet. Pisa *15*:21–37, 1963.

HADLOW, W. J.: Adrenal Cortical Atrophy in the Dog. Amer. J. Path. *29*:353–361, 1953.

HAMILTON, L. H., and HORVATH, S. M.: Immediate Blood Cell Count Response to Epineph-rine in Splenectomized Dogs. Amer. J. Physiol. *178*:58–62, 1954.

KRAL, F.: Epileptiform Manifestations of Endocrine Disturbances Associated with Adrenal Tumors. J. Am. Vet. Med. Assn. *118*:235–239, 1951.

LIEBISCH, H.: Die Histologie der Nebennierenrinde bei verschiedenen Erkrankungen des Hundes. (Ein Beitrag zum Stress-Problem.) Wein tierärztl. Monatschr. *41*:257–279, 1954.

LINDT, S.: Über die Pathologie der Nebenniere des Hundes. Deutsche tierärztl. Wchnschr. *69*:586–588, 1962.

LUKE, D.: The Effect of Adrenocorticotrophic Hormone and Adrenal Cortical Extract on the Differential White Cell Count in the Pig. Brit. Vet. J. *109*:434–436, 1953.

MESCHINI, S., and MESCHINI, M.: Su di un caso di insufficienza cortico-surrenale di una boyina. Analogie col morbo di Addison dell'uomo. Zooprofilassi *2*:8–11, 1947.

MOLL, F. C., and HAWN, C. VAN Z.: The Effect of Adrenocorticotropic Hormone, Cortisone and Adrenalectomy on the Serological and Histological Responses in the Rabbit Following Injections of Foreign Proteins. J. Immunol. *70*:441–449, 1953.

Ross, M. A., Gainer, J. H., and Innes, J. R. M.: Dystrophic Calcification in the Adrenal Glands of Monkeys, Cats, and Dogs. Arch. Path. *60*:655–662, 1955.

Sybesma, W.: Die Pathologie der Nebenniere des Rindes. Arch. Exper. Veterinaermed. *16*: 205–210, 1963.

Trapp, A. L.: Cushing's Syndrome in the Dog. Iowa State Col. Vet. *20*:16–18, 1958.

Wada, M.: Sudorific Action of Adrenalin on the Human Sweat Glands and Determination of Their Excitability. Science *111*:376–377, 1950.

Webber, A. F., McNutt, S. H., and Morgan, B. B.: Structure and Arrangement of Zona Glomerulosa Cells in the Bovine Adrenal. J. Morphol. *87*:393–395, 1950.

Weber, A. F., *et al.*: Studies of the Bovine Adrenal Gland. I. The Production of Lipid Accumulation and Other Histological and Cytological Changes in the Zonae Glomerulosae of Calves. Am. J. Vet. Res. *17*:402–409, 1956.

THE THYROID

In the thyroid, as in the other endocrine glands, we are principally concerned with diseases which lead to insufficient or excessive production of the specific hormone, hypothyroidism or hyperthyroidism, respectively.

The essential feature of **hypothyroidism** is an abnormally low basal metabolic rate. This can be measured by appropriate clinical techniques, but the disorder is commonly recognizable by a characteristic symptomatology. There is a disinclination to vigorous movement and a tendency to obesity, accompanied, in humans, and doubtless in animals also, by an attitude of mental complacency. In cases of much severity, there is, in the young, retardation of growth as regards total stature, sexual development and (in the human) mental acuity. The condition is called **cretinism,** and affected persons, even after they reach the stunted maturity which is their lot, are called cretins (Fr. *cretin*, an idiot). When the thyroid deficiency arises in an adult human, myxedema is the outstanding symptom. This is the accumulation in the subcutaneous and other connective tissues of a mucoid, or myxomatous, semi-fluid substance, essentially mucoid degeneration (p. 52), which gives the face and other body surfaces a puffy and

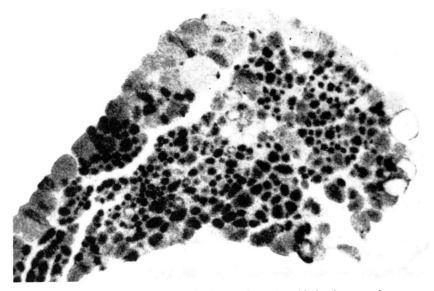

Fig. 27–4.—Autoradiograph of normal rat thyroid gland prepared twelve hours following injection of I-131.

edematous appearance. Hypothyroidism is an infrequent clinical problem in dogs. Loss of hair and of muscular strength are among the signs observed and elevated cholesterol levels in the blood serum are usual. The morphologic changes in the thyroid have not been well studied. In other animal species, adult hypothyroidism is rarely recognized clinically, but in the offspring of hypothyroid animals congenital goiter may be encountered. (See p. 1360.)

In **hyperthyroidism,** an opposite syndrome is present. The individual is unusually active and alert, does not store fat in spite of a vigorous appetite and is often of an irritable or excitable disposition. The heart rate is unusually rapid (tachycardia), and there may be palpitation. The basal metabolic rate, a measure of oxidative processes, is above the normal. In the young, growth may be somewhat accelerated and maturity comes early. The bulging of the eyeballs known as exophthalmos appears to be only an indirect effect of the hyperthyroid state.

Goiter, or enlargement of the thyroid gland as a whole, may be accompanied by either hypo- or hyperthyroidism. The enlargement may be due to an increase of thyroid tissue, which is hyperplasia, or to an increased amount of colloid, distending the lumens of the acini, or, much less commonly, to inflammatory proliferation. Hyperplasia of the thyroid is manifested, as in other glandular organs, by (1) an increase in the height of each individual columnar epithelial cell and (2) by an increase in the number of these epithelial cells. As explained in the study of hyperplasia in general (p. 94), this results in the formation of complicated folds in the epithelial lining of the acini. Hyperplasia of the glandular epithelium does not mean hyperthyroidism, but quite the opposite. Neither does a large amount of colloid in distended acini have this significance. These facts are better understood if we consider the accepted explanations of thyroid function. The morphological and functional activity of the thyroid is induced and sustained by a thyrotropic hormone which the circulating blood brings from the pituitary. The thyroid then releases into the blood its own secretion, thyroxin or a derivative thereof. In accordance with a principle which seems well established in the case of estrogen (folliculin) and the follicle-stimulating hormone (FSH), of progesterone and the luteinizing hormone (p. 1299) and of various other hormonal combinations, there is a reciprocal relationship between the pituitary-activating hormone and the product of its activity. The thyrotropic hormone from the pituitary stimulates the production of thyroxin; the presence of thyroxin inhibits the production of more thyrotropic hormone. Normally the two are in balance and thyroid effect is held at the proper level. But if something, like an absence of the essential ingredient, iodine, arises to prevent successful achievement of the thyroxin-making process, there is no thyroxin to inhibit the generation of pituitary thyrotropic hormone. The result is a continued, and even greater, stimulation of the thyroid cells, which react in the strongest way open to them, by proliferation. Thus develops the hyperplastic thyroid, a reaction to the organ's own impotency.

Certain other adverse influences besides lack of iodine can prevent the proper culmination of thyroid synthesis and lead similarly to hyperplasia. Developmental anomalies of morphological or functional nature doubtless occur rarely in the thyroid mechanism, as elsewhere, and may account for occasional cases of cretinism which appear unrelated to deficiency of iodine. We are principally concerned, however, with a number of substances which have this effect when

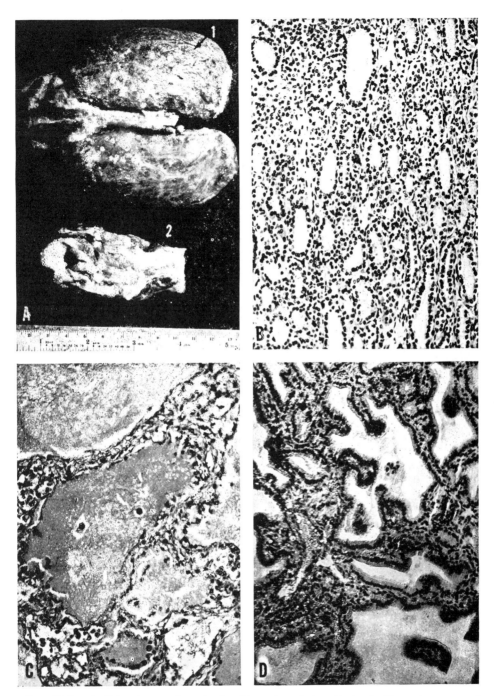

Fig. 27–5.—*A*, Goiter in a newborn lamb. The enlarged thyroid glands (*1*) can be compared with those of a normal lamb (*2*). *B*, Normal thyroid (× 195) of the newborn lamb. Same specimen as in *A* (*2*). *C*, Goitrous thyroid of lamb (× 195), same specimen as (*1*) in *A*. Note large acini of irregular size. *D*, Thyroid of cretinism in a young calf (× 195). Tall cells line large, irregularly shaped acini. (*A-C*, Courtesy of Armed Forces Institute of Pathology.) Contributor: Dr. C. L. Davies.

ingested and are known as **goitrogenic substances.** Among these are thiouracil, which is used therapeutically to reduce hyperthyroidism, thiourea, cyanides, sulfocyanates, or thiocyanates, and even, to a lesser degree, sulfonamides. Certain plants are known to be goitrogenic when eaten in sufficient amount by man or animal. Soybeans are notable in this respect; cabbage and its near relatives, rape and kale, as well as turnips, are less potent goitrogens. Goitrogenic substances from weeds of these and related families have been transmitted through milk, at least in the ovine species. Cooking or heating (and the usual processing of soybean meal) destroys the goitrogenic substance in these plants. Most, and probably all, of these goitrogenic substances are neutralized by unusually liberal supplies of iodine in the diet. Evidence indicates that they act by interfering with the elaboration of the thyroid hormone. The resulting low level of the hormone not only causes the symptoms characterized as hypothyroidism, but also permits unrestrained stimulation by the pituitary thyrotropic hormone to institute hyperplastic enlargement of the gland.

Goiter, a clinical term applicable to any non-malignant gross enlargement, is by far the most frequent disease of the thyroid gland. While there is still obscurity in respect to the cause of some forms, it will be helpful to classify goiters under the following four types:

(1) **Hyperplastic Goiter.**—Hyperplasia is the first morphologic response to iodine deficiency. With reduced thyroxin production the pituitary releases increased levels of thyrotropic hormone which is the stimulus for hyperplasia leading to goiter. The hyperplastic gland may and usually does compensate for the reduced availability of iodine, thus goiter is not synonymous with hypothyroidism. Microscopically the follicles are lined with tall columnar epithelium which forms, papillary projections into the lumens. Colloid is scant and often absent. Hyperplastic goiter is not common, the usual goiter of animals is a colloid goiter (see below). An exception is seen in congenital goiter or the **goiter of cretinism.** Cretinism has already been described as a severe hypothyroidism of the young. Actually, the disorder begins in prenatal life. The classical cretins were children of the Swiss Alps, a region where the soil and water are highly deficient in iodine, but the same effects of unrelieved iodine deficiency occur in other parts of the world. This is the type of goiter that has been common in newborn colts, calves, lambs and pigs in the iodine-deficient territories, which, in the United States, are the regions of the Great Lakes and the Pacific Northwest. As the disease is readily prevented by supplying minute amounts of iodine to the pregnant mother, it is no longer common.

The thyroid is always enlarged, and in these newly born animals the massive lobes may protrude prominently on each side of the neck. Microscopically, there is typically an extreme degree of hyperplasia. The epithelium is tall and the acini, devoid of colloid, are perhaps almost filled with the papillary infoldings characteristic of hyperplasia of glands in general. Such extreme degrees of hyperplastic changes are differentiated from papillary carcinoma by the fact that the individual cells are not anaplastic (p. 97), the basement membrane is not violated and the epithelial layer can, perhaps with difficulty, be followed back to the wall of the acinus. In some species, particularly sheep, the goitrous change is more inclined to manifest itself by a "piling up" of more than one layer of epithelial cells without so much change in the architecture of the acini. There is in severe cases an accompanying lack of hair, especially in pigs, and of wool in lambs

(p. 1016). Subcutaneous edema, possibly akin to myxedema, has been described in the neck region. If only mildly affected, the young animal may be helped to a normal existence and eventual resolution of the goiter, but many are born dead or die soon after birth. There is said to be a certain dwarfing of animals that survive but, if this is true, the condition is not to be confused with the too-frequent occurrence of hereditary dwarfs in certain artificially selected strains of beef cattle.

Familial goiter is a form of hyperplastic goiter that is not related to dietary deficiency of iodine, but rather to inborn errors of the enzyme systems involved in thyroxin synthesis. In man 5 types of familial goiter have been recognized, each with a distinct metabolic basis. In animals congenital goiter is occasionally seen which cannot be traced to iodine deficiency and it seems most probable that certain of these goiters are analogous to familial goiter. Evidence of the existence of inherited goiter in swine, cattle, goats and sheep has been reviewed by Rac and colleagues (1968). In their studies with sheep, the disorder appeared to be inherited as a recessive factor.

(2) **Colloid Goiter (Simple Goiter).**—This form of goiter is characterized by marked enlargement and distention of the acini, which are filled with colloid. The walls are stretched and the epithelium flattened. While the colloid is abundant, it may stain weakly and unevenly. It contains little iodine and little thyroxin, and any symptoms are those of hypothyroidism. Frequently, there are no symptoms beyond the increased size of the gland. The cause is ordinarily a mild deficiency of iodine. The milder goitrogenic agents, such as soy beans, are likely to produce this type of goiter. The pathogenesis of colloid goiter has long been a mystery. As indicated the response of the thyroid to iodine deficiency is hyperplasia mediated by thyrotropic hormone. How then does iodine deficiency result in colloid goiter? Experimental evidence (Follis 1959) indicates that colloid goiter represents an involutional stage of hyperplastic goiter which results when iodine is returned to the diet, or when iodine deficiency is periodic or when iodine deficiency is marginal. Severe deficiency of iodine in man and animals leads to hyperplastic goiter.

(3) **Adenomatous Goiter (Nodular Goiter).**—This form is characterized by nodules of thyroid tissue, more or less spherical in shape, highly variable in size and usually several in number, dispersed through the original tissue of the gland. As a rule, no two nodules show the same histologic appearance, there being all gradations between the colloid goiter with large, colloid-filled acini and low, inactive epithelium, on the one hand, and the hyperplastic, cretinic type, on the other. The picture within a given nodule is, however, usually rather constant. The nodules are often regarded as adenomas. It is idle to speculate on the accuracy of this conception until we have a precise definition of what constitutes an adenoma. The other view is that these forms represent merely a lobular distribution of what is essentially one of the other types of goiter. They frequently resemble Graves' disease in being accompanied by unexplained lymphoid tissue. But, at least, it may be said that, like adenomas in other organs, they grow expansively at the expense of the surrounding tissue, which is easily seen, under the microscope, to be compressed.

Some of the nodules or adenomas are inert functionally, others actively secrete thyroid hormone, producing the usual symptoms of hyperthyroidism. The latter constitute the "toxic adenomas" of clinical terminology. Those adenomas seen in animals, chiefly horses and dogs, have seldom caused noticeable signs of toxicity (hyperthyroidism).

(4) **Exophthalmic Goiter (Goiter of Hyperthyroidism; Toxic Goiter).**—This disorder of humans is also known as Graves' disease or Basedow's disease. It may well be that this condition does not occur in animals, the occasional case of exophthalmos having a nervous or other cause. (Retrobulbar neoplasms produce exophthalmos, usually unilateral, and are not rare.) In man, exophthalmic goiter is the most formidable type. It produces hyperthyroidism which may be alleviated temporarily by iodine, only to be made worse in the course of a few weeks.

The thyroid may or may not be much enlarged; the enlargement may extend around to the dorsal side of the trachea, constituting the so-called "inward goiter." Microscopically, there is hyperplasia but not the extreme degree seen in the thyroid of cretinism. The epithelium is tall, but infolding papillae are absent or few. The colloid is usually present but thin and pale-staining. There is often a row of rounded vacuoles in the colloid where it adjoins the epithelial cells. This has been interpreted as resorption of colloid into the epithelial cells. New acini of small size may be formed. In company with the changes in the thyroid acini, there are almost always to be found areas of lymphoid tissue somewhere in the gland. Active germinal centers are usually present. The superabundance of lymphoid tissue extends to other organs, including the thymus. A tendency toward degenerative changes is described in various locations. Exophthalmos, or protrusion of the eyeballs with a white ring of sclera showing around the cornea, constitutes a startling aspect of the disease but, as stated previously, is thought to be due to some other derangement than the excess of thyroid hormone.

The cause of the condition is unknown, although an excess of pituitary thyrotropic hormone is presumed to be part of the mechanism. Surgical removal of part of the gland or "internal irradiation" by the administration of radioactive iodine usually relieves the condition. Untreated, the disease may lead to death from degenerative changes in an overstimulated heart or, rarely, to practically complete destruction of the exhausted thyroid and a consequent myxedema.

Myxedema.—The subcutaneous accumulation of mucoid material in this hypothyroid state has been described in the general discussion of hypothyroidism. The reason for the severe shortage of hormone is the result of goiter with hypothyroidism, or destruction of the gland by any inflammatory or neoplastic processes. In one form of hypothyroidism the thyroid is all but nonexistent. Compressed islets of thyroid parenchyma, buried in fibrous tissue, are the rule, perhaps with lymphocytes or other inflammatory cells still present. The term Riedel's struma is sometimes used to describe thyroid changes of this nature. The cause of this fibrous atrophy of the thyroid may or may not be readily apparent but is usually the end result of some destructive inflammatory process of infectious origin, centered in either a neighboring or a distant area of the body. Accidents to the blood supply or damage from excessive use of goitrogenic drugs (thiocyanates) are other possibilities. Some cases are the terminal exhaustive phase of exophthalmic goiter. Myxedema, now rare because of therapy with artificial thyroid products, is principally a disease of human beings, but it would be a mistake to say that it cannot occur in animals. The same susceptibility to thyroid deficiency exists and tissue reactions paralleling those of humans are not unknown in domestic animals.

Other changes occasionally possible in the thyroid include hemorrhages, necroses, amyloidosis and metastatic infections, all of which are rare. A tendency to form abnormally small acini with little or no colloid has been reported as occurring in dogs with various infections including experimental Chagas' disease. There were free cells in the acini, suspected of being phagocytes, but there was no inflammatory change. Toxins from the infections were presumed to be causative.

Aberrant thyroid tissue is relatively frequent in most animal species. Most aberrant thyroids result from the failure of all or part of the thyroid anlage to descend from the floor of the pharynx to its normal cervical position or from its descending beyond its normal adult position. In the first case, aberrant thyroid tissue may occur at any median point from the tongue to its normal position and in the second case it occurs caudal to the normal position to include its location within the thoracic cavity. Another form of aberrant thyroid is the result of an anomaly of development of fetal tissue as a whole. In man the most common example is thyroid tissue in the ovary. Aberrant thyroid responds to the same physiological stimuli as the cervical gland.

Lymphocytic Thyroiditis.—In dogs of the beagle breed a lymphocytic thyroiditis, remarkably similar to Hashimoto's disease of man, is a frequently encountered lesion, though rarely associated with clinical disease. The microscopic features consist of diffuse or nodular infiltration of the gland by lymphocytes and lesser numbers of plasma cells and macrophages. Lymphocytic nodules may have prominent germinal centers. There can be marked displacement and destruction of the follicles with colloid gaining entrance to the interstitium where it is engulfed by macrophages and occasionally giant cells. Nodules of hyperplastic interstitial or parafollicular cells often accompany the lesion. In addition to its similarity to Hashimoto's disease, the thyroiditis is also indistinguishable from experimental autoimmune thyroiditis in dogs and other experimental animals. Further studies are necessary to elucidate the pathogenesis of the spontaneous disease in dogs but it would appear to represent an example of an autoimmune disease. Lymphocytic thyroiditis is occasionally seen in old dogs of any species, but the relationships to the disease in beagles has not been established.

Hajdu and Rona (1969) have reported spontaneous lymphocytic thyroiditis in laboratory rats which is also similar to Hashimoto's disease.

Neoplasms primary in the thyroid have been discussed (p. 255). Metastatic neoplasms occasionally invade the thyroid, the malignant lymphoma being the least rare.

A **thyroglossal cyst** is a developmental anomaly arising in the thyroglossal duct. This duct, in early embryonic life, reaches out from the lower pharyngeal mucosa to form the primitive thyroid, normally disappearing before birth. When it persists, a sinus tract or a cyst commonly develops. The cyst is always in the mid-line and is lined either by stratified squamous or simple columnar epithelium or by a mixture of the two. This is anything but a frequent anomaly in animals, but developmental anomalies are not reported with a regularity that permits statistical conclusions.

Thyrocalcitonin (Calcitonin).—Although there is no clear evidence which indicates that altered release of thyrocalcitonin plays a significant role in animal diseases, it is probably only a matter of time before primary disorders of thyrocalcitonin release are documented. Its participation in diseases of the skeleton is assuredly important and Capen and Young (1967) have presented data suggesting that depletion of thyrocalcitonin is the primary disorder in milk fever (p. 1003).

Thyrocalcitonin is a polypeptide, probably a hormone, which occurs in the thyroid gland or ultimobranchial body. The biological action of thyrocalcitonin is to induce hypocalcemia and hypophosphatemia by directly inhibiting bone resorption. In the thyroid thyrocalcitonin is produced by the parafollicular cells (light cells, C cells). Tumors of parafollicular cells occur in cattle (ultimobranchial tumors), dogs (medullary carcinomas) and rats (light-cell tumors) but there is no evidence to suggest they are functional.

Thyroid

BEIERWALTES, W. H., and NISHIYAMA, R. H.: Dog Thyroiditis: Occurrence and Similarity to Hashimoto's Struma. Endocrinology *83*:501–508, 1968.
BLAXTER, K. L.: Severe Experimental Hyperthyroidism in the Ruminant: Metabolic Effects: Physiological Effects. J. Agric. Sci. *38*:1–19, and 20–27, 1948.
CAPEN, C. C., and YOUNG, D. M.: The Ultrastructure of the Parathyroid Glands and Thyroid Parafollicular Cells of Cows with Parturient Paresis and Hypocalcemia. Lab. Invest. *17*:717–737, 1967.
————: Thyrocalcitonin: Evidence For Release in a Spontaneous Hypocalcemic Disorder. Science *157*:205–206, 1967.
CARE, A. D.: Goitrogenic Properties of Linseed. Nature *173*:172–173, 1954.
————: Goitrogenic Activity in Linseed. New Zealand J. Sci. Tech. (Sect. A.) *36*: 321–327, 1955.
CLEMENTS, F.: A Goitrogenic Factor in Milk. Med. J. Austr. Nov. 2:645–646, 1957. Abstr. Vet. Bull., No. 213, 1960.
COFFIN, D. L., and MUNSON, T. O.: Endocrine Diseases of the Dog Associated with Hair Loss. Sertoli-cell Tumor of Testis, Hypothyroidism, Canine Cushing's Syndrome. J. Am. Vet. Med. Assn. *123*:403–408, 1953.
COLE, W. H., and WOMACK, N. A.: The Thyroid in Infections and Toxemias. Proc. Soc. Exper. Biol. and Med. *25*:188–191, 1927–28.
DÄMMRICH, K.: Die Beeinflussung des Skeletts durch die Schilddrüse bei Tieren. Berl. u. Münch. Tierarzte. Wochen *76*:31–34, 53–56, 1963.
EICKHOFF, W.: Zur Histologie und Pathologie der Wildschilddrüse. Archiv. f. Exp. Veterinaer-med. *16*:211–228, 1963.
FALCONER, I. R.: Effect of Thyroid Deficiency in the Ewe on Lamb Viability. Nature *205*: 703, 1965.
FOLLIS, R. H.: Experimental Colloid Goitre Produced by Thiouracil. Nature *183*:1817–1818, 1959.
————: Studies on the Pathogenesis of Colloid Goiter. Trans. Assn. Amer. Physicians *72*:265–274, 1959.
GILMORE, J. W., VENZKE, W. G., and FOUST, H. L.: Growth Changes in the Thyroid of the Normal Dog. Am. J. Vet. Res. *2*:66–72, 1940.
GOBLE, F. C.: Thyroid Changes in Acute Experimental Chagas' Disease in Dogs. Amer. J. Path. *30*:599–611, 1954.
GRIEM, W.: Die Nebennierenveränderungen beim enzootischen Herztod der Schweine. Deutsche tierärztl. Wchnschr. *61*:417–424, 1954.
GRIESBACH, W. E., KENNEDY, T. H., and PURVES, H. D.: Thyroid Adenomata in Rats on Brassica Seed Diet. Brit. J. Exper. Path. *26*:18–24, 1945.
GROTH, W.: Die Pathologie der Strumen und Schilddrüsengeschwülste der Haustiere. Deutsch. tierarzl. Woch. *69*:707–713, 1962.
HAJDU, A., and RONA, G.: Spontaneous Thyroiditis in Laboratory Rats. Experimentia *25*: 1325–1327, 1969.
HARE, T.: Three Cases of Heterotopic Deposits of Thyroid Tissue in the Dog. Proc. Royal Soc. Med. *25*:(2):1496–1499, 1932.
————: Fusion of the Thyroid Glands in a Dog. Proc. Royal Soc. Med. *25*(2):1500, 1932.
HUNT, R. D.: Aberrant Thyroid Tissue in the Mouse. Science *141*:1054–1055, 1963.
JAMIESON, S., and HARBOUR, H. E.: Congenital Goitre in Lambs. Vet. Rec. *59*:102, 1947.
JUBB, K. V., and McENTEE, K.: The Relationship of Ultimobranchial Remnants and Derivatives to Tumors of the Thyroid Gland in Cattle. Cornell Vet. *49*:41–69, 1959.

JUHN, M.: A History of Six Years' Thiouracil Treatment in a Brown Leghorn Hen. J. Endocrinol. 9:155–159, 1953.

KALKUS, J. W.: Goitre and Associated Conditions in Domestic Animals. Exper. Sta. Bull. 156, State College of Washington, Pullman, 1920.

KRACHT, J., and KRACHT, U.: Zur Histopathologie und Therapie der Schreckthyreotoxikose des Wildkaninchens. Virchows Arch. 321:238–274, 1952.

LUCKE, V. M.: An Histological Study of Thyroid Abnormalities in the Domestic Cat. Small Anim. Pract. 5:351–358, 1964.

MATOUSEK, J.: Štitna zláza cervenostrakatého skotu behem ontogenese. (The Thyroid Gland of Cattle.) Ann. Acad. tchécosl. Agric. 27:251–266, 1954.

McQUILLAN, M. T., TRIKOJUS, V. M., CAMPBELL, A. D., and TURNER, A. W.: The Prolonged Administration of Thyroxine to Cows. Brit. J. Exper. Path. 29:93–106, 1948.

MAWDESLEY-THOMAS, L. E., and JOLLY, D. W.: Autoimmune Disease in the Beagle. Vet. Rec. 80:553–554, 1967.

MUSSER, E., and GRAHAM, W. R.: Familial Occurrence of Thyroiditis in Purebred Beagles. Lab. Anim. Care 18:58–68, 1968.

NORFELDT, S., GELLERSTEDT, N., and FALKMER, S.: Studies on Rape-Seed Meal and Its Goitrogenic Effects on Pigs. Acta path. et. micro. biol. Scandinav. 35:217–236, 1954.

OBEL, A. L., SJOBERG, K., and SANDSTEDT, H.: Om medfödd struma hos kalv i Sverige. (Congenital Goitre in Calves in Sweden.) Nord. vet.-med. 2:491–507, 1950.

OSTERTAG, H. G.: Schilddrüsen befunde bei totgeborenen und verendeten Kälbern. Berl. u. Münch. tierarztl Wochschr. 76:253–255, 1962.

PALMER, J. G., CARTWRIGHT, G. E., and WINTROBE, M. M.: Experimental Production of Leukopenia in Rats by Thyroid Feeding. Amer. J. Physiol. 171:385–390, 1952.

PANTIC, V., and JOVANOVIC, M.: Histology of the Thyroid in Endemic Goitre in Domestic Animals. (English summary and title.) Acta Vet., Belgrade 5:13–32, 1955. Abstr. Vet. Bull. No. 2970, 1955.

PELTOLA, P.: Goitrogenic Effects of Cow's Milk from the Goitre District of Finland. Acta Endocrinol. Copenhagen 34:121–128, 1960.

RAC, R., et al.: Congenital Goitre in Merino Sheep Due to an Inherited Defect in the Biosynthesis of Thyroid Hormone. Res. Vet. Sci. 9:209–223, 1968.

SCACCINI, A.: I muscoli della ghiandola tiroide negli equini. Nuova vet. 30:211–217, 1954.

SCHLOTTHAUER, C. F.: Diseases of the Thyroid Gland of Adult Horses. J. Am. Vet. Med. Assn. 78:211–218, 1931.

SCHLOTTHAUER, C. F., McKENNEY, F. D., and CAYLOR, H. D.: The Incidence of Goiter and Other Lesions of the Thyroid Gland in Dogs of Southern Minnesota. J. Amer. Vet. Med. Assn. 76:811–819, 1930.

SCHLUMBERGER, HANS G.: Spontaneous Goiter and Cancer of the Thyroid in Animals. Ohio J. Science 55:24–43, 1955.

SINCLAIR, D. P., and ANDREWS, E. D.: Goitre in New-born Lambs (Fed Kale). New Zealand Vet. J. 2:72–79, 1954.

STEYN, D. G., and SUNKEL, W.: Goitre in Animals in the Union of South Africa. J. So. African Vet. Med. Assn. 25:9–18, 1954.

TASHJIAN, A. H., JR.: Soft Bones, Hard Facts and Calcitonin Therapy. N. E. J. of Med. 283:593–594, 1970.

TUCKER, W. E., JR.: Thyroiditis in a Group of Laboratory Dogs. Amer. J. Clin. Nutrition 38:70–74, 1962.

UOTILA, U., and KANNAS, O.: Quantitative Histological Method of Determining the Properties of the Principal Components of Thyroid Tissue. Acta endocrinol. Copenhagen 11:49–60, 1952.

WARTHIN, A. S.: The Pathology of Goiter. Inter-State Postgrad. Med. Assn. of North Am. Proceedings. 1929, pp. 383–385.

WRIGHT, E., and ANDREWS, E. D.: Availability of Iodate Iodine to Sheep. New Zealand J. Sci. Tech., Sect. A. 37:83–87, 1955.

WRIGHT, E., and SINCLAIR, D. P.: The Goitrogenic Effect of Thousand-Headed Kale (Brassica oleracea, var. acephala) on Adult Sheep and Rabbits. N.Z. J. Agric. Res. 1:477–485, 1958.

ZWART, D.: Struma bij de geit op Nederlands Nieuw-Guinea (Goiter in Goats in Dutch New Guinea). Tijdschr. Diergeneesk. 84:550–559, 1959.

The Parathyroid Glands

As with the other ductless glands, the disorders of the parathyroids are principally those concerned with insufficient or excessive secretion of the specific hormone. Since most of these disorders have received attention in connection with fibrous osteodystrophy (p. 1063) and parathyroid adenoma (p. 257), little more than a summary is needed here. The function of the parathyroid hormone is to maintain a proper level of calcium in the blood, which it accomplishes by stimulating bone resorption. Parathormone may also stimulate intestinal absorption of calcium and possibly renal tubular resorption of calcium, but its most important activity is to increase the rate of bone resorption. Parathyroid hormone causes an increase in urinary loss of phosphorus.

Deficiency of parathyroid secretion causes **parathyroid tetany,** in which the musculature is in more or less continuous tonic (or tetanic) spasms. Due to an imbalance of calcium ions there is hyperirritability, probably in the nerve-endings, and spinal reflexes (see spinal reflex arc, p. 1376) are continuously exaggerated. This condition almost always arises as the result of experimental or accidental removal of the parathyroids surgically. Less than two days is sufficient for the effects to become apparent. The inability of some experimenters to produce parathyroid tetany in the bovine can in all probability be attributed to failure to find and remove all parathyroids. While there are occasional variations in the anatomy of this region, most bovine animals have an anterior parathyroid which is detached and at some little distance from the thyroid lobe, necessitating a very precise anatomical knowledge.

Hyperparathyroidism is characterized by extraction of calcium from the bones. In the bones, fibrous osteodystrophy classically results (p. 1063); at the other end of the process, there may be deposition of excess calcium in urinary calculi (p. 1286) and in the walls of the lower renal tubules and other soft tissues (Metastatic Calcification, p. 56). The amount of calcium in the circulating blood is

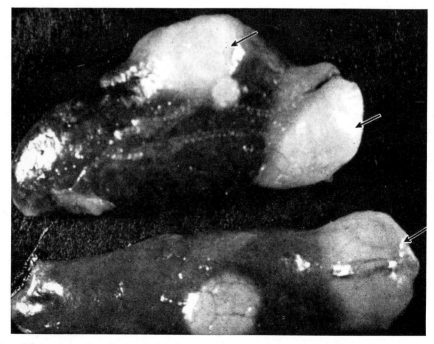

Fig. 27–6.—Secondary hyperplasia of parathyroids in a seven-year-old male airedale with chronic interstitial nephritis. The enlarged gray-colored parathyroids (arrows) stand out against the dark-brown-colored thyroids.   Courtesy of Angell Memorial Animal Hospital.)

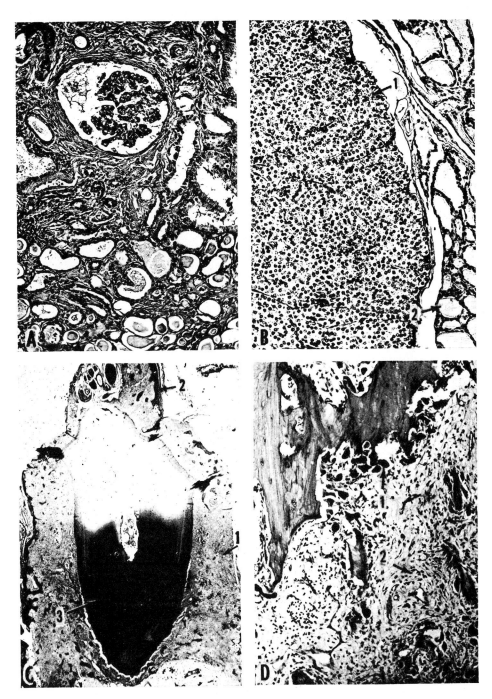

FIG. 27–7.—Renal hyperparathyroidism in a dog. *A*, The kidney (× 110). *B*, The enlarged parathyroid (*1*) compressing adjacent thyroid (*2*). *C*, A tooth (× 11) poorly supported by soft spongy bone. Note absence of bone trabeculae (*1*). Gingival epithelium (*2*), dentine of the root of the tooth (*3*). *D*, The mandible (× 145). Note many osteoblasts (*1*), fibrous marrow (*2*) and irregular spicules of bone. (Courtesy of Armed Forces Institute of Pathology.) Contributor: Dr. Joseph M. Stoyak.

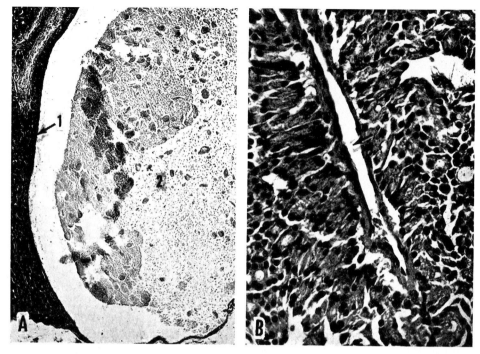

Fig. 27–8.—*A*, Cyst of the parathyroid of a dog (× 60). This cyst, found incidentally, was lined by columnar epithelium (*1*) and contains eosinophilic material (*2*). Contributor: Dr. Elihu Bond. *B*, Adenocarcinoma of parathyroid of a dog (× 305). Intimate relationship of cells to blood vessels (arrow) is a feature of neoplasms of endocrine organs. (*A* and *B*, Courtesy of Armed Forces Institute of Pathology.) Contributor: Dr. M. M. Mason.

traditionally high also. The usual cause of classical human osteitis fibrosa cystica is a functioning parathyroid adenoma. Another group of cases is attributable to hyperplasia of the parathyroids in connection with renal insufficiency. These are represented by the "rubber jaw" syndrome of dogs. Owing to renal damage, there is in this disorder impaired ability to excrete phosphorus, whose ions in the blood reach a very high level causing a lowering of serum calcium (p. 1064). To overcome this, the parathyroids increase their function and their size (hypertrophy by our definition but commonly called hyperplasia) and take large amounts of calcium from the bones, producing the form of fibrous osteodystrophy known in dogs as "rubber jaw." In these cases, the blood calcium appears to be habitually low; the phosphate, high (p. 1064). A third mechanism resulting in hyperparathyroidism involves dietary imbalance in calcium and phosphorus, as occurs in "big head" in horses (p. 1065). Similar to renal insufficiency the dietary induced hypocalcemia results in parathyroid hyperplasia leading to fibrous osteodystrophy.

Other lesions, chiefly inflammatory or circulatory, have been described in the parathyroids but are of slight importance unless, by destruction of functional tissue, they cause hypoparathyroidism and tetany.

Parathyroid

Albright, F., and Reifenstein, E. C.: *The Parathyroid Glands and Metabolic Bone Disease.* Baltimore, The Williams & Wilkins Co., 1948.

CAPEN, C. C., COLE, C. R., and HIBBS, J. W.: Influence of Vitamin D on Calcium Metabolism and the Parathyroid Glands of Cattle. Fed. Proc. 27:142–152, 1968.

CAPEN, C. C., KOESTNER, A., and COLE, C. R.: The Ultrastructure and Histochemistry of Normal Parathyroid Glands of Pregnant and Nonpregnant Cows. Lab. Invest. 14:1673–1690, 1965.

————: The Ultrastructure, Histopathology, and Histochemistry of the Parathyroid Glands of Pregnant and Non-pregnant Cows Fed a High Level of Vitamin D. Lab. Invest. 14: 1809–1825, 1965.

CAPEN, C. C., and ROWLAND, G. N.: The Ultrastructure of the Parathyroid Glands of Young Cats. Anat. Rec. 162:327–331, 1968.

CAPEN, C. C., and YOUNG, D. M.: The Ultrastructure of the Parathyroid Glands and Thyroid Parafollicular Cells of Cows with Parturient Paresis and Hypocalcemia. Lab. Invest. 17: 717–737, 1967.

DERIVAUX, J.: Variations pondérales des parathyroïides chez le chien normal. Compt. rend. Soc. de biol. 138:879–880, 1944.

FORDHAM, C. C., III, and WILLIAMS, T. F.: Brown Tumor and Secondary Hyperparathyroidism. New Eng. J. Med. 269:129–131, 1963.

LOTZ, W. E., TALMAGE, R. V., and COMAR, C. L.: Effect of Parathyroid Extract Administration in Sheep. Proc. Soc. Exper. Biol. and Med. 85:292–295, 1954.

MATHIEU, F.: Excrétion urinaire du calcium et du phosphore chez le chien en insuffisance parathyroïdienne chronique. Arch. internat. de. physiol. 51:278–289, 1941.

PLATT, H.: The Parathyroid Glands with Particular Reference to the "Rubber Jaw" Syndrome. The Skeletal System in "Rubber Jaw." J. Comp. Path. & Therap. 61:188–196, and 197–214, 1951.

SNAPPER, I.: Parathyroid Hormone and Mineral Metabolism. Bull. New York Acad. Med. 29:612–624, 1953.

THE HYPOPHYSIS OR PITUITARY GLAND

The pituitary is morphologically divisible into two distinct components, the anterior pituitary or adenohypophysis (pars distalis) and the posterior pituitary or neurohypophysis. The adenohypophysis is embryologically derived from Rathke's pouch, whereas the neurohypophysis arises from the diencephalon. In most species Rathke's pouch remains as a narrow cleft within the adenohypophysis, a cleft which separates the bulk of the adenohypophysis from that portion in immediate contact with the neurohypophysis, known as the pars intermedia of the adenohypophysis.

The adenohypophysis, despite its small size, secretes a minimum of seven hormones; these are follicle-stimulating hormone (FSH), luteinizing hormone (LH), thyroid-stimulating hormone (TSH), adrenocorticotropic hormone (ACTH), growth hormone (somatotropic hormone; STH), luteotropic hormone (prolactin; LTH) and melanocyte-stimulating hormone (MSH). The neurohypophysis releases two hormones, antidiuretic hormone (ADH) or vasopressin and oxycytocin. Within the adenohypophysis there is probably a specific cell type responsible for the production of each hormone. With special staining techniques at least six distinct cell types can be demonstrated, but with hematoxylin and eosin only three cellular populations are evident. These are the basophils which produce FSH, TSH, LH and MSH, acidophils which produce STH and LTH and chromophobes which lack stainable granules. Chromophobes are thought to represent resting cells or basophils and acidophils which have released their granules. However, newer evidence suggests that at least in some species chromophobes produce ACTH. In man and possibly other species, the role of the chromophobe in ACTH production is not firmly established, and the basophil is considered the origin of this hormone. Production and release of anterior pituitary hormones are under control of the hypothalamus which, in response to the negative feedback mechanisms, produces release and inhibitory factors which pass down nerve fibers to the stalk of the pituitary, enter capillaries and are carried to the anterior pituitary by way of the portal blood vessels. The posterior pituitary hormones are produced in the hypothalamus (principally in the supraoptic and paraventricular nuclei) and pass down nerve fibers in the hypothalamohypophyseal tract as "neurosecretory material" to the neurohypophysis where they are released.

The pathology of the pituitary gland involves the study of a congeries of syndromes and functional abnormalities based on disturbances of its various endocrine functions. They will be reviewed briefly, being of limited frequency in animals. The essence of **hyperpituitarism,** an excess of the predominant endocrine influence, is overgrowth of bones and, to a lesser degree, of the fibrous connective tissues. In the immature individual, this results in **gigantism.** A human being grows to extreme tallness, the long bones reach unusual length. If the hyperpituitarism arises after ossification of the bones has been completed, they grow heavier, wider and thicker, rather than appreciably longer. The result, in the human, is **acromegaly,** characterized by abnormally large hands and feet, thick heavy and often crooked fingers and toes. The face is coarse and deformed because of thickening of the facial bones and subcutaneous tissues. Other abnormalities that may go with hyperpituitarism include increase in amount and coarseness of the hair, increased sweating, intermittent glycosuria and perhaps increased sexual activity and lactation.

Hypopituitarism is characterized by clinical abnormalities which are, in a general way, the opposite of those just described for hyperpituitary function. The usual manifestations are well indicated by the name **dystrophia adiposo-**

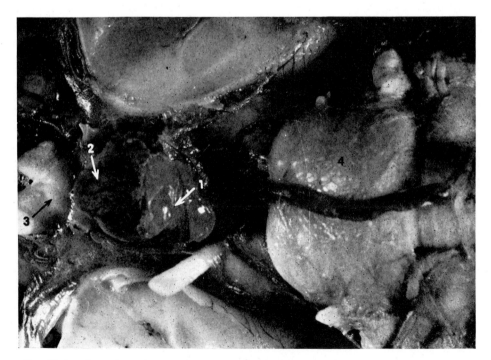

Fig. 27–9.—Cyst of the intermediate lobe of the pituitary of a mongrel terrier, spayed female aged twelve years. An incidental finding. The cyst (*1*), anterior lobe of pituitary (*2*), optic chiasma (*3*), pons (*4*). (Courtesy of Angell Memorial Animal Hospital.)

genitalis. In addition to a tendency to accumulate subcutaneous fat, there are depression or loss of sexual function and atrophy of the sexual organs. The hair is scanty and fine, the skin thin and delicate, quite the opposite of what prevails in the acromegaly of hyperpituitarism. For the male, the disorder is not only demasculinizing but, in effect, feminizing. Even the accumulated fat has a feminine distribution. This is dystrophia adiposo-genitalis, also known as Froelich's syndrome. There are a number of variations in the human, which go by other names. Some involve mental deficiency, a spectacular premature senility, dwarfism with a delicate and childish form quite different from that of cretinism, or adiposis dolorosa, in which the accumulations of fat form painful subcutaneous masses. In view of the obvious effect of pituitary hormones on the reproductive organs, there have been numerous attempts to trace certain types of reproductive failure, particularly in the bovine, to pituitary dysfunction. It cannot be said that these efforts have been successful; any possible connection between the ordinary forms of sterility and the pituitary remains elusive. Jubb and McEntee have recently reviewed magnificently the functional cytology of the gland in the bovine.

The **lesions** of the hypophysis which produce the symptoms of hyperpituitarism always involve an increase of cells, usually of only one of the three histological kinds. In some instances, this increase can be classed as hyperplasia, more often it is to be considered neoplastic, an adenoma, of which chromophobe adenomas are the more frequent, acidophile (eosinophil) adenomas much less so and basophile adenomas the rarest. The neoplastic aspects of these growths have been

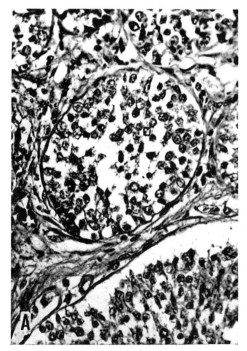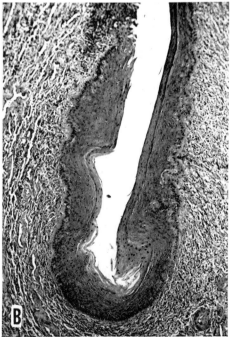

Fig. 27–10.—Feminizing effect of Sertoli-cell tumor. *A*, Sertoli-cell tumor ($\times$ 350) of the testis of a dog. *B*, Squamous metaplasia of the urethra ($\times$ 70) of the same dog, one of the effects of hyperestrogenism. (Courtesy of Armed Forces Institute of Pathology.) Contributor: Rowley Memorial Animal Hospital.

discussed (p. 257). There is no infallible distinction between hyperplasia and neoplasia in the pituitary and in neither case are the causes known. Reciprocal relations with other endocrine glands probably play a part and have received considerable study. For instance, the basophilic cells have been noted to increase during estrus. Changes in the proportions of cells have been described in pregnancy and following castration, but findings have not always been in agreement. The administration of thyroid or anterior pituitary hormones or epinephrine has been found to increase the number of acidophiles.

The pituitary lesions causing deficiency of the hormones are, as would be expected, in the nature of atrophic changes. Thrombosis and embolism are causes of infarction and necrosis, which occur rarely. There is suspicion that the pituitary may suffer degenerative changes in the course of severe infectious diseases (diphtheria, puerperal sepsis), but it must be remembered that tumors, even of the pituitary itself, put pressure on surrounding cells and structures, thereby causing their atrophy. The most frequent cause of such pressure is the craniopharyngioma (p. 240) which encroaches upon the hypophysis as well as the adjacent hypothalamus, but some cases of hypopituitarism prove to be due to a chromophobe adenoma. The chromophobe cells are largely or entirely without endocrine effect in themselves, but the growth destroys the functioning cells of the surrounding normal gland. Certain chromophobe adenomas secrete ACTH which results in hyperadrenalism (p. 1353). Whether adiposity develops is believed to depend upon whether pressure is exerted upon hypothalamic tissues; in the case of a tumor entirely within the sella turcica, such pressure is absent and, likewise, any marked degree of adiposity. Any extensive increase in size of the gland causes gradual enlargement of the bony sella turcica. If the gland later should chance to atrophy, the tell-tale bony changes persist and reveal the previous condition. If the neurohypophysis is damaged, diabetes insipidus results (p. 1020).

Cysts, which arise from remnants of the craniopharyngeal duct (remnant of Rathke's pouch), are occasionally found in or adjacent to the pituitary They are lined by a ciliated columnar epithelium and contain mucin. Similar cysts may arise from the opposite end of the duct in the roof of the pharynx.

Prolonged gestation is now recognized as a dysfunction of the fetal pituitary. Abnormally long pregnancies were first recorded in cattle over seventy-five years ago, but only recently have syndromes in cattle and sheep been characterized and linked to abnormalities of the fetal pituitary. In cattle two distinct forms of prolonged gestation occur. Both are controlled by a single autosomal recessive gene. In Holstein-Friesian and Ayrshire cattle, the disease is characterized by a gestation period of up to 380 days and a calf that is abnormally large but lacks obvious deformities. The pituitary is present but there is marked degranulation of the acidophils. Adrenal cortices are hypoplastic, but other endocrine glands are normal. The calf dies in utero and is born dead (if physically possible) or if delivered by cesarean section may be viable but is weak, unable to nurse and dies in six to twelve hours. Death is associated with severe hypoglycemia, but based on the frequent presence of meconium staining of the skin, other factors associated with intrauterine distress probably contribute.

A second type of prolonged gestation occurs in Jersey and Guernsey breeds where the gestation periods may exceed four hundred seventy-five days. Normal parturition does not occur, though a dead fetus may be expelled. Even if delivered by cesarean section viable calves only survive a few minutes. The calf is small, has hypotrichosis and facial abnormalities such as hydrocephalus, anencephalus and cyclopia. There is aplasia of the anterior pituitary and often hypoplasia of the neurohypophysis. The adrenal glands and thyroid gland are also hypoplastic.

Types of prolonged gestations have been observed in cattle which do not clearly fit into the two syndromes described, however, the fetuses have not been studied with the detail necessary to reach any conclusion regarding pathogenesis.

In sheep, prolonged pregnancy has been described in Karakul ewes in Southwest Africa. Gestation exceeds two hundred days, the lambs are abnormally large, and if delivered survive only a few hours. The abnormally large lambs resulted in the name Grootlamsiekte (big lamb disease) The anterior pituitary is present, but acidophils are degranulated. The adrenal cortices and thymus are hypoplastic. This form of prolonged gestation is caused by consumption of the plant *Salsola tuberculata*. Although the condition most frequently occurs in the Karakul breed, because they are raised where the plant is common, other breeds are susceptible.

Prolonged gestation has also been described in sheep following ingestion of *Veratrum californicum* (p. 971). Ingestion of this plant in early pregnancy results in severe cranial malformations which includes aplasia of the pituitary.

Pituitary

CAPEN, C. C., and KOESTNER, A.: Functional Chromophobe Adenomas of the Canine Adenohypophysis. An Ultrastructural Evaluation of a Neoplasm of Pituitary Corticotrophs. Path. Vet. *4*:326–347, 1967.

CAPEN, C. C., MARTIN, S. L., and KOESTNER, A.: Neoplasms in the Adenohypophysis of Dogs. A Clinical and Pathologic Study. Path. Vet. *4*:301–325, 1967.

————: The Ultrastructure and Histopathology of an Acidophil Adenoma of the Canine Adenohypophysis. Path. Vet. *4*:348–365, 1967.

GUSTON, K., and GIER, H. T.: An Anatomical Description of a Hydrocephalic Calf from Prolonged Gestation and the Possible Relationships of These Conditions. Cornell Vet. *48*: 45–53, 1958.

HOLM, L. W.: Prolonged Pregnancy. Adv. Vet. Sci. *11*:159–205, 1967.

JENSEN, E. C.: Hypopituitarism Associated with Cystic Rathke's Cleft in a Dog. J. Am. Vet. Med. Assn. *135*:572–574, 1959.

JUBB, K. V., and McENTEE, K.: The Bovine Pituitary Gland: I. Adenohypophyseal Functional Cytology; II. Architecture and Cytology with Special Reference to Basophil Function. Cornell Vet. *45*:576–641, 1955.

KENNEDY, P. C.: Interaction of Fetal Disease and the Onset of Labor in Cattle and Sheep. Fed. Proc. *30*:110–113, 1971.

KENNEDY, P. C., LIGGINS, G. C., and HOLM, L. W.: Prolonged Gestation. *Comparative Aspects of Reproductive Failure*. K. Benirschke, Ed. New York, Springer-Verlag, 1967.

KENNEDY, P. C., KENDRICK, J. W., and STORMONT, C.: Adenohypophyseal Aplasia, an Inherited Defect Associated with Abnormal Gestation in Guernsey Cattle. Cornell Vet. *47*: 161–178, 1957.

LEOB, W. F., CAPEN, C. C., and JOHNSON, L. E.: Adenomas of the Pars Intermedia Associated with Hyperglycemia and Glycosuria in Two Horses. Cornell Vet. *56*:623–629, 1966.

THE PINEAL GLAND

Although the pineal gland has long been thought to have an endocrine function, only recently has evidence been gathered which warrants placing it with the endocrine organs in mammals. Embryologically, the organ is thought to be a vestige of a "third eye" which exists in certain reptiles and amphibians. It has been demonstrated that the amphibian and mammalian pineal secretes a hormonelike compound known as **melatonin.** In amphibians, melatonin synthesis is controlled by photoreceptors within the pineal and the hormone causes skin lightening. In mammals photoreceptor cells are not present and the pineal does not respond directly to light. Instead the pineal responds to light received by the retina; increased light depressing melatonin synthesis and decreased light stimulating melatonin synthesis. In mammals melatonin inhibits gonadotropic hormone synthesis or release by the pituitary and is believed to play a major role in the seasonal reproductive activity exhibited by many species.

The known pathology of the pineal is minimal in extent. Necrosis, calcification, cystic degeneration, hyaline degeneration, deposition of hemosiderin, hyperemia and petechiae have been described in the equine pineal body but were asymptomatic. Tumors of the pineal body have been reported in a fox (p. 264), in a horse and in a rat. Hyperplastic enlargement to four times the normal, with consequent pressure on surrounding nervous structures, has been reported as causing a circling syndrome in a mule.

Pineal

LÁSZLO, F.: Beiträge zur pathologischen Anatomie und Histologie der Zirbel. Deutsche. tierärtzl. Wchnschr. *42*:685–689, 1934.
————: Weitere Beiträge zur vergleichenden pathologischen Anatomie der Zirbel. Deutsche. tierärtzl. Wchnschr. *43*:245–247, 1935.
NOBEL, T. A.: Circling Syndrome in a Mule Due to Hyperplasia of the Pineal Gland. Cornell Vet. *45*:570–575, 1955.
RIETER, R. J., and SORRENTINO, S., JR.: Reproductive Effect of Mammalian Pineal. Amer. Zoologist *10*:247–258, 1970.
SANTAMARINA, E., and VENZKE, W. G.: Physiological Changes in the Mammalian Pineal Gland Correlated with the Reproductive System. Am. J. Vet. Res. *14*:555–562, 1953.

28

The Nervous System

GENERAL CONCEPTS

While the general laws of pathology are by no means abrogated in the nervous system, certain peculiar characteristics of the nervous tissues have led to a number of names and concepts which, whether necessary or not, have to be added to the list of those encountered in the study of other bodily systems. Before concerning ourselves with these, we should like to examine briefly the functional aspects of some nervous disorders.

By a precise understanding of neuro-anatomy and neurophysiology it is commonly possible to predict from such symptoms as paralysis or other disturbances of function the particular structures of the brain or spinal cord in which lesions will be found. Details of this very useful science are not within the scope of the present work, although a few outstanding generalizations cannot be denied attention. Fundamental to an interpretation of many nervous symptoms involving the limbs or external parts of the body is the "spinal reflex arc." By virtue of this arc, if an external part of the body is injured or irritated, that part instantly reacts in a way designed as well as possible to offer protection, usually by a sudden movement or jerk. While a sensation of pain passes up the spinal cord to the brain in the cases of irritations that are at all severe, pain is not essential. For instance, a dog (or a man) scratches himself subconsciously where a louse is crawling among his hairs, and a horse stamps his foot to drive off flies that are crawling on his leg; yet these irritations are too mild to cause pain, or even itching, which is the mildest approach to pain. Physiologists have repeatedly shown that such responses occur even though connection with the brain and consciousness is severed by cutting the spinal cord. The impulse for the reflex jerk, scratching or stamping originates in the neurons of the cord itself, at the level where the afferent nerves from the part concerned enter the cord and the corresponding motor nerves depart. The reflex arc being thus constituted, a stimulus traverses the circuit from the site of irritation to the dorsal root, to the ventral root, to the motor nerve, to the part which is to move. Not all such reactions involve movement, as is seen from the cleansing flow of tears which promptly follows contact of irritant substances with the cornea or conjunctiva. These reflexes, of course, occur when necrosis, degeneration, pressure or other disease processes are responsible for severing connection to the cerebral neurons, as well as when it is accomplished by experimental procedures.

On the other hand, suppose one is picking berries. When the finger encounters a thorn there is a reflex impulse to jerk the finger away. But if the anticipated berry is sweet enough and the desire to possess it is great enough, the reflex withdrawal is overruled by the will (the neurons higher in the central nervous tissue of the brain) and the berry is acquired. The same is true of a dog (for some dogs do pick berries) or of a pig, which will squeeze his way through a narrow opening to get food even though he is at the same time squealing with pain. The point is that, while the reflexes of the spinal arc are initiated locally and can be consummated independently, they normally are more or less effectively held in control by the higher centers of the brain, a fact which brings us to some fundamentals of functional neuropathology. If a limb or given external part has completely lost the function of muscular contraction there is disease or injury somewhere in the muscle itself, or in the spinal reflex arc, that is, in the peripheral nerve or nerve-endings, or in the synapses or neurons situated locally in the particular segment of cord concerned. Since afferent and efferent nerve fibers usually run together in the same nerve trunk, sensation and the power of movement are lost together if the fault is in the nerve itself. The condition described is known as **lower-neuron paralysis.** Because of the flabby condition of the affected part it is also called **flaccid paralysis.**

Paralysis from disease or injury in the brain or in the upper cord through which impulses must pass on their way to the brain is known as **upper-neuron paralysis.** Here, sensation in the part is lost or abnormal, depending on the extent of damage, but the part has not lost its power of muscular contraction. The muscles can be caused to contract by stimuli acting locally upon the particular afferent (sensory) nerves involved, and this is exactly what happens. Furthermore, since the local reflex arc is now disconnected from the control of the master switch-board in the upper brain, very slight and ordinarily imperceptible stimuli, unavoidable in view of changes in position, air-pressure and various other ambient influences, continually stimulate the involved musculature to contraction, in which state it remains. This condition of **upper-neuron paralysis** is known clinically as **spastic paralysis**—paralyzed as far as response to the will is concerned and without normal sensation (if any) but by no means flaccid. If unrelieved, the continued contraction of the musculature in the same position leads to fibrosis, as well as atrophy, and permanent "contractures" are the result. (Passive movement and massage are used to avoid this, in treatment.) Coupled with the fact that spastic paralysis goes with disease of the brain or cord and flaccid paralysis with disorder somewhere in the spinal reflex arc, we have another diagnostic aid in the general tendency of neurologic dysfunction, sensory or motor, to be less complete when of high central origin. Abnormal postures and movements, including curving of the body, nystagmus, ataxic and trembling movements, almost always mean disease of the brain stem or cerebellum, although detectable change in the malfunctioning tissue is not necessarily present.

Convulsions (clonic spasms) are usually of cerebral origin but demonstrable lesions often are absent. In fact, convulsions commonly result from surprisingly intangible nervous disorders and are thought to be based upon loss of central control over peripheral reflexes not altogether unlike that which is responsible for spastic paralysis **(tonic spasm).**

Before considering the histopathological changes which can be detected in diseases of the central nervous tissues it will be profitable to review certain anatomical, histological and biochemical features which cause reactions here to differ somewhat from lesions of corresponding etiological basis in other locations. Enclosed in unyielding bony cavities, the brain and spinal cord are encompassed by the thin but dense and fibrous dura mater, which in most places forms a tough, white sheet, suspended, with few attachments, between the bony wall and the organ itself. The brain and cord proper are bounded by a thin limiting membrane, the pia-arachnoid, whose few cell layers are intimately joined with the underlying soft parenchyma, following the convolutions of its surface into the depths of the sulci and over the summits of the gyri. In the sulci especially, the pia-arachnoid thickens slightly to form a matrix through which pass most of the blood and lymph vessels. Between the dura and the pia-arachnoid is the sub-dural space; its surfaces are lined with flat mesenchymal or endothelial cells, according to the terminology used. With the exception of these membranes, known collectively as the meninges, and of a very limited number of adventitial and perivascular fibroblasts accompanying the vessels which ramify into the parenchyma, there is no fibrous connective tissue in the brain and spinal cord. Instead, a soft but densely homogeneous supporting tissue called neuroglia (*glia*, a glue-like substance) constitutes the bulk of these organs and forms a matrix in which lie imbedded the nerve-cell bodies and their dendritic and axonal fibers. In this mass two varieties of tissue are grossly recognizable, the "white matter," which forms the bulk of the inner substance, and the "gray matter," which constitutes the cortical layer of the cerebrum and cerebellum and also composes certain islands of gray matter within the white, called "nuclei," including the basal ganglia.

The white matter is composed principally of nerve fibers with their myelin sheaths and a minimum of supporting tissue which is largely made up of oligo-dendroglia (see below). The gray matter is composed of neuroglia with numerous nerve-cell bodies imbedded in it. The neuroglia consists of an irregular reticulum of fine, criss-crossing fibrils which stain pink by hematoxylin and eosin but which are much better and more completely seen when stained by special methods, such as silver impregnation. The cells have little cytoplasm and are not clearly connected to the fibrils when viewed in ordinary preparations, but suitable methods reveal the unity of the nuclei and the cytoplasmic fibrils, as well as other details. None of their nuclei have nucleoli, a fact which distinguishes them from nearly all the nerve cells. With some difficulty in ordinary preparations but more clearly by the appropriate techniques, three kinds of neuroglial cells can be distinguished. Of these, the **astrocytes** comprise the bulk of the neuroglia in most regions. Their nuclei are usually elliptical, somewhat pale and vesicular in tinctorial properties and of a size somewhat smaller than the nucleus of a monocyte. Special preparations show that each nucleus has a star-like (*astro*, star) network of fibrils around it with at least one of these connected to a "footpad" at the wall of a nearby blood vessel. In sections stained by ordinary methods, they are usually distinguishable from the smaller nerve cells by their less spherical and more vesicular (pale, without internal structure but with a distinct nuclear wall) nuclei and from the other neuroglial nuclei by the fact that the latter are still smaller, darker and of denser appearance. The **oligodendroglial** cells (*oligo*, few; *dendro*, branches) have, as just implied, regularly round, darkly staining nuclei, comparable in size to the nuclei of lymphocytes. Their short and scanty fibrils are revealed only by special techniques, but the fact that a majority of these cells occur in the fiber tracts of the white matter and appear in straight rows between the fibers facilitates their recognition. The **microglial** cells have very small, round and dark nuclei; many of them are found in the vicinity of a nerve cell. Their fibrils are minimal in both number and length and, as usual, require special techniques for their demonstration. They are considered to be of mesenchymal rather than neuro-ectodermal origin, as is the case with the other components of the neuroglia.

The nerve-cell bodies (neurons), which, with the neuroglia, comprise the gray matter, may be those of large multipolar nerve cells or of the less conspicuous bipolar and unipolar nerve cells. The two latter have a practically spherical form unless cut through the origin of their one or two processes, vary from moderately large to a size no larger than astrocytes and are usually provided with a visible nucleolus, as well as some cytoplasm around the nucleus.

The white matter consists exclusively of nerve fibers separated from each other by myelin and a small amount of neuroglia. The fibers have a tendency to lie evenly spaced and parallel to each other as a number of them follow the same intercommunicating path from one area of gray matter to another. Such parallel groups are called fiber tracts; their particular functions are ascertainable and usually well known in human neurology.

The blood vessels within the central nervous parenchyma have the peculiarity of being surrounded by a zone of appreciable width in which the cells and fibers are so scanty as to be limited to a bare supporting framework. This encircling zone constitutes what is known as the Virchow-Robin space or, since it serves for the drainage of lymph, as the perivascular lymph space. In infectious inflammations lymphocytes commonly accumulate in it, constituting perivascular lymphocytic infiltrations ("cuffing") (p. 173).

General Concepts

BERNSTEIN, J., and LANDING, B. H.: Extraneural Lesions Associated with Neonatal Hyperbilirubinemia and Kernicterus. Amer. J. Path. *40*:371–392, 1962.

BLACKWOOD, W., *et al.*: *Greenfield's Neuropathology*. 2nd ed., London, Edward Arnold, 1963.

CROFT, P. G.: Fits in Dogs: A Survey of 260 Cases. Vet. Rec. *77*:438–445, 1965.

EAGER, R. P., and EAGER, P. R.: Glial Responses to Degenerating Cerebellar Corticonuclear Pathways in the Cat. Science *153*:553–554, 1966.

FANKHAUSER, R.: Zur Frage des Hirnoedems beim Rind. Schweiz. Arch. Tierheilk. *104*: 261–274, 1962.

FISCHER, K.: Herdförmige symetrische Hirngewebsnekrosen bei Hunden mit epileptiformen Krampfen. Path. Vet. *1*:133–160, 1964.

Fox, M. W.: Gross Structure and Development of the Canine Brain. Am. J. Vet. Res. *24*: 1240–1247, 1963.

FRANSEN, J. M., and ANDREWS, F. N.: Cerebrospinal Fluid Pressure in Dwarf and Normal Cattle. Am. J. Vet. Res. *19*:336–337, 1958.

FRAUCHIGER, E., and FANKHAUSER, R.: *Die Nervenkrankheiten unserer Hunde.* Bern, Hans Huber, 1949.

————: *Vergleichende Neuropathologie.* Berlin, J. Springer, 1957.

INNES, J. R. M., and SAUNDERS, L. Z.: Diseases of the Central Nervous System of Domesticated Animals and Comparisons with Human Neuropathology. In *Advances in Veterinary Science.* Vol. III. New York, Academic Press, Inc. (Extensive Bibliography). 1957, pp. 33–196.

KAPPERS, C. U. A., HUBER, G. C., and CROSBY, E. C.: *The Comparative Anatomy of the Nervous System of Vertebrates, Including Man.* New York, The Macmillan Co., 1936.

LIM, R. K. S., LIU, C. N., and MOFFITT, R. L.: *A Stereotaxic Atlas of the Dog's Brain.* Springfield, Charles C Thomas, 1960.

LUGINBUHL, H.: (Angiopathies of the CNS in Animals.) Schweiz. Arch. Tierheilk. *104*: 694–700, 1962.

————: Comparative Aspects of Tumors of the Nervous System. Ann. New York Acad. Sci. *108*:702–721, 1963.

McGRATH, J. T.: *Neurological Examination of the Dog,* 2nd Ed., Philadelphia, Lea & Febiger, 1960.

O'DALY, J. A., and IMAEDA, T.: Electron Microscopic Study of Wallerian Degeneration in Cutaneous Nerves Caused by Mechanical Injury. Lab. Invest. *17*:744–766, 1967.

PENFIELD, W.: *Cytology and Cellular Pathology of the Nervous System.* New York, Paul B. Hoeber, Inc., 1932.

SAUNDERS, L. Z.: A Check List of Hereditary and Familial Diseases of the Central Nervous System in Domestic Animals. Cornell Vet. *42*:592–600, 1952.

————: Cerebrovascular Siderosis in Horses. A.M.A. Arch. Path. *56*:637–642, 1953.

SCHERER, H. J.: *Vergleichende Pathologie des Nervensystems der Säugetiere,* Leipzig, Georg Thieme, 1944.

SYKES, J. F., and MOORE, L. A.: The Normal Cerebro-spinal Fluid Pressure and a Method for Its Determination in Cattle. Am. J. Vet. Res. *3*:364–367, 1942.

TISSUE CHANGES

Post-mortem autolysis becomes evident early in the central nervous system and, like necrosis, soon leads to liquefaction. It is not unusual for brains to be almost completely liquefied in three or four days at mild summer temperatures (70 to 90° F., 21 to 32° C.). The differentiation between the two forms of death is made according to the principles already outlined (p. 15).

Necrosis ranges from slow death of an occasional neuron to softening and liquefaction of considerable volumes of central nervous tissue, the former occurring soonest and from milder causes. The usual causes of necrosis in the brain or cord are toxic substances, either "chemical," of plant or fungal origin or dependent upon infectious or abnormal metabolic processes. Included in one group or another are cyanides in repeated small doses (p. 921), mercury (chronic) (p. 961), lead (chronic) (p. 956), manganese (p. 1004), carbon monoxide (p. 921), and alcohol, as well as various other organic and inorganic substances.

Anoxia is a frequent cause of death of nerve cells, usually in a limited area. The disorder results from interference with the blood supply, even though quite transient, the neurons being very susceptible. It is probable that many of the poisons really act through an anoxic mechanism. Massive deprivation of blood through cerebral embolism and infarction, arteriosclerotic changes or hemorrhage are, however, rare in domestic animals.

Necrosis involves some forms of change that are peculiar to nervous tissue and have not been discussed previously. This is particularly true with respect to necrosis of individual neurons, which occurs upon slight provocation of certain sorts. It is difficult to determine in these cells the exact point where various peculiar degenerative (and reversible) changes become (irreversible) necrosis. Since the former regularly lead to the latter, the several consecutive stages will be considered together.

Necrosis of Neurons (Nerve Cell Bodies).—Changes in the neurons themselves which indicate their death or approaching death take several forms. The dendritic processes of multipolar cells tend to disappear, leaving the outline of the cell unduly smooth and rounded. The **Nissl substance** in a normal and perfectly preserved neuron should appear as a sharply granular, basophilic substance in the cytoplasm, giving the latter an appearance like the markings of a tiger, whence the synonym, **tigroid substance.** Under a pathogenetic environment, such as anoxia, these Nissl granules lose their sharpness and, in just a few hours, disappear first centrally and then completely, usually by fading, occasionally by a general blackening of the cytoplasm (known by some neurologists in their own exclusive dialect as "pyknosis"). Concomitantly with the cytoplasmic loss of Nissl granules and loss of the normal cell outline, the nucleus tends to swell and the nucleolus within the nucleus enlarges even more. The more or less swollen nucleus is commonly displaced from its central to an eccentric position, even to lie against the cell wall. Then, by a process of liquefaction, it disappears from view. The whole neuron tends to swell at first, then shrinks into some angular and unrecognizable form and likewise disappears. Incidental to this swelling and shrinking, the axone, if it chances to be visible, swells and is distorted into a writhing, twisting form and then passes from the scene. All this transpires in the course of a day or two. Exceptionally, as in the viral disease called "scrapie," slow dissolution and liquefaction of the neuron involve the formation of one or two large, clear vacuoles which eventually displace practically all of the cytoplasm.

Meantime, even while the hapless cell is dying, arrangements are already being made for disposal of its remains. Little densely staining cells, which apparently may be either oligodendroglial or microglial, gather about the dying neuron, as a magpie sits upon the back of a moribund horse in order to be present at the moment the animal's flesh becomes available to him. While vulture cells might be a better name, these clustering cells are politely called satellite cells and the process is called **satellitosis.** As the neuron dies they not only surround, but enter the cell, engulfing bits of its cytoplasm, and their true phagocytic nature becomes evident. They are then known as neuronophages and the process is designated as **neuronophagia.** Satellitosis and neuronophagia are then indirect but no less reliable signs of necrosis of a neuron. Satellitosis is reported as developing within a matter of minutes after anoxic injury; neuronophagia within a few hours. Satellitosis is a reversible change; in other words, the neuron is injured but not dead. These two processes, unlike the intracellular regressive changes, do not occur in post-mortem autolysis, but only in necrosis.

Necrosis in the neuroglia is also a process of liquefaction but it develops more slowly and, in the case of some of the milder injurious agents it may not occur at all, even though the nerve cells of the area have been killed. Close observation and a precise knowledge of the normal histology of the area are necessary to detect accurately the absence of a few neurons under such circumstances. If an area of neuroglia (and the contained nerve cells and fibers) undergoes necrosis, it is at first (two to five days) softened grossly, a condition known as **encephalomalacia** (or myelomalacia) and, in from one to two weeks, disappears through a process of liquefaction, leaving an empty space of no characteristic shape, size or type excepting its frayed and indefinite borders. Such an area may be difficult to distinguish from an artifact caused by imperfect cutting of the section, but the distinctions mentioned in connection with Liquefactive Necrosis (p. 21) apply. Where appreciable areas of central nervous tissue are destroyed (undergo necrosis) there may be after two or three weeks an increase of neuroglial tissue surrounding the vacant space, called gliosis, and an accumulation of macrophagic cells. These are discussed further in connection with proliferative inflammation in the nervous system (p. 1388).

Necrosis of nerve fibers, whether in the peripheral nerves or in the fiber tracts of the brain or cord, first becomes discernible through fatty change (p. 34) of the myelin sheaths of the affected fibers, a number or group of which are usually involved. Especially within the brain and cord the change is usually called **demyelination.** The axones or nerve fibers eventually disappear, as well as, perhaps, much of the interstitial tissue (neuroglia), but loss of the myelin sheaths alone is sufficient to render the nerves non-functional (although regeneration may be possible). Demyelination in the central nervous tissue is recognizable with some uncertainty in ordinary hematoxylin-eosin sections by the presence of an excessive number and size of holes in an area of white matter. The axon may still be visible in some of them, but there may be difficulty in deciding whether one is dealing with demyelination or spaces due to edema or to excessive shrinkage in the preparation of the tissue. Since the lipoid of the myelin goes through stages involving the presence of free neutral fats, it is possible to demonstrate demyelination by the usual stains for fats (p. 35) or more particularly by Marchi's method, to be described shortly. However, since, in the central nervous system, whole fiber tracts usually share the same fate, it is often preferable to demonstrate the disorder by staining methods (myelin-sheath stains) which directly color normal myelin. Demyelination is then detected by a blank area, usually viewed under low magnification, in the midst of the more darkly staining healthy tissue. Such areas are usually only relatively colorless, for the remaining neuroglial cells and fibers absorb a minimal amount of stain.

In the peripheral nerves, destruction of myelin (and of the functioning fiber) may be detected by similar means but Marchi's method is often used, in spite of a certain reputed inconstancy of action. This involves the use of the oxidizing agent osmic acid (osmium peroxide) to stain the fat separated from the myelin a deep black. Since osmic acid would have the same effect on the lipoids of myelin, the tissue is first exposed to a milder oxidizing agent, potassium dichromate, which oxidizes normal myelin without coloring it but leaves the fatty, injured myelin still susceptible to the osmic acid. Theoretically, at least, a delicate differentiation is obtainable. About two weeks must elapse between the injury to a peripheral nerve and the stainability of injured nerves by this method. Since, unless the injury be very close to the nerve-cell body, the latter does not die, this process is not usually necrosis but, rather, a degeneration. It is known as **wallerian degeneration** (p. 184). The part of the neuron distal to the point of injury (which may well be mechanical severance) dies, undergoing wallerian degeneration throughout its length. It is commonly regenerated by growth from the surviving proximal portion of the neuron, a process requiring a few months. While, as stated, the cell body seldom dies because of injury to its axon, it may suffer transiently a certain degree of degeneration, particularly a rounding of the cell, displacement of the nucleus and fading of the Nissl granules. This is known as Nissl's degeneration. Recovery usually occurs. Demyelination of nerve fibers results from a variety of types of injury including mechanical pressure, brief or prolonged, and deficiency of thiamin and the vitamin-B complex (p. 984).

Calcification and, less frequently, some of the **other degenerative changes** described in Chapter 2 may occur in the central nervous system, but usually in relation to the vessels or meninges. They are of little importance.

Passive congestion of these tissues, most prominent in the pia-arachnoid, accompanies severe passive congestion of the rest of the body. It is readily recognized by virtue of the dark, distended veins which cover the meningeal surfaces and is usually acute and terminal. Hyperemia is a part of the picture of inflammation. **Hemorrhages** of petechial size are frequent in those numerous acute infections and toxemias which injure capillaries in other parts of the body. However, pin-point spots of blood seen on the cut surface when the brain is freshly sliced often mark, not hemorrhages, but the cut ends of congested capillaries. Severe blows to the head may result in fracture of the skull, rupture of one or more branches of the meningeal arteries and hemorrhage into the space between dura and bone. This **epidural hemorrhage** is uncommon in the young or old due to close adherence between the dura and bone. When it does occur, the dura is compressed over the brain and may lead rapidly to hemiplegia, convulsions and death unless relieved surgically. **Subdural hemorrhage** on the other hand usually results from rupture of veins and the blood is mixed with cerebrospinal fluid. The signs may be delayed as bleeding continues. It is possible for large areas of the cerebrum to be compressed by the resulting hematoma which also could become organized, leading to increasing pressure on the brain. The location of the hemorrhage is not necessarily at the site of the blow; it may be at the opposite side owing to the inertia of the brain within the cranium and its elasticity, propensity to rebound strongly and rupture of vessels on the opposite side (*contrecoup*). If the animal survives the immediate injury of the blow, the effects are those of pressure and depend upon the size of the clot. Death from such a blow may then follow the accident by hours or days. In man, a massive hemorrhage into the brain substance is an all too frequent complication of arteriosclerotic and hypertensive disease. The sudden unconsciousness is known as apoplexy; the result, if the patient lives, is paralysis of such parts as are innervated from the portion of the brain that undergoes pressure necrosis. Commonly this is one side of the body, the condition being known popularly as a "paralytic stroke." (Infarction from embolism or occlusion also causes such "strokes.") Hemorrhages of this nature and "strokes" in general are infrequent in animals, doubtless because arteriosclerotic disease is rare, except in aged swine. (See Concussion, p. 1389).

Edema of the brain occurs as a diffuse accumulation of fluid in the tissue, especially in the perivascular (Virchow-Robin) spaces, in the subarachnoid spaces and in spaces that form around the neurons (Fig. 10–41*B*, p. 460). Grossly, the gyri are swollen and flattened and the sulci partly obliterated. The cut surface is moist and shiny; the parenchyma is softened. The causes are the same as the causes of edema elsewhere, either general or local (p. 137).

Tissue Changes in Nervous System

INNES, J. R. M., and SAUNDERS, L. Z.: *Comparative Neuropathology*. New York, Academic Press, 1963.
NEWBERNE, J. W., *et al.*: Granular Structures in Brains of Apparently Normal Dogs. Am. J. Vet. Res. *21*:782–786, 1960.
SIGURDSSON, B., and PALSSON, P. A.: Visna of Sheep. A Slow, Demyelinating Infection. Brit. J. Exp. Path. *39*:519–528, 1958.
SMITH, A. D. M., DUCKETT, S., and WATERS, A. H.: Neuropathological Changes in Chronic Cyanide Intoxication. Nature (Lond.) *200*:179–181, 1963.

Hydrocephalus is the slow accumulation of excessive cerebrospinal fluid in the lateral and other ventricles and sometimes in the subarachnoid spaces, due to obstruction of the lymph drainage. Normally there is a continual secretion of fluid from the choroid plexus of vessels located principally in the lateral ventricles. This drains through the aqueduct of Sylvius into the fourth ventricle. Thence it passes through some minute openings in the roof of that ventricle known as the foramina of Luschka into rather indefinite compartments called the basal cisterns in the subarachnoid space. Some of the fluid finds its way into the spinal canal as cerebrospinal fluid. The overflow continues from the basal cisterns anteriorly

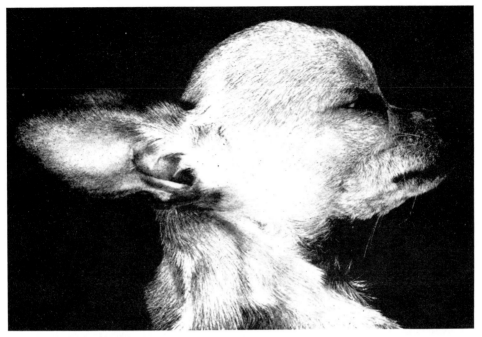

FIG. 28–1.—Hydrocephalus in a three-year-old male Chihuahua.
(Courtesy of Angell Memorial Animal Hospital.)

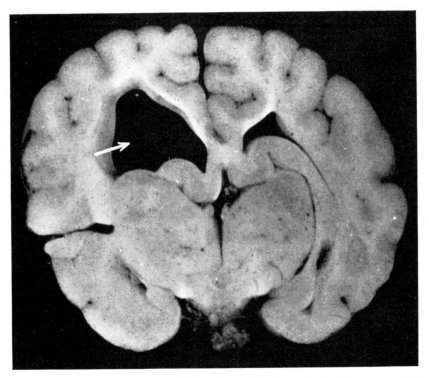

FIG. 28–2.—Hydrocephalus involving left lateral ventricle (arrow) of a fifteen-year-old female
Boston terrier. An incidental finding at necropsy. (Courtesy of Angell Memorial Animal Hosp.)

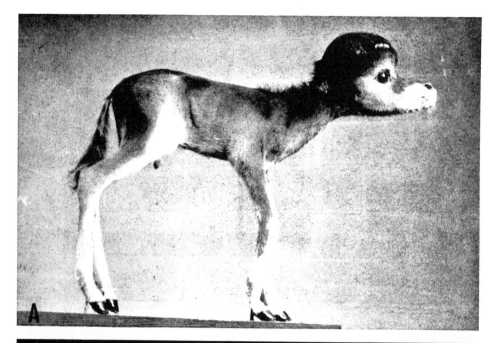

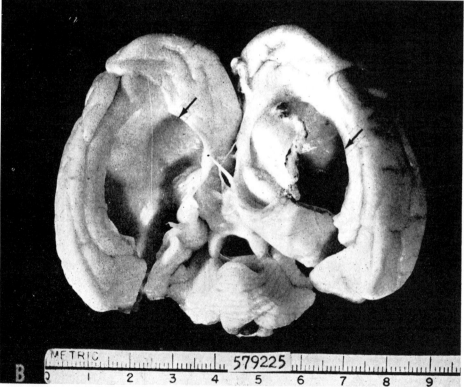

Fig. 28–3.—Hydrocephalus. *A*, A mounted specimen of a newborn colt. Mark Francis Collection. Texas School of Veterinary Medicine. *B*, The brain of a newborn puppy with hydrocephalus. Arrows indicate the dilated lateral ventricle. (*B*, Courtesy of Armed Forces Institute of Pathology.) Contributor: Dr. Russell B. Oppenheimer.

through the intercommunicating subarachnoid spaces, whence it is reabsorbed into the venous circulation, especially through the arachnoid villi, which project into the venous sinuses to afford increased absorptive surface.

The possibility of some obscure derangement of the resorptive process in the subarachnoid villi or elsewhere cannot be entirely excluded, but the causes of hydrocephalus are considered to lie ordinarily in some mechanical obstruction to the outflow of lymph. There are several obvious sites where such obstruction could easily occur and a variety of local disorders which could initiate the stoppage. The slender aqueduct of Sylvius is easily closed by external pressure and the foramina of Luschka which lead from the fourth ventricle are still more vulnerable. Inflammatory exudates, tumors, parasitic cysts (*Coenurus cerebralis*) and similar structures are ready sources of pressure in this region. Another potential barrier is the tentorium cerebelli; not only is the cranial cavity sharply narrowed here, facilitating obstruction of the subarachnoid passageways, but the same interference with flow is also achieved by slight displacement of the brain either forward or backward, its soft mass acting as a plug in the narrow incisura tentorii as a stopper plugs a bottle. Such displacement of the brain can be produced by inflammatory or other swelling in either compartment of the cranial cavity. The brain is also occasionally forced backward into the foramen magnum until escape of fluid into the spinal canal is cut off.

While the preceding statements on causative mechanisms appear to be perfectly valid and are widely accepted, it must be admitted that there are very many cases of hydrocephalus in man and animals in which the exact etiology and manner of development have been impossible of demonstration. In spite of the occasional development of hydrocephalus in connection with tumors and otherwise under the circumstances just outlined, the usual occurrence of hydrocephalus is as a disease of the new-born and the cause is to be attributed to maldevelopment of some of the minutely formed drainage structures.

Margolis and Kilham (1969) have shown that Reovirus type I inoculated into suckling ferrets, hamsters, mice and rats, regularly results in hydrocephalus. The virus specifically attacks ependymal cells leading to destruction of those cells, ulceration and healing by gliovascular proliferation which results in obstructive hydrocephalus. It seems plausible that this viral mechanism may also account for natural cases of hydrocephalus.

The effect of the obstructed drainage, indeed, the essence of the disease, morphologically speaking, is pressure atrophy of the cerebral parenchyma. The ventricles, in the usual "internal hydrocephalus" due to obstruction in the flow of the fluid, enlarge gradually at the expense of the parenchyma until the cerebral hemispheres are reduced to mere hollow rims around the lateral ventricles. In the less frequent "communicating hydrocephalus" in which the interference with return flow is somewhere in the subarachnoid course of drainage, pressure atrophy proceeds also from the exterior of the brain. The eventual outcome of hydrocephalus is death, although, since the primitive vital centers are located in the less accessible mid-brain and hind-brain, it is surprising how long the young animal can survive with almost no cerebrum.

Hydrocephalus

HALSTEAD, J. R., and KIEL, F. W.: Hydrocephalus in a Bear. J. Am. Vet. Med. Assn. *141*: 367–368, 1962.

HYDE, R. R.: An Epidemic of Hydrocephalus in a Group of Experimental Rabbits. Amer. J. Hyg. *31*:1–8, 1940.

JOHNSON, R. T., JOHNSON, K. P., and EDMONDS, C. J.: Virus-induced Hydrocephalus: Development of Aqueductal Stenosis in Hamsters after Mumps Infection. Science *157*: 1066–1067, 1967.

KILHAM, L., and MARGOLIS, G.: Hydrocephalus in Hamsters, Ferrets, Rats, and Mice Following Inoculations with Reovirus Type I. I. Virologic Studies. Lab. Invest. *21*:183–188, 1969.

MARGOLIS, G., and KILHAM, L.: Hydrocephalus in Hamsters, Ferrets, Rats, and Mice Following Inoculations with Reovirus Type I. II. Pathologic Studies. Lab. Invest. *21*: 189–198, 1969.

————: Experimental Virus-induced Hydrocephalus. Relation to Pathogenesis of the Arnold-Chiari Malformation. J. Neurosurg. *31*:1–9, 1969.

MILHORAT, T. H., CLARK, R. G., and HAMMOCK, M. K.: Experimental Hydrocephalus II. Gross Pathological Findings in Acute and Subacute Obstructive Hydrocephalus in the Dog and Monkey. J. Neurosurg. *32*:390–399, 1970.

SCHLOTTHAUER, C. F.: Internal Hydrocephalus in a Dog. J. Am. Vet. Med. Assn. *85*: 788–794, 1934.

WILLIAMS, W. L., and FROST, J. N.: Subdural Hydrocephalus in a Calf. Cornell Vet. *28*: 340–345, 1938.

Inflammation and Inflammatory Disease.—The same general laws of inflammation apply in the brain and spinal cord as elsewhere, but the manifestations of an inflammatory process are restricted in accordance with the kinds of cells and tissues present and by anatomical limitations. (1) Since there are no mucous membranes, catarrhal inflammation does not occur. (2) Serous inflammatory reactions probably do not occur; if they do they are not differentiated from edema (see above). (3) Hemorrhagic exudates are seldom, if ever, encountered, although hemorrhages, by themselves, are frequent, as stated in a preceding paragraph. (4) Fibrinous inflammation is limited practically to the meninges and to penetrating wounds. (5) Purulent, lymphocytic and proliferative inflammations are the types regularly encountered in the central nervous system.

Purulent inflammation occurs as the result of infection by pyogenic microorganisms, to the usual list of which must be added *Listeria* (*Listerella*) *monocytogenes*. Listerellosis is the most frequent cause of a purulent reaction in the brains of farm animals. The accumulations of pus involve both the pia-arachnoid and the parenchymal tissue but are microscopic in amount. While diffuse in a given area, the distribution of the areas of neutrophilic infiltration is limited and variable. Lymphocytic infiltration is also prominent. If other pus-formers reach the brain, as they do occasionally as blood-borne metastases, the infection is usually confined, one or more abscesses being the result. The *Pasteurella* organism has been known to cause formation of intracranial abscesses in the bovine. A limited amount of purulent exudation accompanies some forms (Eastern strain) of equine encephalomyelitis, although the reaction in this disease is fundamentally lymphocytic. Diffuse suppurative or fibrino-purulent meningitis occurs as a wound infection in the rare event of trauma which pierces the bony covering without being immediately fatal. It does not appear that animals have a copiously suppurative meningitis comparable to that caused by the meningococcus of man.

Subacute lymphocytic inflammation (p. 163) is a characteristic type in the central nervous tissues, the cells being trapped in the Virchow-Robin spaces as they leave the vessels and progress further only with difficulty. The cause is usually, but not invariably, one of the neurotropic viruses. It may be said that infiltrations of lymphocytes, which may be only perivascular, constitute the most conspicuous lesions in the viral infections. They may or may not be accompanied by petechial hemorrhages and notable hyperemia. In the earlier stages of some of the viral diseases, such as rabies (p 351), practically no visible lesions may exist. Such infections as toxoplasmosis (p. 684) and even torulosis (cryptococcosis, p. 657) also result in limited infiltrations of lymphocytes, usually perivascular, when they involve the nervous tissues. Practically speaking, without the presence of other exudates, and without other apparent explanation, lymphocytic infiltrations may be considered indicative of an infectious disease, quite likely a viral disease. The localization of lesions and other features of viral diseases are discussed in Chapter 10, page 348.

While the toxic degenerative and necrotic changes described earlier in this chapter might be considered comparable to what we have called alterative inflammation, they are not ordinarily accompanied by any of the usual signs of inflammation and this concept is seldom entertained. A reaction that is both striking and unique does, however, accompany softening and necrosis of appreciable amounts of central nervous tissue. This is the appearance, at the necrotic site, of what are called **scavenger cells,** also known as **compound granular corpuscles, Hortega cells** or **gitter cells** (German, *gitterzellen*). These are large, lipid-filled phagocytes which, in the course of a few days, infiltrate the injured area in large numbers. Evidence indicates that they arise by proliferation and differentiation of the microglial cells, and probably also of the scanty connective-tissue cells which accompany the vascular network. At any rate, they are entirely comparable to the reticulo-endothelial cells found in many inflammations elsewhere. The gitter cells phagocytize and assist in the removal of the large amount of lipoid which is characteristic of central nervous tissue, slowly disappearing when this task has been completed. They thus represent a form of proliferative inflammation. Concurrently, the oligodendroglial cells swell and remain swollen throughout the period of active reaction.

With a little more time (two to three weeks) another proliferative change develops, which is comparable to the formation of fibrous granulation tissue. It differs in that the proliferating cells are the fibrillary astrocytes of the neuroglia, hence the name, **gliosis.** Unlikely to be detected grossly, gliosis has the appearance microscopically of an area of neuroglia which is markedly denser than the surrounding normal areas, with which it gradually blends. There occurs early a marked increase in the number of glial nuclei, but the increased density is due to the larger number of fibrils per unit of area and also to a somewhat greater diameter of some of the individual fibrils. The increase of glial tissue is mainly around the perimeter of the defect when there has been a complete loss of substance (liquefaction necrosis); the new glial tissue does not fill the empty space as would be done by proliferating fibrous granulation tissue. The glia-encircled empty space sometimes remains filled with clear fluid, constituting a cyst.

Proliferation of numerous small capillaries often accompanies proliferation of the glial cells, or the former may occur without the latter in an area which otherwise shows but little change. This constitutes another form of proliferative inflammatory reaction. It first becomes conspicuous about a week after an anoxic or toxic injury.

Sometimes accompanying these several reactive phenomena is a change in the microglia consisting in the formation of **"rod cells."** These are microglial nuclei which elongate until their length is three or four times their diameter. They stain very darkly.

Proliferation of fibrous connective tissue is limited to the immediate vicinity of blood vessels and to the meninges, where a parent fibrous tissue of mesodermal origin exists. Granulation tissue of this kind is rarely extensive except in the case of traumatic injury to the perivascular and meningeal fibroblastic tissues. Scars, be they glial or fibroblastic, tend to contract as they grow older and, in doing so, place unnatural strains and pressures on the neighboring tissue. In human beings, who are more likely than animals to live on after an anoxic, toxic or traumatic injury of the brain, malfunction of the distorted brain tissue some-

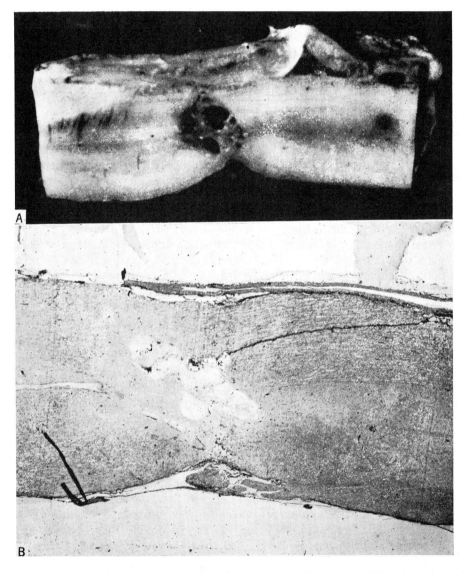

Fig. 28–4.—Compression of spinal cord of an eight-month-old female dachshund as result of dislocation of the first and second cervical vertebrae. *A*, The gross specimen incised after formalin fixation. *B*, Low power of a histologic section. H & E × 4. (Courtesy of Angell Memorial Animal Hospital.)

times leads to periodic convulsive seizures or lapses of consciousness known as traumatic epilepsy. However, animals seldom experience, and still more rarely survive, injuries of these kinds.

Concussion of the brain results from a non-fatal blow on the head, the cranial bones being fractured or not. It produces instant, though transient, unconsciousness; hence it constitutes a humane procedure in putting an animal to death. The concussion causes a sudden, violent displacement of the subarachnoid and other fluid in the brain and the unconsciousness is believed to be due to a transient anemia as a certain amount of blood is jarred prematurely from the capillaries into larger vessels. The same sudden movement of intravascular blood and perivascular lymph (cerebrospinal fluid) may cause numerous hemorrhages of petechial size or lacerations of superficially placed tissues with more extensive hemorrhage into the subarachnoid spaces. These lesions are often on the side opposite to that of the blow, the injury then being caused as the somewhat movable brain, suspended in the cranial cavity, comes to a sudden stop against the opposite wall. It becomes apparent from these considerations that the interpretation of cephalic hemorrhages must be guarded in necropsy of an animal killed by a blow on the head. The fact remains, however, that this factor has seldom, if ever, been a significant cause of diagnostic error.

Diffuse compression of the brain or cord results from the pressure of extensive hemorrhages, tumors, abscesses or edema. The symptoms may at first be manifested as hyperirritability, perhaps with convulsions, but, as the pressure grows, mental depression, somnolence and coma supervene. There may be paralyses as the effect of compression of motor centers. Headache is severe in humans and the same is doubtless true in animals. This is one, and possibly the principal, reason for the tendency of horses and cattle to press the forehead against objects (in various illnesses). It is difficult to evaluate this sign precisely (p. 1241). Vomiting in the absence of any digestive disorder is prominent in those species which vomit. The lesions are obviously those which belong to the individual causative disorder. Edematous swelling has been described (p. 1382). In a localized area of compression, softening and liquefaction necrosis develop if the patient survives a few days.

Pressure upon the cord leads to paralysis of the parts supplied from segments below the point of compression (for instance, a fractured vertebra), perhaps initiated with local hyperirritability. It is of the upper motor-neuron type, that is, spastic. Flaccid paralysis involves parts which happen to be innervated directly from the injured segment. Sensation ceases from the parts below the lesion. As in the brain, the lesion resulting from local pressure is softening and liquefaction necrosis. Myelin stains show demyelinization and loss of fibers in the motor tracts below and the sensory tracts above the injured segment; however the development of this change requires several days.

Incidental Findings

A few incidental findings in the central nervous system deserve mention. Deposits of iron pigment are common in the cerebral blood vessels of the horse and less frequent in the cow. This "cerebrovascular siderosis" has been well described by Saunders (1953). It is apparently a normal process and the amount of iron pigment increases with age.

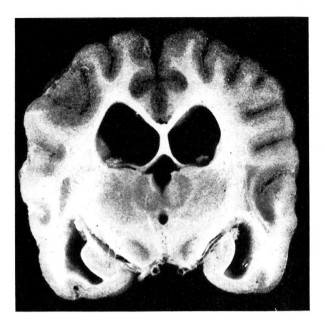

FIG. 28–5.—Brain of an 18-
year-old dog. Ventricles are
enlarged, gyri narrowed and
blood vessels fibrotic. (Courtesy
of Dr. H. Wisniewski and *Laboratory Investigation*.)

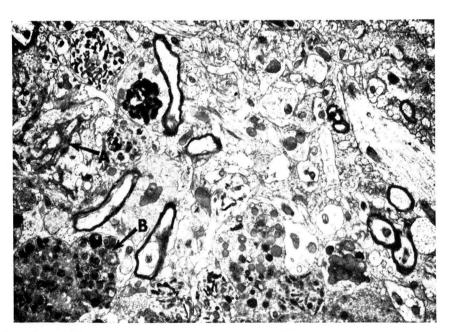

FIG. 28–6.—Senile plaque, brain of aged dog ($\times$ 4,800). Aggregates of degenerating neurites
(B) and small amounts of amyloid (A). (Courtesy of Dr. H. Wisniewski and *Laboratory Investigation*.)

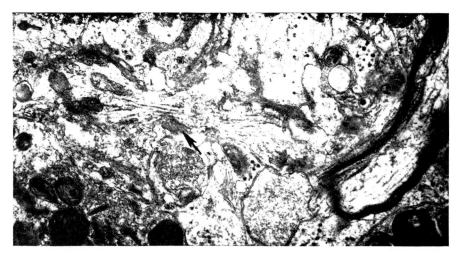

FIG. 28–7.—Senile plaque, brain of aged dog. Higher magnification of Fig. 28–6 (× 25,000). Note normal neurotubules, above amyloid (arrow). (Courtesy of Dr. H. Wisniewski and *Laboratory Investigation*.)

Irregular plaques of melanin-laden cells are often seen grossly and microscopically in the meninges of cattle and sheep. These are considered incidental.

In the brains of senile dogs Braunmühl (1956) has described "Kongophile Angiopathie," characterized by the accumulation of lipoid material in the walls of small arteries and veins. This writer also described focal glial scars designated as "senile plaques" in the cerebral cortex of aged dogs.

Wisniewski *et al.* (1970) have studied these **senile plaques** and **cerebral amy-**

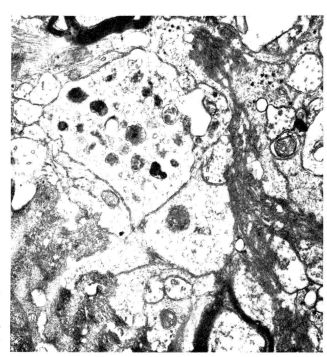

FIG. 28–8.—Senile plaque, brain of an aged dog × 16,000. Perimeter of amyloid (left) from a large plaque. (Courtesy of Dr. H. Wisniewski and *Laboratory Investigation*.)

loidosis in aged dogs with light and electron microscopy. These changes are of interest in comparison with the lesions in Alzheimer's presenile dementia and in aged human patients. The plaques were recognized in histologic preparations stained with acid phosphatase-Congo red preparations as small groups of rounded clusters of acid-phosphatase reactive elements resembling distended neurites. Small foci of Congo-red positive, green birefringent materials were also mixed with linear and globular acid-phosphatase reaction products. A third type consisted of a rounded mass containing congophilic and green birefringent materials. Large macrophages containing acid-phosphatase reactive materials were often seen near small blood vessels. The ultrastructural features described by Wisniewski *et al.* consisted of aggregations of abnormal neurites, amyloid and reactive cells. The enlarged neurites contained normal and degenerating mitochondria, laminated electron-dense bodies, vesicles, profiles of smooth membranes, and clusters of 100 Å filaments and 240 Å tubules. Amyloid was generally scattered as small wisps among the processes of the plaques (Figs. 28–6, 7, 8).

Organized hemorrhages in the choroid plexus are not uncommon in horses. These may reach rather large size (sometimes resulting in nervous signs) and because of their cholesterol content are called **cholesteatomas** (p. 264) but which preferably should be known as cholesterinic granulomas.

Incidental Findings

BRAUNMÜHL, A. VON: "Kongophile Angiopathie" und "senile Plaques" beim greisen Hunden. Arch. f. Psychiat. *194*:396–414, 1956.
WISNIEWSKI, H., *et al.*: Senile Plaques and Cerebral Amyloidosis in Aged Dogs. Lab. Invest. *23*:287–296, 1970.

DISEASES OF UNCERTAIN ETIOLOGY AFFECTING THE NERVOUS SYSTEM

In the foregoing part of this chapter the general neurophysiologic aspects of diseases of the nervous system have been discussed and changes which constitute the reactions of nervous tissue to injury have been described. Important viral diseases affecting the nervous system specifically, such as rabies, equine, avian, ovine and porcine encephalomyelitis, Aujeszky's disease, Borna disease, scrapie, mouse polioencephalitis and others are discussed in Chapter 10; bacterial diseases affecting the nervous system, in Chapters 12 and 13. Cerebrospinal nematodiasis, a parasitic disease of the nervous system, is included in Chapter 15. Neoplasms of the brain and spinal cord are given a place with other neoplasms in Chapter 7. The neurological aspects of certain poisonings are presented in Chapter 17, under the heading of the poison concerned. The bracken fern, mercury, cyanides and especially the yellow star thistle are prominent in this category. Still requiring attention are diseases of the nervous system which, although of uncertain etiology, have distinguishing clinical or pathological features. Certain diseases of animals which fulfill these criteria will be described briefly. Since a number of the nervous disorders are at least suspected of being due to dietary deficiencies, further data on these will be found under the appropriate titles in Chapter 18.

Congenital Anomalies of the Nervous System

The nervous system of animals and man is subject to many anomalies which originate during embryonic life. Some of these have been described separately.

In sections cut parallel to the length of the tract, the axons will appear thickened at some points, absent at others. Glial cells are increased in number and eventually replace the destroyed nerve fibers, giving the affected column a scarred appearance (gliosis). This change is best demonstrated microscopically by means of Weil's stain.

The **diagnosis** of equine incoordination may be established at necropsy by demonstration of characteristic gross and microscopic lesions in the spinal column and spinal cord.

Equine Incoordination

FRASER, H., and PALMER, A. C.: Equine Incoordination and Wobbler Disease of Young Horses. Vet. Rec. *80*:338–355, 1967.

JONES, T. C., DOLL, E. R., and BROWN, R. G.: The Pathology of Equine Incoordination (Ataxia or "Wobbles" of Foals). Proc. 91st Ann. Meeting Am. Vet. Med. Assn., 1954, pp. 139–149.

MATTHIAS, D., DIETZ, O., and RECHENBERG, R.: (Clinical Features and Pathology of Spinal Ataxia in Foals.) Arch. Exp. Vet. Med. *19*: Heinz-Rohrer-Heft (supplement) 43–72, 1965. V.B. *36*:1528, 1966.

ROONEY, J. R.: Equine Incoordination. I. Gross Morphology. Cornell Vet. *53*:411–422, 1963.

Focal Symmetrical Poliomalacia of Sheep

A singular paralytic disease of sheep seen on a farm located in the Rift Valley of Kenya, Africa, has been described by Innes and Plowright (1955). The disease was first noticed between February and April 1952, in 10 of 40 lambs two to four months of age. The following year, 60 of 240 animals in the flock died from the disease and this outbreak also involved older animals. The disease apparently

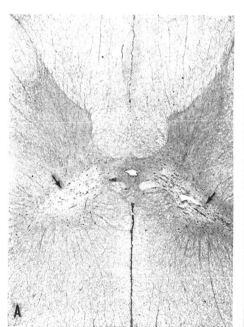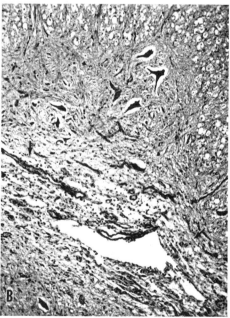

FIG. 28–14.—Symmetrical poliomalacia of sheep. *A*, Spinal cord (× 16). Note symmetry of lesions in each of the ventral horns of gray matter (arrows). *B*, Higher magnification (× 110) of the malacic lesion in the gray matter (arrows). (*B*, Courtesy of Armed Forces Institute of Pathology.) Contributor: Dr. J. R. M. Innes.

did not spread to other farms, but the unusual clinical and pathologic features it displayed justify its inclusion in this chapter.

The disease was sudden in onset, only a few sheep exhibiting premonitory signs such as motor weakness or incoordination of the forelimbs. Flaccid paralysis usually developed rapidly in all limbs, but in some instances spasticity was a feature. Only the forelimbs of some sheep were involved and animals thus affected hopped about on their hind legs like kangaroos during the days or weeks they survived. The muscles of the fixed, adducted front limbs usually underwent atrophy if the animal survived for some time, but most of them died within three weeks. The disease was afebrile and apparently not transmissible from one sheep to another. Cattle in the same pasture did not contract the disease.

The **lesions** were limited to the spinal cord and could be recognized only upon microscopic examination. Symmetrical malacic lesions in the ventral gray columns—never in the dorsal columns—were limited to certain segments in the cervical enlargement, except for a few cases in which the lesions were confined to segments of the lumbar enlargement. In a typical case the lesions in the gray columns started at the level of the fourth cervical vertebra (C4), disappeared at C6 and appeared again at the level of C7 and the first thoracic vertebra (T1). In another case lesions were found between C4 and C6 as well as in the lumbar enlargement.

Bilateral symmetry was particularly striking, the lesions in one ventral column being a mirror image of those in its opposite. These sharply delimited foci of malacia did not evoke a significant surrounding inflammatory reaction, but a rim of well-preserved gray matter, containing neurons, was often evident around them and the commissural gray matter was intact. The involved areas of ventral gray matter were sharply demarcated, pale staining, with the neurons replaced by a ragged, spongy appearing lesion in which capillaries and glial fibers were predominant. In early lesions "gitter cells" were numerous, while in later stages astrocytes and newly proliferated capillaries filled the area of softening. Neither vascular lesions nor demyelination were observed in white columns.

The significance of this disease is not clear at this time, but it is an interesting addition to the growing list of pathologic entities which result in neurologic disturbances in sheep.

The **diagnosis** may be made upon demonstration of the bilaterally symmetrical malacic lesions in the spinal cord of sheep which exhibit characteristic symptoms.

Ovine Symmetrical Poliomalacia

INNES, J. R. M., and PLOWRIGHT, W.: Focal Symmetrical Poliomalacia of Sheep in Kenya. J. Neuropath. and Exp. Neurol. *14*:185–197, 1955.
PIENAAR, J. G., and THORNTON, D. J.: Focal Symmetrical Encephalomalacia in Sheep in South Africa. J. S. Afr. Vet. Med. Assn. *35*:351–358, 1964. V.B. *35*:1051, 1965.

Congenital Demyelinating Disease of Lambs
("Swayback," "Enzoötic Ataxia")

Newborn or young lambs are not infrequently affected with a specific demyelinating disease, known among shepherds in England, Scotland and Wales as "swayback." The disease has also been reported from Australia as "enzoötic ataxia" and is known colloquially in South Africa as "Lamkruis." It has also been reported in the United States. The disease is manifest in suckling or new-born lambs by severe ataxia; affected animals show incoordinated movements; they are unable to walk but able to nurse and they do not exhibit flaccid paralysis. Blindness is sometimes observed; fever is absent, and death usually results from starvation or exposure, frequently accompanied by bronchopneumonia. Affected lambs, as a rule, are sacrificed by the owner.

The disease is most prevalent among lambs born of ewes which have been maintained on a diet low in copper. Many but not all such ewes manifest anemia, some have "stringy" wool, and most have lowered copper levels in blood and liver. It is believed therefore that the disease is related to copper deficiency, but the mechanism of its action is not known.

The **lesions** are limited to the central nervous system and are characterized by diffuse symmetrical destruction of subcortical white matter in the cerebrum accompanied by descending destruction of certain myelinated tracts in the spinal cord. In severe, acute cases the destruction of cerebral white matter leads to grossly visible gelatinous softening in the subcortical white matter with formation of large symmetrical cavities. This cavitation may be followed by secondary internal hydrocephalus. Chromatolysis in neurons of the red nucleus has been observed. The affected myelinated tracts appear spongy microscopically, and in early cases may be bordered by areas containing globules of myelin and col-lections of "gitter cells." All evidence of tissue reaction usually disappears shortly and inflammatory cells are rare in the adjacent viable parenchyma.

Congenital Demyelinating Disease of Lambs

ALLCROFT, R., CLEGG, F. G., and UVAROV, O.:   Prevention of Swayback in Lambs.   Vet. Rec. *71*:884–889, 1959.
BARLOW, R. M.:   Recent Advances in Swayback.   Proc. Roy. Soc. Med. *51*:748–752, 1958.
BARLOW, R. M., *et al.*:   Swayback in Southeast Scotland.   Field, Clinical, Pathological and Biochemical Aspects.   J. Comp. Path. *70*:396–428, 1960.
BARLOW, R. M.:   Further Observations on Swayback.   I. Transitional Pathology.   II. Histo-chemical Localization of Cytochrome Oxidase Activity in the Central Nervous System. J. Comp. Path. *73*:51–60, 61–67, 1963.
BARLOW, R. M., and CANCILLA, P. A.:   Structural Changes of the Central Nervous System in Swayback (Enzootic Ataxia) of Lambs.   Acta. Neuropath. *6*:175–180, 1966.
BENNETTS, H. W., and BECK, A. B.:   Enzootic Ataxia and Cooper Deficiency of Sheep in Western Australia.   Australian Council Sci. and Indust. Res. Bull. *147*:55, 1942.
BENNETTS, H. W., and CHAPMAN, F. E.:   Copper Deficiency in Sheep in Western Australia: A Preliminary Account of the Aetiology of Enzootic Ataxia of Lambs and Anaemia of Ewes. Australian Vet. J. *13*:138–149, 1937.
BUTLER, E. J., BARLOW, R. M., and SMITH, B. S. W.:   Copper Deficiency in Relation to Swayback in Sheep.   II. Effect of Dosing Young Lambs with Molybdate and Sulphate. J. Comp. Path. *74*:419–426, 1964.
CANCILLA, P. A., and BARLOW, R. M.:   Structural Changes of the Central Nervous System in Swayback (Enzootic Ataxia) of Lambs.   IV. Electron Microscopy of the White Matter of the Spinal Cord.   Acta Neuropath. *11*:294–300, 1968.
————:   Structural Changes of the Central Nervous System in Swayback (Enzootic Ataxia) of Lambs. V. Electron Microscopic Observations of the Corpus Callosum. Acta Neuro-path. *12*:307–313, 1969.
HOWELL, M. McC.:   Observation on the Histology and Possible Pathogenesis of Lesions in the Central Nervous System of Sheep with Swayback.   Proc. Nutr. Soc. *27*:85–88, 1968.
INNES, J. R. M., and SHEARER, G. D.:   I. "Swayback": A Demyelinating Disease of Lambs with Affinities to Schilder's Encephalitis in Man.   J. Comp. Path. & Therap. *53*:1–41, 1940.
JENSEN, R., MAAG, D. D., and FLINT, J. C.   Enzootic Ataxia from Copper Deficiency in Sheep in Colorado.   J. Am. Vet. Med. Assn. *133*:336–340, 1958.

ROBERTS, H. E., WILLIAMS, B. M., and HARVARD, A.: Cerebral Oedema in Lambs Associated with Hypocuprosis and Its Relationship to Swayback. I. Field, Clinical, Gross Anatomical and Biochemical Observations. II. Histopathological Findings. J. Comp. Path. 76:279–290, 1966.

SCHULZ, K. C. A., VAN DER MERWE, P. K., VAN RENSBURG, P. J. J., and SWART, J. S.: Studies in Demyelinating Diseases of Sheep Associated with Copper Deficiency. Onderstepoort, J. Vet. Res. 25:35–78, 1951.

Lipodystrophy of the Central Nervous System

An apparently rare disease of dogs, reported by Hagen (1953), and by Ribelin and Kintner (1956) has been shown to have certain similarities with amaurotic familial idiocy (Tay-Sachs disease) of human infants. The human disease occurs in infantile and juvenile forms, with muscular weakness, amaurosis, mental retardation and paralysis. A peculiar cherry-red spot occurs in the retina and optic atrophy often accompanies the blindness. The infantile form of the disease is more common among infants of Jewish descent and tends to be familial in incidence. The characteristic feature recognizable histologically is the deposition of lipid (lecithin) in the cytoplasm of neurons. In this respect the disease appears to be related to the human dystrophies in which lipid is deposited in other tissues of the body (Niemann-Pick disease, Gaucher's disease, Hand-Schüller-Christian syndrome and xanthomatosis) (Anderson, 1953).

The canine disease occurs in mature animals and is characterized by gradual onset of blindness, weakness and incoordination, followed in some cases by hysteria and paralysis. The cerebellum is described as most severely affected. Cerebellar atrophy follows accumulation of lipid droplets in the cytoplasm of Purkinje cells, with gradual destruction of these cells. The cells of the granular layer are largely lost and replaced by astrocytic glia. Myelinated fibers remain intact and leukocytic infiltration does not occur. Purkinje cells which remain in the cerebellum and neurons of the pontine, red and oculomotor nuclei invariably contain cytoplasmic droplets of lipid. These droplets are usually unstained by hematoxylin and eosin and are for the most part removed from the tissue by the usual fat solvents. Some residual material remaining in the cells gives a positive reaction for carbohydrates (periodic acid-Schiff reaction). This material stains deep red with Gomori's trichrome stain but is negative for desoxypentose nucleic acid and pentose nucleic acid as indicated by its failure to stain with the Feulgen reaction and toluidine blue stain. Frozen sections are necessary to demonstrate the lipid component of the affected neurons.

A similar neuronal lipodystrophy has been reported in one bull from a herd of inbred cattle (Read and Bridges, 1969). Neurons in this animal contained cytoplasmic lipid material in fine droplets which ultrastructurally were demonstrated to consist of membrane-bound inclusions containing granular and crescentic linear materials. These suggested the multilamellar cytosomes and curvilinear bodies considered to be characteristic of late infantile amaurotic idiocy of man.

Cerebrospinal lipodystrophy in Yorkshire swine has been described by Read and Bridges (1968) as a disease in which neurons generally contain lipid bodies in their cytoplasm. Ultrastructural features of these bodies include membranous arrays quite similar to those found in human Tay-Sachs disease.

Lipodystrophy (Amaurotic Idiocy)

FANKHAUSER, R.: Degenerative Lipoidosis of the Central Nervous System in Two Dogs. Schweiz. Arch. Tierheilk. 107:73–87, 1965.

HAGEN, L. O.: Lipid Dystrophic Changes in the Central Nervous System in Dogs. Acta Path. Microbiol. Scand. *33*:32–35, 1953.

KARBE, E., and SCHIEFER, B.: Familial Amaurotic Idiocy in Male German Shorthair Pointers. Path. Vet. *4*:223–232, 1967.

KOPPANG, N.: (Familial Glycosphingolipoidosis or Juvenile Amaurotic Idiocy in the Dog.) Ergebn Allg. Path. Path. Anat. *47*:1–45, 1966. V.B. *36*:3638, 1966.

————: Juvenile Amaurotic Idiocy by English Setter in Norway. Acta Path. Microbiol. Scand. *64*:158–159, 1965. V.B. *35*:4344, 1965.

READ, W. K., and BRIDGES, C. H.: Cerebrospinal Lipodystrophy in Swine. A New Disease Model in Comparative Pathology. Path. Vet. *5*:67–74, 1968.

————: Neuronal Lipodystrophy. Occurrence in an Inbred Strain of Cattle. Path. Vet. *6*:235–243, 1969.

RIBELIN, W. E., and KINTNER, L. D.: Lipodystrophy of the Central Nervous System in a Dog. A Disease with Similarities to Tay-Sachs Disease of Man. Cornell Vet. *45*:532–537, 1956.

Globoid-cell Leukodystrophy

This familial, apparently hereditary, disease in children was described by Krabbe (1916) as a type of diffuse sclerosis of the central nervous system. The principal lesion is a disseminated failure of myelination with the accumulation of large "globoid" phagocytic cells around blood vessels in the vicinity of the altered myelin. A very similar disease was originally reported by Fankhauser, Luginbuhl, and Hartley (1963) in dogs. Several other canine cases have subsequently appeared in the literature. Of the 9 cases reported to this writing, 5 were Cairn terriers, 3 were West Highland white terriers and 1 was of unknown breed. Four were female and 5 male. The pedigrees point toward recessive, autosomal mode of inheritance.

The signs appear usually at about four to six months of age but may be recognized earlier. Impairment is usually evident first in the hind legs with incoordination and slight diminution of placing reflexes. This progresses to motor incoordination, generalized tremor, twitching of head and neck, eventually paraplegia. The lesions may be found in white matter throughout the central nervous system. They are usually bilaterally symmetrical with loss of myelin and in severe lesions, of axons. Associated with these lesions of altered myelin, and grouped around blood vessels, are many large globoid cells with cytoplasm filled with material which compresses the nucleus to one side of the cell. This material stains readily with periodic acid-Schiff (PAS) reagent but is not metachromatic (with Giemsa's or toluidin blue), and stains gray with Sudan black B. Hypertrophied astrocytes are also numerous in the immediate vicinity.

It appears that this disease may be due to the lack of one or more enzymes necessary for synthesis of myelin but further evidence is needed. The histochemical and biochemical features of the human disease are discussed further by Wallace, Aronson and Volk (1964).

Globoid-Cell Leukodystrophy

FANKHAUSER, R., LUGINBUHL, H., and HARTLEY, W. J.: Leukodystrophie vom Typhus Krabbe beim Hund. Schweiz. Arch. Tierheilk. *105*:198–207, 1963.

FLETCHER, T. F., KURTZ, H. J., and LOW, D. G.: Globoid Cell Leukodystrophy (Krabbe Type) in the Dog. J. Am. Vet. Med. Assn. *149*:165–172, 1966.

HIRTH, R. S., and NIELSEN, S. W.: A Familial Canine Globoid Cell Leukodystrophy ("Krabbe Type"). J. Small Anim. Pract. *8*:569–575, 1967.

JORTNER, B. S., and JONAS, A. M.: The Neuropathology of Globoid-Cell Leucodystrophy in the Dog. A Report of Two Cases. Acta Neuropath. *10*:171–182, 1968.

KRABBE, K.: A New Familial, Infantile Form of Diffuse Brain Sclerosis. Brain *39*:74–114, 1916.
McGRATH, J., *et al.*: A Morphologic and Biochemical Study of Canine Globoid Leuko-dystrophy. J. Neuropath. Exp. Neurol. *28*:171, 1969.
WALLACE, B. J., ARONSON, S. M., and VOLK, B. W.: Histochemical and Biochemical Studies of Globoid Cell Leucodystrophy (Krabbe's Disease). J. Neurochem. *11*:367–376, 1964.

Metachromatic Leukodystrophy

Another metabolic defect in synthesis of lipids, known as a familial disease of infants, has also been recognized in mink (Brander and Palludan, 1965). The features shared by the human and mink disease are degeneration of myelin sheaths, disorganization of myelin and the presence of metachromatic lipid mate-rial in macrophages. The evidence points toward an autosomal, recessive mode of inheritance in the mink.

Leukodystrophy in Mink

ANDERSON, H. A., and PALLUDAN, B.: Leucodystrophy in Mink. Acta Neuropath. *11*: 347–360, 1968.
BRANDER, N. R., and PALLUDAN, B.: Leucoencephalopathy in Mink. Acta Vet. Scand. *6*: 41–51, 1965.
CHRISTENSEN, E., and PALLUDAN, B.: Late Infantile Familial Metachromatic Leuco-dystrophy in Mink. Acta Neuropath. *4*:640–645, 1965.

"Allergic" Encephalitis

(Postvaccination Encephalitis, Disseminated Encephalomyelitis)

It was observed many years ago that a few persons or animals suddenly exhibit paralytic symptoms several days after the administration of suspensions of nervous tissue (*e.g.*, rabies vaccine). This "postvaccinal encephalitis" has since been reproduced experimentally by repeated parenteral injections of suspensions of normal brain tissue or by single injections of such tissue mixed with certain "adjuvants" which delay absorption. The causal relationship between injection of suspensions of brain tissue and the paralytic symptoms is quite evident, al-though the exact mechanism involved in the phenomenon is not clearly under-stood. It does appear that the process represents a type of induced autoimmune disease and the experimental disease fits into the category of delayed (cellular) hypersensitivity (p. 311). In spite of considerable search for the provoking antigen, it has not been isolated and identified. It occurs only in tissue of the central nervous system, is deficient, but present, in the fetal brain of mammals but is absent in the frog. It is found in the protein fraction of the myelin, is heat stable and not destroyed by formalin or autolysis (Rowe, 1969). A small polypeptide is currently suspected as the most likely antigen.

The signs in this disease usually start with motor paralysis of one or more limbs, which gradually extends to involve most of the body. Death is the usual outcome in animals with a severe form of the disease. Dogs are most commonly affected, presumably because antirabies vaccination is most frequent in this species, but many other species are susceptible.

The **lesions** are most evident upon microscopic examination of the brain and spinal cord. In the brain, the lesions are rather sharply limited to the white matter, destruction of myelinated tracts being the dominant feature. Tracts at all levels may be involved, although the largest lesions are usually seen in the

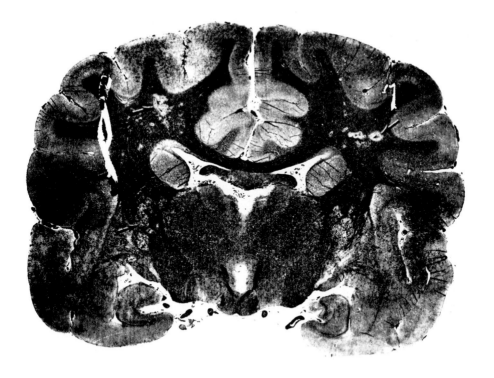

FIG. 28–15.—Demyelinization in allergic encephalitis in a dog. Transverse section of brain. Weil's stain. Arrows indicate pale areas of demyelination in white matter. (Courtesy of Armed Forces Institute of Pathology.) Contributor: Dr. C. P. Zepp, Jr.

cerebellar peduncles, internal capsule and pyramids. Subcortical white matter is often affected and occasionally the corpus callosum is involved. The lesions appear as irregular, nonsymmetrical areas of malacia with destruction of myelin followed by the usual glial and leukocytic response. Perivascular accumulation of lymphocytes is often intense in regions adjacent to foci of malacia. In the spinal cord, tracts in the myelinated white columns are similarly affected, but accumulation of lymphocytes around blood vessels is a more striking feature.

The **diagnosis** of "allergic encephalitis" can usually be based upon the history and on the demonstration of characteristic microscopic lesions in brain and cord.

Allergic Encephalitis

INNES, J. R. M.: Experimental "Allergic" Encephalitis: Attempts to Produce the Disease in Sheep and Goats. J. Comp. Path. & Therap. *61*:241–251, 1951.

JERVIS, G. A., BURKHART, R. L., and KOPROWSKI, H.: Demyelinating Encephalomyelitis in the Dog Associated with Antirabies Vaccination. Amer. J. Hyg. *50*:14–26, 1949.

JERVIS, G. A., and KOPROWSKI, H.: Encephalomyelitis of Possible Allergic Etiology in Mice Injected with Rabies Vaccine. Canad. J. Comp. Med. *13*:116–121, 1949.

LEVINE, S., and SOWINSKI, R.: Reduction of Allergic Encephalomyelitis Incubation Period to Five Days. Amer. J. Path. *56*:97–110, 1969.

OLDSTONE, M. B. A., and DIXON, F. J.: Immunohistochemical Study of Allergic Encephalomyelitis. Amer. J. Path. *52*:251–263, 1968.

PURDY, C. W., and LOAN, R. W.: Induction of Experimental Allergic Encephalomyelitis in the Goat. Amer. J. Vet. Res. *30*:85–89, 1969.

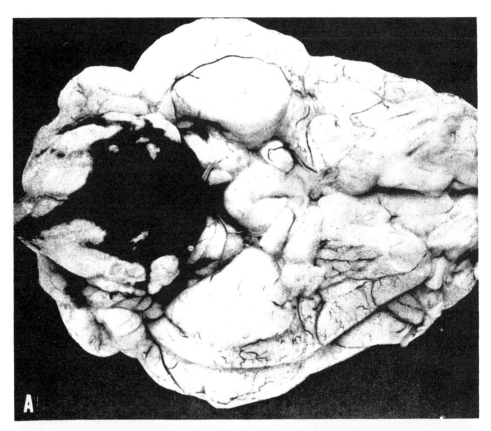

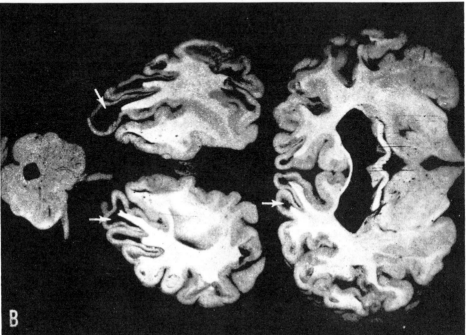

FIG. 28–16.—*A*, Hemorrhage from the basilar artery, brain of a pig which was struck a blow on the forehead. *B*, Polioencephalomalacia in a young calf. Note cavities (arrows) in subcortical **zones** in the cerebrum.

Rowe, M. J., III: Experimental Allergic Encephalomyelitis. A. Review. Bull. Los Angeles Neurol. Soc. *34*:55–56, 1969.

Sherwin, A. L., *et al.*: Myelin-binding Antibodies in Experimental "Allergic" Encephalomyelitis. Science *134*:1370–1372, 1961.

Waksman, B. H., and Adams, R. D.: A Histologic Study of the Early Lesion in Experimental Allergic Encephalomyelitis in the Guinea Pig and Rabbit. Amer. J. Path. *41*:135–162, 1962.

Polyradiculoneuritis

An interesting syndrome in dogs, known colloquially as "coonhound paralysis," has been associated for years with a prior bite by a raccoon. Cummings and Haas (1967) have demonstrated the lesions to consist of inflammation and segmental demyelination of ventral roots and spinal nerves and to resemble the Landry-Guillain-Barre syndrome of man. The clinical features involve acute ascending flaccid paralysis of the coonhound, starting seven to fourteen days following the bite of a raccoon. A viral etiology is suspected, perhaps operating on an allergic basis (Waksman and Adams, 1955, 1956). The suspected antigen has not been identified.

Axonal degeneration in the nerve roots and spinal nerves is accompanied by perivascular infiltration of leukocytes, mostly lymphocytes. Plasma cells may predominate in some sections. The peripheral nerves (sciatic) may be affected but lesions are most consistent in the ventral nerve roots.

Polyradiculoneuritis

Cummings, J. F., and Haas, D. C.: Coonhound Paralysis: A Polyradiculoneuritis in Dogs Resembling the Landry-Guillain-Barre Syndrome. J. Neurol. Sci. *4*:51–81, 1967.

Waksman, B. H., and Adams, R. D.: Allergic Neuritis: An Experimental Disease of Rabbits Induced by Injection of Peripheral Nervous Tissue and Adjuvants. J. Exp. Med. *102*:213–236, 1955.

————: A Comparative Study of Experimental Allergic Neuritis in the Rabbit, Guinea Pig and Mouse. J. Neuropath. Exp. Neurol. *15*:293–314, 1956.

Polioencephalomalacia of Cattle and Sheep

The lesions of a noninfectious nervous disease of cattle and sheep, known in certain western states as "forage poisoning" or "blind staggers," have been characterized by Jensen, Griner and Adams (1956) as necrotizing destruction of cortical gray matter, therefore the disease was named "polioencephalomalacia." These authors estimated that the incidence of this disease in cattle reached 100 per thousand animals in some regions of Colorado. The disorder was more frequently observed in cattle from twelve to eighteen months of age; sheep of all ages were less often affected. The incidence increased during January among cattle in feedlots, while the incidence among those in pasture was highest in July. A similar if not identical disease has been recognized in cattle and sheep in Great Britain, where it is usually referred to as "cerebro-cortical necrosis." The disease is also reported in ruminants in Australia.

The dramatic response of certain clinical cases, diagnosed as polioencephalomalacia, to administration of thiamine has suggested that this vitamin might be involved in some way in the etiology. Some other indirect evidence points toward decreased thiamine levels in liver and cerebral cortex of affected animals. This currently appears to be the most important factor but the pathogenesis and definite etiologic role of thiamine has not been incontrovertibly established.

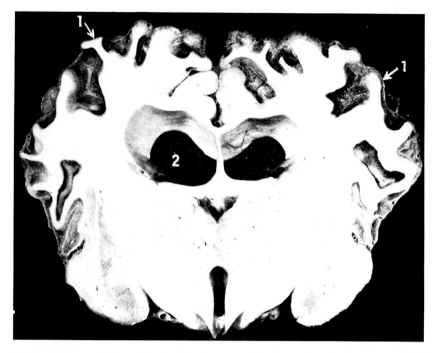

FIG. 28–17.—Polioencephalomalacia, brain of a cow. Note loss of cortical gray matter (*1*) and hydrocephalus (*2*). (Courtesy of Drs. Jean C. Flint and Rue Jensen, Colorado State University.)

The **clinical manifestations** in severely affected animals started with muscular tremors, twitching of the ears, eyelids and facial muscles, followed in some instances by convulsions. Affected animals were unable to see, although no lesions could be detected in the eyes. Visible mucous membranes became injected; respiration and pulse rates accelerated, and temperature sometimes elevated. Mildly affected animals, seen more frequently during the summer months among those in pastures, separated themselves from the herd and occasionally pushed their heads against solid objects. They were unable to see, were apathetic, and often exhibited purposeless masticatory movements accompanied by excessive salivation and, occasionally, twitching of facial or ear muscles. Death occurred in 50 to 90 per cent of affected animals, depending upon the severity of the disorder.

The specific **lesions** were limited to the central nervous system, the changes in the cerebrum being most striking in the cortex, where focal, later diffuse, liquefaction necrosis destroyed most of the gray matter. The adjacent white matter was spared. The cerebral convolutions thus collapsed and gave the appearance in cross section of having been sculptured away, appearing in bas relief against the underlying white matter. This gave the impression that the brain had decreased in size. Internal hydrocephalus was often recognized in severely affected brains.

This selective malacia was seen microscopically to affect only the gray matter, subcortical white matter showing only vascularization, a few "gitter cells" and occasional perivascular lymphocytic aggregations in regions adjacent to affected gray cortex. Neurons were first to become necrotic, but all cells were eventually involved in the areas of necrosis. In the cerebellum, necrosis of the granular layer preceded loss of Purkinje cells. Occasional cystic cavities were observed, but in most cases debris was removed promptly by "gitter cells." Gliosis, with gemistocytic astrocytes predominating, was the usual change adjacent to cortical areas from which all viable tissue had been removed by liquefaction necrosis.

Polioencephalomalacia

ANONYMOUS: Thiamine Deficiency in Ruminants? Nutrit. Rev. 27:176–178, 1968.

EDWIN, E. E., LEWIS, G., and ALLCROFT, R.: Cerebrocortical Necrosis: A Hypothesis for the Possible Role of Thiaminases in Its Pathogenesis. Vet. Rec. 83:176–177, 1968.

FENWICK, D. C.: Polioencephalomalacia of Sheep. Response to Thiamine in a Single Case. Aust. Vet. J. 43:484, 1967.

JENSEN, R., GRINER, L. A., and ADAMS, O. R.: Polioencephalomalacia of Cattle and Sheep. J. Am. Vet. Med. Assn. 129:311–321, 1956.

MARKSON, L. M., TERLECKI, S., and LEWIS, G.: Cerebrocortical Necrosis in Calves. Vet. Rec. 79:578–579, 1966.

MARKSON, L. M., and TERLECKI, S.: The Aetiology of Cerebrocortical Necrosis. Brit. Vet. J. 124:309–315, 1968.

PILL, A. H.: Evidence of Thiamine Deficiency in Calves Affected with Cerebrocortical Necrosis. Vet. Rec. 81:178–181, 1967.

Spinal Demyelination of Rats

Pappenheimer (1952) has described a spontaneous demyelinating disease in adult rats exhibiting progressive flaccid paralysis. The lesions were limited to the spinal cord where ventral and lateral white columns underwent severe demyelination. The lesions were bilaterally symmetrical and appeared as sharply demarcated, spongy areas, replacing most of the white matter. Dorsal columns were generally less severely affected. The cause remained unknown and attempts to transmit the disease and to demonstrate any relation to a viral disease of mice were unsuccessful. The significance of this disease is not clear, although if it were reproducible or occurred spontaneously with more frequency it might be useful as a tool for investigation of demyelinating diseases.

Spinal Demyelination, Rats

PAPPENHEIMER, A. M.: Spontaneous Demyelinating Disease of Adult Rats. Amer. J. Path. 28:247–255, 1952.

Progressive Myoclonus Epilepsy

Although the clinical signs of epilepsy may be initiated by many underlying factors, a specific type in man has been distinguished by Lafora and Glueck (1911) on the basis of accumulation of a complex glycoprotein within neurons and sometimes other tissues. The nature of this material suggests the possibility of an underlying metabolic defect. Two cases in dogs have been reported by Holland, et al. (1970), one in a three-year-old male bassett hound, another in a male miniature poodle, eight years of age. In the first case, progressive depression, prolonged sleep periods, lethargy and stiffness were noted. In the second case, no neurologic manifestations were noted prior to death.

The characteristic Lafora bodies were found in both of these dogs in neurons, especially in Purkinje cells, cerebral cortex, motor nuclei, molecular layer of the cerebellum and retina. These bodies were round, laminated, basophilic in H & E stains, up to 32 microns in diameter and located in the cytoplasm or processes of neurons. They were isotropic to polarized light and did not exhibit any auto-fluorescence. Histochemical and ultrastructural features of these bodies in dogs support the thesis that they consist of complex glycoprotein essentially similar to that reported in the human disease.

Progressive Myoclonus Epilepsy (Lafora)

COLLINS, G. H., COWDEN, R. R., and NEVIS, A. H.: Myoclonus Epilepsy with Lafora Bodies. An Ultrastructural and Cytochemical Study. Arch. Path. 86:239–254, 1968.

HOLLAND, J. M., *et al.*: Lafora's Disease in a Dog; a Comparative Study. Amer. J. Path. 58:509–529, 1970.

LAFORA, G. R., and GLUECK, B.: Beitrag zur histopathologie der myoclonischen epilepsy. Z. Ges Neurol Psychiat. 6:1–14, 1911.

UNVERRICHT, H.: *Die Mycoclonie.* Franz Deuticke, Leipzig u. Wien., 1891.

29
Organs of Special Sense

THE EYE

The eye is a wondrously complex structure whose parts perform a function which even the most blasé must consider miraculous. The eyes of each animal or bird are remarkably adapted to its environment and habits. The hawk can spot his tiny prey from fantastic heights and the cat can see his victim on the darkest night. Such functional adaptations are dependent upon specific structural developments which are different in each species. This alone makes the study of diseased ocular structures in animals both difficult and fascinating.

Not only is the eye the organ of sight, but it also serves as a window through which some disease processes can be observed. With slit-lamp illumination and the corneal microscope, leukocytes or erythrocytes can be seen escaping from the iris, floating in the aqueous, and settling to the bottom of the anterior chamber. Capillaries in the retina can be studied with the ophthalmoscope, and sometimes they yield clues as to the condition of capillaries in the rest of the body. It is unfortunate that the general pathologist often avoids the study of the eye, because this organ follows the general laws of biology in its response to injury and can teach much to the observant. This is not to disclaim the necessity for the special knowledge and interest of ophthalmic pathologists, whose contributions are vital, but rather to encourage veterinary pathologists to cultivate a deeper interest in this important organ in their animal patients.

The eye must be studied carefully in the living animal, the gross specimen approached systematically, and properly fixed for microscopic examination if the best evaluation is to be made. Some things are best detected in the living animal: These would include: The luster of the cornea, size, shape and response of the pupil to light, opacities in the media-cornea, aqueous, lens and vitreous, intra-ocular tension, intraocular masses, etc. The importance of systematic clinical evaluation and record of findings is especially important to the pathologist in this system.

THE ADNEXA

The **eyelids,** having cutaneous and conjunctival surfaces and containing both tear and sebaceous glands (*i.e.* meibomian glands), may be subject to lesions of any of these structures. Any lesion of the skin (Chapter 19) may involve the cutaneous part of the eyelid. The **conjunctiva** is frequently subject to nonspecific inflammation which may at times result in hypertrophy and hyperplasia of sub-epithelial lymphocytic nodules. This may give the conjunctiva a grossly evident roughened, cobblestone appearance. Neoplasms of the conjunctiva are not infrequent, the most common being the squamous cell carcinoma of the bovine eye (p. 225). This neoplasm most frequently originates in the conjunctiva but may arise from the skin of the eyelid. Basal cell carcinomas, cutaneous horns and papillomas may also arise from the conjunctival or cutaneous portions of the eyelids. Adenomas of the **meibomian glands** occur quite frequently in dogs.

The **membrana nictitans,** or nictitating membrane, is particularly well developed in most domestic animals, although vestigial in man. This membrane invests the nasal aspect of the globe and is usually barely visible at the medial canthus. It can be protruded like a "third eyelid" by voluntary or involuntary action to cover most, if not all, of the corneal surface. This is presumed to give the eye additional protection and may have a cleansing function. The membrane is covered by conjunctiva and is richly supplied with simple and compound tubular lacrimal glands. Rigidity is given the structure by a central core of cartilage which is of concave shape to fit the eyeball.

Inflammation of the lacrimal glands (dacryoadenitis), may come to the attention of the veterinary pathologist. The superficial and deep glands of the membrana nictitans of the dog are most commonly involved. This inflammation results in congestion and enlargement of the gland, which, in turn, causes the third eyelid to protrude, usually necessitating its ablation. The microscopic findings in surgical specimens of the third eyelid are usually limited to inflammatory changes in the stroma and the connective tissue surrounding the tubular glands of the eyelid. The ducts of the glands are often dilated, occasionally filled with leukocytes, and the acinar elements are hypertrophic. Frank neoplastic changes in the glands are rare, but adenomas may occur.

The Eye, General

ANDERSON, D. R.: Ultrastructure of Human and Monkey Lamina Cribrosa and Optic Nerve Head. Arch. Ophthal. *82*:800–814, 1969.

COGAN, M. J., and ZIMMERMAN, L. E.: *Ophthalmic Pathology,* 2nd ed., Philadelphia, W. B. Saunders Co., 1962.

COHRS, P.: *Studien zur normalen und pathologischen Anatomie und Histologie des inneren Gehororganes vom Pferde (Equus caballus).* Leipzig, F. C. W. Vogel, 1928.

DUKE-ELDER, W. S.: *Textbook of Ophthalmology,* Vols. I-VI, St. Louis, C. V. Mosby Co., 1938–1954.

MAGRANE, W. G.: *Canine Ophthalmology.* 2nd ed., Philadelphia, Lea & Febiger, 1971.

MANN, I. C.: *The Development of the Human Eye.* 2nd ed., New York, Grune and Stratton, 1950.

MILLER, M. E., and HABEL, R. E.: Harder's Gland in the Dog. J. Am. Vet. Med. Assn. *118*:155–156, 1951.

PRINCE, J. H., DIESEM, C. D., EGLITIS, I., and RUSKELL, G. L.: *Anatomy and Histology of the Eye and Orbit in Domestic Animals.* Springfield, Charles C Thomas, 1960.

SAUNDERS, L. Z.: *Pathology of the Eye of Domestic Animals.* Berlin, Paul Parey, 1968.

SHIVELY, J. N., and EPLING, G. P.: Fine Structure of the Canine Eye: Iris. Am. J. Vet. Res. *30*:13–26, 1969.

SHIVELY, J. N., EPLING, G. P., and JENSEN, R.: Fine Structure of the Canine Eye. Am. J. Vet. Res. *31*:1339–1359, 1970.

WOLFF, E.: *The Anatomy of the Eye and Orbit.* 3rd ed., Philadelphia, Blakiston, 1951.

WYMAN, M., and DONOVAN, E. F.: The Ocular Fundus of the Normal Dog. J. Am. Vet. Med. Assn. *147*:7–26, 1965.

THE CORNEA AND SCLERA

Some of the important anatomic differences between species will be mentioned as the specific anatomic structure is considered. The sclera is the relatively avascular tunic which gives the globe the structural rigidity to maintain its shape. In birds it normally contains cartilage which may ossify to bone.

The cornea of animals of most species is subjected to a wide variety of deleterious influences but has a good capacity for recovery. Unfortunately, healing of lesions in the cornea may result in scarring, which is not objectionable in other structures, but may destroy sight by making all or part of the cornea opaque. Wounds, particularly when accompanied by penetrating foreign bodies, are a common cause of inflammation which may leave opacities in the cornea. Injuries which perforate the cornea are of serious import, often leading to loss of sight in the involved eye. Perforation of Descemet's membrane permits escape of aqueous humor followed by collapse of the cornea, with prolapse of the iris and dislocation of the lens further possibilities. Secondary infection often causes inflammation of the entire globe (panophthalmitis) which may cause permanent loss of sight.

Infectious keratitis, keratoconjunctivitis, so-called pink eye, of sheep, goats and cattle, may result in diffuse inflammation of the cornea, producing temporary blindness. Diffuse scarring with loss of transparency is a common sequel of this infection. The cause is not firmly established although many organisms have been recovered from infected conjunctival sacs and in some cases specific organisms have proved to be pathogenic. *Moraxella bovis* has been isolated most often from affected cattle and, in the presence of sunlight (or a sunlamp), instillation of the organism into the conjunctival sac of normal animals if followed by severe keratitis. *Mycoplasma* have also been recovered from infected sheep and cattle. Viruses, such as bovine rhinotracheitis have also been recovered, sometimes in association with *Moraxella bovis*. A similar organism has been recovered from horses with conjunctivitis. *Rickettsia* have also been demonstrated in infected conjunctiva. The problem of etiology or etiologies is still quite confused— apparently many organisms may cause this clinical disease.

Pigmentary Keratitis.—In some instances, for reasons poorly understood, keratitis in dogs not only is accompanied by deep and superficial vascularization of the cornea, but also is followed by deposition of melanin pigment in the corneal epithelium and the underlying stroma. This may involve much of the cornea, giving it a brown or black color and rendering it opaque. Pigmentary keratitis is difficult to treat and often destroys sight in the affected eye.

Corneal vascularization may follow trauma to the cornea, especially any injury resulting in ulceration of the corneal epithelium, or may be a manifestation of dietary deficiency of certain vitamins (riboflavin) or amino acids (tryptophane). Capillaries which extend into the cornea toward an ulcer usually arise from the vessels in a small zone at the point in the limbus nearest the lesion. **Superficial vascularization,** *i.e.*, formation of new capillaries in the stroma adjacent to the epithelium, usually is first to occur. Proliferation of blood vessels deeper in the stroma, **deep vascularization,** usually follows more prolonged effects on the cornea. Vascularization based upon nutritional deficiency is characterized by proliferation of new capillaries from the corneo-scleral junction (limbus) all around the circumference of the cornea. These extend centripetally toward the centrum of the cornea, may occur in the absence of significant corneal opacity, and do not radiate toward or terminate in an ulcer or opacity of the cornea. Grossly, newly formed vessels in the cornea may appear as vascular arborizations, but microscopic study reveals that each blood vessel does not terminate blindly but forms a capillary loop through which the blood can return to the venules at the limbus (Fig. 29–2).

Pannus (*pannus degenerativus*) is the term applied to a lesion of the cornea

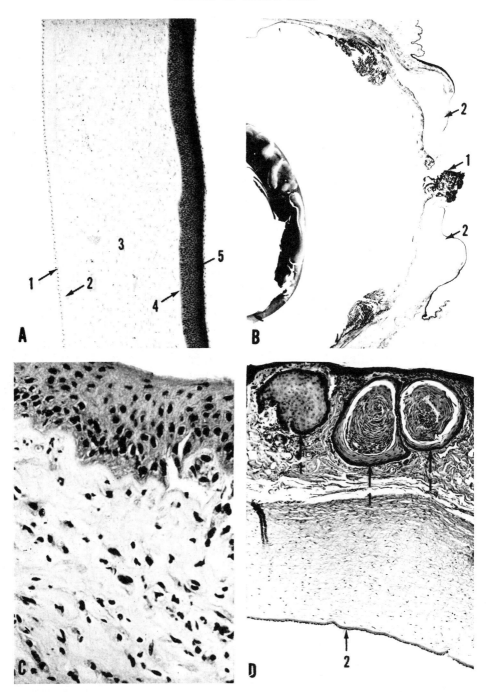

FIG. 29–1.—*A*, Normal equine cornea (× 55). Corneal endothelium (*1*); Descement's membrane (*2*); corneal stroma (substantia propria) (*3*); Bowman's membrane (*4*); and corneal epithelium (*5*). Contributor: Army Veterinary Research Laboratory. *B*, Rupture of the equine cornea following trauma (× 2½). The iris (*1*) has prolapsed through the opening in the cornea (*2*). Contributor: Army Veterinary Research Laboratory. *C*, Keratitis, bovine eye (× 330). Note leukocytes in substantia propria of the cornea. Contributor: Dr. C. L. Davis. *D*, Corneal dermoid, eye of a lamb (× 70). Islands of pigmented epithelium (*1*), between the corneal epithelium and stroma. Corneal endothelium (*2*). (*A-D*, Courtesy of Armed Forces Institute of Pathology.) Contributor: Dr. Robert D. Courter.

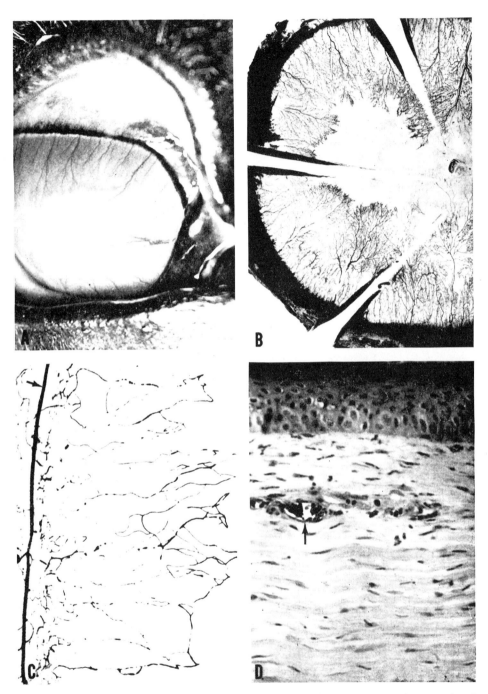

FIG. 29–2.—Corneal vascularization. *A*, Eye of a horse during an acute recrudescence of periodic ophthalmia. *B*, Cornea of a horse with periodic ophthalmia. The fixed cornea was mounted flat on a slide. The limbus is black because of its pigment. *C*, Cornea of a rat with riboflavin deficiency (× 36). Loops of capillaries extend into the cornea from the vessels at the limbus (arrow). *D*, New blood vessel (arrow) in the lamina propria of the cornea of a horse with periodic ophthalmia (× 300).

in which vascular granulation tissue extends from the limbus over the cornea. This tissue, often containing leukocytes, lies between the corneal epithelium and Bowman's membrane, which at times may become duplicated. The granulation tissue may remain as scar tissue, may undergo calcification, and the overlying corneal epithelium is often disorganized and thickened. This condition is frequently associated with glaucoma (p. 1442).

Corneal Dermoid.—A congenital lesion observed in newborn animals may involve one or both eyes. The affected cornea appears to be covered over part of its surface with haired, usually pigmented skin. Microscopically, the affected part of corneal epithelium is replaced with dermal epithelium having skin adnexa in its underlying stroma. Hair follicles, sebaceous glands and cysts lined with epithelium and filled with keratin are common. The corneal stroma may be thickened and vascularized but is otherwise unaffected.

The Cornea and Conjunctiva

BAKER, J. R., FAULL, W. B., and WARD, W. R.: Conjunctivitis and Keratitis in Sheep Associated with *Moraxella* (*Haemophilus*) organisms. Vet. Rec. 77:402–406, 1965.
BERNIS, W. O.: Partial Penetrating Keratoplasty in Dogs. Southwest. Vet. 15:30–44, 1961.
BESSEY, O. A., and WOLBACH, S. B.: Vascularization of the Cornea of the Rat in Riboflavin Deficiency, with a Note on Corneal Vascularization in Vitamin A Deficiency. J. Exp. Med. 69:1–12, 1939.
COOPER, B. S.: Contagious Conjunctivokeratitis (C.C.K.) of Sheep in New Zealand. N. Z. Vet. J. 15:79–84, 1967.
DAVIS, C. L.: An Unusual Occurrence of Corneal Dermatoma in Newborn Lambs. J. Am. Vet. Med. Assn. 85:679–682, 1934.
DYML, B.: (Isolation of a Virus of the Psittacosis-Lymphogranuloma Group from Cattle with Infectious Keratoconjunctivitis.) Vet. Med. Praha. 7:385–392, 1965. V.B. 36:173, 1966.
ECONOMON, J. W. SILVERSTEIN, J. W., and ZIMMERMAN, L. E.: Band Keratopathy in a Rabbit Colony. Invest. Ophthal. 2:361–368, 1963.
FAIRLEE, G.: The Isolation of a Haemolytic Neisseria from Cattle and Sheep in the North of Scotland. Vet. Rec. 78:649–650, 1966.
GLEESON, L. N., and GRIFFIN, R. M.: A Study of Infectious Kerato-Conjunctivitis (I.K.C.). Irish Vet. J. 19:163–182, 1965. V.B. 36:1397, 1966.
HUGHES, D. E., PUGH, G. W., JR., and MCDONALD, T. J.: Ultraviolet Radiation and *Moraxella bovis* in the Etiology of Bovine Infectious Kerato-Conjunctivitis. Am. J. Vet. Res. 26:1331–1338, 1965.
————: Experimental Bovine Infectous Keratoconjunctivitis Caused by Sunlamp Irradiation and *Moraxella bovis* Infection: Determination of Optimal Irradiation. Am. J. Vet. Res. 29:821–827, 1968.
————: Experimental Bovine Infectious Keratoconjunctivitis Caused by Sunlamp Irradiation and *Moraxella bovis* Infection: Resistance to Re-exposure with Homologous and Heterologous *Moraxella bovis*. Am. J. Vet. Res. 29:829–833, 1968.
HUGHES, D. E., and PUGH, G. W., JR.: Isolation and Description of a *Moraxella* from Horses with Conjunctivitis. Am. J. Vet. Res. 31:457–462, 1970.
JONES, F. S., and LITTLE, R. B.: An Infectious Ophthalmia of Cattle. J. Exp. Med. 38:139–148, 1923.
LANDON, J. C., and BENNETT, D.G.: Viral Induced Simian Conjunctivitis. Nature (Lond.) 222:683–684, 1969.
LANGFORD, E. V., and DORWARD, W. J.: A Mycoplasma Isolated from Cattle with Infectious Bovine Keratoconjunctivitis. Canad. J. Comp. Med. 33:275–279, 1969.
LIVINGSTON, C. W., MOORE, R. W., and HARDY, W. T.: Isolation of an Agent Producing Ovine Infectious Keratoconjunctivitis (Pink Eye). Am. J. Vet. Res. 26:295–302, 1965.
MOHANTY, S. B., and LILLIE, M. G.: Relationship of Infectious Bovine Keratoconjunctivitis Virus to the Virus of Infectious Bovine Rhinotracheitis. Cornell Vet. 60:3–9, 1970.
MONLUX, A. W., ANDERSON, W. A., and DAVIS, C. L.: The Diagnosis of Squamous Cell Carcinoma of the Eye (Cancer Eye) in Cattle. Am. J. Vet. Res. 18:5–34, 1957.
MORENO, G., *et al.*: (Infectious Keratoconjunctivitis of Cattle Caused by *Neisseria* [*Neisseria ovis n. sp.* Lindqvist, 1960]). Arqs. Inst. Biol. S. Paulo 35:173–179, 1968. V.B. 39:2363, 1969.

NICHOLS, C. W., and YANOFF, M.: Dermoid of a Rat Cornea. Path. Vet. 6:214–216, 1969.

OLITSKY. P. K., SYVERTON, J. T., and TYLER, J. R.: Studies on the Etiology of Spontaneous Conjunctival Folliculosis of Rabbits. J. Exp. Med. 60:107–118, 1934.

PAVLOV, P., MILANOV, M., and TSCHULEW, D.: Studies on Rickettsial Keratoconjunctivitis in Sheep. Zentbl. Bakt. I. (Orig.) 194:439–442, 1964. V.B. 35:1788, 1965.

PUGH, G. W., JR., and HUGHES, D. E.: Experimental Bovine Infectious Keratoconjunctivitis Caused by Sunlamp Irradiation and Moraxella bovis Infection: Correlation of Hemolytic Ability and Pathogenicity. Am. J. Vet. Res. 27:835–839, 1968.

PUGH, G. W., JR., HUGHES, D. E., and McDONALD, T. J.: Keratoconjunctivitis Produced by Moraxella bovis in Laboratory Animals. Am. J. Vet. Res. 29:2057–2061, 1968.

PUGH, G. W., JR., HUGHES, D. E., and PACKER, R. A.: Bovine Infectious Keratoconjunctivitis: Interactions of Moraxella bovis and Infectious Bovine Rhinotracheitis Virus. Am. J. Vet. Res. 31:653–662, 1970.

ROBERTS, S. R.: The Nature of Corneal Pigmentation in the Dog. J. Am. Vet. Med. Assn. 124:208–211, 1944.

RUSSELL, W. O., WYNNE, E. S., and LOQUVAM, G. S.: Studies on Bovine Ocular Squamous Carcinoma ("Cancer Eye"). Cancer 9:1–52, 1956.

SURMAN, P. G.: Cytology of "Pink-eye" of Sheep, Including a Reference to Trachoma of Man, by Employing Acridine Orange and Iodine Stains, and Isolation of Mycoplasma Agents from Infected Sheep Eyes. Aust. J. Biol. Sci. 21:447–467, 1968.

SYKES, J. A., et al.: Experimental Induction of Infectious Bovine Keratoconjunctivitis. Tex. Rep. Biol. Med. 22:741–755, 1964.

WAGNER, J. E., et al.: Spontaneous Conjunctivitis and Dacryoadenitis of Mice. J. Am. Vet. Med. Assn. 155:1211–1217, 1969.

WILCOX, G. E.: Infectious Bovine Kerato-conjunctivitis: A Review. Vet. Bul. 38:349–360, 1968.

—————: Isolation of Adenoviruses from Cattle with Conjunctivitis and Keratoconjunctivitis. Aust. Vet. J. 45:265–270, 1969.

THE IRIS AND CILIARY APPARATUS

Each species has its own peculiar pupillary outline. The contracted pupil of the cat is vertically slit-shaped; in the horse this slit is horizontal. In both these species the dilated pupil is smoothly circular. In the horse, along the dorsal margins of the pupil the iris bears one or more black nodules which may attain a diameter of nearly a centimeter. These structures, the **corpora nigra,** or **granula iridis,** one or more in number, are made up of pigmented cells from the epithelium of the iris and have been mistaken for neoplasms. Similar but smaller structures occur in the bovine eye. The amount and distribution of pigment in the iris are highly variable between different species as well as individuals. True albinos, of course, do not have any pigment in the iris.

The iris and ciliary apparatus (ciliary body and ciliary processes) are intimately associated in structure and function and thus are frequently involved simultaneously in disease. It is pertinent therefore to consider these structures together. The anterior segment of the vascular tunic, the **uvea,** is formed by the iris and ciliary apparatus, hence **anterior uvea** is often used as a collective term for these structures. The posterior segment of the uvea consists of the choroid.

Neoplasms.—Primary neoplasms of the iris and ciliary apparatus are seldom recorded although their incidence is probably higher than published reports indicate. Malignant melanomas may arise from the iris or ciliary body, and hemangiomas have been observed in the iris. Adenomatous new growths (adenomas of ciliary epithelium) apparently arise from the non-pigmented ciliary epithelium and sometimes displace most of the internal structures of the eyeball (Saunders and Barron, 1958). Metastatic neoplasms may occur in the anterior uvea but are rare.

Anterior synechia is the term used to designate adhesion between the anterior

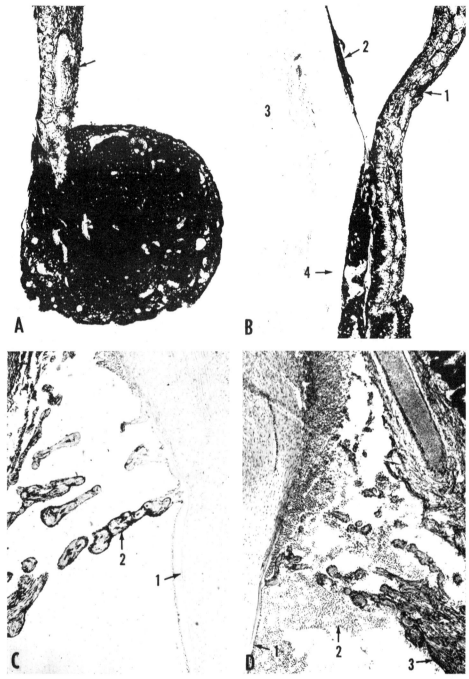

Fig. 29–3.—*A*, Normal iris of the horse (× 35) with the large corpora nigra on the dorsal pupillary margin. *B*, Posterior synechia, a sequel of periodic ophthalmia in the horse. The iris (*1*) is torn away from the lens but leaves pigment upon it at one point (*2*). The cortical lens fibers are disorganized (*3*) (cataract) and the anterior lens capsule (*4*) is firmly adherent to the iris in one zone. *C*, Normal filtration angle, eye of a horse (× 55). Descemet's membrane (*1*) and pectinate ligament (*2*), may be used as landmarks. *D*, The filtration angle in acute equine periodic ophthalmia (× 55). Descemet's membrane (*1*), leukocytes and plasma in anterior chamber (*2*) root of the iris (*3*). (*D*, Courtesy of Armed Forces Institute of Pathology.) Contributor: Army Veterinary Research Laboratory.

surface of the iris and the posterior corneal surface, *i.e.*, the corneal endothelium. This lesion may affect the movement of the iris profoundly, and when the iris is completely adherent all around the perimeter of the cornea (peripheral anterior synechia) an increase in intraocular pressure will be the sequel of occlusion of the filtration angle (see Glaucoma). Anterior synechia will result from iritis when the anterior chamber is collapsed, or in other situations in which the inflamed iris is forced forward to lie in contact with the posterior corneal surface. In some instances the causative factors are obscure.

Posterior synechia means adhesion between the posterior surface of the iris and the anterior lens capsule. This is an even more frequent sequel of iritis than anterior synechia, because the iris normally lies in contact with the anterior lens capsule, at least when the pupil is partially or completely closed, thus has a greater opportunity to adhere. Tenacious posterior synechiae may cause permanent closure of the pupil, or if the adhesions are forcibly torn loose by contraction of the iris, bits of iris pigment may be left clinging to the lens and cause the pupil to appear torn or ragged. Posterior synechia firmly fixed to the lens around the margin of the pupil (so-called ring synechia) and closing the pupillary orifice blocks the flow of aqueous from the posterior chamber. As a result, aqueous fluid accumulates behind the iris, causing it to bulge forward (*iris bombé*).

Posterior synechia may be indicated grossly by failure of the pupil to dilate with mydriatics; or, if it does dilate, by the ragged pupil or by iris pigment clinging to the anterior lens capsule. Microscopically, the iris is adherent to the lens and some fibrinous or, less often, leukocytic exudate is seen in the zone of adhesion. Usually the anterior lens capsule in this area is thickened or bits of iris pigment may be tightly fixed to its surface.

Iridocyclitis.—Inflammation of the iris and ciliary apparatus, or **anterior uveitis,** is not unusual in animals and may have numerous different causes, not all of which are known. The classic example of iridocyclitis in animals is found in recurrent iridocyclitis or periodic ophthalmia of Equidae. The description of this disease which follows immediately will cover all the manifestations of iridocyclitis in any species and from any cause.

EQUINE PERIODIC OPHTHALMIA (RECURRENT IRIDOCYCLITIS)

A specific disease of Equidae, periodic ophthalmia, is the most common cause of blindness in horses and mules. It is characterized clinically by the sudden onset in one or both eyes of severe acute iridocyclitis which gradually abates in a week or more, to become quiescent for a period varying from a few days to many months. Acute exacerbations then follow at irregular intervals, each attack augmenting the damage to the eye. Repeated bouts of acute iridocyclitis usually end in complete loss of vision in the affected eye.

The significant **clinical signs** in the acute stage of the disease include: A tightly contracted pupil (myosis) which fails to dilate in darkness and only slowly after installation of mydriatics; an iris that is yellowish instead of the normal brown; filling of the anterior chamber with finely particulate opacities (leukocytes) which usually settle to the ventral half of the chamber; severe congestion of the sclera and conjunctiva with tiny capillaries entering the cornea from the limbus (corneal vascularization). This is particularly evident (Fig. 29–2) in acute exacerbations. Photophobia is severe, lacrimation excessive and intra-ocular tension diminished.

The acute signs abate rather quickly, usually within a week or so, leaving the disease in a quiescent stage, which, however, can be identified by the careful observer. Evidences of the disease during this period are posterior synechiae, indicated by iris pigment clinging to the anterior lens capsule, and tiny opacities in the vitreous humor on ophthalmoscopic examination. The fluorescein test (Jones, Roby and Maurer, 1946) performed at this time will reveal increased intraocular vascular permeability.

Repeated acute attacks result in posterior synechiae, subcapsular and diffuse cataracts, extensive corneal vascularization, opacities in the vitreous, detached retina and decrease in the size of the globe (*phthisis bulbi*).

The etiology of periodic ophthalmia has been a matter of speculation over the years since the fourth century A.D. when the disease was first described by Vegetius. Ancients ascribed the periodic recrudescences of the disease to the lunar cycle, hence the term "moon blindness."

Studies over the past twenty years have produced some reliable data relative to the etiology, but many facets remain to be elucidated. Good evidence has been obtained to show that affected horses frequently have a high serum titer of agglutinin-lysis antibodies to *Leptospira pomona*, but recovery of this organism from affected horses and reproduction of the disease have not been convincingly demonstrated. It has been shown that under certain circumstances addition of riboflavin to the ration of normal horses will prevent the appearance of new cases of the disease. More evidence is needed before it can be stated unequivocally that the causative factors are known. The status of knowledge of this disease has most recently been summarized by Bryans (1955).

The **microscopic lesions** can be readily correlated with the gross changes, most of which can be seen in the living animal. During the acute stage, the changes are referable largely to the anterior uvea. The iris and ciliary body are severely congested and intensely infiltrated with leukocytes, among which neutrophils predominate at first but are soon replaced by lymphocytes. These cells, along with plasma, escape from the iris and ciliary processes into both the anterior and posterior chambers. A few leukocytes may gain access to the vitreous from the ciliary processes. The anterior choroid and sclera are congested and corneal vascularization is a constant feature. These new vessels start as tiny capillary loops extending from the scleral vessels at the limbus into the lamina propria adjacent to the epithelium, but in later stages well-developed vessels may be demonstrable deeper in the lamina propria of the cornea.

Affected eyes in the quiescent stage exhibit characteristic although subtle microscopic lesions even after only one acute attack. Nodules of lymphocytes in the ciliary body and iris are the most constant finding. It may be possible to detect some collections of lymphocytes and bits of fibrin on the surface of the ciliary processes, iris or lens capsules. Similar exudates may sometimes be found in the vitreous humor.

Repeated acute attacks of periodic ophthalmia usually leave the eye partially or completely blinded. Posterior synechiae commonly interfere seriously with vision, either by occlusion of the pupil or by leaving iris pigment and exudates on the anterior lens capsule. Exudates on both the anterior and posterior lens capsule produce capsular opacities which may eventuate in cataracts. The in-

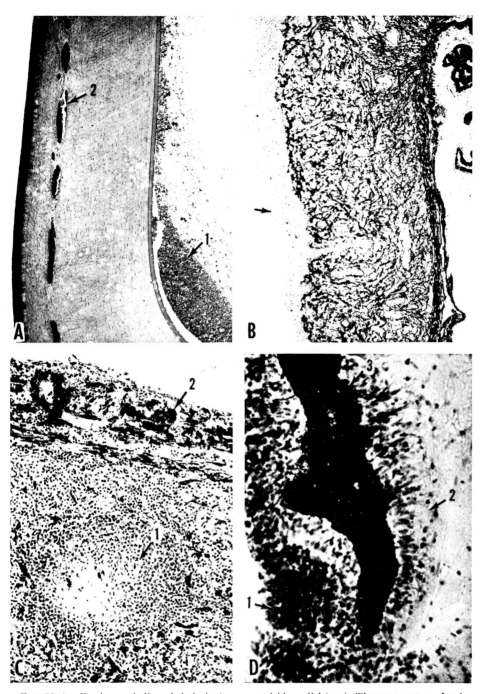

FIG. 29–4.—Equine periodic ophthalmia (recurrent iridocyclitis). *A*, The acute stage. Leukocytes (*1*) in anterior chamber, corneal vascularization (*2*) (× 45). *B*, Leukocytes in anterior chamber (arrow) and iris in the acute stage (× 50). *C*, The iris in the acute stage (× 150). Circumscribed (*1*) and diffuse (*2*) collections of leukocytes in the iris. *D*, Ciliary process in the acute stage (× 240). Collections of leukocytes (*1*), disorganized ciliary epithelium (*2*) and pigment (*3*). (*D*, Courtesy of Armed Forces Institute of Pathology.) Contributor: Army Veterinary Research Laboratory.

flammatory changes in the anterior uvea eventually interfere with the nutrition of the lens, and it becomes opaque with a fused-quartz appearance. Occasionally the lens may be luxated. Exudates accumulate in the choroid and retina, and after a time cause their separation. The pigment layer of the retina usually remains attached to the choroid, while exudate accumulating between it and the layer of rods and cones detaches the retina and forces it into the vitreous. Often the atrophic retina will come to lie in contact with the posterior lens capsule, but it remains attached at the optic papilla and the ora ciliaris retinae. The entire globe becomes smaller in size (*phthisis bulbi*) and the sclera thickened. Secondary degeneration may occur in the optic nerve as a consequence of destruction of the neurons in the retina.

Ectropion Uveae.—One of the specialized terms of ophthalmic pathology, ectropion uveae, applies to the extension of the pigmented layer of epithelium from the posterior surface of the iris, around the margin of the pupil, to the anterior surface of the iris. This results from scarring of the iris with eversion of the pupillary margin by contraction of the scars. It is seen following iritis, in glaucoma and occasionally as a congenital anomaly. Contraction of the iris which inverts the pupillary margin is known as **entropion uveae.**

Iris and Ciliary Apparatus

BALL, R. F.: A Histopathological Study of Depigmented Irises from Single Comb White Leghorns. Cornell Vet. *36*:31–40, 1946.

BRYANS, J. T.: Studies on Equine Leptospirosis. Cornell Vet. *45*:16–50, 1955.

HEUSSER, H., *et al.*: Die periodische Augenentzundung der Pferde als Leptospirenerkrankung. Schweiz. Med. Wchnschr. *78*:756–758, 1948.

JONES, T. C.: Equine Periodic Ophthalmia. Am. J. Vet. Res. *3*:45–71, 1942.

JONES, T. C., MAURER, F. D., and ROBY T. O.: The Role of Nutrition in Equine Periodic Ophthalmia. Am. J. Vet. Res. *6*:67–80, 1945.

JONES, T. C., ROBY, T. O., and MAURER, F. D.: The Relation of Riboflavin to Equine Periodic Ophthalmia. Am. J. Vet. Res. *7*:403–416, 1946.

REESE, A. B.: *Tumors of the Eye*. New York, Paul B. Hoeber, Inc. 1951.

ROBERTS, S. R.: Fundus Lesions in Equine Periodic Ophthalmia. J. Am. Vet. Med. Assn. *141*:229–239, 1962.

ROBY, T. O., and JONES, T. C.: The Blood in Equine Periodic Ophthalmia. Am. J. Vet Res. *8*:145–152, 1947.

SAUNDERS, L. Z., and BARRON, C. N.: Primary Pigmented Intraocular Tumors in Animals. Cancer Res. *18*:234–245, 1958.

TREVINO, G. S.: Canine Blastomycosis with Ocular Involvement. Path. Vet. *3*:652–658, 1966.

WILDER, H. C., and PAUL, E. V.: Malignant Melanoma of the Choroid and Ciliary Body. A Study of 2535 Cases. Mil. Surgeon *109*:370–378, 1951.

YAGER, R. H., GOCHENOUR, W. S., JR., and WETMORE, P. W.: Recurrent Iridocyclitis (Periodic Ophthalmia) of Horses. I. Agglutination and Lysis of Leptospiras by Serums Deriving from Horses Affected with Recurrent Iridocyclitis. J. Am. Vet. Med. Assn. *117*: 207–209, 1950.

The Vitreous

The vitreous body is that part of the transparent media which occupies the largest chamber of the eye. It may become distorted by luxation of the lens, persistence of the hyaloid artery or detachment of the retina. Cells, pigment and tissue debris may become suspended in the vitreous as opacities as a result of iridocyclitis or retinitis. During embryologic development of the lens, the primary vitreous is well vascularized. This vasculature and the hyaloid artery eventually atrophy under normal circumstances but may rarely persist, leaving the artery which terminates in a mass of fibrous, vascular tissue on the posterior capsule of the lens. Congenital cataract (p. 1427) may accompany this anomaly.

Vitreous

GRIMES, T. D., and MULLANEY, J.: Persistent Hyperplastic Primary Vitreous in a Greyhound. Vet. Rec. *85*:607–611, 1969.

THE LENS

The adult lens is composed entirely of epithelium without stroma or vasculature. It receives nourishment from the aqueous humor in which it is bathed. Its simple composition and structure sharply limit the range of morphologic changes which it can undergo, regardless of the type of injury to which it may be subjected. It is surrounded by a tough capsule within which is found the growing layer of epithelium (at the poles and on the anterior surface) whose inner layer of cells mature to become the lens fibers. These fibers are laid down in a concentric manner, the oldest being at the center, or nucleus of the lens. The morphologic changes that the lens itself can exhibit are limited to (1) abnormal growth changes in the epithelium, (2) deterioration of the lens protein with coagulation and disorganization of the lens fibers, and (3) rupture of the capsule which exposes the lens substance to external forces which may lead to liquefaction, organization or dissolution. The lens may be dislocated from its normal position (see Luxation) but if still in contact with normal aqueous humor may not be significantly altered.

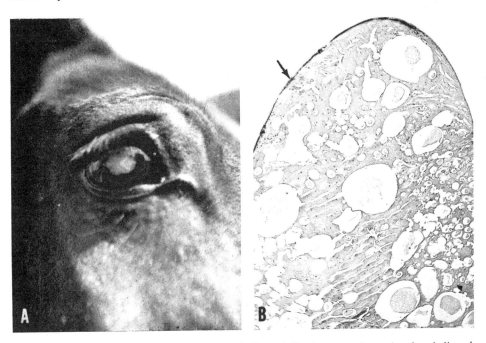

FIG. 29–5.—*A*, Mature cataract in the eye of a horse following several attacks of periodic ophthalmia. *B*, Congenital cataract (× 40) in the eye of a newborn puppy. Anterior lens epithelium is indicated by the arrow. Note large vacuoles, disorganization of lens protein and retention of nuclei. (*B*, Courtesy of Armed Forces Institute of Pathology.) Contributor: Dr. Leo L. Lieberman.

The lens may be damaged by exposure to various toxic substances (naphthalein, ergot) or by nutritive or metabolic disturbances, especially in young animals (riboflavin deficiency, diabetes mellitus). The exact mode of action of substances harmful to the lens is not always clear, although it seems likely that changes in the aqueous probably precede any effect upon the lens.

Luxation.—The lens is held in place by its ligaments which are attached to the ciliary body. A severe blow to the eyeball or a less severe one following damage to the suspensory ligaments may dislocate the lens from its normal position. The luxated lens may be displaced into the anterior chamber, into the ventral part of the posterior chamber, or into the vitreous (Fig. 29–6). The pathologist is sometimes faced with the problem of deciding whether a displaced lens in a specimen is actually luxated or is an artifact in sectioning the eye. This can usually be determined with certainty by careful gross and microscopic study to determine the status of the ocular tissue adjacent to the lens in its new site. Exudates around the lens, particularly if organized, are indications of luxation.

The luxated lens may be resorbed (*phacolysis*) if its capsule is ruptured, may remain intact in its new site, or may become opaque and partially surrounded by leukocytic and fibrinous exudates which may become organized.

Cataract.—A cataract is an opacity of the lens. It may be classified on the basis of its morphologic appearance, its etiology, or both. Opacities on the anterior or posterior lens capsule, usually resulting from iridocyclitis, may interfere with transparency of the lens but are not considered cataracts, nor are they believed to lead, *per se*, to cataracts.

The principal locations of cataracts are (1) the subcapsular epithelium, (2) the cortex, and (3) the nucleus of the lens. **Subcapsular cataracts** occurring under

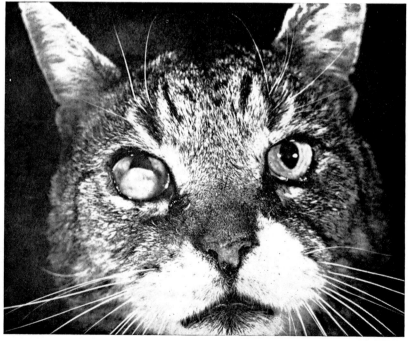

FIG. 29–6.—Luxation of the lens into the anterior chamber of a fifteen-year-old castrated male cat. (Courtesy of Angell Memorial Animal Hospital.)

the anterior capsule (*i.e.*, **anterior polar cataract**) are the result of abnormal proliferation of the lens epithelium at this site. The epithelial cells become redundant, disorganized, or laminated to form an opacity. This lesion may follow prolonged injury to the anterior segment of the lens as the result of a persistent posterior synechia. **Posterior polar cataract,** located under the capsule at the posterior face of the lens, also results from abnormal growth of lens epithelium. However, the absence of epithelium on the posterior surface in the normal adult eye means that epithelial cells must grow into this area from the equator in order to form a cataract.

Cortical cataracts result from disorganization of the lens fibers, presumably following altered metabolism of the lens epithelium. The lens fibers lose their normal concentrically laminated structure to become disorganized and aggregated into irregularly spherical masses of material (*morgagnian globules*).

Nuclear cataracts are the result of changes in the transparency of the oldest lens fibers—those at the nucleus. These central fibers apparently become more dense and appear gray or (more often) yellowish in the center of the lens. It is this type which appears most often in, but is not limited to, senile animals. The **morgagnian cataract** is characterized by complete liquefaction of cortical substance within which the sclerotic nucleus floats. It is a type that to our knowledge has not been described in animals.

Congenital cataracts are observed occasionally in newborn animals. This defect is often attributable to failure of closure of the primary lens vesicle, hence such lesions are most likely to be found near the lens periphery toward the posterior lens surface, at the point where evidence of the lens vesicle is last demonstrable in the normal eye. Congenital cataracts occur with frequency in chicks from hens fed diets low in vitamin E. Puppies, particularly of the collie breed, occasionally have congenital cataracts but the cause in this species is unknown. Genetic factors may be the underlying cause in some congenital cataracts (Rubin, Koch and Huber, 1969) but other factors may also be important. Infection with a virus during early stages of pregnancy is one likely cause (rubella in man, *Herpesvirus canis* in dogs). The evidence is not completely satisfactory at this writing but it appears that autosomal recessive or dominant genes may control hereditary cataracts in dogs.

Lens

ALBANESE, A. A., and BUSCHKE, W.: On Cataract and Certain Other Manifestations of Tryptophane Deficiency in Rats. Science *95*:584–586, 1942.

ANDERSON, A. C.: Inherited (Congenital) Cataracts in the Dog. Amer. J. Path. *34*:965–975, 1958.

CLARK, H. F.: Suckling Mouse Cataract Agent. J. Infect. Dis. *114*:476–487, 1964.

FARMSTON, C.: Observations on Subluxations and Luxations of the Crystalline Lens in the Dog. J. Comp. Path. & Therap. *55*:168–184, 1945.

KOCH, S. A., and RUBIN, L. F.: Probable Nonhereditary Congenital Cataracts in Dogs. J. Am. Vet. Med. Assn. *150*:1374–1376, 1967.

LAPOLLA, L., and MASTRONARDI, M.: Cataract in Young Dogs. Acta Med. Vet. Napoli *8*: 311–321, 1962.

PRINCE, J. H., DIESEM, C. D., EGLITIS, I., and RUSKELL, G. L.: *Anatomy and Histology of the Eye and Orbit in Domestic Animals.* Springfield, Charles C Thomas, 1960.

RIBELIN, W. E., *et al.*: Development of Cataracts in Dogs and Rats from Prolonged Feeding of Sulfaethoxypyridazine. Toxicol. Appl. Pharmac. *10*:557–564, 1967.

RUBIN, L. F., KOCH, S. A., and HUBER, R. J.: Hereditary Cataracts in Miniature Schnauzers. J. Am. Vet. Med. Assn. *154*:1456–1458, 1969.

SMITH, R. S., HOFFMAN, H., and CISAR, C.: Congenital Cataract in the Cat. Arch. Ophthal. *81*:259–263, 1969.

Totter, J. R., and Day, P. L.:   Cataract and Other Ocular Changes Resulting from Trypto-
phane Deficiency.   J. Nutrition 24:159–166, 1942.
Warkany, J., and Schraffenberger, E.:   Congenital Malformations of the Eyes Induced in
Rats by Maternal Vitamin A Deficiency.   Proc. Soc. Exp. Biol. & Med. 57:49–52, 1944.

THE RETINA

The retina is the light-sensitive inner coat that lines the posterior segment of the eyeball.   Its inner surface is in contact with the vitreous and its outer surface with the choroid.   The retina terminates anteriorly near the ciliary body to form a border which, though serrated in man (*ora serrata*), is usually smooth in most animals (*ora ciliaris retinae*).   The retina is firmly attached at this anterior border as well as around the margin of the optic disc, but is more likely to be separated from its pigment epithelium which coheres closely to the adjacent choroid.

In many animals a specific laminated structure, the **tapetum,** lies between the retina and choroid; in some species it is partially pigmented and then is called the **tapetum nigrum**; if unpigmented, the **tapetum lucidum.**   In the horse, for example, a horizontal line in the globe just below the level of the optic disc separates the greenish iridescent tapetum lucidum above from the dark brown, nearly black, tapetum nigrum below.   In some species, as the dog, the tapetum can be detected microscopically or with the ophthalmoscope and the overlying regions of the retina are designated as "tapetal" or "non-tapetal."   These two areas of the retina sometimes respond differently in disease.

The retinal vessels of each species have distinctive anatomic features which must be understood in order to interpret deviations from normal.   In Equidae, for instance, the arteries and veins cannot be distinguished from one another with the ophthalmoscope and they emerge from the margins of the optic disc in a uniform radial manner which gives the disc the appearance of a conventionalized rising sun.   In the dog and cat, as in many other species, veins and arteries are readily differentiated as they emerge from the center of the optic disc and follow a tortuous, branching course into the retina.   The embryonic hyaloid artery, which extends from the optic disc to the posterior lens capsule, may still be present at birth in vestigial form.   This persistence of the hyaloid may be normal in some species (dog, ox), abnormal in others.

The retina may be considered as having two components, the pigment epithelium (which develops from the outer layer of the embryonic cup) and the sensory retina (from the inner layer of the optic cup).   The sensory retina has a complex structure consisting of nine layers which, from the innermost toward the outermost, are: (1) the inner limiting membrane; (2) layer of optic nerve fibers; (3) layer of ganglion cells; (4) inner plexiform layer; (5) inner nuclear layer; (6) outer plexiform layer; (7) outer nuclear layer; (8) outer limiting membrane; and (9) layer of rods and cones (bacillary layer).   These layers vary in thickness in different regions in the retina and between species, but further consideration of these differences lies outside the scope of this book.   It is important to recall that the layer of optic nerve fibers contains the axones of the neurons of the layer of ganglion cells; these axones assemble at the optic papilla and continue as the fibers within the optic nerve.   Thus it is apparent that lesions in the layer of ganglion cells or of nerve fibers could easily result in changes in the optic nerve.

The blood supply of the retina comes from two sources: (1) the chorio-capil-

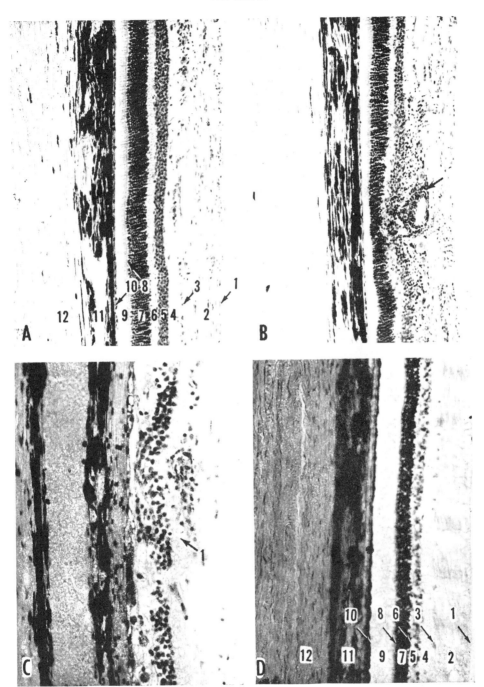

FIG. 29–7.—*A*, Normal canine retina (× 130). Section from non-tapetal zone. Inner limiting membrane (*1*); layer of optic nerve fibers (*2*); layer of ganglion cells (*3*); inner plexiform layer (*4*); inner nuclear layer (*5*); outer plexiform layer (*6*); outer nuclear layer (*7*); outer limiting membrane (*8*); layer of rods and cones (*9*); pigment epithelium (*10*); choroid (*11*); and sclera (*12*). Contributor: Dr. Claude S. Perry. *B*, Early retinitis in a dog with toxoplasmosis (× 130). Leukocytes around blood vessels (arrow); layers of retina distorted. Contributor: Dr. Claude S. Perry. *C*, Retinal atrophy, tapetal zone of retina of a dog. Note atrophy of inner and outer nucleur layers (arrow) as well as layer of rods and cones. Note especially swollen cells of pigment epithelium adjacent to the tapetum. *D*, Normal equine retina (× 165). Numbers indicate same structures as *A*. (*A* and *B*, Courtesy of Armed Forces Institute of Pathology.)

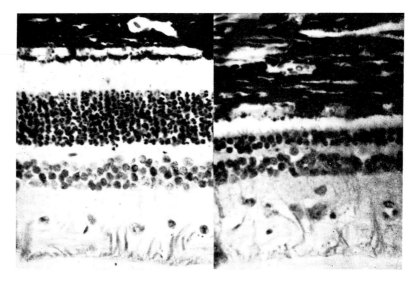

FIG. 29–8.—Hereditary progressive retinal atrophy. Retina of two three-and-one-half-month-old dogs, normal on the left ($\times$ 270). Note reduction in width of outer nuclear and bacillary layers in the affected retina. The rod nuclei are almost completely lost, leaving only cone nuclei. The inner layers are not affected. (Courtesy of Dr. H. B. Parry and *British Journal of Ophthalmology.*)

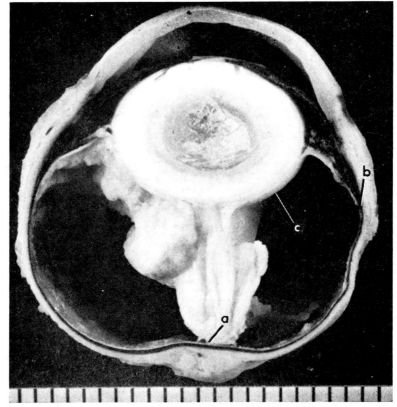

FIG. 29–9.—Detachment of the retina, eye of a spayed female beagle, five years old. Note that the retina remains attached around the margins of the optic disc (*a*) and at the *ora ciliaris retinae* (*b*) and is collapsed over the posterior surface of the lens (*c*). (Courtesy of Angell Memorial Animal Hospital.)

laris, which nourishes the pigment epithelium, the layer of rods and cones and the outer nuclear layer, and (2) the retinal artery which emerges within or adjacent to the optic papilla and continues in the retina within the nerve-fiber layer, dividing dichotomously as it spreads out toward the *ora ciliaris retinae*. The capillaries from this arterial system anastomose only with each other and join only the retinal venous system. The retinal artery supplies the inner layers of the retina (nerve fiber, ganglion cell, inner plexiform and inner nuclear layers).

The retinal artery grows out from the papilla into the retina toward the *ora ciliaris retinae* during embryonic life. In the human fetus, these vessels start growing from the papilla during the fourth month and reach the ora serrata during the eighth month *in utero*. In some animals (dog, cat, rat) this development is slower, newborn kittens, puppies, or four-day-old rats have retinal vessels which reach about halfway to the *ora ciliaris retinae*, a stage of development reached by the human fetus during the seventh month of gestation. This species difference has been used in the experimental reproduction of retrolental fibroplasia or retinopathy of prematurity, a disease of premature infants. In an atmosphere which is high in oxygen (as in an incubator or oxygen tent) the immature retinal vessels of the newborn fail to grow normally, the endothelial cells forming nonfunctional nodules resembling glomerular tufts; this leads to retinal detachment, retinal edema and hemorrhages, and vitreous disorganization—features which closely simulate the lesions of retrolental fibroplasia of infants.

The retina may be affected by a large variety of injurious factors, not all of

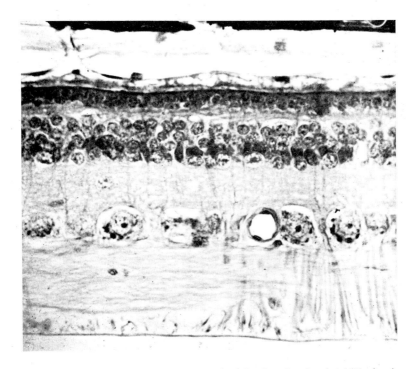

FIG. 29–10.—Hereditary progressive retinal atrophy. Section of retina ($\times$ 450) of a six-month-old dog with a later stage of atrophy than shown in Fig. 29–8. Note complete loss of rod nuclei. Remnants of the cones form a thin layer between the atrophic pigment epithelium and the thickened external limiting membrane. (Courtesy of Dr. H. B. Parry and the *British Journal of Ophthalmology*.)

which are known. It is commonly involved in severe cases of iritis, iridocyclitis and choroiditis—in fact, it is so intimately related to the choroid that inflammation of one usually involves the other. **Chorioretinitis** is therefore not an uncommon pathologic finding. Exudates which accumulate in the retina as a consequence of inflammation, especially in recurrent iridocyclitis (p. 1421), are usually found adjacent to the pigment epithelium. The presence of such exudates results in **detachment of the retina.** The accumulation of edema in the retina may dislodge it from its normal position and in extreme cases force it into the vitreous, sometimes to lie in contact with the posterior lens capsule where it becomes incorporated in an organized **cyclitic membrane.** The recognition of the presence of exudate is essential in order to differentiate between true retinal detachment and detachment as an artifact produced in preparation of the specimen. In either event, the retina remains attached at the optic papilla and *ora ciliaris retinae.*

The secondary changes in the retina resulting from glaucoma are described on page 1444. In some specific diseases, *i.e.*, canine distemper (p. 440), toxoplasmosis (p. 684), and coccidioidomycosis (p. 646), lesions may occur in the retina. Atrophic and degenerative changes in the retina have been described from time to time in animals, but their etiology is usually unknown and it is difficult to classify them in relation to one another. The most thorough attempt to classify and distinguish retinopathies has been made by Parry, whose work will be summarized in the following paragraphs relative to retinopathy in the dog.

Hereditary Progressive Retinal Atrophy.—Retinal atrophy in certain families of Red Irish Setter dogs has been described by Parry (1953) and attributed by him to recessive inherited factors. By utilizing this information concerning the mode of inheritance in test mating prospective stud dogs to known carriers and using only those dogs for breeding which produce only normal pups, the frequency of this defect in the red Irish setter breed has been markedly reduced (Barnett, 1965). The canine lesion appears to differ in some respects from retinitis pigmentosa of man, but similar retinal changes have been described in the cat, rat

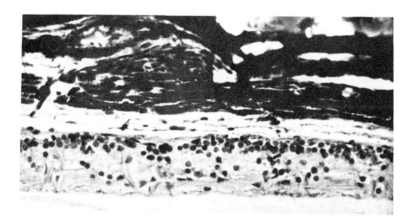

FIG. 29–11.—Hereditary progressive retinal atrophy. Late stage in a six-year-old dog which had been blind for four years (× 240). The retina is completely disorganized, most nuclei have disappeared and the pigment epithelium is missing. The remains of the atrophic retina are in direct contact with the tapetum. (Courtesy of Dr. H. B. Parry and the *British Journal of Ohpthalmology.*)

and mouse. Hereditary retinal atrophy results in progressive, bilaterally symmetrical atrophy of the retina, which starts early in life as night blindness and progresses to complete loss of vision in early adulthood.

Cogan and Kuwabara (1965) have described the clinical and pathologic features of a similar, or identical, disease in Norwegian elkhounds and suggest that it be called "retinal abiotrophy." These authors present evidence indicating that the disease is controlled by a single recessive gene. Electron microscopy was also used to demonstrate fragmentation of the outer segments of the photoreceptors with disorientation of their laminated plates, followed by pleating of the inner surface of the pigment epithelium. These features were all recognized before any changes could be seen with the light microscope.

Familial Progressive Retinal Atrophy.—Parry (1954) described progressive retinal atrophy, not related to the red Irish setter gene, in a family of Afghan dogs and in a yellow Labrador retriever. The lesions in these cases are similar to those of hereditary progressive retinal atrophy except that the retinal changes are associated with cataract formation and fibrosis of the terminal retinal arterioles. The cause is unknown but a vascular origin is suggested. The lesions start in the outer layers of the retina with loss of rods, cones and their nuclei, followed by disappearance of the inner layers. The disease terminates in total sclerosis of the retina.

Three stages of the disease have been recognized and are of value in studying the lesions. During the first stage, two to nine months in duration, there is uniform, bilaterally symmetrical loss of rods and their nuclei, resulting in night blindness without detectable effect upon day vision. In the second stage, lasting three to twenty-four months, retinal cones and cone nuclei are lost, causing progressive failure of day vision. The other layers of the retina remain normal.

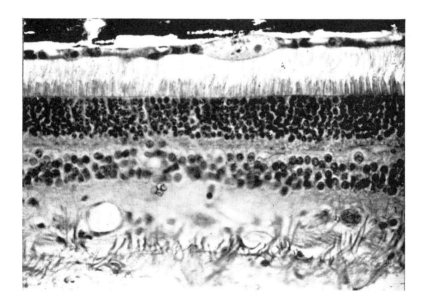

Fig. 29–12.—Progressive central retinal atrophy with pigment epithelial dystrophy. Retina of a two-year-old red Irish setter dog ($\times$ 330). Section near ventral edge of tapetal fundus near papilla. Giant cell in pigment epithelium and gliosis of optic nerve fiber layer. (Courtesy of Dr. H. B. Parry and the *British Journal of Ophthalmology*.)

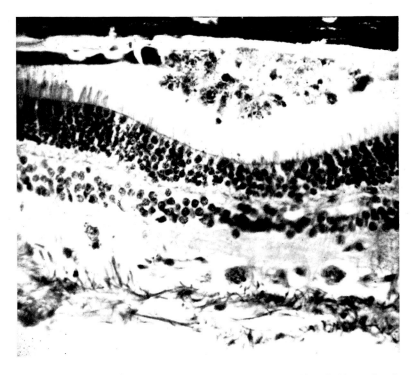

FIG. 29–13.—Progressive central retinal atrophy. Same case as Fig. 29–12, section from mid-tapetal fundus near papilla. Note hypertrophied pigment epithelium which displaces the adjacent layer of rod and cones. There is gliosis in the nerve fiber layer and atrophy of ganglion cells. Courtesy of Dr. H. B. Parry and *British Journal of Ophthalmology.*)

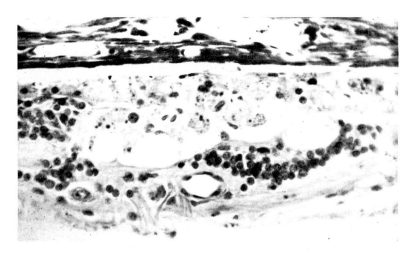

FIG. 29–14.—Progressive central retinal atrophy. Retina of a three-year-old border collie dog ($\times$ 330). Note giant multicellular nest in pigment epithelium, cavities where rods and cones should be, atrophy and sclerosis of most of the retina. (Courtesy of Dr. H. B. Parry and the *British Journal of Ophthalmology.*)

When the third stage is reached, both day and night blindness are complete as a result of the disorganization of all layers of the retina, glial proliferation and diffuse sclerosis of the retina. The pigment layer of the retina is atrophied and a few pigment-laden cells are dispersed in the sclerotic retina. Accumulations of pigment cells are not seen, as they are in human retinitis pigmentosa.

Progressive Central Retinal Atrophy. — Progressive atrophic changes in the central portion of the retina are distinguished by Parry (1954) from hereditary progressive retinal atrophy by the central distribution of the lesions and the occurrence of pigment aggregates which can be detected with the ophthalmoscope. The etiology of this lesion is unknown. The syndrome is recognized clinically by the appearance of small irregular foci of pigmentation in the tapetal fundus of middle-aged or old dogs, with bilateral impairment of central vision but with normal peripheral day and night vision. The lesions apparently start in the central part of the retina with swelling and proliferation of pigment epithelial cells, loss of adjacent rods and cones, and gliosis of the ganglion cell layer. As it progresses, nodular proliferation of the pigment epithelium increases, with displacement and sclerosis of all retinal layers. The final result is complete sclerosis of the retina around the papilla even though peripheral zones are unaffected.

Central Ganglion Cell Degeneration of Retina. — An ocular syndrome has been described by Parry (1955) in a strain of Cocker Spaniels in which a central scotoma results from an anomaly of ganglion cells and optic nerve fibers of the central retina. These non-progressive changes arise in puppyhood and are often associated with congenital cataracts, suggesting that the lesions develop in late intrauterine or early post-natal life. The cause is unknown.

The lesions are limited to the central part of the retina, usually extending a short distance from the papilla to involve the middle of the non-tapetal zone

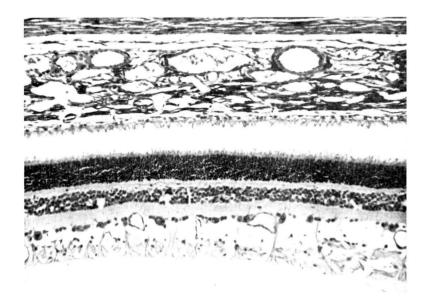

FIG. 29–15.—Central ganglion cell degeneration of the retina. Retina of an eight-week-old cocker spaniel (× 120). Cavitation of optic nerve fiber and ganglion cell layers. Separation of the rod and cone layers from the pigment epithelium is an artifact. (Courtesy of Dr. H. B. Parry and *British Journal of Ophthalmology*.)

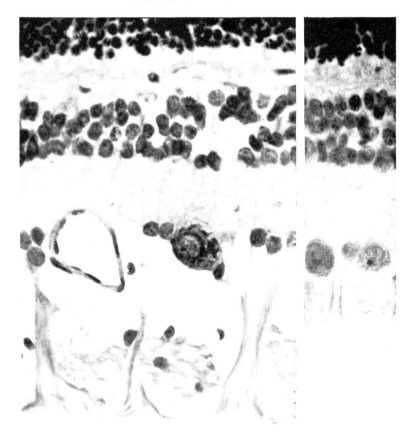

Fig. 29–16.—Central ganglion cell degeneration of the retina. Same case as Fig. 29–15 ($\times$ 590) with normal retina on the right for comparison. Note large vacuoles in the outer portion of the optic nerve fiber layer, with only a few fibers near the internal limiting membrane. The conspicuous strands transcending the cavities are Müller's fibers. (Courtesy of Dr. H. B. Parry and *British Journal of Ophthalmology.*)

ventrally and, to a smaller extent, the tapetal fundus dorsally. The outer layers of the neuroepithelium are normal and the choroid, sclera and tapetum are unaffected. In the diseased central zone of the retina, the optic nerve fiber layer is seen microscopically to be much thickened and to contain many large vacuoles. Across these cavities run heavy strands of Müller's fibers, which fan out and terminate in the internal limiting membrane. The ganglion cells probably are fewer and the Nissl substance of those remaining is agglomerated into large clumps and stains deeply with basic dyes. The retinal vessels are not affected except that many are located rather deep in the thickened ganglion cell layer, and this may explain the apparent disappearance of central subsidiary vessels upon ophthalmoscopic examination.

Retinopathy Associated With Canine Distemper.—Blindness has often been described during or following outbreaks of distemper in dogs. It is difficult to obtain critical proof of the effect of the virus of Carré (p. 440) upon ocular structures, but much indirect evidence points toward such an effect, particularly in animals with involvement of the central nervous system. Parry (1954) has described changes in the choroid and retina of dogs which he believes are the direct result of distemper virus. He has seen this retinopathy in peracute, subacute and chronic forms but all are characterized by generalized destruction of all layers of the retina with foci of more intense damage. These changes first involve the outer and inner layers, progressing toward the middle retinal layers. The damage is more severe over the peripheral than in the central fundus. Early lesions consist of disorganization of the ganglion cell layer with loss of neurons and distortion of the layer of rods and cones. At first the intervening layers of the retina are not affected, but later they are also destroyed, the inner nuclear layer being the last to disappear. In some cases, intranuclear and cytoplasmic inclusion bodies have been observed in the ganglion cell layer. At the end stage, the retina is completely sclerotic, the choroid is thinned and has lost some pigment. The retinal pigment epithelium can no longer be distinguished, but numerous large cells laden with melanin may remain in the sclerosed retina. More study is needed on the possible effect of the distemper virus upon ocular and nervous structures. Correlation of data concerning the presence of virus and its effect upon recognizable lesions is especially necessary to solve this enigma.

Inherited retinopathies in the mouse have been reported by several authors (Keeler, 1970, Sidman and Green, 1965, Sorsby, *et al.*, 1954, and Tansley, 1951).

The Retina

BARNETT, K. C.: Canine Retinopathies. I. History and Review of the Literature. II. The Miniature and Toy Poodle. III. The Other Breeds. IV. Causes of Retinal Atrophy. J. Small Anim. Pract. 6:41–55, 1965. II. 6:93–109, 1965. III. 6:185–196, 1965. IV. 6:229–242, 1965.
————: Retinal Atrophy. Vet. Rec. 77:1543–1552, 1965.
BOURNE, M. C., CAMPBELL, D. A., and TANSLEY, K.: Hereditary Degeneration of Rat Retina. Brit. J. Ophth. 22:613–623, 1938.
COGAN, D. G., and KUWABARA, T.: Photoreceptive Abiotrophy of the Retina in the Elkhound. Path. Vet. 2:101–128, 1965.
KEELER, C.: A New Hereditary Degeneration of the Mouse Retina. J. Hered. 61:62–63, 1970.
PARRY, H. B.: Degenerations of the Dog Retina. I. Structure and Development of the Retina of the Normal Dog. Brit. J. Ophth. 37:385–404, 1953. (Abstr.) Vet. Rec. 68:77, 1956.
————: Degenerations of the Dog Retina. II. Generalized Progressive Atrophy of Hereditary Origin. Brit. J. Ophth. 37:487–502, 1953. (Abstr.) Vet. Rec. 68:77, 1956.
————: Degenerations of the Dog Retina. III. Retinopathy Secondary to Glaucoma. Brit. J. Ophth. 37:670–679, 1953. (Abstr.) Vet. Rec. 68:77, 1956.
————: Degenerations of the Dog Retina. IV. Retinopathies Associated with Dog Distemper-Complex Virus Infections. Brit. J. Ophth. 38:295–309, 1954. (Abstr.) Vet. Rec. 68:78, 1956.
————: Degenerations of the Dog Retina. V. Generalized Progressive Atrophy of Uncertain Aetiology. Brit. J. Ophth. 38:545–552, 1954. (Abstr.) Vet. Rec. 68:78, 1956.
————: Degenerations of the Dog Retina. VI. Central Progressive Atrophy with Pigment Epithelial Dystrophy. Brit. J. Ophth. 38:653–668, 1954.
————: Degeneration of the Dog Retina. VII. Central Nonprogressive Degeneration Due to an Anomaly of Ganglion Cells and Their Axons. Brit. J. Ophth. 39:29–36, 1955. (Abstr.) Vet. Rec. 68:78, 1956.
————: Degeneration and Pigment Cell Dystrophies of the Dog Retina. Excerpta Medica, Sect. VII, Neurology and Psychiatry 8:866–868, 1955.
PARRY, H. B., TANSLEY, K. and THOMSON, L. C.: Electroretinogram During Development of the Hereditary Retinal Degeneration in the Dog. Brit. J. Ophth. 39:349–352, 1955.
RUBIN, L. F.: Atrophy of Rods and Cones in the Cat Retina. J. Am. Vet. Med. Assn. 142:1415–1420, 1963.
SIDMAN, R. L., and GREEN, M. C.: Retinal Degeneration in the Mouse. J. Hered. 56:23–29, 1965.
SORSBY, A., *et al.*: Retinal Dystrophy in the Mouse: Histological and Genetic Aspects. J. Exp. Zool. 125:171–197, 1954.
TANSLEY, K.: Hereditary Degeneration of the Mouse Retina. Brit. J. Ophth. 35:573–582. 1951.

Retinal Dysplasia

Retinal dysplasia has been reported in young children, puppies (Sealyham terriers) and rats as a congenital lesion, apparently present at birth. In children it may be associated with multiple anomalies, in puppies and rats it may be associated with microophthalmia. Blindness is usually evident as soon as the behavior of the animal reaches a stage where detection is possible. In microscopic sections the retina is detached and thrown into disorganized folds and small rosettes. The rosettes may well be the folds of retinal epithelium cut in cross section. A similar if not identical disease in Bedlington terriers has been described by Rubin (1968) who presented evidence that it was caused by a single recessive gene.

Retinal Dysplasia

Ashton, N., Barnett, K. C., and Sachs, D. D.:   Retinal Dysplasia in the Sealyham Terrier. J. Path. Bact. *96*:269–272, 1968.
Rubin, L. F.:   Heredity of Retinal Dysplasia in Bedlington Terriers.   J. Am. Vet. Med. Assn. *152*:260–262, 1968.

THE CHOROID

The choroid is the posterior part of the middle, vascular tunic of the eye. It occupies the entire posterior part of the globe lying behind the *ora ciliaris retinae* except for the space containing the optic papilla. The retina lies on its inner surface except in those areas where the two are separated by the tapetum (p. 1428). The sclera surrounds the choroid and gives it support and the entire globe its relative rigidity. The blood vessels of the choroid penetrate the sclera at various points, the locations depending upon the species.

The vascular nature of the choroid determines the kind of lesions to which it is subject. Metastatic neoplasms and bacterial emboli often lodge in the choroid, and leukocytes may readily escape the blood vessels to invade the choroidal stroma. The retina is commonly involved in inflammatory processes of the choroid, and to these the name **chorioretinitis** may be applied. The causes of chorioretinitis in animals are incompletely understood, but some of the infectious agents which have been demonstrated in chorioretinal lesions are: *Toxoplasma gondii*, *Coccidioides immitis*, and *Mycobacterium tuberculosis*. Too few eyes of animals have been studied following or during the course of generalized infections to determine how often the choroid is involved, but it probably is more frequent than the literature indicates.

THE OPTIC NERVE

Atrophy of the optic nerve has been reported in animals, usually secondary to retinopathy involving the ganglion cell layer. Congenital hypoplasia of the optic nerve has been reported by Saunders (1952) in purebred merle blue collie puppies. In his cases one or both of the optic nerves were grossly atrophic or absent and the optic nerve layer and ganglion cell layer of the retina were also atrophied. These changes were interpreted as resulting from degeneration in the retina, and no proof was found that they were inherited. Complete agenesis of the optic nerve has been observed in rats and in swine with congenital anophthalmos; obviously the optic nerve would not develop in the absence of ganglion cells of the retina.

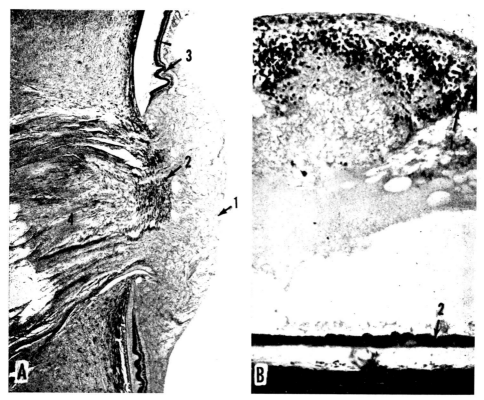

Fig. 29–17.—A, Papilledema (× 17), eye of a ten-month-old Holstein calf which had been fed a ration low in vitamin A since birth. The optic papilla is elevated (1); the pigmented cribriform plate (2) is deflected inward; the retina folded (3); and the optic nerve edematous (4). Contributor: Dr. Louis L. Madsen. B, Detachment of the retina in equine periodic ophthalmia (× 165). Serous exudate in the layer of rods and cones and outer nuclear layer separates the latter (1) from the pigment epithelium (2). (A, Courtesy of Armed Forces Institute of Pathology.)

Papilledema, or choked disc, is the term that denotes edema of the optic papilla and the adjacent retina. This lesion is sometimes associated with internal hydrocephalus but cannot always be explained on this basis. It has been observed in cattle maintained on diets deficient in vitamin A, but its pathogenesis in animals is by no means fully explained.

Optic Nerve

GELATT, K. N., LEIPOLD, H. W., and COFFMAN, J. R.: Bilateral Optic Nerve Hypoplasia in a Colt. J. Am. Vet. Med. Assn. *155*:627–631, 1969.
MOORE, L. A., HUFFMAN, C. F., and DUNCAN, C. W.: Blindness in Cattle Associated with Constriction of Optic Nerve and Probably of Nutritional Origin. J. Nutrition *9*:533–551, 1935.
SAUNDERS, L. Z.: Congenital Optic Nerve Hypoplasia in Collie Dogs. Cornell Vet. *42*: 67–80, 1952.
STUBBS, E. L.: Blindness with Papilledema in Calves. J. Am. Vet. Med. Assn. *105*:209–211, 1944.

OTHER HEREDITARY AND CONGENITAL ANOMALIES

Coloboma, as it pertains to the eye, is defined as a congenital defect in the continuity of one of the tunics of the eye, usually the iris. The defect is seen as a cleft in the iris, and is believed to be the result of incomplete fusion of primordial parts in the optic vesicle during embryonic life.

Congenital anophthalmos, absence of the eye, has been observed in some animals. This defect has been associated with maternal vitamin A deficiency in swine (Hale, 1935). It has been observed in rats, but in this species no satisfactory etiologic explanation has been established (Warkany and Schraffenberger, 1951). One of us (Jones) has seen this condition in young kittens. Not only are the eyes absent, but also as should be expected, the optic nerve and optic tract.

Congenital microphthalmos, decreased size of the eyes, has also been observed in rats, cattle, cats and swine and is possibly related to the same factors that result in anophthalmos.

The Collie Eye Anomaly, first reported by Magrane (1953), has been referred to by many names which have resulted from the diverse clinical manifestations of the syndrome. Some of the names which have been applied: collie ectasia syndrome, congenital anomaly of optic nerve, congenital posterior ectasia of the sclera, ocular fundus anomaly, chorioretinal dysplasia, juxtapapillary staphyloma, retinal detachment, coloboma of optic disc and excavated optic disc. This syndrome is now recognized as widespread in collies, less frequent in other breeds. Present evidence indicates that it is controlled by a single autosomal recessive gene with some variation in its expression (Yakely, *et al.*, 1968).

The lesions vary but may include any one or all of the following: Staphyloma or ectasia of the sclera near the optic disc (a defect in the sclera which allows the choroid and retina to dip into it), dysplasia of retina and choroid, detached retina, and intraocular hemorrhage. Some degree of microphthalmos may be present and pigmentary defects in the retina may be associated.

Collie Eye Anomaly

BARNETT, K. C.: The Collie Eye Anomaly. Vet. Rec. *84*:431–434, 1969.
LATSHAW, W. K., WYMAN, M., and VENZKE, W. G.: Embryologic Development of an Anomaly of Ocular Fundus in the Collie Dog. Am. J. Vet. Res. *30*:211–217, 1969.
MAGRANE, W. G.: Congenital Anomaly of the Optic Nerve in Collies. North Amer. Vet. *34*:646, 1953.
ROBERTS, S. R.: The Collie Eye Anomaly. J. Am. Med. Assn. *155*:859–865, 1969.
WYMAN, MILTON, and DONOVAN, E. F.: Eye Anomaly of the Collie. J. Am. Vet. Med. Assn. *155*:866–870, 1969.
YAKELY, W. L., *et al.*: Genetic Transmission of an Ocular Fundus Anomaly in Collies. J. Am. Vet. Med. Assn. *152*:457–461, 1968.

Hemeralopia (day-blindness) has been reported in two breeds of dogs, Alaskan malamute and poodles. Test crosses with clinically-identified dogs indicate that this characteristic is inherited under the control of a single autosomal recessive gene. The lesions have not been reported.

Retinal lesions related to apparent hereditary or congenital factors are discussed on page 1432. Although such lesions as aplasia of optic nerves, albinism, and other defects have been reported in different species, it is not often that both the anatomic basis for the ocular defect and the evidence for their genetic background are entirely unequivocal. Much is still to be done by pathologists and geneticists to develop sound knowledge of this subject.

Other Anomalies

GELATT, K. N., HUSTON, K., and LEIPOLD, H. S.: Ocular Anomalies of Incomplete Albino Cattle: Ophthalmoscopic Examination. Am. J. Vet. Res. *30*:1313–1316, 1969.

HERRON, W. L., *et al.*: Retinal Dystrophy in the Rat—A Pigment Epithelial Disease. Invest. Ophthal. *8*:595–604, 1969.

LEIPOLD, H. W., and HOUSTON, K.: Congenital Syndrome of Anophthalmia Microphthalmia with Associated Defects in Cattle. Path. Vet. *5*:407–418, 1968.

ROBERTS, S. R., and BISTNER, S. I.: Persistent Pupillary Membrane in Basenji Dogs. J. Am. Vet. Med. Assn. *153*:533–542, 1968.

RUBIN, L. F., BOURNS, T. K. R., and LORD, L. H.: Hemeralopia in Dogs: Heredity of Hemeralopia in Alaskan Malamutes. Am. J. Vet. Res. *28*:355–357, 1967.

ÜBERREITER, O.: (Retinochorioiditis maculosa disseminata in the dog.) Wien Tierarztl Mschr. *55*:707–725, 1968. V.B. *39*:2182, 1969.

NEOPLASMS

Neoplasms are discussed more fully in Chapter 7, but here some mention should be made of the types encountered in the ocular regions in animals. Extraocular neoplasms of the orbit include squamous cell carcinoma and basal cell carcinoma of the eyelid, adenomas of the tear gland (particularly of the third eyelid), and sebaceous adenomas. Benign and malignant melanomas may occur in this region. Secondary neoplasms, such as malignant lymphoma, may at times infiltrate the orbit and cause serious damage to the eye.

The most common neoplasm of the globe itself is the squamous cell carcinoma of the bovine eyeball (p. 225). This tumor most frequently arises from the corneal epithelium at the limbus and may invade and destroy the entire orbital contents. These neoplasms may also originate from the eyelids. Sebaceous adenomas, basal cell carcinomas and papillomas may also arise from the conjunctival or corneal epithelium.

Reports on intraocular tumors in animals have been reviewed by Saunders and Barron (1958), who described fifteen additional cases in dogs. According to these authors, primary intraocular tumors, consisting of "diktyomas," adenomas and adenocarcinomas of ciliary epithelium and melanomas of the uveal tract, have been observed in horses, cattle, sheep, cats, dogs, fish, a rabbit and a hen. Among the fifteen canine cases described in detail by these authors, four were considered to be adenomatous tumors arising from the epithelium of iris or ciliary body, the remaining eleven were malignant melanomas. Three of these melanomas involved the iris, one the ciliary body and two the choroid. Three others replaced both iris and ciliary body to such an extent that the exact site of origin could not be determined. This was also the situation in the final two cases in which the tumors completely filled the globe by the time they were studied.

In two cases, malignant melanomas of the oral mucosa were present in addition to the ocular tumors, and it was not possible to be certain about the origin of several metastases. It is possible that these tumors may have been multicentric in origin. The biologic behavior of these canine tumors appeared to be correlated with their histologic appearance in much the same way that the behavior of human intraocular tumors have been shown to be related to their histologic appearance (Wilder and Paul, 1951). For example, the melanomas made up of epithelioid type cells, with scant reticular fibers and areas of necrosis, were most likely to metastasize. The tumors with fascicular arrangement of the neoplastic cells and abundant reticular fibers were more apt to remain localized.

Neoplasms

BARRON, C. N., *et al.*: Intraocular Tumors in Animals. V. Transmissible Venereal Tumor of Dogs. Am. J. Vet. Res. *24*:1263–1269, 1963.

BELLHORN, R. W., and HENKIND, P.: Adenocarcinoma of the Ciliary Body. A Report of 2 Cases in Dogs. Path. Vet. 5:122–126, 1968.
BLODI, F. C., and RAMSEY, F. K.: Ocular Tumors in Domestic Animals. Amer. J. Ophthal. 64:627–633, 1967.

GLAUCOMA

The term *glaucoma* appeared in the writings of Hippocrates but its present day meaning has evolved over many centuries, and is much broader than indicated by its derivation. Glaucoma is not a specific disease entity but a composite of the clinical and pathological manifestations that result from persistent increase in intraocular pressure. Although the disease in the human subject has been studied for many centuries, many aspects of its causation and pathogenesis remain unknown. For example, the changes which initiate the intraocular hypertension often can not be demonstrated. Although occlusion of the filtration angle is believed to be the basis for the hypertension, even this is uncertain in some instances. Because most glaucomatous eyes become available for pathological study only after prolonged involvement, little is known of the early changes. The advantages of careful study of spontaneous glaucoma in animals would appear to be obvious, but little has been done to attack the problem from this approach.

Certain classifying terms concerning glaucoma in the human eye are well entrenched in the literature. For example, if the apparent underlying cause is demonstrable (anterior synechia following iridocyclitis or trauma to the eyeball, deformities of the lens, detachment of the retina, intraocular hemorrhage, intraocular neoplasms, or circulatory stasis), the condition is called **secondary glaucoma.** If a possible underlying pathologic process is not demonstrated, the term **primary glaucoma** is used. **Absolute glaucoma** is used to describe the distended, turgid, hopelessly blind eye that is the consequence of prolonged intraocular hypertension.

Glaucoma may be unilateral, or, more often, bilateral, and is recognized in early stages by increased intraocular tension which eventually enlarges the globe (buphthalmos), sometimes with apparent exophthalmos. Initially the cornea is edematous and opaque, and in later stages this opacity is accentuated by a degenerative pannus (p. 1415).

The underlying feature usually considered basic to the development of glaucoma is interference with the circulation of the intraocular fluid (aqueous). It will be recalled that the aqueous is secreted into the posterior chamber by the ciliary epithelium. From the posterior chamber, this fluid moves through the pupil into the anterior chamber. The aqueous humor drains from the anterior chamber at the filtration angle near the limbus, where it passes through the spaces of Fontana and eventually reaches the veins at the limbus through the canals of Schlemm. If the filtration angle is occluded—for example, by peripheral anterior synechiae—and aqueous continues to enter the posterior chamber, the fluid pressure must increase. If the pupil is occluded for any reason, aqueous will accumulate behind the iris and force it to bulge forward into the anterior chamber (*see iris bombé*).

Lesions.—The findings on pathologic study of the affected eye can be correlated with those of the clinical examination. The globe is enlarged, increasingly

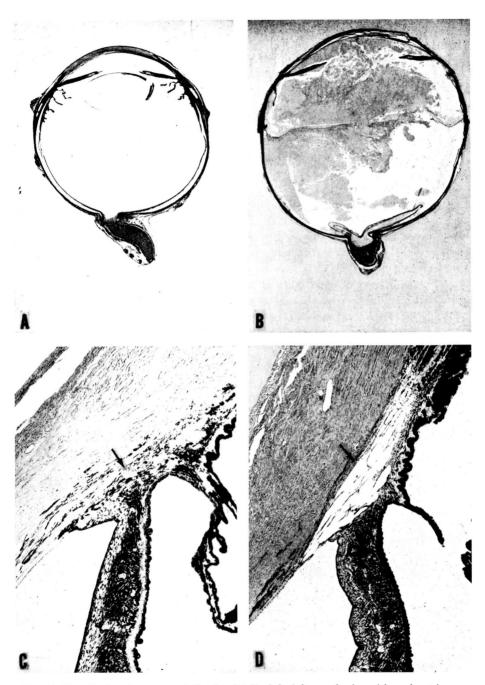

FIG. 29–18.—Canine glaucoma. *A*, Section (× 2) of the left eye of a dog with moderately severe glaucoma. Note spherical outline of the eye, occlusion of the filtration angle and cupping of the optic disc. *B*, Absolute glaucoma in the right eye of the same dog as *A* (× 2). Buphthalmos, severe cupping of the optic disc, disorganization of contents of globe. *C*, Filtration angle (× 35) of same eye as in *A*. Note occlusion (arrow). Contributor: Dr. Leon Z. Saunders. *D*, Normal filtration angle, eye of a dog (× 35). Compare with *C*. (*C*, Courtesy of Armed Forces Institute of Pathology.)

spherical and turgid. The cornea is opaque, as also may be the lens and vitreous. Microscopically evident changes may be found in most of the ocular structures, depending upon the stage in which the eye is studied. In two human cases examined in the very early stages, obliteration of one or more of the vortex veins by thrombosis, endophlebitis or periphlebitis has been reported but this undoubtedly important feature has not been noted in animals. Edema in the corneal epithelium is usually seen in the form of small vacuoles which may coalesce to produce small bullae. It is thought that increased pressure in the anterior chamber forces this fluid through the corneal stroma and into the epithelium.

Significant changes are usually found at the filtration angle. Peripheral anterior synechiae may occlude the filtration angle (Fig. 29–18). The iris is usually thin and atrophic and its blood vessels sometimes are sclerotic. The ciliary processes are thin, compressed and atrophic. The choroid may be similarly compressed and atrophied, eventually appearing only as a thin pigmented membrane containing some thick-walled hyaline vessels. The retina undergoes degenerative changes after prolonged intraocular hypertension, an effect believed to be due to retinal ischemia.

In the dog, Parry (1956) has described glaucomatous retinopathy which results in complete blindness and is characterized histologically by atrophy which is more severe in the inner than the outer layers of the retina. Ganglion cells are lost early, followed by disappearance of optic nerve fibers. The bipolar cells of the inner nuclear layer are next to disappear, but the outer nuclear layer and the layer of rods and cones are only slightly damaged. This degeneration is usually more advanced in the non-tapetal areas of the retina, the tapetal fundus and central fundus are relatively spared. In the peripheral fundus the retina usually exhibits the most advanced sclerosis. There is little or no disturbance of the retinal pigment.

The optic nerve undergoes pathologic changes which are typical of glaucoma. In the advanced stages, the intraocular hypertension causes depression of the optic disc into the characteristic cup shape (cupping of the disc). This change starts with atrophy of the nerve fibers in the area where they go through the lamina cribrosa. The fibers of the lamina cribrosa are also deflected outward to form the cup-shaped space which is usually filled with vitreous. It must be remembered that in some animals (*e.g.*, the elephant) the disc is normally cupped, hence the normal histologic features must be considered in interpreting this change. Cupping of the disc is usually considered to be the direct result of pressure upon the nerve fibers, but a divergent view holds that the pressure first affects the blood supply to the disc, the neuritic atrophy following secondarily.

Diagnosis of glaucoma may be based upon the clinical and pathologic evidences of increased intraocular tension which have been described.

Glaucoma

BECKH, W.: A Case of Spontaneous Glaucoma in a Rabbit. Amer. J. Ophth. *18*:1144–1145, 1935.

JOURDAN, R. J.: Pathogenesis of Canine Glaucoma. J. Am. Vet. Med. Assn. *117*:419–422, 1950.

LOVEKIN, L. G., and BELLHORN, R. W.: Clinicopathologic Changes in Primary Glaucoma in the Cocker Spaniel. Am. J. Vet. Res. *29*:379–385, 1968.

PARRY, H. B.: Degenerations of the Dog Retina. III. Retinopathy Secondary to Glaucoma. Brit. J. Ophth. *37*:670–679, 1953.

THE EAR

The ears of animals do not often come to the pathologist's attention as separate organs but are usually studied in connection with generalized lesions or because of some incidental finding. It seems desirable to describe the few specific lesions which have been recognized in ears of animals, and to recapitulate briefly some of the systemic diseases in which the ear may become involved. These lesions may be conveniently described in connection with the anatomic divisions of the ear, *i.e.*, the external, middle and inner ear.

External Ear.—The external ear consists of the external auricular appendage (auricula) with its cartilage covered by skin, its muscles, and the external auditory meatus which is supported by the cartilage and surrounded by epidermis richly supplied with sebaceous glands, and specialized apocrine glands (ceruminous glands). The external ear is limited in its deepest aspect by the tympanic membrane (*tympanum*). The anatomic details (such as size and position of the auricular appendage, depth and course of the external auditory meatus) in each species are different, hence must be considered individually, but only those features which influence the nature of lesions will be discussed here.

Inflammation of the external ear, **otitis externa,** is not uncommon in animals and may result from a variety of causes. Among the specific infectious agents is *Actinomyces bovis* (p. 616) which may produce a specific granulomatous inflammation of the external ear of swine. This infection usually involves the auricular appendage only, giving it a very thick, indurated appearance. Histologically, a granulomatous tissue reaction, characteristic of actinomycosis, is found in the subcutis around the cartilage and sometimes involving the cartilage. In other species, specific infections are uncommon, but nonspecific infections may result from wounds (usually caused by bites) of the external ear.

Parasitic infestations of the external ear are quite common in most animals and are usually due to parasites which have a specific affinity for the ear. The ear mites of rabbits, sheep, cattle and horses, *Psoroptes communis* (var. *cuniculi, ovis,* etc.) have an obligate affinity for the external ear (p. 821). These acarid (mite) parasites are specific for each species; the variety which infests the rabbit is particularly common. These mites burrow into the epidermis lining the external auditory meatus and cause profuse exudation with accumulation of tenacious, brown, waxy material in the meatus and, in severe cases, over the inner surface of the external ear. Parasitic otitis externa may in some cases cause rupture of the tympanum and involve the middle ear.

Ticks may also attack the external ear, the most common being the spinose ear tick, *Otobius megnini*, of cattle.

Dermatomycosis (p. 673) is often particularly severe in, or limited to, the external ear. The lesions are not significantly different from those in the skin elsewhere in the body, but the term **otomycosis** may be used to designate infection of this type when limited chiefly to the ear.

Yeasts are often associated with chronic otitis externa in the dog but it is not known whether these organisms are actually the cause of the inflammation.

Of particular interest among the causes of severe otitis are the awns of certain grasses (particularly foxtail grass) which may lodge in the external ear. Otitis of this etiology is especially frequent in dogs in certain western states. When these bearded grasses penetrate deep into the external meatus, it is difficult to withdraw them. Severe otitis externa develops and the awns may even break through the tympanum to set up severe inflammation in the middle and internal ear.

Of interest is the occurrence, in cats and sometimes dogs, of **inflammatory polyps** which are attached by a thin pedicle to, or in the region of, the tympanum. These polyps may become relatively large, filling the external auditory meatus and in some cases may be connected through the eustachian tube with a similar polyp which lies in the nasopharynx (Fig. 21–1). These polyps are seen histologically to consist of richly cellular connective tissue, liberally supplied with blood vessels and usually infiltrated by leukocytes, particularly when the squamous epithelium covering the mass is eroded. The cause and exact nature of these polyps is unknown. Although they may recur after surgical excision, they do not appear to be neoplastic.

Neoplasms (p. 190) which are likely to be encountered in the external ear include any new growth of the skin, its adnexa, or the cartilage. Adenomas of the ceruminous gland (p. 233) are specific tumors which have been reported from the ears of man, dogs and cats. The specific neoplasm of horses and mules, **equine sarcoid** (p. 196), appears at the base of the ear or even on the auricula. Chondromas and chondrosarcomas may arise from the auricular cartilage, but only a few have been reported.

Middle Ear.—The middle ear includes the tympanic cavity with its contents and the auditive (eustachian) tubes. In the horse, two large diverticula of the eustachian tubes, the guttural pouches, are also part of the middle ear. The tympanic cavity is lined with epithelium which is continuous with that of the nasal mucosa through the eustachian tubes. The contents include the chain of auditory ossicles (malleus, incus, os lenticulare, and stapes) which communicate vibrations of the tympanum to the inner ear. This tympanic cavity is located within the tympanic and petrous parts of the temporal bone.

Infection of the middle ear **(otitis media)** may reach the tympanic cavity from the external ear by rupture of the tympanum, or may extend from the nasal cavity by way of the eustachian tubes. Extension of otitis externa to involve the middle ear is not infrequent in ear mite infestation and with penetrating foreign bodies (grass awns). Spread of infection from the middle or internal ear sometimes leads to meningitis.

Inner Ear.—The inner ear consists of two parts: (1) the membranous labyrinth in which are found the auditory cells and the peripheral ramifications of the auditory nerve, and (2) the osseous labyrinth, a series of cavities in the petrous temporal bone which enclose the membranous labyrinth. The osseous labyrinth is divided into three parts, the vestibule, the cochlea and the semicircular canals. The membranous labyrinth, which occupies, but does not completely fill, the osseous labyrinth, is surrounded by the perilymphatic space. The labyrinth contains four divisions: the auricle, the saccule, the semicircular ducts and the cochlear duct. The inner ear is concerned not only with hearing but with the sense of equilibrium.

Involvement of the inner ear **(otitis interna)** in the presence of otitis media, is manifested clinically by disturbances in equilibrium. Examples are the otitis interna of rats and mice, presumably resulting from spread of otitis media caused by "pleuropneumonia-like organisms" (PPLO). One of the few studies on the pathologic anatomy of the inner ear of domesticated animals is by Cohrs (1928) who described the histologic features of the inner ear in the horse, and also atrophy of the cochlear apparatus of horses in which no clinical signs were recognized.

Congenital deafness occurs in several species; cat, mink and dog. In the mink and cat, deafness is the result of degenerative changes in the organ of Corti which are associated with white coat color. The deaf white cat was observed and commented upon by Darwin more than one hundred years ago and the histologic features of the affected organ of Corti have been known since the turn of the twentieth century. It appears to be established that the defect is associated with the white coat color (which is due to the Dominant White gene [W] in the cat, not albino) and may occur in the presence of blue, yellow or "odd-eyed" (heterochromia iridis) iris color. The mode of inheritance of the deafness and eye color appears to be complex and is not completely understood. The deafness is more frequent, in our experience, in blue-eyed white cats but may occur in dominant white cats of any iris color.

The lesions may be seen histologically in kittens after they reach four days of age. Starting with degeneration of the hair cells of the organ of Corti, ultrastructure of the organ of Corti in deaf white mink has been studied by Hilding, Sugiura and Nakai (1967).

The Ear

ADAMS, E. W.: Hereditary Deafness in a Family of Foxhounds. J. Am. Vet. Med. Assn. *128*:302–303, 1956.

ALEXANDER, G.: Zur vergleichenden, pathologishen anatomie des gehororganes. I. Gehororgan und Gehirn einer unvollkommen albino-tischen weissen Katze. Archiv. f. Ohrenheilkunde *50*:159–181, 1900.

ALTMAN, F.: Histologic Picture of Inherited Nerve Deafness in Man and Animals. Arch. Otolaryng. *51*:852–890, 1950.

BAMBER, R. C.: Correlation Between White Coat Colour, Blue Eyes and Deafness in Cats. J. Genet. *27*:407–413, 1927.

BOSHER, S. K., and HALLPIKE, C. S.: Observations on the Histological Features, Development and Pathogenesis of the Inner Ear Degeneration of the Deaf White Cat. Proc. Roy. Soc. Ser. B. *162*:147–170, 1965.

FERNANDO, S. D. A.: Certain Histopathologic Features of the External Auditory Meatus of the Cat and Dog with Otitis Externa. Am. J. Vet. Res. *28*:278–282, 1967.

FRASER, G., WITHERS, A. R., and SPREULL, J. S. A.: Otitis Externa in the Dog. J. Small Anim. Pract. *2*:32–47, 1961.

FRASER, G.: Aetiology of Otitis Externa in the Dog. J. Small Anim. Pract. *6*:445–452, 1965.

GETTY, R., FOUST, H. L., PRESLEY, E. T., and MILLER, M. E.: Microscopic Anatomy of the Ear of the Dog. Am. J. Vet. Res. *17*:364–375, 1956.

HILDING, D. A., SUGIURA, A., and NAKAI, Y.: Deaf White Mink: Electron Microscopic Study of the Inner Ear. Ann. Otol. Rhin. & Laryngol. *76*:647–663, 1967.

HUDSON, W. R., and RUBEN, R. J.: Hereditary Deafness in Dalmatians. Arch. Otolaryng. *75*:213–216, 1962.

OLSON, L. D., and MCCUNE, E. L.: Histopathology of Chronic Otitis Media in the Rat. Lab. Anim. Care *18*:478–485, 1968.

SAUNDERS, L. Z.: The Histopathology of Hereditary Congenital Deafness in White Mink. Path. Vet. *2*:256–263, 1965.

SMITH, J. M. B.: The Association of Yeasts with Chronic Otitis Externa in the Dog. Aust. Vet. J. *44*:413–415, 1968. V.B. *39*:1518, 1968.

STRICKLAND, J. H., and CALHOUN, M. L.: The Microscopic Anatomy of the External Ear of *Felis domesticus*. Am. J. Vet. Res. *21*:845–850, 1960.

THOONEN, J., and HOORENS, J.: Infection of the Bulla Tympanica and Adjacent Parts of the Ear in Pigs. Vlaams Diergeneesk. Tijdschr. *31*:237–243, 1962.